JRCALC
Clinical Guidelines 2025
Reference Edition

JRCALC
Clinical Guidelines 2025

Reference Edition

Edited for JRCALC and AACE by

Dr Simon N Brown, Dr Alison Walker,
Cathryn James and Elizabeth Roebuck

On behalf of the National Ambulance Service Medical Directors Group

Dr Katherine Noble and Dr Simon Walsh
and medical director colleagues

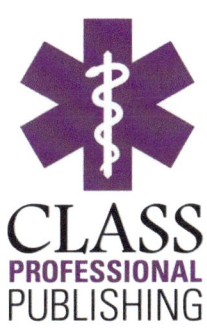

CLASS
PROFESSIONAL
PUBLISHING

© Association of Ambulance Chief Executives (AACE) 2025

All rights reserved. Without limiting the rights under copyright reserved above, no part of this publication may be reproduced, stored in or introduced into a retrieval system, or transmitted, in any form or by any means (electronic, mechanical, photocopying, recording or otherwise) without the prior written permission of the above publisher of this book.

The information presented in this book is accurate and current to the best of the authors' knowledge. The authors and publisher, however, make no guarantee as to, and assume no responsibility for, the correctness, sufficiency or completeness of such information or recommendation.

Printing history

First edition published 2000, second edition 2004, third edition 2006
Fourth edition published 2013, reprinted 2014, 2015 (twice, Version 1.3)

The content for Reference Edition 1.3 and Pocket Book 1.2 was updated in January 2015
2016 edition published 2016, reprinted 2016 (Version 1.5)
JRCALC Clinical Practice Supplementary Guidelines 2017 published 2017. Reprinted 2018
2019 edition published 2019. Reprinted twice in 2019.
2022 edition published in 2022. Reprinted 2022
2025 edition published in 2025. Reprinted 2026

Cover images

Top left: BrianAJackson/iStock
Middle left: Reframe Image Library
Middle right: Jaromir Chalabala/Shutterstock
Bottom left and right: Reframe Image Library

The authors and publisher welcome feedback from the users of this book.
Please contact the publisher:
Class Professional Publishing,
The Exchange, Express Park, Bristol Road, Bridgwater TA6 4RR
Telephone: 01278 427 800
Email: apps@class.co.uk
Website: www.classprofessional.co.uk

Class Professional Publishing is an imprint of Class Publishing Ltd

A CIP catalogue record for this book is available from the British Library
This edition: JRCALC Clinical Guidelines 2025 ISBN 9781801611800
ISSN 2514-6084

Also available: JRCALC Clinical Guidelines 2025 (eBook) ISBN 9781801611824

Printed in the UK by Hobbs the Printers Ltd.

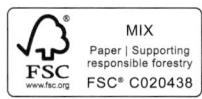

Contents

Disclaimer	vii
Foreword	viii
Guideline Developers and Contributors	ix
Guideline Development Methodology	xiii
Update Analysis – 'What's changed?'	xiv
List of Abbreviations	xxi

Section 1 – General Guidance — 1

Clinical Considerations in Relation to Diversity and Equality	2
Conditions Requiring Specific Prehospital Clinical Management	11
Consent in Pre-hospital Care	22
Domestic Abuse	23
Duty of Care	27
End of Life Care	30
Human Factors	45
Intravascular Fluid Therapy in Adults	47
Intravascular Fluid Therapy in Children	54
Mental Capacity Act 2005	56
Pain Management in Adults and Children	63
Patient Confidentiality	74
Patients with Communication Difficulties	79
Safeguarding Adults at Risk	82
Safeguarding Children	87
Sexual Assault	99
Staff Health and Wellbeing	106

Section 2 – Resuscitation — 109

Out-of-Hospital Cardiac Arrest: Overview	110
Advanced Life Support	115
Basic Life Support in Adults	134
Basic Life Support in Children	137
Emergency Tracheostomy and Laryngectomy Pre-Hospital Management	142
Foreign Body Airway Obstruction	151
Return of Spontaneous Circulation	156
Termination of Resuscitation and Verification of Death in Adults	160
Termination of Resuscitation and Verification of Death in Children	169

Section 3 – Medical Emergencies — 175

Medical Emergencies in Adults – Overview	176
Medical Emergencies in Children – Overview	185
Abdominal Pain	194
Acute Behavioural Disturbance (ABD)	205
Acute Coronary Syndrome	214
Adrenal Insufficiency Patients	221
Agitated Patients	226
Alcohol-use Disorders	231
Allergic Reactions including Anaphylaxis	236
Altered Level of Consciousness	243
Asthma in Adults and Children	251
Behavioural Emergencies	258
Cardiac Arrhythmia and Sudden Cardiac Death	262
Chronic Obstructive Pulmonary Disease	271
Delirium	277
Dyspnoea	285
Febrile Illness in Children	294
Gastrointestinal Bleeding	302
Glycaemic Emergencies in Adults and Children	306
Headache	320
Heart Failure	325
Heat Related Illness	333
Hyperventilation Syndrome	338
Hypothermia	345
Implantable Cardioverter Defibrillator	350
Low Back Pain (Non-traumatic)	356
Management and Resuscitation of Patients with Left Ventricular Assist Devices (LVADs)	365
Meningococcal Meningitis and Septicaemia	379
Mental Health Presentations	385
Non-Traumatic Chest Pain/Discomfort	409
Overdose and Poisoning in Adults and Children	412
Paediatric Gastroenteritis	419
Pulmonary Embolism	425
Respiratory Illness in Children	430
Seizures in Adults	437
Seizures in Children	450
Sepsis	457
Sickle Cell Disease	472
Stroke and Transient Ischaemic Attack	477
Vascular Emergencies	484

Section 4 – Trauma — 499

Trauma Emergencies in Adults – Overview	500
Trauma Emergencies in Children – Overview	511
Abdominal Trauma	518
Burns and Scalds	522
Drowning	528
Electrical Injuries	534
Falls in Older Adults	538
Head Injury	550
Limb Trauma	559
Pelvic Trauma	569
Spinal Injury and Spinal Cord Injury	574
Thoracic Trauma	581

Contents

Section 5 – **Maternity Care** — **589**

Maternity Care (including Obstetric Emergencies Overview)	590
Breech Birth	601
Care of the Newborn	607
Cord Prolapse	613
Imminent Birth	616
Management of Post-partum Haemorrhage (PPH)	628
Maternal Resuscitation	632
Newborn Life Support	638
Pre-eclampsia and Eclampsia	645
Shoulder Dystocia	650
Trauma in Pregnancy	655
Vaginal Bleeding during Pregnancy up to 20 weeks Gestation	657
Vaginal Bleeding during Pregnancy after 20 weeks Gestation	660
Vaginal Bleeding: Gynaecological Causes	662

Section 6 – **Special Situations** — **665**

Atropine for CBRNE	666
Chemical Biological Radiological Nuclear (CBRN) Incidents Including Hazardous Materials	669
Major, Complex and High-Risk Incidents	677
Police Incapacitants	692
Index	697

Disclaimer

Using these Guidelines

The Association of Ambulance Chief Executives and the Joint Royal Colleges Ambulance Liaison Committee have made every effort to ensure that the information, tables, drawings and diagrams contained in these guidelines are accurate at the time of publication. However, the guidelines are advisory and have been developed to assist healthcare professionals, and patients, to make decisions about the management of the patient's health, including treatments. This advice is intended to support the decision making process and is not a substitute for sound clinical judgement. The guidelines cannot always contain all the information necessary for determining appropriate care and cannot address all individual situations; therefore, individuals using these guidelines must ensure they have the appropriate knowledge and skills to enable suitable interpretation.

JRCALC has referenced NICE in these guidelines. NICE guidance is prepared for the National Health Service in England and is subject to regular review and may be updated or withdrawn. NICE has not checked the use of its content in these guidelines to confirm that it accurately reflects the NICE publications from which it is taken.

Users of these guidelines must always be aware that alterations after the date of publication cannot be incorporated into the printed edition.

The Association of Ambulance Chief Executives and the Joint Royal Colleges Ambulance Liaison Committee do not guarantee and accept no legal liability of any nature arising from or connected to, the accuracy, reliability, currency or completeness of the content of these guidelines.

Although some modification of the guidelines may be required by individual ambulance services, and approved by the relevant local clinical committees, to ensure they respond to the health requirements of their local communities, the majority of the guidance is universally applicable to NHS ambulance services.

JRCALC acknowledge the benefits of research and is supportive of innovation and to the promotion, conduct and use of research to improve the current and future health and care of our patients. Research can lead to patients benefitting from earlier access to new treatments and technologies. Paramedics may be involved in research as part of their clinical practice and may engage patients in research.

Modification of the guidelines may occur when participating in research that has been approved by a research ethics committee.

Whilst these guidelines cover a range of paramedic treatments available across the UK they will also provide a valuable tool for a range of care providers. Many of the assessment skills and general principles will remain the same. All clinical staff must practise within their level of training and competence and registered health care professionals are accountable for their own clinical practice. These guidelines are aimed at supporting clinical practice. In some circumstances, particularly because of the nature of prehospital care and the types of situations that are encountered, variation from standard clinical practice as described in these guidelines may be needed. Any deviation from standard practice and the reason for deviation must always be documented in the patient care record.

Throughout these guidelines, we have used the term 'woman, women or mother' in relation to the gynaecological and pregnancy related conditions that ambulance clinicians may be called to assess and manage. We would like to acknowledge that this term does not reflect the diverse range of patients that you may see with these conditions including those who identify as non-binary or transgender, and we commit to continually reviewing the use of language within the guidance to ensure inclusive language is used. We encourage clinicians to consider the terms they use when assessing all patients and to be mindful of drawing erroneous conclusions related to perceived gender related diagnoses.

The Further Resources section contains links to websites owned and operated by third parties. The links are provided for your information, however JRCALC is not responsible for the content held within these sites.

Updates to these guidelines will be published on the JRCALC apps which will always contain the most current content.

Foreword

Welcome to the JRCALC Clinical Guidelines 2025. It is three years since the last full print publication of JRCALC guidelines. During this time, we continued work to ensure guidance was reviewed, updated and newly developed guidance was issued so that we continue to provide the best possible care to our patients. We are aware that the majority of people now access guidance and information via the JRCALC apps, iCPG and JRCALC Plus, and this remains the preferred way of accessing current clinical guidance, particularly when needing guidance for direct patient care. However, we understand that people still want access to printed material, in particular students and for general use as a reference book.

In this 2025 print edition, we have removed the medicines section. New guidelines are being added regularly and existing guidelines expanded, which, on a practical level, means the size of the book is constantly growing; we want to keep the book a manageable size for users, and for it to reflect how the book is mostly used. Furthermore, it supports our recommendation that students and clinicians access the most current information for medicines via the apps. For all references to medicines with the book, please refer to the relevant medicine on the apps.

The apps give us the ability to publish updates to guidance in real-time and in the three years since the previous print edition, we have released a total of ten clinical updates, all of which are included in this book.

We have engaged with a number of patients, patients' representatives and patient organisations who have supported us and provided a new focus on the patient perspective when updating guidance. These include The Sickle Cell Society, The Addison's Disease support group, Parkinsons UK, MND Association and the National Poisons Information Service (NPIS-Toxbase).

Updated guidance has also been included following our support to the responses of a number of Coroners' Preventing Future Death (PFD) rulings; and in response to recommendations from the Health Services Investigation Branch (HSSIB), including specific guidance around AAA herald bleeds and the inclusion of common cardiac arrhythmias.

Building on the updated guidance for the clinical assessment of people with dark skin tones included in the previous edition, we now have a whole new guideline addressing Clinical Considerations in Relation to Diversity and Equality, which also includes further guidance on skin tone as well as guidance on disability, gender and sexual orientation and cultural differences.

New for this edition are significant updates in the Maternity section. There are now standalone guidelines for Breech Birth, Cord Prolapse, Shoulder Dystocia, and bleeding up to and after 20 weeks' gestation. We have also introduced the Prehospital Maternity Decision Tool to be used when assessing patients who are pregnant and up to 4 weeks' post-partum. We have expanded our guidance on behavioural emergencies, with three new guidelines, Behavioural Emergencies, Delirium and Agitated Patients. These are intended to be used in conjunction with one another to aid paramedic decision-making. There have also been significant updates to trauma guidelines; overdose and poisoning, sepsis and pain management. Many more updates have been made across medical, trauma and general guidance, often in response to queries being raised and new evidence becoming available.

Throughout these guidelines, we have used the term 'woman, women or mother' in relation to the gynaecological and pregnancy related conditions that ambulance clinicians may be called to assess and manage. We would like to acknowledge that this term does not reflect the diverse range of patients that you may see with these conditions including those who identify as non-binary or transgender, and we commit to continually reviewing the use of language within the guidance to ensure inclusive language is used. We encourage clinicians to consider the terms they use when assessing all patients and to be mindful of drawing erroneous conclusions related to perceived gender and any related diagnoses.

On behalf of JRCALC, NASMeD and AACE, we would like to thank all those that have contributed to our guidelines, the committee members who acted as lead authors and the groups of expert and enthusiastic healthcare professionals who all gave so willingly of their time. We thank the many paramedics who are passionate about a particular condition and have been motivated and willing to assist us with our work. Our special thanks to Class Professional Publishing, in particular Rebecca Spatuzzi and Evie Coley for their considerable expertise, knowledge and energy.

Dr ALISON WALKER
Chair, Joint Royal Colleges Ambulance Liaison Committee

Dr SIMON BROWN
JRCALC Clinical Guidelines Development Lead

CATHRYN JAMES
Senior Clinical Support Manager for AACE and JRCALC

ELIZABETH ROEBUCK
Clinical Support Manager for AACE and JRCALC

Guideline Developers and Contributors

The authors and editors would like to thank everyone who has contributed to the JRCALC guidelines. Many people have given freely and generously of their time and expertise to help draft, develop and improve the guidelines. In particular, we wish to acknowledge the work of the members of the Joint Royal Colleges Ambulance Liaison Committee, the National Ambulance Service Medical Directors group, the Ambulance Lead Paramedics group, Ambulance Pharmacists Network and national groups for End of Life, Safeguarding and Maternity. Other contributors have come from a variety of multidisciplinary groups which include healthcare professionals, educators and patients.

EDITORIAL LEADS

Dr Simon Brown, *GP and Assistant Medical Director, South Central Ambulance Service, JRCALC guideline lead*

Cathryn James, *Senior Clinical Support Manager for NASMeD and JRCALC, AACE*

Elizabeth (Lizzy) Roebuck, *Clinical Support Manager for NASMeD and JRCALC, AACE*

JRCALC Chair: Dr Alison Walker, *Honorary Medical Director, West Midlands Ambulance Service and Consultant in Emergency Medicine, Harrogate & District NHS FT*

NASMeD Chairs: Katherine Noble, *Medical Director, North East Ambulance Service and Simon Walsh, Medical Director, East of England Ambulance Service*

JRCALC COMMITTEE MEMBERS

Mark Baxter, *The Royal College of Physicians of London*

John Black, *NASMeD and Medical Director South Central Ambulance Service*

Dave Bywater, *Ambulance Lead Paramedic Group*

Charles D Deakin, *The Royal College of Anaesthetists*

Rachel Drain, *The Royal College of Midwives*

Christopher (Toby) Edmunds, *The Royal College of Emergency Medicine*

Timothy Edwards, *Ambulance Lead Paramedic Group*

Paul Ferguson, *The Royal College of Pathologists*

Joanna Girling, *The Royal College of Obstetricians and Gynaecologists*

Charlotte Haldane, *Faculty of Pre Hospital Care (RCSEd)*

Phil Hill, *The Royal College of Nursing*

Kim Hinshaw, *The Royal College of Obstetricians and Gynaecologists*

Matt Inada-Kim, *The Royal College of Physicians of London*

Dawn Kerslake, *The Royal College of Midwives*

Dhushy Surendra Kumar, *The Royal College of Anaesthetists*

John Madar, *The Royal College of Paediatrics and Child Health*

Stuart Maitland-Knibb, *The Royal College of General Practitioners*

Louise Maunick, *The Royal Pharmaceutical Society/ Ambulance Pharmacists Network*

Elizabeth Miller, *The Royal Pharmaceutical Society/ Ambulance Pharmacists Network*

Fionna Moore, *Emeritus member*

Julian Sandell, *The Royal College of Paediatrics and Child Health*

Carl Smith, *College of Paramedics*

Richard Steyn, *The Royal College of Surgeons*

Simon Stockley, *The Royal College of General Practitioners*

Ian Teague, *National Education Network of Ambulance Services*

Matt Thomas, *NASMeD and Medical Director South West Ambulance Service*

Darren Walter, *The Royal College of Emergency Medicine*

Julia Williams, *The College of Paramedics*

Claire Woolcock, *The Royal College of Psychiatrists*

Thanks to the Library and Knowledge Service for NHS ambulance services in England: Matt Holland

Class Publishing – Rebecca Spatuzzi, Evie Coley

JRCALC CONTRIBUTORS

Peter Aitken

Paul Aitken-Fell

Waqas Akhtar

Tasnim Ali

Belinda Allan

Lisa Anderson

Mark Anderson

Dorothy Antrim

Sally Arnold-Jones

Chris Ashton

Shyam Balasubramanian

Jay Banerjee

Jack Barrett

Lucy Bates

Helen Beaumont-Waters

Richard Berry

Christopher Bowles

Annmarie Breslin

Alice Breton

Nova Bridge

Chris Brooker

Marcus Brooks

Cherylene Camps

Claire Capito

Sonia Chand

Simon Chase

Stephen Clarke

Coralie Colburn

Alexander Coldrick

Robert Cole

Andy Collen

Keith Colver

Rosie Conmy

Guideline Developers and Contributors

Christian Cooper
Richard Corrall
Steven Cosh
Simon Da Costa
James Coulson
Phil Cowburn
Louise Cox
Paul Dargan
Shirmilla Datta
Jenna Davies
Jon M Dickson
Tim Draycott
Matthew Dunn
Mark Durham
Sean Edwards
Selwa Elrouby
Ed England
Lewis Ewington
Mark Faulkner
David Fitzpatrick
Craig Garner
Dawne Garrett
Joanna Garrett
Paul Gibbs
Les Gordon
James Gough
Simon Grant
Richard Grunewald
Claire Hall
Rhys Hancock
Sara Harris
Juliet Harrison
Jon Harvey
Nikki Harvey
Robert Harvey
Charlotte Hawkins
Dave Hawkins
Daniel Haworth
Claire Henderson
Stephanie Henry
Amanda Hensman-Crook
Liz Herrieven
Simon Hester
Stephanie Heys
Mark Hodkinson
Daniel Holland
Matthew House
Andrew Humber
Aimee Humphries
Chris Humphries
Kate Humphries
Kirsty Irvine
Mike Jenkins

Bethan Jones
Tim Jones
Sharon Jordan
Paul Kelly
Michelle Knight
Vicky Kypta
Colville Laird
Samantha Laws
Nat Le Blancq
Paul Lewis
Jaqualine Lindridge
Carly Lynch
Denice Mace
Steven Magee
Tom Mallinson
Stephanie Michaelides
Ian Maconochie
Camella Main
Julian Mark
Alan Martin
Chris Martin
John McAnaw
Alistair McCleary
Graham McClelland
Mark Millins
Jane Mitchell
Patrick Morgan
Scott Munro
Barry Murphy-Jones
Georgina Murphy-Jones
Ann Murray
Stephen Murray
Ian Mursell
Joanne Nevett
Roger Neuber
Tracy Nicholls
Helen Nicholson
Nicky Nicol
Tim Nutbeam
Edward O'Brian
Sue Oakley
Menai Owen-Jones
Martin Parkinson
Lorna Pearson
Gavin Perkins
Richard Pilbery
Keith Porter
Carl Powell
Larissa Prothero
Sue Putman
Markus Reuber
Susan Rhind
Ashley Richardson

Guideline Developers and Contributors

Duncan Robertson
Simon Rose
David Rovardi
Amy Sainsbury
Alex Sharp
Gary Shaw
James Short
Steven Short
Nick Sillett
Esther Silva
Neil Sinclair
Nicholas Spence
Niro Siriwardena
Mike Smyth
Gary Spurway
Simon Standen
Tony Stone
Joanne Stonehouse
Binta Sultan
Alan Taylor
Robert Taylor
Lee Thompson
Sam Thompson
Sarah Thompson
Charles Till
Sarah Todd
Jacqui Tomkins
Philip Tremewan
Eddie Tunn
Joseph Tunn
Aarti Ullal
Louise Walker
Matthew Ward
John Wass
Kevin Webb
James Wenman
Damon Wheddon
Dawn Whelan
Mark Whitbread
Katherine White
Dave Whitmore
Jason Wiles
Kirsten Willis-Drewett
Ian Wilmer
Caitlin Wilson
Mark Wilson
Cathy Winter
David Wood
Tholi Wood
Fenella Wrigley
Jonathan Wyllie
Aswinkumar Vasireddy
Aimee Yarrington

CONTRIBUTORS PRIOR TO 2016

Rob Andrews
Marcus Bailey
Andy Carson (posthumous)
Kyee Han
Brendan Lloyd
Kevin Mackway-Jones
Andrew McIntyre
David McManus
Rory McCrea
David Radcliffe
Andy Smith
Bob Winter
Richard Appleton
Louis Appleby
Martin Berry
Mike Brooke
Will Broughton
Daniel Butterworth
Adele Dean
Lucy Derwin
Steve Dick
Kuda Dimbi
Mike Jackson
Paul Jefferies
Andrew Jenkins
Gregory Lloyd
Will Murcott
Andy Newton
Dave Partlow
Gary Richardson
Adrian Robinson
Rashid Sohail
Adrian South
Clare Sutton
Andrew Swinburn
Dahrlene Tough
Roger Watson
Bartholomew Wood
Mark Ainsworth-Smith
Lesley Altoft
Sarah Black
Robin Beal
Wim Blancke
Tony Bleetman
Mark Bloch (posthumus)
Gillian Bryce
Paul Cassford
Shaun Carter
Adrian Castle
Colin Cessford
Ravi Chauhan
Tom Clarke

Guideline Developers and Contributors

James Coe
Mick Colquhoun
Matthew Cooke
Stuart Cooper
Stef Cormack
Ron Daniels
Jonathan Dermott
Alan Dobson
Andrew Downes
Jonathan Ellis
Chris Evans
Geraint Farr
Bob Fellows
Nicky Fothergill
Rodger Gadsby
Paul Grant
James Gray
Rodger Gregson
Henry Guly
Phil Hallam
David Halliewell
Pam Hardy
Katie Hawkins
Emma Hines
Stephen Hines
Tim Hodgetts
Chris Horswell
Rose Jarvis
Fiona Jewkes (posthumous)
Paul Johnson
Christopher Jones
Carl Keeble
Elizabeth Kershaw
Alex Knight
Robin Lawrenson
Caroline Leech
Victoria Leeson

Martin Lewis
Yenushka Llangakoon
Iain McNeil
Bill Mason
Graham Mattison
Jeremy Mayhew
Sean Mitchell
Quen Mok
Steve Mortley
Donal O'Donaghue
Sam Oestreicher
Vicky O'Leary
Matthew O'Meara
Tom Quinn
Steven Rawstorn
Andy Rosser
Rob Russell
Rachel Ryan
Helen Simpson
John Stephenson
Dan Staines
Gary Strong
Lee Styles
Fizz Thompson
Russell Thornhill
Dominic Tolley
Mike Ward
James Webster
Richard Whitfield
Richard Williams
David Wilmot
Malcolm Woollard
Jane Worthington
Matthew Wyse
Tullie Yeghen
Adam Zenkner

Guideline Development Methodology

The methodology used by JRCALC (Joint Royal Colleges Ambulance Liaison Committee) to develop the UK Ambulance Services Clinical Practice Guidelines is designed to comply with the criteria used by the AGREE II (Appraisal of Guidelines for Research and Evaluation in Europe) instrument. This process is a leading academic tool to identify good quality guidelines: http://www.agreetrust.org/

The purpose of the AGREE II, is to provide a framework to:

- assess the quality of guidelines
- provide a methodological strategy for the development of guidelines
- inform what information and how information ought to be reported in guidelines.

By adopting these principles, guidelines are developed that support safe decision making and high quality patient care.

Guideline Selection

JRCALC, NASMeD (National Ambulance Service Medical Directors) and the ALPG (Ambulance Lead Paramedic Group) will advise on those clinical guidelines which need updating and those clinical conditions which need a new guideline developing. These are then prioritised and assessed with regard, to urgency and risk. Clinical topics can be identified through a variety of means including the monitoring of serious incidents within individual UK Ambulance Service Trusts, preventing future death reports issued by coroners and national service reconfigurations. In addition JRCALC provide extensive clinical expertise and advice on potential new developments to ensure that the guidelines capture latest best practice and future innovations and encourage further research into pre hospital care.

Feedback is welcome via JRCALC@AACE.org

Editorial Independence

No external funding has been received for the development of these guidelines and no competing or conflicting interests have been declared by those involved in their development.

Citing the JRCALC Guidelines

The JRCALC Guidelines are cited as:

Joint Royal Colleges Ambulance Liaison Committee, Association of Ambulance Chief Executives (2025) JRCALC Clinical Guidelines 2025. Bridgwater: Class Professional Publishing.

Update Analysis – 'What's changed?'

General Guidance		
Guideline Title	**Last Update**	**Notes**
Clinical Considerations in Relation to Diversity and Equality	April 2025	New wording added around pulse oximetry in dark skin, and also regarding terminology in the disability section.
Conditions Requiring Specific Prehospital Clinical Management	July 2024	New guideline covering a number of clinical presentations where specific pre-hospital clinical considerations are needed.
Consent in Pre-hospital Care	September 2021	Reviewed and updated.
Domestic Abuse	September 2022	Revised and updated with current legislation.
Duty of Care	May 2021	Reviewed and updated.
End of Life Care	May 2021	Reviewed and updated and includes the Macmillan/UKONS tool.
Human Factors	September 2022	New guideline. A short section on human factors will remain in 'Out-of-Hospital Cardiac Arrest: Overview'.
Intravascular Fluid Therapy in Adults	April 2025	A new table for Adrenal Crisis and update to the Sepsis table.
Intravascular Fluid Therapy in Children	May 2021	The duration over which non-shocked patients with DKA should be given an initial 10 ml/kg bolus has been decreased to 30 minutes (was previously 60 minutes). Figure 7.3 (Intravascular Fluid Therapy in Children algorithm) has been removed for clarity.
Mental Capacity Act 2005	September 2022	Revised and updated with current legislation. New flowchart for assessing mental capacity included with information around causative nexus.
Pain Management in Adults and Children	July 2025	Previously separate guidelines for adults and children have now been unified into a single guideline. The updated guideline provides age-specific treatment recommendations and incorporates the PAINAD scale for assessing pain in patients with cognitive impairment. The treatment section has been revised and includes a table outlining pre-hospital analgesia options.
Patient Confidentiality	June 2019	Reviewed and updated.
Patients with Communication Difficulties	April 2025	Amended wording following feedback around patients who are deaf.
Safeguarding Adults at Risk	September 2022	Revised and updated with current legislation.
Safeguarding Children	September 2022	Revised and updated with current legislation.
Sexual Assault	March 2024	Fully revised and updated. Emphasis on use of Sexual Assault Referral Centres (SARCs).
Staff Health and Wellbeing	June 2019	Reviewed and updated.

Update Analysis – 'What's changed?'

Resuscitation		
Guideline Title	**Last Update**	**Notes**
Advanced Life Support	April 2025	An amendment in section 10.3 to confirm that intra-osseous (IO) obtained blood may be used to check blood sugar.
Basic Life Support in Adults	September 2022	Reviewed and updated in line with RCUK. New wording added.
Basic Life Support in Children	September 2022	Reviewed and updated in line with RCUK. New wording added.
Emergency Tracheostomy and Laryngectomy Pre-hospital Management	September 2022	Reviewed in line with RCUK. Revised management algorithms.
Foreign Body Airway Obstruction	September 2022	Reviewed in line with RCUK. All reversible causes should be considered.
Out-of-Hospital Cardiac Arrest: Overview	September 2022	Reviewed and updated in line with RCUK. New wording added.
Return of Spontaneous Circulation	September 2022	Reviewed and updated in line with RCUK. New wording added.
Termination of Resuscitation and Verification of Death in Adults	September 2022	Reviewed and updated in line with RCUK. New section on advance care planning included and more guidance added to clarify decisions around ADRT, lasting power of attorney and DNACPR, expected and unexpected deaths.
Termination of Resuscitation and Verification of Death in Children	September 2022	New title replacing 'Death of a Child' guideline. Reviewed in line with RCUK. Includes guidance for children with care plans and for expected deaths.

Medical		
Guideline Title	**Current Update**	**Notes**
Abdominal Pain	April 2025	Revised and updated. The common causes table for adults and children has been revised and symptom indicators added to aid working diagnosis. Includes diagram of abdominal regions.
Acute Behavioural Disturbance (ABD)	February 2021	Additional wording to emphasise close monitoring of a restrained patient.
Acute Coronary Syndrome	January 2023	Small change to wording about health inequalities, regarding women and ACS.
Adrenal Insufficiency Patients (formerly called Steroid-dependent Patients)	April 2025	Reviewed and updated in line with NICE guidanace NG24. Note new title (previously called Steroid-dependent Patients).
Agitated Patients	January 2023	New guideline to sit alongside ABD.
Alcohol-Use Disorders	September 2023	A new paragraph is included on alcoholic ketoacidosis.

(continued)

Update Analysis – 'What's changed?'

Allergic Reactions including Anaphylaxis	September 2021	Reviewed and updated in line with RCUK guidance. Emphasis on repeat IM adrenaline doses.
Altered Level of Consciousness	July 2025	In response to user feedback, the term "coma" has been replaced with "reduced level of consciousness" throughout the guideline. A new section has been added around sudden cardiac death.
Asthma in Adults and Children	March 2024	Revised colour-coded table of features for the assessment of asthma severity. Amended algorithm.
Behavioural Emergencies	April 2025	New guideline that should be used in conjunction with other existing guidelines including: agitation, delirium and acute behavioural disturbance.
Cardiac Arrythmia and Sudden Cardiac Death	July 2025	This guideline has been revised and now includes a new section on sudden cardiac death. The bradycardia management algorithm has been updated to include the consideration of adrenaline in cases unresponsive to atropine. An appendix has been added, featuring descriptions of common cardiac arrhythmias and their associated treatment pathways to aid clinical decision-making.
Chronic Obstructive Pulmonary Disease	February 2022	Reviewed and updated.
Delirium	September 2023	New guideline to sit alongside ABD.
Dyspnoea	March 2024	Fully reviewed and revised in line with NICE guidance. Includes CRB-65 score.
Febrile Illness in Children	July 2019	Reviewed and updated.
Gastrointestinal Bleeding	July 2019	Reviewed and updated.
Glycaemic Emergencies in Adults and Children	July 2025	Section 3.1, which covers hypoglycaemia in patients without diabetes, has been updated following a review of the evidence. Since no absolute blood glucose threshold was identified in the literature, symptomatic patients with a blood glucose level (BM) of less than 3.9 mmol/L can now be considered hypoglycaemic.

Update Analysis – 'What's changed?'

Headache	May 2023	Bullet point removed from Table 3.69 concerning the use of morphine to treat patient's condition.
Heart Failure	January 2024	Information in 'Key Points' has been revised.
Heat Related Illness	September 2023	A full review and update. New table of medications predisposing to heat related illness.
Hyperventilation Syndrome	June 2019	Reviewed and updated.
Hypothermia	January 2024	Contra-indications and cautions reviewed and revised and new wording in ALS section 10.4.
Implantable Cardioverter Defibrillator	January 2024	Revised and updated. Amended wording on DNACPR and ReSPECT and use of ring magnets.
Low Back Pain (Non-traumatic)	September 2022	Guidance on the assessment and management of this common presentation.
Management and Resuscitation of Patients with Left Ventricular Assist Devices (LVADs)	April 2025	Revised and updated. Small changes include: If possible, anterior-posterior pad positioning would be preferable based on the LVAD position within the chest wall. LVAD centre emergency contacts numbers were checked for accuracy.
Medical Emergencies in Adults – Overview	February 2022	New wording around frailty scoring added; consider using the clincial frailty scale, as per local pathways.
Medical Emergencies in Children – Overview	February 2021	New reference added, linking to an interactive education tool.
Meningococcal Meningitis and Septicaemia	July 2019	Reviewed and updated.
Mental Health Presentations	May 2023	Completely revised guideline.
Non-Traumatic Chest Pain/Discomfort	July 2019	Reviewed and updated.
Overdose and Poisoning in Adults and Children	October 2024	Revised and updated guideline with support from the National Poison Information Service (NPIS) and RCEM toxicologists. New algorithm included. Substance management table removed.
Paediatric Gastroenteritis	July 2019	Reviewed and updated.
Pulmonary Embolism	January 2024	Reviewed and updated in line with NICE. Changes to use of Wells score.

(continued)

Update Analysis – 'What's changed?'

Respiratory Illness in Children	September 2022	Removal of modified Taussig croup score as not advised by NICE. Dexamethasone is now indicated for children with croup.
Seizures in Adults	July 2025	Renamed and comprehensively updated. It now includes the use of Midazolam for the treatment of seizures, with additional guidance on redosing protocols.
Seizures in Children	July 2025	Renamed and comprehensively updated. It now includes the use of Midazolam for the treatment of seizures, with additional guidance on redosing protocols.
Sepsis	April 2025	Guideline reviewed and updated in line with NICE guidance NG51. Note that JRCALC are not advising pre-hospital antibiotics for suspected sepsis.
Sickle Cell Disease	February 2022	Alignment to advise oral, intramuscular, or subcutaneous administration rather than IV.
Stroke and Transient Ischaemic Attack	May 2021	Reviewed and updated.
Vascular Emergencies	July 2025	This guideline has been updated in response to recent clinical feedback and now includes a new section addressing 'other vascular bleed' considerations.

Trauma		
Guideline Title	**Last Update**	**Notes**
Abdominal Trauma	July 2024	Reviewed and updated, placing emphasis that when managing critically ill or injured patients, early consideration should be given to the requirement for additional critical care resources.
Burns and Scalds	November 2019	Reviewed and updated.
Drowning	October 2024	Reviewed, updated and new name (previously called Immersion and Drowning). Revised submerged person tool (JESIP) included and simplified terminology relating to drowning.
Electrical Injuries	July 2024	Reviewed and updated. Additional wording around conveyance decisions, tasers, implantable cardioverter defibrillator and importance of 12-lead ECG monitoring.
Falls in Older Adults	February 2022	New wording around frailty scoring added; consider using the clinical frailty scale, as per local pathways.

Update Analysis – 'What's changed?'

Head Injury	July 2024	Reviewed and updated. Revised guidance around conveyance decisions, and in relation to patients taking anti platelets.
Limb Trauma	September 2023	New guidance and images on fracture reduction and management of patella dislocation. More detail on hip fractures.
Pelvic Trauma	July 2024	Emphasis placed on early consideration for the requirement of additional critical care resources, while still considering the advantage of moving towards hospital care.
Spinal Injury and Spinal Cord Injury	April 2025	Small wording update to reflect current trust practices around use of collars for immobilisation.
Thoracic Trauma	July 2024	Emphasis placed on early consideration for the requirement of additional critical care resources, while still considering the advantage of moving towards hospital care. New guidance on rib fractures.
Trauma Emergencies in Adults – Overview	April 2025	Small wording update to reflect current trust practices around use of collars for immobilisation.
Trauma Emergencies in Children – Overview	February 2022	New guidance around assessment and management of hanging added. New reference added.

Maternity		
Guideline Title	**Last Update**	**Notes**
Breech Birth	September 2023	Revised standalone guideline with new algorithm.
Care of the Newborn	October 2024	Removal of APGAR score.
Cord Prolapse	October 2024	New standalone guideline. Management algorithm can also be found on the algorithms tab in the app.
Imminent Birth	October 2024	Fully reviewed and revised. New wording about identifying if birth is imminent and when to consider conveying to hospital. Inclusion of free birth, water birth, home birth and en caul birth. Revised management algorithm. New table of high-risk pregnancy features. Photos included to show estimates of volumes of blood loss.
Management of Post-partum Haemorrhage (PPH)	January 2024	New guideline. Includes a new algorithm.
Maternal Resuscitation	July 2019	Reviewed and updated.
Maternity Care (including Obstetric Emergency Overview)	October 2024	Includes a new Prehospital Maternity Decision Tool to be used for pregnant patients and up to 4 weeks post-partum.
Newborn Life Support	September 2022	Revised and updated, algorithm revised in line with RCUK.
Pre-eclampsia and Eclampsia	July 2025	This guideline has been fully revised, including the development of a new management algorithm. The updated guidance aligns with NICE NG133 recommendations regarding the use of Magnesium Sulfate for the management of pre-eclampsia and eclampsia.

(continued)

Update Analysis – 'What's changed?'

Shoulder Dystocia	July 2025	The management approach for shoulder dystocia has been revised, with the inclusion of a new algorithm. This is now a standalone guideline following feedback we received.
Trauma in Pregnancy	July 2019	Reviewed and updated.
Vaginal Bleeding: Gynaecological Causes	March 2020	Reviewed and updated.
Vaginal Bleeding During Pregnancy after 20 Weeks Gestation	January 2024	New standalone guideline.
Vaginal Bleeding During Pregnancy up to 20 Weeks Gestation	January 2024	New standalone guideline.

Special Situations		
Guideline Title	**Last Update**	**Notes**
Atropine for CBRNE	October 2022	Reviewed and updated.
Chemical Biological Radiological Nuclear (CBRN) Incidents Including Hazardous Materials	March 2024	Revised and updated by NARU. Revised CRESS tool. Step 123 removed and new: Recognise, Assess and React figure included.
Major, Complex and High-Risk Incidents	January 2024	Reviewed and updated by NARU. Includes the new major incident triage tool algorithm (MITT). Includes the Ten Second Triage (TST), a new primary scene triage tool that has been developed for use by all first responders to any incident with multiple casualties.
Police Incapacitants	October 2022	Reviewed and updated by NARU. Updated guidance on Conducted Energy Devices (Tasers). Updated assessment and management of irritant/incapacitant sprays, attenuating energy projectiles and batons.

List of Abbreviations

The glossary of terms listed below is designed to assist reading ease and is **NOT** provided as a list of shorthand terms. The Joint Royal Colleges Ambulance Liaison Committee reminds the user that abbreviations are not to be used in any clinical documentation.

Term	
AAA	Abdominal Aortic Aneurysm
ABCDE	**A** – Airway
	B – Breathing
	C – Circulation
	D – Disability
	E – Exposure and environment
ABD	Acute behavioural disorder
AC	Alternating Current
ACS	Acute Coronary Syndrome
ADHD	Attention Deficit Hyperactivity Disorder
ADRT	Advance Decision to Refuse Treatment
AED	Automated External Defibrillation
AHF	Acute Heart Failure
ALoC	Altered level of consciousness
ALS	Advanced Life Support
AMHP	Approved Mental Health Professional
APC	Antero-Posterior Compression
ARDS	Acute Respiratory Distress Syndrome
ATMIST	**A** – Age
	T – Time of incident
	M – Mechanism
	I – Injuries
	S – Signs and symptoms
	T – Treatment given/immediate needs
ATP	Anti-Tachycardia Pacing
AV	Atrioventricular
AVPU	**A** – Alert
	V – Responds to voice
	P – Responds to pain
	U – Unresponsive
BBB	Bundle branch block
BG	Blood Glucose
BIA	Best Interest Assessors
BiPAP	Bilevel Positive Pressure Ventilation
BLS	Basic Life Support
BM	Stick Measures blood sugar
BMI	Body mass index

Term	
BP	Blood Pressure
bpm	Beats per minute
BR	Breech
BTCS	Bilateral Tonic-Clonic Seizures
BTS	British Thoracic Society
BVM	Bag-Valve-Mask
<C>ABCDE	**<C>** – Catastrophic haemorrhage
	A – Airway
	B – Breathing
	C – Circulation
	D – Disability
	E – Exposure and environment
CAMHS	Child and Adolescent Mental Health Services
CBRNE	Chemical, Biological, Radiological, Nuclear and Explosive
CBT	Cognitive Behavioural Therapy
CCF	Congestive cardiac failure
CCS	Central Cord Syndrome
CES	Cauda Equina Syndrome
CEW	Controlled Electrical Weapon
CFR	Community first responder
CMHT	Community Mental Health Team
CMI	Combined Mechanical Injury
CNS	Central Nervous System
CO	Carbon monoxide
CO$_2$	Carbon dioxide
COP	Code of Practice
COPD	Chronic Obstructive Pulmonary Disease
CPAP	Continuous Positive Airway Pressure
CPN	Community Psychiatric Nurse
CPP	Cerebral Perfusion Pressure
CPP	Coronary perfusion pressure
CPR	Cardiopulmonary Resuscitation
CPR-IC	CPR-induced consciousness
CRT	Capillary Refill Test
CRT	Cardiac Resynchronisation Therapy
CSA	Child Sexual Abuse
CSE	Child Sexual Exploitation
CSE	Convulsive status epilepticus

List of Abbreviations

Term	
CT	Computerised Tomography
DBS	Disclosure and Barring Service
DC	Direct Current
DKA	Diabetic Ketoacidosis
DM	Diabetes Mellitus
DNA	Deoxyribonucleic Acid
DNACPR	Do Not Attempt Cardio-Pulmonary Resuscitation
DoLS	Deprivation of Liberty Safeguards
DPA	Data Protection Act
DVT	Deep Vein Thrombosis
ECG	Electrocardiograph
ECT	Electro-convulsive therapy
ECMO	ECMO Extra-corporeal membrane oxygenation
ED	Emergency Department
EDD	Estimated Date of Delivery
EF	Ejection fraction
EOC	Emergency Operations Centre
ERC	European Resuscitation Council
ESC	European Society of Cardiology
ET	Endotracheal
EtCO$_2$	Exhaled (end-tidal) carbon dioxide
FAST	**F** – Face
	A – Arms
	S – Speech
	T – Test
FBAO	Foreign Body Airway Obstruction
FGM	Female genital mutilation
FLACC	**F** – Face
	L – Legs
	A – Activity
	C – Cry
	C – Consolability
FII	Fabricated or Induced Illness
FGM	Female Genital Mutilation
g	Grams
GBS	Group B Strep Infection
GCS	Glasgow Coma Scale
GDPR	General Data Protection Regulations 2018
GP	General Practitioner
GTN	Glyceryl Trinitrate
GUM	Genito-urinary medicine
HART	Hazardous Area Response Team

Term	
HCP	Healthcare Professional
HFpEF	Heart failure with preserved ejection fraction
HFrEF	Heart failure with reduced ejection fraction
HIV	Human Immunodeficiency Virus
HME	Heat moisture exchanger
HPV	Human papillomavirus
HR	Heart Rate
HVS	Hyperventilation Syndrome
IA	Impaired awareness
IBS	Irritable Bowel Syndrome
ICD	International Classification of Diseases
ICD	Implantable Cardioverter Defibrillator
ICE	Infant Cooling Evaluation
ICP	Intracranial Pressure
IHD	Ischemic Heart Disease
ILCOR	International Liaison Committee on Resuscitation
IM	Intramuscular
IMCA	Independent Mental Capacity Advocates
IN	Intranasal
IO	Intraosseous
IPAP	**I** – Intent
	P – Plans
	A – Actions
	P – Protection
IN	Intranasal
ITD	Impedance threshold device
ITU	Intensive Care Unit
IV	Intravenous
IVC	Inferior Vena Cava
J	Joule
JESIP	Joint Emergency Services Interoperability Programme
JRCALC	Joint Royal Colleges Ambulance Liaison Committee
JVP	Jugular Venous Pressure
kg	Kilogram
kPa	Kilopascal
LBBB	Left Bundle Branch Block
LC	Lateral Compression
LMP	Last Menstrual Period
LOC	Level of Consciousness

List of Abbreviations

Term	
LPA	Lasting Power of Attorney
LVAD	Left ventricular assist device
LVF	Left Ventricular Failure
LVSD	Left ventricular systolic dysfunction
MAOI	Monoamine Oxidase Inhibitor antidepressant
MAP	Mean Arterial Pressure
MBRRACE	Mothers and Babies: Reducing Risk through Audits and Confidential Enquiries
MCA	Mental Capacity Act
mcg	Microgram
mCPR	Mechanical chest compression devices
MDMA	Methylene Dioxymethamphetamine
MECC	Making Every Contact Count
mg	Milligram
MHA	Mental Health Act
MI	Myocardial Infarction
MINAP	Myocardial Ischaemia National Audit Project
ml	Millilitre
mmHG	Millimetres of Mercury
mmol	Millimoles
mmol/l	Millimoles per Litre
MOI	Mechanisms of Injury
MSC	**M** – Motor
	S – Sensation
	C – Circulation
msec	Millisecond
MTC	Major Triage Centre
NARU	National Ambulance Resilience Unit
NEET	Not in Education, Employment or Training
NEWS	National Early Warning Score
NG	Nasogastric
NHS	National Health Service
NICE	National Institute for Health and Care Excellence
NLS	Newborn Life Support
NPA	Nasopharyngeal airway
NPIS	National Poisons Information Service
NSAID	Non-Steroidal Anti-inflammatory Drug
NSTEMI	Non-ST Segment Elevation Myocardial Infarction
O_2	Oxygen

Term	
OHCA	Out of Hospital Cardiac Arrest
OOH	Out of Hours
OPA	Oropharyngeal Airway
ORS	Oral Rehydration Salt
P	Parity
PCO_2	Measure of the Partial Pressure of Carbon dioxide
PE	Pulmonary Embolism
PEaRL	Pupils Equal and Reacting to Light
PEA	Pulseless Electrical Activity
PEF	Peak Expiratory Flow
PEFR	Peak Expiratory Flow Rate
PHECG	Pre-hospital 12-lead electrocardiogram
PNES	Psychogenic non-epileptic seizures
PPCI	Primary Percutaneous Coronary Intervention
PPE	Personal Protective Equipment
PPH	Post-Partum Haemorrhage
pr	Per Rectum
PTSD	Post-traumatic Stress Disorder
PRESS	Prehospital Recognition of Severe Sepsis
PSP	Patient specific protocol
prn	When required medication
PV	Per Vaginam
pVT	Pulseless ventricular tachycardia
RBBB	Right bundle branch block
RCT	Randomised Controlled Trial
ReSPECT	Recommended Summary Plan for Emergency Care and Treatment
ROLE	Recognition Of Life Extinct
ROSC	Return of Spontaneous Circulation
RR	Respiratory Rate
RSV	Respiratory Syncytial Virus
RTC	Road Traffic Collision
RVF	Right Ventricular Failure
RVP	Rendezvous Point(s)
SARC	Sexual Assault Referral Centre
SBAR	**S** – Situation
	B – Background
	A – Assessment
	R – Recommendation
SBI	Serious Bacterial Infection
SBP	Systolic Blood Pressure

List of Abbreviations

Term	
SC	Subcutaneous
SCENE	**S** – Safety
	C – Cause including MOI
	E – Environment
	N – Number of patients
	E – Extra resources needed
SCI	Spinal Cord Injury
SGA	Supraglottic airway
SOB	Shortness of breath
SOBOE	Shortness of breath on exertion
SOCRATES	**S** – Site
	O – Onset
	C – Character
	R – Radiation
	A – Associated symptoms
	T – Time
	E – Exacerbation
	S – Severity
SOP	Standard operating procedure
SORT	Special Operations Response Team

Term	
SpO$_2$	Oxygen Saturation Measured With Pulse Oximeter
SSRIs	Selective Serotonin Re-Uptake Inhibitors
STEMI	ST Segment Elevation Myocardial Infarction
SVT	Supraventricular Tachycardia
TARN	Trauma Audit Research Network
TBI	Traumatic Brain injury
TBSA	Total Body Surface Area
TIA	Transient Ischaemic Attack
TLoC	Transient loss of consciousness
URTI	Upper Respiratory Tract Infection
UTI	Urinary Tract Infection
VF	Ventricular Fibrillation
VS	Vertical Shear
VT	Ventricular Tachycardia
VTE	Venous Thromboembolism
WHO	World Health Organisation

1

General Guidance

Clinical Considerations in Relation to Diversity and Equality

1. Introduction

- The people we care for come from a diverse set of heritages and with individual needs and expectations from their healthcare providers. There is an expectation that the care they receive is delivered in a sensitive and respectful manner and in a manner that is accessible to them.
- The JRCALC guidelines seek to set out the clinical practice and approach to the people who seek help from ambulance services. In a diverse society we need to understand how our clinical practice needs to flex and adapt to ensure an equity of care for all.
- The JRCALC guidelines of their nature are subject to change and are never static as they manage often incomplete scientific knowledge and changes in society and behaviour.
- This section is no different and reflects a starting point in an area where societal custom and attitudes are changing rapidly and where scientific evidence regarding best approaches and clinical practice are incomplete.
- There is a commitment as with all guidelines that where there is new evidence or changes to consensus on approach these will be reflected.
- This section contains the background and underpinning information to support an inclusive approach. Individual guidelines will contain the accommodations or flexing of clinical practice that may help ensure the best assessment and delivery of care to an individual.

2. Why do we Need to Flex our Clinical Practice?

- The purpose of this work is to create best clinical practice within a diverse society and optimise patient care. Failure to recognise when care or clinical practice needs to be flexed or adapted can result in poor outcomes for the individual.
- Different patient groups and individuals will have different needs to others, and illness and diseases may present differently or need additional consideration if we are to manage them appropriately and equally.
- The skill and requirement to be able to flex our practice is therefore a clinical, professional, and ethical outcome.
- Additionally, for many of these groups there is a legal requirement to adapt care and approach where required.

2.1 Equality Act 2010

- The Equality Act 2010 sets out nine protected characteristics of individuals and places a requirement on those providing services to them to do so without discrimination and to make reasonable adaptions where required to provide equal access to those services.

Protected Characteristics (Equality Act 2010)
- age
- gender reassignment
- being married or in a civil partnership
- being pregnant or on maternity leave
- disability
- race including colour, nationality, ethnic or national origin
- religion or belief
- sex
- sexual orientation

2.2 Health Inequality and Cognitive Bias

- There are strong correlations between some of the protected characteristics and health inequalities with certain groups.
- The causes for this are multifactorial and where bias or discrimination are contributing factors this should be recognised and minimised.
- At an individual level practitioners should be aware that their preconceptions and liability to cognitive bias can influence how they perceive and care for patients and actively minimise their impact.[1]

2.3 Inadvertent Bias and Preconceptions in the Initial Approach to Patients

- It is important to achieve rapport and mutual respect with the people we care for in order for them to be best able to confide in us with the confidence that they will be respected.
- This enables them to receive the most appropriate care and for the practitioner to carry out the best possible assessment.
- The words we use can impact on how people respond to us and how they feel about the care they are given, but importantly, it is good practice when approaching a patient to ask them how they would like to be known.
- A patient's recorded name on medical records may be different to what they would like to be called.
- Clinicians should use and record the patient's chosen name, especially when handing over care of the patient to other health care professionals so as to ensure the correct name is used for the patient further down the chain of care. Clinicians should ask patients what pronouns they use in much the same way we ask what patients would like to be called. This could be especially important for certain groups of people, for example people with gender dysphoria.

2.4 Direct and Indirect Discrimination

Direct discrimination is said to have occurred when a person is treated unfairly as a result of their protected characteristic. This can occur

Clinical Considerations in Relation to Diversity and Equality

because that person has a protected characteristic, or is perceived to have that characteristic, or be connected to a person with that characteristic.

Indirect discrimination arises when circumstances are applied equally to a population, but this disproportionately discriminates against a proportion of that population with a shared protected characteristic leading to personal disadvantage.

3. Ethnicity and Race

- We refer to ethnicity and not race to reflect the heritage and cultural identity of an individual. We should recognise and reflect in our practice the different cultural differences and concerns regarding health and wellbeing.
- Consent to examination and/or treatment may legitimately be restricted by cultural, religious or ethnic expectations. Care should be taken to be respectful of the restrictions the individual may place on their care. Refer to **Consent in Pre-Hospital Care**.
- Consideration should be given to how reasonable adjustments may be made to overcome such difficulties by either modifying the treatment offered or offering examination by a same sex practitioner. (Local practice and guidance should be followed.) Consent where communication is limited and or comprehension not clear, such as where there are language barriers or learning difficulties, should be handled sensitively and in line with the Mental Capacity Act 2005.[2]

4. Skin Colour and Tone

General principles

- Skin tone refers to the individual combination of pigmentation in a person's skin, whilst skin colour can change when a person is unwell.
- Assess for skin changes closely using natural light if possible (or non-fluorescent light to avoid a blue tinge). Lighting conditions can affect how you see changes in skin colour.
- Palpate the skin for a raised rash or swelling and/or local changes in skin temperature.
- Consider moistening the skin (if unbroken) to enhance the visibility of skin changes.
- If erythema is identified, it may be pink, purple or red, or the skin may become darker than the surrounding area.
- Contusions may only be seen as an area of skin that is darker than its surroundings. They could alternatively be a purple/maroon or green/yellow colour.
- Peripheral cyanosis may be difficult to detect. Use natural light (or non-fluorescent light to avoid a blue tinge) and examine the lips, mucous membranes and tongue for central cyanosis.
- Pallor may be difficult to detect in dark toned skin and may present as ashen or grey. In brown toned skin, the skin will present more yellowish in colour. An alternative method for identifying pallor in dark skin tones can be assessing the palmar surface which can appear paler. Also consider the mucosal membranes and conjunctiva which may be grey, white or ashen.
- Heightened skin colour (flushing) relating to increased blood flow may not be easily detected in dark skin tones. Palpate for local skin temperature changes to support this assessment.
- References to 'darker skin' are to be discouraged as this suggests that light skin is the default.
- Skin colour can change in illness, but appropriate words need to be used to describe those changes. For example, using pallor or a decrease/reduction in skin colour instead of pale. Heightened colour relating to increased blood flow, instead of flushed. Mottling or 'blue' cannot be seen easily on dark skin.
- Pulse oximetry can over-estimate oxygen levels, and this inaccuracy is more likely to occur in patients with a dark skin tone than a light skin tone. The SPO_2 reading may misleadingly suggest the patient is within a normal oxygenation range despite oxygen saturations being low. Use caution and a wide clinical assessment to assess for possible hypoxia, particularly respiratory rate.

5. Disability

- Disability is a condition or impairment that limits an ability to perform certain activities, often the result of a physical, sensory, cognitive or developmental condition. A disability may be present from birth or have been acquired at any point.
- Disability results from the interaction between the individual condition, personal and environmental factors. The extent to which an individual is impacted by disability will vary considerably.
- When referring to disability it encompasses temporary and permanent, visible and non-visible conditions and impairments, physical and psychological, mental health conditions and neurodivergent conditions. It is accepted that disability is different for everyone and can result in varying levels of disruption to daily life. Not everyone will be comfortable with the term disability or impairment (or other disability related terminology) being used to refer to a particular condition, and some conditions may be labelled as 'differences'. The term disability is used, however it is recognised and accepted that there are different positions, perspectives and views on this terminology and (we) wish to acknowledge this.

Clinical Considerations in Relation to Diversity and Equality

5.1 Learning Disability

- A learning disability (LD) is a reduced intellectual ability and difficulty with everyday activities, e.g. household tasks, socialising or managing money, that affects someone for their whole life. The level of impairment can vary from mild to severe in all conditions.
- A learning disability is different from a learning difficulty, as a learning difficulty does not affect general intellect. Examples of learning difficulties include attention deficit-hyperactivity disorder (ADHD) and dyslexia.
- People with learning disabilities are likely to die 20 years earlier than people without them. Reasons include increased comorbidities, challenges with accessing healthcare, difficulties in assessment and inappropriate or delayed care.[3, 4]
- People with LD are up to 5 times more likely to die of something treatable compared to others.[3]
- The top three causes of death in people with LD are respiratory illness, cardiovascular disease and cancer.[4]
- 2.16% of adults and 2.5% of children have a learning disability.[5]
- People with dementia, frailty needs, mental health problems and other communication needs are also at higher risk of ill health. This is for similar reasons to people with learning disabilities, such as difficulties accessing healthcare, multiple comorbidities, medications and assessment challenges.
- Communication is vital to assessment.
- Be aware of polypharmacy. This needs to be taken into consideration when assessing a patient. Consider drug interactions, potential accidental overdoses or toxicity, and side effects.
- Complete any assessments you would usually complete, including NEWS2. Note, however, that some patients may be very unwell but actually have normal vital signs and a low NEWS2. For example, some patients with certain neurological conditions may not mount a tachycardia or pyrexia and some may not be able to sustain an increased respiratory rate, so their NEWS2 score may be falsely reassuring.
- For more information on learning disability and autism take a look at the Oliver McGowan Training on Learning Disability and Autism for healthcare staff.

5.2 Neurodivergence

- Neurodiversity: this term means that some people's brains work in a way that is unique to them. The general population is neurodiverse, with a wide range of variation in how people's brains work.
- Neurotypical: this is a term used to broadly describe how the majority of people's brains work.
- Neurodivergent: this includes autistic people, those with ADHD or dyslexia, and those with other types of neurodivergence including forms of learning difficulty (as opposed to learning disability).
- There are many different types of learning difficulty. Some of the more well-known are dyslexia, ADHD, dyspraxia and dyscalculia. A person can have one, or a combination.
- Some neurodivergent people will have a learning disability too, although most will not.
- Some neurodivergent people will face challenges with communication.
- Autism is a form of neurodivergence. Every autistic patient is different, with different strengths and challenges.
- Autism is a lifelong developmental condition that affects how people perceive the world and interact with others. Each autistic person will have their own strengths and challenges. Areas of challenge might include social communication and social interaction, repetitive and restrictive behaviour, over- or under-sensitivity to sensations such as sound, light, taste or touch, highly focused interests or activities, anxiety and meltdowns or shutdowns.
- Autistic patients are more likely to suffer mental illness and more likely to face health inequalities and poor outcomes with regards to physical health.[6]
- Autistic patients face higher mortality rates for all illness.
- Autistic patients are more than twice as likely to die during an inpatient stay following an emergency presentation (likely related to delayed presentation after previous poor experience, and delayed diagnosis and treatment due to diagnostic overshadowing).
- 32% of autistic adults in a study in 2022 did not seek help for potentially severe symptoms, due to a fear of not being believed or a previous poor experience.
- Consider Autistic SPACE for autistic patients:[7]
  - **Sensory**: autistic patients might have challenges with sensory processing, so may need a quieter environment, altered lighting, time to get used to BP cuffs, etc. Others may have sensory needs and so may need to self-stimulate to reduce anxiety (this may look like hand-flapping, fidgeting, teeth grinding, for example).
  - **Predictability**: routine and structure can help to alleviate anxiety for some people. Explain what is happening and how long things will take.

Clinical Considerations in Relation to Diversity and Equality

- **Acceptance**: accept that everyone is different with different needs, challenges and strengths. Find out about your patient as an individual.
- **Communication**: be clear, avoid jargon or metaphors and listen to answers. Non-verbal cues may be difficult for some patients to exhibit or to interpret, but when present can be very useful. Do not assume the lack of non-verbal cues means that someone is not in pain or distress. Remember that behavioural changes can also be a form of communication. Do not assume someone is being aggressive – are they anxious, in pain, or trying to convey a frustration or need?
- **Empathy**: contrary to popular belief, autistic patients do not lack empathy. Some patients may be hyper-empathic and pick up on emotions to such an extent as to overwhelm them. Remember to also show empathy for your patient, even if they do not communicate in a way you are used to.

5.3 General Principles

- Be cautious of assumptions based on a patient's disability e.g.: level of activity/ability.
- There are challenges in understanding pain in patients with chronic conditions/disability.
- Pain is subjective and individuals who experience chronic pain (and thus disability) may report this in different ways compared to those experiencing an acute onset of pain. Chronic pain and disability present challenges in terms of multiple symptoms impacting different body systems and most pain assessment tools do not take the holistic view into consideration. Patients who are unable to verbally articulate their pain levels in a way that corresponds with the clinician's understanding are at risk of being treated incorrectly. This increases the risk that clinician bias overly influences decision making regarding treatment.
- Where possible, establish the regular parameters for the individual e.g.: GCS, Pain score, level of activity etc, this may differ to non-disabled patients. Compare if/how this is different to regular parameters.
- Not every disability is synonymous with illness: a presenting condition may not necessarily be directly linked to a pre-existing disability.
- Treatment plans should, where possible, consider the impact to a pre-existing condition/disability.
- Ensure the patient has access to their assistance aids such as electronic communication aids, assistance dogs, mobility aids or anything that supports communication, treatment and transportation.
- The literature indicates that:
  - Healthcare provider/clinician's characteristics, beliefs and personal assumptions impact on the clinician's decision making[8]
  - Conflict commonly exists between the patient's reported experience of pain and the clinician's observations and expectations of pain[9]
  - Pain interventions are primarily based on the clinician's knowledge rather than the patient's experience and not evidence based[10]
- A patient with a physical or learning disability may have communication difficulties (refer to **Patients with Communication Difficulties**).

6. Maternity and Gender Related Conditions

- The maternity section in the guidelines, uses the term 'woman, women or mother' in relation to the gynaecological and pregnancy related conditions that ambulance clinicians may be called to assess and manage.
- This is consistent with where other conditions traditionally associated with males are considered and the term 'man and men' are used.
- It is acknowledged that these terms do not reflect the diverse range of patients that you may see with such conditions including those who identify as non-binary or transgender.
- We will keep this language under review and acknowledge that there is as yet a lack of consensus in clinical practice as how best to reflect these issues and challenges.
- Language aside it is important that when assessing all patients to be mindful of drawing erroneous conclusions related to perceived gender related diagnoses.
- Where clinically appropriate gender-neutral descriptions will be adopted.

7. Sexual Orientation

7.1 Overview

- In 2021 1.5 million people (3.2% of the population aged 16 years and over) identified as having a sexuality other than heterosexual.[11]
- Conditions such as depression, anxiety, self-harm and substance misuse including alcohol are found with greater frequency amongst the LGBT+ community than in the general population.[12]
- These can have a basis in their experience of hostility and discrimination because of their sexual orientation.
- Clinicians should be aware of these often-hidden health issues and reflect these in their clinical assessment and practice.

Clinical Considerations in Relation to Diversity and Equality

7.2 Consent to Sharing Sexual Orientation with Other Health Professionals

- Clinicians taking a social history from patients and asking about family and support structures must not make assumptions as to sexuality.
- Where relevant information regarding a patient's sexuality has been obtained, this information should be recorded and handed over to other health care professionals with the patient's consent, to ensure this information is available for those caring for the patient further along the chain of care.
- Patients may be reluctant to consent to this information being shared. Where the regarding sexual orientation is relevant to possible diagnosis and could alter or influence care, it is expected that the professional will encourage the individual patient to allow sharing of this sensitive information.

8. Gender

8.1 What is transgender/non-binary?

- The sex of all children born in the UK is observed, confirmed and recorded at birth. This is usually based on their genitalia and traditionally that child is then raised in a way which matches this assigned sex. A minority find that how they view themselves and their gender does not match with the sex they were assigned. Identifying as a different gender to that recorded at birth is what makes someone transgender.
- If someone finds that their gender identity does not fit with the male/female binary and they identify more as someone else or in-between, then they commonly will identify as non-binary.
- There is no one size fits all approach to the provision of care for transgender/non-binary patients. Some patients may identify in ways not covered in these guidelines. If in doubt – ask. The patient is the expert on their own experiences and will be able to clarify how they would like you to refer to them.

8.2 Transitioning

- Some patients who discover that their gender identity is not that which they were assigned at birth, may decide to begin transitioning to their actual gender.

> - **Social transitioning** occurs when the individual has begun to inform others – also known as coming out.
> - **Medical transitioning** involves individuals taking steps to change their appearance in a more permanent way.

- Some acts of Social Transitioning:
  - Changing their names either legally or socially
  - Using pronouns in their preferred gender
  - Using the bathroom of their preferred gender
  - Adopting the traditional clothing and hairstyle of their gender
  - Using binders to reduce the appearance of breasts or implants to increase breast size
  - Using packers to replicate the appearance of male genitalia through underwear or tucking to conceal genitalia.
- Some acts of Medical Transitioning:
  - Taking hormones to induce endocrinological changes.
  - Gender confirmation surgery on genitalia (sometimes referred to as bottom surgery)
  - Breast removal/breast augmentation (sometimes referred to as top surgery)
  - Facial surgery
  - Laser hair removal

8.3 Considering Transition when Providing Emergency Care

- Always consider the gender of a patient might not be obvious or what they were assigned at birth. While it is preferred that patients are referred to by their names and pronouns, consideration as to both their gender assigned at birth and their current stage of transition is essential for the provision of good medical care. Male and non-binary patients may need to be screened for medical emergencies such as ectopic pregnancy, while female and non-binary patients may need to be screened for medical emergencies such as testicular torsion.
- Clinicians should consider undertaking a relevant history of transition including any social, hormonal and surgical elements of the individual's transition. These should be recorded, and any relevant details noted, then handed over to other relevant health care professionals as required.[13]
- Patients may be reluctant to consent to this information being shared, so it is important that clinicians ensure the patient understands the importance of this information to the provision of proper medical care. Patients should be reassured that their current name, pronouns and gender identity will also be handed over alongside their assigned gender identity and birth and transitional history.

8.4 Disorders of Sex Development

- There are also people that do not fit the binary physical classification of male or female, these people were previously known as Intersex.[14]
- Due to the complexity of the various conditions that may be considered intersex (e.g. Klinefelter syndrome, Turners syndrome, XXX, XYY, X0, XXYY to name only a few), the clinician may

Clinical Considerations in Relation to Diversity and Equality

need to ask their patient about how the condition affects them and if they have any particular treatment requirements.

8.5 Gender Dysphoria

- Gender dysphoria (GD) is a term that describes a sense of unease that a person may have because of a mismatch between their biological sex and their gender identity.
- Gender dysphoria is a constellation of symptoms experienced by most trans/non-binary people. This can be experienced as physical discomfort, and psychological and emotional distress. Deadnaming an individual or using the wrong pronouns can trigger dysphoria in patients. Clinicians should use the right pronouns and name for a patient.
- People with gender dysphoria may have a range of feelings and behaviours that show discomfort or distress. The level of distress can be severe and affect all areas of their life.
- Gender dysphoria is not a mental illness, but some people may develop mental health problems because of gender dysphoria.
- WHO and its International classification of disease (ICD) 11th edition redefined gender identity-related health as gender incongruence, reflecting current knowledge that trans-related and gender diverse identities are not conditions of mental ill-health.

Statistics	- People with an incongruent gender identity are over 4 times more likely than the general population to suffer from mental health problems. - Transgender-identified youth are prone to elevated rates of depression and/or anxiety and are more likely to suffer from eating disorders. - Around 1 in 8 LGBT+ people have experienced unequal treatment from healthcare staff because they are LGBT+. One in seven have avoided treatment for fear of discrimination.
Risk factors	- Isolation or rejection from family or friends based on their identity. - Those with known GD or who are in the process of being diagnosed are at higher risk of mental health problems. - Barriers to accessing healthcare. - Bullying and harassment. - Victimisation and hate crimes.
Signs and symptoms	**Children** - A diagnosis of gender dysphoria in childhood is rare. **Adolescent and Adult** - If feelings of gender dysphoria began in childhood, by now there may be a much clearer sense of a gender identity and how to deal with it. - Certain that their gender identity conflicts with their biological sex. - Comfortable only when in the gender role of your preferred gender identity (may include non-binary). - A strong desire to hide or be rid of physical signs of your biological sex, such as breasts or facial hair. - Having or suppressing these feelings affects their emotional and psychological wellbeing.
Assessment and Management	Assess for any physical or physiological concerns (self-harm, suicide attempt, hypoxia secondary to binding, infection from surgery) and refer to the Mental Health team if necessary. If there are no life-threatening concerns you should - Refer the patient to their GP for consideration of referral to a Gender Dysphoria clinic (GDC) where an assessment by a specialist team can be undertaken.

Clinical Considerations in Relation to Diversity and Equality

9. Cultural Differences

- The ways people express themselves is variable (louder, stand closer to people, express pain, how people present when distressed, or bereaved).
- Practitioners should be conscious not to misinterpret such behaviours according to their own cultural biases.
- Cultural, ethnic and religious practice around illness, particularly death and dying may need to be considered when managing the patients and their families.
- Some of the products used in health care may come from sources that some faith groups find difficult, such as blood or porcine derived products. Whilst not in common paramedic practice, practitioners should be familiar and respectful with the issues and be able to respond to questions about the products they use.

10. Talking about People

- It is easy to give unintended offence by referring to an individual using insensitive, inappropriate or outdated language.
- Similarly, not understanding an unfamiliar term used by an individual about their needs or protected characteristics can make providing appropriate adjustments challenging.
- This section does not cover all such terms, but it includes some of the more frequently used terms and examples of preferred approaches.

10.1 Gender and Sexuality

Some useful terms when caring for transgender/non-binary patients, writing notes and handing over care.	
Assigned male at birth (AMAB)	Someone who was assigned male sex and gender identity at birth
Assigned female at birth (AFAB)	Someone who was assigned female sex and gender at birth
Transgender	Those who were assigned a gender at birth that is incongruent with their actual gender identity
Trans	An acceptable and commonly used term, short for transgender
Non-binary	People who identify neither as male, nor female – outside of the traditional gender binary
Transitioning	The process of social, medical or surgical interventions to live in one's true gender identity, rather than the one assigned at birth.
Deadname	The name assigned to an individual at birth, which has been discarded by the individual
Deadnaming	The act of using a deadname to refer to someone, which can be a painful reminder of past traumatic experiences
Binder	A piece of clothing/wrapping/bandage placed around the chest to reduce the appearance of breasts. Binders can be made for this purpose or improvised.
Packer	A prosthetic penis and/or testicles placed in the underwear. Packers can be made for this purpose or improvised
Gender confirmation surgery	Surgical interventions and procedures which alter the patient's body to better reflect their gender identity

10.2 Person Centred Language

- Person centred language reflects good manners and helps develop empathy facilitating good communication and care.
- The general approach should be to describe the person with a disease or impairment not as a condition or disability. i.e. Person with diabetes, not a diabetic.
- It may be more appropriate to describe the adjustment that needs to be considered rather than the specific condition, i.e. John has some communication difficulties and finds it easier to lip read. This is important as many conditions and impairments produce different levels of disability for people, i.e. restricted vision and uses visual aids may have different needs to someone with little or no vision who needs written material in a different format or uses an electronic reading device.
- The table produced below is for illustration rather than a complete list.[28]

Clinical Considerations in Relation to Diversity and Equality

Use	Avoid
Disabled	(the) handicapped, (the) disabled
Has (a condition) e.g. has diabetes Person with epilepsy	Afflicted by, suffers from, victim of.
Wheel-chair user	Confined to a wheelchair
Uses British sign language/lip-reads	Deaf, Deaf Mute
Person with a hearing impairment	
Person with restricted growth	Dwarf, Midget
Person with a visual impairment	Blind

11. Current Areas for Development not Completely within the Remit of JRCALC

- As stated at the start of this chapter, promoting equality and removing particularly inadvertent or indirect bias is a continuing challenge for organisations. JRCALC references national standards of practice which reflect the current limitations of evidence and policy, but where we feel there are opportunities to reflect if the science and practice of medicine allows us to remove bias, we will undertake to do this.
- With this in mind we are having conversations regarding skin tone and colour in currently widely used tools.
- Tools under discussion include:
  - NICE Fever in Children guidance
  - APGAR scoring
  - CRESS tool
  - Pulse oximetry

References

1. HCPC. 2023. The Standards of Proficiency of a Paramedic Clause 5.3. Available from: https://www.hcpc-uk.org/standards/standards-of-proficiency/paramedics/. Accessed 15/3/2024.
2. Mental Capacity Act 2005. https://www.legislation.gov.uk/ukpga/2005/9/contents
3. HQIP. *Confidential Enquiry into Deaths of People with Learning Disabilities CIPOLD 2013*. 2013. Available from: https://www.hqip.org.uk/resource/confidential-enquiry-into-deaths-of-people-with-learning-disabilities-cipold-2013/#.Xbya1fZ2vIU.
4. NHS England. *Learning from lives and deaths – People with a learning disability and autistic people (LeDeR)*. 2024. Available from: https://www.england.nhs.uk/learning-disabilities/improving-health/learning-from-lives-and-deaths/
5. Mencap. *How Common Is Learning Disability?* 2020. Available from: https://www.mencap.org.uk/learning-disability-explained/research-and-statistics/how-common-learning-disability
6. Barriers to healthcare and self-reported adverse outcomes for autistic adults: a cross-sectional study – PubMed (nih.gov)
7. Autistic SPACE: a novel framework for meeting the needs of autistic people in healthcare settings | British Journal of Hospital Medicine (magonlinelibrary.com)
8. Aronowitz SV et al. Mixed studies review of factors influencing receipt of pain treatment by injured black patients. *Journal of Advanced Nursing 2020*, 76(1): 34–46. doi: 10.1111/jan.14215.
9. Ahluwalia SC et al. "Sometimes you wonder, is this really true?": Clinician assessment of patients' subjective experience of pain. *Journal of evaluation in clinical practice* 2020, 26(3): 1048–1053. doi: 10.1111/jep.13298.
10. De Vaal, A et al. Pain assessment and management: An audit of practice at a tertiary hospital. *Health SA Gesondheid 2020*, 25(1): 1–7. doi: 10.4102/hsag.v25i0.1281
11. Office for National Statistics (ONS), released 6 January 2023, ONS website, statistical bulletin, Gender identity, England and Wales: Census 2021
12. Backmann CL, Gooch B. 2018. Pub Stonewall LGBT in Britain Health Report 2018. Available from: https://www.stonewall.org.uk/system/files/lgbt_in_britain_health.pdf. Accessed 15/3/2024.
13. National Ambulance LGBT Network, 2020. The Ambulance Service Trans Toolkit - Book 2 Better Care to Trans Patients.
14. Office of the United Nations High Commissioner for Human Rights. 2016. "Free & Equal Campaign Fact Sheet: Intersex. Available from: https://www.unfe.org/wp-content/uploads/2017/05/UNFE-Intersex.pdf
15. Frietas LD. Psychiatric disorders in individuals diagnosed with gender dysphoria: A systematic review. *Journal of Psychiatry and clinical neurosciences* 2019, 74(2): 99–104.
16. Gender dysphoria – NHS (www.nhs.uk)
17. Gender dysphoria – Signs – NHS (www.nhs.uk)
18. Government Equalities Office. 2018. National LGBT survey summary report [online]. London: Government Equalities Office.

Clinical Considerations in Relation to Diversity and Equality

19. Equality Act, 2010. Available from: https://www.legislation.gov.uk/ukpga/2010/15/contents

20. Gender Identity Clinic (GIC), 2023. *Gender dysphoria* [online]. London: The Tavistock and Portman NHS Foundation Trust. Available from: https://gic.nhs.uk/info-support/gender-dysphoria/. Accessed 10 February 2023.

21. NHS England, NHS England/medical directorate. 2013. Interim Gender Dysphoria Protocol and Service Guideline 2013/14. London: NHS England.

22. Sax, L. 2010. How common is Intersex? A response to Anne Fausto-Sterling. https://doi.org/10.1080/00224490209552139

23. Council of Europe Commissioner for Human Rights. 2016. Human rights and intersex people. Retrieved from https://rm.coe.int/16806da5d4

24. Intersex. https://en.wikipedia.org/wiki/Intersex.

25. Office of the United Nations High Commissioner for Human Rights. 2019. Background Note on Human Rights Violations against Intersex People. Retrieved from https://www.ohchr.org/en/documents/tools-and-resources/background-note-human-rights-violations-against-intersex-people

26. NHS England. What are health inequalities? Available from: https://www.england.nhs.uk/about/equality/equality-hub/national-healthcare-inequalities-improvement-programme/what-are-healthcare-inequalities/

27. Knight M, Bunch K, Tuffnell D, Shakespeare J et al. (eds). MBRRACE (2020) Saving Lives, Improving Mothers' Care: Lessons learned to inform maternity care from the UK and Ireland Confidential Enquiries into Maternal Deaths and Morbidity 2016–18. Available from: https://www.npeu.ox.ac.uk/assets/downloads/mbrrace-uk/reports/maternal-report-2020/MBRRACE- UK_Maternal_Report_Dec_2020_v10_ONLINE_VERSION_1404.pdf.

28. GOV.UK. 2021. Inclusive language: words to use and avoid when writing about disability. Available from: https://www.gov.uk/government/publications/inclusive-communication/inclusive-language-words-to-use-and-avoid-when-writing-about-disability. Accessed 20/3/24.

Conditions Requiring Specific Prehospital Clinical Management

1. Introduction

- This document aims to provide both guidance on conditions that are less frequently encountered in the out-of-hospital environment, and conditions that may require additional considerations further to the standard JRCALC guidance.
- It is important to remember that patients experiencing chronic or rare diseases are often experts in their own condition. This knowledge should be respected and will often heavily influence your decision-making regarding both treatment and transportation decisions.
- As clinicians we appropriately have a lower threshold for wanting to convey these clinically complex patients to hospital, however careful consideration must be given to whether this really is the best option for the patient both medically and holistically. The constantly evolving community healthcare services available may better fit the patient's overall needs.
- Many patients with long-term conditions will have personalised advance care plans or ReSPECT plans (Recommended Summary Plan for Emergency Care and Treatment) in place. These outline recommendations for a person's clinical care and treatment in a future emergency in which they are unable to make or express choices.
- Finally, it must be recognised that some of these conditions may be undiagnosed. Consequently, arrangements for formal diagnosis should be pursued, incorporating appropriate safety-netting measures as needed.

2. Autonomic Dysreflexia

Overview

Autonomic dysreflexia (AD) is a potentially life-threatening condition experienced by those with spinal cord injuries. It is characterized by an uninhibited sympathetic nervous system response to stimuli below the level of spinal cord injury. It primarily affects individuals with spinal cord injuries at T6 or above, and the most common trigger for autonomic dysreflexia are bladder and bowel distension.

Presentation/Signs & Symptoms/Disease Characteristics

- Hypertension: Greater than 20 mmHg above baseline for both systolic and diastolic.
- Severe bilateral pounding headache.
- Diaphoresis or flushing above the level of the spinal cord lesion (diaphoresis can be profuse).
- Nasal congestion.
- Visual changes or disturbances.
- Bradycardia or tachycardia (bradycardia at onset, tachycardia may follow).
- Pallor or gooseflesh below the level of the spinal cord lesion.
- Respiratory distress or bronchospasms.
- Anxiety (apprehension over impending physical problem to fear of death is common).
- Metallic taste in mouth.
- Significantly elevated BP with minimal or no symptoms (Silent Autonomic Dysreflexia).

Assessment & Management

Refer to **Medical Emergencies in Adults – Overview** for general assessment and management.

Specific management / key points:

- Identify and where possible remove the trigger. Common triggers include urinary retention, faecal impaction, tight clothing, pressure sores or any other noxious stimulus below the level of the spinal cord injury.
  – For patients with a catheter – empty the leg bag and note the volume. Check the tubing is not blocked or kinked.
  – Loosen or remove any tight clothing.
- Where possible, sit the patient upright.
- Review patient treatment plan and support the patient to take medication they have been prescribed for AD. This may include sublingual Nifedipine or GTN.

References

Autonomic Dysreflexia. Royal National Orthopaedic Hospital https://www.rnoh.nhs.uk/services/spinal-cord-injury-centre/clinical-resources-advice/autonomic-dysreflexia

Autonomic Dysreflexia. Spinal Injuries Association. https://spinal.co.uk/get-support/body-matters/autonomic-dysreflexia/

3. Cauda Equina Syndrome

For Cauda Equina Syndrome (CNS), also refer to **Spinal Injury and Spinal Cord Injury** and **Low Back Pain (Non-traumatic)**.

Overview

Cauda Equina Syndrome (CES) is a serious neurological condition where the nerve roots at the bottom of the spinal cord become compressed. CES is considered an acute surgical emergency, as delayed treatment can lead to permanent nerve damage, resulting in long-term consequences like incontinence and paralysis. The condition is typically treated with surgery to relieve the pressure on the nerves. Causes of CES include herniated discs, spinal stenosis, tumours, infections, or spinal injuries. Early diagnosis and treatment are crucial for the best outcomes.

Conditions Requiring Specific Prehospital Clinical Management

Presentation / Signs & Symptoms / Disease Characteristics

Cauda Equina Syndrome (CES) presents with a range of signs and symptoms, which may develop rapidly or gradually.

Key symptoms include:

- Severe lower back pain
  - Often the first symptom, this pain can be intense and persistent.
- Sciatica
  - Sharp, stabbing pain radiating from the lower back down to one or both legs. Bilateral sciatica is a red flag for CES.
- Saddle anaesthesia
  - Loss of sensation in the areas that would touch a saddle when sitting – inner thighs, back of legs, and around the rectum.
- Bladder and bowel dysfunction
  - This can range from difficulty in urinating, loss of bladder control (urinary retention or incontinence), to bowel incontinence.
- Motor weakness or loss of reflexes in lower limbs
  - This includes heaviness in the legs, difficulty walking, or a marked decrease in reflexes.
- Sensory deficits
  - Numbness, tingling, or loss of sensation in the lower limbs or genital region.
- New onset sexual dysfunction
  - Erectile dysfunction, or loss of sensation.

Assessment & Management

Clinical diagnosis of CES is not easy. Most cases are of sudden onset and progress rapidly within hours or days. However, CES can evolve slowly, and patients do not always complain of pain. Roughly 50–70% of patients present late with urinary retention.

Use the GIRFT National Suspected Cauda Equina Syndrome Pathway to support decision making: https://girft-interactivepathways.org.uk/cauda-equina-1/

Manage the patients pain (refer to **Pain Management in Adults and Children**).

If the cause of CES is due to trauma (rare) – consider spinal immobilisation of the patient (refer to **Spinal Injury and Spinal Cord Injury**).

Recognition and conveyance for further assessment is the priority for CES.

References

- https://caudaequinaawareness.co.uk/
- https://www.nhs.uk/conditions/lumbar-decompression-surgery/why-its-done/
- https://spinal.co.uk/get-informed/cauda-equina-syndrome/
- https://girft-interactivepathways.org.uk/cauda-equina-1/

4. Cerebral Palsy

Overview

Cerebral palsy (CP) is a group of permanent movement disorders that appear in early childhood. It's primarily characterized by poor coordination, stiff muscles, weak muscles, and tremors. There may also be problems with sensation, vision, hearing, swallowing, and speaking. Other symptoms include seizures and problems with thinking or reasoning, which can occur in about one-third of cases.

Cerebral palsy is caused by abnormal development or damage to the parts of the brain that control movement, balance, and posture.

There is no cure for cerebral palsy, but supportive treatments, medications, and surgery can help many individuals improve their motor skills and ability to communicate.

Assessment & Management / Key Points

During acute medical emergencies:

- Airway management – be cautious as patients with CP may have abnormal airway anatomy or reflexes. They may also be at an increased risk of aspiration. Have a low threshold for escalation of care in case of airway compromise.
- Seizure control – refer to **Seizures in Children** and **Seizures in Adults**.
- Have a low threshold for conveyance of patients with CP who present with signs of infection due to increased risk of deterioration.
- Family / caregivers will often be familiar with the patients baseline condition, and therefore their concerns should be carefully considered when making transport / admission decisions.

References

Cerebral Palsy Overview. NHS. https://www.nhs.uk/conditions/cerebral-palsy/

http://www.cerebralpalsy.org.uk/

https://www.scope.org.uk

5. Diabetes Insipidus

Overview

Diabetes Insipidus (DI) is a rare condition characterised by intense thirst and the production of large amounts of urine. It is different to the more common diagnosis of diabetes mellitus in that it involves antidiuretic hormone (ADH) dysfunction rather than a problem with blood sugar regulation. Patients with DI will usually have normal blood glucose levels.

It's crucial for patients with DI to maintain adequate hydration.

Conditions Requiring Specific Prehospital Clinical Management

Presentation / Signs & Symptoms / Disease Characteristics

In severe cases or if left untreated, Diabetes Insipidus can lead to dehydration and an electrolyte imbalance, which may present with symptoms such as dry mouth, hypotension, muscle pains or cramps, and in extreme cases, arrhythmias, shock, or coma.

Assessment & Management

If any major <C>ABCD problems, refer to **Medical Emergencies in Adults** and **Medical Emergencies in Children**.

Assess for signs of dehydration – administer fluid therapy as required. Oral hydration is an option if the patient is conscious and able to drink without the risk of aspiration. See **Intravascular Fluid Therapy in Adults** and **Intravascular Fluid Therapy in Children**.

A 12-lead ECG should be undertaken in all cases to help identify arrythmias. This may also identify electrolyte imbalance. See **Cardiac Arrhythmia and Sudden Cardiac Death**.

Unwell patients with DI require blood testing at hospital.

References

Diabetes Insipidus Overview. NHS. https://www.nhs.uk/conditions/diabetes-insipidus/

6. Epiglottitis

For epiglottitis also refer to **Foreign Body Airway Obstruction**, **Medical Emergencies in Children** and **Medical Emergencies in Adults** and **Dyspnoea** guidance.

Overview

Epiglottitis is a potentially life-threatening condition characterized by inflammation and swelling of the epiglottis, a small cartilage lid that covers the trachea. This swelling can cause upper airway occlusion. It's most commonly caused by a bacterial infection, although it can also result from other factors like injury.

Epiglottitis can develop rapidly and requires immediate medical attention. Symptoms include severe sore throat, fever, a hoarse or muffled voice, difficulty swallowing, and, in severe cases, difficulty breathing. Since the widespread introduction of Haemophilus Influenza type B (Hib) vaccination, acute epiglottitis is now extremely rare in children.

Can occur in all age groups and is becoming more prevalent in adults due to decreased uptake of Hib Vaccine. May present with 2–3 days of worsening symptoms followed by acute airway obstruction.

Presentation / Signs & Symptoms / Disease Characteristics

- Rapid onset
  - Symptoms develop quickly, often over hours
- High fever
- Severe sore throat
- Difficulty breathing
- Muffled or hoarse voice
- Stridor
  - A high-pitched wheezing sound during breathing.
- Drooling
- Anxious or agitated behaviour
- Sitting upright or leaning forward ("tripoding")
- Cyanosis

The main symptoms of epiglottitis in young children are breathing difficulties, stridor and a hoarse voice.

In adults and older children, swallowing difficulties and drooling are the main symptoms.

Assessment & Management

Recognition is the most important factor in the management of epiglottitis. Unrecognised epiglottitis may quickly become life-threatening.

Assess and manage these patients, refer to **Medical Emergencies in Children – Overview**, **Respiratory Illness in Children** and **Medical Emergencies in Adults – Overview**, with particular attention to addressing Airway and Breathing compromise.

- Try to keep the patient calm to prevent agitation worsening the airway obstruction.
- If possible, sit the patient upright to aid with breathing.
- Rapidly transport the patient to the Emergency Department.
- Avoid unnecessary procedures that may further irritate the airway.
- Prepare for escalating airway management as required. Consider specialist / advanced support.

References

Epiglottitis. NHS. https://www.nhs.uk/conditions/epiglottitis/

7. Factor V Leiden

Overview

Factor V Leiden is a genetic disorder characterised by a mutation in the Factor V gene. This mutation leads to an increased tendency for blood to clot, a condition known as thrombophilia. People with Factor V Leiden are at a higher risk of developing abnormal blood clots, which can include deep vein thrombosis (DVT) and pulmonary embolism (PE).

The risk of thrombosis can be influenced by other factors such as surgery, pregnancy, and the use of oral contraceptives.

Conditions Requiring Specific Prehospital Clinical Management

Assessment & Management

In patients with known Factor V Leiden be aware of their increased risk of venous thrombosis when undertaking patient assessment and formulating differential diagnosis.

Assess particularly for:

- Deep vein thrombosis
  - Swelling in one leg (rarely both legs).
  - Pain or tenderness in one leg (rarely both legs); often felt only when standing or walking.
  - Increased warmth in the leg that is swollen or painful.
  - Red or discoloured skin around the painful area.
  - Swollen veins that are hard or sore when touched.
  - IMPORTANT: DVTs may also occur in the patient's upper leg, pelvis / abdomen and arms.
  - Consider Wells criteria for DVT.
- Pulmonary embolism
  - See Pulmonary Embolism.
  - See Dyspnoea.
- Stroke
  - See Stroke and Transient Ischaemic Attack.

The fact that patients with Factor V Leiden are at an increased risk of developing thrombus must be considered in all patient assessment and diagnosis.

References

https://thrombosisuk.org/

https://www.mkuh.nhs.uk/patient-information-leaflet/factor-v-leiden-information

8. Guillian-Barre Syndrome

Overview

Guillain-Barre syndrome is a rare inflammatory condition that affects the nerves. It most commonly occurs after a recent viral infection, but not always. This causes muscle weakness, pain, and sometimes paralysis. The onset of Guilian-Barre Syndrome is gradual and progressive over several days. 20–30% of patients with this condition go on to require non-invasive or invasive ventilatory support. Most patients make a full recovery with treatment.

Presentation / Signs & Symptoms / Disease Characteristics

Signs and symptoms of Guillain-Barre:

- Muscle weakness
- Paraesthesia
- Speech problems
- Areflexia/hyporeflexia (decreased reflex reaction of muscles)
- Diplopia
- Dysarthria
- Dysphagia
- Dysautonomia

Signs and symptoms of respiratory muscle fatigue in patients with GB:

- Tachypnoea
- Sweating
- Tachycardia
- Asynchronous movements of the chest and abdomen
- Use of accessory muscles

Assessment & Management / Key Points

- If any major <C>ABCD problems, treat as per **Medical Emergencies in Adults** and **Medical Emergencies in Children**.
- Consider pre-hospital specialist / advanced support if needed.
- Transfer to a hospital, ideally with ICU capabilities.

References

Guillain-Barre syndrome – Symptoms, diagnosis and treatment | BMJ Best Practice

Diagnosis and treatment of Guillain-Barré Syndrome in childhood and adolescence: An evidence- and consensus-based guideline.

R Korinthenberg[1], R Trollmann[2], U Felderhoff-Müser[3], G Bernert[4], A Hackenberg[5], M Hufnagel[6], M Pohl[7], G Hahn[8], H J Mentzel[9], C Sommer[10], J Lambeck[11], F Mecher[12], M Hessenauer[13], C Winterholler[14], U Kempf[15], B C Jacobs[16], K Rostasy[17], W Müller-Felber[18]

Diagnosis and management of Guillain–Barré syndrome in ten steps.

Sonja E. Leonhard,[1] Melissa R. Mandarakas,[1] Francisco A. A. Gondim,[2] Kathleen Bateman,[3] Maria L. B. Ferreira,[4] David R. Cornblath,[5] Pieter A. van Doorn,[1] Mario E. Dourado,[6] Richard A. C. Hughes,[7] Badrul Islam,[8] Susumu Kusunoki,[9] Carlos A. Pardo,[5] Ricardo Reisin,[10] James J. Sejvar,[11] Nortina Shahrizaila,[12] Cristiane Soares,[13] Thirugnanam Umapathi,[14] Yuzhong Wang,[15] Eppie M. Yiu,[16,17,18] Hugh J. Willison,[19] and Bart C. Jacobs[20]

9. Haemophilia

Overview

Haemophilia is a rare condition that affects the blood's ability to clot. It's usually inherited and most people who have it are male.

There are two main types: Haemophilia A, caused by a deficiency of clotting factor VIII, and Haemophilia B, caused by a deficiency of clotting factor IX. Regardless of type, the overall principles of management are the same for all bleeding disorders.

Conditions Requiring Specific Prehospital Clinical Management

BLEEDING DISORDER INFORMATION CARD

Name: Forename Surname
Date of Birth: 01 June 1995   CHI No: 1234567890
Diagnosis: Information 2
Level   Information 3   Current Inhibitor: YES/NO
Usual Treatment Product: Information 8
Hospital   Address 1
Tel: Information 5   Out of Hours No: Information 6
2nd line treatment: Information 7

ATTENTION!

If this patient presents with head injury or trauma, contact Haematology immediately and assess / treat the bleeding disorder without delay under the supervision of an experienced haematologist

In the event of any presentation to casualty the Haemophilia team should be contacted without delay

Before any surgery is carried out the managing Haemophilia Centre must be consulted

WWW.UKHCDO.ORG

Trauma patients with haemophilia are at an increased risk of bleeding for an extended period of time; this bleeding may be concealed (internal). Bleeding may also occur spontaneously. Ongoing and unmanaged bleeding may result in a threat to life.

Presentation / Signs & Symptoms / Disease Characteristics

The patient may carry a Bleeding Disorder Alert Card (as below) or have a MedicAlert device.

Assess carefully for signs and symptoms of internal and external bleeding in all patients with haemophilia.

The following may be considered as time-critical emergencies:

- Suspected intracranial bleed or history of head trauma.
- Oropharyngeal bleed or neck bleed that may threaten the airway.
- Suspected spinal bleed.
- GI bleed.
- Intra-abdominal/retroperitoneal bleed.
- Muscle or soft tissue bleed with compartment syndrome.
- Haemorrhage in and around the eye.

There's a small risk of patients with haemophilia experiencing subarachnoid haemorrhage. However, spontaneous bleeding inside the skull is uncommon and usually only caused by a head injury. Refer to **Stroke and Transient Ischaemic Attack**.

The symptoms of a brain haemorrhage include (refer to **Headache**):

- Severe, sudden onset (thunderclap) headache.
- Neck stiffness.
- Vomiting.
- Change in mental state, such as confusion.
- Difficulty speaking, such as slurred speech.
- Changes in vision, such as double vision.
- Loss of co-ordination and balance.
- Paralysis of some or all of the facial muscles.

Conditions Requiring Specific Prehospital Clinical Management

Assessment & Management / Key Points

If any major <C>ABCD problems, treat as per **Medical Emergencies in Adults** and **Medical Emergencies in Children** guidelines or **Trauma Emergencies in Adults** and **Trauma Emergencies in Children** as appropriate.

Do not underestimate the potential for apparently minor trauma to cause serious bleeding.

If bleeding is suspected *from any trauma*, have a low threshold for administering Tranexamic Acid, even if there is no major trauma. Refer to **Tranexamic Acid**. Also, consider fluid replacement therapy as required. Refer to **Intravascular Fluid Therapy in Adults** and **Intravascular Fluid Therapy in Children**. Care should be taken when IV cannulation is attempted.

Ensure information regarding the patient's bleeding disorder is shared at any subsequent handover of care. If possible, transport the patient to a receiving hospital that hosts a haemophilia centre.

Ask the patient or a carer to administer their Factor Concentrate if the patient is on a home treatment programme.

References

Haemophilia. NHS. https://www.nhs.uk/conditions/haemophilia/

Dr Lishel Horn. Consultant Haematologist. *Haemophilia and Pre-Hospital Care*. UK BASICS Conference.

10. Kawasaki Disease

Overview

Kawasaki Disease is an acute, usually self-limiting inflammatory condition mainly affecting children, most commonly under the age of five. The cause of Kawasaki Disease isn't fully understood.

The disease is characterized by a high fever lasting at least five days, alongside other symptoms such as rash, swollen lymph nodes, red eyes, lips, and tongue, and swelling in the hands and feet.

It's critical to diagnose and treat Kawasaki Disease early to prevent complications such as coronary artery aneurysms. Kawasaki Disease is treated in hospital.

Presentation / Signs & Symptoms / Disease Characteristics

A child with Kawasaki disease has a high temperature that lasts for five days or longer, and possibly one or more of the following symptoms:

- Rash
- Swollen lymph nodes in the neck
- Dry, red cracked lips
- Swollen, bumpy, red tongue ("strawberry tongue")
- Red inside the mouth and at the back of the throat
- Swollen and red hands and feet
- Red eyes

It is important to recognise that some of the above symptoms may be difficult to recognise in patients with dark skin tones, particularly black and brown skin. Careful examination and parental / carer feedback may aid diagnosis. See https://www.blackandbrownskin.co.uk/for further information.

Assessment & Management / Key Points

The definitive diagnosis and treatment of Kawasaki Disease occurs in the hospital setting. Patients with suspected Kawasaki Disease must be transported for further assessment.

References

Kawasaki Disease. BMJ best practice. https://bestpractice.bmj.com/topics/en-gb/236

Kawasaki Disease. NHS. https://www.nhs.uk/conditions/kawasaki-disease/

11. Marfan Syndrome

Overview

Marfan Syndrome is an uncommon inherited disorder of connective tissue characterised by loss of elastic tissue, resulting in musculoskeletal deformities, lens subluxation (dislocation), aortic dissection, and aortic root aneurysms.

These patients are at high risk of acute aortic dissection/rupture, either spontaneously or through traumatic injury (refer to **Vascular Emergencies**).

Assessment & Management / Key Points

Marfan Syndrome may be undiagnosed. It should be considered in patients who are tall and slim with long, thin arms, legs, and fingers.

If a dissection is suspected:

Refer to **Vascular Emergencies**, **Aortic Dissection**.

Transfer immediately to the Emergency Department, and ideally to a hospital with a vascular centre for immediate intervention. Consider prehospital critical care team for support.

References

Heart and Blood Vessels – Marfan Foundation

Marfan syndrome – Symptoms, diagnosis and treatment | BMJ Best Practice

12. Motor Neurone Disease

Overview

Motor Neurone Disease (MND), also known as Amyotrophic Lateral Sclerosis (ALS), is a neurodegenerative condition that affects the brain and nerves. It causes weakness that worsens over time. The disease primarily impacts motor neurons, which are nerve cells responsible for controlling voluntary muscle activities like walking, speaking, breathing, and swallowing. As MND progresses, these neurons deteriorate and die, leading to muscle weakness and atrophy.

Conditions Requiring Specific Prehospital Clinical Management

The exact cause of MND is unknown, but it's believed to involve a combination of genetic and environmental factors. Symptoms vary but often start with slurred speech or weakness in the arms and legs. Unfortunately, there is no cure for MND, and treatment focuses on relieving symptoms and improving quality of life. The progression of the disease is different for each individual, but it can significantly shorten life expectancy.

Assessment & Management / Key Points

Common ambulance service presentations for people with MND:

- Breathing difficulties
- Choking or swallowing problems
- Falls and injuries
- Severe weakness or mobility issues
- Infection

People with MND are at higher risk of infections, such as pneumonia, due to weakened respiratory muscles and potential difficulties with coughing or clearing the lungs. Have a low threshold for seeking early intervention.

There is a subset of MND patients who are at risk of loss of hypoxic drive when high concentrations of oxygen are provided, oxygen should be administered with caution in this group.
Click here for more information on a short 3 minute video clip.

Many patients with MND will have a specific clinical management plan and/or a specialist nursing team. Wherever possible these resources should be considered.

References

MND for acute, urgent and emergency care staff. Motor Neurone Disease Association. https://www.mndassociation.org/professionals/management-of-mnd/management-by-specific-professions/acute-urgent-and-emergency-care-staff

Motor neurone disease

First contact with a patient with MND?

Motor neurone disease (MND) is a fatal, rapidly progressing disease that effects the brain and spinal cord. It has no cure.

Make sure you find out how they communicate

Never lie them flat even if breathless

Don't allow them high flow oxygen (unless in their care plan)

- Consult their care plan
- Avoid A&E wherever possible
  - contact their district nursing team and local care team
  - speak to their local palliative care coordinator or their GP

People experience MND differently.
Please take your time with these patients, and their carers/relatives.

You may come across a patient with MND. These patients have complex needs. This tool card is to help you understand their condition and to give brief guidance on appropriate treatment for these patients.

Key points

People with MND could have a high NEWS score however this could be normal for them. They will have a normal increased respiratory rate and also a lower SpO_2 that needs to be taken into account. Establish if this has changed.

Do they have an emergency health plan (EHA), an advance care plan (ACP), or an advance decision to refuse treatment (ADRT)?

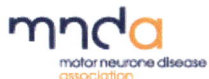
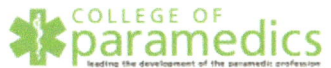

Conditions Requiring Specific Prehospital Clinical Management

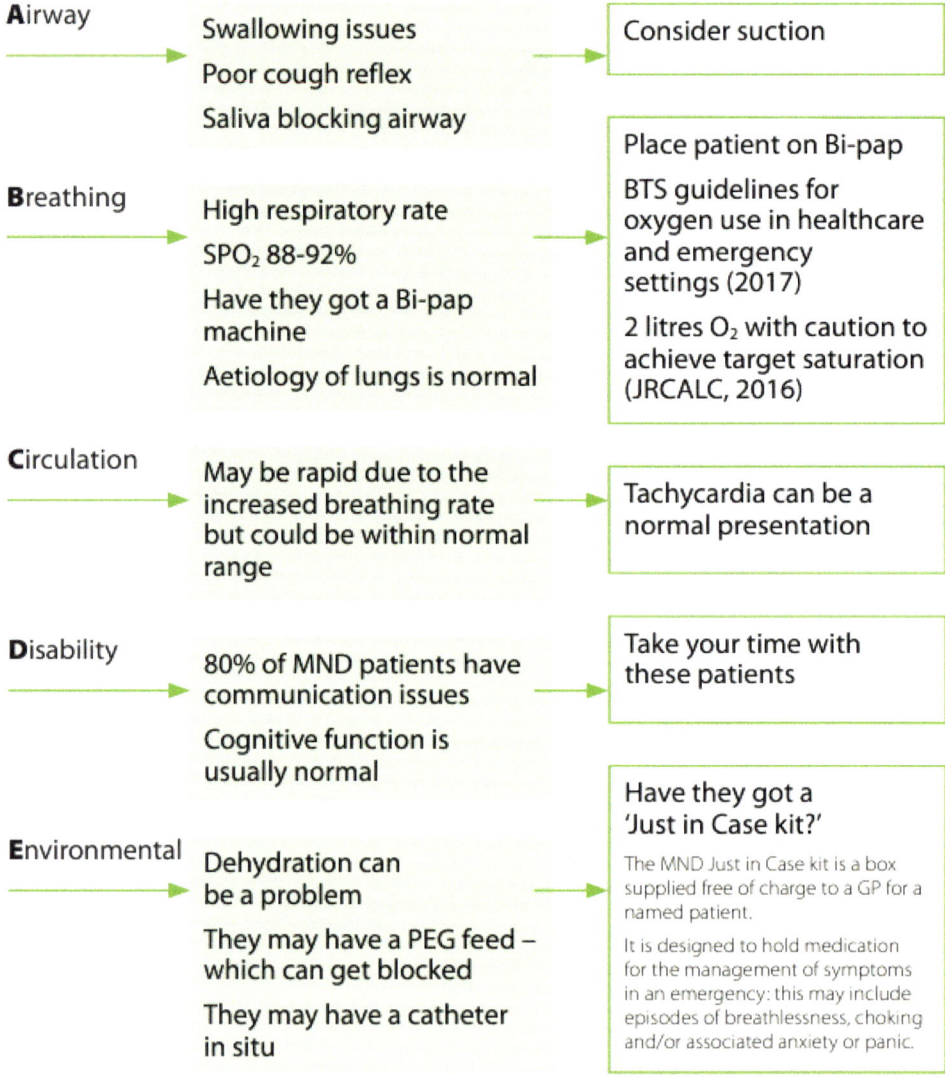

For more information about MND see NICE guideline NG42 and visit www.mndassociation.org

13. Multiple Sclerosis

Overview

Multiple Sclerosis (MS) is an idiopathic, inflammatory demyelinating disorder of the brain and spinal cord. It is a chronic and potentially highly disabling disorder.

The symptoms of MS vary widely from person to person and can affect any part of the body. MS is characterised by episodes of multiple neurological dysfunction, e.g. vision and sensory disturbances, limb weakness, gait problems and bladder and bowel symptoms followed by incomplete recovery.

Patients with an established diagnosis of MS may present with acute complications for which treatment needs to be instituted promptly in order to minimise complications.

The treatments for acute episodes of MS are those that modify the inflammatory process and immune system are used in an attempt to minimise this demyelination and this often includes administration of high-dose cortico-steroids.

Assessment & Management / Key Points

Two-thirds of MS patients die of complications of the disease, particularly pulmonary complications.

Be aware of the following –

- **Fever:** Fever must be reduced to minimise the increased weakness caused by even a small elevation of core temperature.
- **Infection:** It is vital to identify and treat any cause of infection. Urinary tract infections and pyelonephritis must be excluded in any acute exacerbation of MS.

Conditions Requiring Specific Prehospital Clinical Management

- **Urinary retention:** Especially in patients with symptoms of UTI, a post-voiding residual volume may require clinical intervention.
- **Respiratory function:** Respiratory infections must be managed aggressively and may be more frequent due to the higher risk of aspiration.
- **Seizures:** Seizures should be treated according to **Seizures in Adults**.

References

mstrust.org.uk

www.nice.org.uk/guidance/ng220

14. Muscular Dystrophy

Overview

Muscular dystrophy defines a group of genetic muscle conditions with progressive skeletal muscle weaknesses. This wasting is caused by degeneration of muscle cells. This eventually affects the respiratory muscles and even the heart muscle. These conditions vary in severity and affect about 8000 to 10000 people in the UK.

As the condition progresses, these patients are at increased risk of respiratory failure as the lung muscles become weaker.

Assessment & Management / Key Points

Try to ascertain which type of MD the patient has. Some patients may carry alert cards. Treatment differs slightly between conditions.

Patients with MD may present without the usual signs of respiratory distress.

Duchenne muscular dystrophy and Becker muscular dystrophy –

- Consider supplementary O_2 for patients with oxygen saturations of <95%
- Lung volume recruitment (air stacking) may be indicated – patients may respond to a self-inflating manual ventilation bag. BVM.
- Patients may benefit from NIV – consider prehospital advanced / critical care services.
- Suspect arrhythmias in patients with palpitations – ECG.

Facioscapulohumeral muscular dystrophy-

- Carefully titrate oxygen saturations to maintain 88–92%.
- Patients may benefit from NIV – consider prehospital advanced / critical care services.

Congenital muscular dystrophy –

- Titrate supplementary oxygen to achieve saturations of 94–98%.

All patients with MD are at risk of rhythm abnormalities – refer to **Cardiac Arrhythmia and Sudden Cardiac Death**.

Have a low threshold for conveyance of medically unwell patients with MD. MD patients will normally have individual care plans.

Patient may have an alert card: Muscular Dystrophy UK has created condition-specific alert cards for different muscle-wasting conditions. The wallet-sized alert cards contain key recommendations and precautions that a non-specialist clinician should know during a health crisis. They address a range of symptoms and scenarios to ensure their effectiveness. The cards also include space for the contact information of an individual's specialist neuromuscular team, making it easier to access expert advice.

References

Management of respiratory complications and rehabilitation in individuals with muscular dystrophies: 1st Consensus Conference report from UILDM – Italian Muscular Dystrophy Association (Milan, January 25–26, 2019) – PMC (nih.gov)

Muscular dystrophies – Symptoms, diagnosis and treatment | BMJ Best Practice

Muscular Dystrophy UK | Muscular Dystrophy UK

Diagnosis and management of Duchenne muscular dystrophy, part 2: respiratory, cardiac, bone health, and orthopaedic management – ClinicalKey

15. Myasthenia Gravis

Overview

Myasthenia Gravis (MG) is a rare autoimmune disorder resulting from binding of autoantibodies to components of the neuromuscular junction, most commonly the acetylcholine receptor. This leads to muscular weakness with excessive fatigue, which is worse on exercise and improves with rest.

Acute illness, medications, pregnancy, and hypokalaemia can all exacerbate weakness and may swiftly precipitate a myasthenic crisis and respiratory inadequacy.

In severe cases, this can result in life-threatening respiratory failure.

Presentation / Signs & Symptoms / Disease Characteristics

Some of the common signs and symptoms of MG may include:

- Muscle weakness, which may be worse with exercise or later in the day
- Fatigue
- Drooping eyelids
- Double vision
- Difficulty speaking, chewing or swallowing
- Weakness in the limbs or neck

Conditions Requiring Specific Prehospital Clinical Management

Assessment & Management / Key Points

If a patient with MG presents with respiratory distress or difficulty breathing, it is important to act quickly and provide immediate support. This may involve providing supplemental oxygen and assisting with ventilation if necessary (consider advanced / specialist care for NIV if required).

In addition, it is important to be aware that some medications commonly used in pre-hospital care, such as neuromuscular blocking agents and certain antibiotics, can exacerbate MG symptoms.

JRCALC Medication Cautions: (all can cause worsening exacerbation of symptoms)

- Midazolam
- Diazepam
- Morphine
- Atropine (CBRNE only)

References

Myasthenia Gravis: Causes, Symptoms, and Treatment | Doctor | Patient

Myasthenia gravis – NHS (www.nhs.uk)

16. Parkinson's Disease

Overview

Parkinson's is a progressive, fluctuating condition that affects all aspects of daily living including talking, swallowing and writing. Every person's symptoms are different. People with Parkinson's often find it hard to move freely and may be subject to 'freezing'. People describe this as feeling like their feet are 'glued' to the ground. There may also be other issues including anxiety, depression, dementia, hallucinations, pain and continence problems. The severity of symptoms can fluctuate from day to day and people can experience rapid changes in functionality over the course of the day.

Patients may have deep brain stimulation to relieve their symptoms – fine wires are implanted into the brain with a battery pack often under the skin on the chest. An ID card with model number and contact details should be present.

Common complications of Parkinsons:

- Postural hypotension and falls – check meds and BP for postural changes
- Chest infection, especially aspiration pneumonia
- Urinary Tract Infections
- Constipation
- Delirium (acute confusion due to drugs or infection)

Assessment & Management / Key Points:

In the pre-hospital setting there are some considerations related to medications:

- It is important to recognise the significance of regular medication to patients with Parkinsons. Missing doses of Parkinson's medication increases care needs and can cause serious complications, including rare but potentially fatal neuroleptic-like malignant syndrome – DO NOT STOP PARKINSON'S MEDICATION.
- Impaired swallow may make the oral route of medication administration unsuitable due to increased risk of aspiration.
- Anti-emetics – AVOID metoclopramide as this can worsen Parkinson's symptoms.

References

www.parkinsons.org.uk

https://www.parkinsons.org.uk/sites/default/files/2017-12/pk0135_emergencymanagement.pdf

NICE Guideline NG71 – Parkinson's disease in adults (2017)

17. Spinal Metastases and Metastatic Spinal Cord Compression

Overview

Cancer that has spread to the spine is known as 'spinal metastases'. Without treatment, spinal metastases can press on the spinal cord. This is called metastatic spinal cord compression (or MSCC). If it isn't treated quickly, MSCC can lead to serious disability, including permanent paralysis.

MSCC is rare, but very serious. About 3 to 5 in 100 people with cancer develop it. Any type of cancer can lead to spinal cord compression, but it is more common in people with breast cancer, lung cancer, prostate cancer, lymphoma or myeloma.

Presentation / Signs & Symptoms / Disease Characteristics

Think about the possibility of spinal metastases or MSCC in people with any of the factors below:

Cancer:

- Past or current diagnosis of cancer
- Suspected diagnosis of cancer

Pain characteristics suggesting spinal metastases:

- Severe unremitting back pain
- Progressive back pain
- Mechanical pain (aggravated by standing, sitting or moving)

Conditions Requiring Specific Prehospital Clinical Management

- Back pain aggravated by straining (for example, coughing, sneezing or bowel movements)
- Night-time back pain disturbing sleep
- Localised tenderness
- Claudication (muscle pain or cramping in the legs when walking or exercising)

Symptoms and signs suggesting cord compression:

- Bladder or bowel dysfunction
- Gait disturbance or difficulty walking
- Limb weakness
- Neurological signs of spinal cord or cauda equina compression
- Numbness, paraesthesia, or sensory loss
- Radicular pain

Assessment & Management / Key Points

MSCC is an oncological emergency.

Spinal Immobilisation:

Start immobilisation without delay (including for transfer to hospital) for people with:

- Suspected or confirmed MSCC

and

- neurological symptoms or signs suggesting spinal instability.

Consider spinal immobilisation for people with:

- suspected or confirmed spinal metastases or MSCC

and

- moderate to severe pain associated with movement.

Ensure adequate pain relief is provided promptly for people with suspected or confirmed spinal metastases or MSCC. See **Pain Management in Adults and Children** and **End of Life Care** guidelines.

References

Spinal metastases and metastatic spinal cord compression. NICE guideline [NG234] Published: 06 September 2023.

Consent in Pre-hospital Care

1. Consent in Pre-hospital Care

- The laws and guidance that relate to consent to assessment, treatment, care and other interventions are different in the countries and/or jurisdictions that constitute the UK.
- Therefore, these guidelines do not offer guidance on obtaining consent beyond the general advice in this statement; the Joint Royal Colleges Ambulance Liaison Committee (JRCALC) advises strongly that readers should seek specific guidance on consent from their ambulance services, Trusts or other relevant employers.
- JRCALC advises that obtaining consent in ways that are lawful in the jurisdiction in which each reader works is fundamental to meeting patients' legal and ethical rights in determining what happens to them and to their own bodies. Therefore, it is important to ensure that you always act in the patient's best interest and that you have legally valid consent to conduct assessments, treatments or interventions, and provide care.
- Consent must be obtained from each patient or their legally valid representative (defined according to the law in the relevant country or jurisdiction) prior to conducting examinations or treatment, or providing care.
- Ensure that you provide patients with the appropriate information to enable them to comprehend the assessment, treatment or interventions being proposed. This means that in order for the patient to provide informed consent, they must be able to understand not only the assessment, treatment and interventions to be carried out, but also the consequences of such actions.
- In pre-hospital situations, it is not uncommon for patients to refuse assessment, care or treatment. Although patients may refuse, there may be, depending on the circumstances, continuing moral duties and legal responsibilities for ambulance clinicians to provide further intervention, particularly if life-threatening risk is involved. Again, ambulance clinicians are advised to obtain advice from their employers about circumstances of this nature so the actions they take are appropriate to the legal jurisdiction in which they are working.
- When communicating with other healthcare professionals, discussion should include information about the patient's ability to consent.

Domestic Abuse

1. Introduction

- Domestic violence and abuse is any incident or pattern of incidents of controlling, coercive or threatening behaviour, violence or abuse between those aged 16 or over who are or have been, intimate partners or family members regardless of gender or sexuality. The abuse can encompass, but is not limited to, psychological, physical, sexual, financial and emotional harm.
- Controlling behaviour is a range of acts designed to make a person subordinate and/or dependent by isolating them from sources of support, exploiting their resources and capacities for personal gain, depriving them of the means needed for independence, resistance and escape and regulating their everyday behaviour.
- Coercive behaviour is an act or pattern of acts of assault, threats, humiliation and intimidation or other abuse that is used to harm, punish or frighten the victim.
- Domestic abuse is the most prevalent form of violence against women and girls.
- Pre-hospital healthcare practitioners are in a key position to identify domestic abuse and to initiate support and safety for victims.
- Domestic abuse is extremely distressing; managing such cases demands sensitive, non-judgemental medical and emotional care and an awareness of the forensic requirements.
- In December 2015, a new criminal offence of domestic abuse, 'coercive and controlling behaviour', came into force, making all domestic abuse a reportable crime. In April 2021, the Domestic Abuse Act 2021 came into force recognising children as victims and economic abuse as a form of domestic abuse, and introducing new measures to support victims.
- Patients are likely to be very distressed about the events surrounding domestic abuse. They may not want to involve anybody else, and may not consent to disclosure of information to other parties such as the police. Do not judge or give the appearance of judging the patient. Be kind and considerate, and allow the patient space and as much choice as possible about options for their treatment.
- There can be a complex but significant relationship between alcohol and drug use and domestic abuse perpetration.
- **Further care** – it is important to encourage all victims of domestic abuse to seek medical helpand inform the police. Both will be able to provide physical, medical and emotional support.
- In cases of domestic abuse in adults with needs for care and support, refer to **Safeguarding Adults at Risk**.
- In cases of domestic abuse where children are present, involved or potentially affected by the emotional impact of domestic abuse, refer to **Safeguarding Children**.

2. Incidence

- In 2020, 5.5% of adults aged 16 to 74 years experienced domestic abuse in the 12 months prior. 18% of all offences recorded by the police in the year ending March 2021 were domestic abuse-related crimes. There were 362 domestic homicides recorded in the three-year period between year ending March 2018 and year ending March 2020.
- Women are significantly more likely than men to be victims and survivors of domestic abuse.

3. Severity and Outcome

- The severity of the abuse can vary from verbal abuse to sustaining life-threatening injuries or death. The outcome of the abuse can lead to long-term psychological and physical effects.
- Exposure to domestic abuse during childhood can have a profound effect on children's development and wellbeing.

4. Pathophysiology

- Domestic abuse is an incident or pattern of incidents of controlling, coercive or threatening behaviour, violence or abuse to those aged 16 or over. These types of abuse include: psychological, physical, sexual, financial and emotional harm..
- Domestic abuse also includes 'honour'-based violence, forced marriage and female genital mutilation (FGM); for FGM, also refer to **Safeguarding Adults at Risk** and **Safeguarding Children**.

5. Consent

- Clinicians should seek the consent of the adult to share information, unless doing so would increase the risk of harm. Whilst a capacitated adult is free to make an unwise or bad decision, the local authority and/or the police can take steps to protect them if they are at risk of abuse if they are being unduly influenced, coerced or intimidated.
- Information can be shared with other professionals, without the adult's consent, if the following apply:
  - There is an immediate risk of harm.
  - Other people are being put at risk (for example, letting friends who are abusive or exploitative into a shared living environment, where they may put other residents at risk).
  - A child is involved.
  - The alleged person causing harm has care and support needs and may also be at risk.
  - A crime has been committed.
  - Staff are implicated.

Domestic Abuse

- There will be times when an adult who has mental capacity decides to accept a situation considered as harmful or neglectful. Where this is the situation and they do not want any action to be taken, this does not preclude the sharing of information with relevant professional colleagues. This is to enable professionals to assess the risk of harm and be confident that the adult is not being unduly influenced, coerced or intimidated and is aware of all the options.
- Poor handling of the consent process may result in a breakdown of trust between patients and clinicians, may result in opportunities to safeguard patients being missed and may also result in complaints from patients through the NHS complaints procedure or to professional bodies.
- Where a person lacks the capacity to make a decision for themselves, any decision must be made in that person's best interests.
- Remember that GDPR applies and you should only share relevant information to the safeguarding concern. Medical information not relevant should not be shared.
- If the concern is a care concern and not safeguarding, then consent must be obtained. All consent discussions and decision should be recorded using your trust's reporting processes.

6. Assessment and Management

For the assessment and management of domestic abuse, refer to Table 1.1.

TABLE 1.1 – ASSESSMENT and MANAGEMENT of: Domestic Abuse

Assess <C>ABCDE

If any **TIME-CRITICAL** features present major ABCDE problems:

- Start correcting **<C>ABCDE** problems.
- Undertake a **TIME-CRITICAL** transfer to nearest receiving hospital.
- Continue patient management en route.
- Provide an ATMIST information call.

Assess

- Limit questions to those identifying the need for medical treatment, but allow the patient to talk and document what is said. **NB** It is not appropriate to probe for details of the abuse and it could affect the outcome of criminal investigations.
- Manage according to condition:
  – Acute injury – refer to **Trauma Emergencies in Adults** and **Trauma Emergencies in Children**.
  – Acute illness – refer to **Medical Emergencies in Adults** and **Medical Emergencies in Children**.

Indicators in the patient:

- Seems afraid or anxious to please their partner.
- Agrees with everything their partner says.
- Checks everything first with their partner.
- Talks about their partner's temper or jealousy.
- Has frequent injuries, often described as 'accidents'.
- Dresses in clothing designed to hide bruises or scars.
- Is restricted from seeing family and friends.
- Has limited access to money, credit cards etc.
- Has low self-esteem.
- Is depressed, anxious or has suicidal thoughts/action.

Approach

- Know and recognise risk factors, signs and presenting patterns of behaviour associated with domestic abuse.
- Facilitate privacy and do not do anything which could place the victim at further risk, such as making enquiries in earshot of the perpetrator.
- Use a sensitive and respectful manner but ask direct questions about relationships, risks and safety factors.
- Focus on your care but be mindful of your surroundings and the information that is being passed to you, both verbal and non-verbal.
- Consider cultural/religious issues.
- Where possible, accommodate the patient's requests.

Domestic Abuse

TABLE 1.1 – ASSESSMENT and MANAGEMENT of: Domestic Abuse *(continued)*

Remember that this may be the first time the victim has felt able to disclose risk to a professional, or even the only time they have ever had the opportunity.

- Where possible, avoid disturbing the scene.
- Where possible, and safe to do so, gain consent from the victim for referral to the police or a specialist domestic abuse service approved by your organisation's safeguarding lead.
- Multiagency input and assessment is essential in reducing the risk of domestic abuse. Follow your local protocols when referring to external agencies. If your local protocol recommends that you complete a DASH risk assessment, then always complete this face to face with the victim rather than retrospectively after the episode of contact has concluded.
- Obtain a safe contact number for the victim for other agencies to use to contact them without risk of alerting the perpetrator.

Criminal Offence/Forensic Examination

- Many forms of domestic violence are criminal offences and staff must report all serious crimes to the police, particularly if:
  - The patient has suffered from abuse involving a weapon/strangulation/smothering or has sustained a significant injury
  - The patient is in fear of the perpetrator
  - The abuse is escalating
  - The perpetrator is stalking the patient and/or
  - There is an immediate risk to the patient or any children in the household.
- Always attempt to gain consent from the victim to report to the police, but consent is not required if there is a public interest of other legal justification.
- Forensic examination may be required if a physical assault has taken place. Domestic abuse is a criminal offence and the police must be informed immediately (refer to **Sexual Assault**).

Transfer[1]

- Encourage all patients to attend further care.
- Refer the victim to an appropriate external service.
- Transfer patients to further care according to local guidelines.
- Where a patient is competent and refuses hospital treatment, advise them to seek further medical attention.
- If safe to do so, provide information on where the patient may seek further support in relation to domestic abuse.
- If children are involved, a safeguarding notification of concern must be made using local ambulance procedures.
- If the patient is transported to hospital, do not leave children in the care of the alleged perpetrator.
- Always try to speak to the patient alone to avoid placing them at further risk.
- Remember that consent is not always required from the patient to report the crime, particularly if the patient remains at risk.
- Share concerns at the receiving hospital.

[1] *In some areas, arrangements exist for patients to be examined and interviewed in police or other facilities.*

Documentation

- Complete the clinical record in great detail contemporaneously and document:
  - only facts, not personal opinion
  - what the patient says and in their own words
  - clinical findings with relevant timings
  - the ambulance identification number.
- A police statement may be required later.
- Consideration must be given with regard to leaving any documentation (such as a clinical record) with a victim, which could potentially increase the risk of harm.

Domestic Abuse

> **KEY POINTS!**
>
> **Domestic Abuse**
> - If staff suspect a crime has been committed resulting in harm to the patient, the police must be called.
> - Always attempt to obtain consent from the patient before making a referral for them but recognise when consent is not required.
> - Listen closely to the patient for disclosure, and document this on the patient record.
> - If possible, take the patient away from the scene.
> - Treatment should avoid disturbing evidence where possible.
> - Take into account any information that is disclosed by children.
> - Never leave a child with an alleged perpetrator if transporting the patient to hospital.
> - Accommodate patient wishes where possible.

Further Reading

Other useful resources include:

Department of Health: Domestic violence and abuse. Professional guidance. https://www.gov.uk/government/uploads/system/uploads/attachment_data/file/211018/9576-TSO-Health_Visiting_Domestic_Violence_A3_Posters_WEB.pdf.

Women's Aid: Support for women to escape abuse. www.womensaid.org.uk.

Mankind Initiative: Information and support for male victims of domestic abuse or violence. https://www.mankind.org.uk.

LGBT+ Domestic Abuse Helpline: Support for LGBT+ people who have experienced abuse and violence. 0300 999 5428, www.broken-rainbow.co.uk.

Refuge. National helpline: 0808 2000 247, email: helpline@refuge.org.uk.

Foreign and Commonwealth Office: Forced marriage. www.fco.gov.uk/en/travel-and-living-abroad/when-things-go-wrong/forced-marriage.

Bibliography

1. HM Government. *Tackling Domestic Abuse Plan*. 2022. Available from: https://assets.publishing.service.gov.uk/government/uploads/system/uploads/attachment_data/file/1064427/E02735263_Tackling_Domestic_Abuse_CP_639_Accessible.pdf.

2. House of Common Library. *Briefing Paper 9233: The Role of Healthcare Services in Addressing Domestic abuse*. 2021. Available from: https://researchbriefings.files.parliament.uk/documents/CBP-9233/CBP-9233.pdf The role of healthcare services in addressing domestic abuse (parliament.uk).

3. Department of Health. *Responding to Domestic Abuse: A resource for health professionals*. 2017. Available from: https://www.gov.uk/government/publications/domestic-abuse-a-resource-for-health-professionals.

4. National Institute for Health and Clinical Excellence. *Domestic Violence and Abuse: Multi-agency working* (PH50). London: NICE, 2014. Available from: https://www.nice.org.uk/guidance/ph50/chapter/introduction.

5. Office for National Statistics. *Domestic Abuse Prevalence and Trends, England and Wales: Year ending March 2021*. 2021. Available from: https://www.ons.gov.uk/peoplepopulationandcommunity/crimeandjustice/articles/domesticabuseprevalenceandtrendsenglandandwales/yearendingmarch2021.

6. Home Office. *Multi-agency Statutory Guidance for Dealing with Forced Marriage*. 2022. Available from: https://www.gov.uk/government/publications/the-right-to-choose-government-guidance-on-forced-marriage/multi-agency-statutory-guidance-for-dealing-with-forced-marriage-and-multi-agency-practice-guidelines-handling-cases-of-forced-marriage-accessible#page25.

7. Edelson JL. The overlap between child maltreatment and women battering. *Violence Against Women* 1999, 5(2): 134–154.

8. Home Office, *Female Genital Mutilation: Resource pack*. 2021. Available from: https://www.gov.uk/government/publications/female-genital-mutilation-resource-pack/female-genital-mutilation-resource-pack.

9. McAfee RE. *Domestic Abuse as a Woman's Health Issue*. Chicago: Elsevier Science Inc, 2001.

10. McWilliams M, McKiernan S. *Bringing It Out in the Open*. Belfast: HMSO, 1999.

11. NSPCC. *Domestic Abuse*. 2022. Available from: https://www.nspcc.org.uk/what-is-child-abuse/types-of-abuse/domestic-abuse.

Duty of Care

1. Introduction

- It is obvious that ambulance clinicians have a duty to provide care to their patients but establishing exactly how that duty applies during high-risk emergency situations can be challenging.
- The duty of care represents moral, professional and legal obligations. The moral obligation to provide care is a matter of individual and social conscience. The professional obligation arises from a clinician's professional registration and organisational procedures or national best practice guidelines. The legal obligation arises from several sources which are summarised below.
- It is particularly hard for ambulance clinicians to discharge their duty of care correctly at incidents where patients need clinical interventions but hazards expose responders to considerable risk.

2. Application

The duty of care applies to ambulance clinicians and managers in two fundamental ways:

1. Staff safety: The duty to keep yourself and your team safe.

2. Patient care: The duty to provide a reasonable standard of care to your patient.

Whilst the United Kingdom has three separate jurisdictions – England and Wales, Scotland and Northern Ireland – the duty of care principles are broadly consistent throughout.

3. Health and Safety Duties

- The Health and Safety at Work Act 1974 and associated regulations require ambulance clinicians to have a safe system of work. NHS ambulance services have a legal duty to implement and maintain safe systems of work for their employees, and in turn employees have a legal duty to comply with these systems.
- A safe system of work is usually achieved through:
  - Effective operating procedures
  - Staff competence (qualifications and training)
  - Fit for purpose equipment
  - Effective risk assessments.
- This means ambulance clinicians should:
  - Ensure they and their colleagues engage in approved activities which have procedures and controls in place to mitigate the risks
  - Ensure that they are competent to perform those activities (i.e. they have been suitably trained to do it and that training is up to date or current)
  - Ensure that they have the necessary equipment for those activities and the equipment being used is fit for purpose (i.e. appropriately maintained). This includes personal protective equipment (PPE)
  - Ensure that staff are aware of pre-existing generic risk assessments for the specific activity being undertaken and that subsequent dynamic risk assessments are used just prior to committing to the activity so that specific situational hazards and risks are considered.
- A safe system of work does not necessarily mean one which is free of risk. It is one where the risk is being appropriately managed or controlled. Given the nature of pre-hospital ambulance work, a level of risk exposure will need to be accepted.
- Safe systems of work must also be reviewed periodically and/or when the work activity or risk changes. NHS ambulance services must also implement appropriate monitoring/supervision to ensure compliance with the safe system of work.

4. The Tort of Negligence

- The emergency services (including police and fire and rescue services) do not generally owe a legal duty of care to individual members of the public except in certain, limited circumstances (*Hill v Chief Constable of West Yorkshire* [1989] AC 53 (HL)). Their duty is focused more on protecting the public 'at large'.
- The law will recognise a breach of duty by Police or Fire and Rescue Services if they have acted in a certain way in certain specific situations (*Caparo Industries Plc v Dickman* [1990] 2 AC 605).
- However, the NHS Ambulance Service has an established legal duty to provide a reasonable standard of care to patients without unreasonable delay. This is a positive duty which engages from the point at which the Ambulance Service accepts the emergency call and agrees to attend (*Kent v Griffiths* [2001] QB 36).
- A reasonable standard of care relates to clinical care that can be supported by a responsible body of medical opinion (*Bolam v Friern Hospital Management Committee* [1957] 2 All ER 118). The opinion relied upon must have a logical basis (*Bolitho v City and Hackney Health Authority* [1998] AC 232). With regard to the clinical practice of ambulance staff, these standards are set out in approved clinical practice guidelines and the standards set by relevant professional bodies.
- This puts the ambulance service in a position where the care provided or any unreasonable delay in the provision of care may need to be explained and legally justified to avoid liability. Failure to discharge this duty could expose the ambulance service to a charge of clinical negligence.

5. Article 2 – The Right to Life

- It has been recognised that Article 2 of the Human Rights Act 1998 creates a positive duty on public sector organisations, including the NHS

Duty of Care

- ambulance services, to do all they reasonably can to protect those they know, or ought to know, are at real and immediate risk (*Van Colle v CC of Hertfordshire* [2007] EWCA Civ 325).
- However, there may be occasions where it is justifiable not to act immediately to save someone's life. For example, ambulance clinicians are not under a duty to sacrifice their own life to save a patient.
- If you manage to effectively balance two fundamental duties of care by putting a safe system of work in place and avoiding any unreasonable delay in providing care to patients, then you will invariably discharge your obligations under Article 2.

6. Appendix – Duty of Care Aide Memoire

- The aide memoire depicted in Table 1.2 has been developed to assist you in applying the duty of care correctly.

TABLE 1.2 – Duty of Care Aide Memoire

Duty of Care Requirement		Steps to Take	Explanation
Duty of care to staff	• Take all reasonable and practical steps to keep employees safe.	• Perform approved activities and apply the controls specified in procedures. Ensure there is a generic risk assessment already in place. • Ensure you are trained and competent to undertake the activity. • Ensure the minimum equipment mandated by procedures is available and used (including your Personal Protective Equipment (PPE).	• These are statutory duties under the Health and Safety at Work Act 1974 and associated regulatory provisions. • These steps will help ensure you have a safe system of work. Most of these provisions should already be established prior to the incident.
Duty of care to the patient	• Provide a reasonable standard of care without any unreasonable delay.	• Undertake a dynamic risk assessment and determine the action you need to take as quickly as possible. Continually review the position and deliver care as soon as possible. • If you need specialist support, make sure you request it as soon as possible.	• This is an established duty at common law. It is a positive duty on the ambulance service to provide a reasonable standard of care without unreasonable delay. This duty is unique to healthcare professionals. The police and fire services have duties to the public at large but their duty to individual patients is largely discretionary (*Kent v Griffith* [2001] QB 36).
Article 2 right to life	• Take steps to protect people from harm which may lead to loss of life.	• Balance the two duties set out above.	• If the correct balance is achieved (staff safety but also avoiding unreasonable delay in treating patients), this duty will be discharged. If the rescue is too dangerous for the responders, Art. 2 positive duties can be temporarily avoided.

Duty of Care

TABLE 1.2 – Duty of Care Aide Memoire *(continued)*

Duty of Care Requirement		Steps to Take	Explanation
Risk-assess the activity	• Assess the risks for both staff and patients.	• Supplement the pre-existing generic risk assessment with a dynamic risk assessment at the scene considering the situation and hazards. Mitigate the risks as best you can. The risk to patients must be included in that assessment. Regularly review the risk assessment.	• If the activity is likely to result in death or serious injury to you or a member of your team despite the controls, do not commit. Statutory health and safety obligations provide justification for the temporary delay of care. • If the risk of death or serious injury to you or your team can be mitigated by a safe system of work, making the likelihood low but accepting some residual risk, you must avoid unreasonable delay in committing and providing emergency care. • For complex or major incidents, ambulance commanders are responsible for balancing these principles.
Multi-agency Joint Doctrine	• Contribute to the joint risk assessment as part of JESIP and ensure a common understanding of the risks.	• For complex incidents involving a multi-agency response, ensure there is a joint risk assessment using the JESIP tools. • Ensure the ambulance service duty of care is considered as part of this joint risk assessment.	

KEY POINTS!

Duty of Care

- The duty of care requires ambulance clinicians to achieve a careful balance. They must take reasonable steps to ensure they are as safe as is realistically possible, but they must also be prepared to accept some risk to deliver effective care to patients in the pre-hospital setting. They must also be sufficiently trained and experienced to act quickly where life is at risk.
- **To do this they must:**
  - **Implement an approved safe system of work and associated procedures.**
  - **Avoid any unreasonable delays in providing emergency care to patients that require it.**

End of Life Care

1. Introduction

- Approximately 1% of the population of the UK die each year, which is about half a million people, and around 75% of these deaths are expected. This presents an opportunity to plan for an individual's death, to improve the quality of life remaining, to support those close to the patient, to provide symptom control and to establish preferences for care as an illness progresses.

- Palliative care is for people living with a progressive terminal illness where a cure is no longer possible. In addition to cancers, this encompasses conditions secondary to end organ failure, e.g. COPD, renal failure, liver failure, dementia, heart failure and motor neurone disease. Patients with progressive incurable illnesses may receive palliative care for weeks, months or years and include end of life care planning as their condition deteriorates.

- End of life care is considered for patients within the last year of life. As illness trajectories differ for each condition, end of life care may refer to the last few months, weeks or days of life.

- Ambulance clinicians increasingly encounter patients who are palliative and approaching their end of life, either whilst facilitating planned transfers or providing an emergency response to a sudden crisis.

- Due to an ageing population and an expected 17% increase in annual deaths by 2030, there will be an increasing demand for high-quality end of life care. This will be reflected in the workload of ambulance services.

- Unlike conventional areas of pre-hospital care, such as cardiac arrest and trauma, which aim to save life and rely on algorithms and clear parameters, end of life care seeks to provide supportive care using a holistic approach tailored to each individual. This presents unique challenges to ambulance clinicians insofar as there is no pre-existing relationship with the patient, there is limited or no knowledge of either their condition or treatment preferences and, based on limited information, **TIME-CRITICAL** decisions have to be made.

- People at the end of life may have contact with ambulance services on several occasions, for example when a complication occurs which creates a sudden health crisis or for an unrelated event such as a fall. Be aware of the underlying condition(s) and any advance care planning decisions that may be in place when administering care or seeking a referral or admission.

- Increasingly, calls to ambulance services may indicate that a person's condition is deteriorating; for example, in a person with COPD who is experiencing increased difficulty in breathing, ambulance clinicians may be the first point of contact for this individual. Ambulance clinicians need to be able to recognise signs, signals and clues that suggest it may be time to initiate discussions about end of life care and relay this information to the patient's GP, hospital or other appropriate health professional or organisations so that appropriate action can be taken.

2. Severity and Outcome

- The focus in managing end of life care situations should always be to enable a person to achieve care according to their preferences.

- For those who are nearing the terminal phase of illness, the aspirational outcome would be for that person to have a 'good death'; to die in a place of their choosing, with dignity and respect, without pain, in a calm and familiar atmosphere, surrounded by loved ones.

- Several acute presentations are reversible and require urgent treatment including transfer to the Emergency Department (ED) in order to improve an individual's prognosis or quality of life. However, sometimes a potential reversible condition may have been discussed previously between the patient and their care provider and following these discussions a 'ceiling of treatment' may have been agreed. If a ceiling of treatment has been set, remember the ceiling is for a certain treatment only: there is never a ceiling to care. Where possible, check that any previously agreed ceiling of treatment is still what the patient wants. Any patient with capacity is allowed to change their mind.

3. Management – Patients Who Are Not Expected to Die Within 72 Hours

- Establish the patient's wishes for their care, including their desire for interventions and preferred place of care.

- If the patient does not have the capacity for decision making, establish if an advance care plan, a Recommended Summary Plan for Emergency Care and Treatment (ReSPECT) or an Advance Decision to Refuse Treatment (ADRT) exists.

- Establish if a family member has Lasting Power of Attorney (LPA) for Health and Welfare. An LPA for Health gives a family member the legal right to refuse a treatment for the patient that has lost capacity, if they deem it not in that patient's best interests at that time. It does not however allow the Attorney to insist on any forms of treatment or conveyance to hospital.

- Consult with family members and carers but remember that the patient's best interests take precedence.

End of Life Care

- Access personalised care plans and follow directions where appropriate.
- **If not in the active stage of dying, determine:**
  - if there is a reversible cause for symptoms and manage as per guidance
  - if the patient's symptoms can be managed in their home environment or if hospital/hospice admission is required
  - if the patient has psychological, emotional or spiritual needs that would benefit from specialist support
  - if the patient requires additional social support at home or if hospital admission is necessary: Are family members exhausted? Can they manage to provide care? Is physical equipment required to support care at home? Seek out local services that may be able to assist with support.

3.1 Care Pathways

- Unless the patient clearly requires urgent hospital conveyance for a reversible condition, seek specialist advice to support decision making.
- Be aware of any wishes regarding future care that may have been recorded on an advance care plan, especially patients receiving palliative care and those with long-term conditions, such as COPD and dementia, however be aware that patients can change their mind and contradict what's in their care plan, if they have capacity, and then their current preference takes priority.
- Be prepared to ask the person/carer about possible end of life care planning and related issues.
- Contact the palliative care team using contact details in a personalised care plan.
- Contact the patient's GP, an out-of-hours GP or district nurse.
- Contact local palliative care pathways (e.g. rapid response teams or hospice-at-home services).
- Consider contacting a religious leader if appropriate.
- Consider referral to social services if appropriate.
- Consider contacting senior clinical support within your Trust.

3.2 Shared Decision Making

- Ambulance clinicians often become involved in the complex care of patients with whom they have had no prior contact. In managing end of life situations, where there may be a need to administer medicines for symptom control or facilitate the patient's preference with regard to the place of care, remember that the patient's existing care team will hold more information about them and have met them in person in the past. Shared decision making by contacting and discussing cases with the patient's GP, an out-of-hours GP or local palliative care teams is invaluable.

3.3 Palliative Emergencies

Metastatic Spinal Cord Compression

Background

- Spinal cord compression due to direct pressure or collapse of a vertebral body due to spinal metastases can result in vascular injury, cord necrosis and neurological disability.

Signs and Symptoms

- Pain in thoracic or cervical spine and/or progressive, severe lumbar spinal pain.
- Pain aggravated by straining (passing stools, coughing or sneezing) or nocturnal pain preventing sleep.
- Limb weakness.
- Difficulty walking.
- Sensory loss or bladder or bowel dysfunction.
- Localised spinal tenderness.

Management

1. If any of the following **TIME-CRITICAL** features are present, undertake a **TIME-CRITICAL** transfer to nearest Emergency Department:
   - major ABCD problems
   - neurological deficit in lower limbs.
- Undertake a **TIME-CRITICAL** transfer to nearest Emergency Department.
- Provide patient management en route.
- Provide an alert/information call.

2. Measure and record a pain score.
- Offer analgesia (refer to **Pain Management in Adults and Children**).

3. Position supine with neutral spine alignment for patients with severe pain, neurological symptoms or signs of compression. Exceptions to this would be patients with severe COPD or heart failure who, due to co-morbidity, are unable to tolerate lying supine. In these cases the patient should be transferred in the most comfortable position for them.

NB There are no clear guidelines and there is a lack of evidence to advise the correct position for patients – adopt NICE guidelines, as in the pre-hospital phase it seems prudent to manage as if the spine is unstable until an MRI can confirm this.

4. Transfer to the nearest Emergency Department or to a specialist unit if advised by expert team.

Superior Vena Cava Compression

Background

- Occlusion of the superior vena cava due to either external compression or internal obstruction. This is most commonly caused by a tumour of the bronchus or lymphomas, or cancers of the breast,

End of Life Care

colon or oesophagus. Patients with lung, prostate and breast cancer are at the greatest risk, with the thoracic spine most commonly affected.

- Severity of symptoms varies depending on the degree of obstruction but reflects the underlying venous congestion, laryngeal and cerebral oedema.

Signs and Symptoms

- Facial, neck or arm swelling, worse on lying down or bending over.
- Dilated veins on neck, chest and arms.
- Dyspnoea.
- Cough or hoarseness.
- Headache.
- Dizziness, confusion or lethargy.

Management

1. If any of the following **TIME-CRITICAL** features are present, undertake a **TIME-CRITICAL** transfer to the nearest Emergency Department:
   - major ABC problems
   - stridor or severe difficulty in breathing.
- Start correcting A and B problems.
- Undertake a **TIME-CRITICAL** transfer to the nearest Emergency Department.
- Provide patient management en route.
- Provide an alert/information call.

2. Sit the patient upright or elevate the head.

3. If the patient is hypoxaemic, administer supplemental oxygen and aim for a target saturation within the range of 94–98% (refer to **Oxygen**).

(**NB** – Points 2 and 3 provide symptomatic relief.)

4. Transfer to the nearest Emergency Department or to a specialist unit if advised by an expert team.

Neutropenic Sepsis

NB Neutropenic sepsis can occur in patients who are undergoing treatment for curative cancer as well as patients receiving palliative care.

Background

- Neutropenic sepsis is a potentially fatal complication of treatments for cancer, such as chemotherapy or immunotherapy. Such treatments can suppress the ability of bone marrow to respond to infection.
- Patients that have received chemotherapy and anti-cancer treatments in the past 8 weeks are at particular risk (the highest risk is within the first 10 days after treatment).
- Consider use of the UKONS/Macmillan Primary Care Triage Pocket Tool to help identify patients at risk of deterioration

Disclaimer: Clinicians using the UKONS/ Macmillan Primary Care Triage Tool are expected to use independent clinical judgement in the context of the presenting clinical circumstances to determine any patient's care or treatment. UKONS and Macmillan do not guarantee, and accept no legal liability of whatever nature arising from or connected to, the accuracy, reliability, currency or completeness of the content of the above UKONS/Macmillan Primary Care Triage Tool.

Signs and Symptoms

- Classic signs of sepsis may be absent. A neutropenic patient at risk of sepsis can look deceptively well but deteriorate rapidly. A high index of suspicion is necessary, particularly in a patient who has recently undergone chemotherapy and has an increased temperature.
- Neutropenic patients are unable to produce the pus normally associated with skin infections.
- Minor illness or feels unwell.
- Vomiting and/or diarrhoea.
- Raised temperature. Fever may be absent in some infected patients who are dehydrated, severely shocked or taking steroids or NSAIDs.

Management

1. Treat suspected neutropenic sepsis as an acute medical emergency.

2. Manage as per sepsis guidelines.

3. Identify a patient alert card and contact local acute oncology team. Consider the patient's advance care plan, ReSPECT plan or ADRT. They may wish to remain at home. Otherwise, transfer to the nearest Emergency Department or to a specialist unit if advised by an expert team.

Hypercalcaemia

Background

- Hypercalcaemia (high calcium level) occurs in 20–30% of patients with cancer (most commonly in patients with bone secondaries from their cancer). Some patients may have repeated episodes of hypercalcaemia; ask them if they have had this before.

Signs and Symptoms

- Too much calcium in the blood interferes with brain function, resulting in alterations in mental status, confusion, fatigue, headache and lethargy. If left to accumulate, this can lead to unconsciousness, coma and ultimately death.
- Frequent urination and excessive thirst.
- Nausea, vomiting, diarrhoea/constipation.
- Palpitations and fainting.

Management

1. Transfer to the nearest Emergency Department or to a specialist unit if advised by an expert team. In some areas, treatment can be provided at home or in a day-hospice setting, therefore contact the acute

End of Life Care

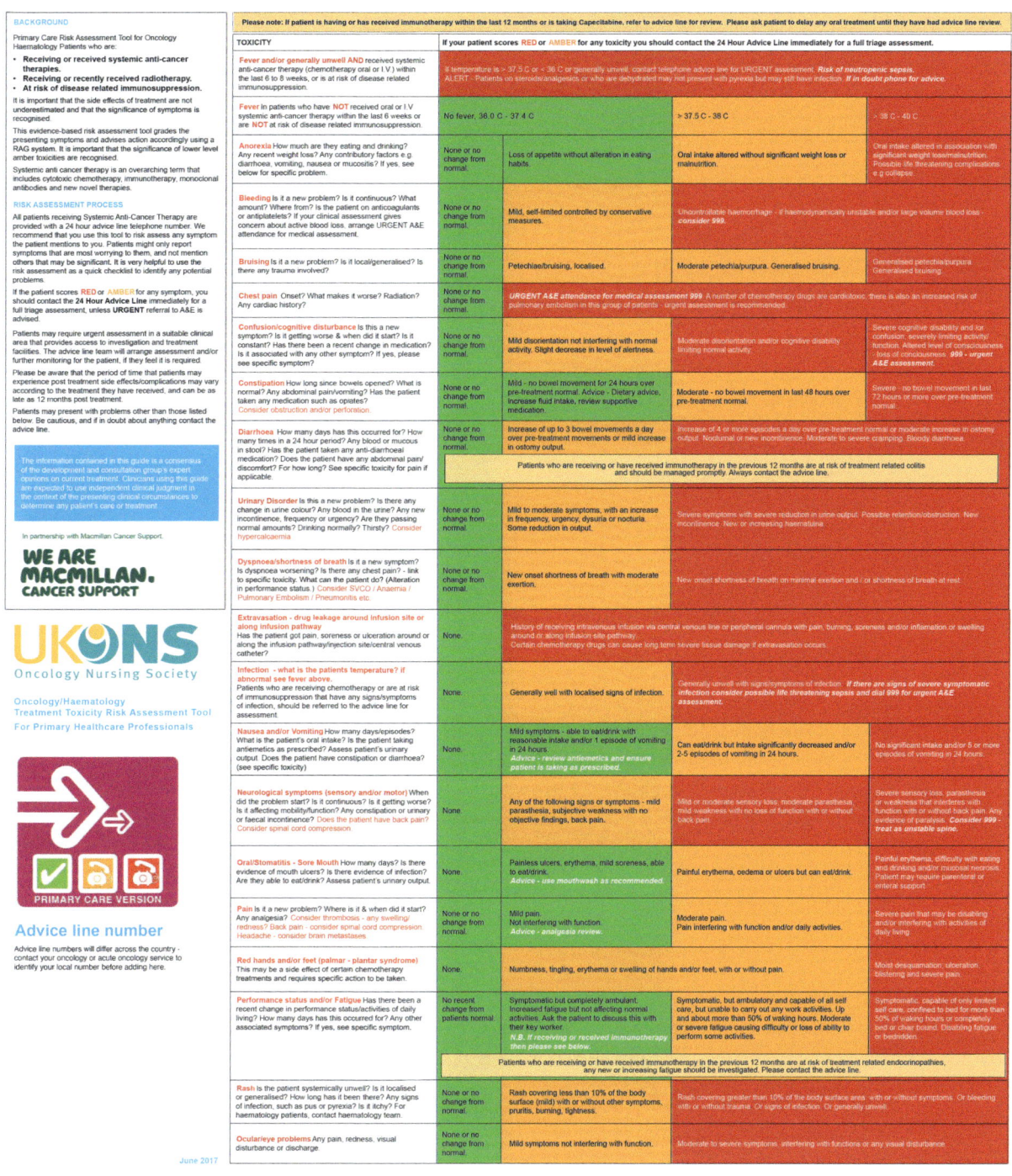

Figure 1.1 – UKONS/Macmillan Primary Care Triage Pocket Tool. Reproduced with kind permission from UKONS and Macmillan.

oncology helpline or palliative care helpline for advice (if patient receiving palliative as opposed to curative treatment).

3.4 Recognising the Last Year of Life

- End of life care is defined as care of a patient with any disease process who is thought to be in their last year of life. Care should always be delivered in accordance with a person's cultural, spiritual or religious beliefs wherever possible and where clinically appropriate.

- There are different tools used within palliative care to help identify patients that may be in their last year of life: these include the Gold Standards Framework (GSF) and the Supportive and Palliative Care Indicators Tool (SPICT). These tools include prompts such as use of the surprise question (GSF): 'Would you be surprised if this patient were to die in the coming months, weeks or days?'. It also provides both general indicators of decline and disease-specific indications that a patient may be in the last year of life.

End of Life Care

The SPICT tool asks the question 'Are there clinical indicators that the health of this person who has one or more progressive conditions is deteriorating?'. If yes, it is time to assess the person's holistic care needs and start planning future care with them.

- **General indications of the last year of life may include:**
  - Decreasing activity: functional performance status declining, limited self-care, in bed or a chair for half of the day and increasing dependence during most activities of daily living
  - Co-morbidity: this is regarded as the biggest predictive indicator of mortality and morbidity
  - General physical decline and increasing need for support
  - Advanced disease: unstable, deteriorating and complex symptom burden
  - Decreasing response to treatments and decreasing reversibility
  - Choice of no further active treatment
  - Progressive weight loss >10% in the past 6 months
  - Repeated unplanned and crisis admissions
  - Sentinel event, for example a serious fall, bereavement or transfer to nursing home.
- **Specific indicators may include:**
  - Cancer: metastatic disease. The Gold Standard Framework explains that 'the single most important predictive factor in cancer is performance status and functional ability'
  - COPD: disease is severe, recurrent hospital admissions, i.e. at least three in the last 12 months due to COPD, fulfils long-term oxygen therapy criteria, Medical Research Council (MRC) Dyspnoea Scale grade 4/5, shortness of breath after 100 metres and confined to house
  - Dementia: unable to walk without assistance, urinary and faecal incontinence, no consistently meaningful conversation and unable to undertake Activities of Daily Living (ADLs).

3.5 Care in the Last Few Days of Life

- A point comes when the person enters the 'dying phase'. Ambulance services are frequently called upon at this stage. This may be for planned transport, such as the rapid transfer of a person from clinical settings to their preferred place of death.
- Ambulance services are also frequently called during the dying phase because of an unexpected complication or a sudden deterioration in condition. Good call-handling procedures can help ascertain what outcome the person or carer wants and expects from ambulance services – to make the person comfortable, for example, and avoid unwanted hospital admission or attempts at resuscitation.
- Families and carers may sometimes wish for ambulance services to be called even where the patient themselves has indicated a preference to die at home or in their usual care setting, such as a care home. The reasons for this may be multi-factorial.
- At the scene, the focus must at all times be on providing the patient with the care and treatment that is in their best interests. Families and carers can be valuable sources of knowledge and expertise on this and should be kept informed. Ambulance clinicians must at the same time be alert to the possibility of differing views and/or resistance to following an agreed care plan or stated preference among families and carers, including GPs, and be prepared to manage these. Be aware that relatives and carers may be distressed by the situation, especially in the case of unexpected complications or sudden deterioration.

Management

- Focus on care and treatment that is in the patient's best interests.
- Try and establish the wishes of the patient but be aware of differing views or resistance to follow an agreed care plan among families and carers.
- Seek clinical decision support, i.e. shared decision making with medical colleagues, e.g. GP or palliative medicine team; or follow the patient's care plan (if appropriate).
- Recognise the signs that a patient is at the end of life and that lifesaving skills, interventions and clinical observations may not be appropriate.

3.6 Signs That a Patient Is at the Very End of Life

- It can sometimes be difficult to decide when someone is in the last few days or hours. However, some of the signs below may become noticeable:
  - Abnormal clinical observations
  - Breathing may become irregular (shallow with deep sighs), with pauses (apnoeic episodes)
  - Reduced conscious levels; sleeping more and at times being difficult to waken
  - Impaired vision and may develop a fixed stare
  - Confusion or agitation
  - Restlessness, pulling at the bed linen and having visions or hallucinations of persons or things that are not present
  - Loss of appetite
  - Loss of control of urine or bowels. The amount of urine may decrease or stop as death approaches
  - Occasionally after death there may be a 'last sigh' or gurgling sound particularly on

End of Life Care

  moving or rolling a patient. There is no need to become alarmed about this, as it is the normal pattern
- Secretions collect at the back of the throat that sound like a rattle. Respiratory secretions are common and often occur in the last 24–48 hours of life. These secretions may be the reason for the 999 call as family members fear their loved one is drowning or choking. It can be useful to explain when offering reassurance that secretions are a small amount of fluid (saliva) at the top of the larynx or voice box and that breathing through the secretions is therefore amplified; that the sound is not a build-up of fluid within the lungs; and that the patient is no longer able to clear their throat, hence the pooling of saliva
- Cool arms and legs as the circulation slows down. The face may become pale, and the feet and legs take on a purple-blue mottled appearance.

3.7 Care at and After Death

- Ambulance clinicians will often be on the scene at or shortly after the point of death. There may be occasions where it is clear that the patient is in the final stages of dying. If all reversible causes have been considered, then supportive care for the patient and the relatives/carers may be all that is required. If a DNACPR or ReSPECT form is not present, ambulance clinicians are not obliged to commence CPR where the person is known to be in the final stages of an irreversible condition and where CPR would be both inappropriate and unsuccessful. Refer to **Termination of Resuscitation and Verification of Death in Adults** and **Termination of Resuscitation and Verification of Death in Children**.

4. Symptom Management in End of Life Care

- There are several common symptoms that may present at the end of life; these are often referred to as breakthrough symptoms. Symptoms will vary for each individual and may be controlled through non-pharmacological and/or pharmacological approaches.
- If the patient has their own medicines present, these should always be used in preference to ambulance service medicines to manage breakthrough symptoms. Using a patient's own medicines at the prescribed dose is a safe course of action to assist with symptom relief.
- The use of communication skills should not be underestimated when providing good symptom management. Acknowledging a patient's situation along with explanation, reassurance and a calm approach are all beneficial.

4.1 Pain – Introduction

- Adequate pain management at the end of life is a right of the dying patient and the duty of all clinicians. This provides one of the most challenging tasks that the clinician will face and requires the treatment of the 'whole person' as well as the physical pain by adopting a biopsychosocial approach.
- Pain is present in approximately 70% of patients with advanced cancer, and 65% in patients with a non-malignant disease. However, due to the longevity and nature of the dying process it is likely that most patients nearing the end of life will feel pain at some stage. In 10% of patients, the pain is described as 'difficult' and may require a more in-depth investigation and pain management programme.
- Most of these patients who are suffering with complex pain have input/support from a palliative care team/clinic who, along with the patient's GP, have the responsibility of monitoring for changes in pain intensity and character, and adjusting the management strategy accordingly. For those not under the guidance of a pain specialist/clinic, it is advisable for the clinician to make a referral or to make contact with a doctor so that a long-term plan to manage the pain can be sought.
- Of patients in the last week of life, 35% describe their pain as 'severe' or 'intolerable', and should be treated as a medical emergency where the challenge is to provide comprehensive pain management in order to alleviate suffering.
- Be aware that not all people in the last days of life experience pain. If pain is identified, manage it promptly and effectively. Identify and treat any reversible causes of pain; examples of this may include urinary retention requiring catheterisation or patient repositioning/turning.

4.2 Assessment of Pain

- Pain is a complex, subjective and dynamic phenomenon, which is affected by the emotional context in which it is endured. In line with current JRCALC guidelines set out in **Pain Management in Adults and Children**, clinicians should pay particular attention to any psychological and sociological factors. Wherever possible, a patient self-assessment strategy should be used and only substituted when the patient is unable to do so. A patient-centred approach should take into account the patient's needs and preferences so that they may be able to make an informed decision about their care. For this, good communication and understanding is essential.

End of Life Care

TABLE 1.3 – Types of Assessment	
Medical assessment	• It is important to take the time to thoroughly assess patients at the end of life as there may be other underlying issues that need addressing. • As well as the usual assessments carried out in line with clinical training and local protocols, it is advisable to also check for pressure ulcers and review dressings as these may need attention. If the patient is catheterised, it may be worth asking if it is fitted comfortably or causing any issues. If possible, advise the patient to maintain a degree of movement as this helps to prevent muscle atrophy and joint stiffness.
Sociological assessment	• A sociological assessment builds upon the premise that no illness is experienced in isolation; in fact, the assumption is that people will rationalise what is happening to them within a social model and create a social construction that is based on their relationships, past experience and language. The sociological assessment should look at how the individual makes sense of the illness and the physical and social interactions that are affected as a result. This 'individualism' of the disease combined with the social factors cannot, and does not, fit into the biomedical model which lends its intellect mainly to the giving of drugs to treat a specific dysfunction. If left untreated, the sociological aspect of dying will affect both the medical and psychological states of the patient.
Psychological assessment	• For many patients nearing the end of life, the dying process will lead to various psychological problems, especially disorders such as depression and anxiety. These have long since been known to accompany chronic pain and long-term illness, with research showing that increased pain perception contributes to the variables seen in the development of the symptomatology of psychological disorders. • The general assumption is that pain perception, alongside cognitive behavioural traits, plays an important part in the symptomatology of chronic pain, and therefore patients suffering from more intense, more frequent and longer-lasting painful episodes are more likely to suffer severe depression. • A lack of treatment will only serve to increase the level of depression, which acts as a vicious circle that is degenerative in nature and contributes to, or even exacerbates, the psychological problems encountered.

- Many patients nearing the end of life live with a degree of persistent pain for which they may already be receiving treatment. This is termed 'background pain'. If a new pain or an increase in the severity of the background pain occurs, then this should be treated as a new condition and assessed as such. An increase in severity of background pain or a new pain is termed as 'breakthrough' or 'breakout' pain.

4.3 Management of Pain

Non-pharmacological Management of Pain

- Non-pharmacological treatment of end of life pain involves addressing many different issues.
- Patient position: As many palliative care patients spend considerable lengths of time in the same position it may be possible to help reduce levels of pain through movement and pillow placement. Always be aware of pressure areas and treat if required.
- Psychological, social and spiritual concerns: Although the clinicians' time with the patient is limited, studies have shown that addressing these areas will help to provide comfort for the patient. The mental state is very important and will affect pain levels if left untreated.
- A good bed-side manner: Calm and reassurance may be all that the patient needs in some circumstances, and this plays a big role in caring for end of life patients.

Pharmacological Management of Pain

- Where pain is intense and opioids are already prescribed, morphine should be the first-line treatment for breakthrough pain (unless a patient has an anticipatory prescription chart for other analgesics). This should be administered in line with local protocols and as part of a multi-modal pain management strategy (i.e. to be administered alongside other analgesics like NSAIDs or paracetamol). Where the new pain is not intense, the WHO analgesic ladder should be followed. It is important that the baseline medication is checked FIRST before administering any medication. If morphine is not the baseline medication then it should not be used as a breakthrough; there may be a reason why another opioid has been chosen and morphine should be avoided. Use the opioid of choice for breakthrough.

End of Life Care

TABLE 1.4

Step 1 – (<3/10) non opioid +/– adjuvant

Step 2 – (3–6/10) opioid for mild to moderate pain +/– non opioid +/– adjuvant

Step 3 – (>6/10) opioid for moderate to severe pain +/– non opioid +/– adjuvant

- The use of subcutaneous morphine should be considered in end of life care patients not wishing to attend hospital. It is important to administer morphine cautiously so as to achieve a stable and satisfactory level of pain relief without any adverse effects. The use of intravenous paracetamol may also be used by the clinician and has shown to be good at relieving symptoms of bone pain (a pain which is often difficult to fully control using morphine alone). Refer to **Morphine Sulfate** and **Paracetamol**.
- Do not dilute the morphine, as more than 2 ml of fluid injected subcutaneously into the site of administration is not recommended.
- The effects of IM/SC morphine are evident after 15–20 minutes.
- For pain in the last days or hours of life when the patient is in the dying phase, morphine may be given with caution for patients with a systolic blood pressure of 90 mmHg or less.
- It is important to check for prior paracetamol and opioid use before administration (including transdermal analgesic patches) to avoid overdosing the patient. The minimum dose of paracetamol should not be less than 4 hours apart (6 hours in patients with renal impairment).
- Paracetamol should be administered over a 15-minute period.
- Check that if the patient has a syringe driver in situ:
  - it is connected to the patient
  - where it is infusing into the patient the infusion site is not red/inflamed and therefore likely to be affecting the absorption and effect of the opioid
  - the syringe driver or tubing is not leaking
  - it is 'running to time', as if the delivery of medication is slow then breakthrough symptoms may become evident, e.g. an increase in pain if an opioid syringe driver is leaking or running slowly.
- After any drug has been administered, it is good practice to inform the patient's own GP or palliative team.
- Be cautious if the patient is on a syringe driver. In such cases contact the patient's care provider prior to the administration of any analgesic. However, if the patient is written up for and has their own anticipatory prescription or 'just in case' (JIC) medications, and they are on a syringe driver, the prescribed PRN dose has likely been calculated taking the syringe driver dose into account, meaning the PRN dose is safe to administer whilst the syringe driver is running.
- Where pain relief medication is administered, the ambulance clinician should check the patient's response after each dose. If further analgesia is required and the anticipatory prescription allows, this should be administered according to the drug chart. Shared decision making with the patient's GP or palliative care team is recommended when giving repeat doses of analgesia.

4.4 Managing Breathlessness

- Breathing discomfort varies in intensity and may not be associated with hypoxia, tachypnoea or bradypnoea.
- Be aware that severe breathlessness often causes anxiety, which can then increase breathlessness further.
- Identify and, if appropriate, treat reversible causes of breathlessness in the dying person, for example pulmonary oedema or pleural effusion.
- Consider patient positioning.
- Consider non-pharmacological management of breathlessness in a person in the last days of life.
- Do **NOT** routinely start oxygen to manage breathlessness. Only offer oxygen therapy to people known or clinically suspected to have symptomatic hypoxia.
- Medications to manage breathlessness may include:
  - an opioid, e.g. Oramorph® or low-dose morphine sulphate.
  - a benzodiazepine, e.g. lorazepam or midazolam
  - a combination of an opioid and benzodiazepine.

Oxygen Administration

- There is no evidence that oxygen therapy relieves breathlessness, unless the patient suffers hypoxia. Considering its disadvantages, namely an invasive intervention requiring tubing and tanks, the risk of nosebleeds and the patient's psychological addiction to this 'umbilical cord', it cannot be recommended for routine use.[1] The British Thoracic Society (2017) has published guidelines on the use of oxygen in adults, which includes a review of oxygen use for the patient with breathlessness associated with palliative illness in the emergency care setting:[2]
  - 'Oxygen therapy for the symptomatic relief of breathlessness in palliative care patients is more complex than the simple correction of hypoxia.

End of Life Care

- Consider the following issues:
- Consider early involvement of palliative care specialists and physiotherapists.
- As breathlessness is a multifactorial sensation— a comprehensive assessment of contributing factors (such as anxiety) should be carried out.
- Low-dose opioids should be considered because they are effective for the relief of breathlessness in palliative care patients. Remember, oxygen is a cure for hypoxia, it is **NOT** a cure for breathlessness.
- A trial of a hand held fan or sitting by an open window to help relieve breathlessness is recommended prior to trial of oxygen.
- Oxygen use has to be tailored to the individual and a formal assessment made of its efficacy for improving quality of life for that person.
- Oxygen therapy should not be continued in the absence of patient benefit or where its disadvantages (e.g. discomfort of masks or nasal cannulae, drying of mucous membranes) outweigh any likely symptomatic benefit'. (BTS, 2017)

- As an ambulance clinician it is vital that you are mindful of the evidence which concludes that the use of a fan and low-dose opiates is as effective, if not more effective, than the administration of oxygen. The disadvantages often outweigh the benefit of administering oxygen in that if a patient feels that they cannot breathe and an ambulance clinician attends and administers oxygen, the patient may believe that they need oxygen therapy each time thereafter that they feel breathlessness. Even worse, the patient may fear that the thing they need to breathe is being taken away when you leave the house. This may result in the person feeling that they need an emergency response whenever they feel breathless.

Non-pharmacological Management of Breathlessness

- Positioning (various advice depending on position: sit upright, legs uncrossed, let shoulders droop, keep head up; lean forward).
- Relaxation techniques.
- Pursed-lips breathing. In pursed-lips breathing, people inhale through their nose for several seconds with their mouth closed, then exhale slowly through pursed lips for 4–6 seconds. This can help to relieve the perception of breathlessness during exercise or when it is triggered.
- Reduce room temperature.
- Cooling the face by using a cool flannel or cloth.
- Portable fan use or sitting near an open window. **NB** Portable fans are not recommended for patients with suspected or confirmed COVID-19.

Pharmacological Management of Breathlessness

- Oxygen (no evidence of benefit in the absence of hypoxia).
- Opioids may reduce the perception of breathlessness.
- Oramorph® if present. If patient has own Oramorph® refer to patient's prescribed dose on drug chart. If using ambulance service morphine, refer to dosage table 'Breathlessness End of Life – Oral' in the **Morphine Sulfate** guideline.
- Morphine SC/IM. If patient has own JIC medication, refer to patient's prescribed dose on drug chart. If using ambulance service morphine, refer to dosage table 'Breathlessness End of Life – SC/IM' in the **Morphine Sulfate** guideline.
- Other medications may also need to be administered for breathlessness and anxiety, such as lorazepam or midazolam.

4.5 Managing Nausea and Vomiting

- Consider likely causes of nausea or vomiting in the dying person. These may include:
    - Certain medicines that can cause or contribute to nausea and vomiting
    - Recent chemotherapy or radiotherapy
    - Psychological causes
    - Biochemical causes, e.g. hypercalcaemia
    - Raised intracranial pressure
    - Gastrointestinal motility disorder
    - Ileus or bowel obstruction.
- If the patient had previous, well-controlled nausea and vomiting using medicines via a syringe driver, consider reviewing the syringe driver to confirm it is not leaking and the infusion site is not inflamed (inflammation at the infusion site which might reduce absorption and therefore effectiveness of medication).
- Discuss the options for treating nausea and vomiting with the dying person and those important to them.
- Consider non-pharmacological methods for treating nausea and vomiting. For people in the last days of life with obstructive bowel disorders who have nausea or vomiting, medications used include:
    - Hyoscine butylbromide
    - Octreotide
    - Cyclizine
    - Haloperidol
    - Levomepromazine.
- See 4.8 – Patient's Own Medications.

End of Life Care

Non-pharmacological Management of Nausea and Vomiting

- Avoid eating or preparing food when patient feels sick or nauseous.
- Avoid fried foods or foods with strong smells.
- Small meals.
- Sip drinks slowly.

Pharmacological Management of Nausea and Vomiting

- Patient's own JIC medication prescribed for nausea/vomiting as per their medication chart.

4.6 Managing Anxiety, Delirium and Agitation

- Explore the possible causes of anxiety or delirium with the dying person and those important to them. Be aware that agitation in isolation is sometimes associated with other unrelieved symptoms or bodily needs, such as unrelieved pain, their positioning, medications, a full bladder or rectum, organ failure or infection.
- Consider non-pharmacological management of agitation, anxiety and delirium in a person in the last days of life, e.g. care for the patient in a well-lit room to avoid misinterpretation of shadow, ensure spectacles if used are clean, use short sentences. Consider calming music and environmental changes that may help.
- Consider any reversible causes of agitation, anxiety or delirium, for example psychological causes or certain metabolic disorders, such as renal failure or hyponatraemia.
- Medications used include:
    - Benzodiazepine to manage anxiety or agitation, e.g. lorazepam and midazolam
    - An antipsychotic medicine to manage delirium or agitation, e.g. haloperidol and levomepromazine.
- Seek specialist advice if the diagnosis of agitation or delirium is uncertain, if the agitation or delirium does not respond to antipsychotic treatment or if treatment causes unwanted sedation.
- See 4.8 – Patient's Own Medications.

Non-pharmacological Management of Managing Anxiety, Delirium and Agitation

- Identify and manage the possible underlying cause or combination of causes (pain, urinary retention, constipation, anxiety, breathlessness).
- Ensure effective communication and reorientation (for example explaining where the person is, who they are and what your role is) and provide reassurance for people diagnosed with delirium.
- Consider involving family, friends and carers to help with this.
- Where possible, ensure people at risk of delirium are cared for by family or carers who are familiar to the patient.
- Avoid moving people within and between rooms unless absolutely necessary.
- Ensure adequate lighting and consider environmental factors.

Pharmacological Management of Managing Anxiety, Delirium and Agitation

- Patient's own JIC medication prescribed for delirium as per their medication chart.
- Ambulance Service JIC Midazolam (**NB** This is only applicable to Trusts that have either a PGD that specifically allows Midazolam use in EoLC, or if a verbal order process is set up and authorised that allows for its use in EoLC). Refer to local guidance.

4.7 Managing Noisy Respiratory Secretions

- These can be associated with the disease process, or a result of excessive weakness in the patient and an inability to maintain their own airway through normal physiological procedures, such as coughing or clearing of the throat, resulting in a pooling of saliva.
- Assess for the likely causes of noisy respiratory secretions in people in the last days of life. Establish whether the noise has an impact on the dying person or those important to them. The noise associated with respiratory secretions can be a source of distress for carers.
- Ambulance clinicians may need to provide additional explanation and reassurance that although the noise can be distressing, it will not cause discomfort or distress to the patient.
- Repositioning the patient such that they are sitting up a little or laying on their side to aid postural drainage can be effective in managing secretions. Suctioning is not usually used or recommended.
- Be prepared to talk about any fears or concerns the patient or carers may have.
- Consider non-pharmacological measures to manage noisy respiratory or pharyngeal secretions, to reduce any distress in people at the end of life.
- Medications include:
    - Glycopyrronium bromide
    - Hyoscine butylbromide
    - Hyoscine hydrobromide.
- It is important to note that medications will not dry up existing secretions; positioning is the primary treatment to aid this. Medications may then be administered to help prevent a further build-up of secretions.
- See 4.8 – Patient's Own Medications.

End of Life Care

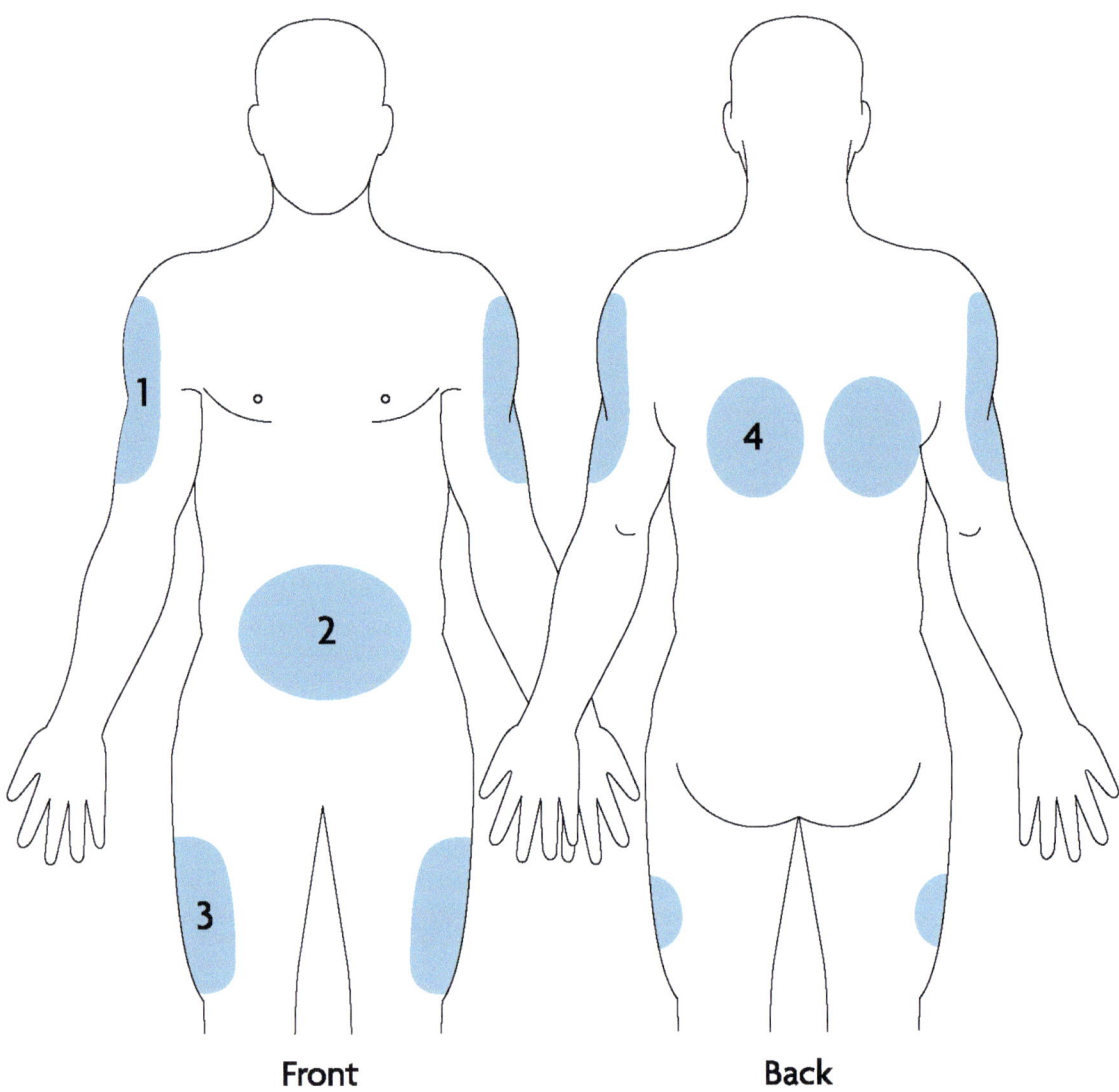

1. The deltoid (upper arm)
2. The abdomen (avoid the umbilicus)
3. The thigh
4. The scapula

Figure 1.2 – Sites for injection of intramuscular and subcutaneous administrations.

Non-pharmacological Management of Respiratory Secretions

- Positioning (sit up slightly if lying flat or onto side – postural drainage).
- Explanation/reassurance to relatives that noise is not causing distress or pain to patient.

Pharmacological Management of Respiratory Secretions

- Patient's own JIC medication prescribed for respiratory secretions as per their medication chart.
- Ambulance Service JIC Glycopyrronium or Hyoscine (if available).

4.8 Patients' Own Medications

Many more patients nearing the end of life are cared for at home in their final days/weeks with the express wish to remain at home. As part of their end of life care plan, they may have 'anticipatory' or 'just in case' medications.

Clinicians are permitted to administer these medications provided that:

- The clinician is competent in the method of administration. A person who administers a prescribed medicine is accountable for their own practice.

End of Life Care

- A signed Medication Administration and Authorisation Record (MAAR) chart is present and authorised by an independent prescriber. (In some Trusts, local guidelines specific to EoLC medication administration are in place. Refer to local guidance.)
- The clinician has access to the relevant paperwork supplied with the 'just in case' medication, providing the necessary information on each drug's indication, dosage, adverse effects, signs and treatments for overdose.
- In law, anyone may follow a Patient Specific Direction (PSD), but some organisations may extend or limit those who are authorised to administer medicines under a PSD within their local medicines policies and governance arrangements. Always check local policy.
- Follow this best practice advice when working with 'just in case' medications:
  - Establish what medication the patient has already received, including drug name, dosage and time of administration.
  - Use shared decision making if appropriate; see 3.2 –Shared Decision Making.
  - Only administer via the prescribed route and the prescribed dose.
  - Consider reversible causes.
  - Consider if the patient is opioid naïve (not on regular opioids). Start on the lowest dose prescribed.
  - Check for and leave transdermal patches in situ.
  - Never alter syringe driver settings.
  - Talk to the patient, family and caregivers. Ask what helps ease their discomfort and what does not.

4.9 Documentation

- Ambulance clinicians **MUST** complete the administration chart that accompanies a patient's medication in addition to completing their own Trust documentation following the use of anticipatory or 'just in case' medications. This enables the specialist palliative team, district nurse or GP to see what medications have been administered. There are some self-explanatory pages at the back of the administration chart which should be filled in and signed to show the use of certain controlled medications, and also the current stock level. Always be mindful of the stock balance; fill out on the form when a medication is administered and arrange a GP follow-up if the stock is sufficiently depleted. Be particularly mindful of this when approaching a weekend or bank holiday when medication prescriptions can be harder to source. Proactive care ensures crisis management is minimised and makes a great deal of difference in the patient's experience in their last days or hours of life.

5. Considerations Relating to Medicine Administration Near the End of Life

- When administering medications at the end of life, there are additional factors that should be considered; this applies to both the patient's own and ambulance service medications. Shared decision making should always be considered prior to administration. Follow Trust guidelines relating to shared decision making.

5.1 Management of Opioid Overdose in End of Life Patients

- Opioid reversal in end of life patients is a specialist skill and should never be undertaken without advice and guidance from specialist palliative care teams.
- If the patient is opioid naïve, (not on regular opioids) then it is safe to reverse the opioid effect immediately (refer to **Naloxone Hydrochloride**). This is unlikely in end of life patients.
- It is important in the management of patients in pain that the signs of advanced progressive disease are not confused with those of opioid overdose.
- If the patient is taking regular opioids, the aim is to reverse the respiratory depression only:
  - Stop the opioid.
  - Administer oxygen if saturations <94%.
  - Give Naloxone until the respiratory status is satisfactory (>8 respirations per minute) – ensure the cannula is flushed after each administration. Refer to **Naloxone Hydrochloride**.
  - If IV access cannot be established or is not permitted (due to clinical grade of ambulance clinician), carry out IM administration. Refer to **Naloxone Hydrochloride**. Shared decision making should always be considered prior to administration.
  - The aim is for slow administration of the drug to avoid a surge of pain from complete antagonism of opioid.
  - If there is no response, consider other causes.

5.2 Naloxone Use in End of Life Care

- The use of naloxone in palliative care is not routinely practised and is only indicated in circumstances where a clinician suspects opioid-induced toxicity, from intentional or unintentional

End of Life Care

overdose. The aim is to reverse life-threatening respiratory depression only, e.g. if the respiratory rate is <8 breaths per minute and the patient is unconscious and/or cyanosed.

- Do not give Naloxone for opioid-induced drowsiness or reduced level of conscious if the respiratory rate is satisfactory or the patient is in the final dying stage.
- If the respiratory rate is ≥8 breathes per minute and the patient is easily rousable/not cyanosed, adopt a wait-and-see approach; consider reducing or omitting the next regular dose or discontinuing continuous parenteral administration.
- Patients on regular opioids for pain and symptom control can be physically dependent; naloxone given in too large a dose or too quickly can cause an acute withdrawal reaction and an abrupt return of pain that is difficult to control; this is also extremely distressing for patients with cancer or advanced progressive illness.

5.3 Opioid Administration in the Last Hours of Life

- The BMA Medical Ethics Today (2012) explains the use of opioids and sedatives in end of life care and the principle of double effect as follows: 'the principle of double effect allows doctors to provide medical treatment that has both good and bad effects, as long as the intention is to provide an overall good effect. They can give sedatives and analgesics with the intention of and in proportion to the relief of suffering, even if as a consequence the patient's life risks being shortened. The moral distinction is between intending and foreseeing harm. The intention of giving the drugs is to relieve pain and distress; the harmful but unintended effect is the risk of shortening life, which the doctor may foresee but not intend'.[49]

5.4 Death After Medicine Administration

- It must be recognised that the prognosis for patients receiving palliative care is poor and death is an expected consequence of their condition. It is entirely possible that a patient may die whilst in our care or shortly after an intervention we have provided. As ambulance clinicians we should be prepared for this, but it is also important to explain to any relatives or carers present that the purpose of any intervention, whether pharmacological or not, is to relieve symptoms, not advance death.

5.5. Renal Failure

- Prescribing at the end of life for patients with renal failure is complex, and advice should always be sought from the renal and palliative care specialists. Many of the medicines used for symptom control in end of life care are eliminated by the kidney to a greater or lesser degree. Morphine and diamorphine accumulate in even modest degrees of renal impairment; great care is needed to avoid opioid toxicity.

5.6. Syringe Drivers and Transdermal Patches

- If the patient has a syringe driver or transdermal patch in situ and suddenly experiences an increase in pain then some problem-solving is required.
- Assess:
  - When was the patch (Fentanyl or Buprenorphine) last changed and when should it have been changed? Some patches need to be changed every 7 days, whereas others require changing every 3 days.
  - Is the patch fully adherent to the skin? The dose of the drug depends on the surface area of the patch. If the patch is falling off, the dose of drug administered/absorbed will be reduced. Sometimes the patch can become dislodged due to body hair, sweating or movement. Take advice if the patch has been dislodged. Ensure safe disposal of any patches (these can be disposed of in a sharps box).
  - Is the syringe driver running properly? Is the battery light flashing? Is the battery still in? If not, take advice.
  - Is the syringe driver site (subcutaneous butterfly cannula) intact? Is there any evidence of it becoming dislodged or a significant amount of unabsorbed fluid being present around the cannula site? If so, take advice.

6. Staff Wellbeing and End of Life Care

- Managing a patient at the end of their life and supporting their families and carers is very distressing for all those involved. Opportunities for debriefing and/or counselling should be available for ambulance clinicians. Follow local procedures for post-critical incident debriefing and refer to **Staff Health and Wellbeing** for more guidance.

End of Life Care

> **KEY POINTS!**
>
> **End of Life Care**
>
> - Providing adequate pain management at the end of life is a right of the dying patient and the duty of all clinicians.
> - Acute or escalating pain is a medical emergency requiring a prompt response.
> - Wherever possible, a patient self-assessment strategy should be used and only substituted when the patient is unable to do so.
> - Pain is easier to prevent than to relieve.
> - Where pain is intense and opioids are already prescribed, morphine should be the first line treatment for breakthrough pain.
> - The presence (or absence) of a DNACPR order must not direct treatment options or discussion in a patient who is actively dying. In the absence of a valid DNACPR form, any ambulance clinician who has diagnosed a patient as dying is not obliged to commence CPR at the point of death. Remember that a DNACPR is not a legally binding document; it is a decision support tool to help guide clinicians as to whether CPR is appropriate. Refer to local guidelines on DNACPR orders, as many Trusts have clear guidance to help clarify queries such as forms from different areas, photocopies, etc.
> - Patients' own just in case (JIC) medication may be administered by a trained clinician (refer to local guidance).
> - Just in case medication carried by registered ambulance clinicians can be administered via a valid Patient Specific Direction or via a verbal order depending on your Trust. Local guidelines and policies must be adhered to.

Further Resources

Visit https://www.respectprocess.org.uk for more information on caring for people when they do not have capacity to make or express choices.

Further important information and evidence in support of this guideline can be found in the Bibliography.

Bibliography

1. Kloke M, Cherny N. Treatment of dyspnoea in advanced cancer patients: ESMO Clinical Practice Guidelines. *Annals of Oncology* 2015, 26: 5.
2. British Thoracic Society. *Guidelines*. 2017. Available from: www.brit-thoracic.org.uk/standards-of-care/guidelines.
3. British Thoracic Society Emergency Oxygen Guideline Development Group. BTS guideline for oxygen use in adults and healthcare and emergency settings. *Thorax* 2017, 72(1): 1–90. Available from: https://www.brit-thoracic.org.uk/document-library/clinical-information/oxygen/2017-emergency-oxygen-guideline/bts-guideline-for-oxygen-use-in-adults-in-healthcare-and-emergency-settings/.
4. Colvin L, Forbes K, Fallon M. ABC of palliative care: difficult pain. *British Medical Journal* 2006, 332(7549): 1081–1083.
5. Vantafridda V, Ripamonti C, DeConno F, et al. Symptom prevalence and control during cancer patients' last day of life. *Journal of Palliative Care* 1990, 6: 7.
6. McCaffery M, Pasero CL. Assessment: underlying complexities, misconceptions, and practical tools. *Pain Clinical Manual*. 2nd edn. St Louis: Mosby, 1999, 35–102.
7. World Health Organization. *Cancer Pain Relief: With a Guide to Opioid Availability*. 2nd edn. Geneva, 1996.
8. Freidman DP. Perspectives on the medical use of drugs of abuse. *Journal of Pain Symptom Management* 1990, 51 suppl: S2–5.
9. Scottish Intercollegiate Guidelines Network. *Control of Pain in Adults with Cancer*. SIGN, 2008. Available from: https://www.sign.ac.uk/assets/sign106.pdf.
10. Quill TE, Brady RV. "You promised me I wouldn't die like this." A bad death as a medical emergency. *Arch Interim Med* 1995, 155: 1250.
11. Rudy TE, Kerns RD, Tuerk DC. Chronic pain and depression: toward a cognitive-behavioural medication model. *Pain* 1988, 35: 129–140.
12. Tan G, Jensen MP, Robinson-Whelen S, Thornby JI, Monga TN. Measuring control appraisals in chronic pain. *The Journal of Pain* 2002, 3(5): 385–393.
13. Turner JA, Dworkin SF, Manel LL, Huggins KH, Truelove EL. The roles of beliefs, catastrophizing, and coping in the functioning of patients with temporomandibular disorders. *Pain* 2001, 92: 41–51.
14. Fishbain DA, Cutler R, Rosomoff HL, Rosomoff RS. Chronic pain-associated depression: antecedent of consequence of chronic pain? A review. *Clinical Journal of Pain* 1979, 13(2): 116–137.
15. Poole H, White S, Blake C, Murphy P, Bramwell R. Depression in chronic pain patients: prevalence and measurement. *World Institute of Pain* 2009, 9(3): 173–180.
16. Morley S, Williams AC, Black S, A confirmatory factor analysis of the Beck Depression Inventory in chronic pain. *Pain* 2009, 99: 289–298.

End of Life Care

17. Leeds-Hurwitz W. Social construction of reality. In Littlejohn S, Foss, K. *Encyclopedia of Communication Theory*. Thousand Oaks, CA: SAGE Publications, 2009.

18. Bury M. Chronic illness as biographical disruption. *Sociology of Health and Illness* 1982, 4: 167–182.

19. Gonzales MJ, Pantilat SZ. Pain at the end of life. *Hospital Medicine Clinics* 2012, 1(1): 109–123.

20. National Institute for Health and Clinical Excellence. *Supportive and Palliative Care: The manual*. NICE, 2004. Available from: http://guidance.nice.org.uk/CSGSP/Guidance/pdf/English.

21. Patient UK. *Palliative Care*. Available from: http://patient.info/doctor/palliative-care.

22. Department of Health. *End of Life Care Strategy – Promoting high quality care for all adults*. DOH, 2008. Available from: https://www.gov.uk/government/publications/end-of-life-care-strategy-promoting-high-quality-care-for-adults-at-the-end-of-their-life.

23. Beauchamp TL, Childress JF. *Principles of Biomedical Ethics*. 6th edn. Oxford University Press, 2008.

24. European Court of Human Rights. *Convention for the Protection of Human Rights and Fundamental Freedoms (European Convention on Human Rights, as amended)* (ECHR), Article 2.

25. European Court of Human Rights. *Convention for the Protection of Human Rights and Fundamental Freedoms (European Convention on Human Rights, as amended)* (ECHR), Article 3.

26. European Court of Human Rights. *Convention for the Protection of Human Rights and Fundamental Freedoms (European Convention on Human Rights, as amended)* (ECHR), Article 8.

27. South Western Ambulance Service Trust. *Palliative Care Clinical Guideline*, 2014.

28. South Western Ambulance Service Trust. *Palliative Care Clinical Guideline*. 2014. Available from: http://www.swast.nhs.uk/.../Clinical%20Guidelines%20SWASFT%20staff/CG29.

29. Scottish Palliative Care Guidelines. Palliative Emergencies. 2014. Scotland: NHS Scotland View. Available from: https://www.palliativecareguidelines.scot.nhs.uk.

30. Health and Care Professions Council. *Standards of Conduct, Performance and Ethics: Your Duties as a Registrant*. London: Health Professions Council, 2003.

31. Blackmore S, Pring A, Verne J. *Predicting Death: Estimating the Proportion of Deaths That Are 'Unexpected'*. London: National End of Life Intelligence Network, 2011.

32. Department of Health. *End of Life Care Strategy. Promoting High Quality Care for All Adults at the End of Life*. London: HMSO, 2008.

33. Office for National Statistics. *Mortality in the United Kingdom*, 2010. London: Crown Copyright, 2012.

34. NHS England. *Actions for End of Life Care: 2014–16*. London: NHS England, 2014.

35. Gomes B, Higginson I. Where people die (1974–2030): past trends, future projections and implications for care. *Palliative Medicine* 2008, 22: 33–41.

36. National End of Life Care Programme. *The Route to Success in End of Life Care – Achieving quality in ambulance services*. London, 2012.

37. Leadership Alliance for the Care of Dying People. *One Chance to Get it Right. Improving people's experience of care in the last few days and hours of life*. London: Leadership Alliance for the Care of Dying People, 2014.

38. Robson P. Metastatic spinal cord compression: a rare but important complication of cancer. *Clinical Medicine* 2014, 14(5): 542–545.

39. Sui J, Fleming JS, Kehoe M. An audit of current practice and management of metastatic spinal cord compression at a regional cancer centre. *The Irish Medical Journal* 2011, 104(4): 111–114.

40. McLinton A, Hutchison C. Malignant spinal cord compression: a retrospective audit of clinical practice at a UK regional cancer centre. *British Journal of Cancer* 2006, 94: 486–491.

41. National Institute for Health and Care Excellence. *Metastatic Spinal Cord Compression. Diagnosis and management of adults at risk of and with metastatic spinal cord compression*. Manchester, 2008.

42. Watson M, Lucas C, Hoy A, et al. (eds). *Palliative Adult Network Guidelines*. Anglia, Kent and Medway, Mount Vernon, Northern Ireland, South East London, Surrey, West Sussex and Hampshire, Sussex Cancer Networks and Palliative Care Cymru Implementation Board, 2011.

43. McCurdy M, Shanholtz CB. Oncological emergencies. *Critical Care Medicine* 2012, 40(7): 2212–2222.

44. Samphao S, Eremin JM, Eremin O. Oncological emergencies: clinical importance and principles of management. *European Journal of Cancer Care* 2010, 19: 707–713.

45. Walji N, Chan AK, Peake DR. Common acute oncological emergencies: diagnosis, investigation and management. *Postgraduate Medical Journal* 2008, 84: 418–427.

46. Abner A. Approach to the patient who presents with superior vena cava obstruction. *Chest* 1993, 103: 394–397.

47. National Institute for Health and Care Excellence. *Neutropenic Sepsis: prevention and management of neutropenic sepsis in cancer patients*. Manchester, 2012.

48. Royal College of General Practitioners. *The National GSF Centre's Guidance for Clinicians to Support Earlier Recognition of Patients Nearing the End of Life*. 2011. Available from: https://www.goldstandardsframework.org.uk/cd-content/uploads/files/General%20Files/Prognostic%20Indicator%20Guidance%20October%202011.pdf.

49. BMA. *Medical Ethics Today*. 2012. Available from: https://www.bma.org.uk/advice/employment/ethics/medical-ethics-today.

50. Welsh Ambulance Service NHS Trust Clinical Guidelines. *Palliative Symptom Control Guidance for Welsh Ambulance Service Staff*, 2020.

Human Factors

1. Introduction

- Team resource management, a component of human factors, is a discipline that seeks to understand the interaction of humans, their work and the systems and environment they inhabit in order to utilise **ALL** available resources, both human and technological, to achieve safe and efficient clinical best practice.
- Effective leadership skills are vital when it comes to ensuring maximal efficiency, particularly at critical and life-threatening incidents, but most of the errors occur when there is a failure to establish leadership in the first place (refer to Table 1.5).

TABLE 1.5 – Leadership Skills: Good Practice

States own position and acknowledges lead role	Supports team awareness
Coordinates and manages the scene	Actively listens to and acknowledges team suggestions
Motivates and coaches	Active and approachable
Guidelines and standard operating procedure (SOP) compliant	Adheres to Guidelines, SOPs or evidence base
Challenges deviation	Recognises and addresses errors
Encourages and utilises team around them	Shares tasks
Uses clear and inclusive communications	Involves the team in changes in the clinical and operational plans
Maintains situational awareness	Recognises own capacity to lead and manages this through delegation to increase 'band width' or hands over leadership to others appropriately
Maintains team focus and role allocation	Oversees task completion

2. Situational Awareness

- Situational awareness is made up of three elements:
  1. **Perception** – the understanding of where you and your team are in the environment around you.
  2. **Comprehension** – how this will impact on your ability to undertake the task at hand.
  3. **Projection** – what is likely to happen next.
- Although effective team resource management requires that everyone is situationally aware, the team leader will be best placed to focus on these three elements, sharing and implementing this mental model with the team.
- Failure to appreciate and act on any one of those elements within a critical situation may lead to situational awareness errors occurring.

3. Communication

- As well as strong leadership and shared situational awareness, an important indicator of team function is the extent and quality of communication. Effective leaders will utilise and encourage those around them, fostering an environment of respectful communications.
- In the early stages of a life-threatening situation or critical incident, team members' bandwidth may be predominantly utilised for technical tasks. As the team grows, its capacity for simultaneous activity increases. So too does the need for the team leader to establish a shared model of what the team must achieve and how it will go about doing so.
- This is where the need for clear and concise communications is vital. Effective communications should have clarity, brevity, empathy and an element of feedback for confirmation of instructions passed or decisions being made.
- There is strong evidence to support the use of checklists to improve clinical management and patient safety. No one can remember everything in every situation.

4. Clinical Decision Making

- Clinical decision making involves the assimilation of information leading to an appropriate course of action.
- There are many barriers to effective decision making, including time, incomplete facts, stress and seniority. These barriers can be overcome by utilising tools such as checklists and SOPs. Using the Page for Age, for example, will save time and reduce workload when calculating drug doses, and ensure accurate calculations.
- Trying to do too much yourself will only lead to cognitive overload – a high risk when dealing with life-threatening incidents.
- Stress can have positive and negative effects on our performance and, ultimately, some level of stress is necessary to achieve an ideal mental state for performance. However, very high levels

Human Factors

of stress are associated with disordered thinking and reduced motor control, which will hinder performance.

- Human factors can greatly influence the clinical effectiveness and efficiency of incident and patient management. Only by understanding these factors and applying principles of their management can the efficiency and effectiveness of patient care be optimised, leading to improved patient outcomes.

5. Managing Behaviours

- Clinically demanding situations can involve differing opinions on the right course of action. As discussed above, good communication, shared decision making and good situational awareness will aid in successful delivery of clinical interventions.
- Professional standards and behaviours in modern clinical practice should welcome and encourage challenge as part of a shared decision making model. Only by challenging the ideas of others in a structured and positive way can we learn as individuals and perform well as a team.
- Good team resource management (TRM) will respect that every individual has a voice, an opinion and should be heard. Good leaders will foster and empower staff to speak up and challenge interventions and actions being undertaken. Three steps for effective challenge for patient advocacy are:
  - **Clarify** – Simply ask for clarification of the course of action being undertaken. Each clinician should be able to articulate at any time clinical rational for what they are doing and why, which will improve team situational awareness.
  - **Advocate** – If any course of action is deemed unjustified or if a more suitable alternative needs to be made apparent, any team member should feel empowered to speak up, advocate an alternative and initiate a professional conversation about the course of action being undertaken.
  - **Intervene** – If during an incident, despite clarification and advocation being undertaken, the course of action is still unnecessary or dangerous (e.g. a clinician attempting to defibrillate a non-shockable rhythm), an intervention is required, whether physical or verbal, to prevent patient or clinician harm.
- With challenge comes potential conflict; the good aspects of correctly focused challenge will be beneficial:
  - Challenge is the root of change.
  - People learn and grow as a result of appropriate challenge.
  - Challenge can provide diagnostic information about problem areas to improve.
  - After challenge, a sense of achieved partnership working can be established.
- The key is maintaining sustained professional behaviours in the face of stress, and understanding that limiting conflict to that of positive challenge in all situations (fact based, SOP and clinical rationale driven) can lead to resolution avoiding interpersonal conflict (emotional, personality and frustration driven) which could lead to negative scene management or patient outcome.

Bibliography

1. Resuscitation Council (UK). *Acute Care – Quality standards for CPR (2010)*. London: Resuscitation Council UK, 2021. Available from: https://www.resus.org.uk/quality-standards/acute-care-quality-standards-for-cpr/#team.

2. Resuscitation Council (UK). *ALS Course. Chapter 2: Human factors and quality in resuscitation*. Available from: https://lms.resus.org.uk/modules/m40-v2-decisions/10346/resources/chapter_2.pdf.

Intravascular Fluid Therapy in Adults

1. Introduction

- Despite a lack of evidence demonstrating any significant beneficial effects, pre-hospital fluid therapy has become an established practice.
- There is, however, a significant body of evidence that indicates that routine pre-hospital intravascular fluid therapy may, in fact, be detrimental.
- Adverse effects may be attributed to prolonged on-scene times delaying time to definitive surgical intervention, thrombus disruption, dilution of clotting factors and other coagulopathies.

2. Pathophysiology

- The objective of fluid therapy is to improve end-organ perfusion and, as a consequence, oxygen delivery.
- By increasing the circulating volume, cardiac output and blood pressure are increased by the Bainbridge Reflex and Frank–Starling Law of the Heart.
- The speed with which a given fluid will produce its effect will largely be determined by how it is distributed throughout the body and how long it remains in the vascular space.

2.1 pH buffering

- Reduced perfusion leads to acidosis as a result of anaerobic metabolism producing lactic acid, phosphoric acids and unoxidised amino acids.
- This acidosis can depress cardiac function (negative inotropic effect) and cause arrhythmias.

2.2 Oxygen transport

- Crystalloid fluids currently used in the pre-hospital environment have no oxygen carrying capacity.
- However, the administration of fluids reduces blood viscosity which in turn may lead to improved peripheral blood flow and hence oxygen delivery.

2.3 Haemostasis

- In general, administration of fluid has a detrimental effect on haemostasis and a tendency to increase bleeding.
- The administration of fluid raises intravascular pressures and usually causes vasodilation, both of which may precipitate disruption of the primary haemostatic thrombus.
- Furthermore, supplemental administration of fluid reduces blood viscosity and dilutes clotting factors both of which can be detrimental to haemostatic mechanisms.
- Finally, in order to minimise hypothermia-induced coagulopathies, the use of cold fluids should be avoided if possible.

3. General Considerations

3.1 Pulse versus blood pressure as a threshold for treatment

- Within the guidelines references are made to the use of central and peripheral pulses as a surrogate marker to determine perfusion and the thresholds on which to base decisions relating to intravascular (IV) fluid therapy. Reference is also made to systolic blood pressure.
- Wherever possible, decisions pertaining to initiating or withholding IV therapy should be based on systolic BP and an assessment of cerebral perfusion (denoted by conscious level). Where early implementation of non-invasive blood pressure monitoring has not been possible or in the event that readings appear inaccurate (i.e. they do not reflect the clinical condition of the patient based on assessment) then central and peripheral pulses should be used as a surrogate marker.

3.2 Patients with pre-existing hypertensive disease

- Many patients encountered by ambulance clinicians will have a known diagnosis of hypertensive disease, however determining the point at which they are considered hypotensive is dependent on knowing the grade of their disease and normal baseline BP and as such may be challenging.
- There is a paucity of evidence relating to the identification of hypotension in patients with an underlying diagnosis of hypertensive disease or the impact this may have on clinical outcomes in those with acute illness or injury.
- Have a high index of suspicion for serious underlying illness or injury when a patient with chronic hypertension exhibits a systolic blood pressure significantly lower than their estimated or known baseline – this is a concept referred to as 'relative hypotension'.
- Currently, there is no consensus regarding the targets for systolic blood pressure on which to base IV fluid therapy decisions specifically in this patient group.
- Mean arterial pressure, or MAP, is significant because it measures the pressure necessary for adequate organ perfusion and is often considered a better indicator of perfusion than systolic blood pressure. In adults, a MAP of at least 60 mmHg is required to ensure adequate blood supply to the coronary circulation, kidneys and brain.
- Whilst a theoretical risk exists that patients with a poorly controlled or chronically high baseline BP may become significantly hypotensive before meeting the thresholds for IV fluid therapy defined within the guideline, there is a greater

Intravascular Fluid Therapy in Adults

risk of excessive fluid administration and its associated iatrogenic complications.

- Determining the threshold for treatment in patients with haemorrhagic emergencies and a history of hypertensive disease should be based on objective evidence of impaired major organ perfusion and clinicians should pay particular attention to the development of an altered level of consciousness suggestive of poor cerebral perfusion.

4. Haemorrhagic Emergencies

TABLE 1.6 – Early Indicators of Impaired Major Organ Perfusion

SIGNS	CAUSE
Tachypnoea	↑ Metabolic acidosis
Tachycardia	↓ Cardiac output
Hypotension	↓ Vascular volume
↓ Consciousness	↓ Cerebral perfusion

- Haemorrhage may occur as a result of traumatic or medical aetiologies and may be classified as:
  - **apparent** (external) blood loss
  - **concealed** (internal) blood loss.
- Current thinking suggests that fluids should **ONLY** be administered when there are signs of impaired major organ perfusion (refer to Table 1.6).
- Control of external haemorrhage must be achieved before administering fluids.

4.1 Trauma

4.1.1 Penetrating trauma to the trunk

- Penetrating trauma to the trunk carries the risk of significant disruption of major vessels that, due to their location, are not amenable to compression or other methods of haemorrhage control.
- As a consequence of this inability to control further bleeding, the general aim of fluid therapy is to maintain a good volume central pulse (carotid or femoral) **OR** systolic BP of 60 mmHg, along with adequate cerebral perfusion (denoted by level of consciousness).

4.1.2 Penetrating trauma to the limbs

- Penetrating trauma to the limbs also carries a risk of significant disruption of major vessels; however, these vessels are both fewer and more amenable to compression or other methods of haemorrhage control.
- As a consequence of this ability to control further bleeding, the general aim of fluid therapy is to maintain a palpable peripheral pulse (radial) **OR** systolic BP of 90 mmHg.

4.1.3 Blunt trauma to trunk or limbs

- Blunt trauma to the trunk carries a lower risk of major vessel disruption; consequently, the trigger point for fluid administration is different from penetrating trauma.
- In cases of blunt trauma to the trunk or limbs, the aim of fluid therapy is to maintain a palpable peripheral pulse (radial) **OR** systolic BP of 90 mmHg.

4.1.4 Limb crush injuries and crush syndrome

- Crush injury is a term used to describe the direct injury resulting from crush and in of itself does not require fluid resuscitation unless the patient is exhibiting signs of hypovolaemia, which should be managed in line with the guidance for fluids in blunt trauma. Crush syndrome is the systemic manifestation of muscle cell damage resulting from pressure or crushing and its severity is largely dependent on the magnitude and duration of the compressing force combined with the bulk of muscle/tissue involved.
- Patients at risk of developing crush syndrome or who are exhibiting clinical signs of crush syndrome should receive intravenous fluids; however, the identification of patients at risk may be challenging and requires the clinician to consider the mechanism, duration of crush or entrapment and degree of injury present.
- Patients identified at risk of developing crush syndrome should receive 2 litres of Sodium Chloride 0.9% irrespective of systolic BP reading. Patients experiencing cardiac arrhythmias associated with crush syndrome may require intravenous Calcium Chloride according to locally agreed guidelines.

TABLE 1.7 – Dosages for Fluid Therapy – Crush Syndrome

INITIAL DOSE	REPEAT DOSE / REPEAT INTERVAL	REPEAT INTERVAL	MAXIMUM DOSE
2 litres	ONCE ONLY	NOT APPLICABLE	2 litres

Intravascular Fluid Therapy in Adults

4.1.5 Trauma to the head (all types)
- Significant head injury results in raised intracranial pressure (ICP) as cerebral tissues swell within the enclosed skull; to ensure adequate cerebral perfusion pressure (CPP) the body compensates and raises the mean arterial blood pressure (MAP).

CPP = MAP − ICP

- As a result of this compensatory mechanism, significant head injuries are usually associated with hypertension and NOT hypotension.
- Hypotension in the setting of significant head injury indicates not only significant blood loss but also CRITICALLY IMPAIRED CEREBRAL PERFUSION.
- In order to support cerebral perfusion the administration of fluids may be required.
- In the setting of significant head injury with evidence of other blunt trauma and hypotension, fluid therapy should be titrated to maintain a palpable peripheral pulse (radial) OR systolic BP of 90 mmHg unless penetrating trunk trauma is felt to be the dominant cause of hypotension, in which case aim for a good volume central pulse (carotid or femoral) OR systolic BP of 60 mmHg.
- Patients with significant head injury whom are hypotensive but have no other objective signs of blunt or penetrating injury (i.e. apparent isolated head injury) should have intravenous fluid therapy titrated to maintain a systolic BP of 110 mmHg.
- Hypertensive head injury does not normally require fluid therapy unless the patient demonstrates signs of cerebral herniation. Patients with significant head injury and evidence of developing cerebral herniation may benefit from the administration of an osmotic fluid (i.e. hypertonic saline); follow locally agreed clinical guidelines.

4.2 Medical conditions
- Principles of fluid therapy in medically related haemorrhage are fundamentally no different from those of blunt trauma.
- Generally, the aim of fluid therapy is to maintain a palpable peripheral pulse (radial) OR systolic BP of 90 mmHg.
- Medically related haemorrhage may also be complicated by vascular disease, coagulopathies or the presence of tumours.

4.3 Fluid therapy following haemorrhage
- **DO NOT** delay at scene to obtain vascular access or to commence fluid replacement; wherever possible obtain vascular access and administer fluid **En route TO HOSPITAL**.
- If the clinician determines that there is a definite need for fluid therapy they should obtain vascular access.
- Clinicians should attempt to gain intravenous access in the first instance; however, they may consider intraosseous access where intravenous access fails or is unlikely to be successful.
- Vascular access devices should be flushed with 5 ml of 0.9% sodium chloride for injection to confirm patency prior to administering large volumes of fluid.
- Once patent vascular access is confirmed, administer an initial bolus of 250 ml of crystalloid, further boluses will be dependent on pulse / BP assessment (refer to Table 1.8).
- Where the need for intravascular fluid therapy is less certain, clinicians should still obtain vascular access and flush to confirm patency.
- **Do not connect any fluids to the cannula unless intravascular fluid therapy is indicated.**

NB The slow administration of fluids to keep a vein open (TKO/TKVO) should not be practised to avoid inadvertent excess fluid administration.

TABLE 1.8 – Dosages for Fluid Therapy – Haemorrhagic Emergencies

INITIAL DOSE	REPEAT DOSE	REPEAT INTERVAL	MAXIMUM DOSE
250 ml	250 ml	PRN	2 litres

5. Non-Haemorrhagic Emergencies

5.1 Trauma
- The loss of bodily fluids other than blood, as a result of trauma, is rare. Burn injuries are notable exceptions (see exceptions and special circumstances below).

5.2 Medical conditions
- Patients suffering medical emergencies may experience fluid loss as a result of dehydration (e.g. heat related illness, vomiting or diarrhoea) and/or redistribution of fluid from the vascular compartment (e.g. as a result of anaphylaxis or sepsis).
- The volume of fluids lost to such processes can easily be underestimated.
- Such patients may be significantly dehydrated resulting in reduced fluid volumes in both the vascular and tissue compartments which has usually taken time to develop and will take time to correct.

Intravascular Fluid Therapy in Adults

- Rapid fluid replacement into the vascular compartment can compromise the cardiovascular system particularly where there is pre-existing cardiovascular disease and in the elderly.
- In cases of dehydration, fluid replacement should be aimed at gradual re-hydration over many hours rather than minutes. Oral electrolyte solutions may be an appropriate consideration in some patients (e.g. heat illness). To that end, intravenous fluids should not be initiated in the pre-hospital setting solely for the purposes of rehydration. Fluid therapy should be initiated based on evidence of circulatory compromise.

5.3 Fluid therapy

- **DO NOT** delay at scene to obtain vascular access or to provide fluid replacement; wherever possible obtain vascular access and administer fluid **EN ROUTE TO HOSPITAL**.
- If the clinician determines that there is a definite need for fluid therapy, they should obtain vascular access.
- Clinicians should attempt to gain intravenous access in the first instance; however, they may consider intraosseous access where intravenous access fails or is unlikely to be successful.
- Vascular access devices should be flushed with 5 ml of 0.9% sodium chloride for injection to confirm patency prior to administering large volumes of fluid.
- Once patent vascular access is confirmed, administer an initial bolus of 250 ml of crystalloid and review the need for continued fluids based on re-assessment of circulation (i.e. peripheral pulse assessment/systolic BP), refer to Table 1.9.
- Where the need for intravascular fluid therapy is less certain, clinicians should still obtain vascular access and flush to confirm patency.
- Do not connect any fluids to the cannula unless intravascular fluid therapy is indicated.

NB The slow administration of fluids to keep a vein open (TKO/TKVO) should not be practised to avoid inadvertent excess fluid administration.

TABLE 1.9 – Dosages for Fluid Therapy

INITIAL DOSE	REPEAT DOSE	REPEAT INTERVAL	MAXIMUM DOSE
250 ml	250 ml	PRN	2 litres

- Monitor the physiological response, re-assess perfusion, pulse, respiratory rate and blood pressure wherever possible.
- If these observations improve, suspend any further administration.
- If there is no improvement, administer further 250 ml boluses, reassessing for improvement after each fluid bolus (refer to Table 1.9).
- The maximum cumulative fluid dose is usually 2 litres (refer to Table 1.9).
- If the patient remains hypotensive despite repeated 250 ml boluses OR the patient is likely to remain on scene for a considerable time (e.g. due to extrication difficulties), request senior clinical support (according to local procedures).

5.4 Exceptions and Special Circumstances

5.4.1 Burns

- <15% do not administer fluid.
- ≥15 – <25% and time to hospital is greater than 30 minutes, then administer 1 litre sodium chloride 0.9% (refer to Table 1.10).
- ≥25% administer 1 litre sodium chloride 0.9% (refer to Table 1.10).

NB If fluid therapy is indicated **DO NOT** delay transfer to further care but continue fluid therapy en route – stopping if practicable to insert the cannula.

- Exercise caution in patients who are elderly or who have heart failure; consider the use of fluids judiciously and observe for early signs of circulatory overload.
- In order to minimise the risk of hypothermia, the use of cold fluids should be avoided if possible.

TABLE 1.10 – Dosages for Fluid Therapy – Burns

INITIAL DOSE	REPEAT DOSE	REPEAT INTERVAL	MAXIMUM DOSE
1 litre over 1 hour	NONE	N/A	1 litre

Intravascular Fluid Therapy in Adults

5.4.2 Sepsis
- Refer to **Sepsis**.

TABLE 1.11 – Dosages for Fluid Therapy – Sepsis

INITIAL DOSE	REPEAT DOSE	REPEAT INTERVAL	MAXIMUM DOSE
250 ml over 10–15 minutes	Repeat up to 1000 ml	PRN	1 litre

5.4.3 Anaphylaxis
- Large volumes of fluid may leak from the patient's circulation during an anaphylactic reaction. There will also be vasodilation, a low blood pressure and signs of shock. If there is intravenous access, infuse intravenous fluids immediately. Give a rapid IV fluid challenge (500–1000 ml) and monitor the response; give further doses as necessary. If intravenous access is delayed or impossible, the intra-osseous route should be used. Do not delay the administration of IM adrenaline attempting intra-osseous access.

TABLE 1.12 – Dosages for Fluid Therapy – Anaphylaxis

INITIAL DOSE	REPEAT DOSE	REPEAT INTERVAL	MAXIMUM DOSE
500–1000 ml	500–1000 ml	PRN	2 litres (if further fluids required, seek senior clinical advice)

5.4.4 Diabetic Ketoacidosis (DKA)
- Formal diagnosis of DKA in the pre-hospital setting may be challenging, however, a clinical history and examination may identify DKA as a likely cause for current clinical state. Patients with suspected DKA may benefit from early administration of intravenous crystalloids which help to restore circulating volume, clear ketones, reduce blood sugar and correct electrolyte disturbances. However, caution should be applied when considering IV fluid therapy for patients in DKA who are elderly, pregnant, suffering heart/renal failure or who have additional co-morbidities.

TABLE 1.13 – Dosages For Fluid Therapy — DKA

INITIAL DOSE	REPEAT DOSE	REPEAT INTERVAL	MAXIMUM DOSE
If clinically shocked 500 ml over 15 minutes	Repeat ONCE over 15 minutes if patient remains hypotensive, OR continue repeat dose over 45 minutes if blood pressure restored	PRN	1 litre
If dehydrated 1000 ml (1 L) over 60 minutes	N/A	N/A	1 litre

5.4.5 Young Adults with low BMI – Diabetic Ketoacidosis (DKA)

Young adults (18–25 years of age) with a low BMI should be given IV fluids if there is significant evidence of hypovolaemic shock. Establish IV/IO access and commence fluids if shocked, giving an initial fluid bolus of 20 ml/kg (over 15 minutes) whilst undertaking an urgent transfer and pre-alerting the ED. Further fluid may be required, using smaller volumes (a 10 ml/kg bolus), but only after discussion with a senior clinician. If these patients deteriorate during fluid administration, stop administering fluid immediately. When intravenous fluids are felt to be indicated In NON-SHOCKED patients with DKA, an initial 10 ml/kg bolus should be given (over 60 minutes).

5.4.6 Adrenal Crisis

TABLE 1.14 – Dosages for Fluid Therapy — Adrenal Crisis

INITIAL DOSE	REPEAT DOSE	REPEAT INTERVAL	MAXIMUM DOSE
1 litre over 30 minutes	NONE	N/A	1 litre

Intravascular Fluid Therapy in Adults

> **KEY POINTS!**
>
> **Intravascular Fluid Therapy in Adults**
> - Current research shows little evidence to support the routine use of IV fluids in adult acute blood loss.
> - Current consensus is that fluids should only be administered when major organ perfusion is impaired in the majority of cases (with the exception of some non-haemorrhagic indications).
> - **DO NOT** delay on scene for vascular access or fluid replacement; wherever possible obtain vascular access and administer fluid En route TO HOSPITAL stopping if practicable to insert the cannula.

Bibliography

1. Revell M, Porter K, Greaves I. Fluid resuscitation in pre-hospital trauma care: a consensus view. Emergency Medicine Journal 2002, 19(6): 494–498.
2. Bickell WH, Wall MJJ, Pepe PE, Martin RR, Ginger VF, Allen M K, et al. Immediate versus delayed fluid resuscitation in patients with trauma. New England Journal of Medicine 1994, 331: 1105–9.
3. Consensus Working Group on Pre-hospital Fluids. Fluid resuscitation in pre-hospital trauma care: a consensus view. Journal of the Royal Army Medical Corps 2001, 147(2): 147–52.
4. Cotton BA, Jerome R, Collier BR, Khetarpal S, Holevar M, Tucker B, et al. Guidelines for pre-hospital fluid resuscitation in the injured patient. Journal of Trauma 2009, 67(2): 389–402.
5. Dalton AM. Pre-hospital intravenous fluid replacement in trauma: an outmoded concept? Journal of the Royal Society of Medicine 1995, 88(4): 213P–216P.
6. Gausche M, Tadeo RE, Zane MC, Lewis RJ. Out-of-hospital intravenous access: unnecessary procedures and excessive cost. Academic Emergency Medicine 1998, 5(9): 878–82.
7. Henderson RA, Thomson DP, Bahrs BA, Norman MP. Unnecessary intravenous access in the emergency setting. Prehospital Emergency Care 1998, 2(4): 312–16.
8. Mitra B, Cameron PA, Mori A, Fitzgerald M. Acute coagulopathy and early deaths post major trauma. Injury 2012, 43(1): 22–5.
9. Roberts K, Revell M, Youssef H, Bradbury AW, Adam DJ. Hypotensive resuscitation in patients with ruptured abdominal aortic aneurysm. European Journal of Vascular & Endovascular Surgery 2005, 31(4): 339–44.
10. Kaweski SM, Sise MJ, Virgilio RW. The effect of pre-hospital fluids on survival in trauma patients. Journal of Trauma 1990, 30(10): 1215–18; discussion 1218–19.
11. Spahn D, Cerny V, Coats T, Duranteau J, Fernandez-Mondejar F, Gordini G, et al. Management of bleeding following major trauma: a European guideline. Critical Care 2007, 11(1): R17.
12. Eckstein M, Chan L, Schneir A, Palmer R. Effect of pre-hospital advanced life support on outcomes of major trauma patients. Journal of Trauma 2000, 48(4): 643–8.
13. Honigman B, Rohweder K, Moore EE, Lowenstein SR, Pons PT. Pre-hospital advanced trauma life support for penetrating cardiac wounds. Annals of Emergency Medicine 1990, 19(2): 145–50.
14. National Institute for Clinical Excellence. Pre-hospital Initiation of Fluid Replacement Therapy in Trauma (TA74). London: NICE. Available from: https://www.nice.org.uk/guidance/ta74, 2004.
15. Bulger EM, May S, Brasel KJ, Schreiber M, Kerby JD, Tisherman SA, et al. Out-of-hospital hypertonic resuscitation following severe traumatic brain injury: a randomized controlled trial. Journal of the American Medical Association 2010, 304(13): 1455–64.
16. Chung KK, Wolf SE, Cancio LC, Alvarado R, Jones JA, McCorcle J, et al. Resuscitation of severely burned military casualties: fluid begets more fluid. Journal of Trauma 2009, 67(2): 231–7; discussion 237.
17. Cooper DJ, Myles PS, McDermott FT, Murray LJ, Laidlaw J, Cooper G, et al. Pre-hospital hypertonic saline resuscitation of patients with hypotension and severe traumatic brain injury: a randomized controlled trial. Journal of the American Medical Association 2004, 291(11): 1350–7.
18. Holcroft JW, Vassar MJ, Turner JE, Derlet RW, Kramer GC. 3% NaCl and 7.5% NaCl/dextran 70 in the resuscitation of severely injured patients. Annals of Surgery 1987, 206(3): 279–88.
19. Maningas PA, Mattox KL, Pepe PE, Jones RL, Feliciano DV, Burch JM. Hypertonic saline-dextran solutions for the pre-hospital management of traumatic hypotension. American Journal of Surgery 1989, 157(5): 528–33; discussion 533–4.
20. Thompson R, Greaves I. Hypertonic saline-hydroxyethyl starch in trauma resuscitation. Journal of the Royal Army Medical Corps 2006, 152(1): 6–12.
21. Vassar MJ, Perry CA, Gannaway WL, Holcroft JW. 7.5% sodium chloride/dextran for resuscitation of trauma patients undergoing helicopter transport. Archives of Surgery 1991, 126(9): 1065–72.
22. Vassar MJ, Perry CA, Holcroft JW. Pre-hospital resuscitation of hypotensive trauma patients with 7.5% NaCl versus 7.5% NaCl with added dextran: a controlled trial. Journal of Trauma 1993, 34(5): 622–32; discussion 632–3.
23. Carney N, Totten AM, O'reilly C, Ullman JS, et.al. Brain Trauma Guidelines: Guidelines for the Management of Severe Traumatic Brain Injury, Fourth Edition. Neurosurgery 2016. 0:0:2016
24. Greaves I, Porter K, Smith JE. Consensus statement on the early management of crush injury and prevention of crush syndrome. J R Army Meds Corps 2003; 149: 255–259. DOI: 10.1136/jramc-149-04-02
25. Allison K, Porter K. Consensus on the pre-hospital approach to burns patient management. Emergency Medicine Journal 2004, 21(1): 112–14.

Intravascular Fluid Therapy in Adults

26. Williams G, Dziewulski P. Intravascular fluid therapy in burns injury. In Group. TJRCALGD, editor, 2011.

27. Greaves I, Porter K, Smith JE. Consensus statement on the early management of crush injury and prevention of crush syndrome. Journal of the Royal Army Medical Corps 2003, 149(4): 255–9.

28. Holcomb JB. Fluid resuscitation in modern combat casualty care: lessons learned from Somalia. Journal of Trauma 2003, 54(suppl.): S46–51.

29. Treharne LJ, Kay AR. The initial management of acute burns. Journal of the Royal Army Medical Corps 2001, 147(2): 198–205.

30. Mattox KL, Maningas PA, Moore EE, Mateer JR, Marx JA, Aprahamian C, et al. Pre-hospital hypertonic saline/dextran infusion for post-traumatic hypotension: the U.S.A. Multicenter Trial. Annals of Surgery 1991, 213(5): 482–91.

31. Smith JE, Hall MJ. Hypertonic saline. Journal of the Royal Army Medical Corps 2004, 150(4): 239–43.

32. Pons PT, Moore EE, Cusick JM, Brunko M, Antuna B, Owens L. Pre-hospital venous access in an urban paramedic system: a prospective on-scene analysis. Journal of Trauma 1988, 28(10): 1460–3.

33. Jones SE, Nesper TP, Alcouloumre E. Pre-hospital intravenous line placement: a prospective study. Annals of Emergency Medicine 1989, 18(3): 244–6

34. Minville V, Pianezza A, Asehnoune K, Cabardis S, Smail N. Pre-hospital intravenous line placement assessment in the French emergency system: a prospective study. European Journal of Anaesthesia 2006, 23(7): 594–7.

35. Sampalis JS, Tamim H, Denis R, Boukas S, Ruest SA, Nikolis A, et al. Ineffectiveness of on-site intravenous lines: is pre-hospital time the culprit? Journal of Trauma 1997, 43(4): 608–15; discussion 615–17.

36. Daniels R. Surviving Sepsis Campaign: indications for fluid administration in patients with sepsis. Personal communication, 2011.

37. Dellinger RP, Levy MM, Cadet JM, Bion J, Parker MM, Jaeschke R, et al. Surviving Sepsis Campaign: international guidelines for management of severe sepsis and septic shock 2008. Critical Care Medicine 2008, 36(1): 296–327: doi 10.1097/01.CCM.0000298158.12101.41.

38. NICE. Diabetic Ketoacidosis: Management. Online summary guidance by NICE (2013). Available from: https://bnf.nice.org.uk/treatment-summary/diabetic-ketoacidosis.html.

39. Dhatariya K, Savage M, et al. The Management of Diabetic Ketoacidosis in Adults: Second Edition 2013. Joint British Diabetes Society Inpatient Care Group. Available from: http://www.diabetologists-abcd.org.uk/JBDS/JBDS_IP_DKA_Adults_Revised.pdf.

Intravascular Fluid Therapy in Children

1. Introduction

- There has been no significant research in paediatric fluid administration in the literature and thus advice is dependent on that of adult studies and expert consensus.

2. Pathophysiology

- Although the basic pathophysiology is similar to adults, children have one very important difference. Their relatively healthy hearts and vasculature make the compensatory mechanisms very efficient. This means that only subtle signs of circulatory failure (shock) may be evident even in children with severe intravascular fluid depletion. When compensatory mechanisms start to fail, the child is in extremis and will deteriorate very quickly.

3. Assessment

- It is crucial that children with shock are treated before decompensation occurs whenever possible. There is no one sign that reliably dictates the state of shock a child may be in and a combination of all the markers of shock, along with an assessment of the mechanism of the shock (the history) must all be taken into account when deciding how shocked a child is.

- Blood pressure drops late in children for the reasons given above, and therefore is not a good indicator of the degree of volume depletion of the child. It is therefore of limited use in the pre-hospital setting, but if it is taken and found to be low (for the age of the child), this can be regarded as a pre-terminal sign.

- The following should be assessed:
  - pulse rate and volume
  - capillary refill measured on the forehead or sternum
  - respiratory rate
  - colour (pallor ect.)
  - cold peripheries
  - conscious level (AVPU) including drowsiness.

These must be considered as a whole in the light of what is known about the mechanism (i.e. volume of blood or fluid lost).

Only when all these are taken together can a rough estimate of the degree of shock be made. Each one of these is not reliable when measured on its own.

NB Children have compensatory physiological mechanisms that maintain "normal' blood pressures even in the face of significant blood loss; as a result, 'permissive hypotension' is neither recommended or practised in paediatric trauma. Small boluses (5 ml/kg) of fluid are administered and repeated (as needed) following frequent clinical reassessment (titrated against response/improvement) – see below.

NB There is NO evidence that the absence of the radial pulse correlates with the blood pressure or degree of shock in a consistent manner in children. Do not monitor the need for fluids against the presence of the radial pulse.

4. Management

4.1 Medical causes of shock

It is usually difficult to measure volumes of fluid lost in children with medical causes of shock.

- 10 ml/kg is used as standard medical fluid replacement (equates to 12.5% of the child's blood volume).
- This can be given intravenously or intraosseously and is given as a bolus.
- The exact volume given must be documented.
- The child must be re-assessed after each bolus.
- It may be repeated once – total 20 ml/kg.

4.2 Exceptions

Diabetic Ketoacidosos (DKA)

Children and young adults with DKA may also present with significant dehydration. Establish IV/IO access at scene, and commence fluids if shocked, giving an initial fluid bolus of 10 ml/kg (over 15 minutes) whilst undertaking an urgent transfer and pre-alerting the ED. Further fluid may be required, using smaller volumes (a 5 ml/kg bolus), but only after discussion with a senior clinician. When intravenous fluids are felt to be indicated in **NON-SHOCKED** patients with DKA, an initial 10 ml/kg bolus should be given (over 30 minutes).

Anaphylaxis

Large volumes of fluid may leak from the patient's circulation during an anaphylactic reaction. There will also be vasodilation, a low blood pressure and signs of shock. If there is intravenous access, infuse intravenous fluids immediately. Give a rapid IV fluid challenge (10 ml/kg) and monitor the response; give further doses as necessary. If intravenous access is delayed or impossible, the intra-osseous route can be used. Do not delay the administration of IM adrenaline attempting intra-osseous access.

Heart or Renal Failure

If a child has heart failure or renal failure give a 5 ml/kg bolus but stop if the patient deteriorates. Transfer to hospital as a priority.

4.3 Trauma: hypovolaemic shock

Fluid overload should be avoided. For ease and because all trauma patients should not be overloaded, it is not necessary to distinguish between compressible and non compressible haemorrhage.

5 ml/kg aliquots of fluid should be given.

Re-assessment should be undertaken after each 5 ml/kg dose, using the signs described above.

Intravascular Fluid Therapy in Children

The 5 ml/kg dose can be repeated until the child is **significantly** improved. The vital signs (e.g. pulse) need not be normalised, but the child must be obviously more stable. There is no absolute upper dose.

The child must be constantly re-assessed during transport.

Clinical deterioration should be addressed with further 5 ml/kg fluid bolus(es), until the child improves clinically.

4.4 Burns

- Children lose fluids rapidly from severe burns and scalds and should have intravenous sodium chloride 0.9% started early.
- If the child has a >10% but <20% burn and the hospital time is more than 30 minutes, fluids should be started, and if greater than 20% burn fluid should be given regardless of the time to hospital.

Where burn surface area is:

- <10% do not administer fluid.
- ≥10 – <20% and time to hospital is greater than 30 minutes then administer sodium chloride 0.9% 10 ml/kg over an hour.
- ≥20% administer sodium chloride 0.9% 10 ml/kg over an hour.
- The total dose must be calculated and given as regular, tiny portions of this to aim to have infused the correct amount over the hour.
- If fluid therapy is indicated DO NOT delay transfer to further care but continue fluid therapy en route – stopping if practicable to insert the cannula.
- Vascular access also means analgesia can be administered.

4.5 Cardiac Arrest

In children where hypovolaemia is thought to be a contributory factor, give a fluid bolus of 10 ml/kg (N.saline (0.9%) or Hartmann's solution), repeated once if indicated. Seek appropriate medical opinion if further boluses are thought to be indicated.

KEY POINTS!

Intravascular Fluid Therapy in Children

- **Children compensate well for shock.**
- **Once decompensated, they deteriorate very rapidly.**
- **All physiological signs must be taken in combination to diagnose shock.**
- **10 ml/kg is the standard bolus for medically caused shock.**
- **5 ml/kg is the standard bolus for traumatic shock.**
- **10 ml/kg over 1 hour should be given to children with burns ≥20% and also to children with burns of ≥10 and <20% whose journey time will be more than 30 minutes. This procedure must not delay the time to hospital admission.**
- **Re-assessment after each bolus is vital to avoid fluid overload.**
- **Fluids should be used with extreme caution in renal failure and cardiac failure.**

Mental Capacity Act 2005

1. Introduction
- The Mental Capacity Act 2005 (MCA) was implemented in England and Wales to provide protection and powers to individuals aged 16 years and over who may lack capacity to make some (or all) decisions for themselves. It is also for people working with or caring for them. It applies to public and private locations.

2. What Is the MCA?
- The MCA empowers individuals to make their own decisions where possible and protects the rights of those who lack capacity. Where an individual lacks capacity to make a specific decision at a particular time, the MCA provides a legal framework for others to act and make that decision on their behalf, in their best interests. This includes decisions about their care and/or treatment.

3. What Is Mental Capacity?
- 'Capacity' is 'the ability of an individual to make decisions regarding specific elements of their life' (MCA, 2005) and it is crucial within the pre-hospital emergency care environment since everything done to/for a conscious patient requires their consent. Patients must have mental capacity in order to give (or withhold) consent and, apart from situations where the Mental Health Act 1983 (MHA) applies, mental capacity is central to determining whether treatment and care can be given to someone who refuses.
- The MCA defines a lack of capacity as:

  'For the purposes of this Act, a person lacks capacity in relation to a matter if at the material time he is unable to make a decision for himself in relation to the matter because of an impairment of, or a disturbance in the functioning of, the mind or brain' (MCA, 2005).

- For the person's wishes to be overridden there must be evidence that some impairment or disturbance of mental functioning exists, rendering the person unable to make an informed decision at the time it needs to be made. In simple terms, 'capacity' is the ability to a make a decision at the time it needs to be made.

4. Responsibilities under the Act
- Ambulance staff have a formal duty of regard to the Act and the Code of Practice, and every ambulance trust should, as best practice, have a formal process (i.e. a policy/protocol) for establishing the capacity of patients to give, or withhold, consent for assessment, treatment and/or being transported for further care, when required.
- There must always be a presumption of capacity. In every situation, staff must assume that a person can make their own decision(s) unless it is found, on balance of probabilities, that they are unable to do so.
- Doubts about mental capacity may arise for many reasons, including the person's behaviour, their circumstances or concerns raised by someone else. Approximately 2 million people in England and Wales may lack capacity to make decisions for themselves because of:
  - dementia
  - learning disabilities
  - mental health problems
  - stroke and brain injuries
  - temporary impairment due to medication, intoxication, injury or illness.
- Staff must always act in the best interests of any person who lacks capacity; but if the impairment is temporary you should consider if it is safe to wait until the patient regains capacity before acting on their behalf.

5. Key Principles
- The MCA has five Key Principles which emphasise the fundamental concepts and core values of the Act. These must be considered and applied when you are working with, or providing care or treatment for, people who lack capacity.
- They are:

1. Every person must be assumed to have capacity unless it is proved otherwise.

   This means that you cannot assume that someone is unable to decide for themselves just because they have a particular medical/neurological condition, disability or because of their age. The Human Rights Act protects individuals' autonomy and the threshold for over-riding this is high.

2. People must be supported as much as possible to make a decision before anyone concludes that they cannot make their own decision.

   This means that you should make every effort to encourage and support the person to make the decision for themselves. If a lack of capacity is established, it is still important that you involve the person as much as possible in making decisions.

3. A person should not be considered as unable to make a decision solely because they make an unwise decision.

   This means that capacity should not be confused with an assessment of the reasonableness of the person's decision. A person is entitled to make a decision that others might perceive to be unwise, eccentric or irrational, *as long as they have the capacity to do so*.

   However, it is important to note that when an apparently irrational decision is based on a misperception of reality (e.g. someone

Mental Capacity Act 2005

experiencing hallucinations/delusions/disordered thinking), rather than a different *value system* to that held by the assessor, then the patient may not truly be able to understand. This would lead to doubts about their ability to make a decision and an assessment should be completed.

4. Any act done, or decision made, on behalf of someone who lacks capacity must be done, or made, in their best interests.

   This means that anything done for, or on behalf of, a person who lacks mental capacity must be done in their best interests, which should be assessed by the decision maker, drawing upon all reasonably ascertainable and relevant information.

5. Before making a decision, or acting on behalf of someone who lacks capacity, a decision maker must consider if the outcome could be achieved effectively in a less restrictive manner.

   The Act does not mandate the use of the 'least-restrictive' option; instead, you must consider options that interfere less with the patient's rights and freedom of action while still achieving the objective of the decision/Act in hand. Make sure that whatever you do, you do not limit their freedom of movement any more than is necessary.

6. Helping People to Make Decisions for Themselves

- When a person in your care needs to make a decision, you must start from the assumption that the person has capacity to make the decision in question (Principle 1). You should make every effort to encourage and support the person to make the decision themselves (Principle 2) and you will have to consider a number of factors to assist in the decision making process.
- These could include:
  - Does the person have all the relevant information needed to make the decision? If there is a choice, has all the information been given on the alternatives? This should include information about the nature of the decision, the risks and benefits of choosing either way and the implications of not making a decision.
  - Could the information be explained or presented in a way that is easier for the person to understand? Help should be given to communicate information wherever necessary. For example, a person with a learning disability might find it easier to communicate using pictures, photographs or sign language.
  - Where it is safe to defer a decision, are there particular times of the day when a person's understanding is better, or is there a particular place where they feel more at ease and able to make a decision? For example, if a person becomes drowsy soon after they have taken their medication, this would not be a good time for them to make a decision.
  - Can anyone else help or support the person to understand information or make a choice? For example, a relative, carer, friend or advocate.
- When there is reason to believe that a person lacks capacity to make a decision, you should consider the following:
  - Has everything been done to help and support the person to make the decision?
  - Does the decision need to be made without delay?
  - If not, is it possible to wait until the person does have the capacity to make the decision for him/herself?

7. Assessing Capacity

- There are several questions to consider when you are assessing a person's capacity:
  - What is the decision that needs to be made?
  - Is the person able to make that decision? (Functional Test)
  - Is there an impairment of, or disturbance in the functioning of, the person's mind or brain (this can be temporary or permanent)? (Diagnostic Test)
  - Is the impairment or disturbance sufficient to cause the person to be unable to make that particular decision at the relevant time? (Causative Nexus)
- A person may be mentally incapable of making the decision in question either because of a long-term mental disability or because of temporary factors such as unconsciousness, confusion or the effects of fatigue, shock, pain, anxiety, anger, alcohol or drugs (or drug withdrawal). When possible, attempts should be made to enhance capacity by, for example, pain management.
- Assessments of capacity are 'functional', and are related to the individual decision that needs to be made – at the time it needs to be made (i.e. can the person complete the functions required to make the decision, thus demonstrating they have capacity?). The more serious or complex the decision, the greater the level of capacity required. If an adult is mentally capable of making the decision, then his or her decision about whether to receive treatment or care must be respected, even if a refusal may risk permanent injury to that person's health or even lead to premature death (unless he or she is mentally disordered and can be treated under the MHA). Refusals of treatment can vary in importance. Some may involve a risk to life or of irreparable damage to health; others may not. What matters is whether, at the time in question, the patient has capacity to make that decision.
- Causative nexus refers to a direct link between the inability to make a decision and the

Mental Capacity Act 2005

impairment/disturbance identified. For example, a patient may not be able to understand information because they are unconscious. Such determinations help to support and evidence a reasonable belief that at the time of the assessment, the patient lacked capacity. The absence of causative nexus can also help to identify where the patient is under undue external influence, or simply making an unwise decision.

- Remember that an unwise decision made by a person does not itself indicate a lack of capacity. Most people will be able to make most decisions, even when they have a diagnosis that may seem to imply that they cannot. This is a general principle that cannot be over-emphasised. The more complex the decision is, the greater the level of capacity required to make it.
- When consent is refused by a competent adult, the least you should do is:
  – Respect the patient's refusal as much as you would their consent.
  – Make sure that the patient is fully informed of the implications of refusal.
  – Involve other members of the healthcare team (as appropriate).
  – Ensure this is clearly and fully documented in the patient's records.
- Local policy may require additional elements. **If there is uncertainty as to the consequences of an act of self-harm, then it should be assumed that the consequences will be serious.**
- When an individual is reasonably believed to lack capacity to make the decision required, ambulance staff have a legal duty to act in that person's best interests – unless a valid and applicable Advance Decision to Refuse Treatment (ADRT) is in place.
- Figure 1.3 outlines the assessment process. Assessors must be able to show how their assessment was completed if required later on and details must be included in the patient's clinical record.

7.1 Alcohol and Substance Use

- When determining if there is an impairment of the mind or brain, the consumption of alcohol or use of illicit substances is often a complicating factor. This does not necessarily mean that the patient is not aware of their behaviour, or aware of the decisions they make, but it may mean that they are less aware/concerned about the consequences than they would otherwise be. Judging capacity in such circumstances is difficult and subjective, but the patient's safety is paramount, so consideration should be given to balancing the risk of getting the determination of capacity wrong against the clinical risk of non-intervention.

8. Best Interests and Decision Making

- If a person has been assessed as lacking capacity, then any action taken or any decision made for – or on behalf of – that person must be made in their best interests (Principle 4).
- 'Best Interest Assessors' (BIA) are appointed to assist in making complex decisions for those who are unable to do so for themselves (e.g. when deciding on long-term treatment for a medical condition, or on where to live).
- There is a significant difference between making a 'best interest' decision involving a BIA and making a decision that is in the best interests of the patient in an emergency. BIAs are required to consider a wide range of elements when making such a decision on someone else's behalf. In emergencies, where there is limited or no information available, it will often be in a patient's best interests for urgent treatment to be provided without delay.
- Key factors which you must consider when working out what is in the best interests of a person who lacks capacity (whenever possible) include:
- *Identify all relevant circumstances.*
- Try to identify all the things that the person would consider if they were making the decision or acting for themselves.
- *Find out the person's views.*
- Try to find out the views of the person who lacks capacity, including:
  – Their past and present wishes and feelings – these may have been expressed verbally, in writing or through behaviour or habits (e.g. an ADRT).
  – Any beliefs and values (e.g. religious, cultural, moral or political) that would be likely to influence the decision in question.
  – Any other factors the person themselves would be likely to consider if they were making the decision or acting for themselves.
- Relatives/friends/carers may be able to assist with this.
- *Avoid discrimination.*
  – Do not make assumptions about someone's best interests simply based on the person's age, appearance, condition or behaviour.
- *Assess whether the person might regain capacity.*
  – Consider whether the person is likely to regain capacity. If so, can the decision wait until then? It may be that the person lacks capacity to make a decision to accept initial treatment but, having received that treatment, regains capacity to refuse further treatment/intervention (including transport to hospital).

Mental Capacity Act 2005

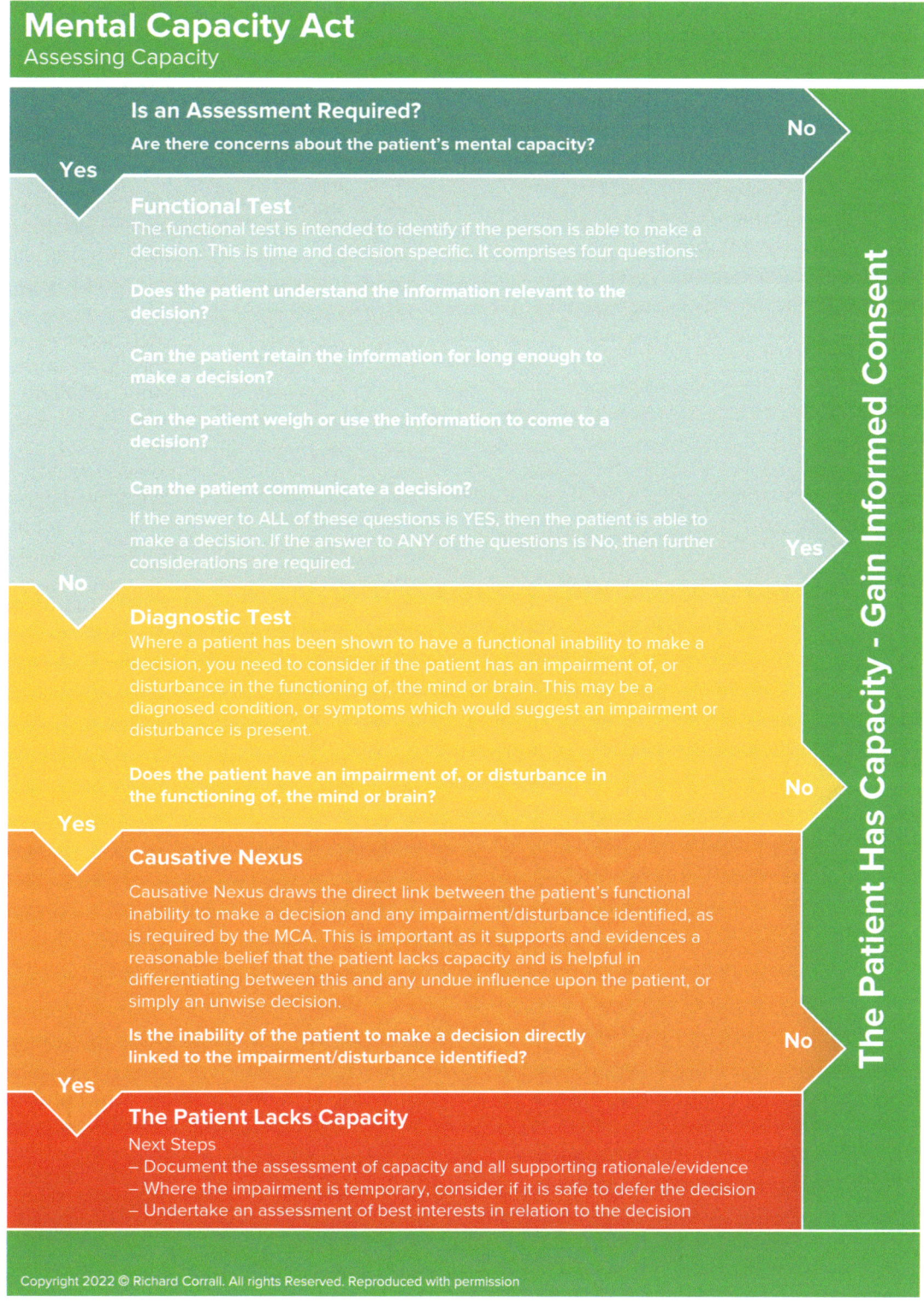

Figure 1.3 – Flow chart outlining MCA assessment of capacity for ambulance staff. Reproduced with permission of R Corrall.

- *If the decision concerns life-sustaining treatment.*
  - This should not be motivated in any way by a desire to bring about the person's death.
  - Always check for an advance decision to refuse treatment – if the person has previously made arrangements for withholding life-sustaining treatment (when they had capacity to do so) this should be recorded in an ADRT. If a **valid and applicable** ADRT is found, it must be respected, and treatment withheld.
- *Consult others.*
  - As far as possible, the decision maker must consult other people (e.g. family, friends, carers, Lasting Power of Attorney) if it is

Mental Capacity Act 2005

appropriate to do so, and take into account their views as to what would be in the best interests of the patient lacking capacity.

- *Avoid restricting the person's rights.*
  - Use the least-restrictive intervention.
- *Take all of this into account.*
  - Whenever possible, weigh up all of these factors in order to work out what is in the person's best interests.
- Section 5 of the MCA Code of Practice (CoP) outlines specific actions taken by ambulance staff (and others) that will be protected from liability and includes the following:
  - Carrying out diagnostic examinations and tests (to identify an illness, condition or other problem).
  - Providing professional medical, dental and similar treatment.
  - Giving medication.
  - Taking someone to hospital for assessment or treatment.
  - Providing nursing care (whether in hospital or the community).
  - Carrying out any other necessary medical procedures (e.g. taking a blood sample) or therapies (e.g. physiotherapy or chiropody).
  - Providing care in an emergency.

9. Restraint and Deprivation of Liberty

- In some cases, restraint, or restriction of the person's liberty, may be necessary to carry out acts of care or treatment under Section 5. Section 6 of the MCA, however, imposes some limitations on how Section 5 can be applied.
- Restraint is defined in Section 6 of the MCA as:
  - the use, or threat, of force where an incapacitated person resists, and any restriction of liberty or movement, whether or not the person resists.
- Restraint, or restrictions, on an incapacitate individual's liberty can be justified under the MCA, provided:
  - The person lacks capacity and restraint is in their best interests.
  - Restraint is used to prevent harm to the person.
  - It is proportionate to the seriousness of the harm.
- The least-restrictive method must be used for the shortest amount of time.
- Any power to restrain a person as a result of the MCA does not interfere with any other existing powers of arrest for criminal offences or powers under the Mental Health Act 1983.
- Deprivation of liberty is defined in case law (known as the acid test) as being any person who is subject to continuous control or supervision and is not free to leave. The nature and degree of any restriction, as well as the length of time it is applied, will impact on what may be considered a deprivation of liberty.
- However, the distinctions between restraining or restricting an individual, and depriving them of their liberty, are not always easy to identify. For example, it is possible to 'deprive' someone of their liberty not just by physical confinement, but also by virtue of the level of control exercised over an individual's movements.
- The concepts of restraint, restriction and deprivation of liberty are best understood as existing on the same continuum, with deprivation of liberty involving a higher degree or intensity of restrictions over that individual. Ultimately, the concept is one to be interpreted in view of the specific circumstances of that individual at the time.
- Deprivation of liberty without lawful justification is prohibited under Article 5 of the European Convention on Human Rights. There is a distinction between restraining or *restricting* an individual's movements and depriving that individual of their liberty.
- Most patients within the pre-hospital environment will not require any form of deprivation of liberty; however, in some cases the nature of their need for emergency life-sustaining treatment, or treatment to prevent a serious deterioration in the condition, may require it. In such situations, Section 4b of the MCA may provide a framework to deprive a person of their liberty in an emergency, subject to some pre-requisite conditions.
- Within hospital and care home settings, DoLS exist to protect the human rights of people who lack capacity to consent to arrangements for their care or treatment, and who might need to be deprived of their liberty (e.g. a person who has dementia may need to have doors locked to prevent them walking away from where they live and getting lost or coming to harm as a result).
- In simple terms, any person who is subject to regular and recurrent restrictions of their liberty should be considered for DoLS. Under this process, safeguards are put in place to keep the person safe; this includes regular review of the need for restriction. DoLS only apply to an individual at a stated location (address). If the person moves to another address (e.g. goes into hospital), then a new DoLS application will be required by the agency caring for them; DoLS authority will not be required during transit from one place to another.

Mental Capacity Act 2005

10. Use of Restraint by Ambulance Staff

- Ambulance staff are obliged under the MCA to act in the best interests of/for patients who lack capacity, even when the patient refuses treatment or is abusive, threatening or violent.
- The MCA also protects carers from liability when 'reasonable force' is required to ensure that patients lacking capacity receive care that is in their best interests, or to protect them from further harm. As stated previously, Section 6 of the Act defines restraint as the use or threat of force where an incapacitated person resists, and any restriction of liberty or movement, whether or not the person resists.
- Ambulance staff have limited training in this aspect. Minimal restraint (i.e. reasonable force) can be used in cases where patients lack capacity and there is no perceived risk of harm to the ambulance crew. If the behaviour of the patient exceeds what the crew can safely manage, then assistance must be requested in line with local policy (this does not necessarily have to be police).
- A dynamic risk assessment should always be completed prior to the use of any form of restraint, recording decisions and actions in the patient clinical record.
- Ambulance staff should always monitor the physical well-being of the patient and should be familiar with the information elsewhere in this guidance pertaining to **Acute Behavioural Disturbance**, which may result after prolonged forcible restraint.

11. Record-keeping

- Decision-makers should ensure that where a capacity assessment is undertaken, this is recorded in the individual's care and treatment record in line with local policy. This should include as a minimum:
  - The reasons an assessment of capacity was required.
  - What decision the assessment of capacity relates to.
  - The information provided to the person to support their understanding of the decision.
  - Any functional inability to make a decision identified and evidence to support this.
  - The nature and severity of any impairment/disturbance identified.
  - Evidence supporting the link between the inability to make a decision and the impairment/disturbance.
  - A clear statement as to whether you reasonably believe the patient to have capacity or not in light of the assessment.
- Where a patient lacks capacity:
  - Whether a valid and applicable ADRT exists.
  - The factors considered as part of the best interests decision.
  - The names and relationships of those you consult with as part of a best interests decision making process.
  - The identified decision or action.
- If the person was restrained or deprived of their liberty, the following should also be recorded:
  - Why restraint/deprivation of liberty was required.
  - An assessment of the restraint (including any force used), that this was in the person's best interests, that less-restrictive options were considered and how long any restraint/deprivation lasted.
  - Who was involved.
- It is recognised that it may not be possible to complete full details in an emergency situation, but do remember that it is not sufficient to say a patient does not have capacity without detailing how that decision was reached. A written record of the ambulance crew assessment and outcome must be made at the earliest opportunity.
- Ambulance trusts should monitor and audit capacity assessments, best interest assessments and any restraint or deprivation of liberty to ensure compliance with legislation, statutory codes of practice and national guidance.

12. Transfer and Continuing Care of the Patient

- Ambulance staff must complete a clinical record (in line with local policy) with the normal clinical information, including full details of the capacity assessment, risk factors and – where relevant – actions agreed with others, such as the transport method and a description of any restraint applied by either ambulance staff or others.
- Consider if a pre-alert to the receiving hospital/unit is required, and complete if necessary.
- Ambulance staff must provide a full clinical handover at hospital and a copy of the completed patient clinical record. Emergency department (ED) staff must be informed that the patient has been brought to ED using the provisions of the MCA. ED staff may need to re-assess the patient's capacity to make a decision regarding staying for further care, assessment and/or treatment.

13. Other Mental Capacity Act Safeguards

- The MCA includes other safeguards to protect vulnerable people who have reduced capacity and those using the Act to care for them.

Mental Capacity Act 2005

- Briefly, these include (amongst others):
  - **Lasting Power of Attorney (LPA)**
- An individual can give another person the authority to make a decision on their behalf if/when they become unable to do so. This is achieved by establishing a LPA. Once activated, the LPA can make decisions that are as valid as one made by the person. There are two types – Health and Wellbeing and Property and Financial Affairs. The LPA should always act in the best interests of the person.
  - **Advance Decisions to Refuse Treatment (ADRT)**
- Allow people to refuse treatment, providing that the decision to do so was made when the person had capacity.
- To make a valid ADRT the person must:
  - Be at least 18 years of age.
  - Have capacity to make the decision.
  - Make a decision that is specific and able to be complied with (i.e. outline in detail what they want to refuse and the circumstances in which it can be refused).
- The ADRT doesn't need to be in writing, unless it relates to life-sustaining treatment – in which case it must be in writing and witnessed.
- An ADRT is only valid and applicable when all of the conditions described are met and the person lacks capacity to make the decision themselves.
- If ambulance staff are not aware of an ADRT's existence when caring for someone who lacks capacity, then they should continue to act in the best interests of the patient.
  - **Court of Protection**
- Makes decisions on financial or welfare matters for people who can't make decisions at the time they need to be made and have no one appropriate to do this for them. Most cases are heard by district judges and a senior judge, but they are sometimes heard by High Court judges.
  - **Court Deputies**
- People who are appointed by the Court of Protection to act on behalf of a person with reduced capacity when there is no LPA. Court Deputies have similar powers to those of an LPA.
  - **Independent Mental Capacity Advocates (IMCAs)**
- IMCAs are a legal right for people over 16 who lack capacity and do not have an appropriate family member or friend to represent their views. An IMCA can be used to assist with decisions regarding serious medical treatment or a change of accommodation.
- The position taken in this guideline is that staff of the ambulance services should refer to their employers any questions or concerns they might have as regards gaining lawful consent from their patients or regarding the application of the relevant legislation (and associated codes of practice) that applies in the jurisdiction in which they work for assessing, caring for and treating apparently incapacitous persons.
- Readers should be aware that there are different laws relating to capacity and consent, and there is different mental health primary and secondary legislation in England and Wales, Northern Ireland and Scotland. This guideline cannot cover in detail any of that legislation, the associated codes of practice and governmental guidance. Therefore, it provides a very brief overview of some facets of the process in England and Wales.

Bibliography

1. Department of Constitutional Affairs. *The Mental Capacity Act 2005*. London: The Stationery Office, 2005.
2. Parliament of the United Kingdom. *The Mental Health Act 1983 (amended 2007)*. London: The Stationery Office, 2007.
3. Department of Constitutional Affairs. *Mental Capacity Act Code of Practice*. London: The Stationery Office, 2007.
4. Department of Health. *Reference Guide to Consent for Examination or Treatment*. 2nd edition. London: The Stationery Office, 2009.
5. S Willis, R Dalrymple. *Fundamentals of Paramedic Practice: A Systems Approach*. Oxford: Wiley-Blackwell, 2015.
6. National Collaborating Centre for Mental Health. *Self-Harm: The Short-Term Physical and Psychological Management and Secondary Prevention of Self-Harm in Primary and Secondary Care*. Leicester: British Psychological Society, 2004.
7. Department of Health. *Positive and Proactive Care: Reducing the Need for Restrictive Interventions*. London: The Stationery Office, 2014.
8. Ministry of Justice *The Human Rights Act 1998*. London: The Stationery Office, 1998.
9. Ministry of Justice. *Mental Capacity Act 2005: Deprivation of Liberty Safeguards – Code of Practice to Supplement the Main Mental Capacity Act 2005 Code of Practice*. London: The Stationery Office, 2008.

Pain Management in Adults and Children

1. Introduction

- Pain is "An unpleasant sensory and emotional experience associated with, or resembling that associated with, actual or potential tissue damage":
  - Pain is always a personal experience that is influenced by biological, psychological, and social factors.
  - Through their life experiences, individuals learn the concept of pain.
  - A person's report of an experience as pain should be respected.
  - Although pain usually serves an adaptive role, it may have adverse effects on function and social and psychological well-being.
  - Verbal description is only one of several behaviours to express pain; inability to communicate does not negate the possibility that a person experiences pain.
- Pain management is an essential and basic humanitarian standard. The provision of adequate analgesia is becoming recognised as a basic human right by the World Health Organisation. Our aim is to relieve pain as early and as completely as possible.
- When pain is not recognised, assessed and treated effectively, several short and long-term consequences may arise which can have a lifelong impact, including:
  - Development of a harmful catabolic state, characterised by increased oxygen consumption, tachycardia, hypercoagulability and immunosuppression.
  - Delayed healing
  - Increased risk of developing chronic pain syndromes - if poorly managed, acute pain can result in nervous system changes, commonly described as 'plasticity', predisposing to the development of chronic pain
  - Post-traumatic stress disorder
  - Poor functional outcomes
- Clinicians should be aware of the risks of unconscious bias and should not manage any patient based on a stereotype based on age, gender, sexuality, ethnicity or any other characteristic. There are a wide range of expressed emotions in patients from all backgrounds. Care must be taken not to treat an individual in pain as 'stoical' or 'highly expressive' based on any characteristic as this may lead to either ineffective or excessive pain relief.
  - Research indicates that patients from Black and Mixed ethnic groups are less likely to be offered pain relief; this may lead to harm.
  - Pain management in women is often inadequate. Research shows women are more likely to have their pain dismissed as emotional or exaggerated.
- A patient's memory of pain is an important consideration. The "peak-end" effect states that patients will remember the most intense pain, and the final moments of the pain. Therefore:
  - Good pain management should occur before movement or manipulation (where possible) to minimise the "peak" pain.
  - Aim to reduce the pain severity towards the end of the phase of care.

2. Assessment

- Having a calm and relaxed approach will ease patient, relative, and bystander fear and anxiety, reducing the perceived severity of pain. Wherever possible, speaking directly to your patient is the "gold standard" for assessing pain. It is accepted that this may not always be possible due to age, language barriers or other clinical reasons. If the communication barrier is purely due to language, make use of a locally available translation service and/or pre-hospital phrase book, guide or app.

2.1 Assessment of pain

- An assessment of pain should be made immediately after the primary survey, with minimal impact on other aspects of the patient's management. Knowledge of exacerbating and relieving factors can complement pain management.
- A commonly used mnemonic in acute pain assessment is SOCRATES:
  - **S**ite (e.g. calf pain due to deep venous thrombosis; associated chest pain may be due to pulmonary embolism).
  - **O**nset (acute onset or progressive worsening of an underlying condition).
  - **C**haracter (aching pain with movements can be musculoskeletal; burning pain, pins and needles can be neuropathic).
  - **R**adiation (back pain radiating to legs can be due to nerve root irritation; chest pain with radiation to the left arm can be due to angina).
  - **A**ssociated symptoms (fever, chills, nausea may be due to infectious cause).
  - **T**ime/duration.
  - **E**xacerbation and relieving factors (pain with movement may be musculoskeletal, pain associated with bowel and bladder disturbance may be due to abdominal problems).
  - **S**everity (scoring tools to assess baseline intensity and monitor progress).
- The patient is the most reliable sources of information about their pain. Open communication is essential for accurate assessment. Pain assessment allows for personalised care plans tailored to the patient's unique pain experience. What works for one person may not be effective for another, and pain

Pain Management in Adults and Children

assessment helps clinicians choose the most suitable interventions.

- **Non-verbal cues:** Clinicians can use non-verbal cues (facial expressions, body language) to assess pain in individuals who cannot communicate verbally, like adults with dementia, children, and individuals with intellectual disabilities.
- **Cultural considerations:** Be aware that cultural beliefs and practices may influence how people experience and express pain. Healthcare providers should be sensitive to cultural differences.

Refer to **Maternity Care (including Obstetric Emergencies Overview)** and **Imminent Birth** for women in labour.

2.1.1 Chronic pain

- Chronic pain is not prolonged acute pain. The experience of pain is influenced by 'bio-psycho-social' factors, such as medical condition, mood, sleep, beliefs and behaviour, as well as cultural and social factors.
- Patients with chronic pain may have heightened sensitivity of the nervous system and are prone to develop exacerbation episodes necessitating a call for urgent help.
- The prevalence of persistent pain in older adults is high, with the main causes originating because of degenerative changes. In both sexes, the incidence of arthritis increases with age. Both osteoarthritis and osteoporosis are more common in women. Managing pain in older adults is often suboptimal due to a combination of unmet healthcare needs, other concurrent medical conditions or poor compliance with medication. This has adverse effects on mood, sleep and activity. Ageing-related alteration to pharmacokinetics (what the body does to the drug), pharmacodynamics (what the drug does to the body) and polypharmacy also contributes to poorly controlled pain.

2.1.2 Patients taking other analgesics agents

- Patients may be taking analgesics for a range of other conditions:
  - acute pain, for example post-operative pain or muscular skeletal pain
  - chronic pain, for example osteoarthritis
  - palliative care
- Examples include:
  - Paracetamol
  - Non-Steroidal Anti-Inflammatory Drugs (NSAID) – e.g. naproxen and ibuprofen
  - Opioids – e.g. codeine, morphine or oxycodone
  - Gabapentinods - e.g. gabapentin and pregabalin
  - Antidepressants – e.g. amitriptyline

- Patient's requirement for analgesia may relate to an exacerbation of an existing condition or a new presentation such as trauma.
- In chronic pain, a patients' reaction to and perception of pain will differ to that for acute pain.
- Patients on existing medication may be more tolerant to analgesics used in acute pain and this should be taken into consideration when selecting both analgesic agent and dose.
- For palliative care please refer to **End of Life Care**.

2.2 Measuring pain severity

- All patients with pain should have at least two pain scores taken, the first one before treatment and subsequent measurements afterwards.
- Scoring and systematic assessment increases awareness of pain management, reveals previously unrecognised pain, and improves analgesic administration.
- There is no gold standard objective measurement of pain severity. It is important to remember that the pain experienced cannot be objectively validated in the same way as other vital signs.

2.2.1 Patients with severe trauma

- In patients with obvious traumatic injuries appearing in significant pain, formal pain scoring may not be appropriate. In these cases, an initial pain score of "severe" or "10/10" may be documented, with a comment in the clinical record citing the assumed nature of the initial pain score.

2.2.2 Pain scales for children and young people

- Given that pain is strongly influenced by emotions such as fear and anxiety, it is important to gain the child's trust:
  - Get down to the child's level
  - Adjust your communication to the child's current level of cognition
  - Use play and distraction techniques. Identify and discuss the child's interests (favourite cartoon or sport for example)
  - Be honest - even about causing more pain through cannulation or manipulation
  - Empower the child to be part of the decision making (where possible)
- Involve the parents at an early stage
- Remove unnecessary bystanders from the scene (other children, friends, members of the public)

2.2.2.1 Children Under 3

- For children under 3 years of age or children with reduced cognitive function, the behavioural pain scale FLACC (Face, Legs, Activity, Crying, Consolability) should be used by the clinician to provide an indication of pain severity, see Table 1.15.

Pain Management in Adults and Children

TABLE 1.15 – The FLACC Scale

Criteria	Score: 0	Score: 1	Score: 2
Face	No particular expression or smile	Occasional grimace or frown, withdrawn, uninterested	Frequent to constant quivering chin, clenched jaw
Legs	Normal position or relaxed	Uneasy, restless, tense	Kicking, or legs drawn up
Activity	Lying quietly, normal position, moves easily	Squirming, shifting back and forth, tense	Arched, rigid or jerking
Cry	No cry (awake or asleep)	Moans or whimpers, occasional complaint	Crying steadily, screams or sobs, frequent complaints
Consolability	Content, relaxed	Reassured by occasional touching, hugging or being talked to, distractible	Difficult to console or comfort

2.2.2.2 Children 3 to 8 years

- For children aged 3 years and above, the Wong and Baker FACES® pain scale should be used for those who are able, see Figure 1.4.

Instructions: Point to each face using the words to describe the pain intensity. Ask the child to choose the face that best describes their own pain and record the appropriate number.

Explain to the child that each face is for a person who feels happy because they have no pain (hurt) or sad because they have some or a lot of pain.

- Face 0 is very happy because they don't hurt at all
- Face 2 hurts just a little bit
- Face 4 hurts a little more
- Face 6 hurts even more
- Face 8 hurts a whole lot
- Face 10 hurts as much as you can imagine, although you don't have to be crying to feel this bad

Please note: The clinician must allow the child to choose the face that most represents their perceived level of pain. The clinician must not use this scale to judge the patient's pain themselves.

2.2.2.3 Children over 8 years

- For children and young people aged 8 years and above, the Numeric Pain Rating Scale (zero to ten numbers) or the Adjective Response Scale (No Pain, Mild, Moderate or Severe Pain) should be used for those who are able.

2.2.3 Pain scales for adults

- For adults, the Numeric Pain Rating Scale (zero to ten) or the Adjective Response Scale (No Pain, Mild, Moderate or Severe Pain) should be used. The following is generally accepted for the purpose of equivalence:
  - No Pain = 0
  - Mild Pain = 1–3
  - Moderate Pain = 4–6
  - Severe Pain = 7–10

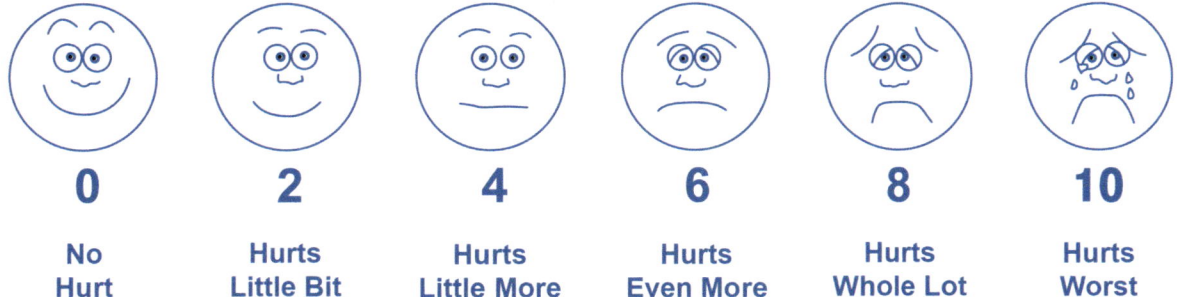

Figure 1.4 – Wong-Baker FACES pain rating scale (for children aged 3 to 8 years)

Pain Management in Adults and Children

The Abbey Pain Scale
For measurement of pain in people who cannot verbalise.

How to use scale: While observing the patient, score questions 1 to 6.

Q1. Vocalisation
e.g. whimpering, groaning, crying
Absent 0   Mild 1   Moderate 2   Severe 3

Q1 [ ]

Q2. Facial expression
e.g. looking tense, frowning, grimacing, looking frightened
Absent 0   Mild 1   Moderate 2   Severe 3

Q2 [ ]

Q3. Change in body language
e.g. fidgeting, rocking, guarding part of body withdrawn
Absent 0   Mild 1   Moderate 2   Severe 3

Q3 [ ]

Q4. Behavioural change
e.g. increased confusion, refusing to eat, alteration in usual patterns
Absent 0   Mild 1   Moderate 2   Severe 3

Q4 [ ]

Q5. Physiological change
e.g. temperature, pulse or blood pressure outside normal limits, perspiring, flushing or pallor
Absent 0   Mild 1   Moderate 2   Severe 3

Q5 [ ]

Q6. Physical changes
e.g. skin tears, pressure areas, arthritis, contractures, previous injuries
Absent 0   Mild 1   Moderate 2   Severe 3

Q6 [ ]

Add scores for Q1 to Q6 and record here → Total pain score [ ]

Now tick the box that matches the Total Pain Score →

0–2 No pain	3–7 Mild	8–13 Moderate	14+ Severe

Finally, tick the box which matches the type of pain →

Chronic	Acute	Acute on chronic

Abbey J, De Bellis A, Piller N, Esterman A, Gilles L, Parker D, Lowcay B. The Abbey Pain Scale. Funded by the JH & JD Gunn Medical Research Foundation 1998–2002. (This document may be reproduced with this reference retained.)

Figure 1.5 – The ABBEY pain scale.

2.2.4 Pain scales for older adults and those with cognitive impairment

- Assessing pain can be challenging in any patient but is made more so if your patient has communication difficulties (refer to **Patients with Communication Difficulties**).
- These communication difficulties are often compounded by the fact that trying to use an adjectival / numerical grading system can be difficult to achieve with your patient.
- In such cases the use of a scale such as the ABBEY scale or the PAINAD scale may be more

Pain Management in Adults and Children

1. Observe your patient for 5 minutes in totality before scoring them on their **five behaviors**.
2. **Breathing**: Normal (0); little labored breathing (1); Noisy labored breathing (2).
3. **Negative vocalization**: None (0); Occasional moan (1); Loud moaning (2).
4. **Facial expression**: Smiling (0); Sad (1); Frimacing (2).
5. **Body language**: Relaxed (0); Tense (1); Rigid (2).
6. **Consolability**: No need to console (0); Distracted (1); Unable to console (2).
7. Total all scores above: **1-3 = Mild pain; 4-6 = Moderate pain; 7-10 = Severe pain**

Figure 1.6 – The PAINAD pain scale

useful. Both these scales allow the practitioner to observe and assess for themselves signs and symptoms that the patient may not be able to clearly articulate or describe adequately to you.

- Although both scales are designed primarily for patients with dementia, it is suggested that they can be applied to a wider range of patients experiencing communication difficulties.

3. Treatment

- Patients should be informed about all reasonable pain treatment options, including pharmacological, non-pharmacological, and integrated approaches.
- Whenever possible, treat the cause (for example, glyceryl trinitrate sublingual spray for angina or oxygen for sickle cell crisis). When the cause is not readily treatable or if it is not apparent, then other analgesic interventions are necessary.

3.1 Non-pharmacological treatments

- Clinicians should aim to provide as many non-pharmacological methods of pain relief as appropriate, in addition to providing pharmacological pain relief. See Table 1.16.

TABLE 1.16 – Non-Pharmacological Methods of Pain Relief

Biological/Physical

- Temperature management:
  - Cooling of burns reduces pain. Burns should not be cooled for longer than 20 minutes total time and care should be taken with large burns to avoid hypothermia.
  - Heat can relax muscles and reduce discomfort, while cold can numb pain and reduce swelling. Use warm (not hot) for muscle aches or stiffness. Use cool (not freezing) compresses for sprains, bruises or swelling.
- Immobilisation and positioning:
  - Reduction in movement provides pain relief as well as minimising ongoing tissue damage, bleeding and other complications in fractures and dislocations.
  - Move the patient into the most comfortable position.
- Dressings:
  - Lacerations, abrasions, and burns should be dressed appropriately to minimise pain and reduce risk of infection.

Psychological

- Emotional support and reassurance:
  - Provide verbal reassurance, maintain a calm demeanour, and show empathy. Be kind and communicate appropriately. Allow caregivers to provide support.
- Distraction:
  - Makes pain easier to tolerate; simple conversation is the simplest form of distraction.
  - With children - storytelling, singing, playing with toys, blowing bubbles, using stickers, watching cartoons, or using a flashlight or colourful objects to capture the child's attention.
- Relaxation:
  - Helps to calm and reduce anxiety. Breathing exercises, guided imagery (like imagining a favourite place or activity) or listening to soothing sounds or music.

(continued)

Pain Management in Adults and Children

TABLE 1.16 – Non-Pharmacological Methods of Pain Relief *(continued)*

Social
- Proximity of relatives:
  - Having a relative or friend nearby, who can provide emotional support.
  - For children, holding, swaddling, or cuddling young children, using pillows for support, or allowing the child to sit on a caregiver's lap.
- Pacification:
  - Allow infants to breastfeed or use a comforter (dummy).

NB These should be used with all other methods of pain relief.

3.2 Pharmacological treatments

- Since different classes of analgesics work at different sites along the pain pathway (see Figure 1.7), using combinations of analgesics can:
  - improve effectiveness
  - reduce side effects
  - reduce opiate need (when morphine and paracetamol are combined, for example)
- Any pain relief must be accompanied by careful explanation, involving the patient, where possible, and relatives as appropriate. Include details of the patient's condition, the pain relief methods being used, and any possible side effects.
- Always consider non-pharmacological treatments when planning, preparing and administering pharmacological treatments (see Table 1.16).
- Always check for previously administered analgesics prior to your arrival on scene.
- When a patient believes an analgesic will improve their pain, an additional psychological effect will occur during analgesic administration (like the placebo effect), triggering a physiological response and improved analgesic effect.[24]

3.2.1 Choice of Analgesics

- The choice of analgesic(s) should reflect the patient's pain severity and wishes (see Figure 1.8).
- For patients suffering mild to moderate pain:
  - introduce simple analgesics first, adding analgesics incrementally to effect.

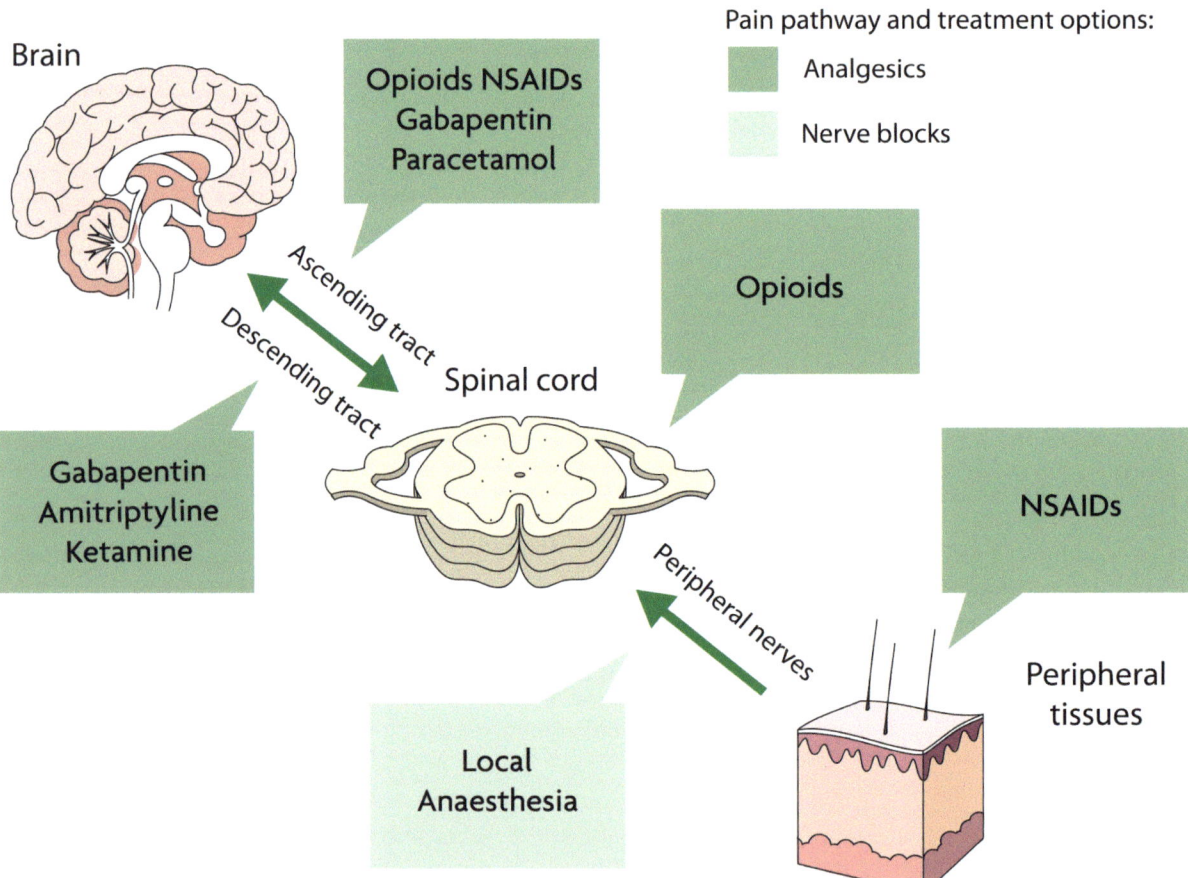

Figure 1.7 – Pain Pathway

Pain Management in Adults and Children

- For patients suffering moderate to severe pain:
  - it may be appropriate to start with stronger analgesics first.
  - consider administering an inhaled analgesic first, whilst other analgesics are prepared and administered.
- Clinician discretion should be used for patients suffering moderate pain.

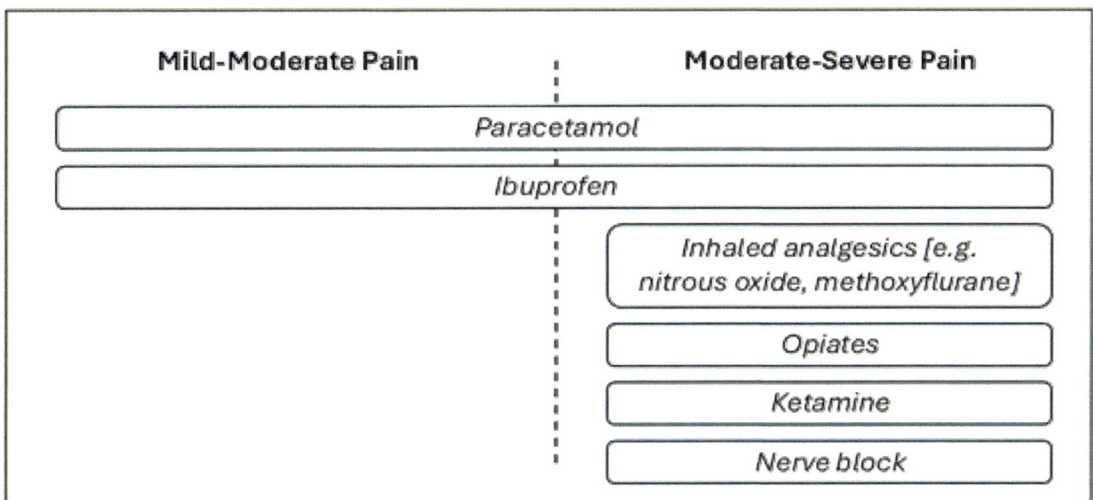

Figure 1.8 – Choice of analgesics (caution: not all of these are available in paediatric practice).

3.2.2 Pharmacokinetics

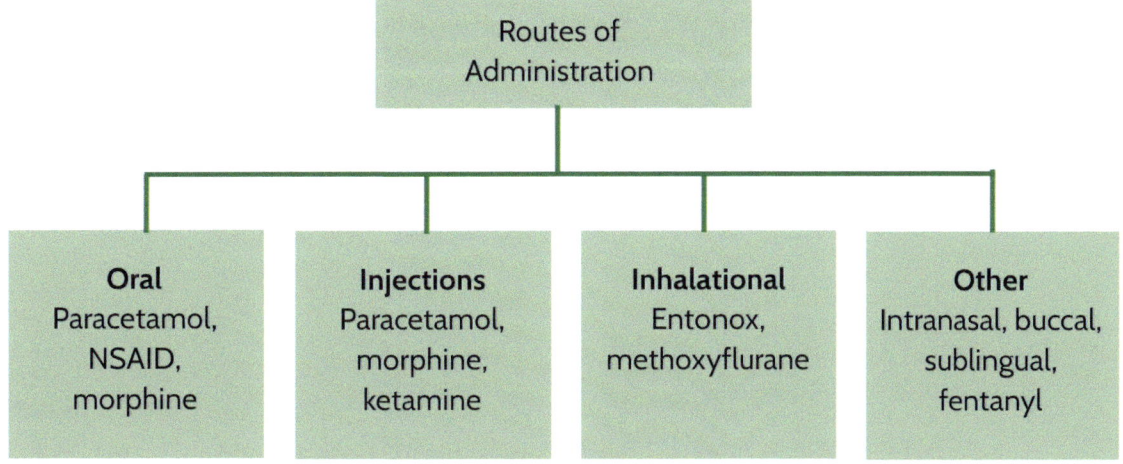

Figure 1.9 – (caution: not all of these are available in paediatric practice).

3.2.2.1 Oral Analgesics

- Oral analgesia has the advantage of ease of administration, however due to gastric transit time and dissolution of tablets in the GI tract often results in a slower onset of analgesic effect compared to parenteral routes of administration.
- Oral analgesia is not recommended for patients who are immobilised, who have or may vomit, or with a reduced GCS.
- Certain conditions such as shock, migraine and trauma may result in gastric stasis significantly delaying onset of action.
- Paracetamol, ibuprofen and morphine can be administered orally.

3.2.2.2 Parenteral analgesia (intravenous (IV), intramuscular (IM), subcutaneous (SC), intraosseous (IO))

- IV medication has the advantage of rapid onset of action and allows more accurate dose titration.
- Obtaining IV access can be both painful and distressing in certain patient groups i.e. paediatrics.
- Obtaining IV access in patients that are peripherally shut down or with large body habitus can be challenging.
- IM injections are generally slower acting and more painful than IV, however can allow for faster medicines administration.

Pain Management in Adults and Children

- IM is preferred in sickle cell crisis due to difficulty and increased pain in IV access and potential vascular occlusion leading to therapeutic failure.
- In hypothermic patients and patients in shock, IM injections can lead to "dose dumping" increasing the risk of undesirable drug reactions such as respiratory depression with morphine.
- SC injections are usually reserved for specialist conditions such as palliative care.
- IO route can be used for rapid access if indicated. Flushing of the IO cannulation can be very painful and should be reserved for high acuity cases only.
- Morphine can be administered IV / SC/ IM and IO.
- Paracetamol can be administered IV and IO.

3.2.2.3 Inhalational analgesia

- Inhalation agents are easily administered, have a rapid onset of action and allow compliant patients to self-administer, according to effect.
- Disadvantage for patients with limited dexterity or confusion.
- Nitrous oxide and oxygen (Entonox® / Nitronox®) cylinders and giving sets can be heavy and are temperature sensitive.
- Can "offgas" where product is exhaled in a confined spaces (i.e. the back of an ambulance) potentially causing undesirable effects on staff.

3.2.2.4 Other routes of analgesia

Intranasal (IN)

- Intranasal drug administration is a non-invasive method that delivers medications through the nasal mucosa for local or systemic effects.
- The nasal mucosal vasculature enables absorption resulting in rapid onset of action and bypassing gastrointestinal degradation and first-pass metabolism.
- Ideal for emergencies or acute conditions.

Buccal

- Buccal analgesics, particularly opioid formulations like fentanyl, are designed for rapid pain relief.
- Administered between the cheek and gum where the drug dissolves and is absorbed through the oral mucosa.
- The oral mucosal vasculature allows rapid systemic absorption, bypassing gastrointestinal degradation and first-pass metabolism.

Sublingual

- Sublingual analgesics are administered under the tongue for rapid systemic absorption, bypassing gastrointestinal degradation and first-pass metabolism.

TABLE 1.17 – Pre-Hospital Analgesic Drugs – Routes of administration, onset time, maximal effect time and duration of actions

Drug	Route	Pain Severity	Advantages	Disadvantages	Onset of Action (mins)	Maximal Effect Time (mins)	Duration of Action
Paracetamol	Oral	Mild–moderate	Readily accessible, well-tolerated orally, antipyretic, can be opioid-sparing for musculoskeletal pain.	Slow action when given orally, unpredictable levels if given rectally.	30 to 45	60 to 120	4 hours
Paracetamol	IV	Mild–moderate	Rapid onset compared to oral, antipyretic.	Requires IV access.	5 to 10	60	4 to 6 hours
Ibuprofen	Oral	Mild–moderate	Moderately good analgesic, antipyretic, and anti-inflammatory. Can be opioid-sparing for musculoskeletal pain.	Slow onset, may cause bronchospasm in asthmatics, caution with trauma, platelet, renal issues, and drug interactions. Significant cardiovascular/renal cautions.	30	60	6 to 8 hours

Pain Management in Adults and Children

TABLE 1.17 – Pre-Hospital Analgesic Drugs – Routes of administration, onset time, maximal effect time and duration of actions *(continued)*

Entonox	Inhaled	Moderate–severe	Quick, self-regulating, opioid-sparing for musculoskeletal pain, can be supported by parents in paediatric settings.	Fear of mask in children, requires understanding and cooperation, can't use in confined spaces (e.g., ambulances without scavenging).	2	2 to 5	2 mins
Methoxyflurane	Inhaled	Moderate–severe	Rapid-acting, good for trauma pain.	Not for paediatrics or pregnancy/labour pain. Requires understanding, coordination, and cooperation.	1	2	1 hour
Morphine	Oral	Moderate	Good for moderate pain, especially visceral pain.	Reduced bioavailability, slow action, may require dose adjustments if switching to IV.	<30	45	4 to 6 hours
Morphine	IV, IO, IM, SC	Severe	Can be titrated to effect, rapid onset, can be reversed with naloxone, some euphoria.	Respiratory depression, hypotension, allergic reactions, nausea/vomiting, controlled drug, less effective solo for musculoskeletal pain.	IV: 5 to 10 (IM: 10 to 30)	IV: Up to 20 (IM: 45)	4 to 6 hours
Fentanyl	IV, IM, IN, Buccal	Severe	Rapid onset, IN and buccal forms don't require IV access, buccal can be self-administered, less hypotension/allergy risk compared to morphine.	Controlled drug.	IV: <1 (IN: 5) (Buccal: 2)	IV: 2 (IN: 10) (Buccal: 5)	1 to 2 hours (dose dependent for buccal)

(continued)

Pain Management in Adults and Children

TABLE 1.17 – Pre-Hospital Analgesic Drugs – Routes of administration, onset time, maximal effect time and duration of actions *(continued)*

Ketamine	IV, IM, IN	Severe	Can be titrated to effect, effective for musculoskeletal/visceral pain, less respiratory/cardiovascular depression, short-acting.	Unpleasant emergence phenomena, salivation, laryngospasm at higher doses. Higher doses may cause sedation/anaesthesia. Different concentrations can cause patient safety issues.	IV: 30 sec to 1 min (IN: 5)	IV: 1 (IN: 5)	IV: 5 to 15 mins (IN: up to 15 mins)

NB: Refer to individual drug monographs for details on age/weight ranges, pregnancy, breastfeeding and renal/hepatic impairment.

In addition to this list of JRCALC analgesic agents, consideration should be given to the potential need for extended analgesia carried by other teams. The administration of analgesia by the crew on scene should not be delayed awaiting the arrival of a more specialist resource. The guide below is intended to inform crews of other analgesic options which may be available in their area if required.

Request advanced clinical support as per local policy.

- **Ketamine**
  - Rapid onset of action and dose-dependent effect able to produce analgesia, sedation or anaesthesia.
  - Can be useful for re-alignment of limbs / joints and helpful in extraction in patients with severe injuries, due to its amnesic effects.
  - Relatively short duration of action – frequent dosing may be required for analgesic effect.
  - Can cause unpleasant "emergence phenomena" for patients and any bystanders.
  - Can be titrated to effect.
- **Fentanyl**
  - Rapid onset of action and can be given transmucosally or intranasally (avoiding need for IV access).
  - Causes less hypotension than opioid alternatives (morphine).
- **Local anaesthetic blocks**
  - May provide highly effective analgesia without adverse effects.
  - Can be time consuming to administer.
  - Skilled technique requiring training, with risk of neurological injury or systemic local anaesthetic toxicity if misplaced.
- **Prehospital emergency anaesthesia (PHEA) (formally known as RSI)**
  - A general anaesthetic used for both humane reasons and stabilisation in critically ill or injured patients and major trauma. Crews should consider an early request for specialist resources when PHEA is required.
  - Crews can minimise the time PHEA takes by helping to prepare the patient prior to specialist team arrival:
    - **T**wo full bottles O2 – Pre oxygenate via NRBM and nasal cannulae
    - **U**ndress the patient. Skin to scoop with pelvic binder if appropriate
    - **B**ilateral IV/IO access with a bag of fluid run through and attached
    - **E**nsure 360 degree access around the patient
    - **S**uction units – two fully charged.

> **KEY POINTS!**
>
> **Pain Management in Adults and Children**
> - Managed pain has lasting physical and emotional consequences.
> - Children, young people and, those with communication difficulties require a tailored, calm approach.
> - A balanced, multimodal analgesic plan combined with non-pharmacological techniques is considered best practice to increase effectiveness and reduce side-effects.
> - Regular patient reassessment and pain assessment is essential to monitor treatment effects.
> - Always check for previously administered analgesics.
> - Pain relief does not make later diagnosis harder; in fact, it may facilitate it.

Pain Management in Adults and Children

Bibliography

1. Alzheimer's Australia. *Pain and Dementia*. 2011. Available from: https://www.fightdementia.org.au/files/helpsheets/Helpsheet-DementiaQandA16-PainAndDementia_english.pdf.

2. Bendall JC, Simpson PM, Middleton PM. Effectiveness of prehospital morphine, fentanyl, and methoxyflurane in pediatric patients. *Prehospital Emergency Care* 2011, 15(2).

3. Colloca L, Barsky AJ. Placebo and Nocebo Effects. N Engl J Med. 2020 Feb 6; 382(6): 554–561. doi: 10.1056/NEJMra190780PMID: 32023375

4. *Desborough JP: The stress response to trauma and surgery. Br J Anaesth 2000; 85:109–117*

5. Eccleston C, Fisher E, Howard RF, Slater R, Forgeron P, Palermo TM, Birnie KA, Anderson BJ, Chambers CT, Crombez G, Ljungman G, Jordan I, Jordan Z, Roberts C, Schechter N, Sieberg CB, Tibboel D, Walker SM, Wilkinson D, Wood C. Delivering transformative action in paediatric pain: a Lancet Child & Adolescent Health Commission. Lancet Child Adolesc Health. 2021 Jan; 5(1): 47–87. doi: 10.1016/S2352-4642(20)30277-7

6. Guzikevits, M. et al. (2024) Sex bias in pain management decisions | PNAS. Available at: https://www.pnas.org/doi/10.1073/pnas.2401331121

7. *Hedderich R, Ness T: Analgesia for trauma and burns. Crit Care Clin 1999; 15: 167–184*

8. Hewes HA, Dai M, Clay Mann N, Baca T, Taillac P. Prehospital pain management: disparity by age and race. *Prehospital Emergency Care* 2018, 22(2): 189–197.

9. Hockenberry MJ, Wilson D, Winkelstein ML: Wong's Essentials of Pediatric Nursing, ed. 7, St. Louis, 2005, p. 1259. Copyright, Mosby.

10. Kennel J, Withers E, Parsons N, Woo H. Racial/ethnic disparities in pain treatment: evidence from oregon emergency medical services agencies. *Medical Care* 2019, 57(12): 924–929.

11. Lo JC, Kaye DA. Benzodiazepines and muscle relaxants. *Essentials of Pharmacology for Anesthesia, Pain Medicine, and Critical Care*. New York: Springer, 2015: 167–178.

12. Lord B, Deveson M. Assessment and management of chronic pain in adults: implications for paramedics. *Journal of Paramedic Practice* 2011, 3(4): 166–172.

13. Lord B, Khalsa S. Influence of patient race on administration of analgesia by student paramedics. *BMC Emergency Medicine* 2019, 19(1): 32.

14. Malviya S, Voepel-Lewis T, Burke C, Merkel S, Tait AR. The revised FLACC observational pain tool: improved reliability and validity for pain assessment in children with cognitive impairment. *Pediatric Anesthesia* 2006, 16(3): 258–265.

15. Mossey, Jana, Defining racial and ethnic disparities in pain management : *Clinical Orthopaedics and Related Research®, Clinical Orthopaedics and Related Research*. Available at: https://journals.lww.com/clinorthop/abstract/2011/07000/defining_racial_and_ethnic_disparities_in_pain.10.aspx.

16. National Institute for Health and Care Excellence. *Diazepam*. Available from: https://bnf.nice.org.uk/drug/diazepam.html.

17. National Institute for Health and Clinical Excellence. *Analgesia –Mild-to-moderate pain*. London: NICE, 2015. Available from: https://cks.nice.org.uk/analgesia-mild-to-moderate-pain#!scenario.National Institute for Health and Clinical Excellence. *When Using Paracetamol or Ibuprofen in Children with Fever, Do Not Give Both Agents Simultaneously*. London: NICE, 2013. Available from: https://www.nice.org.uk/donotdo/when-using-paracetamol-or-ibuprofen-in-children-with-fever-do-not-give-both-agents-simultaneously.

18. Nixon, R. D., Nehmy, T. J., Ellis, A. A., Ball, S. A., Menne, A., & McKinnon, A. C. (2010). Predictors of posttraumatic stress in children following injury: The influence of appraisals, heart rate, and morphine use. Behaviour research and therapy, 48(8), 810–815.

19. Pak SC, Micalos PS, Maria SJ, Lord B. Nonpharmacological interventions for pain management in paramedicine and the emergency setting: a review of the literature. *Evidence-Based Complementary and Alternative Medicine* 2015 (2015).

20. Raja SN, Carr DB, Cohen M, Finnerup NB, Flor H, Gibson S, Keefe FJ, Mogil JS, Ringkamp M, Sluka KA, Song XJ, Stevens B, Sullivan MD, Tutelman PR, Ushida T, Vader K. The revised International Association for the Study of Pain definition of pain: concepts, challenges, and compromises. Pain. 2020 Sep 1; 161(9): 1976–1982. doi: 10.1097/j.pain.0000000000001939

21. Sabater-Gárriz, A. Molina-Mula, J. Montoya, P., & Riquelme, I. (2024). Pain assessment tools in adults with communication disorders: systematic review and meta-analysis. BMC Neurology volume 24, Article number: 66 (2024)

22. Saxe G, Stoddard F, Courtney D, Cunningham K, Chawla N, Sheridan R, King D, King L. Relationship between acute morphine and the course of PTSD in children with burns. J Am Acad Child Adolesc Psychiatry. 2001 Aug; 40(8): 915–21. doi: 10.1097/00004583-200108000-00013

23. Scottish Intercollegiate Guidelines Network. *Management of Chronic Pain* (SIGN 136). Edinburgh: SIGN, 2013.

24. Sinatra R. Causes and consequences of inadequate management of acute pain. Pain Med. 2010 Dec; 11(12): 1859–71. doi: 10.1111/j.1526-4637.2010.00983.x.

25. Smyth, Micheal. et al. (2025) Paramedic analgesia comparing ketamine and morphine in trauma (Packman): A randomised, double-blind, phase 3 trial, *The Lancet Regional Health - Europe*. Available at: https://www.sciencedirect.com/science/article/pii/S2666776225000572. https://doi.org/10.1016/j.lanepe.2025.101265

26. Von Korff M, Ormel J, Keefe FJ, Dworkin SF. Grading the severity of chronic pain. *Pain* 1992, 50: 133–149.

27. Whitley, G.A., Hemingway, P., Law, G.R. & Siriwardena, A,N. 2022. Improving ambulance care for children suffering acute pain: a qualitative interview study. BMC Emergency Medicine. 22, 96. https://doi.org/10.1186/s12873-022-00648-y

28. Whitley, G.A., Hemingway, P., Law, G.R., Jones, A.W., Curtis, F. & Siriwardena, A.N. 2021. The predictors, barriers and facilitators to effective management of acute pain in children by emergency medical services: A systematic mixed studies review. J Child Health Care. 25(3): 481–503 https://doi.org/10.1177/1367493520949427

29. Young MF, Hern HG, Alter HJ, Barger J, Vahidnia F. Racial differences in receiving morphine among prehospital patients with blunt trauma. *The Journal of Emergency Medicine* 2013, 45(1): 46–52.

Patient Confidentiality

1. Introduction

- Health professionals have a duty of confidentiality regarding patient information. They also have a priority, which is to ensure that all relevant information about their patients, their assessments, examinations and advice is recorded clearly and accurately, and passed to other staff whenever it is necessary for provision of ongoing care.
- Sometimes, aspects of legislation relating to these issues appear to conflict with each other. This guideline provides a brief overview of the relevant legislation.

2. Patient Identifiable Information

- Patient identifiable information is any information that may be used to identify a patient directly or indirectly. It may include:
  - Patient's name, address, postcode or date of birth.
  - Any image or audio/digital recording of the patient.
  - Any other data or information that has the potential, however remote, to identify a patient (e.g. rare diseases, drug regimes, statistical analysis of small groups, IP addresses or biometric data).
  - Patients' record numbers.
  - Combinations of any of the items here that may increase the risk of a breach of confidentiality, that include all verbal, written and electronic disclosure, whether formal or incidental.

3. Data Protection Act 2018

- The main principles of the GDPR should be read in conjunction with this guideline. GDPR describes processes for obtaining, recording, holding, using and sharing information, and forms part of the data protection regime in the UK, together with the DPA 2018.
  - Patients must be informed and give explicit consent to any sharing of their personal information.
  - Only the minimum amount of data should be collected and used to achieve the agreed purpose.
  - Information can only be retained for as long as it is needed to achieve its originally intended purpose.
  - Strict rules apply to sharing information and with whom it may be shared.

4. NHS Policy

- All NHS employees must be aware of and respect a patient's right to confidentiality and protect their personal information. A disciplinary offence may have been committed for any behaviour contrary to their organisation's policy or the *NHS Code of Practice: Confidentiality* (in Scotland, the *NHS COP on Protecting Patient Confidentiality*). Ambulance clinicians should be aware of how to gain access to training, support or information, which they may need, and be able to show that they are making every reasonable effort to comply with the relevant standards.

5. Protecting Patient Information

There are five essential steps that all ambulance clinicians should take to ensure that they comply with the relevant standards of confidentiality. They are listed below:

5.1 Record Information Given By, and About, Patients Concisely and Accurately

- Inaccurate clinical records about patients may contain false information that has been created by, for example, omissions, errors, unfounded comments or speculation. This breaches DPA standards. It also brings the professional integrity of ambulance clinicians and their employing organisations into question. Any comments and opinions, whether verbal, written or electronic, must be justifiable and accurate.

5.2 Keep Patient Information Physically Secure

- Ambulance services have particular difficulties in ensuring that information is not shared accidentally with the public. Not only must patients be treated confidentially, but the information gained must not be disclosed to anyone else unless to do so genuinely promotes patient care. (Comments to the public must be guarded.) Information given to other clinicians when handing over patients' care should not be overheard by or shared with people who are not directly involved in each patient's care. Patients' records, either electronic or written, must be protected against unwarranted viewing: thus, patients' clinical records must be shielded from the view of other people, stored securely after case closure and only handed over to staff who are entrusted with ongoing care of particular patients or other authorised personnel who have legitimate reasons for possessing the information. Personal health data must be destroyed in an approved manner and according to each organisation's policies when they have served their function. Discussions of each patient must not disclose personal information unless there is genuine and provable health benefit.
- Leaders of healthcare and health information systems believe that electronic health information systems, which include computer-based patient records, can improve healthcare. Achieving this goal requires systems to be in place that: protect the privacy of individual persons and data about patients; provide appropriate access; and use data security measures that are adequate.

Patient Confidentiality

Sound policies and practices relating to handling confidential information must be in place prior to deploying health information systems. Strong and enforceable policies on the privacy and security of confidential and patient identifiable information must shape the development and implementation of these systems.

5.3 Follow Guidance Before Disclosing Any Patient Information

- It is not sufficient for ambulance clinicians to understand the basic principles of confidentiality alone. They must also understand and comply with their employing organisations' requirements for information-sharing. Similarly, it is the responsibility of each service to ensure that policies for data-sharing are produced, communicated, monitored, updated and reviewed. Each ambulance service will have a senior advisor available. There must be a Data Protection Officer, Information Governance Manager and/or Caldicott Guardian available to advise ambulance clinicians if they have any doubts about sharing information.

5.4 Conform to Best Practice

- All grades of ambulance clinicians come into contact with the public and other NHS clinicians. Any temptation for ambulance clinicians to share information unnecessarily with other people who are known to them must be avoided, and the responsibility lies firmly with the holder of the data, both personally and in respect of employing organisations. Commitment to best practice should be applied to all information in any form about patients (e.g. patients' records, electronic data, surface mail, email, faxes, telephone calls, conversations that may be overheard and private comments to friends or colleagues).

- If, for any reason, ambulance staff discover that personal data has been lost or has the potential for being viewed by anyone not authorised to view it, they have a duty to immediately:
  - take every action possible to recover the data and/or protect them, and
  - to inform immediately an officer in their employing organisation who has responsibility for data (or their immediate supervisor) that such an event has occurred
  - record the event.

5.5 Anonymise Information Where Possible

- Information about patients is said to be anonymised when items such as those listed in section 2 are removed. It means that patients cannot be identified by any receiver of the information and any possibility of recognition is extremely small.

- Ambulance clinicians are advised to anonymise confidential data about patients wherever possible and reasonable. If information is recorded, retained or transmitted in any way, it should be anonymised unless to do so would frustrate any genuine reasons for its collection/storage that create identifiable benefits to patients' health.

6. Patients' Rights of Access to Personal Health Records

- Patients have a right to see, and obtain a copy of, personal health information held about them. This right in law includes any legally appointed representative and those persons who have parental responsibility for children who are patients. Children also have this right provided they have the capability to understand the information. Services have the right to charge for this information; and there are guidelines on the processes that are to be followed.

- There are exceptions to the rights of patients to see their personal health information. The information is subject to legal restrictions if it could identify someone else and if that information cannot be removed from the record. Also, a request can be refused if there is substantial opinion that access to the information could cause serious harm to a particular patient or to someone else's physical or mental well-being. These instances are extremely rare in ambulance service operations. If there were to be doubt about whether exceptions such as these do exist, staff should consult the Caldicott Guardian, Information Governance Manager or Data Protection Officer and agreement should be reached with each patient's lead-clinician.

- Notwithstanding the exceptions noted here, clinicians should make every effort to support each patient's right to gain access to their personal health information. It is a requirement that this information should be received by a patient who requests it within 30 days of their request. Services should have clear written procedures in place to deal with these requests.

7. Disclosure to Other Bodies and Organisations

7.1 Police

- The police have the right of access via ambulance service systems to personal information (name, address, etc.) in their investigation, detection and prevention of any crime. They also have the right of access to confidential health information (type of illness or injury, etc.) in their investigation, detection or prevention of a serious crime (e.g. rape, arson, terrorism, murder, etc.). This information must go

Patient Confidentiality

through an ambulance service system, as per local pathways.

- They have no right to expect to receive information when criminality, crew safety or public safety are not involved. Generalised information regarding attendance at an incident may be passed to the police through locally agreed procedures, when details of the location of an incident and what is involved **may** be disclosed – but passage of personal or confidential health data **may not**.

7.2 Local Authorities

- A local authority officer may require any person holding health, financial or other records relating to a person whom the officer knows or believes to be an adult at risk to give the records, or copies of them, to the officer, for the purposes of enabling or assisting the authority to decide whether it needs to do anything in order to protect an adult at risk from harm.

7.3 Secretary of State (By Proxy)

- The Secretary of State's '**security management functions**' in relation to the health service mean that their powers to take action for the purpose of protecting and improving the security of health service providers (and persons employed by them) includes releasing documents for the purpose of preventing, detecting or investigating fraud, corruption or other unlawful activities.

7.4 Fire Service and Other Emergency Services

- There is no right of access for emergency service personnel other than the police to patients' personal health information. Situations may occur in which ambulance clinicians feel that such disclosure would be in the best interests of a particular patient, or that, by not disclosing it, other emergency workers could be put at risk. Ambulance clinicians should be fully aware of their obligations towards their patients' confidentiality. Avoidable breaches of confidentiality occur when colleagues and authorities (such as the police and persons in a judicial context) ask for information. On these occasions, ambulance clinicians should follow the best practice advice given in the relevant section of the *NHS Code of Practice on Protecting Patient Confidentiality*; otherwise, access to information should be governed by formal documented requests and consideration by the Data Protection Officer, Information Governance Manager and/or Caldicott Guardian.

7.5 The Media

- There is no basis for disclosure of confidential or patient identifiable information to the media. Services may receive requests for information in special circumstances (e.g. requests for updates on celebrity patients or following large incidents, and when responding to press statements – public interest exemption). In instances such as these, the explicit consent of the persons about whom information is sought should be gained and recorded prior to any disclosure. Occasionally, services or ambulance clinicians can be criticised in the press by patients or by someone else with whom a patient has a relationship. Criticism of this nature may contain inaccurate or misleading details of behaviour, diagnosis or treatment. Services or ambulance clinicians should always seek advice from professional bodies on how to respond (if at all) to press criticism and about any legal redress that may be available. Although these instances may cause frustration or distress, they do not relieve anyone of their duty to respect the confidentiality of any patient.

7.6 For Commercial Purposes

- Ambulance services are not registered to use information for primarily commercial purposes. If such use was permitted, each patient would have to give explicit consent for information given by or about them to be used within the express commercial setting and each patient should be given an opt-out facility. This includes all intended purposes of all parties to the agreement and lists of all persons/groups who would have access to the data. Due to the nature of commercial enterprise, this consent must be explicit (expressly and actively given) as opposed to implied (acceptance without voicing an objection).

8. Research

- All data for research should be anonymised wherever possible. If anonymisation would be contrary to the aims of the research, prior consent must be gained. Formal research guidelines exist for the use of health-related data and they must be adhered to.

9. Consent

- Consent and patients' confidentiality are inextricably linked. In essence, each patient is said to be the owner of their own personal, non-anonymised patient information and/or data. Therefore, each patient should give approval before information provided by or about them is used by other people. There are exceptions to this general rule:
  - There may be legal requirements to disclose data without consent (e.g. due to persons having **notifiable diseases**). Even then, however, each patient must be informed that this situation has arisen.
  - When there is a risk to a patient's well-being by not informing other professionals without consent (e.g. where a child or vulnerable adult, an adult without capacity or a patient

Patient Confidentiality

who is being treated using powers given by the Mental Health Act may be in need of protection) and informing the relevant authorities would appear to be to the patient's wider benefit.

- Inability to consent (e.g. some children, adults who lack capacity or patients who are seriously ill or injured and who could reasonably be expected to give consent if it were otherwise possible to do so). Even in circumstances such as these, information must be used cautiously and anonymised when possible. A proxy, guardian or parent should be consulted if such a person is available.

- Use of personal information without consent may be justified if it is in the **public interest** to do so. This may occur to prevent or detect a serious crime, for example.
- In all the instances described here, the advice of the service's Caldicott Guardian, Information Governance Manager and/or Data Protection Officer should be sought prior to using or releasing any personal health information or data. Each service must advise their own ambulance clinicians in relation to consent, and this advice must be studied by ambulance clinicians.

KEY POINTS!

Patient Confidentiality

- **Health professionals have a duty of confidentiality regarding information about or that may identify patients. They also have a priority to ensure that all relevant information is recorded clearly and accurately, and passed to others when this is necessary for providing ongoing care.**
- **Inaccurate clinical records may contain false information about patients, which is created by, for example, omissions, errors, unfounded comments or speculation. Any comments or opinions, whether verbal, written or electronic, must be justifiable and accurate.**
- **Data Protection Officers, Information Governance Managers and Caldicott Guardians are available to advise and assist ambulance clinicians of the ambulance services.**
- **Consent and confidentiality of information that is held about patients are inextricably linked. In essence, patients are the owners of personal, non-anonymised information that is provided by or about them and they, therefore, are required to give approval before it is used by other people.**
- **Ensure you are aware of the rules in your service regarding patients' confidentiality and follow them – but remember that ongoing care of patients should never be compromised in their application.**

Further Reading

Further important information and evidence in support of this guideline can be found in the Bibliography.[1, 2, 3, 4, 5, 6, 7, 8, 9, 10, 11, 12, 13, 14, 15, 16, 17, 18, 19]

Bibliography

1. Health and Care Professions Council. *Standards of Conduct, Performance and Ethics: Your duties as a registrant*. London: Health Professions Council, 2016. Available from: https://www.hcpc-uk.org/assets/documents/10004EDFStandardsofconduct,performanceandethics.pdf.

2. Gold M, Philip J, McIver S, Komesaroff PA. Between a rock and a hard place: exploring the conflict between respecting the privacy of patients and informing their carers. *Internal Medicine Journal* 2009, 39(9): 582–7.

3. Department of Health. *Confidentiality: NHS Code of Practice*. London: Stationery Office, 2003. Available from: https://www.gov.uk/government/publications/confidentiality-nhs-code-of-practice.

4. NHS Scotland. *NHS Code of Practice on Protecting Patient Confidentiality*. 2010. Available from: https://www2.gov.scot/Publications/2010/04/20142935/0.

5. Department of Health. *Confidentiality: NHS Code of Practice – Supplementary guidance: public interest disclosures*. 2010. Available from: https://www.gov.uk/government/publications/confidentiality-nhs-code-of-practice-supplementary-guidance-public-interest-disclosures.

6. General Medical Council. *Confidentiality: good practice in handling patient information*. London: General Medical Council, 2018. Available from: https://www.gmc-uk.org/ethical-guidance/ethical-guidance-for-doctors/confidentiality.

7. Thomas MG. Team learning: the issue of patient confidentiality. *Work Based Learning in Primary Care* 2004, 2(4): 377–80.

8. Department of Health. *The Caldicott Committee Report on the Review of Patient-Identifiable Information*. London: Stationery Office, 1997. Available from: https://webarchive.nationalarchives.gov.uk/20130123204013/http://www.dh.gov.uk/en/Publicationsandstatistics/Publications/PublicationsPolicyAndGuidance/DH_4068403.

Patient Confidentiality

9. Woodward B. The computer-based patient record and confidentiality. *The New England Journal of Medicine* 1995, 333(21): 1419–1422.

10. Gostin LO. Health information privacy. *Cornell Law Review* 1995, 80(3): 451–528.

11. Brooks J. Caldicott Guardians: driving the confidentiality agenda. *British Journal of Healthcare Computing and Information Management* 2004, 21(3): 20–21.

12. White C, Hardy J. What do palliative care patients and their relatives think about research in palliative care? A systematic review. *Support Care Cancer* 2010, 18(8): 905–911.

13. Department of Health. *The Data Protection Act 2018*. London: HMSO, 2018. Available from: http://www.legislation.gov.uk/ukpga/2018/12/contents/enacted.

14. Griffith R, Tengnah C. Access to health records: the rights of the patient. *British Journal of Community Nursing* 2010, 15(7): 344–347.

15. Wougare J. Patient rights to privacy and dignity in the NHS. *Nursing Standard* 2005, 19(18): 33–37.

16. Ministry of Justice. *The Mental Capacity Act 2005 Code of Practice 2007*. London: The Stationery Office, 2005. Available from: https://www.gov.uk/government/publications/mental-capacity-act-code-of-practice.

17. British Medical Association. *The Mental Capacity Act 2005: Guidance for Health Professionals*. 2009. Available from: https://egret.psychol.cam.ac.uk/medicine/legal/BMA_MCA_2005_guidance_March2007.pdf.

18. Information Commissioner's Office. *Guide to the General Data Protection Regulation (GDPR)*. Cheshire: Information Commissioner's Office. Available from: https://ico.org.uk/for-organisations/guide-to-the-general-data-protection-regulation-gdpr/.

19. NHS Digital. *General Data Protection Regulation (GDPR) guidance*. Leeds: NHS Digital. Available from: https://digital.nhs.uk/data-and-information/looking-after-information/data-security-and-information-governance/information-governance-alliance-iga/general-data-protection-regulation-gdpr-guidance.

Patients with Communication Difficulties

1. Introduction

- This guideline comprises generic guidance intended to be used for any patient interaction where there are communication difficulties, e.g. patients with learning disabilities (LDs), autism, dementia, mental health problems or hearing or speech difficulties. The guidance does not relate directly to any specific patient group or condition. It has been developed without individual direct consultation with specific patient groups, given the number of patient groups that would potentially be involved. This is intentional due to the nature and breadth of out-of-hospital care and the need to ensure all patients receive the most appropriate care in an emergency situation.

2. Background

- A learning disability is a reduced intellectual ability and difficulty with everyday activities, e.g. household tasks, socialising or managing money, that affects someone for their whole life. The level of impairment can vary from mild to severe in all conditions.
- A learning disability is different from a learning difficulty, as a learning difficulty does not affect general intellect.
- There are many different types of learning difficulty. Some of the more well-known are dyslexia, attention deficit-hyperactivity disorder (ADHD), dyspraxia and dyscalculia. A person can have one, or a combination.
- Autism is a lifelong developmental disability that affects how people perceive the world and interact with others. There is a triad of impairment: social interaction, communication and imagination or flexibility of thought.[1]
- People with learning disabilities are likely to die 20 years earlier than people without them. Reasons include increased comorbidities, challenges with accessing healthcare, difficulties in assessment and inappropriate or delayed care.[2,3]
- People with LD are three times more likely to die of a treatable condition.[2]
- The commonest causes of death in people with LD are pneumonia, sepsis and aspiration pneumonia.[3]
- 2.16% of adults and 2.5% of children have a learning disability.[4]
- People with dementia, frailty needs, mental health problems and other communication needs are also at higher risk of ill health. This is for similar reasons to people with learning disabilities, such as difficulties accessing healthcare, multiple comorbidities, medications and assessment challenges.
- Communication is vital to assessment.
- Be aware of polypharmacy. This needs to be taken into consideration when assessing a patient. Consider drug interactions, potential accidental overdoses or toxicity.

3. Communication

Interpretation services may be available to support conversations where required.

Clinicians should undertake appropriate assessments and adapt their communication accordingly to take into account the presenting condition, any communications difficulties and any concerns regarding confidentiality or safeguarding. Consider the following:

- Speak clearly and slowly enough for the patient and keep instructions short and straightforward.
- Help the patient to feel as secure and safe from harm as possible.
- Give your patient time to process information and to reply.
- Try and keep background noise to a minimum.
- Consider light level or the intensity of light.
- Eye contact can help communication with some people, although others with autism may find it very uncomfortable.
- Find out how your patient usually communicates. Can someone help you with sign language? Would pointing to equipment help? Can you use symbols or pictures? Would gestures help?
- BSL is a recognised language in England, Scotland and Wales and qualified interpreters can be accessed through resources such as language line.
- Makaton is a language tool based on a system of signs to support communication. It is usually used by people with a learning disability or speech and language delay. Makaton is simple and easy. You don't have to sign every word, just key words and many signs are similar to everyday gestures.
- Watch out for non-verbal communication for both yourself and your patient.
- Your patient may have an individualised care plan such as a hospital or health passport or an All About Me book, which can give you valuable information.
- Communication and understanding are not the same. Some patients can understand but not communicate. Some can communicate but not understand.
- Ensure your patient has as much choice and control over their treatment as possible.

4. Examination

- Explain things as clearly as you can using the previously established method of communication,

Patients with Communication Difficulties

e.g. via a hospital or health passport, or a family member or care giver.

- You may need to alter the order or structure of your examination — start with less-threatening things and work towards things that are more uncomfortable or scary.
- Your patient may have a sensory processing disorder, where sensations are perceived inappropriately by the body. For example, a light touch may be very painful whilst a firmer touch may be more comfortable. Noises and lights can also present challenges. Find out more from family, carers or the hospital or health passport.
- Your patient may have had very bad experiences of previous healthcare, which can make examining them difficult. Use reassurance and explanation, and consider distraction or altering your examination.
- Some patients may be more settled if distracted by family, videos, books, fidget toys, etc. Others may not be distractible at all. Find out more about this.
- You may need to be opportunistic, flexible and resourceful.
- If possible, conduct the examination in a familiar or calming environment, e.g. in a specific room or sensory room.

4.1 Vital Signs and Scoring Systems

- Some patients may always have abnormal vital signs and NEWS2 — find out their baseline score.
- Some patients may be very unwell but have normal vital signs and NEWS2. For example, some patients with neurological conditions may not mount a tachycardia or pyrexia; some may not be able to sustain an increased respiratory rate.
- The Learning Disabilities Mortality Review (LeDeR)[3] found issues with NEWS2 and patients with LD, including the score not being recorded, or being recorded and not acted upon. These both lead to avoidable deaths.
- Many illnesses may not present in a typical way in patients with underlying conditions such as Down/Down's syndrome.
- Pain scores are also difficult to interpret as some patients with autism or other sensory processing conditions may have a very 'high pain threshold'.

4.2 Soft Signs

- These are signs that vary from patient to patient, which may mean someone is unwell. Families and carers are more likely to notice these than healthcare professionals.
- For example, someone might be unwell if they are refusing their favourite food, not interested in their favourite TV programme, more pale than usual or quieter than usual.
- Pay attention to soft signs as they can indicate serious illness in people with normal vital signs or a normal NEWS2 score.

4.3 Diagnostic Overshadowing

- This occurs when someone already has a pre-existing diagnosis and a healthcare professional puts any new symptoms or signs down to this diagnosis, rather than looking for another cause.
- For example, someone with autism or mental health problems presents with agitation. Rather than looking for a cause such as pain or infection, the healthcare professional assumes the agitation is purely due to the autism or mental health condition.
- Be aware of diagnostic overshadowing; make sure you are thorough and consider other causes for symptoms and signs. Finding out what is normal for your patient from sources such as family, carers or a hospital or health passport can help.

5. Reasonable Adjustments

- These are required by law, under the Equality Act 2010.[5]
- In essence, this means doing your best to make things as easy as possible for your patient, whilst still doing a thorough job.
- Consider things such as the environment you assess your patient in, the language you use, whether you need any help from family or carers and how best to communicate with your patient.
- Do what needs to be done now without delay, making appropriate adjustments. Avoid unnecessary interventions or interventions that could wait until the patient reaches hospital.

Patients with Communication Difficulties

> **KEY POINTS!**
>
> **Patients with Communication Difficulties**
> - The **TEACH** mnemonic may help ambulance clinicians with communication.
>   - **TIME:** you may need to spend more time on your assessment.
>   - **ENVIRONMENT:** consider the impact of your surroundings on your patient. Is it quiet enough? Too distracting? Too unfamiliar? How can you make things better for your patient?
>   - **ATTITUDE:** don't assume anything about quality of life. Be as thorough as you would with anyone else, although you may need to adjust how you work. Admit what you don't know.
>   - **COMMUNICATION:** how can you best communicate with your patient? Using symbols or signs? Checking for understanding? Can family or carers help?
>   - **HELP:** who or what can help you? Family? Carers? A learning disability (LD) nurse? A hospital or health passport? An individualised care plan?

Bibliography

1. National Autistic Society. *About Autism*. 2020. Available from: https://www.autism.org.uk/about.aspx.
2. HQIP. *Confidential Enquiry into Deaths of People with Learning Disabilities CIPOLD 2013*. 2013. Available from: https://www.hqip.org.uk/resource/confidential-enquiry-into-deaths-of-people-with-learning-disabilities-cipold-2013/#.Xbya1fZ2vIU.
3. University of Bristol. *Learning Disabilities Mortality Review (LeDeR)*. 2020. Available from: http://www.bristol.ac.uk/sps/leder/.
4. Mencap. *How Common Is Learning Disability?* 2020. Available from: https://www.mencap.org.uk/learning-disability-explained/research-and-statistics/how-common-learning-disability.
5. Mencap. *Learning Disability Explained*. 2020. Available from https://www.mencap.org.uk/learning-disability-explained.
6. Public Health England. *Reasonable Adjustments: A legal duty*. 2016. Available from: https://www.gov.uk/government/publications/reasonable-adjustments-a-legal-duty/reasonable-adjustments-a-legal-duty.
7. Makaton. *Healthcare Cards*. 2020. Available from: https://www.makaton.org/shop/shopping/freeDownloadDetails/Lanyard-cards.
8. PEM Infographics. *Triaging and Treating Kids with Down's Syndrome*. 2019. Available from: https://www.peminfographics.com/infographics/triaging-and-treating-kids-with-down-s-syndrome.
9. Mencap. *Resources for Healthcare Professionals*. 2020. Available from: https://www.mencap.org.uk/learning-disability-explained/resources-healthcare-professionals.
10. RCEM Learning. *Learning Difficulties in the ED*. 2018. Available from: https://www.rcemlearning.co.uk/foamed/learning-difficulties-in-the-ed/.
11. My PECS. *Communicating PECS*. 2020. Available from: http://www.mypecs.com/Search.aspx?catid=30&isParent=true.
12. O'Dwyer M, Peklar J, McCallion P, et al. Factors associated with polypharmacy and excessive polypharmacy in older people with intellectual disability differ from the general population: a cross-sectional observational nationwide study. *BMJ Open* 2016, 6:e010505.
13. St Oswald's Hospice. *Distress and Discomfort Assessment Tool*. 2020. Available from: https://www.stoswaldsuk.org/how-we-help/we-educate/education/resources/disability-distress-assessment-tool-disdat/.
14. Regnard C, Matthews D, Gibson L, Clarke C & Watson B. Difficulties in identifying distress and its causes in people with severe communication problems. *International Journal of Palliative Nursing* 2003, 9: 173–176.
15. Regnard C, Reynolds J, Watson B, Matthews D, Gibson L, Clarke C. Understanding distress in people with severe communication difficulties: developing and assessing the disability distress assessment tool (DisDAT). *Journal of Intellectual Disability Research* 2007, 51: 277–292.
16. Fuchs-Lacelle S et al. Development and preliminary validation of the pain assessment checklist for seniors with limited ability to communicate (PACSLAC). *Pain Management Nursing* 2004, 5(1): 37–49. Available from: https://www.painmanagementnursing.org/article/S1524-9042(03)00122-X/fulltext.

Safeguarding Adults at Risk

1. Introduction

- Everyone has the right to live their life free from harm. Safeguarding adults at risk from significant harm is reliant on effective joint working and communication between agencies and professionals.
- This guidance is for the management of people aged 18 years and over; for those under 18 years, refer to **Safeguarding Children**.
- Ambulance clinicians are often the first professionals to make contact with an adult at risk and may identify initial concerns regarding abuse. The role of the ambulance service is not to investigate suspicions but to ensure that any suspicion is passed, with the consent of the adult (where no consent, state why), to the appropriate agency (e.g. social care or the police) in line with locally agreed procedures.
- Ambulance clinicians need to be aware of local policies and procedures relating to the abuse of vulnerable adults. The aim of this guideline is to assist ambulance clinicians to recognise and report cases (with consent) of suspected abuse of adults at risk.
- The principles of adult protection differ from those of child protection in that adults have the right to take risks and may choose to live at risk if they have the capacity to make such a decision (refer to **Mental Capacity Act 2005**).
- Anyone can be a victim of abuse.
- An abuser may be anyone, including a friend, family member, carer or professional involved in delivering care to the adult.

The introduction of the Care Act 2014[1] provides a statutory framework to safeguard adults at risk of abuse or neglect. The Care Act puts the wishes and experience of the adult at the centre of safeguarding and is a move away from the previous process-led culture.

2. Making Safeguarding Personal

2.1 'No Decision About Me Without Me'[2]

Under the Care Act 2014 there has been a move away from process-led practice to a person-centred approach that works in partnership with the adult to achieve the outcomes that they need to make them feel safe. In the words of Lord Justice Munby, 'What good is it making someone safer if it merely makes them miserable?'.[3]

2.2 Six Key Principles

There are six key principles underpinning the Care Act guidance that put the patient at the heart of decision-making:

1 **Empowerment:** 'I am asked what I want as the outcome from the safeguarding process, and this directly informs what happens'.

2 **Prevention:** 'I receive clear and simple information about what abuse is, how to recognise the signs and what I can do to seek help'.

3 **Proportionality:** 'I am sure that the professionals will work in my interests, as I see them, and they will only get involved as much as needed'.

4 **Protection:** 'I get help and support to report abuse and neglect. I get help so that I am able to take part in the safeguarding process to the extent that I want'.

5 **Partnership:** 'I know that staff treat any personal and sensitive information in confidence, only sharing what is helpful and necessary. I am confident that professionals will work together and with me to get the best result for me.'.

6 **Accountability:** 'I understand the role of everyone involved in my life and so do they'.

The aim of safeguarding is to:

- Stop abuse or neglect wherever possible
- Prevent harm and reduce the risk of abuse or neglect to adults with care and support needs
- Safeguard adults in a way that supports them in making choices and having control about how they want to live
- Promote an approach that concentrates on improving life for the adult concerned.

3. Definition of Adult at Risk

Not every adult will require safeguarding. To meet the criteria set out in the Care Act 2014, the adult must meet the following criteria:

- Demonstrates a need for care and support (whether or not the local authority is meeting any of those needs) **and**
- Is experiencing, or at risk of, abuse or neglect **and**
- As a result of those care and support needs, is unable to protect themselves from either the risk or the experience of abuse or neglect.

An adult's needs meet the eligibility criteria for care and support if:

1 Their needs arise from, or are related to, a physical or mental impairment or illness

2 As a result of the adult's needs, the adult is unable to achieve two or more of the outcomes

3 As a consequence there is, or is likely to be, a significant impact on the adult's well-being.

The specified outcomes are the adult:

1 Managing and maintaining nutrition
2 Maintaining personal hygiene
3 Managing toilet needs
4 Being appropriately clothed
5 Being able to make use of their home safely
6 Maintaining a habitable home environment

Safeguarding Adults at Risk

7 Developing and maintaining family or other personal relationships

8 Accessing and engaging in work, training, education or volunteering

9 Making use of necessary facilities or services in the local community, including public transport, and recreational facilities or services

10 Carrying out any caring responsibilities they have for a child.

TABLE 1.18 – Types and Signs of Abuse

TYPES OF ABUSE	SIGNS OF ABUSE
Physical: hitting, slapping, misuse of medication, restraint.	• Multiple bruising • Fractures • Burns • Bed sores • Fear • Depression • Unexplained weight loss • Assault (can be intentional or reckless).
Domestic violence: incidents, or pattern of incidents, of controlling, coercive or threatening behaviour, violence or abuse by someone who is, or has been, an intimate partner or family member, regardless of sex or sexuality.	Includes: psychological, physical, sexual, financial, emotional abuse; so-called 'honour'- based violence; female genital mutilation; forced marriage. Note: The age range extended down to 16 (for the purpose of the safeguarding adult arrangements; safeguarding children arrangements would be applied to a person under 18).
Sexual abuse: rape, indecent exposure, subjection to pornography, not consented or pressured to consent.	• Loss of sleep • Unexpected or unexplained change in behaviour • Bruising • Soreness around the genitals • Torn, stained or bloody underwear • Preoccupation with anything sexual • Sexually transmitted diseases • Pregnancy • Rape – e.g. a male member of staff having sex with a mental health client (see Mental Health Act 1983) • Indecent assault.
Psychological abuse: emotional abuse, threat of harm or abandonment, blaming, humiliation, isolation.	• Fear • Depression • Confusion • Loss of sleep • Unexpected or unexplained change in behaviour • Deprivation of liberty could be false imprisonment • Aggressive shouting causing fear of violence in a public place may be an offence against the Public Order Act 1986, or harassment under the Protection from Harassment Act 1997.

(continued)

Safeguarding Adults at Risk

TABLE 1.18 – Types and Signs of Abuse *(continued)*

Financial or material abuse: internet scamming, will issues, inheritance, financial transactions, theft.	• Unexplained withdrawals from the bank • Unusual activity in bank accounts • Unpaid bills • Unexplained shortage of money • Reluctance on the part of the person with responsibility for the funds to provide basic food and clothes etc. • Fraud, theft.
Modern slavery: human trafficking, forced labour, domestic servitude, coerce, deceive and force individual into life of abuse.	Modern slavery is an international crime; it can include victims that have been brought from overseas, and vulnerable people in the UK. Slave masters and traffickers will deceive, coerce and force adults into a life of abuse, callous treatment and slavery.
Discriminatory abuse: slurs, issues of race, gender, disability etc.	Abuse can be experienced as harassment, insults or similar actions due to race, religion, gender, gender identity, age, disability or sexual orientation.
Organisational abuse: neglect or poor care within an institution or care setting. Neglect or poor professional practice as a result of policies and processes.	• Inflexible and non-negotiable systems and routines. • Lack of consideration of dietary requirements. • Name-calling; inappropriate ways of addressing people. • Lack of adequate physical care – an unkempt appearance.
Neglect and acts of omission: ignoring medical, emotional or physical care needs. Failure to provide access to appropriate healthcare.	• Malnutrition. • Untreated medical problems. • Bed sores. • Confusion. • Over-sedation. • Deprivation of meals may constitute 'wilful neglect'.
Self-neglect: wide-ranging neglect for one's personal hygiene, health or surroundings; includes behaviour such as hoarding.	This includes various behaviours: disregarding one's personal hygiene, health or surroundings, resulting in a risk that impacts on the adult's wellbeing – this could consist of behaviours such as hoarding.

Incidents can be a one-off or multiple and may affect one person or more.

- Bruising in dark skin tones may appear as purple or dark brown discolouration, and it may be more difficult to see very recent bruising on dark skin tones (on light skin tones very recent bruising may appear red). It may only become obvious as the colour of the bruising develops into a dark purple, brown or black colour which is then darker than the surrounding skin. Also, the yellow discolouration of older bruises may be more subtle in dark skin tones. Assess for skin changes closely using natural light if possible (or non-fluorescent light to avoid a blue tinge).
- Enquiring about how long the colour change has been there and what might have caused it is important. The colour of the bruising will change over time but it is not possible to reliably date bruising based on appearance alone.
- Note that bruising could also be caused by bleeding disorders or medicines.

4. Wellbeing

- Ambulance clinicians often come across adults who have an unmet or increasing care need. Whilst these are unlikely to meet the threshold for safeguarding, raising an alert is still possible with the patient's consent. Please follow your local reporting procedures.

5. Consent

- Adults at risk should, where possible, be given full information about any concerns for their safety to enable them to give informed consent to the ambulance service raising a safeguarding alert with the local authority or other appropriate agency. Where the adult does not have capacity (refer to **Mental Capacity Act 2005**), or having a discussion may increase the risk to the adult, ambulance clinicians can raise an alert in the patient's best interests.

Safeguarding Adults at Risk

- If there is a risk to others (i.e. other residents in a care setting or an identified fire or public health risk), ambulance clinicians can share information without consent (refer to **Mental Capacity Act 2005**).

6. Mandatory Reporting of Female Genital Mutilation (FGM)

- From 31 October 2015, the FGM Act introduces a mandatory reporting duty which requires health and social care professionals as well as teachers to report known cases of FGM in those under 18 years of age to the police.
- FGM is child abuse and the current procedure is set out below:
  - **Children and vulnerable adults:** if any child (under 18) or vulnerable adult in your care has symptoms or signs of FGM, or if you have good reason to suspect they are at risk of FGM having considered their family history or other relevant factors, they **must** be referred using existing safeguarding procedures as with all instances of child abuse. This will involve referral to police and social care in the usual way.
  - **Adults:** there is no requirement for automatic referral of adult women with FGM to adult services or the police. Ambulance clinicians should be aware that a disclosure may be the first time that a woman has discussed her FGM with anyone. Referral to police must not be introduced as an automatic response when identifying adult women with FGM, and each case must be individually assessed. Ambulance clinicians should seek to assist women by offering referral to community groups for support, clinical intervention or other services as appropriate, for example through an NHS FGM clinic. The wishes of the woman must be respected at all times. If she is pregnant, the welfare of the unborn child or others in her extended family must be considered at this point as they are potentially at risk, and action taken accordingly.
  - In all cases where staff are unsure of their actions, they should seek the advice of the Trust Safeguarding Service.

7. Prevent

7.1 Introduction

- The NHS, including the ambulance service, has a statutory responsibility to comply and engage with *Prevent*.[1]
- This involves the formulation of policy and procedures, the training of staff and, importantly, having appropriate mechanisms in place to ensure that concerns are noted and shared.

The three key objectives of the national *Prevent* strategy are to:

1. Challenge the **ideology** that supports terrorism and those who promote it.
2. Prevent vulnerable **individuals** from being drawn into terrorism, and ensure that they are given appropriate advice and support.
3. Work with sectors and **institutions** where there are risks of radicalisation.

- It remains clear that while the focus is an imminent threat from Al-Qaida or Islamic State (IS), it should be noted that radicalisation of vulnerable individuals can be undertaken by any extremist group. These forms of terrorism include (but are not limited to):
  - Far-right extremists, e.g. English Defence League
  - Al-Qaida-influenced groups
  - Environmental extremists
  - Animal rights extremists.

7.2 Definitions

- The following examples of vulnerability are included within 'Building Partnerships, Staying Safe' (DoH, 2011).
  - **Identity crisis** Adolescents/vulnerable adults who are exploring issues of identity can feel both distant from their parents/family and cultural and religious heritage, and uncomfortable with their place in the society around them. Radicalisers can exploit this by providing a sense of purpose or feelings of belonging. Where this occurs, it can often manifest itself in a change in a person's behaviour, their circle of friends and the ways in which they interact with others and spend their time.
  - **Personal crisis** This may, for example, include significant tensions within the family, which produce a sense of isolation in the vulnerable individual from the traditional certainties of family life.
  - **Personal circumstances** The experiences of migration, local tensions or events affecting families in countries of origin may contribute to alienation from UK values and a decision to cause harm to symbols of the community or state.
  - **Unemployment or under-employment** Individuals may perceive their aspirations for career and lifestyle to be undermined by limited achievements or employment prospects. This can translate into a generalised rejection of civic life and the adoption of violence as a symbolic act.
  - **Criminality** In some cases, a vulnerable individual may have been involved in a

---

[1] Section 26 of the Counter-Terrorism and Security Act 2015 places a duty on certain bodies (including the NHS) in the exercise of their functions to have 'due regard to the need to prevent people from being drawn into terrorism'.

Safeguarding Adults at Risk

group that engages in criminal activity or, on occasion, a group that has links to organised crime, and be further drawn to engagement in terrorist-related activity.

- An additional vulnerability is around young people moving from childhood into adulthood, and, in particular, those children known to children's services as they transition into adult services.

7.3 Duties/Responsibility

- Any member of staff identifying concerns that vulnerable people may be radicalised should report to the safeguarding service, their *Prevent* lead or their line manager in the Trust.

- If the incident occurs outside of office hours, staff should contact police for advice.

8. Assessment and Management

- Identify an adult(s) at risk.
- Report concerns following local guidelines:
  - Ascertain the patient's wishes wherever possible.
  - Gain consent if it is safe and appropriate to do so.
  - Consider the use of the Mental Capacity Act (MCA) if needed.
- Ensure concerns are clearly and concisely documented and jargon free.

KEY POINTS!

Safeguarding Adults at Risk

- Stop abuse and neglect wherever possible.
- Respect the adult's wishes wherever possible.
- Concerns of suspected abuse must be reported as soon as possible following trust policy and procedures.
- Ambulance clinicians must document fully the reasons for concern and any action taken.
- Documentation of consent or the reason it has not been obtained must be clearly recorded.
- Ambulance clinicians should not investigate concerns, but should identify and report appropriately.

Further Reading

Further important information and evidence in support of this guideline can be found in the Bibliography.[4, 5, 6, 7, 8, 9, 10, 11]

Bibliography

1. Department of Health. *Care Act 2014*. London: HMSO, 2014. Available from: http://www.legislation.gov.uk/ukpga/2014/23/pdfs/ukpga_20140023_en.pdf.

2. Department of Health. *Liberating the NHS: No decision about me without me*. London: HMSO, 2012.

3. Munby J. *Safeguarding Adults: Advice and guidance to directors of adult social services*. 2013. Available from: https://www.adass.org.uk/safeguarding-adults/public-content/advice-and-guidance-to-directors-of-adults-social-services-march-2013.

4. Office of the Public Guardian. *Office of the Public Guardian and Local Authorities: A protocol for working together to safeguard vulnerable adults*. London: HMSO, 2008.

5. Office of the Public Guardian. *Safeguarding Policy: Protecting vulnerable adults*. 2015. Available from: https://www.gov.uk/government/publications/safeguarding-policy-protecting-vulnerable-adults.

6. Lord Chancellor's Department. *Who Decides? Making decisions on behalf of mentally incapacitated adults*. London: HMSO, 1997.

7. Department of Health. *Clinical Governance and Adult Safeguarding: An integrated process*. London: HMSO, 2010. Available from: http://webarchive.nationalarchives.gov.uk/20130107105354/http://www.dh.gov.uk/en/Publicationsandstatistics/Publications/PublicationsPolicyAndGuidance/DH_112361.

8. Department of Health. *Safeguarding Adults: Report on the consultation on the review of No Secrets*. London: HMSO, 2009. Available from: http://webarchive.nationalarchives.gov.uk/20130107105354/http://www.dh.gov.uk/prod_consum_dh/groups/dh_digitalassets/documents/digitalasset/dh_102981.pdf.

9. Department of Health. *No Secrets: Guidance on developing and implementing multi-agency policies and procedures to protect vulnerable adults from abuse*. London: HMSO, 2000. Available from: https://www.gov.uk/government/uploads/system/uploads/attachment_data/file/194272/No_secrets__guidance_on_developing_and_implementing_multi-agency_policies_and_procedures_to_protect_vulnerable_adults_from_abuse.pdf.

10. Department of Health. *Safeguarding Adults: The role of health services*. London: HMSO, 2011. Available from: http://www.dh.gov.uk/en/Publicationsandstatistics/Publications/PublicationsPolicyAndGuidance/DH_124882.

11. Biarent D, Bingham R, Eich C, López-Herce J, Maconochie I, Rodriguez-Nunez A, et al. European Resuscitation Council Guidelines for Resuscitation 2010 Section 6: Paediatric life support. *Resuscitation* 2010, 81(10): 1364–1388.

Safeguarding Children

1. Introduction

- Safeguarding is everyone's responsibility and a statutory duty under the Children Act.[1] Ambulance clinicians must be aware of the signs, symptoms and indicators of abuse and neglect that constitute harm. This applies to staff who have direct contact, either face-to-face or on the telephone.
- Throughout this section, reference to a child equates to someone who is not yet 18 years of age.
- Members of staff in an ambulance trust have a **duty of care to report abuse or neglect**. If the abuse is not reported, the victim may be at greater risk. They may also feel discouraged from disclosing again, as they may feel they were not believed. This may put other people at risk.
- All partners who work with children, including local authorities, police, the health service, courts, professionals, the private and voluntary sectors and individual members of local communities, share the responsibility for safeguarding and promoting the welfare of children and young people. It is vital that all partners are aware of, and appreciate, the role that each of them plays in this area.[2]
- Healthcare professionals have a statutory duty to report, while social care and the police have statutory authority to investigate allegations or suspicions of child abuse.
- Ambulance clinicians are often the first professionals on scene and, therefore, may identify initial concerns regarding a child's welfare and alert social care, the police, the GP or another appropriate health professional, in line with locally agreed procedures. Accurate recording of events/actions may be crucial to subsequent enquiries.
- The role of the ambulance service is not to investigate suspicions but to use professional curiosity to identify risk and to ensure that any concern is passed to the appropriate agency (e.g. social care or the police). Ambulance clinicians need to be aware of child abuse issues and the aim of this guideline is to:
  - ensure all staff are aware of, and can recognise, cases of suspected child abuse or children at risk of significant harm, and provide guidance enabling operational and control staff to assess and report cases of suspected child abuse
  - where appropriate, ensure that all staff involved in a case of suspected abuse are aware of the possible outcome and of any subsequent actions.
- Further information on local procedures can be obtained from the safeguarding services within individual ambulance trusts.

2. Significant Harm

- All children have the right:
  - to be protected from harm/ill-treatment
  - to be protected from impairment of their health[1] and development
  - to grow up in circumstances consistent with the provision of safe and effective care.
- The maltreatment of children, physically, emotionally, sexually or through neglect, can have a major impact on their health, well-being and development.
- There are no absolute criteria on which to rely when judging what constitutes significant harm. In some cases, a single traumatic event may constitute significant harm, but more generally it is a compilation of significant events, both acute and longstanding, which interrupt, change or damage the child's physical and psychological development. Considerations include:
  - the degree and extent of physical harm
  - the duration and frequency of abuse and neglect
  - the extent of premeditation
  - the degree of threat, coercion, sadism and bizarre or unusual elements.
- In order to understand and identify significant harm, consider:
  - the nature of harm, in terms of maltreatment or failure to provide adequate care
  - the impact on the child's health and development
  - the child's development within the context of the family and wider environment
  - any special needs, such as a medical condition, communication impairment or disability, that may affect the child's development and care within the family and the capacity of parents/carers to meet adequately the child's needs.
- Take a 'think family' approach to identifying and assessing risk. Consideration is needed towards other siblings and/or vulnerable people living in the household/establishment.
- Abuse and neglect are forms of maltreatment, and children may suffer as a result of a deliberate act or failure on the part of a parent, legal guardian or carer to act to prevent harm (descriptions of abuse and neglect are detailed in Table 1.19).
- Children can be abused in any care or community setting, and abuse can be perpetrated by those known to them or by a stranger.

---

1   Health means physical or mental health.

Safeguarding Children

TABLE 1.19 – Examples of Types of Abuse and Neglect

Emotional abuse

- The persistent emotional maltreatment of a child so as to cause severe and persistent adverse effects on the child's emotional development, which may:
  - involve conveying to the child(ren) that they are worthless or unloved, inadequate or valued only insofar as they meet the needs of another person
  - involve not giving the child opportunities to express their views, deliberately silencing them or 'making fun' of what they say or how they communicate
  - feature age or developmentally inappropriate expectations being imposed on children (e.g. interactions that are beyond the child's developmental capability), as well as overprotection and limitation of exploration and learning, or preventing the child from participating in normal social interaction
  - involve seeing or hearing the ill-treatment of another
  - involve serious bullying (including cyberbullying), causing children frequently to feel frightened or in danger, or the exploitation or corruption of children
  - involve witnessing domestic abuse.
- Some level of emotional abuse is involved in all types of maltreatment of a child, though it may occur alone.
- Emotional abuse alone can be difficult to recognise as the child may be physically well cared-for and the home in good condition. Some common factors that may indicate emotional abuse are:
  - if the child is constantly denigrated/humiliated in front of others
  - if the child is constantly given the impression that the parents are disappointed in them
  - if the child is blamed for things that go wrong or is told they may be unloved/sent away
  - if the parent does not offer any love or attention (e.g. leaves them alone for a long time)
  - if the child is obsessive about cleanliness, tidiness etc.
  - if the parent has unrealistic expectations of the child (e.g. educational achievement/toilet training)
  - if the child is either bullying others or being bullied themselves
  - if there is an atmosphere of domestic abuse, adults or parents with mental health problems or a history of drug or alcohol abuse
  - if there is evidence of self-harm, intentional overdose or the excessive use of alcohol on the part of either the parent(s) or child
  - unusual behaviour of the parents/carers towards the child(ren) in an emergency situation (e.g. are they comforting a distressed child? What is the interaction like between the child and care giver?).

Sexual abuse

- Sexual abuse involves forcing or enticing a child or young person to take part in sexual activities. Both girls and boys of all age groups are at risk.
- The sexual abuse of a child is often planned and chronic. A large proportion of sexually abused children have no physical signs, and it is therefore necessary to be alert to behavioural and emotional factors that may indicate abuse.
- The activities may involve physical contact, including assault by penetration (e.g. rape or oral sex) or non-penetrative acts (e.g. masturbation, kissing, rubbing and touching outside of clothing). They may include non-contact activities, such as involving children in looking at, or in the production of, sexual images, watching sexual activities, encouraging children to behave in sexually inappropriate ways or grooming a child in preparation for abuse (including via the internet).
- Men, women and children perpetrate sexual abuse. However, most abuse is perpetrated by someone known to the child.

Safeguarding Children

TABLE 1.19 – Examples of Types of Abuse and Neglect *(continued)*

Child sexual exploitation/abuse (CSE/CSA)

- Sexual exploitation/abuse of children and young people under 18 can involve gangs or individuals. It is defined when children and young people receive something (such as food, accommodation, drugs, alcohol, cigarettes, affection, gifts or money) as a result of performing, and/or others performing on them, sexual acts. It can occur through direct contact or the use of the internet or mobile phones. Perpetrators have power over the child(ren) because of their age, gender, intellect, physical strength and/or resources. Both girls and boys of all age groups are at risk.

There are four models used to describe CSE:

1. **Peer-on-peer exploitation:** outlines instances when children are sexually exploited by their own peers who could be known to them at school, through mutual friends or in the neighbourhood.
2. **Boyfriend model:** the perpetrator targets children by posing as their boyfriend and showeringthem with attention, which results in them becoming infatuated. The perpetrator then initiates a sexual relationship with the child, who is then expected to return it as 'proof of their love', or they are told they owe money for the gifts, and sexual activities are a way of paying back.
3. **Party model:** organised by groups who lure young people by offering drinks, drugs and car rides often for free and as an introduction to an exciting environment. This often results in incriminating evidence being obtained at e.g. parties, such as photos or videos of sexual acts, that is then used to exploit through fear.
4. **Exploitation through befriending and grooming:** befriending directly by the perpetrator, either in person or online, or through other children or young people.

- All children can be vulnerable to CSE/CSA but those who are most vulnerable are:
  - missing or runaway children
  - children in care
  - those with experience of sexual abuse or violence in the home
  - neglected children
  - children who are homeless/sofa-surfing
  - children who are misusing substances
  - children with mental health issues
  - those with a learning disability
  - unaccompanied children
  - children not in education, employment or training (NEET).

Physical abuse

- Physical abuse may involve hitting, shaking, throwing, poisoning, burning (including cigarette burns or scalding), suffocating, use of restraint, spitting, force-feeding or otherwise causing physical harm. Physical harm may also be caused when a parent or carer fabricates the symptoms of, or deliberately induces, ill-health; this situation is commonly described as 'fabricated or induced illness' (FII).

Neglect

- Neglect is the persistent failure to meet a child's basic physical and/or psychological needs, and is likely to result in the serious impairment of the child's health or development. Neglect may occur during pregnancy as a result of maternal substance abuse.
- A neglected or abused infant may show signs of poor attachment. They may lack the sense of security to explore, and appear unhappy and whining. There may be little sign of attachment behaviour, and the child may move aimlessly around a room or creep quietly into corners.
- Signs of potential neglect include:
  - poor weight gain
  - failure to use prescribed medication or medication withheld by parent/carer
  - severe nappy rash
  - tooth decay
  - failure to immunise

(continued)

Safeguarding Children

> **TABLE 1.19** – Examples of Types of Abuse and Neglect *(continued)*
>
> – poor hygiene and dirty clothes
> – obesity
> – poor growth
> – delayed development
> – failure to attend appointments
> – delayed presentation
> – poor physical condition
> – child not at school
> – child not registered with a GP
> – clothes not consistent with the climate.
>
> - Do not rely on this list when assessing risk. Take a holistic approach and use professional curiosity to identify and assess risk. An absence of identifiable risk factors does not mean that a child is always safe.

2.1 Children in Need

- Children are defined as being 'in need' when:
  - they are unlikely to reach or maintain a satisfactory level of health or development
  - their health and development will be significantly impaired without the provision of services (section 17 (10) of the Children Act 1989)[1]
  - they have a disability.
- Local authorities have a duty to safeguard and promote the welfare of children in need.

3. Recognition of Abuse

- Ambulance clinicians may receive information or make observations that suggest that a child has been abused or is at risk of harm, for example:
  - the nature of the illness/injury
  - observation of hazards in the home (e.g. alcohol or drug paraphernalia, home conditions such as lack of bedding)
  - child(ren) has/have been locked in a room
  - signs of distress shown by other children in the home
  - observations regarding the condition of other children or adults in the household (e.g. an environment where domestic abuse has taken place). In the case of domestic dispute between adults, the presence of children in the household creates a need to notify even if the child(ren) was/were not injured
  - parents or carers who seek medical care from a number of sources.

3.1 Non-accidental/Deliberate Injury

- When assessing an injury in any child, you should be aware of the possibility of the injury being non-accidental/deliberate and you should consider this possibility in every case, even if you promptly dismiss the idea.

- For an injury to be accidental it should have a clear, credible and acceptable history and the findings should be consistent with the history and with the development and abilities of the child.

3.2 Suspicion of Abuse

- Suspicions should be raised by:
  - any injury in a non-mobile (non-independent) baby
  - accidents/injuries in unusual places (e.g. the buttocks, trunk, inner thighs)
  - extensive injuries or signs of both recent and old injuries
  - small, deep burns in unusual places
  - repeated burns and scalds
  - 'glove and stocking' burns
  - poor state of clothing, cleanliness and/or nutrition
  - delayed reporting of the injury
  - inappropriate sexual knowledge for the child's age
  - overt sexual approaches to other children or adults
  - fear of particular people or situations (e.g. bath time or bedtime)
  - drug and alcohol abuse
  - suicide attempts and self-injury
  - running away and fire-setting
  - environmental factors and family situations (e.g. domestic abuse, drug or alcohol abuse, learning disabilities that affect parents, carers and/or child).
- The following symptoms should give cause for concern and further assessment:
  - soreness, discharge or unexplained bleeding in the genital area (including anal area and severe nappy rash)
  - chronic vaginal/anal infections

Safeguarding Children

- bruising, grazes or bites to the genital/anal or breast area
- sexually transmitted infections
- pregnancy, especially when the identity of the father is vague or if it is a concealed or denied pregnancy.

- When assessing an injured child, you should use your clinical knowledge regarding what level of accidental injury would be appropriate for their stage of development. Although stages of development vary (e.g. children may crawl or walk at different ages), injuries can broadly be divided between mobile and non-mobile children.

- Bruising in dark skin tones may appear as purple or dark brown discolouration, and it may be more difficult to see very recent bruising on dark skin tones (on light skin tones, very recent bruising may appear red). It may only become obvious as the colour of the bruising develops into a dark purple, brown or black colour which is then darker than the surrounding skin. Also, the yellow discolouration of older bruises may be more subtle in dark skin tones. Assess for skin tone changes closely using natural light if possible (or non-fluorescent light to avoid a blue tinge).

- Enquiring about how long the colour change has been there and what might have caused it is important. The colour of the bruising will change over time but it is not possible to reliably date bruising based on appearance alone.

- Note that bruising could also be caused by bleeding disorders or medicines.

- Any non-mobile child with skin discolouration that could be attributed to bruising should be seen by a paediatrician.

3.3 Disguised Compliance

- Disguised compliance involves parents and carers appearing to co-operate with professionals to allay concerns and stop professional engagement. This can mean that social workers and other practitioners may be unaware of what is happening in a child's life and the risks they face may be unknown and unassessed by local authorities. Staff should remain professionally curious when engaging with families and ensure that they share safeguarding concerns with the local authority even if they are led to believe this information is already known to them.

4. Extra-Familial Harm

- As adolescents begin to develop their independence and engage more in their local communities in the absence of their parents, they can be at increased risk of experiencing harm from outside the family environment. Extra-familial harm is the term used when children and young people's experience of harm is beyond their home, family or carers. This can include:
  - sexual abuse/exploitation
  - criminal exploitation
  - peer-on peer-pressure
  - gang affiliation
  - trafficking and modern-day slavery
  - serious youth violence
  - radicalisation.

- Professionals will need to remain alert and make a safeguarding referral should they suspect a child is at risk of or is experiencing extra-familial harm.

5. Duty to Report to Police

- The Serious Crime Act 2015 enhances the protection of children from cruelty and abuse and adults at risk. Serious and organised crime includes drug trafficking, human trafficking, organised illegal immigration, child sexual exploitation, high-value fraud and other financial crime, counterfeiting, organised acquisitive crime and cybercrime.

- The Act places a duty on healthcare professionals and others to report serious crime, including and not limited to:
  - Serious domestic abuse (Domestic Abuse Act 2021)
  - Female genital mutilation (FGM) risk or actual (children)
  - Mandatory duty to notify the police – The 2015 Act places a duty on practitioners in regulated professions (health, teaching and social work) to notify the police when they identify that an act of FGM appears to have been carried out on a girl under the age of 18. This applies in cases where the victim discloses the offence to the practitioner or where the practitioner has observed physical signs of FGM. Failing to comply with the duty will be dealt with via existing disciplinary measures, which may include referral to the professional regulator
  - Gang-related activity
  - CSE/CSA
  - Cybercrime

- Depending on individual circumstances, you should either request immediate police support or report via 101. Please refer to own trust safeguarding policies.

6. Non-mobile (Non-independent) Babies

- Babies aged under one year are the most vulnerable group of children, as they cannot speak for themselves and are dependent on their parents/carers. Any injury in a non-mobile baby requires review by a clinician. If there is any doubt, the clinician should speak with the on-call paediatrician in the acute trust and/or the child should be conveyed.

Safeguarding Children

- Healthy babies do not bruise or break their bones easily. They do not bruise themselves with their fists or toys, bruise themselves by lying against the bars of a cot or acquire bruises on the legs when they are held for a nappy change. When in an environment, checks can be made for safety equipment, such as stair gates etc.
- Bruising on the ears, face, neck, trunk and buttocks is particularly suspicious. A torn frenulum (behind the upper lip) is rarely accidental in babies, and bleeding from the mouth of a baby should always be regarded as suspicious. Try to avoid using diagnostic terms such as 'bruise' when writing a referral. Use objective language and descriptive terminology instead.

6.1 Fractures

- Fractures may not be obvious on observation and the baby may present only with crying on handling. Often a fracture will not be diagnosed until an X-ray is performed. Fractures in babies are seldom caused by 'rough handling' or putting their legs through the bars of the cot. Babies rarely fracture their skull after a fall from a bed or a chair. Fractures in non-mobile infants should be assessed by an experienced paediatrician to exclude non-accidental injury (refer to Table 1.20 for types of fractures).
- Children's bones tend to bend rather than break and require considerable force to damage them. There are various kinds of fractures (refer to Table 1.20), depending on the direction and strength of the force that caused them.
- Unless there is an obvious bony deformity, bone injuries may not be apparent on initial clinical assessment. A clear history and appreciation of the mechanism of injury are crucial parts of the initial assessment and must be clearly documented.

TABLE 1.20 – Types of Bone Fractures

Greenstick	
The bones bend rather than break. This is a very common accidental injury in children.	
Transverse	
The break goes across the bone and occurs when there is a direct blow or a direct force on the end of the bone (e.g. a fall on the hand may break the forearm bones or the distal humerus).	
Spiral or oblique	
A fracture line that goes right around the bone or obliquely across it is due to a twisting force, which may be a feature in non-accidental injuries.	
Metaphyseal	
These fractures occur at the extreme ends of the bone and are usually only confirmed radiologically. These are caused by a strong twisting force.	
Skull	
These must be consistent with the history and explanation given. Complex (branched), depressed or fractures at the back of the skull are suspect of abuse.	
Rib	
These do not occur accidentally, except in a severe crushing injury. Any other cause is highly suspicious of non-accidental injury.	

6.2 Shaking Injuries

- When small babies are shaken violently, their head and limb movements cannot be controlled, causing brain damage and haemorrhage within the skull. This can also be caused by being thrown.
- Finger bruising on the chest may indicate that a baby has been held tightly and shaken. These babies usually present with collapse or respiratory problems and the diagnosis is only made on further detailed assessment.

7. Mobile Babies and Toddlers

7.1 Bruising

- It is normal for toddlers to have accidental bruises on the shins, elbows and forehead. Bruises in unusual areas such as the back, upper arms and abdomen do not tend to occur accidentally. Defensive wounds commonly occur on the forearm, upper arm, back of the legs, hands or feet. You may see clusters of bruises on the upper arm, outside of the thigh or on the body. You may see bruises with dots

Safeguarding Children

of blood under the skin. A bruised scalp and swollen eyes may suggest that hair has been pulled violently.

- Bruising caused by a hand slap leaves a characteristic pattern of 'stripes' representing the imprint of fingers. Forceful gripping leaves small round bruises corresponding to the position of the fingertips. 'Tramline' bruising is caused by a belt or stick, and shows as lines of bruising with a white patch in between.

7.2 Burns and Scalds

- Burns and scalds can result from hot liquids, hot objects, flames, chemicals or electricity.
- Burns are caused by the application to the skin of dry heat, and the depth of the burn will depend on the temperature of the object and the length of time it is in contact with the skin.
- Abusive burns are frequently small and deep, and may show the outline of the object (e.g. the soleplate of an iron), whereas accidental burns rarely do so because the child will pull away in response to pain.
- Cigarette burns are not common. They are round, deep and have a red flare around a flat brown crust. These burns usually leave a scar.
- Scalds are caused by steam or hot liquids. Accidental scalds may be extensive but show splash marks unlike the sharp edges of damage done when the child is dunked in hot water (although splash marks may also feature in a non-accidental burn, indicating that the child had tried to escape hot water). The glove and stocking pattern of burns on the arms and legs is typical of non-accidental injury. The head, face, neck, shoulders and front of the chest are the areas affected when a child pulls over a kettle accidentally.

7.3 Bite Marks

- Bites result in small bruises forming part or all of a circle. They are usually oval or circular in shape. There may be visible wounds, indentations or bruising from individual teeth.

7.4 Deliberate Poisoning and Attempted Suffocation

- These are very difficult to assess and may need a period of close observation in hospital. Deliberate poisoning, such as might be found in a child in whom illness is fabricated or induced by carers with parenting responsibilities (fictitious or induced illness), may be suspected when a child has repeated puzzling illnesses, usually of sudden onset. The signs include unusual drowsiness, apnoeic attacks, vomiting, diarrhoea and fits. There may be respiratory problems due to suffocation.

8. Older Children and Adolescents

- If the injury is accidental, older children will give a very clear and detailed account of how it happened. The detail will be missing if they have been told what to say.
- Overdosing and other self-harm injuries must be taken seriously in this age group, as they may indicate sexual or other abuse (such as exploitation).

8.1 Parental Factors

- Parental unavailability for whatever reason increases the risk to the child of all forms of abuse, especially neglect and emotional abuse. Specific consideration of the effects of the parent's problem on the children must be made, whatever the circumstances of presentation. Sources of stress within families may have a negative impact on a child's health, development or well-being, either directly or because they affect the capacity of parents to respond to their child's needs. Sources of stress may include social exclusion, domestic abuse, unstable mental illness of a parent or carer or drug and alcohol misuse. Parents who appear overanxious about their child when there is no sign of illness or injury may be signalling their inability to cope.
- Parental factors that might have a negative impact on parenting capacity include:
  - learning difficulties
  - mental health problems
  - substance abuse
  - domestic abuse
  - chronic ill-health
  - physical disability
  - unemployment or poverty
  - homelessness/frequent moves
  - social isolation
  - young, unsupported parents
  - parents with poor role models of their own
  - lack of, or poor, education
  - criminality
  - unwanted or unplanned pregnancy.

9. Special Circumstances

9.1 Individuals Who Pose a Risk to Children

- Once an individual has been sentenced and identified as presenting a risk of harm to children, agencies have a responsibility to work collaboratively to monitor and manage the risk of harm to others.
- Where an offender is given a community sentence, offender managers or youth offending team workers will monitor the individual's risk

Safeguarding Children

of harm to others and their behaviour, and liaise with partner agencies as appropriate.
- Multi-Agency Public Protection Arrangements (MAPPAs) should be in place to enable agencies to work together within a statutory framework for managing risk of harm to the public.
- There are certain work forces that are exempt from the Rehabilitation of Offenders Act 1974. Patient-facing roles within the ambulance service are part of this. Safer recruitment checks will be undertaken, including an enhanced DBS (Disclosure and Barring Service).

9.2 Disabled Children

- Abuse may be difficult to separate from symptoms of disability (e.g. increase in seizures in a child with epilepsy if anticonvulsants are withheld). Induced and fabricated illness may be even more difficult to recognise because the child may have coexistent diagnoses.
- Important points to remember about abuse of disabled children are:
  - It may be more common than abuse of non-disabled children, but evidence for this is poor.
  - It may be under-reported.
  - Children may have difficulty communicating their abuse.
  - Abuse may compound pre-existing disability, or be the cause of the disability.
  - All forms of abuse are seen, including neglect and sexual abuse.
  - It is easy to fail to recognise abuse in disabled children by making too many allowances for the disability as a cause of problems.
  - Be aware that professionals can be drawn into collusion with families; this is a term known as 'disguised compliance'.
- These children are at risk of achieving poor outcomes. Ambulance clinicians need to be aware of the role they can play in recognition of these children, identifying their particular needs and preventing significant harm. In the current multicultural society of the United Kingdom, it is important to recognise that there may be children and families in need of skilled interpreters, and that differences may exist in child-rearing practices in minority groups.

9.3 Special Circumstances for Consideration

- **Children and young people living away from home** – many looked-after children and young people that live independently have been abused or neglected prior to going into care. This is a particular group where assessment may be made more difficult because of pre-existing symptoms and behaviour. There should be a low threshold for seeking advice from experienced professionals in these circumstances (e.g. designated/named professional).
- **Asylum-seeking children or refugees, both with families and unaccompanied** – the importance of having skilled interpreters in assessment of these children cannot be over-emphasised. The children's behaviour on entering the country may already have been influenced by previous experience. It is important to remember their general health needs and that families will need help in accessing services. It is also important to refer children who are victims of human trafficking.
- **Children with maladjusted parent(s)/carers** (see also Parental Factors) – these include children of substance-misusing parents/carers, children living with domestic abuse, children whose parents/carers have chronic mental or physical health problems, children whose parents/carers have a learning disability, children with a parent/carer in prison and children living in flexi-families. Effects on the child(ren) can be profound and include fearfulness, withdrawal, anxious behaviour, lack of self-confidence and social skills, difficulties in forming relationships, sleep disturbance, non-attendance at school, aggression, bullying, post-traumatic stress disorder and behaviour suggestive of ADHD.

The following children may also have unmet health needs (low immunisation levels, poor dental health and either poor or non-attendance at clinic appointments).

- **Children of Gypsy/Roma/Traveller background** – these children are subjected to the same problems because of frequent moves. They may also suffer from poor health, poor access to primary healthcare and vaccinations, in addition to poor living conditions.
- **Runaway children and exploitation** – many runaway children may already have been the subject of abuse and are at risk of exploitation. They are also at risk of child trafficking for sexual exploitation.
- **Children as young carers** – neglect and emotional abuse may be part of the difficulties of taking on parental responsibilities and a caring role at a young age. Young carers lose out on normal childhood experiences and should be considered at higher risk of abuse, whether intentional or unintentional (e.g. school attendance, peer groups).

Safeguarding Children

10. Parental Consent

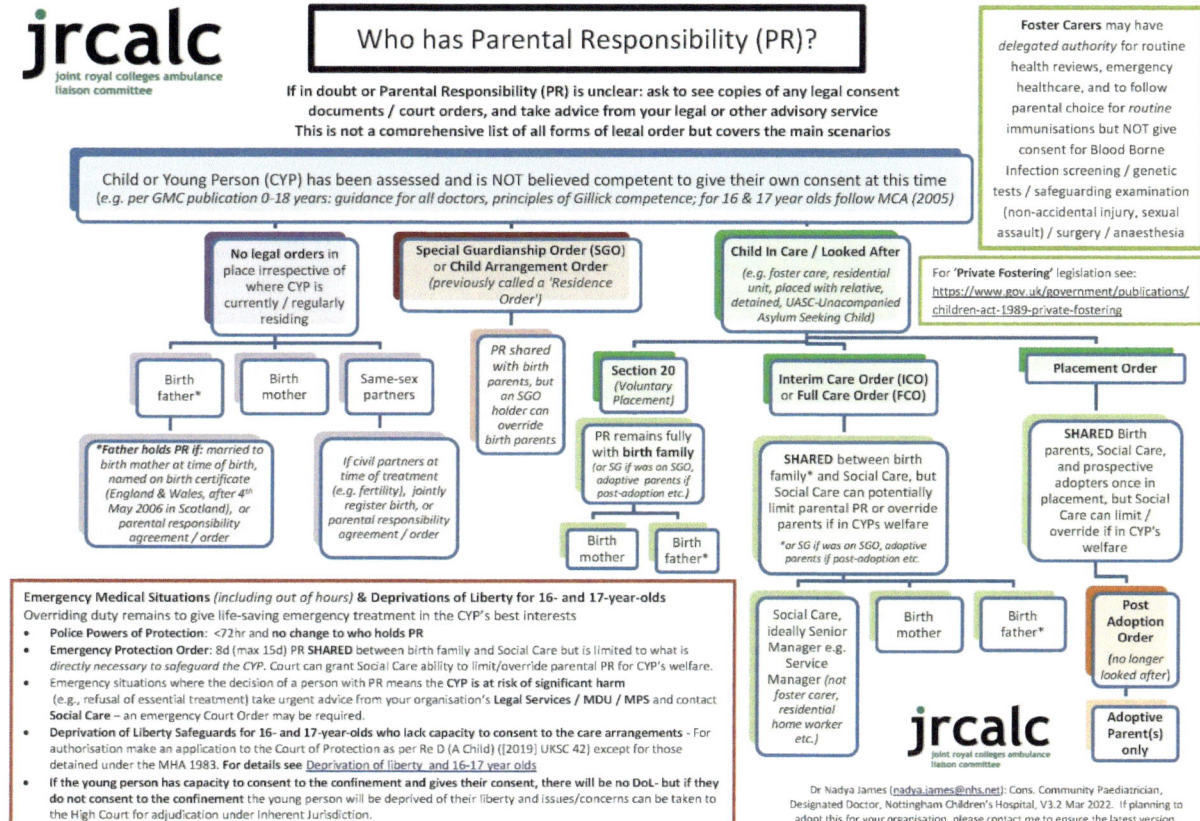

11. Maternity Safeguarding

- For some pregnant women, complex social factors are likely to impact on their engagement with their maternity care (NICE, 2010). Examples of complex social factors in pregnancy include:
  - Trafficked/modern slavery
  - Mental ill-health
  - Substance/alcohol misuse
  - Recent migrant/refugee/asylum-seeker
  - Language barrier
  - Domestic abuse
  - Sexual assault/rape/sexual exploitation
  - Previous child(ren) removed from care
  - Learning disabilities
  - Teenage pregnancy
  - Difficult childhood (ACES)
  - Homelessness/financial difficulties
- Ambulance services are in a very unique position whereby we may be the first point of contact for the pregnant/post-natal woman during her pregnancy.
- Any staff that attend to a woman who has delivered (whether unassisted or attended to by ambulance crew), who presents late in pregnancy and has engaged with little to no antenatal care (whether free-birthing or otherwise) or who has delivered yet declined to convey should undertake a safeguarding risk assessment and use professional curiosity to establish whether there are any safeguarding concerns identified which would warrant further management to protect the unborn/born and mother from harm.
- In the event of a BBA where the mother declines to be conveyed in the absence of a midwife in attendance, or a situation where there are immediate risks of harm to a baby or any other children within the household, staff should contact Children's Social Care and **should not leave the baby/children alone** with the mother until the staff has had a direct discussion with the Duty Social Worker and a plan is put in place. Staff should also consider contacting the police for a PPO (Police Protection Order) **after** a discussion has taken place with the Duty Social Worker, or if the risk of harm is so high, then the police should be contacted immediately.
- For pregnant women who are visiting the UK from abroad, the above recommendations also apply. Staff should be mindful that overseas visitors will not have an NHS number and must be considered as a potential increased risk for absconding, particularly in the event of a BBA.

Safeguarding Children

Maternity Safeguarding Flow Chart

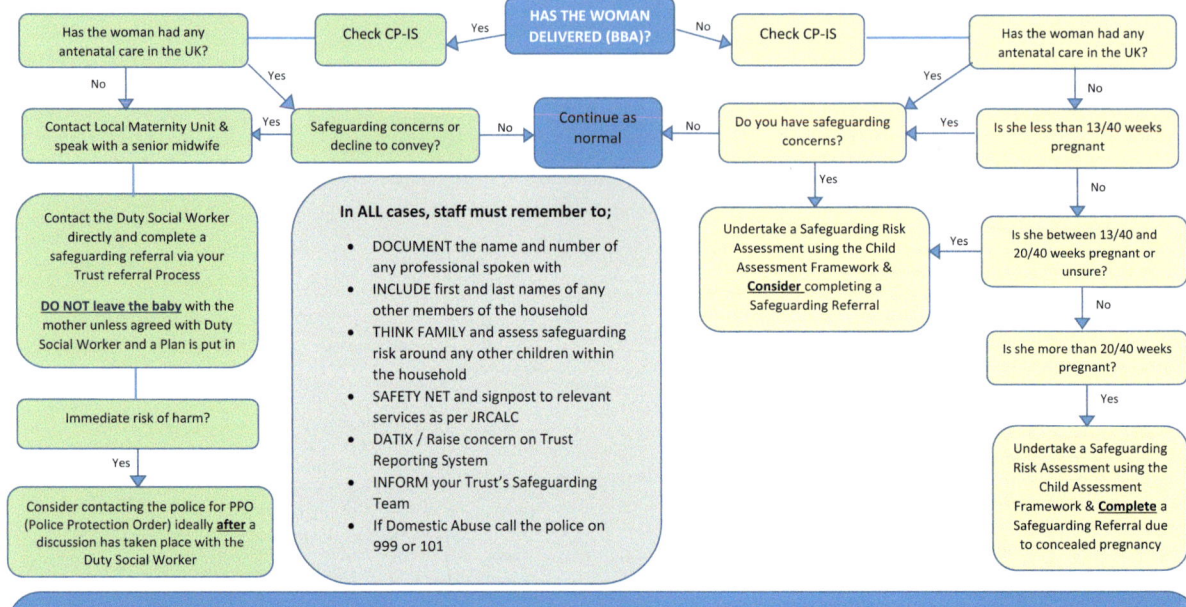

Claire Sidley-Jenkins, RM, PMA, May 2022

- If the pregnant woman speaks limited to no English, then appropriate interpretation services must be used. Staff must not rely on family and friends to translate for the woman.
- If ambulance staff are referring women for antenatal care, then establish whether there is an online booking system in multiple languages.
- If the pregnant woman advises that she has transferred her care from another trust but is unable to share her antenatal records/notes with staff, then this should be considered as a safeguarding concern and a children's safeguarding risk assessment should be carried out with consideration for a safeguarding referral.

12. Mandatory Reporting of Female Genital Mutilation (FGM)

- On 31 October 2015, the FGM Act introduced a mandatory reporting duty that requires health and social care professionals as well as teachers to report known cases of FGM in those under 18 years of age to the police.
- FGM is child abuse and the current procedure is set out below:
  - **Children and vulnerable adults** – if any child (under 18) or vulnerable adult has symptoms or signs of FGM, or if there is good reason to suspect they are at risk of FGM on consideration of their family history or other relevant factors, they **must** be referred using existing safeguarding procedures as with all instances of child abuse. This will involve referral to police and social care in the usual way.
- In all cases where staff are unsure of their actions, they should seek the advice of the Trust Safeguarding Service.

13. Assessment and Management

- If physical, sexual or emotional abuse or neglect is suspected, follow local procedures; information can be obtained from the named professional for safeguarding within individual ambulance trusts. Ambulance clinicians may obtain contact information from ambulance control.

13.1 If the Child Is the Patient

- The first priority is the health and safety of the child. Ambulance clinicians should follow the usual **ABCDE** and **<C>ABCDE** assessment (refer to **Medical Emergencies in Children – Overview** and **Trauma Emergencies in Children – Overview**). Children with significant injury should be transferred to further care without delay.
- Where a child is thought to be at immediate risk, they should be referred to the police as an emergency by contacting ambulance control for a 999 response.

Safeguarding Children

In all circumstances:

- Ensure that no action taken will place the child at further risk of harm.
- Limit questions to those of routine history-taking, asking questions only in relation to the injury or for clarification of what is being said. It is important to stop questioning when suspicions are clarified. Unnecessary questioning or probing may affect the credibility of subsequent evidence.
- Accept the explanations given and do not make any suggestions to the child as to how an injury or incident may have happened.
- Care must be taken not to directly accuse parents or carers of abuse, as this may result in a refusal to transfer to further care and place the child at further risk. Always work in partnership with parents or carers as far as possible, and inform them of concerns and the need to share these with the statutory agencies, unless to do so would put the child or others at greater risk of harm. Professional curiosity and judgement is crucial as to what information should be shared with parents.
- Any allegation of abuse made by a child is an important indicator and should always be taken seriously – it is important to listen to the 'voice of the child' and what they are saying. Do not ask probing questions. Consider what is a 'safe space' for them to talk.
- Adult responses can influence how able a child feels to reveal the full extent of the abuse. Listen and react appropriately to instil confidence. It is important to note that children may only tell a small part of their experience initially.
- It is important to make an accurate record of events and actions. Write down exactly what the child says. Their first language may not be English and care must be taken not to use family members or carers as interpreters in cases of suspected abuse. Take note of any inconsistency in history and any delay in calling for assistance. A child should not be asked to repeat what they have told you to someone else.
- On arrival at hospital, inform the receiving staff and the most senior member of nursing staff on duty of any concerns or suspicions. When reporting suspected abuse, the emphasis must be on shared professional responsibility and immediate communication.
- Complete safeguarding documentation/report as per local procedures; complete in private if possible. Follow local/trust protocols/guidelines.
- Ambulance clinicians must report suspected child abuse to the relevant statutory bodies (e.g. social care and the police), but they do not have a statutory duty to investigate it.
- Where a practitioner feels that their concerns have not been taken up (commonly known as professional challenge), they have a duty to escalate their concerns to a higher level by discussing this with their line manager, a more experienced colleague or named/designated doctor or nurse.

13.2 If the Child Is Not the Patient

- If the circumstances are suspicious, the ambulance clinician(s) should consider the implications of leaving the child.
- If the child is accompanying another person (e.g. a parent/carer) who is being conveyed, the ambulance clinician(s) should inform ED staff of their concerns and remember to report through their own safeguarding services as required.
- If no one is transferred to hospital, follow local/trust protocols/guidelines and inform safeguarding services of the incident/concerns at the earliest opportunity.
- Complete safeguarding documentation/report as per local procedures; complete in private if possible. Follow local/trust protocols/guidelines.

13.3 Allegations Against Ambulance Service Employees and Volunteers

- An allegation made by a child against ambulance service employees and volunteers is no different from an allegation made against any other healthcare professional, and the appropriate procedures should be followed, that is a referral to social care or the police. In other words, a child protection inquiry must follow such allegations.
- No staff, regardless of their position, volunteer, commissioned service or person associated with delivering services on behalf of an NHS Trust must act in any way that constitutes any of the following:
  - Behaviour that harms, or may harm, a child, young person or adult
  - Behaviour that results in a criminal offence against, or related to, a child, young person or adult
  - Behaviour towards a child, young person or adult that indicates they are unsuitable to work in a position of trust.
- The member of staff who is alleged to have abused the child must report the allegation to their line manager/named professional, who should follow employment procedures, that is a possible restriction of practice or suspension while investigations are conducted. There should be close liaison between the police carrying out the investigation and the line manager/named professional, who should be guided by the police as to how much information about the inquiry should be relayed to the member of staff. There will also need to be a support system in place for the member of staff.

Safeguarding Children

> **KEY POINTS!**
>
> **Safeguarding Children**
> - The safety and welfare of the child are paramount.
> - There is a duty to report concerns. Staff should not investigate concerns themselves.
> - Be aware of any special circumstances that the child is in which may increase the risk of abuse.
> - Police should be involved where there may be an immediate risk to the child.
> - Staff should document the circumstances giving rise to their concern as soon as possible.

Further Reading

Further important information and evidence in support of this guideline can be found in the Bibliography.

Other useful resources include:

Barnado's – http://www.barnados.org.uk/

Child Exploitation and Online Protection Command – http://www.ceop.gov.uk

Childline – http://www.childline.org.uk/

Children's Legal Centre – http://www.childrenslegalcentre.com

Family Lives – http://www.familylives.org.uk/

Kidscape – http://www.kidscape.org.uk

NSPCC – http://www.nspcc.org.uk

Samaritans – http://www.samaritans.org http://www.samaritans.org.uk

Victim Support – http://www.victimsupport.org.uk

NSPCC Learning – Recently published case reviews: https://learning.nspcc.org.uk/case-reviews/recently-published-case-reviews

Bibliography

1. Department of Health. *The Children Act 2004*. London: HMSO, 2004. Available from: https://www.legislation.gov.uk/ukpga/2004/31/content.
2. HM Government. *Working Together to Safeguard Children: A guide to inter-agency working to safeguard and promote the welfare of children*. London: HMSO, 2018. Available from: https://assets.publishing.service.gov.uk/government/uploads/system/uploads/attachment_data/file/942454/Working_together_to_safeguard_children_inter_agency_guidance.pdf.
3. National Institute for Health and Clinical Excellence. *Child Abuse and Neglect (NG76)* London: NICE, 2017. Available from: https://www.nice.org.uk/guidance/ng76.
4. NSPCCLearning. *Guidance on Protecting d/Deaf and Disabled Children and Young People from Abuse*. 2022. Available from: https://learning.nspcc.org.uk/safeguarding-child-protection/deaf-and-disabled-children.
5. HM Government. *Information Sharing: Advice for practitioners providing safeguarding services to children, young people, parents and carers*. 2018. Available from: https://assets.publishing.service.gov.uk/government/uploads/system/uploads/attachment_data/file/1062969/Information_sharing_advice_practitioners_safeguarding_services.pdf.
6. Department of Health. *Responding to Domestic Abuse: A resource for health professionals*. London: HMSO, 2017. Available from: https://assets.publishing.service.gov.uk/government/uploads/system/uploads/attachment_data/file/597435/DometicAbuseGuidance.pdf.
7. Home Office. *Adoption and Children Act 2002*. London: HMSO, 2002. Available from: http://www.legislation.gov.uk/ukpga/2002/38/contents.
8. Home Office. *Female Genital Mutilation Act 2003*. London: HMSO, 2003. Available from: http://www.legislation.gov.uk/ukpga/2003/31/pdfs/ukpga_20030031_en.pdf.
9. Royal College of Nursing. *Safeguarding Children and Young People: Roles and competencies for healthcare staff*. 2019. Available from: https://www.rcn.org.uk/-/media/Royal-College-Of-Nursing/Documents/Publications/2019/January/007-366.pdf.
10. Scottish Parliament. *Prohibition of Female Genital Mutilation (Scotland) Act 2005*. Edinburgh: HMSO, 2005. Available from: https://www.legislation.gov.uk/asp/2005/8/contents.
11. WHO. *Fact Sheet: Female Genital Mutilation*. 2022. Available from: https://www.who.int/news-room/fact-sheets/detail/female-genital-mutilation.
12. NICE. *Pregnancy and Complex Social Factors: A model for service provision for pregnant women with complex social factors*. 2010. Available from: https://www.nice.org.uk/guidance/cg110.

Sexual Assault

1. Introduction

- Sexual assault and abuse are serious crimes which continue to have a significant impact on our society. Their devastating consequences can often be misunderstood and neglected.
- Sexual assault is defined by Section 3 of the Sexual Offences Act 2003 (Protection of Children and Prevention of sexual offences (Scotland) Act 2005; Sexual Offences (Scotland) Act 2009) as intentionally touching another person, where the touching is sexual, and the other person has not consented to the touching, and the offender does not reasonably believe that the person consents. This offence covers a wide range of behaviour including, for example, rubbing up against someone's private parts through the person's clothes for sexual gratification.
- It is vital we take a patient centred approach to sexual assaults, enabling patients to feel in control of, and empowered within their pathway by giving them choices where possible.
- Sexual assault (or exploitation) can happen to anyone; men, women and children; at any age, and may be a one-off event or happen repeatedly. In some cases it can involve the use of technology such as the internet or social media which may be associated with grooming, online sexual harassment and trolling.
- Sexual assault of a child (<18 years) is considered Child Sexual Abuse (CSA) and you should follow your organisations Safeguarding Children procedures (Child Protection in Scotland) or Safeguarding Adults at Risk procedures. Remember you have a duty to report it to safeguarding/police.
- In the case of children and young people consider parental responsibility and who should go with the child or young person to hospital (not the parent or sibling that has caused sexual harm).
- Sexual assault can occur in Adults at Risk and you should follow your organisation's Safeguarding Adults at Risk procedures, remembering your duty to report it to safeguarding/police.
- Some people are more at risk of sexual assault and abuse[1] including those:
  - with a history of previous sexual abuse or who have experienced other forms of abuse.
  - with a disability.
  - who are in care (looked after in Scotland) or who have a disrupted home life.
  - known to have Adverse Childhood Experiences (ACE's) or complex trauma experiences.
  - who live without adequate supervision or who are isolated.
- The impacts of sexual assault are hard to spot as there is not a 'standard' or 'universal' diagnostic tool that would definitely identify the person who has been harmed and therefore it requires professional curiosity, cultural competence and trauma informed practice. (If appropriate refer to **Mental Health Presentations** and NHS Guide to Spotting the Signs of CSA).
- It can take many years for an individual to disclose sexual assault or abuse, particularly those people who have been abused or assaulted as a child, or those with a disability, men and sex workers. Non-recent abuse should still be reported and healthcare support offered in consultation with the patient.
- It is important that you take a patient centred approach and that your focus is on achieving the best outcome for the patients, minimising the risk of re-traumatisation and ensuring care and support is delivered to the patient.
- Importantly, patients subject to sexual abuse must be treated equally with compassion, respect and dignity irrespective of either the patient's or the clinician's social status, race, religion, culture, sexual orientation, lifestyle, gender or occupation.
- In September 2023 NHS England launched its first ever sexual safety charter.

Glossary of Sexual Assault	
Sexual abuse	- Rape, includes penetration without consent (in the cases of 'stealthing', using items/objects to penetrate without consent) indecent exposure, sexual harassment, inappropriate looking or touching, sexual teasing or innuendo, sexual photography, subjection to pornography or witnessing sexual acts, indecent exposure and sexual assault or sexual acts to which the individual has not consented or was pressured into consenting. This includes situations where an individual cannot give informed consent to engage in sexual activity, including those affected by alcohol, illicit drugs or a disability.

(continued)

Sexual Assault

Glossary of Sexual Assault *(continued)*	
Sexual exploitation	• Involves exploitative situations, contexts and relationships where individuals at risk (or a third person or persons) receive 'something' (e.g. food, accommodation, drugs, alcohol, cigarettes, affection, gifts, money) as a result of them performing and/or another or others performing on them, sexual activities. It affects everyone - children, men, women and non-binary individuals. • People who are sexually exploited do not always perceive that they are being exploited. • In all cases those exploiting the individual child or adult have power over them by virtue of their age, gender, intellect, physical strength and/or economic or other resources. There is a distinct inequality in the relationship. Signs to look out for are: not being able to speak to the child or adult alone; observation of the child or adult seeking approval from the exploiter to respond; and the person exploiting the child or adult answering for them and making decisions without consulting them.
Sexual consent	• Where an individual has the freedom and mental capacity to agree to sexual activity with other persons. It is important to note that individuals with mental health conditions may appear to consent to activity, but may lack mental capacity due to their mental health condition. • Consent must be given freely and not due to threats or emotional pressure (explicit or implicit). A person cannot be presumed to have consented to sexual activity simply because they are in a relationship with the other person; or because they have had sexual contact with them in the past. • Although the UK's legal age of sexual consent is 16 years, children under the age of 13 years cannot under any circumstance legally consent to any form of sexual or penetrative activity; such acts are considered as a crime of rape.
Sexual incident	• This includes any behaviour of a sexual nature that is unwanted, or makes another person feel uncomfortable or afraid. This includes assault and harassment. It also extends to being spoken to using sexualised language or observing other people behaving in a sexually disinhibited manner, including nakedness and exposure or self-stimulation and "sex texting" or sending images or text of a sexual nature.
Non-fatal strangulation	• Strangulation is the obstruction of blood vessels and/or airway by external pressure to the neck resulting in decreased oxygen supply to the brain and can lead to brain injury, stroke and miscarriage. • Patients may describe a "choking" episode or being "grabbed by the neck" but can be confused secondary to oxygen deprivation at the time and be unable to provide a clear chronological account of events. • It can be: – Non-fatal strangulation (NFS) where the strangulation does not cause death. NFS significantly increases the chance of being killed. – Fatal strangulation when death ensues. • Symptoms vary and can include confusion, sore neck, breathing and swallowing difficulties, voice changes (deeper, husky), headache or vomiting. At the time of the NFS, some will have experienced visual and auditory disturbance, loss or impairment of consciousness and/or urinary/faecal incontinence. • Bruising/abrasions around the neck or head may be seen, but do not be reassured by a lack of physical signs (50% show no visible external injuries). Internal injury, including carotid artery dissection and acquired brain injury can occur without external injuries. • The definition of NFS also includes patients who partake in breath-play (sexual bondage, discipline, dominance and submission, sadomasochism activities) that restrict a person's ability to breathe. Though this may be consensual, it has significant medical consequences and there is no safe way to strangle.

Sexual Assault

Glossary of Sexual Assault *(continued)*	
	• Note that bruising in people with dark skin may appear as purple or dark brown discolouration and it may be difficult on dark skin to see very recent bruising (which would appear red in lighter skin tones). It may only become obvious as the colour of the bruise subsequently develops a dark purple, brown or black colour that is darker than the surrounding skin. Again, in dark skin types the yellow discolouration seen in older bruises may be more subtle.

2. Assessment and Approach

- Initial responders should offer a sensitive and trauma-informed approach, known to help recovery and reduce future health issues and sexual abuse. Patients experiencing sexual assault may wrongly believe they are responsible for what happened to them and should be assured that they are not to blame for what has happened.
- Many people subject to sexual assault cite fear of not being believed as a reason for not reporting sexual assault, and recovery may be hindered when others disbelieve or blame the patient for the assault. Validation of the patient's feelings is thus critical to recovery.[3] Body language, gestures and facial expressions all contribute to conveying an atmosphere of believing the patient's account.
- **This guideline applies to everyone regardless of status and should not be a barrier in receiving treatment.** You need to offer treatment and support both the patients' physical and emotional needs. Your assessment needs a holistic approach and you should be professionally curious.
- Consider any evidence that may be needed at a later date such as clothing, and if possible advise patient not to wash and try and avoid contamination
- It may be appropriate for the patient to be accompanied by another person. The patient may be anxious if left alone with a person of the same sex as the assailant. On the other hand, they may be reassured by the presence of a professional person. The wishes of the patient must be considered and attempts made to reassure them and make them feel safe
- Beware of controlling and coercive behaviours and take steps to ensure that the patient is not left alone or accompanied by the perpetrator or parent/sibling that caused harm (refer to **Domestic Abuse**).
- If transferring to care ensure you hand over all concerns.

For the assessment and management of sexual assault, refer to Table 1.21.

TABLE 1.21 – ASSESSMENT and MANAGEMENT of: Sexual Assault

Assess <C>ABCDE

If any **TIME-CRITICAL** features present major ABCDE problems:

- Start correcting <C>ABCDE problems.
- Undertake a TIME-CRITICAL transfer to nearest receiving hospital.
- Continue patient management en route.
- Provide an ATMIST information call.

Assess

- Your professional curiosity is important to help ensure the patient's ongoing safety. Open questions should be used, limiting questioning primarily to matters related to identifying any immediate medical needs or matters of risk and safety, allowing the patient to talk freely whilst documenting *verbatim* what is said. **NB** do not probe for details of the assault as this can affect later criminal investigation(s), but if volunteered, these need to be accurately recorded.
- Manage according to condition:
  - Acute injury – refer to **Trauma Emergencies in Adults – Overview** and **Trauma Emergencies in Children – Overview**.
  - Acute illness – refer to **Medical Emergencies in Adults – Overview** and **Medical Emergencies in Children – Overview**.

(continued)

Sexual Assault

TABLE 1.21 – ASSESSMENT and MANAGEMENT of: Sexual Assault *(continued)*

Approach
- Rape and sexual abuse is often about power and control, not the sexual act. Listen to the patient with a sensitive and respectful manner and return control to them by giving choice where possible.
- Establish the patient's safety.
- Let the patient know you believe them. Take them seriously, be empathetic and non-judgemental.
- If possible, ensure privacy.
- Consider cultural/religious issues and the shame associated with rape and sexual abuse.
- Where possible accommodate patient's requests.
- Where possible avoid disturbing the scene.
- Where possible avoid being alone with the patient.
- Patients are not required by law to report sexual violence to police.
- Healthcare professionals are not required by law to report cases of sexual violence to police unless:
    - the patient is classed as a child (<18 years) or "An Adult at Risk (Care Act definition)".
    - the patient does not have capacity to consent to referral (refer to **Mental Capacity Act 2005**).
    - there is a clear and present danger of immediate risk to the patient or public.
    - the patient wishes to involve the police.
- Where this is requested, police should be called promptly so the scene may be secured.
- Where patients decline any support or referral, they should be encouraged to contact the local SARC, whilst ensuring their ongoing safety is secured (visit NHS Guide for Help after rape and sexual assault).
- A safeguarding referral should be raised for all children who experience or are at risk of experiencing sexual abuse as well as "Adults at Risk" who are unable to protect themselves from abuse.
- Consider activating your body worn camera (if available and according to local procedures) for protection against any allegations.

Awareness
- Clinicians should be aware of forensics evidence and where this is relevant patients should be informed why and encouraged not to:
    - wash (shower/bathe) or brush their teeth
    - change, throw away or destroy clothes
    - discard nappies or sanitary wear
    - urinate. If the patient needs to urinate if possible try and collect a sample.
    - smoke, eat or drink – a mouth swab and mouth wash may also be requested by the police
    - defecate.
- If a blanket is required for modesty or warmth, a single-use blanket should be used and kept with the patient – the blanket needs to be retained in order to analyse cross-contamination.
- Avoid cleaning any wounds unless clinically absolutely necessary.
- If required, lightly apply dry dressings – retain any used dressing and swabs for forensic examination; also keep the sterile packets in which they were contained in order to examine for cross-contamination.

NB All of these recommendations are vital to conserve forensics evidence, supporting a successful prosecution BUT the need for this approach must be conveyed with great sensitivity to the patient, who may well want to wash and change.

Sexual Assault

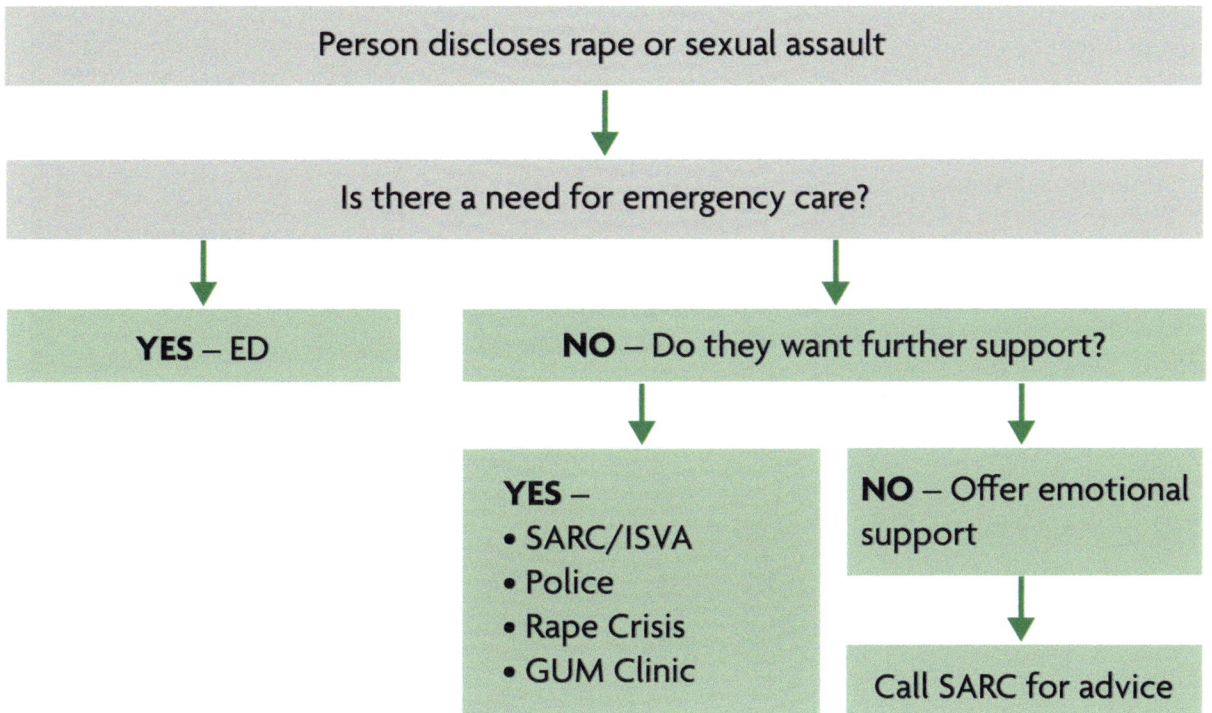

Figure 1.10 – Assessment and management of sexual assault.

3. Care Pathways

As primary caregiver and advocate, clinicians should inform the patient of their options without judgement, bias or coercion. Any physical examination should allow identification of life-threatening injuries and those requiring emergency care only. Genital areas should only be exposed and examined if there is evidence of bleeding requiring immediate treatment (use a chaperone if available).

Allow the patient space and as much choice about options for their treatment as possible. Options for the care of sexual assault victims may be summarised as:

Accident & Emergency or other appropriate health pathway	Sexual Assault Referral Centre (SARC) (Also available in Scotland)	Police and/or Safeguarding
• If the patient has injuries requiring emergency care. • If the patient has injuries and lacks mental capacity to express their wishes.	• SARCs provide people who have been subjected to sexual assault with immediate care and crisis support from specialist staff trained to allow patients to make informed decisions. • They also provide access to acute physical assessment with testing for STIs and provision of post-exposure prophylaxis and emergency contraception. • SARCs can also facilitate access to the criminal justice system. Forensic retrieval may be undertaken regardless of whether the patient reports to police or not. • Where the patient decides not to report, forensic samples may be stored, allowing patients time to consider their options until after the immediate 'crisis period'.[10] • SARCs provide direct access to Independent Sexual Violence Advisers (ISVAs) who provide advice, support and access to follow-up services addressing the patient's medical, safeguarding, psychosocial and ongoing needs. • ISVAs will also support patients through the judicial process; importantly, patients supported by ISVAs are more likely to go through the full course of criminal justice proceedings, again highlighting the importance of encouraging patients to access SARCs wherever possible.[11]	• When it involves a child (<18 years). • Where the patient gives expressed and informed consent. • Where there is a threat to life or severe risk to other members of the public. • Where a patient lacks mental capacity and it is felt to be in their best interests.

Sexual Assault

3.1 Access to SARCs (Refer to local service pathways)

- **Self-referral** – patients may self-refer to SARCs by telephone. Patients can have a conversation with a crisis worker who will help them decide on an immediate plan and makes an appointment for them to attend. Where this appointment is immediate, subject to local protocols, you may transport the patient directly to the SARC or alternatively make certain the patient will be able to be taken there safely by a third party.
- Consider contacting SARC for advice on behalf of the patient. Local SARC contact details may be on your hand held electronic devices or held centrally by ambulance control rooms; they are also available via NHS Help after rape and sexual assault Turn to SARCs (Scotland).

3.2 Refusal of Care

- Patients refusing referral to support services place a duty of care on clinicians to ensure their immediate safety.
- Encouraging patients to call a friend or relative for support is a priority. In these cases, patients should be given details of their nearest SARC, GUM/Sexual Health service or clinic, rape crisis or other voluntary services.
- These conversations require tact and sensitivity, as patients may not have considered the risk of STIs or pregnancy, and this alone may create another crisis.
- In cases of sexual assault in vulnerable adults and children, you have a duty to ensure their safety and to make a referral to refer to **Safeguarding Adults at Risk** and **Safeguarding Children** local authority partners (Adult and Child Protection referrals in Scotland). If you are not able to leave the patient safely consideration should be given to calling the police for support. Be mindful this may trigger a crisis response from the patient.
- Consider informing the GP.

Documentation

- Complete the clinical record in great detail contemporaneously and document:
  - only facts, not personal opinion
  - what the patient says
  - clinical findings with relevant timings
  - identification and documentation of injuries
  - the ambulance identification number
  - list any forensic items have been removed with the patient
- A police statement may be required later.

In cases of sexual assault it is important that ambulance staff are mindful of vicarious trauma and it is important that ambulance services make time and ensure that debriefing the incident takes place in a timely manner.

4. Forensic Timescales

- Within the limits of any immediate care needs, there is a responsibility to preserve evidence. Where police are on scene and injuries do not require emergency care, the police will normally take responsibility for the patient.
- If not being transported and police are called to scene, patients should be kept within the environment in which they present, unless this is unsafe or increasing the patient's distress; if so, they can be moved to the ambulance, seated on a clean sheet and wherever possible discouraged from any activities that jeopardise collection of evidence. This will include cutting, removing or changing clothing, eating or drinking, passing urine or opening bowels.
- Where the patient cannot be dissuaded from the natural need to clean themselves, they should be encouraged to place any tissues or towels along with any body fluids, blood stained clothes into paper (not plastic) bags, which do not destroy biological evidence.
- Where patients are transported to hospital and police action is requested, all blankets, sheets, towels and associated paraphernalia should be passed to police for forensic retrieval.

Sexual Assault

> **KEY POINTS!**
>
> **Sexual Assault**
> - Sexual assault may be concurrent with other injuries that will need urgent medical treatment.
> - Treatment should avoid disturbing evidence where possible.
> - Leave the investigation to the police.
> - Accommodate the patient's wishes where possible. The patient's rights to autonomy should be respected whilst considering safeguarding duties.
> - Contact or connect the patient with their local Sexual Assault Referral Centre (SARC).

Further Resources

NHS Guide for Help after rape and sexual assault

Turn to SARC (Scotland)

Bibliography

1. British Association for Sexual Health and HIV. *UK National Guidelines on the Management of Adult and Adolescent Complainants of Sexual Assault 2022*. Macclesfield: BASHH, 20 11. Available from: http://www.nordhaven.co.uk/BASHH.PDF.

2. NHS England. *National sevice specification for sexual assault referral centres.* London: HMSO, 2023. Available from: https://www.england.nhs.uk/publication/public-health-functions-to-be-exercised-by-nhs-england-service-specification-sexual-assault-referral-centres/

3. Home Office. *The role of the Independent Sexual Violence Adviser (ISVA)* London: Home Office, 2017. Available from: https://www.gov.uk/government/publications/the-role-of-the-independent-sexual-violence-adviser-isva.

4. Sexual Offences Act 2003 updated December, 2023. Available from: https://www.legislation.gov.uk/ukpga/2003/42/contents

5. Protecting Children from Sexual Abuse. Available from: https://learning.nspcc.org.uk/child-abuse-and-neglect/child-sexual-abuse/

6. Care Act 2014. Available from: https://www.legislation.gov.uk/ukpga/2014/23/contents/enacted

7. Working Together to Safeguard Children, 2023. Available from: https://www.gov.uk/government/publications/working-together-to-safeguard-children--2

8. Sexual Assault Referral Centre (SARC). Available from: https://rapecrisis.org.uk/get-help/sexual-assault-referral-centres-sarcs/

9. NHSE Sexual Safety Organisational Charter, 2023. Available from: https://www.england.nhs.uk/publication/sexual-safety-in-healthcare-organisational-charter/

10. Key messages from research on intra-familial child sexual abuse. Centre of expertise on Child Sexual Abuse, Sep 2023. Available from: https://www.csacentre.org.uk/app/uploads/2023/09/Key-messages-from-research-on-intra-familial-child-sexual-abuse-2nd-edition.pdf.

11. Faculty of Forensic & Legal Medicine, 2021. Available from: SARC-Storage-of-Forensic-Samples-and-the-Human-Tissue-Act-Dr-C-White-Jan-2021.pdf (fflm.ac.uk)

Staff Health and Wellbeing

1. Introduction

- The importance of good mental health and wellbeing cannot be underestimated. The World Health Organization defines good mental health as: 'a state of wellbeing in which every individual realizes his or her own potential, can cope with the normal stresses of life, can work productively and fruitfully and is able to make a contribution to her or his community'.[1]

- However, there is evidence to suggest that, for those who work in the emergency services, the risk of experiencing a mental health issue is greater than average.[2] The number and type of significant tragedies and events in the UK in recent years combined with the ever-increasing workload placed upon emergency services has highlighted the difficulties often experienced by staff. As a result, the subject has been looked at from a fresh perspective, with many new and useful resources becoming available.

- The blue light scoping survey undertaken by Mind – the mental health charity – suggested that there are a number of areas that are directly attributable to a change in the mental wellbeing of ambulance service workers.[3] Similarly, it highlighted some worrying trends:
  - Emergency service staff are twice as likely to identify work as the cause of their mental health issue, with over 85% of staff experiencing stress, low mood, anxiety or depression at some point in their career.
  - Over 50% of staff are unaware of services they can access to help them with their mental health needs.
  - Despite the Equality Act (2010) offering protection, only 12% would approach a line manager for help and almost 80% said they would never speak to their HR departments.

- But this need not be the case and there is a wealth of resources at hand. The most common issues around ambulance staff mental wellbeing are centred upon several key themes.[3]

2. Anxiety

- Anxiety is a perfectly normal reaction to a stressful situation and is linked closely to the fight-or-flight response. Anxiety disorders can take several different forms, the most common of which is generalised anxiety disorder and is widely experienced.

- The most commonly experienced symptoms are very much in line with those of PTSD:[3,4]
  - palpitations
  - shortness of breath
  - diarrhoea
  - nausea.

- Once the trigger for the symptoms of anxiety stop, you would expect the anxiety to reduce. However, if the anxiety starts to influence our lives too greatly, we must look for ways to deal with it effectively.

3. Post-traumatic Stress Disorder (PTSD)

- Post-traumatic stress disorder (PTSD) can affect anyone and is closely associated with very intense situations in which someone experiences life-threatening or life-changing events, especially those that involve witnessing death and dying.[5]

- These types of situation are not uncommon for ambulance clinicians, and recognising that you may have been negatively influenced by a single event or accumulation of events should never be considered a weakness. Research points towards the severity, intensity and number of exposures to stressful experiences as being the key reason someone may suffer from PTSD and not because of an individual's personality traits.[6]

- Common symptoms include:
  - flashbacks or reliving traumatic incidents
  - nightmares
  - feeling constantly on edge
  - a numbing of emotions
  - an unwillingness to talk about or visit memories and reminders of an event.

- Other symptoms can include:
  - pain
  - nausea
  - diarrhoea
  - choosing to withdraw and becoming socially isolated
  - increased drug and alcohol use
  - depression
  - low mood
  - anxiety
  - a strong sense of guilt.[7]

4. Low Mood and Depression

- It is estimated one in five people in the UK suffer from depression at some point throughout their lives, making depression amongst the most common of disorders.[8]

- A sense of hopelessness, sadness, loss and reduced interest in your normal life and activities is felt over an extended period. It can affect appetite, sleep, concentration, self-worth and relationships. At its worst it can lead to feelings and thoughts of self-harm and suicide.[9]

- There are a range of services such as talking therapies, self-help and medication which are available to anyone experiencing symptoms and these can be accessed quickly and easily.

Staff Health and Wellbeing

5. Spotting the Signs

- The potential for reduced mental wellness is greater throughout the emergency services in all roles. As clinicians, we often assist the people we encounter by finding the most appropriate source of help for their current situation. Recognising a need in yourself or a colleague is difficult, but research suggests that ambulance personnel are far more likely to confide in each other rather than their own GP.[3]

- Even when we do recognise the need for help, fear of discrimination and stigma still presents a significant concern for many, despite the protection afforded by the 2010 Equality Act.

- Anyone can experience any number of mental health issues at any point in their lives regardless of their history or circumstance. The cause and nature of any individual's issues can be as unique as the individual and can be cumulative in nature, building over time and for any number and combination of reasons.

- It is not unusual in today's workplace for individuals to see concentrating upon work and careers as vital to maintaining professionalism; however, achieving a healthy work–life balance can have a very positive influence upon the stress and productivity experienced by any individual.[10]

- There is a wealth of independent, confidential and high-quality sources of help. Accessing help in a timely manner can have a significant impact upon the speed and quality of an individual's recovery. The benefits of spending time on relationships outside of work, family, hobbies and interests, volunteering, exercising and continued learning all have a role to play in maintaining and improving wellbeing. This in turn can have benefits not only to ourselves, but also to the many people we encounter in our roles.

6. Sources of Help and Signposting

- Ambulance Hub on NHS Employers website – Head First tool. Available from: https://www.nhsemployers.org/headfirst
- HR/work-related sources
- College of paramedics. Available from: https://www.collegeofparamedics.co.uk
- MIND Blue light. Available from: https://www.mind.org.uk/news-campaigns/campaigns/bluelight/
- TASC. Available from: http://www.theasc.org.uk/
- Samaritans. Available from: https://www.samaritans.org/
- CALM. Available from: https://www.calm.com/
- Step change. Available from: https://www.stepchange.org/
- Alcoholics Anonymous (AA). Available from: https://www.alcoholics-anonymous.org.uk/
- TRiM. Available from: http://www.marchonstress.com/page/p/trim

Bibliography

1. World Health Organization. *Mental Health: a state of wellbeing.* 2014. Available from: https://www.who.int/features/factfiles/mental_health/en/.

2. Fjeldheim CB, Nöthling J, Pretorius K, Basson M, Ganasen K, Heneke R, Cloete KJ, Seedat S. Trauma exposure, post-traumatic stress disorder and the effect of explanatory variables in paramedic trainees. *BMC Emergency Medicine* 2014, 14: 11. Available from: https://www.ncbi.nlm.nih.gov/pubmed/24755358.

3. Mind. *Blue Light Scoping Survey.* 2015. Available from: https://www.mind.org.uk/media/4627950/scoping-survey.pdf.

4. Rethink Mental Illness. *What Are Anxiety Disorders.* 2018. Available from: https://www.mind.org.uk/media/4627950/scoping-survey.pdf.

5. Royal College of Psychiatrists. *Post-traumatic Stress Disorder.* 2015. Available from: https://www.rcpsych.ac.uk/healthadvice/problemsanddisorders/posttraumaticstressdisorder.aspx.

6. Javidi H and Yadollahie M. Post-traumatic stress disorder. *International Journal of Occupational and Environmental Medicine*, 2012, 3(1). Available from: http://theijoem.com/ijoem/index.php/ijoem/article/view/127/247.

7. National Health Service. *Post-traumatic Stress Disorder (PTSD).* 2015. Available from: https://www.nhs.uk/conditions/post-traumatic-stress-disorder-ptsd/symptoms/.

8. Royal College of Psychiatrists. *Depression: Key facts.* 2014. Available from: https://www.rcpsych.ac.uk/healthadvice/problemsanddisorders/depressionkey-facts.aspx.

9. World Health Organization. *Depression: Let's talk.* 2018. Available from: https://www.who.int/mental_health/management/depression/en/.

10. Burn SM. *How's Your Work-Life Balance? The importance of work-life balance and how to achieve it.* 2015. Available from: https://www.psychologytoday.com/us/blog/presence-mind/201509/hows-your-work-life-balance.

2

Resuscitation

Out-of-Hospital Cardiac Arrest: Overview

Every five years, the International Liaison Committee on Resuscitation (ILCOR) reviews current resuscitation science from which the European Resuscitation Council (ERC) then draws up evidence-based guidelines. These guidelines then form the basis from which the Resuscitation Council (UK) provides national, NICE-accredited guidelines for both hospital and pre-hospital UK practice.

JRCALC guidelines are based directly on these RC UK guidelines, currently the 2021 iteration (https://www.resus.org.uk/library/2021-resuscitation-guidelines https://www.resus.org.uk/resuscitation-guidelines).

1. Incidence of Cardiac Arrest and Epidemiology

- 2020 NHS England data indicate that ambulance services respond to approximately 94,000 cardiac arrest calls and attempt to resuscitate approximately 32,000 people from out-of-hospital cardiac arrest (OHCA) each year. (https://warwick.ac.uk/fac/sci/med/research/ctu/trials/ohcao/publications/epidemiologyreports/ohca_epidemiological_report_2020_-_england_overview.pdf). This is in addition to the annual 3,200 resuscitation attempts reported by Scotland (https://www.gov.scot/publications/scottish-out-hospital-cardiac-arrest-data-linkage-project-2018-19-results/), 2,800 cardiac arrests reported by Wales and 1,400 resuscitation attempts reported by Northern Ireland.
- Table 2.1 shows the rate of return of spontaneous circulation (ROSC) on arrival at hospital and survival to hospital discharge when resuscitation is attempted.
- The Utstein group is defined as those with witnessed cardiac arrests where the initial rhythm is found to be ventricular fibrillation (VF).
- 2% of cases were children; of the remainder, one third were less than 64 years of age.

TABLE 2.1 – Current Resuscitation Outcomes (2020)

	ROSC on arrival at hospital	Survival to Discharge
All patients	26%	8%
Utstein patients	48%	25%

- The incidence of bystander cardiopulmonary resuscitation (CPR) rates before ambulance arrival is approximately 70%.
- The initial rhythm is VF in approximately 23% and asystole in 51% of cases. The remainder present in pulseless electrical activity (PEA).
- Unless in a specialist role, most paramedics attend cardiac arrests relatively infrequently.
- Anyone involved in the resuscitation of patients in cardiac arrest (including those involved in the training) should have annual competency assessments and regular face-to-face training to include high-quality CPR and associated skills, such as airway management, aligned to their scope of practice. This should include adult and paediatric resuscitation.
- This guideline refers to enhanced care. This includes specialist and advanced practice roles above the paramedic skillset. Refer to local procedures and definitions.

2. Chain of Survival

The Chain of Survival, Figure 2.1, links the critical actions required to treat cardiac arrest, recognising that all links need to be intact and functioning to achieve neurologically intact survival. The links are:

1. Early recognition and call for help.
2. Early CPR to support circulation to the heart and brain until normal heart activity is restored.
3. Early defibrillation to treat cardiac arrest caused by shockable rhythms.
4. Post-resuscitation care to improve survival rates.

The earlier links contribute far more to survival than the later links, because rapid recognition and good-quality basic life support (BLS) with defibrillation are the key factors influencing a good outcome.

3. Human Factors in Out-of-Hospital Cardiac Arrest: Team Resource Management

- A coordinated, well-rehearsed resuscitation attempt, with a team leader and all team members effectively delivering specific roles, will improve the effectiveness of CPR and the overall resuscitation.
- Four people with a minimum skillset of basic life support and defibrillation should attend patients in cardiac arrest where possible. This should include at least one registered healthcare professional with ALS competencies. One person with clinical decision making and leadership skills should form part of the team. Some members of the team may be non-ambulance staff, for example a Community First Responder (CFR) or other emergency service personnel trained in BLS.
- An effective resuscitation attempt requires a series of actions, skills and decisions to be delivered quickly and efficiently, including:
  - scene management
  - clear roles and responsibilities
  - clinical assessment

Out-of-Hospital Cardiac Arrest: Overview

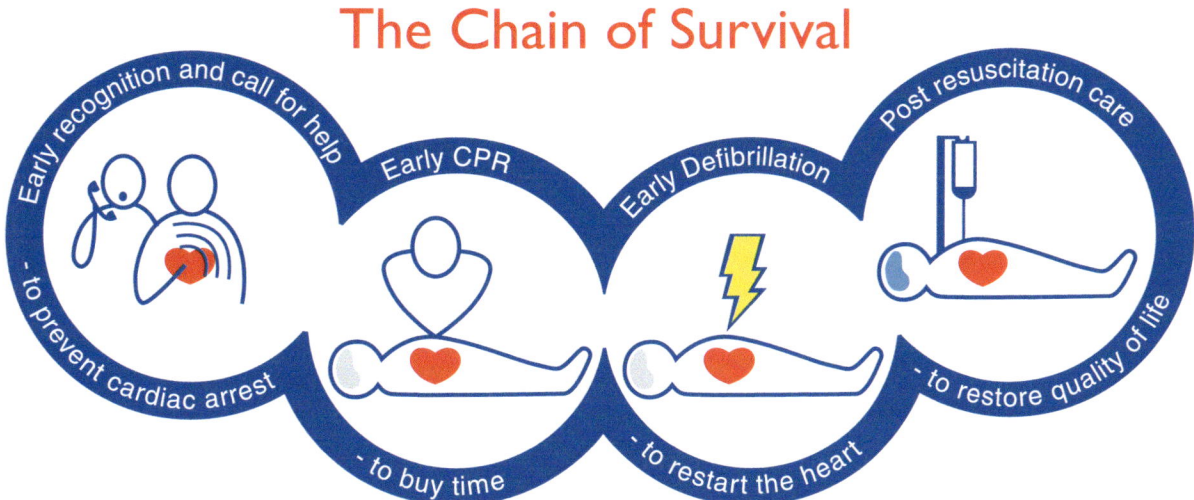

Figure 2.1 – The chain of survival.

- effective delivery of interventions
- teamwork
- communication.
- These often-simultaneous tasks can have a cumulative effect on workload and potentially compromise the overall effectiveness of the resuscitation attempt.

4. Pathophysiology of Cardiac Arrest and Resuscitation

- The pathophysiology of cardiac arrest, due to a primary cardiac cause resulting in ventricular fibrillation, consists of three phases:
  1. **Electrical phase** Constitutes the initial 4–5 minutes during which tissue metabolism is relatively normal and restoration of a perfusing rhythm can lead to a good chance of neurologically intact survival. Early defibrillation in the electrical phase can achieve survival rates in excess of 50%.
  2. **Circulatory phase** From 4–5 minutes to approximately 10–15 minutes after cardiac arrest. Worsening tissue hypoxia and accumulating metabolites reduce the likelihood of successful defibrillation. The most important treatment is to initiate high-quality CPR to optimise tissue oxygenation and to deliver defibrillation. Restoration of a spontaneous circulation requires a coronary perfusion pressure (CPP) >15–20 mmHg, which may require the administration of adrenaline.
  3. **Metabolic phase** Extends beyond approximately 10–15 minutes after cardiac arrest. Survival becomes less likely due to myocardial and cerebral ischaemia. Reperfusion injury is more likely to occur if ROSC is achieved. Defibrillation and drug therapy become less effective in this phase.

- CPR aims to circulate adequate amounts of oxygen to vital organs (particularly the heart and brain) to maintain tissue viability until ROSC is achieved. In the immediate few minutes after cardiac arrest, reserves in the arterial circulation can provide adequate tissue oxygenation through compression-only CPR, although they are rapidly depleted and rescue breaths are then needed to oxygenate the blood.

5. Mechanisms of Forward Blood Flow

- There are three main mechanisms thought to generate forward blood flow:
  - **Cardiac pump theory** Direct compression of the cardiac chambers between the sternum and vertebral column increases intracardiac pressure. This ejects blood from the heart into the pulmonary artery and aorta. Recoil of the sternum generates a negative pressure, which contributes to the passive filling of the ventricles before the subsequent compression.
  - **Thoracic pump theory** Chest compressions increase the pressure in the thorax which raises the pressure in the great vessels. The thinner-walled veins tend to collapse, while the arteries remain patent, and blood flows from the arterial to venous circulation due to the resulting pressure gradient.
  - **Lung pump theory** It has been suggested that neither the heart compression nor thoracic pump hypotheses fully explain blood flow resulting from cardiac compressions. The 'lung pump' model suggests that chest compressions cause a cyclical rise in intrathoracic pressure, which acts to compress the pulmonary vasculature and eject blood from the lungs with each compression (like wringing a sponge).

Out-of-Hospital Cardiac Arrest: Overview

- Chest compressions must generate a coronary perfusion pressure of >15–20 mmHg to create sufficient coronary blood flow for the heart to be re-oxygenated and start contracting. Achieving this coronary perfusion pressure requires high-quality chest compressions. When chest compressions are interrupted, coronary perfusion pressure drops very quickly but takes some time to increase again after compressions are restarted – this may contribute to worse survival and hence the importance of minimising interruptions to chest compressions.
- Adequate cerebral blood flow is also dependent on high-quality chest compressions.

6. Rate and Depth of Chest Compressions

- Chest compressions hold the key to survival. Even when chest compressions are performed optimally, cardiac output is no more than 25–40% of pre-arrest values.
- Every effort must be made to ensure that compressions are carried out correctly and effectively. Rescuer fatigue is well described, with an onset time between 1 and 3 minutes. Ideally no one should perform chest compressions for greater than 2 minutes, wherever practicable.
- Interruptions to CPR are associated with a reduced chance of survival and must be avoided wherever possible.
- Too slow a compression rate fails to generate sufficient circulatory pressure, resulting in inadequate coronary blood flows. An excessive rate reduces the time for passive ventricular filling between compressions and also reduces coronary blood flow.
- Inadequate compression depth fails to generate adequate circulatory pressures, but excessive depth does not increase cardiac ejection and may risk myocardial and other organ damage.
- Allowing complete recoil of the sternum between each chest compression optimises the negative pressures generated inside the thorax during passive chest recoil and draws some blood back into the heart. This assists the passive refilling of the heart and increases the amount of blood ejected with the subsequent compression. Inadvertent leaning on the chest, preventing it from fully recoiling after each compression, reduces the above mechanisms.
- Where a patient presents in a shockable rhythm, chest compressions and defibrillation are the most effective treatment. Do not allow any advanced life support intervention to compromise delivery of high-quality BLS and defibrillation in these patients.
- For the solo responder, over-the-head CPR may be considered until other help arrives.

- Delivering good chest compression means:
  - Interruptions are minimised.
  - Proper depth is ensured (5–6 cm).
  - Full recoil is ensured between compressions.
  - Appropriate rate is maintained (100–120 per minute); metronome or feedback device use is recommended.
  - CPR compressions provider is swapped every 2 minutes.
  - When changing the compressions provider, work as a team, communicate with each other and plan to minimise the time spent with hands off the chest.
  - Be ready to charge the defibrillator after the rhythm check and deliver a shock with no more than a 5-second interruption to CPR. (Charging the defibrillator 5 seconds before rhythm check, and either delivering the shock or dumping the charge as required, is an acceptable alternative.)
  - Recommencing CPR as soon as rhythm check/shock is complete.
  - Minimal interruptions to CPR for airway manoeuvres.
  - No interruptions for IV/IO placement.

7. Ventilation

- Ventilation aims not only to deliver oxygen but also to remove CO_2 from the blood.
- Each positive pressure breath inflates the lungs, enabling oxygenation of pulmonary blood and CO_2 excretion. The ventilation tidal volume should be approximately 6–7 ml/kg (about 600 ml for most adults), delivered as either two breaths after 30 compressions or at a rate of 10/min as asynchronous breaths. Inadequate ventilation rates and/or tidal volumes will not provide sufficient blood oxygenation/CO_2 removal.
- Positive pressure breaths increase intrathoracic pressure, which has the adverse effect of reducing venous return to the heart and therefore reducing cardiac filling. Too much ventilation (excessive rates and/or tidal volumes) has a significant adverse impact on cardiac output.
- Each positive pressure breath also increases intracranial pressure (ICP), thus reducing cerebral blood flow. Optimising cerebral and myocardial oxygen delivery therefore requires no more than gentle ventilation that is sufficient to inflate the lungs and remove CO_2.

7.1 Gasping

- Gasping occurs in about 40% of patients in the first few minutes after cardiac arrest and may also be seen during CPR that is sufficiently effective to oxygenate the brainstem. Gasping during CPR creates negative intrathoracic pressure. This causes inhalation of air, increases

Out-of-Hospital Cardiac Arrest: Overview

venous return to the heart and decreases ICP, facilitating increased cerebral and coronary perfusion. It is this mechanism that is thought to be responsible for the more favourable outcomes that result in patients who have been gasping.

- Do not mistake gasping (slow, deep, irregular breaths) for normal breathing. An unresponsive patient who is gasping requires CPR.

8. Drug Therapy

- **Adrenaline:** Adrenaline acts to stimulate beta-adrenergic receptors to increase the force and rate of contraction and stimulate alpha-adrenergic receptors to cause vasoconstriction.
- Following the publication of the PARAMEDIC-2 trial, the use of adrenaline in cardiac arrest continues unchanged.
- **Amiodarone:** Ischaemic myocardial cells may spontaneously depolarise as they lose the ability to control their internal metabolism. Cumulatively, this may result in wave fronts of depolarisation that spread across the myocardium to cause ventricular ectopic beats, ventricular tachycardia or ventricular fibrillation.
- Antiarrhythmic medicines, primarily amiodarone, are used to:
  – decrease conduction velocity
  – reduce myocyte excitability
  – suppress abnormal automaticity

  which assists in terminating shockable rhythms in conjunction with defibrillation and maintaining a perfusing rhythm.
- **Atropine:** Vagal (parasympathetic) stimulation is not thought to be the cause of cardiac arrest in sustained asystole. That is why atropine is not recommended in the mangament of asystolic cardiac arrest. However, it may be a mechanism that causes peri-arrest bradycardia by slowing the sinoatrial node. Vagal tone may be blocked by atropine in patients where bradycardia is contributing to hypotension.

8.1 Acid–base Balance

- The acid–base balance of the body is carefully regulated to optimise cellular metabolism. During cardiac arrest, the build-up of metabolites and CO_2 may cause an acidosis, which acts to reduce oxygen delivery to cells, reduce myocardial contractility and cause myocardial irritability. This makes ROSC more difficult to achieve. The longer the duration of cardiac arrest, the more severe the acidosis.
- CO_2 build-up that causes respiratory acidosis can be limited by ventilating with the correct rate and tidal volume. The use of sodium bicarbonate is not routinely indicated unless blood gas measurements are available on scene.

9. Ambulance Services Response to Out-of-Hospital Cardiac Arrest

9.1 Checklist Use in Resuscitation

- Cardiac arrest checklists should be used by all responders.
- The out-of-hospital paramedic does not usually function as an individual – they are part of a team, and members usually have varying levels of expertise.
- The checklist may help compensate to some degree for this.
- The purpose of a checklist is to help ensure efficient and effective treatment delivery by individuals and teams, to minimise the risk of elements of care and avoid treatment being omitted, delayed or delivered inappropriately in a stressful situation, as a result of human factors.
- The ERC states that the use of checklists may improve adherence to guidelines as long as they do not cause delays in starting CPR.

9.2 Cardiac Arrest Downloads

- Data downloads should be used to review each cardiac arrest to understand the quality of care and chest compressions for future and real-time improvement.
- Auditing and reviewing data downloads will help determine how quickly shocks are being delivered. Decisions can be made based on local data as to whether to recommend using AED mode for the first shock in order to minimise shock delays. Local audit data can help inform the decision making process.
- Hot debriefs after cardiac arrest incidents should be undertaken wherever possible. There is evidence to suggest that where these downloads are reviewed and an appropriate debriefing session is held, rescuer performance improves.
- Where download summaries are available, paramedics should take advantage of this opportunity to reflect on the resuscitation attempt, critically analysing their performance and planning how they could improve on their next attempt.

9.3 Use of CPR Feedback Devices

- The use of CPR feedback and coaching devices is strongly recommended on all occasions where resuscitation is taking place.
- A number of studies have shown that the quality of CPR during training and in clinical practice is often suboptimal, with inadequate compression depth, interruptions in chest compression, prolonged pre- and post-shock pauses and hyperventilation occurring frequently.
- CPR feedback and prompt devices (e.g. voice prompts, metronomes, visual dials, numerical

Out-of-Hospital Cardiac Arrest: Overview

displays, waveforms, verbal prompts and visual alarms) aim to improve the performance of resuscitation skills.

- These devices enable the CPR provider to receive real-time objective feedback on the quality of CPR, and have been evaluated in several clinical studies that support their use to improve the quality of CPR delivered.

- Devices on the market give prompts (i.e. signal to perform an action, e.g. metronome for compression rate or voice feedback), give feedback (i.e. after-event information based on the effect of an action, such as a visual display of compression depth) or give a combination of prompts and feedback.

9.4 Clinical Handover

- Clinical handover begins with a pre-alert. Concise and appropriate information should be passed to the emergency department using the ATMIST format (or a format as per local protocol).

- The clinical handover with the patient can be challenging to deliver succinctly. Standardised tools such as ATMIST should be used as per locally agreed protocols (refer to Table 2.2).

- Useful information includes the time of collapse, whether bystander CPR was being performed, the time of arrival of the first crew, the initial rhythm and the patient's pre-arrest co-morbidities.

- Try to speak loudly and clearly, be concise and use the template headings before communicating the information for each heading.

TABLE 2.2 – ATMIST

A	Age
T	Time of incident
M	Mechanism of injury
I	Injuries
S	Signs and symptoms
T	Treatment given and immediate needs

Bibliography

1. Resuscitation Council (UK). *Resuscitation Guidelines 2021*. London: Resuscitation Council (UK), 2021. Available from: https://www.resus.org.uk/resuscitation-guidelines.

2. NHS England. *Resuscitation to Recovery: A national framework to improve care of people with out-of-hospital cardiac arrest (OHCA) in England*. London: NHS England, 2015. Available from: https://aace.org.uk/wp-content/uploads/2017/03/FINAL_Resuscitation-to-Recovery_A-National-Framework-to-Improve-Care-of-People-with-Out-of-Hospital-Cardiac-Arrest-in-England_March-2017.pdf.

3. Scottish Government. *Scottish Out-of-Hospital Cardiac Arrest Data Linkage Project: 2018–2019*. Edinburgh: Scottish Government, 2020. Available from: https://www.gov.scot/publications/scottish-out-hospital-cardiac-arrest-data-linkage-project-2018-19-results/.

4. Perkins GD, Brace-McDonnell SJ. The UK Out of Hospital Cardiac Arrest Outcome (OHCAO) project. *BMJ Open* 2015, 5: e008736. Available from: https://bmjopen.bmj.com/content/5/10/e008736.

5. Weisfeldt ML, Becker LB. Resuscitation after cardiac arrest: a 3-phase time-sensitive model. *JAMA* 2002, 288: 3035–3038. Available from: https://www.researchgate.net/publication/10992588_Resuscitation_after_cardiac_arrest_A_3-phase_time-sensitive_model.

6. Georgiou M, Papathanassoglou E, Xanthos T. Systematic review of the mechanisms driving effective blood flow during adult CPR. *Resuscitation* 2014, 85: 1586–1593. Available from: https://www.sciencedirect.com/science/article/abs/pii/S0300957214007400.

7. Lurie KG, Nemergut EC, Yannopoulos D, Sweeney M. The physiology of cardiopulmonary resuscitation. *Anesthesia & Analgesia* 2016, 122(3): 767–783. Available from: http://umanitoba.ca/faculties/health_sciences/medicine/units/anesthesia/media/The_Physiology_of_Cardiopulmonary_Resuscitation.pdf.

8. Perkins GD, Ji C, Deakin CD et al. on behalf of PARAMEDIC2 collaborators. A randomized trial of epinephrine in out-of-hospital cardiac arrest. *New England Journal of Medicine* 2018, 379: 711–721. Available from: https://www.nejm.org/doi/full/10.1056/NEJMoa1806842.

9. Soar J, Berg B, Andersen L et al. Adult advanced life support 2020 international consensus on cardiopulmonary resuscitation and emergency cardiovascular care science with treatment recommendations. *Resuscitation* 2020, 156: A80–119. Available from: https://www.resuscitationjournal.com/article/S0300-9572(20)30460-3/pdf.

10. Olasveengen T, Mancini M, Perkins GD et al. Adult basic life support: international consensus on cardiopulmonary resuscitation and emergency cardiovascular care science with treatment recommendations. *Resuscitation* 2020, 156: A35–79. Available from: https://www.resuscitationjournal.com/article/S0300-9572(20)30458-5/fulltext.

Advanced Life Support

1. Advanced Life Support Overview

1.1 Introduction

- Advanced life support (ALS) may be defined as the use of resuscitation drugs and interventions above and beyond basic life support and AED use. However, if a trained ALS provider attends as a solo responder, they are limited to basic life support (BLS) and defibrillation until other responders arrive.
- The availability of ALS must not affect the provision of high-quality basic life support and appropriate defibrillation.
- Out-of-hospital cardiac arrest (OHCA) management follows similar principles for ALS as in-hospital treatment. It is recognised, however, that the environment, equipment, resources, access to the patient, extrication and transportation of the patient play a pivotal part in the overall clinical management decisions.
- A team approach should be adopted as early as possible and a team leader appointed (resources allowing), who can use cardiac arrest checklists for the overall management of the cardiac arrest and for specific clinical skills, e.g. intubation checklists.

1.2 Stages of Assessment and Management

- The assessment and management of an out-of-hospital medical cardiac arrest includes:
  - Confirmation of the cardiac arrest.
  - Immediate implementation and continuation of effective BLS and defibrillation.
  - The addition of ALS, including IV/IO access, the administration of medicines, advanced airway management and clinical decision making, where appropriate.
  - Early identification and management of reversible causes.
  - Early decision making on:
    - the appropriateness of the resuscitation attempt (ReSPECT, recognition of life extinct, futility and best interests).
    - an early transportation plan if a reversible cause is identified that cannot be treated on scene or if admission to a cath lab is considered appropriate (according to local protocols).
    - requesting enhanced care resources to attend the scene to help with clinical decision making, enhanced assessments (e.g. ultra-sound) and interventions (e.g. blood products)
    - seeking senior remote advice where available through a structured and governed system.
  - Witnessed cardiac arrests generally do not need temperature to be taken as part of cardiac arrest management.
  - If there are any circumstances where hypothermia may be an issue, then consider taking a temperature prior to drug administration e.g. unwitnessed arrests, drowning, those with prolonged exposure to cold. Refer to ALS section 10.4.

2. Advanced Life Support in Adults

Refer to ALS algorithm, Figure 2.2.

Additional Information

- Once adrenaline has been administered, further doses should be given every 3–5 minutes, irrespective of rhythm, while the patient remains in cardiac arrest.
- Peripheral IV access should be established as soon as possible. However, paramedics should attempt intraosseous access if two cannulation attempts have failed (or initially if IV cannulation is unlikely to succeed). External jugular vein access is also acceptable as an alternative for those appropriately trained.
- If a patient who is being **monitored** has a **witnessed** arrest:
  - Confirm cardiac arrest.
  - Request further resources if appropriate.
  - A precordial thump is no longer recommended for initial treatment of shockable rhythms even if a defibrillator is not immediately available.
  - If the rhythm is VF/pVT and a defibrillator is immediately available, give a shock first and immediately commence CPR; treat any recurrence of VF/pVT following the shockable rhythm algorithm.
  - Where the arrest is witnessed but unmonitored, defibrillation pads must be applied immediately.
  - Three stacked shocks may be considered as per local protocols in a witnessed and monitored cardiac arrest, only when the patient is already connected to a manual defbrillator. For the purposes of medicine administration, these three shocks should be treated as the first shock in the ALS algorithm.
  - If VF persists, refer to **Defibrillation**.

ADULT ALS – SUMMARY

- During ALS, the priority remains to deliver high-quality chest compressions and effective ventilations with high-flow (100%) oxygen.
- When indicated, defibrillate and resume chest compressions for two minutes without re-assessing the rhythm or feeling for a pulse.

Advanced Life Support

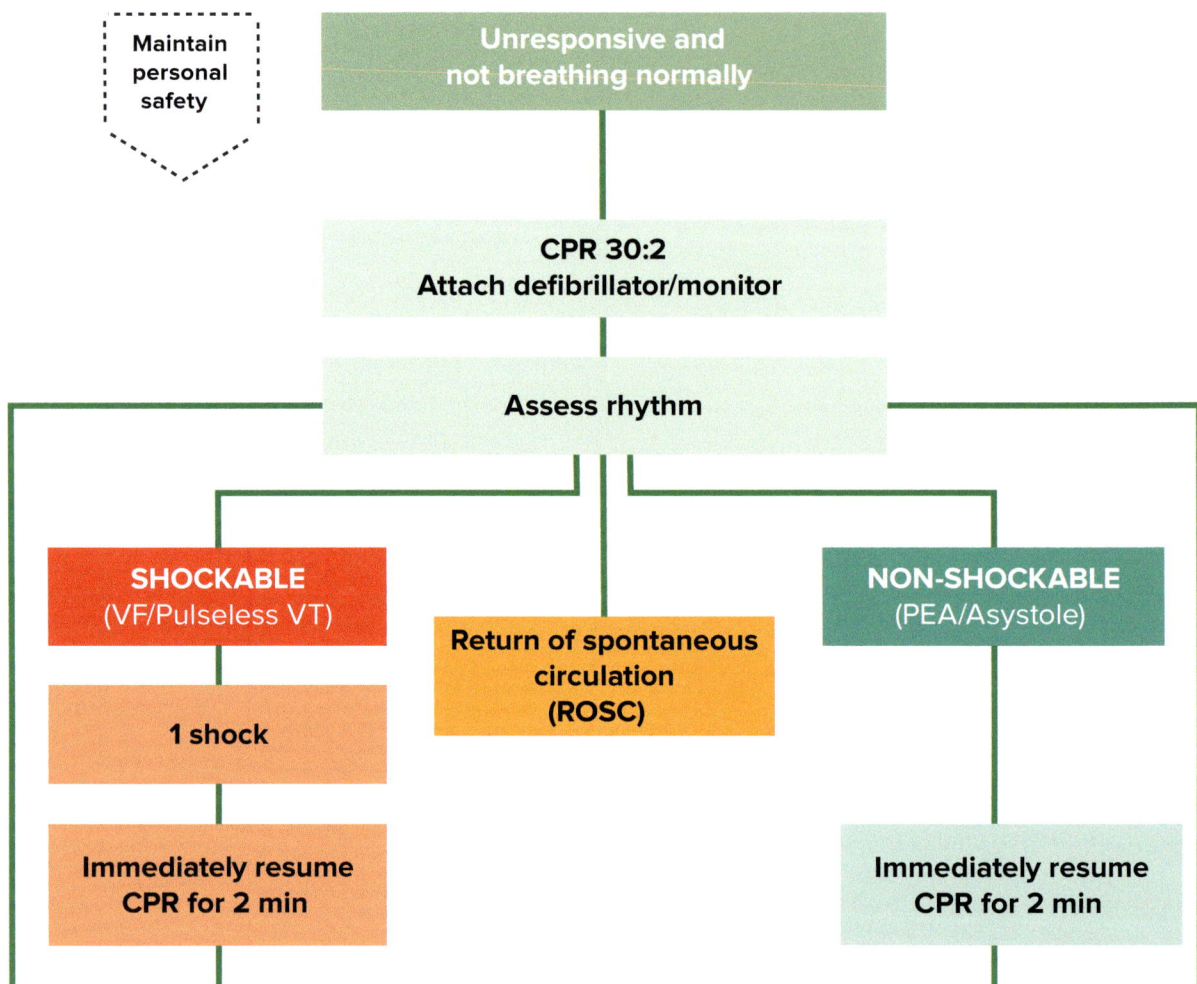

Figure 2.2 – Advanced life support in adults algorithm. Reproduced with permission from the Resuscitation Council (UK) Guidelines 2021 algorithm (www.resus.org.uk).

- Defibrillation energy levels should be at least 150 J for the first shock. Consider escalating energy for subsequent shocks.
- Give amiodarone 300 mg IV/IO after three shocks for VF/pVT, irrespective of whether these are sequential or intermittent shockable rhythms.

Advanced Life Support

- A further 150 mg may be administered after a total of 5 shocks (check dose/volume if using a pre-filled syringe).
- Promptly identify and treat reversible causes (4Hs and 4Ts).
- In most patients where ROSC is not achieved on scene, despite appropriate ALS and treatment of any reversible causes, there is little to be gained from transferring these patients to hospital. The exceptions are:
  - Children – aim for minimum scene time.
  - Refractory/recurrent VF (or pVT) – consider early departure from scene for PPCI, according to local protocols.
  - Cardiac arrest in pregnancy – make plans to undertake a time-critical transfer to hospital – this should be commenced within 5 minutes of arrival at the cardiac arrest (seek senior advice early).
  - Penetrating traumatic cardiac arrest – make plans to undertake a time-critical transfer to hospital – this should be commenced within 5 minutes of arrival at the cardiac arrest. These patients are absolutely time-critical if they are to survive.
  - Possible electrolyte disturbances (e.g. renal dialysis patients, anorexic patients, dehydration, excessive fluid intake, chronic diarrhoea and vomiting etc.).
  - Hypothermia as a contributory factor.
- In cases of **persistent** and **continuous** asystole for 30 minutes in adults, despite ALS and where all reversible causes have been identified and treated, the chances of survival are so unlikely that resuscitation can be ceased.

3. Advanced Life Support in Children

3.1 Introduction

- Paediatric ALS resuscitation broadly follows adult protocols.
  Differences between adult and paediatric resuscitation largely reflect a differing aetiology; paediatric cardiac arrest is most commonly due to hypoxia, whereas adult cardiac arrest is usually due to myocardial disease.
  The definition of a child is between 1 year and 18 years of age. A clinician should use judgement and information from relatives/bystanders to estimate the age and weight of the child. If the rescuer believes the victim to be a child, they should use the paediatric guidelines. If a misjudgement is made, and the victim turns out to be a young adult, little harm will result.
- This guideline covers:
  - infants (defined as under 1 year old)
  - children (defined as between 1 year and 18 years of age).
- In this guideline, the term 'child' includes infants, unless specified otherwise.
- Newborn life support is not covered in this guideline. For newborn babies, refer to **Newborn Life Support**.
- Initiate the delivery of good quality BLS on scene, prioritising oxygen delivery, ventilation and chest compressions. ALS procedures including defibrillation if indicated, airway management and establishing IV/IO access to deliver therapies for reversal of hypovolaemia/hypoglycaemia should be considered where resources, training and skillset permit, but should not inappropriately delay transfer to definitive care.
- Paediatric defibrillation (4 J/kg) should be carried out using paediatric defibrillation pads. However, if these are not available, use adult defibrillation pads. Ensure that the defibrillation pads are not in contact with each other; usually a front-to-back (anterior–posterior) pad placement ensures adequate pad separation.

PAEDIATRIC ALS – SUMMARY

- During ALS, the priority remains the delivery of high-quality chest compressions and effective ventilations with high-flow oxygen. Particular focus should be to ensure reversal of any hypoxia.
- Supraglottic airways (SGAs) may be considered if BVM ventilation is ineffective.
- Intubation is rarely indicated and should only be undertaken by those with appropriate skills, according to local protocols and only when waveform capnography is available.
- Defibrillation should be delivered at 4 J/kg, rounded up to the energy level the defibrillator can deliver.
- As with adults, give amiodarone IV/IO after three shocks and a further dose after five shocks. Refer to **Amiodarone Hydrochloride**, **Page for Age** for children.
- In children where hypovolaemia is thought to be a contributory factor, give a fluid bolus of 10 ml/kg (N.saline (0.9%) or Hartmann's solution), repeated once if indicated. Seek appropriate medical opinion if further boluses are thought to be indicated.

4. Defibrillation

4.1 Principles of Defibrillation

- The purpose of defibrillation is to terminate VF/pVT by passing an electrical current across the heart to depolarise a critical mass of myocardial cells.
- Defibrillation is more likely to be successful if:
  - Time from collapse to shock is minimised.
  - The collapse has been witnessed and the patient has received bystander CPR.

Advanced Life Support

Paediatric advanced life support

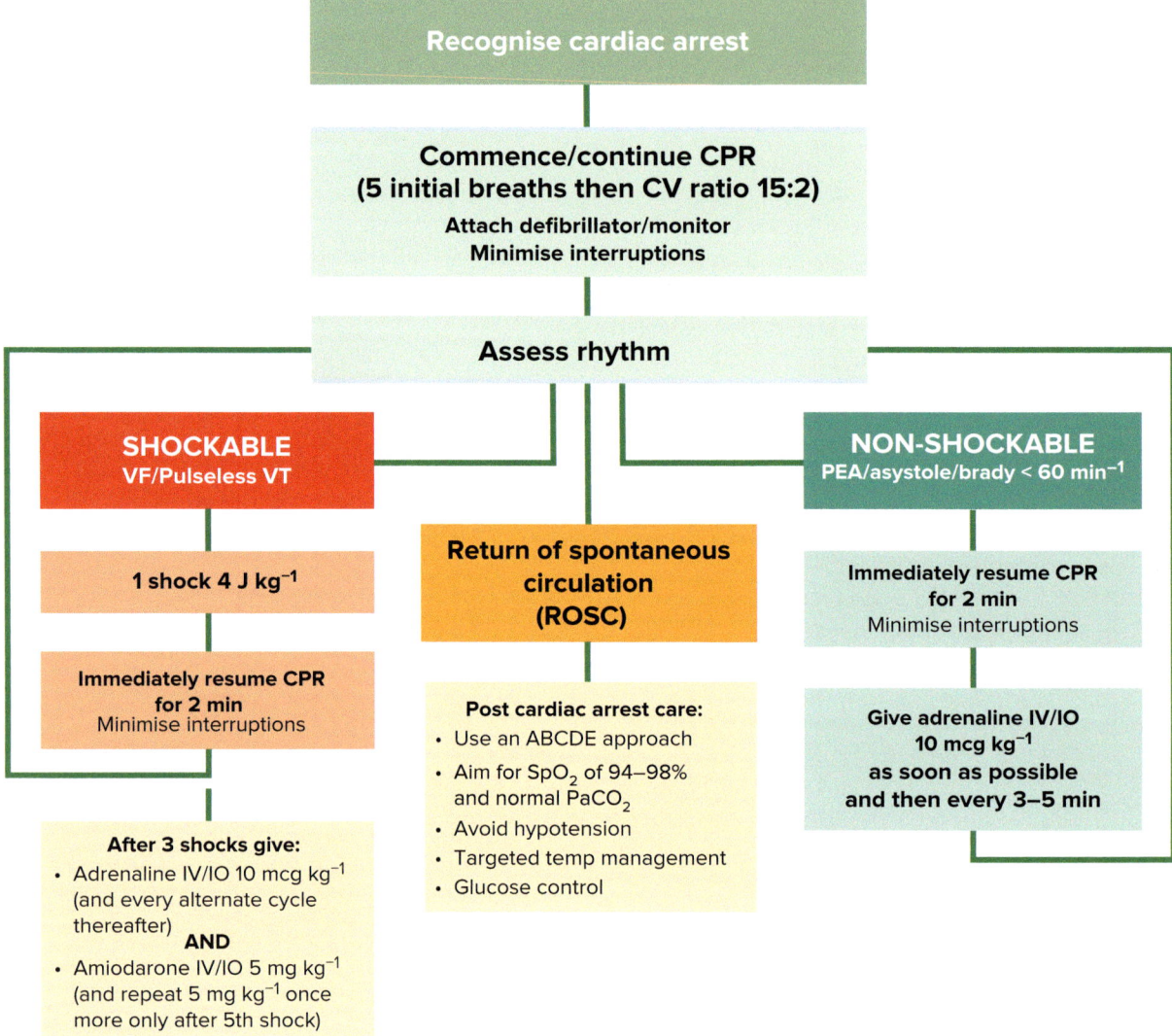

Figure 2.3 – Advanced life support in children algorithm. Reproduced with permission from the Resuscitation Council (UK) Guidelines 2021 (www.resus.org.uk).

- BLS is of good quality (correct rate and depth, complete chest recoil, minimal interruptions and maximal chest compression fraction).
- The pre-shock pause is as short as possible (< 5 secs).
- The defibrillation pads are placed correctly (refer to Figure 2.4).

- Minimise pre-shock pauses, by resuming chest compressions immediately after the rhythm check while the defibrillator charges. It is also acceptable to charge the defibrillator as the end of the 2 minutes of CPR approaches while continuing chest compressions. All team members should stand clear for the rhythm check

Advanced Life Support

so that the shock can be delivered without delay if appropriate, before immediately resuming CPR.

- Current guidelines for biphasic waveforms recommend commencing with an initial shock of at least 150 J if using a manual defibrillator. Consider increasing the energy for second and subsequent shocks if using a manual defibrillator.

- A range of defibrillation energy levels have been recommended by manufacturers and previous guidelines, ranging from 120–360 J. In the absence of any clear evidence for the optimal initial and subsequent energy levels, any energy level within this range is acceptable for the initial shock, followed by a fixed or escalating strategy up to maximum output of the defibrillator. We suggest a starting energy of at least 150 J, escalating to maximum output for refractory rhythms.

- Paediatric defibrillation should be delivered at 4 J/kg, rounded up to the nearest energy level the defibrillator can deliver. (NB Defibrillators that deliver a maximum output of 200 J at least match the current delivered by defibrillators with a 360 J output).

- When using a monitor that filters out ECG movement artefact and the underlying rhythm can be clearly seen without having to pause for a rhythm check, charge the defibrillator with ongoing CPR. If using manual chest compressions, stand clear to then deliver the shock. If using mechanical chest compression, there is no need to stop this when the shock is delivered. Note that the mechanical chest compression device may move when the shock is delivered, therefore it is important to ensure the device remains correctly positioned.

4.2 Priorities in Delivery of Defibrillation

- Delivering the first shock as soon as possible is the priority. Therefore, when attending as a solo responder equipped with a defibrillator, immediate assessment of the rhythm and defibrillation (when indicated) should take precedence over airway or breathing interventions. If possible, use a bystander to start and continue chest compressions while the defibrillator is attached. Although defibrillation is an initial priority, it is important to minimise delays and interruptions in delivering chest compressions.

4.3 Fine VF

- Immediate defibrillation should always be performed in patients where a shockable rhythm is identified on the ECG, irrespective of the amplitude. Automated defibrillators use a low threshold for the recognition of fine VF.

4.4 AED vs Manual Modes

- Most manual defibrillators carried in ambulances can also be used in an AED mode where they

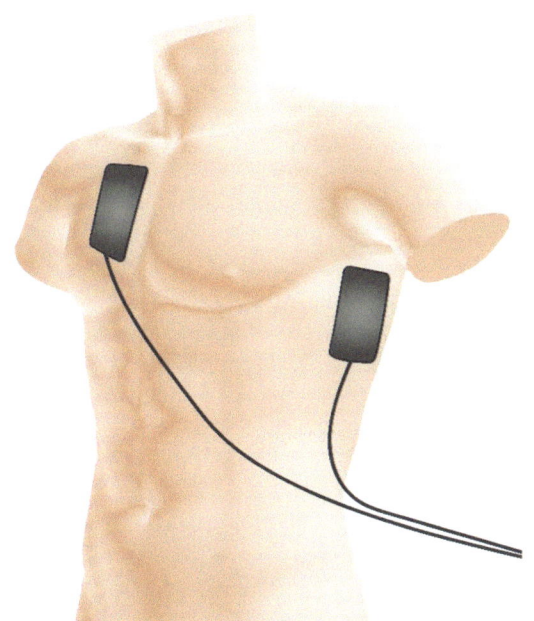

Figure 2.4 – Correct placement of defibrillation pads in the antero–lateral position. Note the relatively high and lateral positioning of the lateral pad (just below the armpit). © Charles D. Deakin. Reproduced with permission.

analyse the ECG and recommend delivery of a shock when appropriate. There are advantages and disadvantages of each mode. Although AED mode may improve the time to first shock, manual mode may reduce pre-shock pauses and increase chest compression fraction, which is associated with increased ROSC. Therefore, although manual defibrillation should be the preferred option for appropriately trained paramedics, it should be recognised that solo responders are potentially in a stressful environment and are attempting to manage multiple complex factors. Therefore, the initial use of the AED function is acceptable in these situations until additional help arrives.

4.5 Defibrillator Pads

- It is important to ensure correct pad positioning so that adequate current traverses the myocardium in order to optimise defibrillation success. In the conventional sternal–apical position the right (sternal) pad is placed to the right of the sternum, below the clavicle. The apical pad is placed in the left mid-axillary line, approximately level with the V6 ECG electrode (i.e. just below the armpit). This pad must be placed sufficiently laterally, as shown in Figure 2.4.

- Other acceptable pad positions include:
  - Anterior–posterior – one pad anteriorly, over the left precordium, and the other pad posteriorly to the heart just inferior to the left scapula and spine.
  - Bi-axillary – one pad placed just below each axilla, in the mid-axillary line (for example in

Advanced Life Support

patients with burns, or where a subcutaneous pacing box may preclude standard pad placement).

- When paediatric defibrillation pads are not available, adult pads can be used as an alternative for children. Ensure that the pads are not in contact with each other; usually a front to back (anterior–posterior) pad placement ensures adequate pad separation.

- Self-adhesive defibrillation pads have a water/electrolyte-based matrix to improve conductivity with the skin. Defibrillation pads do not need to be changed during a resuscitation attempt unless visibly damaged, although they may be replaced if the pads need to be moved for an alternative position.

- Quickly shaving the chest prior to defibrillation not only ensures better electrical contact (and therefore defibrillation success) but is likely to reduce the risk of electrical arcing between pads, which may trigger a fire.

4.6 Hands-on Defibrillation

- Hands-on defibrillation is not recommended by JRCALC. Delivering continuous chest compressions during defibrillation can minimise pre-shock pause and prevent interruption of chest compressions. However, the benefits of hands-on defibrillation are not proven, and further studies are required to assess the safety and efficacy of this technique. Standard clinical examination gloves (or bare hands) do not provide a safe level of electrical insulation.

4.7 Recurrent and Refractory VF

- Recurrent VF refers to VF that is cardioverted following each shock but returns before the next rhythm check. Recurrence of VF after a successful shock is common.

- Refractory VF refers to VF that persists despite several defibrillation attempts. In the out-of-hospital environment, it may be difficult to determine whether persistent VF is recurrent or refractory, as CPR is resumed immediately post-shock.

- Administer 300 mg amiodarone IV after the third shock and give a further 150 mg IV dose after the fifth shock.

- Optimise oxygenation and ventilation and ensure high-quality CPR.

- Ensure that the defibrillation pads are placed correctly and that electrical contact is not impaired by moisture or a hairy chest. If using antero–lateral defibrillation pad placement, ensure that the lateral pad is placed sufficiently laterally, as shown in Figure 2.4.

- Consider early transport to a primary percutaneous coronary intervention (PPCI) centre. Consider requesting enhanced care support.

4.8 Dual Sequential Defibrillation (DSD)

- JRCALC does not support use of dual sequential defibrillation. DSD involves the use of two separate manual defibrillators, delivering shocks at the same time or in rapid succession. Usually the pads from the second defibrillator are placed in an antero-posterior position to deliver a current at a different angle to the antero-lateral pads. A recent study has shown that when used for defibrillation of refractory VF, DSD is no more effective than when compared to antero-posterior pad orientation alone; the latter already being a technique recommended for defibrillation of refractory VF. Additionally, DSD is not recommended practice and it is not licensed or recommended by the defibrillator manufacturers as there is a documented risk of damage to the defibrillators.

- For cases of VF where conventional antero-lateral pad position has failed to successfully defibrillate, check that the pads are correctly positioned before considering changing to antero-posterior pad positioning (a fresh set of pads is not necessary).

4.9 Pacemakers and External Pacing

External pacing is not recommended as a core paramedic competency. If the patient is bradycardic, consider requesting enhanced care teams or clinical advice as per local procedures.

- Pacemakers (and internal defibrillators) are generally positioned below the left clavicle, although on occasion they may be placed on the right side. They appear as a subcutaneous firm mass, approximately 5 x 5 cm, over which is a scar from the insertion. Check the patient for a MedicAlert bracelet.

- In relation to resuscitation, pacemakers may have several different functions:
  - **Pacing only** – to keep the heart rate above a set level (may be ventricular pacing only, but may be set to deliver both atrial and ventricular pacing).
  - **Defibrillation only** (implantable cardioverter-defibrillator – ICD) – to monitor the heart continually and deliver a shock when a shockable arrhythmia is detected. They give no warning when firing and are programmed to give repeated shocks if indicated.
  - **Pacing and defibrillation** – a combination of both functions.

- These devices may be damaged during defibrillation if current is discharged through pads placed directly over the device.

- Place the pad away from the device (at least 8 cm) or use an alternative pad position (anterior–lateral, anterior–posterior, bi-axillary).

- Pacemakers will continue to discharge even in a patient who is deceased. This appears as

Advanced Life Support

very narrow pacing spikes on the ECG and the monitor may even display a heart rate. However, an ECG showing pacing spikes not followed by any ventricular (or atrial) complex is effectively an asystolic trace.

- Placing a magnet over a pacing device will generally result in it pacing at a fixed (asynchronous mode) rate of 50–100/min and does not stop pacemaker function.
- Placing a magnet over an ICD will result in disabling of the defibrillation function and shocks will not be delivered. This may be necessary in some cases of fast atrial arrhythmias, or if the pacing (sensing) lead is faulty, when the ICD may repeatedly discharge erroneously, which is distressing for the patient.

4.10 Safe Use of Oxygen

- Use oxygen safely during defibrillation by:
  - removing any oxygen mask or nasal cannulae and placing them at least 1 m away from the patient's chest during defibrillation
  - leaving the ventilation bag connected to the tracheal tube or SGA.
- Oxygen-powered LUCAS devices discharge large amounts of oxygen over and around the defibrillation pads which may be a significant hazard, particularly in a closed environment (e.g. the back of an ambulance).

5. Airway and Breathing Management

5.1 Introduction

- The Airways2 trial found that the initial approach to airway management is bag-mask ventilation (BVM) for approximately half of all cardiac arrest patients, with the remainder managed with a supraglottic airway (SGA) (20%) or tracheal intubation (25%).
- The most common reason cited by paramedics for changing from BVM was to carry out ALS, followed by regurgitation and inadequate ventilation.
- Inadequate ventilation was the most common reason cited for removing an SGA.
- A stepwise approach to airway management is recommended. This should include a strategy on how and when to progress from one airway technique to another.
- It should be noted that the stepwise approach is not one way. If a technique is failing, then it is sometimes more appropriate to move to a less advanced technique than to attempt techniques that are more advanced.
- However, in the context of out-of-hospital cardiac arrest, it might also be appropriate to move directly to more advanced techniques, depending on the circumstances. For example, the early application of an SGA may be beneficial, rather than attempting oropharyngeal or nasopharyngeal airways. Tracheal intubation as the initial airway is not recommended; use of a BVM or SGA should proceed any attempt at tracheal intubation.
- Laryngoscopy remains an important skill for visually inspecting the oropharynx in choking, and should be part of ongoing competency assessments.
- Staff attending the arrest will need to be trained to provide support to the clinician that is performing the intubation, such as preparing and passing the equipment.

Spinal precautions must be started at the same time as airway management, but these do not take priority. Refer to **Spinal Injury and Spinal Cord Injury**.

5.2 Bag-mask Ventilation (BVM)

- The initial approach to airway management should usually be BVM. An oropharyngeal airway (OPA) or nasopharyngeal airway (NPA) may be used to improve the efficacy of ventilations via the BVM.
- A complication of ventilation with a BVM is gastric inflation, resulting in impaired ventilation and regurgitation, especially where forceful ventilations are delivered. This risk is reduced where gentle ventilations are delivered over 1 second or where an SGA is used. As such, it is reasonable to place a suitable SGA as part of BLS, when trained in its use.

5.3 Airway Sizes

- Table 2.3 provides a guide for airway sizes in children and adults.

5.4 Supraglottic Airways

- There are several SGAs (e.g. iGel and laryngeal mask airway); all sit above the larynx, and are simpler and quicker to insert than a tracheal tube. They can be inserted with minimal interruption to chest compressions.
- A number of case reports exist describing patients who have been found to have foreign bodies deep within their oropharynx. It is therefore recommended that if there is a high degree of suspicion of foreign body airway obstruction, inspection of the oropharynx should be undertaken with a laryngoscope before inserting any SGA.
- Once an SGA has been placed, continuous chest compressions with 10 ventilations per minute are preferred. However, 30 compressions to two ventilations are acceptable if ventilation is inadequate when delivering continuous compressions.

Advanced Life Support

- Waveform capnography should always be used when using a supraglottic device and BVM.
- Air leaks from around the SGA are common. If the chest wall can be seen to be moving, ventilation is generally adequate. However, repositioning or replacement of the airway with a more suitable size may be necessary if the air leak is of sufficient magnitude to prevent the chest rising and falling with each breath.

5.5 Tracheal Intubation

- The tracheal tube is a challenging airway device to insert successfully and requires both adequate initial training and ongoing practice. Paramedics must ensure that they have appropriate competence to undertake it safely and that this skill has been regularly updated and evidenced through maintaining an airway skills log.
- There is no evidence that patient outcome is any better following tracheal intubation compared with any other type of airway.
- When tracheal intubation is undertaken, the availability of a bougie and use of waveform capnography is mandatory.
- Where, as a paramedic, the governance system you work within allows you to intubate, you should only do so if you have maintained your skills and have evidence of self-audit with a success rate of greater than 95% success rate within two attempts.
- Visualisation of the tube entering the trachea, auscultation over both axillae and epigastrium, and observation of chest wall movement should all aid confirmation but are not in themselves 100% diagnostic of correct tube placement. This can only be achieved by using waveform capnography.
- If the capnography trace is flat (or only shows minimal baseline fluctuation), then it must be assumed that the tracheal tube is sited incorrectly and must be removed.
- Once a tracheal tube is in place, continue continuous chest compressions with 10 gentle ventilations per minute. Avoid hyperventilation and high airway pressures during manual ventilation which adversely affect outcome.
- It is important to remember the following for tracheal intubation:
  - Ensure 360° access around the patient where possible. (This may involve rapidly moving the patient to give better access.)
  - Prepare a kit dump of all the necessary equipment close to the patient before starting the process of intubation. This must include suction, a bougie and immediate access to capnography monitoring and any additional airway equipment necessary for a failed intubation.
  - Do not routinely use cricoid pressure for tracheal intubation during CPR.
  - If during laryngoscopy the paramedic needs a better view, use external laryngeal manipulation. Pressure directed to move the trachea backwards, upwards and to the right (BURP manoeuvre) may improve visualisation of the vocal cords.
  - Secure the tracheal tube immediately after insertion, noting length at incisors. This is approximately:
    - adult males: 22–24 cm
    - adult females: 21–23 cm.
  - Listen to any team member who suggests that the attempt has become a 'Can't intubate, can't ventilate scenario', irrespective of clinical grade.
  - Avoid hypoxaemia during intubation: pre-oxygenate the lungs before and between intubation attempts.
  - Where possible, use two team members to attempt intubation, and ensure a failed intubation plan has been communicated to all the team.

5.6 Capnography

- Capnography (measurement of exhaled (end-tidal) carbon dioxide – $EtCO_2$) assists in confirmation and continuous monitoring of tracheal tube placement, can provide feedback on the quality of CPR and can provide an early ROSC.
- Waveform capnography is a real-time waveform display of $EtCO_2$ and is more accurate and reliable than a paper indicator.
- The use of waveform capnography is mandatory in paramedic intubation. Tracheal intubation and subsequent monitoring must only be performed with the assistance of waveform capnography monitoring. Recorded values must be documented on the patient record at 5-minute intervals. In the absence of waveform capnography, an alternative airway technique or device should be employed.
- Any decision to terminate resuscitation should not be based on either the presence or absence of $EtCO_2$ alone.
- Waveform capnography is recommended where an SGA has been placed, as it is useful in providing positive feedback on the quality of CPR.

Advanced Life Support

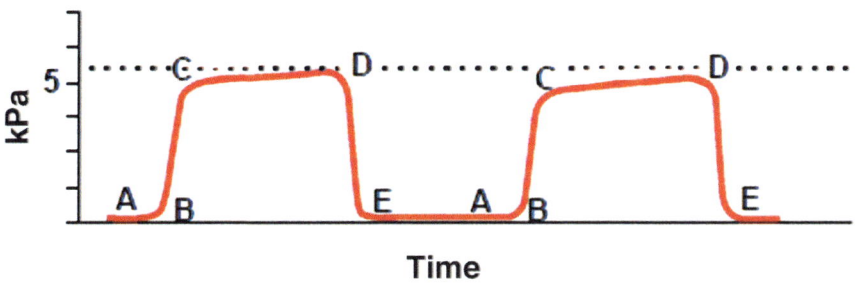

A-B: Baseline
B-C: Expiratory upstroke
C-D: Expiratory plateau
D: EtCO$_2$
D-E: Inspiration

Figure 2.5 – Capnography.

TABLE 2.3 – Airway Sizes by Type			
Age	**Airway Size by Device Type**		
	Oropharyngeal	**SGA**	**Cuffed Tracheal tube** **Internal diameter** **Length at the lips**
Birth	000 (ISO 3.5)	1.0	Diameter: 3.0 mm Length: 10 cm
1 month	00 (ISO 5.0)	1.0	Diameter: 3.0 mm Length: 10 cm
3 months	00 (ISO 5.0)	1.5	Diameter: 3.0 mm Length: 11 cm
6 months	00 (ISO 5.0)	1.5	Diameter: 3.0 mm Length: 12 cm
9 months	00 (ISO 5.0)	1.5	Diameter: 3.0 mm Length: 12 cm
12 months	00 OR 0 (ISO 5.0 or 5.5)	1.5 OR 2.0	Diameter: 3.5 mm Length: 13 cm
18 months	00 OR 0 (ISO 5.0 or 5.5)	1.5 OR 2.0	Diameter: 3.5 mm Length: 13 cm
2 years	0 OR 1 (ISO 5.5 or 6.5)	1.5 OR 2.0	Diameter: 4.0 mm Length: 14 cm
3 years	1 (ISO 6.5)	2.0	Diameter: 4.0 mm Length: 14 cm
4 years	1 (ISO 6.5)	2.0	Diameter: 4.5 mm Length: 15 cm
5 years	1 (ISO 6.5)	2.0	Diameter: 4.5 mm Length: 15 cm
6 years	1 (ISO 6.5)	2.0	Diameter: 5.0 mm Length: 16 cm
7 years	1 OR 2 (ISO 6.5 or 8.0)	2.0	Diameter: 5.0 mm Length: 16 cm
8 years	1 OR 2 (ISO 6.5 or 8.0)	2.5	Diameter: 5.5 mm Length: 17 cm

(continued)

Advanced Life Support

TABLE 2.3 – Airway Sizes by Type *(continued)*

Age	Airway Size by Device Type		
	Oropharyngeal	SGA	Cuffed Tracheal tube Internal diameter Length at the lips
9 years	1 OR 2 (ISO 6.5 or 8.0)	2.5	Diameter: 6.0 mm Length: 17 cm
10 years	2 OR 3 (ISO 8.0 or 9.0)	2.5 OR 3.0	Diameter: 6.5 mm Length: 18 cm
11 years	2 OR 3 (ISO 8.0 or 9.0)	2.5 OR 3.0	Diameter: 6.5 mm Length: 18 cm
Adult >70 kg	4 OR 5 (ISO 10 or 12)	4.0 OR 5.0	Female diameter: 7.0–8.0 mm Length: 21–23 cm Male diameter: 8.0–9.0 mm Length: 22–24 cm

6. Mechanical Chest Compression Devices (mCPR)

- Mechanical chest compression (mCPR) devices are designed to provide consistent high-quality chest compressions to the required depth and frequency for prolonged periods of time.

  mCPR can act as an additional rescuer, enabling uninterrupted chest compressions while attention is focused on delivering other aspects of ALS.

  Delivery of manual chest compressions is often inconsistent and subject to fatigue, particularly when wearing PPE, during prolonged resuscitation. mCPR can be of particular benefit during extrication and transport in a moving vehicle to ensure continuous chest compressions and ensure rescuer safety.

  In patients presenting with a shockable rhythm, mechanical devices should not be used prior to the first shock.

- However, large randomised controlled trials of the routine use of mCPR in the out-of-hospital setting have found no evidence of improved patient outcome compared with manual CPR. Routine use of mCPR is therefore not indicated.

- In particular mCPR should be considered during the extrication and transportation of a patient in cardiac arrest, when prolonged CPR is indicated (e.g. ECMO, hypothermia, refractory VF etc.) or for patients being taken to the cath lab for PCI where manual chest compression during the procedure is not possible.

- mCPR should be deployed by dedicated teams that are regularly drilled, practised and signed off in its deployment to ensure effective use and minimal interruption to CPR during its placement.

6.1 Impedance Threshold Valve

- In the same way that gasping generates negative intrathoracic pressure, mechanical devices that enhance negative intrathoracic pressure during CPR may also increase venous return and enhance forward blood flow.
- Some, but not all, studies have shown that impedance threshold devices (ITDs) may improve outcome; but where they are effective, they appear to be so only in the context of CPR that delivers correct compression rate and depth.
- Further studies are required to understand the possible benefits of this device.

7. Head-up CPR

- A head-up position improves cerebral venous return by facilitating cerebral venous drainage. It also lowers intracranial pressure, which together results in an increase in cerebral perfusion pressure.
- Animal and human cadaver studies have suggested that gradual head and thorax elevation to an angle of 30° while performing CPR, **when combined with** an ITD and active compression–decompression CPR, improves cerebral perfusion pressures.
- In the absence of any clinical studies, the use of head-up CPR must only be undertaken in the context of a closely monitored trial or evaluation, with regular review of neurological outcome in survivors.

Advanced Life Support

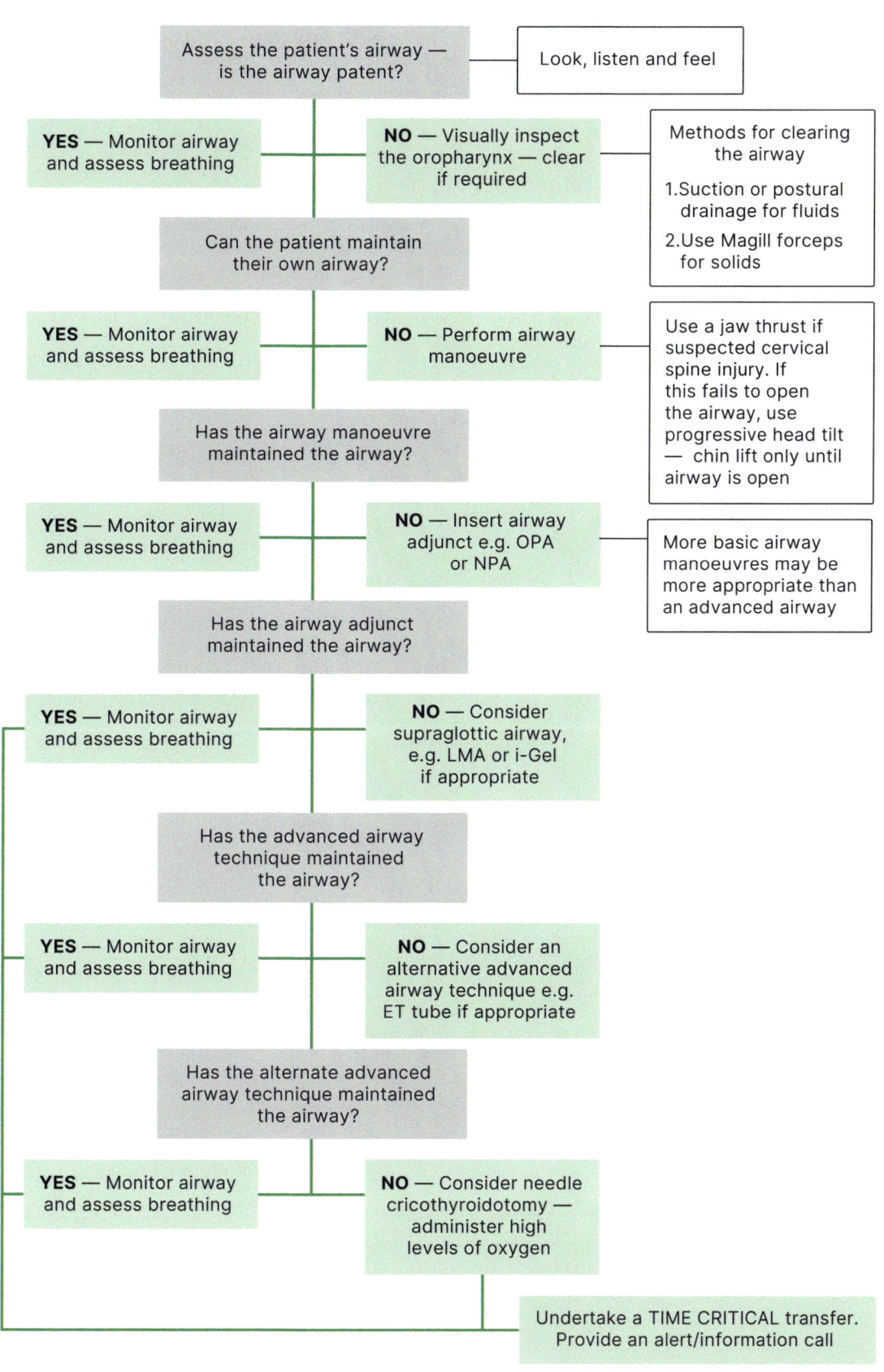

Figure 2.6 – Breathing assessment and management overview.

Advanced Life Support

8. Extra-Corporeal Membrane Oxygenation (ECMO) and Possible Out-of-Hospital Applications

- One area of growing interest is the use of ECMO in refractory cardiac arrest, where survival is poor.
- Conventional cardiopulmonary resuscitation involves chest compressions, which produce a 'low-flow' cardiac output. The longer the period of chest compressions, the greater the likelihood of irreversible organ damage, and the less the chance of an ROSC.
- Because ECMO can match a normal native cardiac output (5.0 litres/min), it is very effective in perfusing the heart and the brain, and preventing on going damage despite a patient being in cardiac arrest.
- When used in this way, it is referred to as extracorporeal cardiopulmonary resuscitation (ECPR). It is normally achieved by placing a large cannula in the femoral vein to drain venous blood, and pumping oxygenated blood back through another large cannula placed in the femoral artery.
- Some ambulance services in Europe and North America have begun trials of pre-hospital ECPR for out-of-hospital cardiac arrest. Trials are shortly planned for the UK.

9. CPR-induced Consciousness

- In some patients, the application of CPR, particularly when using mCPR, may produce sufficient cerebral perfusion for signs of consciousness in the absence of ROSC.

9.1 Characteristics

- Patients may display a variety of signs, including:
  - eye opening
  - increased jaw tone
  - incomprehensible sounds
  - recognisable words or speech
  - limb movement
  - purposeful movements, e.g. localising to pain
  - combative movements, e.g. pushing rescuers away.

9.2 Key Points for CPR-induced Consciousness

- Even if a patient is displaying any of these features, ad hoc rhythm checks are not recommended and paramedics should limit rhythm checks to once every 2 minutes, as per conventional guidance.
- CPR-induced consciousness (CPR-IC) should be recognised at the earliest opportunity. Signs that may help paramedics distinguish CPR-IC from ROSC may include:
  - an absence of palpable pulses
  - a rapid deterioration in consciousness when chest compressions are stopped
  - a cardiac rhythm considered incompatible with life.
- In patients with symptoms that create difficulty in delivering high-quality CPR, or when the patient may be distressed, paramedics may wish to consider requesting enhanced care support or advice as per local procedures/pathways or rapid conveyance to hospital to facilitate ongoing treatment.

10. Reversible Causes and Specialist Circumstances in Cardiac Arrest (4Hs and 4Ts)

10.1 Hypoxia

- All patients in cardiac arrest should be ventilated with high-concentration (100%) oxygen to minimise the risk of hypoxia. Ensure regular checks of the oxygen cylinder and replace it if needed before the cylinder runs empty.

10.2 Hypovolaemia

- Most patients who suffer a cardiac arrest due to a cardiac cause are not hypovolaemic. IV fluids are not indicated in these patients during CPR because excess intravascular filling may worsen coronary perfusion. However, in patients who suffer a cardiac arrest due to blood loss or a depleted intravascular volume (e.g. sepsis or severe dehydration), hypovolaemia may require treatment. Prioritise management of hypovolaemia by controlling any catastrophic haemorrhage. Where hypovolaemia is suspected, intravascular volume should be restored rapidly with IV (or IO) fluid. Up to 2 litres of normal saline should be rapidly infused. Early transportation of these patients should be considered.

10.3 Hypo/hyperkalaemia (and Hypoglycaemia)

- Diagnosing this in the pre-hospital setting is challenging. The patient's medical history or identification of a dialysis fistula may give an indication of dialysis history and potential hyperkalaemia. Patients with a history of diabetic ketoacidosis (DKA) will often also have a high serum potassium. Patients living with frailty, or patients with eating disorders, who have a recent history of gastric disease, may have low serum potassium. On suspicion or identification of any potential reversible metabolic disorder, a time-critical transfer to hospital should be considered.
- Blood sugar should remain an important consideration during cardiac arrest and should be undertaken as soon as practical, commencing during the actual cardiac arrest itself. Hypoglycaemia can cause significant

Advanced Life Support

brain injury, and this will occur if the patient is hypoglycaemic during the actual cardiac arrest itself. Blood sugar should therefore be monitored both during the arrest and in the post-ROSC period. Hypoglycaemia is rarely, if ever, a primary cause of cardiac arrest; hypoglycaemia is usually a result of cardiac arrest itself. However, identification and treatment of hypoglycaemia is important, in order to optimise the chances of neurologically intact survival. When measuring blood sugar during a cardiac arrest, a IV or IO sample should be used where possible (a capillary sample may be less accurate but is acceptable if it is not possible to obtain an IV sample). Blood glucose monitors are not calibrated for IV or IO samples (although they are likely to still be accurate). If hypoglycaemia is identified, IV glucose should be administered as appropriate (refer to **Glycaemic Emergencies in Adults and Children**), and the blood sugar rechecked at regular intervals until normal levels are obtained.

10.4 Hypothermia

- Accidental hypothermia is often under-diagnosed in temperate climates. Generally, hypothermia can develop during exposure to cold environments and in people who have been immobilised or immersed in cold water. In the older/frail person and the very young, where thermoregulation is impaired, hypothermia can follow a very mild insult. The risk of hypothermia is also increased by exhaustion, illness, injury, neglect, reduced level of consciousness or when drugs or alcohol have been ingested.

- Severe hypothermia is associated with the depression of cerebral blood flow and oxygen requirement, reduced cardiac output and decreased arterial pressure. Patients can appear to be clinically dead because of significant depression of brain and cardiovascular function, but the threshold for full resuscitation should remain low, as recovery with intact neurology is possible.

- The patient's peripheral pulses and respiratory effort may be difficult to detect. Therefore, resuscitation should not be withheld based on clinical presentation. Consider whether on the basis of history, hypothermia is believed to be the primary cause of the cardiac arrest. If hypothermia is believed to be the primary cause, follow the guidance below.

- Pre-hospital core temperature measurement can be inaccurate and so should not always be relied upon to confirm hypothermia. In a hypothermic patient, resuscitation should not be withheld unless the cause of the cardiac arrest is clearly attributable to fatal illness, prolonged asphyxia, lethal injury or if the chest is incompressible.

- Because hypothermia itself may produce a very slow, small-volume, irregular pulse and unrecordable blood pressure, signs of life may be so minimal that it is easy to overlook them. Palpate a major artery, obtain an ECG and look for signs of life (pulse, chest rise, breathing efforts, movements, eye opening or shockable rhythm) for up to 1 minute before concluding that there is no cardiac output. Hypothermia can cause stiffness of the chest wall, making chest compressions and ventilations difficult; however, if the patient is pulseless, start chest compressions and ventilations at the same rate as for normothermic patients.

- It is important to prevent further heat loss from the patient's body core, by removing wet garments (providing this does not result in additional exposure) and protecting against heat loss and wind chill by using blankets/heated blankets, head coverings and insulating equipment.

- The hypothermic heart may be unresponsive to cardioactive drugs and defibrillation; therefore, when the temperature is 30–35°C, double intervals between medicines should be used, e.g. adrenaline every 6–10 minutes.

- Where the core temperature is <30°C, no drugs should be administered until the temperature reaches 30°C, at which point double intervals of adrenaline should be used. A maximum of three shocks should be delivered to a patient in a shockable rhythm below 30°C. Double intervals between adrenaline should only be used in cases where hypothermia is thought to be the main or precipitating cause of the arrest.

- Consider hospital bypass to a centre that can provide extracorporeal rewarming and phone ahead to discuss the case, as per local procedures.

10.5 Hyperthermia

- Hyperthermia occurs when the body's ability to thermoregulate fails and core temperature exceeds that normally maintained by homeostatic mechanisms. Either the body's metabolic heat production or environmental heat load exceeds the body's normal heat loss capacity, or heat loss is impaired.

- In addition to heat stroke, patients with acute behavioural disorder (ABD) often present with hyperthermia. Both groups are at risk of hyperthermia, contributing to metabolic disturbance and an ensuing cardiac arrest.

- When managing the hyperthermic patient in cardiac arrest, follow standard procedures for basic and advanced life support and cool the patient by removing excess clothing and

Advanced Life Support

adjusting the surrounding environmental temperature if possible.

- Prognosis is poor when compared to normothermic cardiac arrests. High body temperature is capable of producing irreversible brain damage and the risk of unfavourable neurological outcome increases for each degree of body temperature above 37°C.

10.6 Toxins

- Patients who may have ingested a deliberate or accidental amount of toxin before their cardiac arrest should be transported to the ED, with effective resuscitation delivered en route. Consider mechanical CPR if resuscitation attempts are likely to be prolonged. If possible, communication regarding the suspected ingestion substance should be made with the ED as early as possible. Crew safety regarding cross-contamination must always be a high priority in these situations.
- Where there is suspicion of poisoning of unknown origin (e.g. snake or animal bites), the antidote is required rapidly and will rarely be available in the pre-hospital setting. Paramedics should therefore aim for rapid conveyance with pre-alert.
- Refer to **Overdose and Poisoning in Adults and Children**.

10.7 Tension Pneumothorax

- The diagnosis of a tension pneumothorax in the pre-hospital environment can be challenging. If there is suspicion of tension pneumothorax, supported by clinical findings, the chest should be decompressed using needle thoracentesis. This procedure may not always relieve the tension and even in patients where it does, a tension pneumothorax may recur as the cannula becomes blocked or dislodged. A high index of suspicion should be applied to any re-occurrence of tension pneumothorax.
- Consider enhanced care for insertion of a more definitive thoracostomy incision.

10.8 Thrombosis – Coronary or Pulmonary

- **Coronary** Where the rhythm is shockable, this should be managed as outlined in the ALS algorithm.
- **Pulmonary** This will be challenging to diagnose in the cardiac arrest situation. If available, the patient's history before cardiac arrest may give some indication. If pulmonary thrombosis is suspected, a time-critical transfer to hospital is indicated. In situations where thrombolysis is administered, CPR for as long as 90 mins may be required to break up the clot. In these circumstances, consider mechanical CPR.

Intra-arrest thrombolysis can be considered if available: follow local pathways but do not delay conveyance to hospital.

10.9 Cardiac Tamponade

- Diagnosis of this in the pre-hospital environment is challenging due to its occult nature. Cardiac tamponade compresses the heart, prevents adequate filling and ejection and leads to cardiac arrest; it requires urgent decompression. Therefore, if suspected, a time-critical transfer to hospital is indicated. Consider enhanced care support where available.
- In patients presenting in pulseless electrical activity (PEA), evaluation of the ECG waveform may assist in identifying any reversible causes. Figure 2.7 shows a classification of PEA according to the reversible cause.

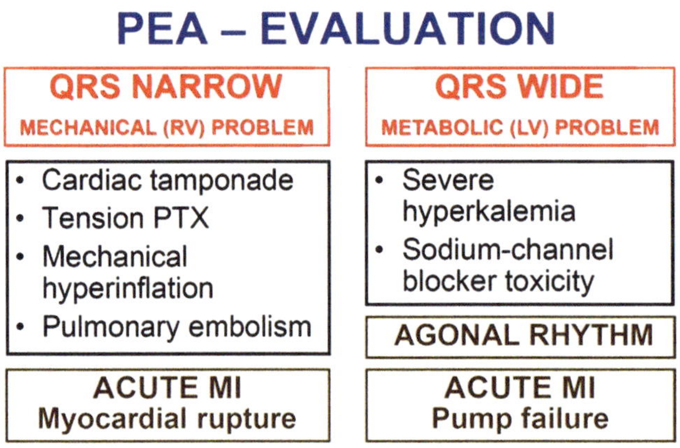

PEA – EVALUATION

QRS NARROW MECHANICAL (RV) PROBLEM	QRS WIDE METABOLIC (LV) PROBLEM
• Cardiac tamponade • Tension PTX • Mechanical hyperinflation • Pulmonary embolism	• Severe hyperkalemia • Sodium-channel blocker toxicity
	AGONAL RHYTHM
ACUTE MI Myocardial rupture	**ACUTE MI** Pump failure

Figure 2.7 – Classification of PEA based on its initial electrocardiographic manifestation. LV = Left ventricular; PTX = pneumothorax; RV = right ventricular. Source: Littmann L et al. Med Princ Pract 2014. Simplified and Structured Teaching Tool for the Evaluation and Management of Pulseless Electrical Activity. Republished with permission.

Advanced Life Support

11. Special Considerations in Cardiac Arrest

Use of Ultrasound

Ultrasound can be a useful tool in supporting and guiding resuscitation practice to help determine the cause of the arrest. It should not be used as the sole determinant to terminate resuscitation. Staff must have had appropriate additional training in order to use it and this is unlikely to be available for core paramedics.

11.1 Pregnancy

- Refer to **Maternal Resuscitation**.
- Establishing effective resuscitation, focusing on delivering ALS to the mother, is the first priority. Specific modifications include:
  - The hand position for chest compressions may need to be slightly higher on the sternum for patients in the third trimester.
  - Hypoxia and hypovolaemia are common causes of maternal cardiac arrest and should be considered early.
  - Tracheal intubation may be considerably more difficult. A tracheal tube may need to be 0.5–1.0 mm smaller than that for a non-pregnant woman of the same size.
  - Manually displace the uterus to the left to ensure that there is adequate venous return to the heart. Add left lateral tilt (ideally 15–30° but even a small amount of tilt may be better than no tilt).
  - Make plans to undertake a time-critical transfer to hospital – this should be commenced within 5 minutes of arrival at the cardiac arrest.
- Advanced life support intervention can be carried out en route. Emphasise the pregnancy at the earliest opportunity during pre-alert to allow for further specialist hospital staff to be available to perform a peri-mortem caesarean section on arrival to resus if indicated.

11.2 Drowning

- Refer to **Drowning**.

11.3 Asthma

- Cardiac arrest in the asthmatic patient is often a terminal event after a period of hypoxaemia and respiratory exhaustion, and is associated with:
  - Severe bronchospasm and mucous plugging leading to asphyxia.
  - Cardiac arrhythmias due to hypoxia, stimulant drug or electrolyte abnormalities.
  - Dynamic hyperinflation where a gradual build-up of pressure occurs which reduces venous return and blood pressure.
  - Tension pneumothorax (sometimes bilateral).
- Consideration of reversible causes (the 4Hs and 4Ts) will help identify these causes of cardiac arrest. Management of cardiac arrest in asthma patients should follow standard ALS guidelines while incorporating the following recommendations:
  - Ventilation may be difficult because of increased airway resistance; a two-person technique may assist.
  - If dynamic hyperinflation is suspected during CPR, manual compression of the chest wall and/or a period of planned apnoea achieved by disconnecting the BVM from the tracheal tube may reduce gas trapping.
  - There is a significant risk of gastric inflation and hypoventilation of the lungs when ventilating a severely asthmatic patient; therefore, consider early tracheal intubation where required.
  - Regularly check for evidence of reversible causes, specifically tension pneumothorax.
- Decompress suspected pneumothoraces and consider enhanced/critical care support to perform a thoracostomy. **NB:** Bilateral needle decompression will not make the situation worse and may reverse the cause of the cardiac arrest.

11.4 Opioid Overdose

- Cardiac arrest following opioid overdose (OD) is usually secondary to a respiratory arrest. If cardiac arrest occurs, follow standard resuscitation guidelines while incorporating the following modifications:
  - Administering naloxone is unlikely to cause harm; it can be given where opioid OD is likely. The usual adult dose is 400 microgram IV/IO, which should be titrated to affect every 60 seconds, with the subsequent doses being 800 microgram IV/IO. Administer incrementally until the patient is breathing adequately and is able to protect their airway.
  - If no response is observed after a total of 10 mg IV/IO naloxone, consider a non-opioid-related drug or other cause.
  - The administration of Naloxone should not compromise the provision of quality CPR, early defibrillation and adequate airway management and effective ventilation.
  - Prolonged resuscitation may be appropriate in this cohort of patients, as good neurological outcome is possible. Cessation of resuscitation should be in consultation with a senior clinician.

11.5 Rhythm-affecting Drugs

- Consider the effect that rhythm-affecting drugs (e.g. beta blockers, tricyclic anti-depressants, cocaine etc.) and non-opiate recreational drugs may have on cardiac output before terminating a resuscitation attempt. Follow normal ALS guidance for these patient groups.

Advanced Life Support

11.6 Bariatric Patients

- While normal ALS guidance and shock protocols should be followed in the resuscitation of bariatric patients, it is recognised that delivery of effective CPR may be challenging. Chest compressions will be difficult to perform in many patients, simply because of suboptimal positioning of rescuers. A step or platform may be required, or compressions can be performed from the patient's head end.

- Additional rescuers may be required to assist due to rescuer fatigue, particularly in relation to the delivery of chest compressions. It may be necessary to change the CPR provider more frequently and mechanical devices may not accommodate this patient group. Although chest compressions are most effective when performed with the patient lying on a firm surface, where it is unsafe to attempt to move the patient they may remain on a mattress, as the heavier torso compresses the surface, leaving less potential for displacement during chest compressions.

- Higher inspiration pressure is needed for positive pressure ventilation due to increased intra-abdominal pressure. In all patients with extreme obesity, difficult intubation must be anticipated, with a clear failed intubation drill if necessary.

- It is important to request additional resources to assist with moving the patient, with consideration for specially adapted vehicles. Weight limits of equipment must be checked before use. Underestimation of the technical aspects of rescue operations may cause trauma or prohibit safe transfer of bariatric patients.

12. Chemical, Biological, Radiological and Nuclear (CBRN) Incidents

- The key priority of the first medical personnel on arrival at a chemical, biological, radiological and nuclear (CBRN) incident is to ensure all emergency service control centres are alerted and specialist resources are summoned early.

- If there is one casualty, rescuers may approach as usual. If there are two casualties, only approach with caution, considering all options. If there are three or more casualties, one should not approach. Instead withdraw, contain the scene, report the situation, self-isolate and await specialist resources.

- A patient in cardiac arrest as a result of a CBRN incident should only be approached and treated once the risk to rescuers is known. A chemical incident may initially present with patients in a peri or actual cardiac arrest. Proper scene management of chemical incidents is crucial for preventing further exposure and incident escalation. Early pattern recognition of chemical agent syndromes is vital, and paramedics should be aware of the constant threat of this type of incident. These can result from terrorist action, or industrial and chemical incidents, as well as isolated cases of toxic exposure.

- The signs of a CBRN incident can often be subtle or delayed, and emergency medical personnel should always be vigilant for abnormal situational or patient factors that raise suspicion of a CBRN incident. Exposure to a CBRN agent can occur through direct contact, inhalation, injection, ingestion or irradiation.

12.1 Personal Protection

- Rescuers must not approach potential casualties unless adequate PPE is worn.

- Personal protection is paramount if a CBRN incident is suspected. If in doubt, the rescuer should withdraw to a place of safety until the CBRN threat can be accurately identified and the necessary PPE brought to the scene.

- Entering a CBRN scene without adequate PPE puts the rescuer at risk of harm and also risks spread of contamination. A CBRN patient will need decontamination before being able to receive advanced medical care.

- There are also an increasing number of individual chemical exposure incidents in the UK, this may occur as a result of suicide or agricultural accidents, for example. There are a number of different agents commonly used, which include:
  - hydrogen sulphide (made by mixing a combination of household chemicals)
  - aluminium phosphide (from rat poison)
  - cyanide salts
  - helium gas
  - nitrogen gas
  - carbon monoxide (e.g. from a disposable BBQ or car exhaust).

13. Trauma

- Establishing the cause of cardiac arrest may not be straightforward. A primary medical arrest can occur before a patient suffers a secondary traumatic insult. Primary medical cardiac arrests resulting in falls from height or while driving are examples that can typically result in rescuers suspecting cardiac arrest of traumatic origin.

- Pay close attention to a witness history and perform an accurate scene assessment to establish the course of events and mechanism of injury. If there is a possibility that the patient has had a primary medical cardiac arrest, follow standard BLS and ALS guidelines. Where trauma is considered to be the primary cause of the arrest, consider early enhanced care support and follow the traumatic cardiac arrest algorithm in Figure 2.8.

Advanced Life Support

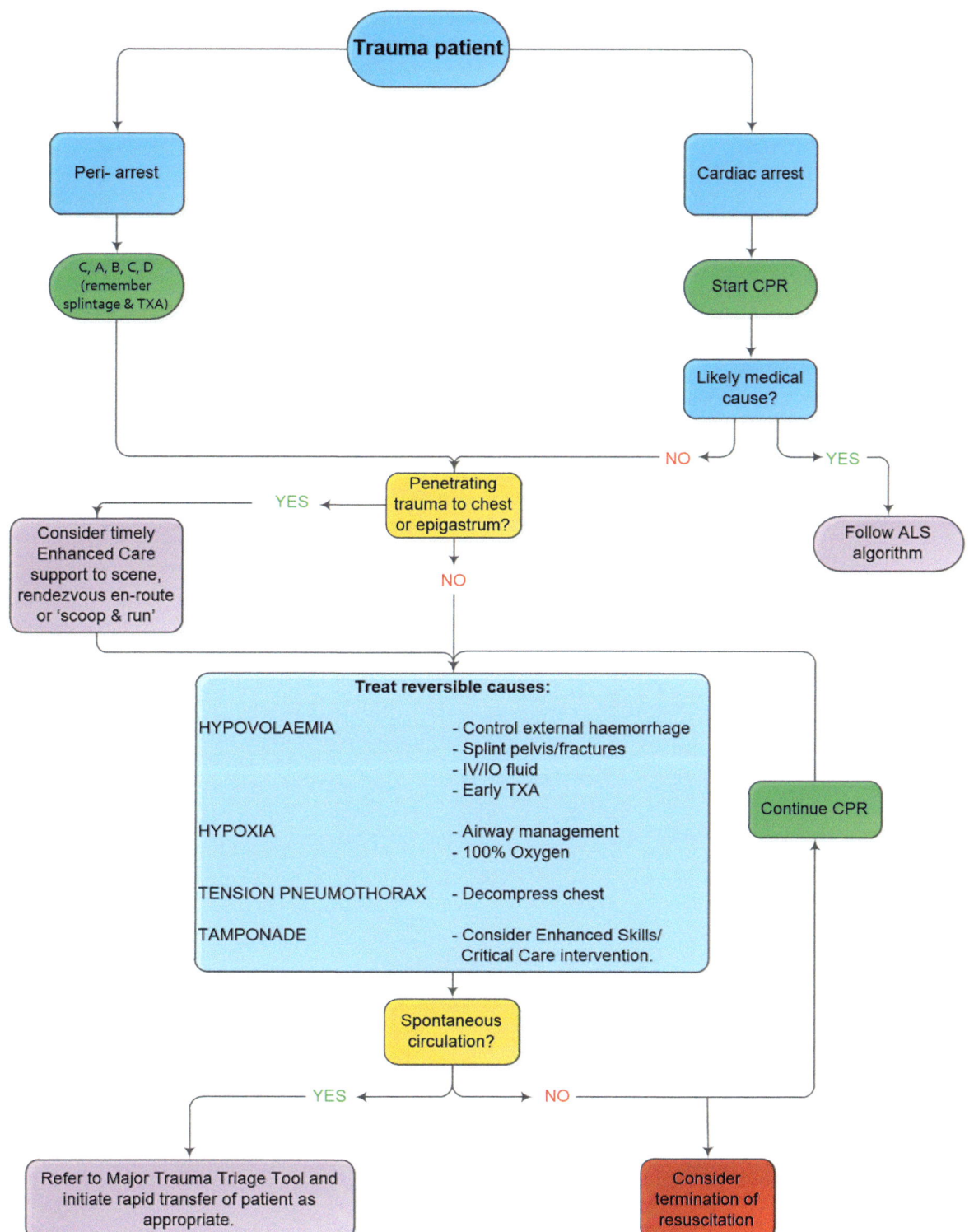

Figure 2.8 – Traumatic cardiac arrest algorithm. Source: Resuscitation Council (UK), 2015.

- Patients who are in cardiac arrest following drowning, hanging or asphyxiation should not automatically be conveyed to a major trauma centre (MTC) (unless there is significant mechanism to trigger TU bypass). However, all patients for whom ROSC has been achieved following traumatic cardiac arrest should be conveyed to an MTC unless airway and/or catastrophic haemorrhage cannot be safely managed, when a pit stop at the nearest Emergency Department is indicated.
- Consider termination of the resuscitative effort if the patient presents in asystole and has not responded to 30 minutes of ALS **with likely reversible causes treated successfully (rapid MTC conveyance is indicated where reversible causes cannot be corrected, or for patients with penetrating trauma)**. The exceptions to

Advanced Life Support

Hypovolaemia	• Control external haemorrhage • Splint pelvis / fractures • IV/IO fluid bolus • Early administration of TXA (IV/IO/IM)
Oxygenation (hypoxia)	• Basic/advanced airway management • Maximise oxygenation
Tension pneumothorax	• Decompress chest

Figure 2.9 – HOT checklist.

termination at 30 minutes are for pregnancy, children and where hypothermia may be a contributory factor. Consider senior advice when appropriate.

13.1 Blunt Trauma

- In the pre-hospital setting, advanced life support and exclusion of reversible causes using the 4Hs and 4Ts or the HOT approach should take priority. The commonest causes of traumatic cardiac arrest are **h**ypovolaemia, **o**xygenation (hypoxia) and **t**ension pneumothorax, which form the mnemonic 'HOT' – a helpful short checklist of reversible causes for the management of these patients.

- Rapid treatment of reversible causes should take priority over chest compressions and ALS drug administration. However, high-quality chest compressions are important and may generate some forward flow, even in cases of severe hypovolaemia or cardiac tamponade; it is therefore important to continue chest compressions as soon as sufficient personnel are available to allocate someone to this task.

- Undertake only essential lifesaving interventions on scene. If the patient has signs of life (pulse, chest rise, breathing efforts, movements, eye opening or shockable rhythm), rapidly transfer to hospital or arrange rendezvous with enhanced/critical care support. Do not delay for spinal immobilisation.

- Effective airway management using a stepwise approach is essential to maintain oxygenation of the severely compromised trauma patient. In low cardiac output conditions, positive pressure ventilation may cause further circulatory depression or even cardiac arrest by impeding venous return to the heart. Monitor ventilation with continuous waveform capnography and adjust rate to achieve normocarbia.

- Consider performing all further interventions en route and administer tranexamic acid early. Refer to **Tranexamic Acid**, **Page for Age** for children.

- Hypovolaemia due to blood loss that is sufficient in volume to cause cardiac arrest is difficult to treat. Gain large bore IV access. Although IV normal saline may restore blood volume (often requiring 2–3 litres), excessive crystalloid causes coagulopathy, acidosis and hypothermia, which in itself worsens outcome. Request enhanced care, particularly if it enables blood and blood products to be brought to scene without delay. Once ROSC is achieved, only give IV fluids to achieve a systolic BP no higher than 80 mmHg.

- Consider whether the patient can be conveyed for early blood or blood product intervention, or whether this can be brought to the scene or to a rendezvous point in a timely manner by enhanced care assets.

- In blunt trauma cases, where ALS (including attempts to address reversible causes) is being delivered, clinical judgement may be applied as to whether enhanced care assets may be accessed, or the patient can be conveyed to an MTC (or TU if necessary) in a timely manner. If likely reversible causes of traumatic cardiac arrest have been treated and there has been no ROSC after 30 minutes of ALS, resuscitation may stop.

13.2 Penetrating Trauma

- In penetrating traumatic cardiac arrest, patients should be transferred rapidly to hospital because surgical intervention is often needed to treat the cause of the arrest. A rapid transport approach is appropriate to the nearest MTU (or TU if necessary), but crew safety should be a consideration where there are prolonged journey times in a moving vehicle.

- Enhanced care assets should be requested early for attendance at the scene (but do not delay departure from scene while waiting for these assets) and/or during conveyance.

- Rapidly address immediate issues:
    - catastrophic haemorrhage (splinting, trauma dressings, tourniquet etc.)
    - airway and breathing (consider tension pneumothorax, sucking chest wound etc.)
    - defibrillation, if indicated.

Advanced Life Support

- Consider performing all further interventions en route and administer tranexamic acid early.
- The principles for volume resuscitation for penetrating trauma are similar to those for blunt trauma. However, the priority for rapid conveyance to hospital often precludes any significant pre-hospital volume being administered. Do not delay on scene to obtain IV access. If IV fluids are administered, a systolic BP no greater than 80 mmHg is adequate. Surgical intervention is often the only intervention that will save the patient's life, and rapid conveyance to hospital is vital to achieve this.

Bibliography

1. Resuscitation Council (UK). *Resuscitation Council Guidelines 2021: Adult advanced life support.* London: Resuscitation Council, 2021. Available from: https://www.resus.org.uk/resuscitation-guidelines/adult-advanced-life-support.

2. Resuscitation Council (UK). *Resuscitation Council Guidelines 2015: Paediatric advanced life support.* London: Resuscitation Council, 2021. Available from: https://www.resus.org.uk/resuscitation-guidelines/paediatric-advanced-life-support.

3. Resuscitation Council (UK). *Resuscitation Council Guidelines 2021: Peri-arrest arrhythmias.* London: Resuscitation Council UK, 2021. Available from: https://www.resus.org.uk/resuscitation-guidelines/peri-arrest-arrhythmias.

4. Resuscitation Council (UK). *Resuscitation Council Guidelines 2021: Prehospital Resuscitation.* London: Resuscitation Council UK, 2021. Available from: https://www.resus.org.uk/resuscitation-guidelines/prehospital-resuscitation/.

5. Soar J, Nolan JP, Bottiger BW et al. European Resuscitation Council Guidelines for Resuscitation 2015: Section 3. Adult advanced life support. *Resuscitation* 2015,95: 100–147. Available from: https://www.resuscitationjournal.com/article/S0300-9572(15)00328-7/fulltext.

6. Truhlar A, Deakin CD, Soar J et al. European Resuscitation Council Guidelines for Resuscitation 2015: Section 4. Cardiac arrest in special circumstances. *Resuscitation* 2015, 95: 148–201. Available from: https://www.resuscitationjournal.com/article/S0300-9572(15)00329-9/fulltext.

7. Maconochie I, Bingham R, Eich C, López-Herce J, Rodriguez-Nunez A, Rajka T, Van de Voorde P, Zideman D, Biarent D. European Resuscitation Council Guidelines for Resuscitation 2015 Section 6: Paediatric life support. *Resuscitation* 2015, 95: 223–248. Available from: https://www.resuscitationjournal.com/article/S0300-9572(15)00340-8/fulltext.

8. Deakin CD, Soar J, Morley P, Drennan I. Double sequential defibrillation for refractory ventricular fibrillation cardiac arrest: a systematic review. *Resuscitation* 2020, 155: 24–31. Available from: https://doi.org/10.1016/j.resuscitation.2020.06.008.

9. Finn J, Jacobs I, Williams TA et al. Adrenaline and vasopressin for cardiac arrest. *Cochrane Database of Systematic Reviews* 2019, 327(15): 1051. Available from: http://doi.org/10.1002/14651858.CD003179.

10. Soar J, Perkin G, Maconochie I et al. European Resuscitation Council Guidelines for Resuscitation: 2018 update —antiarrhythmic drugs for cardiac arrest. *Resuscitation* 2019, 134: 99–103. Available from: https://www.sciencedirect.com/science/article/pii/S0300957218310967/pdfft?md5=22f72cc33ecab-8b1e38130bfb18dc680&pid=1-s2.0-S0300957218310967-main.pdf.

11. Perkins GD, Ji C, Deakin CD et al, on behalf of PARAMEDIC2 collaborators. A randomized trial of epinephrine in out-of-hospital cardiac arrest. *New England Journal of Medicine* 2018,379: 711–721. Available from: https://www.nejm.org/doi/full/10.1056/NEJMoa1806842.

12. Holmberg MJ, Geri G, Wiberg S et al. Extracorporeal cardiopulmonary resuscitation for cardiac arrest: a systematic review. *Resuscitation* 2018,131: 91–100. Available from: https://www.resuscitationjournal.com/article/S0300-9572(18)30373-3/pdf.

13. Benger J, Kirby K, Black S et al. Effect of a strategy of a supraglottic airway device vs tracheal intubation during out-of-hospital cardiac arrest on functional outcome: the AIRWAYS-2 randomized clinical trial. *JAMA* 2018,320: 779–791. Available from: https://www.ncbi.nlm.nih.gov/pmc/articles/PMC6142999/.

14. Poole K, Couper K, Smyth MA et al. Mechanical CPR: Who? When? How? *Critical Care* 2018,22: 140. Available from: https://ccforum.biomedcentral.com/track/pdf/10.1186/s13054-018-2059-0.

15. Dee R et al. The effect of alternative methods of cardiopulmonary resuscitation – cough CPR, percussion pacing or precordial thump – on outcomes following cardiac arrest. A systematic review. *Resuscitation* 2021, 162: 73–81.

Basic Life Support in Adults

1. Introduction

- When there is only one person on scene, resuscitation is limited to providing basic life support (BLS) and defibrillation.
- When available, the first priority is to attach defibrillation pads to reduce the time to first shock and then begin BLS with minimal delay.
- If a bystander is willing and able to provide good-quality chest compressions, utilise their skills until further trained assistance arrives. This is particularly helpful in ensuring that immediate uninterrupted chest compressions are delivered while the defibrillator is attached.
- Once other providers are in attendance, BLS and defibrillation should continue, while advanced life support (ALS) interventions are provided.

2. Assessment and Management

- The assessment and management of a collapsed patient is detailed in Table 2.4. The adult BLS sequence is detailed in Figure 2.10.

TABLE 2.4 – ASSESSMENT and MANAGEMENT of: Basic Life Support in Adults

This sequence is for a single ambulance paramedic; however, when more than one person is present, tasks can be shared and undertaken simultaneously.

Assess Safety

- Ensure that you are safe.

Check Responsiveness

- Check the responsiveness of the patient.
- If there are no signs of life (and the patient is not breathing normally) and it is in the best interests of the patient, begin CPR.
- A pulse check is often inaccurate and may lead to an erroneous diagnosis, delaying CPR.
- Agonal breathing (occasional irregular gasps; slow, laboured, noisy breathing) is common in the early stages of cardiac arrest and should not be confused with signs of life/circulation.

Next Steps

- As a solo responder, the first priority is to attach defibrillation pads to reduce the time to first shock, but commence BLS as quickly as possible with minimal delay. (With two or more responders, chest compressions/ventilations should be commenced immediately while the defibrillator is applied by the second responder).
- Ensure further/enhanced resources are en route.
- BLS should be commenced while obtaining details to inform a best interests decision.
- Every effort should be made to gain 360° access to the patient.
- Start chest compressions at a rate of 100–120 per minute.
- Compression depth should be 5–6 cm.
- Allow the chest to recoil completely after each compression.
- Take approximately the same amount of time for each compression and recoil.
- Use of a CPR feedback device allows optimisation of BLS delivery and assessment of performance.
- Minimise interruptions to chest compressions.
- A palpable pulse (carotid, femoral or radial) during CPR is not a gauge of effective blood flow.

Combine Chest Compressions with Ventilations

Refer to Airway and Breathing Management.

- Maintain patency of the airway during CPR:
  - Consider the use of a laryngoscope and forceps if foreign body airway obstruction (FBAO) is suspected. Refer to **Foreign Body Airway Obstruction**.
  - Establishing a patent airway takes priority over concerns about a potential spinal injury.
- After 30 compressions:
  - Open and inspect the airway
  - Provide two ventilations with the most appropriate equipment available.
  - Use an inspiratory time of 1 second with adequate volume to produce a visual rise of the chest.

Basic Life Support in Adults

TABLE 2.4 – ASSESSMENT and MANAGEMENT of: Basic Life Support in Adults *(continued)*

- Resume chest compressions without delay.
- Add high-flow oxygen as soon as possible; refer to **Oxygen**.
- Continue chest compressions and ventilation in a ratio of 30:2.
- Stop to recheck only if the patient starts breathing normally; otherwise do not interrupt chest compressions and ventilation.
- Performing chest compressions is tiring; try to change the person doing chest compressions every 2 minutes; ensure the minimum of delay during the changeover.
- Ventilate gently 10 times per minute. Hyperventilation and hyperinflation must be avoided. Refer to **Airway and Breathing Management**.
- Do not attempt more than two breaths each time before returning to chest compressions.

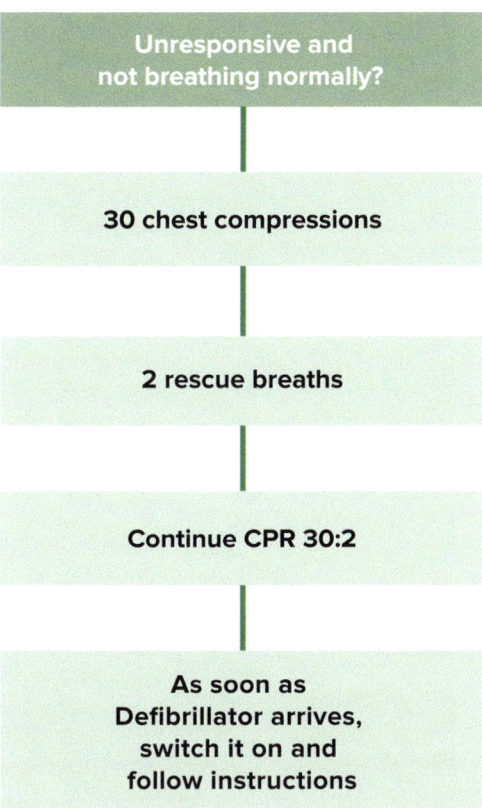

Figure 2.10 – Adult basic life support sequence. Reproduced with permission from the Resuscitation Council (UK) Guidelines 2021 (www.resus.org.uk).

Basic Life Support in Adults

> **KEY POINTS!**
>
> **Basic Life Support in Adults**
> - High-quality basic life support is a key determinant of survival from OHCA. Begin and maintain chest compressions and ventilations without interruption.
> - Chest compressions should be provided at a rate of 100–120 per minute and a depth of 5–6 cm using a ratio of 30:2 compressions to ventilations.
> - Attach defibrillator pads as soon as available, to identify and treat shockable rhythms.
> - Agonal breathing is common in the early stages of cardiac arrest and should not be confused as a sign of life or spontaneous circulation.

Bibliography

1. Olasveengen TM, Semeraro F, Ristagno G et al. European Resuscitation Council Guidelines for Resuscitation 2021: basic life support. *Resuscitation* 2015, 95:81–99. Available from: https://cprguidelines.eu/assets/guidelines/European-Resuscitation-Council-Guidelines-2021-Ba.pdf.

2. Perkins GD, Colquhoun M, Deakin CD et al. Resuscitation Council (UK). *Adult Basic Life Support Guidelines 2021*. London: Resuscitation Council (UK), 2021. Available from: https://www.resus.org.uk/library/2021-resuscitation-guidelines/adult-basic-life-support-guidelines.

Basic Life Support in Children

1. Introduction

- Cardiac arrest in children is different from that of the adult patient in its aetiology and early pathophysiology, with the vast majority of cases being caused by hypoxia.
- It is a rare phenomenon, with an incidence of 9 per 100,000 children. Paramedics are less likely to encounter a paediatric than adult cardiac arrest.
- Proactive dispatch of enhanced care, where available, should be considered. Most calls coded as paediatric cardiac arrest are subsequently found to be post-ictal; unresponsive children with abnormal breathing may also appear blue.
- Due to the prevalence of hypoxia as a cause of paediatric cardiac arrest, paediatric resuscitation focuses primarily on ensuring a patent airway and adequate oxygenation/ventilation.
- A small number of paediatric patients will experience cardiac arrest without warning, often during exertion, and present in a shockable rhythm as a result of an often undiagnosed cardiac abnormality. The possibility of a successful outcome is high if appropriate action is taken promptly in these cases, i.e. rapid defibrillation.

2. Age Definitions

- This guideline covers:
  - infants (defined as under one year old)
  - children (defined as between 1 and 18 years of age).
- In this guideline, the term 'child' includes infants, unless specified otherwise.
- Newborn life support is not covered in this guideline. For newborn babies, refer to **Newborn Life Support**.

3. General Principles

- The priorities should include:
  - effective airway management
  - effective ventilations
  - effective chest compressions
  - early defibrillation, if appropriate.
- Do not delay on scene once these interventions have been attempted.
- Consider conveyance to the most appropriate hospital with early pre-alert.
- In the event of a life-threatening episode for any child, consideration must be given to the need for clinical assessment of other siblings in the property if the cause of illness is unknown.
- In the event of a life-threatening episode for any child, consideration must be given to safeguarding concerns for that child and siblings.

4. Airway Management

- Bag-mask ventilation (BVM) is the recommended first-line method for achieving airway control and ventilation in children.
- Appropriate padding behind the shoulder blades, which also supports the head in children, may aid airway management.
- Gastric insufflation is a complication of paediatric resuscitation, leading to splinting of the diaphragm, vomiting and compression of the vena cava causing diminished venous return. This is best avoided by delivering gentle ventilations over 1 second, just sufficient to cause chest rise.
- Basic airway adjuncts may assist in maintaining an open airway.
- Although bag-mask ventilation remains the recommended first-line method for achieving airway control and ventilation in children, a supraglottic airway is an acceptable airway device for providers trained in its use. It is particularly helpful in airway obstruction caused by upper airway anatomical supraglottic airway abnormalities or if bag-mask ventilation is not possible.

TABLE 2.5 – ASSESSMENT and MANAGEMENT of: Basic Life Support in Children

This sequence is for a solo paramedic; however, when more than one person is present, tasks can be shared and undertaken simultaneously.

Assess Safety
- Ensure that you are safe.

Check Responsiveness
- Check the responsiveness of the patient.
- Agonal breathing (occasional irregular gasps; slow, laboured, noisy breathing) is common in the early stages of cardiac arrest and should not be confused with signs of life/circulation.
- It may be difficult to be certain that there is no pulse. If there is any doubt and it is in the best interest of the patient, begin CPR.

(continued)

Basic Life Support in Children

TABLE 2.5 – ASSESSMENT and MANAGEMENT of: Basic Life Support in Children *(continued)*

Next Steps
- Every effort should be made to gain 360° access to the patient.
- The first priority is to open, inspect and clear the airway and begin effective ventilations using BVM with high-flow oxygen.
- Open the child's airway by tilting the head and lifting the chin:
  – Place your hand on the forehead and gently tilt the head back. Be careful not to hyperextend the neck.
  – At the same time, lift the point of the chin with your fingertip(s). Do not push on the soft tissues under the chin as this may block the airway.
  – If you still have difficulty in opening the airway, try a jaw thrust: place the first two fingers of each hand behind each side of the child's mandible (jawbone) and push the jaw forward.
- Maintain patency of the airway during CPR:
  – Refer to **Airway and Breathing Management**.
- There is a high incidence of choking in children.
  – Consider the use of a laryngoscope and forceps if FBAO is suspected. Refer to **Foreign Body Airway Obstruction**.
  – Establishing a patent airway takes priority over concerns about a potential spinal injury.
- Give five ventilations.

Ventilations – Child
- Ensure head tilt and chin lift.
- Use paediatric BVM (with a mask appropriate to the size of the child) and inflate the chest steadily over 1 second, watching for chest rise.
- Maintaining head tilt and chin lift, watch the chest fall.
- Repeat this sequence 5 times.
- Identify effectiveness by observing the child's chest rise and fall in a similar fashion to the movement produced by a normal breath.

Ventilations – Infant
- Ensure a neutral position of the head and apply a chin lift.
- Use paediatric BVM (with a mask appropriate to the size of the child) and inflate the chest steadily over 1 second, watching for chest rise.
- Maintaining the chin lift, watch the chest fall.
- Repeat this sequence 5 times.
- Identify effectiveness by observing the child's chest rise and fall in a similar fashion to the movement produced by a normal breath.

If There Is Difficulty Achieving an Effective Breath, the Airway May Be Obstructed
- Open the child's mouth and remove any visible obstruction.
- **DO NOT** perform a blind finger sweep.
- Ensure that there is adequate head tilt and chin lift but also that the neck is not over-extended.
- If head tilt and chin lift has not opened the airway, try the jaw thrust method.
- Make up to 5 attempts to achieve effective breaths.
- If still unsuccessful, examine the oropharynx with a laryngoscope and remove any obstruction. If an obstruction is removed, make 5 further attempts at ventilations.
- If still unsuccessful, move on to chest compressions.

Assess the Child's Circulation
- Look for signs of life. This includes checking for a pulse, any movement, coughing or normal breathing (not agonal gasps – these are infrequent, irregular breaths).

NB If you are not sure if there is a pulse, assume there is no pulse.

Basic Life Support in Children

TABLE 2.5 – ASSESSMENT and MANAGEMENT of: Basic Life Support in Children *(continued)*
Pulse Check – Child
• Feel for the carotid pulse in the neck.
Pulse Check – Infant
• Feel for the brachial pulse on the inner aspect of the upper arm.
🚩 **Remember that pulse checks may be unreliable and are prone to errors. The detection of circulation therefore should also include other intra-arrest parameters such as EtCO$_2$, blood pressure and SpO$_2$.**
Where a Pulse Is Present and Breaths Are Absent:
• Continue ventilating, until the child starts breathing effectively on their own.
• Re-asssess the child frequently.
If There Are No Signs of Circulation – OR There Is Any Doubt:
• Start chest compressions.
• Combine ventilations and chest compressions.
NB – For paediatric patients in a collapsed state, with no signs of life and a heart rate <60 beats per minute, compressions must be commenced.
For all children, compress the lower half of the sternum.
• Avoid compressing the upper abdomen, by locating the xiphisternum (i.e. find the angle where the lowest ribs join in the midline) and compressing the sternum one finger's breadth above this point.
• Compressions should be sufficient to depress the sternum by at least one-third of the depth of the chest (approximately 4 cm for an infant and 5 cm for a child).
• Release the pressure, and repeat at a rate of 100–120 per minute.
• After 15 compressions, give two ventilations.
• Continue compressions and ventilations in a ratio of 15:2.
• Solo rescuers may use a ratio of 30:2, particularly if they are having difficulty with the transition between compressions and ventilations.
• The best method for compression varies slightly between infants and children (see below).
Compressions – Child
• Place the heel of one hand over the lower half of the sternum (as above).
• Lift the fingers to ensure that pressure is not applied over the child's ribs.
• Position yourself vertically above the child's chest and, with your arm straight, compress the sternum to depress it by approximately 5 cm.
• In larger children or for small rescuers, this may be achieved most easily by using both hands with the fingers interlocked.
• Ensure complete recoil following each compression.
Compressions – Infant
• The solo rescuer should compress the sternum with the tips of two fingers.
• If there are two or more rescuers, an alternative method would be to use the encircling technique:
– Place both thumbs flat, side by side on the lower half of the sternum (as above) with the tips pointing towards the infant's head.
– Spread the rest of both hands with the fingers together to encircle the lower part of the infant's rib cage with the tips of the fingers supporting the infant's back.
– Press down on the lower sternum with the two thumbs to depress it by approximately 4 cm.
• Ensure complete recoil following each compression.

Basic Life Support in Children

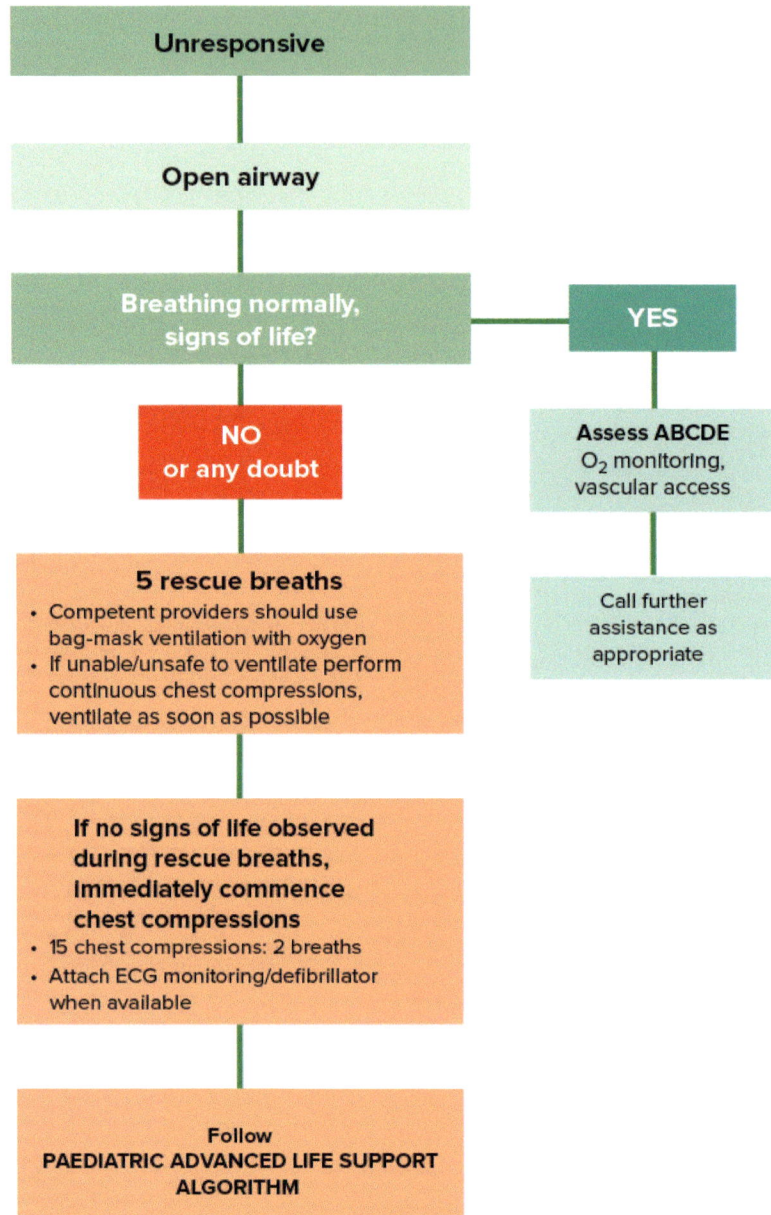

Figure 2.11 – Child basic life support sequence algorithm (modified). Reproduced with permission from the Resuscitation Council (UK) Guidelines 2021 algorithm (www.resus.org.uk).

> **KEY POINTS!**
>
> **Basic Life Support in Children**
> - Hypoxia is the most common cause of cardiac arrest.
> - Some children may present in a shockable rhythm as a result of an often undiagnosed cardiac abnormality.
> - Treatment should focus on rapidly correcting the cause where possible.
> - If the child is not breathing, carefully remove any obvious airway obstruction but DO NOT perform blind finger sweeps.
> - Give five initial ventilations using a BVM, watching for chest rise.
> - Adopt a high index of suspicion of airway obstruction and treat accordingly.
> - The duration of ventilations is about 1 second (comparable with adult practice).

Basic Life Support in Children

- **If there are:**
  - **no signs of life**
  - **or an absent or slow pulse (<60 bpm with poor perfusion)**
  - **or you are not sure**

  start chest compressions at a rate of 100–120 per minute.
- **Continue alternating compressions and breaths at a ratio of 15:2.**

Bibliography

1. Van de Voorde P, Turner NM, Djakow J et al. European Resuscitation Council Guidelines 2021: paediatric life support. *Resuscitation* 2021, 161: 327–387. Available from: https://doi.org/10.1016/j.resuscitation.2021.02.015.

2. Skellett S, Maconochie I, Bingham B et al. *Resuscitation Council (UK). Paediatric Basic Life Support Guidelines 2021*. London: Resuscitation Council (UK), 2021. Available from: https://www.resus.org.uk/library/2021-resuscitation-guidelines/paediatric-basic-life-support-guidelines.

Emergency Tracheostomy and Laryngectomy Pre-Hospital Management

1. Introduction

'*A patient with a tracheostomy or laryngectomy is at risk of death or harm if inappropriate or inadequate care is provided. This patient group requires airway devices to be safely inserted, securely positioned and appropriately cared for, in order to continue to provide the patient with a patent airway. Failure to do so may lead to a displaced or blocked tube, which, if not dealt with immediately, may be fatal within minutes*'.[1]

An increasing number of patients with long-term tracheostomies and laryngectomies are now being managed in the community. Approximately 12,000 tracheostomy procedures are performed each year in the UK.[2] Patients are discharged from hospital once the tracheostomy is stable and the patient or carer is competent with self-care along with support from community nurses.

2. Incidence

- All trusts can expect to see more patients requiring emergency care due to the increase in head and neck cancers. These are the fifth leading cause of cancer and the sixth leading cause of cancer mortality.[3]
- Approximately 34 people receive a diagnosis every day in the UK[4] and this is the most common cause of a laryngectomy.[5]
- There are approximately 15,000–20,000 tracheostomies performed annually throughout the NHS.[6]

3. Severity and Outcome

- Commonly, patients are discharged with all the necessary equipment to manage most emergencies. The majority of patients are also discharged with a hospital passport or digital care plan that provides vital details in relation to the specifics of the patient, their airway management and the history of their condition.
- The most common tracheostomy airway emergencies are displacement, accidental de-cannulation and obstruction.[1]
- Obstruction of the tube is the third most common cause of death in patients with tracheostomies.[4] Maintaining a patent airway is the priority. Clinicians must be able to recognise a blocked tube in the presence of severe difficulty in breathing or apnoea. Tubes can become blocked with plugs of mucous, blood and crusts, and the clinician must be competent and trained in suction techniques. They should also be aware of the different types of tracheostomy tubes in use in order to clear the tube safely and effectively.

4. Physiology

4.1 Laryngectomy

- Laryngectomy is the total removal of the larynx and the separation of the airway from the nose, mouth and oesophagus. In a total laryngectomy, the laryngectomee breathes through an opening in the neck. This becomes the patient's primary airway. Total laryngectomy results in permanent changes to the airway anatomy; the trachea is pulled forward during surgery and stitched to the anterior neck skin, forming a new stoma (Figure 2.12).
- It is vital to recognise that following a laryngectomy, the patient's airway does not communicate with their nose or mouth at all.

4.2 Tracheostomy

- A tracheostomy is an opening in the trachea performed via a surgical incision or a percutaneous technique. A tracheostomy tube is passed into the trachea between the second and third tracheal rings, and a stoma is formed 3–5 days post surgery. The airway is then secured. Tracheostomies can be permanent or temporary (Figure 2.13).

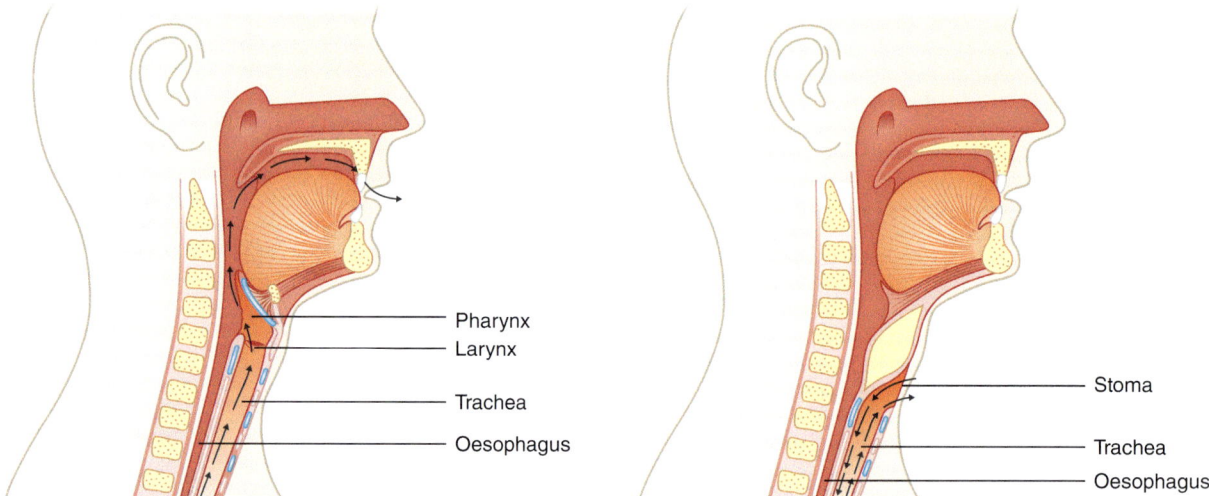

Figure 2.12 – Airway anatomy before and after laryngectomy.

Emergency Tracheostomy and Laryngectomy Pre-Hospital Management

- Tracheostomy tube – this is sometimes referred to as the outer tube, or outer cannula. This is the main tube which secures the airway through the stoma. It may or may not be cuffed, and it may or may not be fenestrated dependent on need and manufacturer.
- Inner cannula – this may or may not be present, dependent on the manufacturer of the tracheostomy tube. It is sometimes known as the inner tube. It is the part of the equipment which can be removed and replaced. Its purpose is secretion management. It should lock into the outer tube by either clicking or twisting into place, to prevent accidental removal.

NB: A fenestrated tube has small holes in the tube shaft.

There will be a code on the flange that will state:
- Fen: Fenestrated
- Non-Fen: Non-fenestrated. Some tubes will allow our equipment such as BVM or $EtCO_2$ to be connected to the main tube, though some makes will only allow connection to the inner cannula.

5. Assessment and Management

For the assessment and management of tracheostomy, and laryngectomy refer to Table 2.6 and Figures 2.13 to 2.15.

TABLE 2.6 – ASSESSMENT and MANAGEMENT of: Suction and Oxygen

ENSURE PPE INCLUDING FACE MASK PROTECTION. REMOVE FENESTRATED TUBES BEFORE SUCTIONING. REMEMBER SUCTION IS A HYPOXIC PROCESS.

Indications for Suction Found on Assessment:
- Excessive secretions not cleared by coughing
- Increase in pulse, BP or respiratory rate
- Decrease in O_2 saturations, prolonged capillary refill
- Difficulty in mechanically ventilating the patient
- Assess the need for oxygen based on reliable saturation readings.

Aims of Suction and Oxygenation:
- Prevent respiratory distress.
- Maintain a patent airway.
- Clear excessive secretions.
- Reassurance.
- Pre-oxygenate* the patient before the suction procedure; aim for 94–98% SpO_2 (88–92% SpO_2 for COPD patients). Explain your actions to the patient.
- Remove the inner cannula and clean it if blocked. Replace and assess for improvement.
- When suctioning, replace a fenestrated inner cannula with a non-fenestrated one; this will reduce the chance of the suction catheter damaging the tracheal wall through the fenestrations.
- Set suction at 150–200 mmHg.
- When using a soft catheter, go no further than 2 cm beyond the tube length; suction on the way out. (Remove the inner cannula from the tube to measure against the suction catheter to get an idea of length.)
- Remember to re-oxygenate* the patient after suctioning.
- If you are unable to pass suction beyond the length of the tube, refer to the conscious patient algorithm.

*High-flow oxygen 15 l/min, tracheostomy O_2 mask at the neck, non-rebreather mask over the nose and mouth.

Emergency Tracheostomy and Laryngectomy Pre-Hospital Management

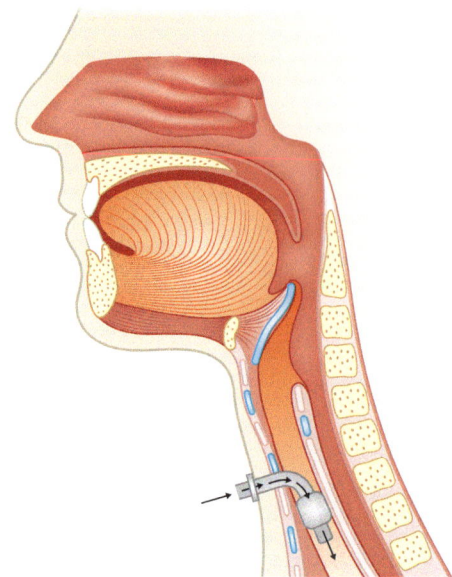

Figure 2.13 – Tracheostomy.

Does the tracheostomy tube appear to be sitting correctly?
- Is it Mid-line?
- Flange is flush to anterior neck?

NO → **Gently re-align,** taking care that re-positioning does not cause further internal damage or create a false passage (placed into the soft tissue surrounding the stoma)

YES ↓

Are there excessive secretions NOT cleared by coughing?

YES → Remove inner cannula (tube), clean it and replace.
If it is a laryngectomy tube it may not have an inner cannula.
Apply suction: 150–200 mmHg. Re-assess. (Before suctioning, replace fenestrated inner cannula with solid inner cannula, if available)

NO ↓

Auscultate for breath sounds. Are there crepitations, signs of respiratory distress or hypoxia?

YES → Apply suction: 150–200mmHg. If unable to pass suction catheter, remove the entire outer tube–give oxygen over the stoma (and if possible also over the face)

Aim for target saturations:

SpO_2 94%–98%
(88–92% SpO_2 COPD)

Prepare to ventilate

Consider:
Could there be another cause for the respiratory distress? i.e. pulmonary embolism?

Figure 2.14 – Steps for confirming tracheostomy patency on the conscious patient.

Emergency Tracheostomy and Laryngectomy Pre-Hospital Management

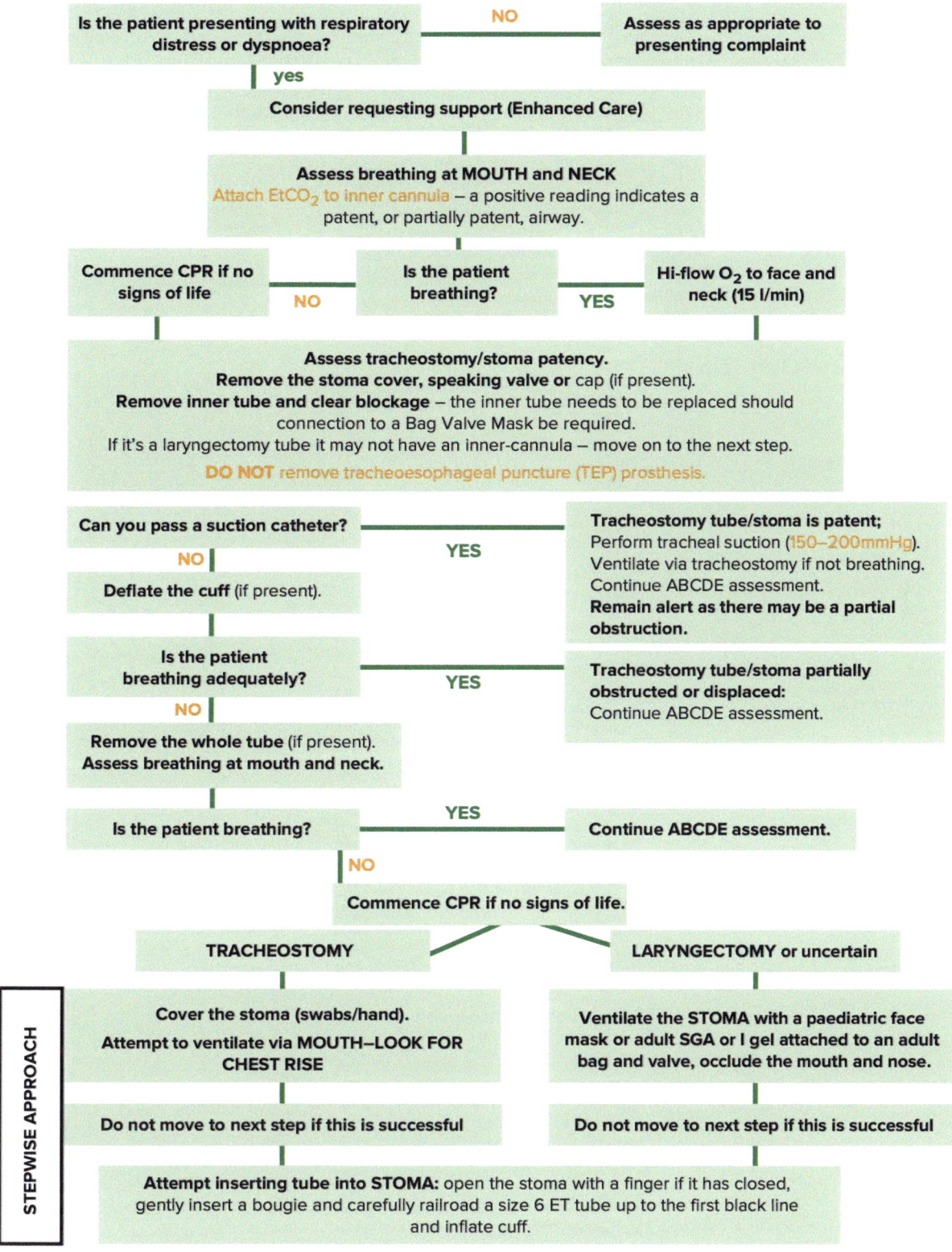

Last resort: If all else fails and airway remains closed you could try inserting a spare tracheostomy tube, attempt to fashion a bougie from a soft suction catheter to allow an ET tube to be placed over or insert finger to open stoma and use as a guide to slide the ET or tracheostomy tube in next to it). Always remember to attach EtCO2.

Be mindful that this is a last resort and will be dependent on what equipment is available to you at the time, i.e. the soft suction catheter will have to be cut off at the top to allow an ET tube to be railroaded meaning you will need another soft catheter to continue suctioning.

Figure 2.15 – Emergency tracheostomy and laryngectomy management.

Emergency Tracheostomy and Laryngectomy Pre-Hospital Management

TABLE 2.7 – Glossary of Commonly used Tracheostomy/Laryngectomy Terms

Term	Definition
Tracheotomy/tracheostomy	Technically, the suffix -otomy means 'to cut into'. The suffix -ostomy means 'opening into'. So a tracheotomy is the surgical procedure to create an opening into the trachea to enable a tracheostomy.
Inner and outer cannula	The inner part of the tracheostomy tube can be removed, cleaned or replaced. The outer part of the tube stays in place.
Cuff 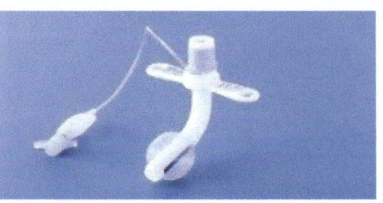 Republished with permission of Fuji Systems.	The balloon at the end of the tracheostomy tube that can be inflated, similar to that of inflatable cuffs on ET tubes.
De-cannulation	Removal or accidental removal of the whole tracheostomy tube.
Fenestrated tracheostomy tube 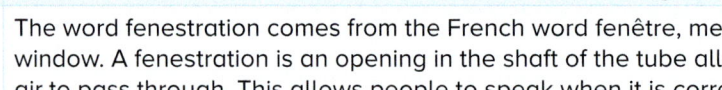 Republished with permission of Kapitex.	The word fenestration comes from the French word fenêtre, meaning window. A fenestration is an opening in the shaft of the tube allowing air to pass through. This allows people to speak when it is correctly fitted. **NB** A fenestrated inner cannula must be removed and replaced with a non-fenestrated inner cannula before suctioning.
Flange 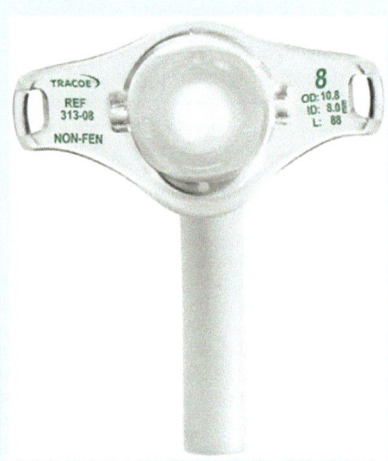 Republished with permission of Kapitex.	The part of the tracheostomy tube that fits against the anterior neck and around the stoma. It also carries written information about the tube. The flange provides anchoring for securing straps and stops the tube from slipping into the stoma.
Laryngectomee	A person who has had a laryngectomy.
Laryngectomy	The surgical removal of the larynx.

Emergency Tracheostomy and Laryngectomy Pre-Hospital Management

TABLE 2.7 – Glossary of Commonly used Tracheostomy/Laryngectomy Terms *(continued)*

Mucus plug	An accumulation of mucus that can obstruct the lumen of the tracheostomy tube.
Speaking valve Republished with permission of Kapitex.	Usually a one-way valve that fits on the tracheostomy tube. It allows air to pass into the tracheostomy, but closes with exhalation, forcing air into the mouth and nose which allows speech. Used only on cuffless tubes or in 'cuff down' mode. This is more commonly known as a 'Passey Muir valve' by patients, family and carers.
Stoma	Translates as 'mouth' in Greek. It refers to the skin around the opening.
Suctioning	Removal of tracheal secretions or blood in the airway.
Heat moisture exchanger (HME) Republished with permssion of Intersurgical.	A device that fits on the tracheostomy tube. It collects exhaled water vapour, allowing it to be inhaled, which aids humidification. Patient or family may know this as a 'Swedish nose'.
Laryngectomy Tube Republished with permission of Kapitex.	This appears very similar to the tracheostomy tubes but with no inner cannula. It is for use in laryngectomies and is placed to support the stoma.

(continued)

Emergency Tracheostomy and Laryngectomy Pre-Hospital Management

TABLE 2.7 – Glossary of Commonly used Tracheostomy/Laryngectomy Terms *(continued)*

Buchanan bibs 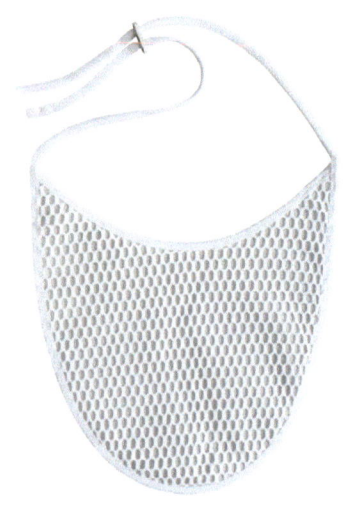 Republished with permission of Kapitex.	Buchanan DeltaNex® is a three-layer system with a hydrolox foam core and a breathable soft cotton outer mesh. It is designed specifically for airway protection, to filter fine particles and allow moisture transfer. It is a bib of plastic foam covered with knitted fabric of honeycomb pattern. The neck band includes Velcro strips for fastening onto the strip on the bib and around the neck.
Phonation	Using the voice.

TABLE 2.8 – Stepwise Approach to Airway Management

A tracheostomy tube in situ with a dressing, neck tie, cuffed tube and a heat moisture exchanger (HME). 1. Any attachment that covers the tube must be removed if the patient is experiencing difficulty in breathing. Ensure that the tube is in neutral alignment.	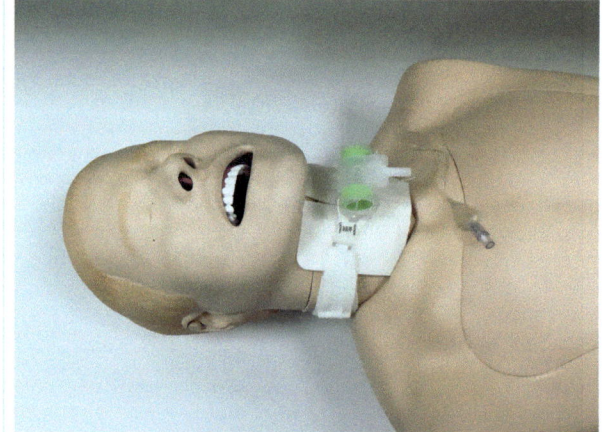
2. Dependant on the manufacturer, the inner part of the tracheostomy tube can be removed either by twisting and gently extracting or by directly pulling out, dependent on the manufacturer. It can then be cleaned or replaced. The outer part of the tube stays in place. The BVM and catheter mount will fit to the inner cannula. They may also fit to some tracheostomy tubes once the inner cannula has been removed, though this is not universally the case and depends on the manufacturer.	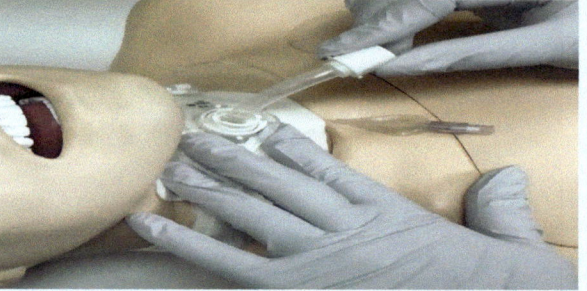

Emergency Tracheostomy and Laryngectomy Pre-Hospital Management

TABLE 2.8 – Stepwise Approach to Airway Management *(continued)*	
3. If there are **no airway problems** and the **airway is patent**, you can use a **CUFFED** tube with the inner tube in place as an advanced airway. The cuff must be inflated to achieve positive pressure ventilations. EtCO$_2$ must be recorded to confirm advance airway. **Look for equal bilateral chest rise.**	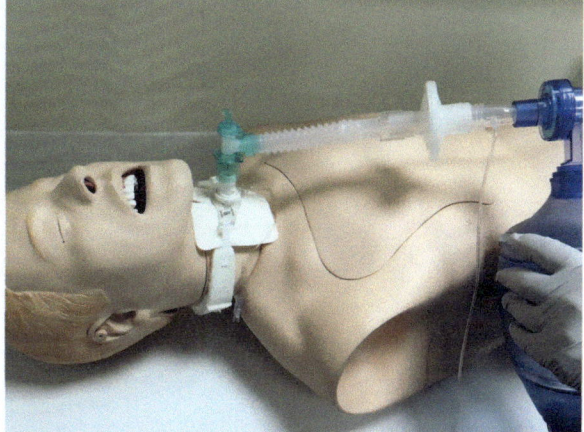
4. If the tube is blocked, it must be removed. As a last resort open the stoma with a finger if it has closed, gently insert a bougie and carefully railroad a size 6 ET tube up to the first black line. Inflate the cuff. This is a two-person procedure; be gentle in your technique and remember the delicate nature of tracheal tissue. Be careful not to create a false passage by inserting the tube into the subcutaneous tissue rather than the stoma.	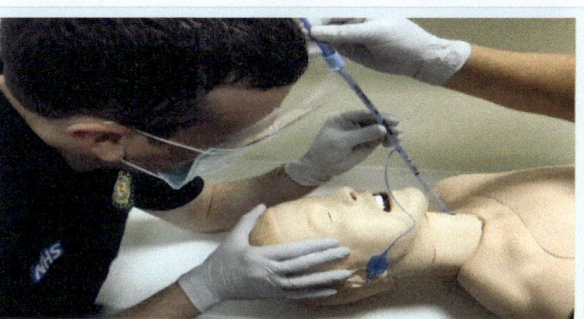
5. Once the cuff is inflated, attach the catheter mount, filter, EtCO$_2$ line and BVM. **Do not let go of the tube, and do not use a Thomas™ tube holder.** Best practice is to appoint someone to hold the tube and monitor the airway constantly. This is a two-person technique. **Look for equal bilateral chest rise.** If there is no chest rise and surgical emphysema develops in the neck, a false passage has been created and the ET tube should be removed.	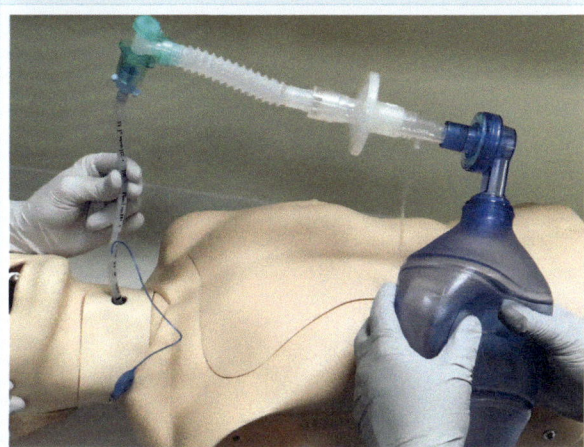
6. If the tracheostomy tube is blocked, it must be removed. The nose and mouth must be occluded to prevent any air escape. Use a small paediatric mask attached to an adult bag and valve, seal over the stoma and ventilate the patient, you can also use an i-Gel to cover the stoma if required. This is best carried out as a two-person technique. **Look for equal bilateral chest rise.**	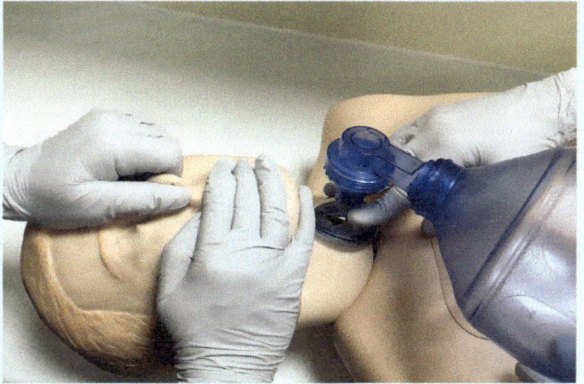

Images republished with kind permission of Dorothy Antrim, London Ambulance Service.

Emergency Tracheostomy and Laryngectomy Pre-Hospital Management

> **KEY POINTS!**
>
> **Emergency Tracheostomy and Laryngectomy Pre-Hospital Management**
> - A third of deaths associated with tracheostomy and laryngectomy patients are due to hypoxia caused by a blocked tube.
> - Early recognition of a blocked tube is vital.
> - Inability to pass suction catheters beyond the tube indicates a blockage.
> - Accidental removal of the whole tracheostomy tube (de-cannulation) is a TIME-CRITICAL emergency.
> - Try to remember to take the patient's emergency box to hospital; it contains their appropriately sized tubes.
> - NEVER reintroduce a tracheostomy tube.
> - Emphasis must be on oxygenation to reverse the hypoxia together with reassurance.
> - Always be prepared to ventilate airway-compromised patients.

Acknowledgements

Acknowledgements to Jacqueline Mitchell, CNS Tracheostomy Specialist at Guy's and St Thomas' NHS Foundation Trust; Lewis Ewington at London Ambulance Service; and Dr Lucy Bates at the National Tracheostomy Safety Project.

Bibliography

1. McGrath BA. Executive summary key recommendations. In BA McGrath, *Comprehensive Tracheostomy Care*. Chichester: John Wiley & Sons Ltd, 2014: xix.
2. Wilkinson KA, Freeth H, Kelly K. On the right trach. A review of care received by patients who underwent a tracheostomy. *British Journal of Hospital Medicine* 2014, 76(3): 163–165.
3. Goon PKC, Stanley MA, Ebmeyer J, Steinsträsser L, Upile T et al. HPV and head and neck cancer: a descriptive update. *Head and Neck Oncology* 2009, 1: 36.
4. Feber T. Tracheostomy care for community nurses: basic principles. *British Journal of Community Nursing* 2016, 11(5): 186–193.
5. Heathline. *Laryngectomy: Purpose, Procedure, and Recovery*. Available from: https://www.healthline.com/health/laryngectomy.
6. McGrath et al. Improving tracheostomy care in the United Kingdom: results of a guided quality improvement programme in 20 diverse hospitals. *British Journal of Anaesthesia* 2020, 125(1): e119–112.

Foreign Body Airway Obstruction

1. Introduction

- Foreign body airway obstruction (FBAO) is an uncommon but potentially treatable cause of accidental death.
- Most cases occur when eating or playing (in children) and are consequently witnessed. Therefore, interventions are usually initiated when the patient is conscious.
- The signs and symptoms vary, depending on the degree of airway obstruction (refer to Table 2.9).
- FBAO is characterised by the sudden onset of respiratory distress associated with coughing, gagging or stridor.
- Similar signs and symptoms may also be associated with other causes of airway obstruction such as laryngitis or epiglottitis, which tend to be of slower onset and require different management.
- This guideline covers:
  - infants (defined as under one year old)
  - children (defined as between one year and 18 years of age)
  - adults (aged >18 years of age).
- In this guideline, the term 'child' includes infants, unless specified otherwise.

2. General Management Principles

- When a foreign body enters the airway, the patient will usually react immediately by coughing in an attempt to expel it.
- A spontaneous cough is likely to be more effective and safer than any manoeuvre a rescuer might perform.
- If coughing is absent or ineffective and the object completely obstructs the airway, the patient will rapidly become asphyxiated.
- Active interventions to remove FBAO are only required when coughing becomes ineffective; but when required, these should be commenced confidently and rapidly.
- A high index of suspicion of airway obstruction must be maintained where airway compromise is noted, and paramedics should examine the oropharynx with a laryngoscope at an early stage if chest rise is not witnessed.
- Finger sweeps are not recommended, particularly when paramedics have the benefit of McGill forceps and suction, as they may drive any foreign body deeper into the airway. If an obstruction is seen and it can be grasped easily, make an attempt to remove it with forceps and/or suction.

TABLE 2.9 – General Signs of Foreign Body Airway Obstruction

Mild airway obstruction	Severe airway obstruction

- The patient is able to:
  – speak
  – cough
  – breathe.
	- The patient is unable to:
	  – speak
	  – breathe.
	- Attempts at coughing are silent.
	- The patient may be unconscious.

Other indicators

- The episode was witnessed.
- The patient may clutch their neck.
- The patient may appear panicked or anxious.
- Coughing or choking may be present:
  - Cough may be ineffective, silent, quiet or loud.
- A stridor or wheeze may be present.
- Onset is sudden.
- There is recent history of playing with, or eating, small objects.
- The patient is cyanosed.
- The patient has a decreasing level of consciousness.
- The patient was able to breathe before coughing.

Foreign Body Airway Obstruction

3. Assessment and Management

For the assessment and management of foreign body airway obstruction, refer to Table 2.10.

TABLE 2.10 – ASSESSMENT and MANAGEMENT of: Foreign Body Airway Obstruction (FBAO)

Assess for Severity of Obstruction

Adult, Child > 1 year and Infant < 1 year

- Consider enhanced care.
- Determine the patient's level of consciousness.
- Refer to Table 2.9.
- Consider severe allergic reaction which can cause airway obstruction (refer to **Allergic Reactions including Anaphylaxis**).

Mild Airway Obstruction

Adult and Child > 1 year

- Encourage the patient to cough but do nothing else.
- Monitor carefully and re-assess frequently.
- Rapid transport to hospital.

Infant < 1 year

- Monitor carefully and re-assess frequently.
- Rapid transport to hospital.

Severe Airway Obstruction – Conscious Patient

Adult and Child > 1 year

- Give up to 5 back blows – after each back blow, check to see if the obstruction has been relieved.
- If 5 back blows do not relieve the airway obstruction, give up to 5 abdominal thrusts.
- These manoeuvres increase intrathoracic pressure and may dislodge the foreign body.
- Alternate these until the obstruction is relieved or the patient loses consciousness.

Infant < 1 year

- Give up to 5 back blows – after each back blow, check to see if the obstruction has been relieved.
- If 5 back blows do not relieve the airway obstruction, give up to 5 **CHEST** thrusts.
- These manoeuvres increase intrathoracic pressure and may dislodge the foreign body.
- Alternate these until the obstruction is relieved or the infant loses consciousness.

Severe Airway Obstruction – Unconscious Patient

Adult, Child > 1 year and Infant < 1 year

- Open the mouth and look for any obvious obstruction.
- Attempt to visualise the vocal cords with a laryngoscope.
- If an obstruction is seen and it can be grasped easily, make an attempt to remove it with forceps, or suction.
- **DO NOT** attempt finger sweeps – these can cause injury and force the object more deeply into the pharynx.
- If the patient is unconscious or becomes unconscious, begin basic life support (refer to **Basic Life Support in Adults** and **Basic Life Support in Children**).
- If all other measures fail and airway remains obstructed, also consider cricothyroidotomy or surgical airway (<u>not</u> infants) where trained and authorised.
- During CPR, the patient's mouth should be checked for any foreign body that has been partly expelled each time the airway is opened.

Foreign Body Airway Obstruction

TABLE 2.10 – ASSESSMENT and MANAGEMENT of: Foreign Body Airway Obstruction (FBAO) *(continued)*

Additional Information

Adult, Child and Infant

- Chest thrusts/compressions generate a higher airway pressure than back blows.
- Following successful treatment for FBAO, foreign material may remain in the upper or lower respiratory tract and cause complications later.
- Patients with a persistent cough, difficulty swallowing or the sensation of an object being stuck in the throat must be assessed further.
- Abdominal thrusts can cause serious internal injuries and all patients who receive them must be assessed for injury in hospital.
- Infants (< 1 year of age): 5 back blows, alternating with 5 chest thrusts. Child (> 1 year of age): 5 back blows, alternating with 5 abdominal thrusts.

Back Blows

Child > 1 year

- Back blows are more effective if the child is positioned head down.
- A small child may be placed across the rescuer's lap.
- If this is not possible, support the child in a forward-leaning position and deliver the back blows from behind.

Infant < 1 year

- Support the infant in a head-down, prone position, to allow gravity to assist the removal of the foreign body.
- Support the infant's head by placing the thumb of one hand at the angle of the lower jaw, with one or two fingers from the same hand at the same point on the other side of the jaw.
- Do not compress the soft tissues under the infant's jaw, as this will exacerbate the airway obstruction.
- Deliver up to 5 sharp back blows with the heel of one hand in the middle of the back between the shoulder blades, aiming to relieve the obstruction with each blow.

Chest/Abdominal Thrusts

Abdominal thrusts – children

- Stand or kneel behind the child. Place your arms under the child's arms and encircle their torso.
- Clench your fist and place it between the umbilicus and the xiphisternum. Grasp this hand with the other hand and pull sharply inwards and upwards.
- Repeat up to 5 times (if required).
- Ensure that pressure is not applied to xiphoid process or lower rib cage (as this may result in abdominal trauma).

Chest thrusts – infants

- Turn the infant into a head-down, supine position (this can be safely achieved by placing the paramedic's arm along the infant's back and encircling the occiput with the hand). Rest this arm against a solid surface or the paramedic's thigh.
- Identify the landmark for chest compression (lower sternum, approximately a finger's breadth above the xiphisternum).
- Deliver 5 chest thrusts (if required).
- These are similar to external chest compressions but sharper in nature and delivered at a slower rate.
- There will be occasions when a patient who has a DNACPR form may have a cardiac arrest that is considered unnatural and not in the envisaged circumstances and has a potentially reversible cause such as choking. All reversible causes should be considered (refer to Section 10, ALS Reversible Causes). In these circumstances, resuscitation and rapid conveyance to hospital should be considered, as the cause of the arrest is unrelated to their main clinical problem(s) and could be reversible.

Foreign Body Airway Obstruction

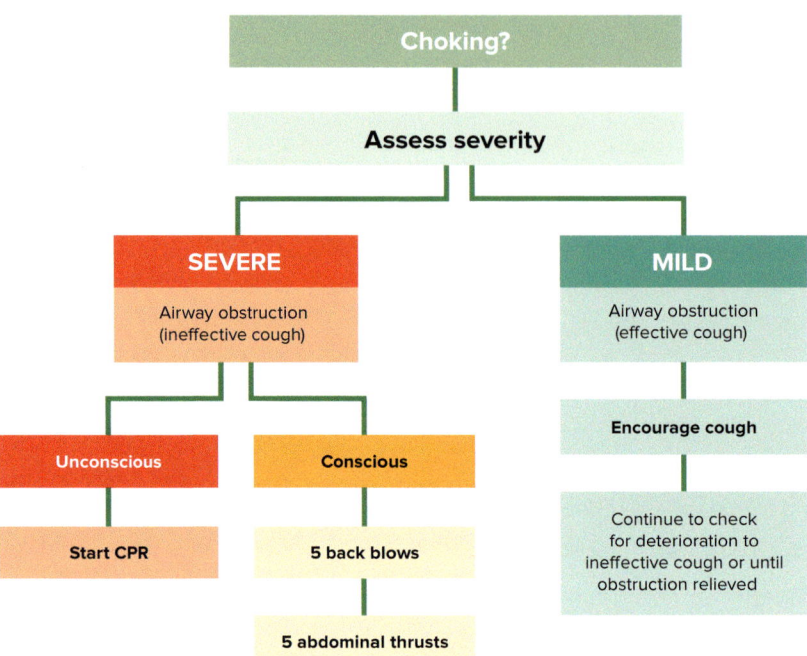

Figure 2.16 – Foreign body airway obstruction in adults. Reproduced with permission from the Resuscitation Council (UK) Guidelines 2021 algorithm (www.resus.org.uk).

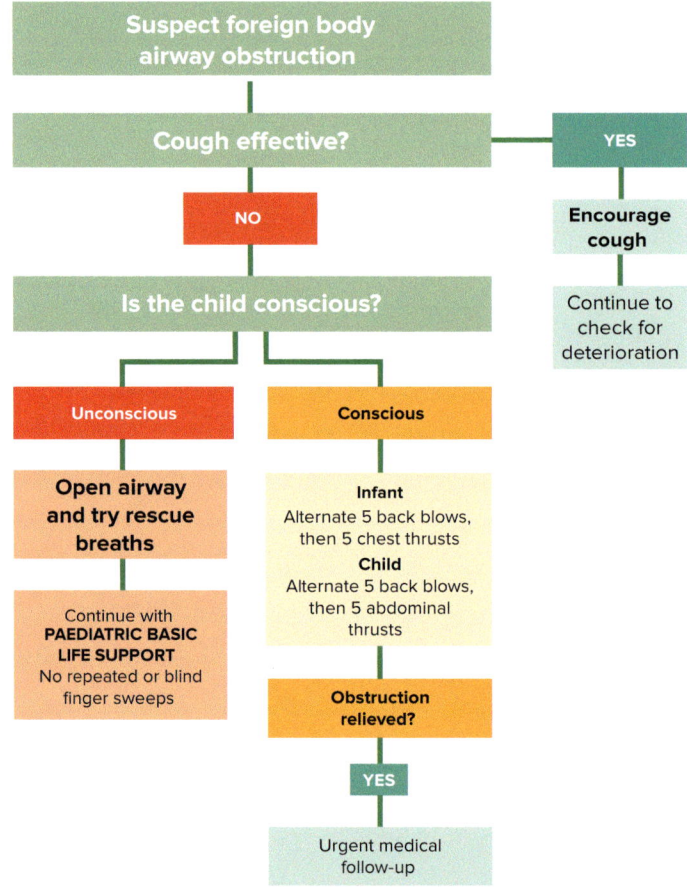

Figure 2.17 – Foreign body airway obstruction in children (modified). Reproduced with permission from the Resuscitation Council (UK) Guidelines 2021 algorithm (www.resus.org.uk).

Foreign Body Airway Obstruction

> **KEY POINTS!**
>
> **Foreign Body Airway Obstruction**
> - FBAO is a potentially treatable cause of death that often occurs while playing or eating. It is more common in children.
> - It is characterised by the sudden onset of respiratory distress.
> - If the patient is coughing effectively, encourage them to cough.
> - If coughing is ineffective, back blows should initially be given.
> - Use chest thrusts in infants and abdominal thrusts in children and adults.
> - Avoid finger sweeps; use suction and/or McGill forceps.
> - Check after each manoeuvre to see if the obstruction is removed.
> - If the object is expelled successfully, assess the patient's clinical condition. It is possible that part of the object may remain in the respiratory tract and cause complications.
> - Abdominal thrusts may cause internal injury – patients who have received abdominal thrusts require further hospital assessment.

Bibliography

1. Perkins GD, Handley AJ, Koster RW, Castrén M, Smyth MA, Olasveengen T et al. European Resuscitation Council Guidelines for Resuscitation 2015: Section 2. Adult basic life support. *Resuscitation* 2015, 95:81–99. Available from: https://www.resuscitationjournal.com/article/S0300-9572(15)00327-5/fulltext https://cprguidelines.eu/sites/573c777f5e61585a053d7ba5/content_entry573c77e35e61585a053d7baf/573c781e5e61585a053d7bd1/files/S0300-9572_15_00327-5_main.pdf.

2. Maconochie I, Bingham R, Eich C, López-Herce J, Rodriguez-Nunez A, Rajka T, Van de Voorde P, Zideman D, Biarent D. European Resuscitation Council Guidelines for Resuscitation 2015: Section 6. Paediatric life support. *Resuscitation* 2015, 95: 223–248. Available from: https://www.resuscitationjournal.com/article/S0300-9572(15)00340-8/fulltext.

3. Resuscitation Council (UK). *Adult Basic Life Support and Automated External Defibrillation 2021.* London: Resuscitation Council (UK), 2021. Available from: https://www.resus.org.uk/resuscitation-guidelines/adult-basic-life-support-and-automated-external-defibrillation.

4. Resuscitation Council (UK). *Paediatric Resuscitation Guidelines 2021.* London: Resuscitation Council (UK), 2021. Available from: https://www.resus.org.uk/resuscitation-guidelines/paediatric-basic-life-support/.

Return of Spontaneous Circulation

1. Introduction

- Gaining return of spontaneous circulation (ROSC) is the initial step towards recovery from out-of-hospital cardiac arrest (OHCA). As such, it is important that paramedics are aware of the critical nature of the post-ROSC patient. A large proportion of patients who have achieved ROSC will re-arrest, the chances of which are minimised by appropriate and timely post-ROSC care.
- Undertake an accurate and complete patient assessment and rapidly provide all interventions to ensure that the patient's condition has been optimised before transfer to hospital, except where an intervention only available in hospital is required or it is unsafe to remain on scene.
- Be prepared for re-arrest; the recurrence rate of a shockable rhythm is at its highest during this period.
- Following ROSC, patients may present with a varying degree of post-cardiac arrest syndrome. Post-cardiac arrest syndrome comprises four key elements:
  – **Brain injury** – coma, seizures, myoclonus, varying degrees of neurocognitive dysfunction and brain death; this may be exacerbated by microcirculatory failure, impaired autoregulation, hypercarbia, hyperoxia, pyrexia, hyper/hypoglycaemia and ongoing seizures.
  – **Myocardial dysfunction** – this is common after cardiac arrest, but usually improves in the following weeks.
  – **Systemic ischemia/reperfusion response** – the whole-body ischaemia/reperfusion that occurs with resuscitation from cardiac arrest activates immunological and coagulation pathways contributing to a systemic inflammatory response syndrome (SIRS).
  – **Persistence of the precipitating pathology.**
- The management of post-cardiac arrest syndrome requires ambulance paramedics to assimilate their clinical assessment and findings, with a view to targeting therapy to the patient's needs.

2. Assessment and Management

TABLE 2.11 – ASSESSMENT and MANAGEMENT of: Return of Spontaneous Circulation

Return of Spontaneous Circulation

- Early recurrence of VF is common; ensure appropriate ongoing monitoring through defibrillator pads.
- Undertake a structured <C>ABCDE assessment that enables appropriate treatment to be applied, as described in the immediate management below. Consider and continue to treat any reversible cause of the initial cardiac arrest. Refer to **Medical Emergencies in Adults – Overview** and **Medical Emergencies in Children – Overview**.
- Measure and record a full set of observations and repeat these at regular intervals.
- Early optimisation of airway, breathing and circulatory support will assist in the heart and brain recovery.
- Forward planning – ensure appropriate resources are on scene or requested to the scene; this may include enhanced care.
- Consider the extrication plan and facilitate preparations for extrication and onward transfer.
- Transfer the patient directly to the nearest appropriate hospital in accordance with local pathways for primary percutaneous coronary intervention (PPCI) or ECMO (where available).
- Provide an ATMIST pre-alert call to the receiving facility.

Airway and Breathing

- Ensure an effective airway; consider enhanced care support for advanced airway insertion or maintenance.
- Maintain oxygen saturations of 94–98%; titrate oxygen to prevent hypoxia or hyperoxia. Refer to **Oxygen**.
- Assist ventilations where required.
- Use of a mechanical ventilator (if available) is preferable to manual ventilation; ensure the settings are appropriate for age, weight and rate (generally a tidal volume of 6–7 ml/kg with a rate of 10/min).
- Monitor waveform capnography.
- Ventilate lungs to normocarbia (4.6–6.0 kPa); consider the reason for readings that fall outside normocarbia, i.e. is this a perfusion, ventilation or metabolic issue?

Return of Spontaneous Circulation

TABLE 2.11 – ASSESSMENT and MANAGEMENT of: Return of Spontaneous Circulation *(continued)*

Circulation

- Perform a 12-lead ECG.

NB Post-ROSC ECGs frequently demonstrate a 'recovering heart'; therefore, ECGs should be obtained at regular intervals.

- Ensure adequate vascular access.
- Following ROSC, patients are often haemodynamically unstable, arrhythmogenic and hypotensive. Aim for a systolic blood pressure (SBP) >100 mmHg. In patients with an adequate heart rate, attempt to achieve this with IV (or IO) fluids, together with IV (or IO) adrenaline (see below for the management of **bradycardia).**
- Most patients who suffer a cardiac arrest due to a cardiac cause are not hypovolaemic, but vasodilation may result in the circulation being relatively underfilled. Administer a 250 ml IV/IO bolus of 0.9% saline, repeated as necessary to a maximum of 500 ml. Patients with sepsis, anaphylaxis, respiratory conditions and dehydration may benefit from larger volumes; seek medical advice in these cases.
- Although 250–500 ml of IV (or IO) fluid may support the circulation, it may take several minutes to administer. If hypotension is present during or after this fluid administration, provide additional circulatory support using careful administration of an adrenaline bolus, repeated as required, every 3–5 mins to maintain the systolic BP >100 mmHg.
    - Initial dose: 50 mcg (0.05 mg) IV/IO. (0.5 ml from a 1:10,000 pre-filled 10 ml adrenaline syringe).
    - Subsequent doses: 50–100 mcg (0.05–0.10 mg). (0.5–1.0 ml from a 1:10,000 pre-filled 10 ml adrenaline syringe).
- Follow each adrenaline bolus with a flush of 20 ml 0.9% normal saline.
- In the event of symptomatic bradycardia in adults (HR <60/min), atropine should be administered.
- In the event of symptomatic bradycardia in children/infants, first ensure that hypoxia has been reversed (the commonest cause of bradycardia). Refer to **Atrophine Sulfate**, **Page for Age** for children.
- If bradycardia persists, external pacing should be considered.

Control Temperature

- There is no evidence that cooling patients post-ROSC is of benefit, but extremes of temperature are harmful. Some patients post ROSC will have a mild hypothermia. Use no more clothing/blankets than is necessary. Vehicle heating is only required to provide a comfortable ambient temperature.
- Aim for a core temperature no higher than 37.5°C.

Blood Glucose Level

- Measure and record blood glucose for hypo/hyperglycaemia (refer to **Glycaemic Emergencies in Adults and Children**).
- Accuracy of blood glucose measurements immediately following ROSC may be impaired by capillary blood stasis. Venous blood glucose is preferred to capillary samples and should be measured and repeated 10 minutes following ROSC.

Combative Patient

- Following ROSC, patients may be cerebrally irritated, agitated or combative, which can make oxygenation difficult.
- Exclude hypoglycaemia and hypoxaemia.
- Try to establish why the patient may be agitated, such as in pain, need for oxygenation or airway device removal.
- If available, request additional support from enhanced care teams to consider the need for anaesthetic management or sedation, as per local procedures.
- This should only be provided by defined teams or individuals in line with robust governance and scope of practice.

(continued)

Return of Spontaneous Circulation

TABLE 2.11 – ASSESSMENT and MANAGEMENT of: Return of Spontaneous Circulation *(continued)*

Pain Relief
- CPR is a painful procedure, therefore the patient is likely to be in pain.
- Consider the provision of analgesia (IV paracetamol, supplemented with small dose of opiates) following resuscitation efforts.
- Observe and manage respiratory function after opiate administration.

Seizure Control
- Seizures that do not self-terminate within 5 minutes may be treated with a benzodiazepine (refer to **Diazepam, Page for Age** for children).
- The administration of diazepam or midazolam (where available) should be carried out in line with clinical practice guidelines or PGD (in the context of midazolam).

3. Disposition

- Acute coronary syndrome (ACS) is a frequent cause of OHCA. Adult patients with a cardiac arrest of presumed primary cardiac aetiology should be transported directly to a hospital with 24/7 coronary angiography capability (this includes both STEMI and non-STEMI patients).
- Adult patients with non-traumatic OHCA should be considered for transport to a recognised centre of care for appropriate specialist treatment, according to local protocols. There is no evidence for a preference for a policy of primarily transporting via ambulance (using bypass protocols) or one of secondary inter-hospital transfer.
- Patients who obtain ROSC following traumatic cardiac arrest should be conveyed in line with the local major trauma pathways, normally to a major trauma centre, assuming criteria for trauma unit bypass are met.

Bibliography

1. Nolan JP, Sandroni C, Bottiger B et al. European Resuscitation Council and European Society of Intensive Care Medicine Guidelines 2021. Post-resuscitation care. *Intensive Care Med* 2021, 47: 369–421. Available from: https://link.springer.com/content/pdf/10.1007/s00134-021-06368-4.pdf.

2. Nolan JP, Neumar RW, Adrie C et al. Post-cardiac arrest syndrome: epidemiology, pathophysiology, treatment, and prognostication: A Scientific Statement from the International Liaison Committee on Resuscitation; the American Heart Association Emergency Cardiovascular Care Committee; the Council on Cardiovascular Surgery and Anesthesia; the Council on Cardiopulmonary, Perioperative, and Critical Care; the Council on Clinical Cardiology; the Council on Stroke. *Resuscitation* 2008, 79: 350–379. Available from: https://www.ilcor.org/data/Post-cardiac_arrest_syndrome.pdf.

3. Dankiewicz J, Cronberg T, Lilja J et al. Hypothermia versus normothermia after out-of-hospital cardiac arrest. *N Engl J Med* 2021, 384: 2283–2294. Available from: https://www.nejm.org/doi/pdf/10.1056/NEJMoa2100591?articleTools=true.

Return of Spontaneous Circulation

Prepare for Transfer
a. Early recurrence of VF is common; ensure appropriate ongoing monitoring through defibrillator pads.
b. Transfer the patient directly to the nearest appropriate hospital in accordance with local pathways.
c. Provide an ATMIST pre-alert call to the receiving facility.

Airway & Breathing
a. Ensure an effective airway; consider enhanced support
b. Record and maintain oxygen saturations of 94–98%, refer to Oxygen.
c. Monitor waveform capnography.
d. Ventilate lungs to normocarbia (4.6–6.0 kPa)

Circulation
a. Record Blood Pressure and aim for SBP > 100 mmHg.
b. First: Fluid (crystalloid) - restore normovolaemia. Refer to Intravascular Fluid in Adults and Intravascular Fluid in Children.
c. Second: Consider small doses of adrenaline to support the circulation if unresponsive to fluid resuscitation – refer to Adrenaline.
d. In the event of symptomatic bradycardia, atropine should be administered, refer to Atropine.

ECG
Perform a 12-lead ECG

Temperature
a. Measure temperature.
b. Patients post-ROSC should be allowed to cool passively.

BM
Measure and record blood glucose for hypo/hyperglycaemia, refer to Glycaemic Emergencies in Adults and Children.

Other
a. Consider the provision of analgesia (small dose opiates or IV Paracetamol) for the management of pain
b. Seizures that do not self-terminate within five minutes may be treated with a benzodiazepine, refer to Diazepam.
c. Combative patients may benefit from anaesthetic management or sedation. Consider enhanced care.

Figure 2.18 – Assessment and management of return of spontaneous circulation (ROSC).

Termination of Resuscitation and Verification of Death in Adults

1. Introduction

Clinical management aims to differentiate between those for whom cardiac arrest is their natural end of life event and for whom resuscitation is not indicated, and those where there is a chance to restore life to a quality acceptable to the patient and in accordance with their wishes, through provision of optimum pre-hospital care.

- Where no explicit decision about CPR has been considered and recorded in advance, there should be an initial presumption in favour of CPR.

- However, in some circumstances where there is no recorded explicit decision regarding CPR, but death is imminent and unavoidable and CPR would not be successful (for example, a person in the advanced stages of an irreversible illness), a decision not to commence CPR should be considered in order to allow a natural death to occur. For patients in whom there is no chance of survival, CPR is not supported; for example:
    - where resuscitation would be both futile and distressing for the patient, relatives, friends and healthcare personnel
    - where time and resources would be ineffective undertaking such measures.

- Every effort should be made to identify patients with a DNACPR decision, Recommended Summary Plan for Emergency Care and Treatment (ReSPECT) form, treatment escalation plan or Advance Decision to Refuse Treatment (ADRT).

- The views of the patient's general practitioner (GP) or relevant third party should be considered. Ask if the patient has a care plan or ADRT in place. Family members may be able to provide verbal information about the patient's wishes, although this is not legally binding in this format.

- CPR should not be attempted, or it should be abandoned if already started by the general public or volunteer responders, if the ambulance clinician is as certain as they can be that a person is dying as an inevitable result of underlying disease (it is therefore their natural end of life event) and CPR would not restart the heart and breathing for a sustained period.

- Where there is uncertainty, it is acceptable to commence basic life support (BLS) while further information is rapidly gathered to enable the decision to be made about whether resuscitation can be stopped.

- On rare occasions, it may be appropriate to continue CPR until patient privacy and dignity can be assured, before stopping the resuscitation attempt.

- Refer to local policies and procedures regarding the clinical grade of ambulance clinician that is permitted to undertake verification of death.

2. Conditions Unequivocally Associated with Death in Adults

The following conditions are unequivocally associated with death in adults (for children, refer to **Termination of Resuscitation and Verification of Death in Children**), and can be used by ambulance clinicians to verify death:

- **Decapitation.**

- **Massive cranial and cerebral destruction.**

- **Hemicorporectomy** or similar massive injury.

- **Decomposition/putrefaction** – where tissue damage indicates that the patient has been dead for some hours, days or longer.

- **Incineration** – the presence of full-thickness burns with charring of greater than 95% of the body surface.

- **Hypostasis** – the pooling of blood in congested vessels in the dependent part of the body in the position in which it lies after death. Initially, hypostatic staining may appear as small round patches looking rather like bruises but later these will combine to merge as the familiar pattern. Above the hypostatic engorgement, there is obvious pallor of the skin.

- The presence of hypostasis is diagnostic of death – the appearance is not present in a live patient. In extremely cold conditions, hypostasis may be bright red in colour, and in carbon monoxide poisoning it is characteristically 'cherry red' in appearance.

- **Rigor mortis** – the stiffness occurring after death from the post-mortem breakdown of enzymes in the muscle fibres.
    - Rigor mortis occurs first in the small muscles of the face, next in the arms, then in the legs, with these changes taking between 30 minutes and 3 hours. The recognition of rigor mortis can be made difficult where, rarely, death has occurred from tetanus or strychnine poisoning.
    - In some, rigidity never develops (infants, cachectic individuals and the aged), while in others it may become apparent more rapidly, i.e. in conditions in which muscle glycogen is depleted, e.g. exertion (which includes struggling), strychnine poisoning and local heat (e.g. from a fire, hot room or direct sunlight).
    - Rigor should not be confused with cadaveric spasm (sometimes referred to as instant rigor mortis), which develops immediately after death without preceding flaccidity following intense physical and/or emotional activity. Examples include death by drowning or a fall from a height. In contrast with true rigor mortis, only one group of muscles is affected and **not** the whole body. Rigor mortis will develop subsequently.

Termination of Resuscitation and Verification of Death in Adults

— Rigor is also distinct from trismus (spasm of the muscles around the jaw which may occur in those with a reduced level of consciousness). Rigor mortis is not isolated to jaw muscles alone.

Note:

In cases that do not meet these criteria, where it is thought that CPR is futile or inappropriate, do not withhold or terminate resuscitation until senior clinical advice has been sought.

If access to the patient is restricted and it is believed that one of the conditions above may exist, then a multi-agency decision (Fire, Police, Coast Guard etc.) should be made on whether ongoing rescue should continue or whether the incident becomes that of body recovery. The JESIP principles should be followed and include factors such as risks posed to the rescue teams.

3. Other Conditions Where Resuscitation May Be Withheld or Discontinued

- In addition to the conditions above, there are other criteria which can be used to confirm death, and which indicate that resuscitation should not be attempted, or may be discontinued:

  A) The presence of a DNACPR (do not attempt cardiopulmonary resuscitation) decision or ReSPECT form that advises resuscitation is not to be attempted.

  B) A valid Advance Decision to Refuse Treatment (ADRT), which refuses cardiopulmonary resuscitation, or a Lasting Power of Attorney (LPA) for Health and Welfare that includes decisions related to life-sustaining treatments and where CPR is refused by the attorney.

  C) If a person is known to be in the final stages of an advanced, irreversible condition, in which attempted CPR would be both inappropriate and unsuccessful, CPR should not be started or can be stopped if already commenced. Even in the absence of a recorded DNACPR decision, ambulance clinicians may be able to recognise this situation and make an appropriate decision, based on clear evidence that they should document. Examples of clear evidence include the presence of anticipatory medications, hospice or palliative care notes and advance care plans, but always refer to local guidance. While seeking evidence or where there is doubt, it is appropriate to start BLS and seek senior clinical advice. The relatives/carers should be included in the decision making process.

NB: An advanced and irreversible condition is an illness or injury that can no longer be cured and care is refocused to promote quality of life, comfort and symptom control. Examples of conditions are not confined to cancer, but also include organ failure (e.g. heart, respiratory, renal and liver), neurological illness (e.g. motor neurone disease, Parkinson's, Dementia) and advanced frailty in older people.

When identifying patients near end of life, it is useful to utilise available screening tools, such as the Gold Standards Framework (GSF) or the Supportive and Palliative Care Indicators Tool (SPICT). They offer insight into a patient's pattern of deterioration and an overall impression of their stage of illness. Further information to support this can also be gleaned from the patient's history, medical notes and any completed advance personalised care plan.

  D) Submersion (refer to **Drowning**).

  E) There is no realistic chance that CPR would be successful if **ALL** the following exist together:
  - >15 minutes has elapsed since the onset of cardiac arrest.
  - No evidence of bystander CPR in the 15 minutes before the arrival of the ambulance.
  - Exclusion factors are absent (drowning, hypothermia, poisoning/overdose, pregnancy, child/neonate).
  - Asystole for >30 seconds on the ECG monitor screen. CPR should only be paused for a 30-second asystole check if all other criteria are met.

- Whenever possible, a confirmatory ECG demonstrating asystole should be documented as evidence of death. In this situation, a 3- or 4-electrode system using limbs alone will cause minimum disturbance to the deceased. If a paper ECG trace cannot be taken, it is permissible to make a diagnosis of asystole from the screen alone (**NB** due caution must be applied in respect of electrode contact, gain and, where possible, using more than one ECG lead).

- It is important that in order to confirm death, the rhythm is unequivocally persistent and continuous asystole. If CPR is stopped when any other rhythm is present (i.e. agonal rhythm or PEA), it is important to wait until all cardiac electrical activity has ceased and the ECG shows asystole. Only at this stage should the patient be declared life extinct and the family/relatives informed that this is the case. This is because there have been well-documented cases where spontaneous ROSC has occurred following termination of resuscitation.

Termination of Resuscitation and Verification of Death in Adults

4. Advance Care Planning

- Advance care planning is a voluntary process involving a person-centred discussion that helps an individual in understanding choices and sharing their preferences and priorities for future care.
- The aim of advance care planning is to ensure that individuals receive medical care that is appropriate and consistent with their values, goals and preferences, when they no longer have the mental capacity to make such decisions.
- The outcome of advance care planning discussions may include an ADRT, or context-specific recommendations such as emergency care plans or treatment escalation plans. A trusted person/s may also be nominated as an LPA with legal power to make medical treatment decisions, including life-sustaining treatment.
- A DNACPR decision is a part of advance care planning but differs as it is clinician led, in discussion with the patient and their family members wherever possible. The decision is based on a clinical assessment that the person is dying as an inevitable result of an advanced, irreversible disease and that CPR would not be successful and should not be attempted.
- Ambulance clinicians should be familiar with these documents and their legal standing; they are critical elements of resuscitation decision making.

4.1 Advance Decision to Refuse Treatment (ADRT)

- An ADRT enables a person over 18 years of age to refuse specified medical treatment in advance of a time where they are unable to consent or refuse treatment following the loss of mental capacity. **It is legally binding.**

An ADRT in Scotland is known as an Advance Directive; they do not have the same legal recognition as in England and Wales but are widely recognised under common law and by healthcare professionals. In Northern Ireland, they are not legally recognised. Refer to local policies regarding use of these documents.

- ADRTs are defined within the Mental Capacity Act 2005 (MCA). Providing ADRTs meet all the requirements of the MCA, they are legally binding for health and social care professionals. This makes ADRTs quite distinct from other aspects of advance care planning.
- An ADRT must be valid and applicable to current circumstances. If it is, it has the same effect as a decision that is made by a person with capacity: healthcare professionals (including ambulance clinicians) must follow the decision.
- ADRTs are only valid if the patient is unconscious or lacks capacity. If the patient has capacity, their decision and wishes should be followed.
- Paramedics will be protected from liability if they:
  - stop or withhold treatment because they reasonably believe that an ADRT exists, and that it is valid and applicable
  - treat a person because, having taken all practical and appropriate steps to find out if the person has made an ADRT, they do not know or are not satisfied that a valid and applicable ADRT exists.
- There is no official form for recording an ADRT, although there are several well-known versions for completion. It can be informal, e.g. a hand-written paper copy; the important issue is that it fulfils the criteria for validity.
- If the advance decision refuses life-sustaining treatment, it **must**:
  - be in writing (if the patient cannot write it themselves, it is acceptable to have someone else write it but this must be signed and witnessed by an independent person)
  - be signed by the patient or another in their presence if they are unable to sign it themselves
  - specify the exact treatment being refused; this can be written in layperson's terms
  - specifically acknowledge an intention to refuse treatment even if this puts the patient's life at risk, and must include a statement to this effect
  - be witnessed and dated (there are no legal requirements on who should be a witness, except being over 18 years of age) and it is not necessary to involve a solicitor in this process.
- To establish whether an advance decision is valid and applicable, ambulance clinicians must take reasonable steps to find out if the person:
  - has done anything that clearly goes against their advance decision
  - has withdrawn their decision
  - has subsequently conferred the power to make that decision on an LPA
  - would have changed their decision if they had known more about the current circumstances.
- If any of these apply, then the ADRT is not considered to be valid or applicable. The ADRT would additionally not apply in cases of attempted suicide or suicide. In these cases, seeking urgent senior clinical support is advised.
- If there is any genuine doubt about the validity of an ADRT, ambulance clinicians must act in the patient's best interests. When an advance decision is not followed, the reasons must be clearly documented.
- In Scotland and Northern Ireland, ADRTs are not covered by statute but it is likely that they are binding under common law. Although no cases have been taken to court in Scotland or Northern Ireland, it is likely that the principles that emerged from consideration of cases by the

Termination of Resuscitation and Verification of Death in Adults

English courts (before the MCA) would also guide decision making in these jurisdictions.

- An advance refusal of CPR is likely to be legally binding in Scotland and Northern Ireland if:
  - the person was an adult at the time the decision was made (16 years old in Scotland and 18 in Northern Ireland)
  - the person had capacity when the decision was made
  - the circumstances that have arisen are those that were envisaged by the person
  - the person was not subjected to undue influence in making the decision.
- If an ADRT does not meet these criteria but appears to set out a clear indication of the person's wishes, it will not be legally binding but should be taken into consideration in determining the person's best interests.

4.2 Lasting Power of Attorney (LPA)

- An LPA is a **legally binding** document which allows someone to nominate another person (or persons) to make decisions on their behalf after they lose mental capacity. The document is completed in advance of that person losing capacity, during which time the person continues to make their own decisions.
- The document must be registered with the Office of the Public Guardian (England and Wales) or the Public Guardian (Scotland) and include their official stamp or crest. The original document or a certified copy must be viewed physically or digitally; in England and Wales, an LPA can be viewed online using an access code at www.gov.uk. In Northern Ireland, the Health and Welfare Power of Attorney does not exist.
- In England and Wales, there are two types of LPA: property and financial affairs and health and welfare. Only a health and welfare LPA allows healthcare decisions to be made on the person's behalf when they lack capacity. In Scotland, a Welfare Power of Attorney or Combined Power of Attorney allows an attorney to make decisions related to the person's health.
- An LPA can include decisions relating to life-sustaining treatment. If the donor wishes the attorney to be able to consent to or refuse life-sustaining treatment, it will be clearly included in the document. An attorney cannot insist on any treatment which is inappropriate, including resuscitation.
- The document should be viewed before basing a decision on information provided by the named individual.
- Where both an ADRT and LPA exist for a patient; if the ADRT is dated after the LPA, and is valid, then the ADRT should be followed. If the ADRT is dated prior to the LPA, then the decision of the attorney should be followed if the LPA applies in the specific situation and is in the patient's best interests.
- If there is any genuine doubt about the validity of an LPA, ambulance clinicians must act in the patient's best interests.

4.3 Do Not Attempt Cardiopulmonary Resuscitation (DNACPR) Decision

- A DNACPR decision is an advance clinical assessment, recorded to guide immediate decision making in the event of a cardiac arrest. DNACPR decisions are made when a person is near the end stage of an advanced, irreversible condition (or on some occasions sooner), to ensure that the individual is not exposed to the trauma and indignity of CPR, which has no realistic prospect of benefit.
- A DNACPR decision is **not legally binding** but is one of a number of elements to inform decision making regarding CPR. The final decision regarding whether or not attempting CPR is clinically appropriate lies with the healthcare professional who is responsible for their care at the time.
- The majority of DNACPR decisions are made for adults. Children with advanced irreversible conditions may have recorded within their care plan text stating that, following discussions with family and the child's healthcare team, CPR is not considered appropriate. (Refer to **Termination of Resuscitation and Verification of Death in Children**.)
- DNACPR decisions are only made for advanced, irreversible physical health conditions. Learning Disabilities and/or autism are not physical health conditions and should never be used as rationale for a DNACPR decision.
- A DNACPR decision applies solely to cardiopulmonary resuscitation. All other treatment and care that a patient requires is not precluded or influenced by a DNACPR decision.
- DNACPR documents should, ideally, move with patients as they are transferred from one setting to another – particularly when death is expected (e.g. an end of life patient being discharged home to die). It is anticipated that the senior clinician responsible for the patient in each setting (e.g. the GP after patient discharge from hospital) will review the patient at the earliest opportunity. This may not always be possible and although processes can vary by locality, in principle the DNACPR decision remains valid.

4.4 Resuscitation Decision Making and DNACPR Decisions

- DNACPR recommendations and similar decisions are often recorded on a form approved by the organisation providing the care for the patient. The design and content of these forms can vary significantly.

Termination of Resuscitation and Verification of Death in Adults

- Care-planning documents can often contain DNACPR sections, or the decision may be documented in a letter, hospital discharge summary or as an entry in the patient's health records. Formal letters can also be used to communicate resuscitation instructions to other professionals. These are often communicated to ambulance control and logged against the patient's address, or the decision is available to access via an electronic care record database.
- It is important to note that all of the above are acceptable methods for recording and communicating resuscitation decisions. Documentation of the decision includes:
  - Patient identification (e.g. name, DOB, NHS number).
  - The decision, including the date it was made.
  - Rationale for making the decision
  - Name and position of the clinician making the decision
  - Information of any discussions about the decision with the patient and/or those close to them.
- If a review date is specified, expiry of that date DOES NOT invalidate the DNACPR. Many DNACPR forms/records will not have a review date; this is acceptable and indicates that the patient's condition is not expected to improve. A decision must be made and recorded by the ambulance clinician (with senior clinical advice if appropriate) as to whether the document is still considered valid.
- In the absence of the original copy, a photocopy can be considered valid. Refer to local policy as to whether additional verification is required, for example seeking confirmation that the photocopy is the most up-to-date version of the decision.
- Where a DNACPR exists, ambulance clinicians should support dying patients, provide appropriate comfort measures and support relatives and carers. Contact should be made with the patient's GP, district nursing team or specialist team, to arrange the provision of ongoing care and effective symptom control and to ensure the death is managed appropriately.
- Ambulance staff will be protected from liability if they stop or withhold resuscitation because they reasonably believe that a DNACPR exists, and that it is valid and applicable.
- Where there are concerns regarding the validity of the DNACPR decision and its authenticity cannot be confirmed, any evidence obtained should be taken into consideration in determining the person's best interests. This may require paramedics to provide BLS while they seek senior clinical advice.
- There will be occasions when a patient who has a DNACPR decision may have a cardiac arrest that is considered unnatural and not in the envisaged circumstances and has a potentially easily reversible cause (e.g. patient has taken an overdose, is choking or has anaphylaxis). All reversible causes should be considered (refer to Section 10 of **Advanced Life Support**). In these circumstances, resuscitation and rapid conveyance to hospital should be considered, as the cause of the arrest is unrelated to the patient's main clinical problem(s) and could be reversible. In these potentially reversible situations, it is vital to seek urgent senior clinical advice as per local policy. Documented DNACPR decisions are not valid in cases of suicide.

4.5 Recommended Summary Plan for Emergency Care and Treatment (ReSPECT)

- A ReSPECT form summarises treatments to be considered and those that would not be wanted or would not work for the patient in an emergency. It might include recommendations of when transfer to hospital would be desirable or not.
- ReSPECT is a summary of recommendations to help the ambulance clinician make immediate decisions about the patient's care and treatment. It contains recommendations about whether CPR should be attempted.
- A ReSPECT form contains more than a CPR decision: it is not just a replacement for a DNACPR form. It is to promote recording an emergency care plan by many people, and may recommend active treatment, including attempted CPR if it should be needed.
- Like a DNACPR form, it is **not legally binding**; clinical judgement must still be applied and ambulance clinicians may decide not to follow the recommendations on a ReSPECT form. However, paramedics should be prepared to justify valid reasons for overriding the recommendations on a ReSPECT form, remembering the information contained reflects that the patient's wishes and preferences. An example of such a decision would be treating an immediately reversible emergency such as choking if it was believed that this was not the circumstance envisaged when the decision was made for resuscitation not to be attempted.
- The ReSPECT form should be with the person and be readily available; in some areas it may be accessed electronically.

4.6 Best Interests Decision Making

- Ambulance clinicians must consider any evidence as an expression of previous wishes when establishing the person's best interests. This may involve the provision of clinical treatment, including resuscitation.
- It is the most senior member of the ambulance team in charge of a patient's care and treatment who must decide what is in the patient's best

Termination of Resuscitation and Verification of Death in Adults

interests. However, joint decision making by the entire team is considered best practice.

- Ambulance clinicians should be guided by advice from those close to a patient regarding the patient's previously expressed wishes and beliefs, even though the patient's spouse, family, friends or colleagues may not be entitled to give or withhold consent to treatment on the patient's behalf.
- Decisions must not be based on assumptions made solely on factors such as the person's age, disability or a professional's subjective view of a person's quality of life.
- Refer to the Mental Capacity Act Code of Practice (2007) for guidance on making best interests' decisions. In a resuscitation situation where there is uncertainty about what is in the patient's best interests, gather information rapidly and seek senior clinical support and/or advice from the patient's care team/GP.

5. Termination of Resuscitation

- If there is a realistic chance that CPR could be successful, then resuscitation should continue to establish the patient's response to ALS interventions (ALS is defined in **Advanced Life Support**).
- If, following ALS interventions, the patient has been **persistently and continuously** asystolic for 30 minutes and all reversible causes have been identified and corrected, resuscitation may be discontinued, except in the following cases:
  - pregnancy
  - hypothermic patients (where hypothermia is the primary cause of the cardiac arrest)
  - suspected drugs overdose/poisoning
  - infants, children and adolescents (i.e. all those <18 years of age). (Refer to **Termination of Resuscitation and Verification of Death in Children**.)
- These patients should be transported to the nearest facility with on going resuscitation, unless the circumstances would make transport futile.

5.1 Pulseless Electrical Activity

- Pulseless electrical activity (PEA) is a scenario that presents challenges to decision making about cardiac arrest management.
- Although there is ongoing myocardial electrical activity, the outcome is often poor.
- An early decision around the need for rapid removal to hospital should be considered.
- The use of cardiac ultrasound, if available, may enable more guided therapy or decision making.
- Senior clinicians may be asked to advise on situations where the patient remains in PEA following 30 minutes of resuscitation, and where paramedics on scene believe continuing the resuscitation is futile. Refer to local senior clinician guidance.
- There is limited evidence to support when one should terminate a PEA cardiac arrest; however, the following factors are important to consider when making this decision:
  - the interval of time in arrest without life support
  - the absence of reversible causes
  - the presence of comorbidities
  - the rate/width of the QRS complexes
  - the trend and absolute value of $EtCO_2$.
- Some patients undergoing prolonged CPR can survive with good outcome.

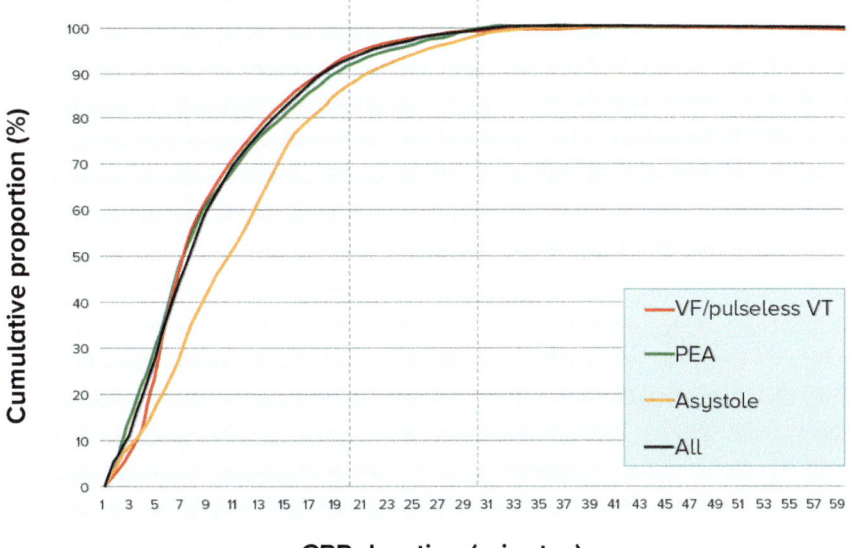

Figure 2.19 – Relationship between the duration of cardiopulmonary resuscitation and favourable neurological outcomes after out-of-hospital cardiac arrest.[13] Extending the duration of resuscitation from 20 to 30 minutes will result in a small but significant number of additional survivors.

Termination of Resuscitation and Verification of Death in Adults

- Young age, myocardial infarction and potentially reversible causes of cardiac arrest, such as hypothermia and pulmonary emboli, are associated with a better outcome, especially when the arrest is witnessed and followed by prompt and effective resuscitative efforts.

5.2 Refractory ventricular fibrillation (VF)

- A significant number of patients may present in ventricular fibrillation (VF) that is unresponsive to repeated defibrillation shocks and amiodarone.
- Many cases of VF are secondary to myocardial ischaemia as a result of myocardial infarction, which is potentially reversible with primary percutaneous coronary intervention (PPCI). Resuscitation should not therefore be stopped in cases of refractory or persistent VF.
- Where practical, transport patients with persistent/refractory VF or pulseless VT to a cardiac arrest centre with ongoing CPR, because further in-hospital treatment may occasionally be successful.

5.3 Agonal Rhythm

- As resuscitation progresses, organised QRS complexes often deteriorate to wide, low-amplitude, irregular complexes, known as an idioventricular or agonal rhythm. This is typically at a rate <10 bpm and is not associated with effective cardiac output.
- This rhythm is usually a prelude to asystole.
- A persistent agonal rhythm can be treated as asystole and resuscitation can be terminated if it has **persisted continuously** for more than 30 minutes.

6. Deaths During a Major Incident

- In a major incident scenario, deceased patients **MUST** have a mass casualty assessment/triage card attached to them with the following details recorded:
  - That the patient is identified as dead.
  - The time the patient was identified as dead.
  - The identity of the paramedic making the decision.
- Deceased patients should only be moved if they are obstructing an evacuation route for other casualties, as the location is to be treated as a crime scene. Follow major incident protocols.

7. Action to Be Taken after Death Has Been Established

- Following termination of a resuscitation attempt and verification of death, repositioning of the body and removal of advanced airways and/or indwelling cannulae should be in accordance with local protocol.
- Complete documentation, including the factors that influenced resuscitation decision making and those relating to DNACPR decisions/ADRTs/LPAs/ReSPECT forms.
- Actions taken after verification of death by ambulance clinicians will depend on whether the death was believed to be expected or unexpected.
  - **Expected death** This occurs where a death was anticipated, expected and predicted and there are no unusual circumstances, and the person has been assessed by a doctor or healthcare professional either remotely or in person during their last illness and within the last 28 days of life (currently, under the Coronavirus Act). In the majority of cases, the patient's GP will certify the death and issue a Medical Certificate of Cause of Death (MCCD).
  - **Unexpected death** This is where a death is not clinically expected or has occurred in suspicious, unnatural, violent or otherwise unexpected circumstances. These deaths will be referred to HM Coroner's office.
- It is not necessary for a medical practitioner to attend to confirm the fact of death. Subsequent actions to be taken by ambulance clinicians will vary by location; refer to local policies and procedures.
- Services should be encouraged, in conjunction with their Coroner's service (or Procurator Fiscal in Scotland), to develop a local procedure for handling the body once death has been verified by ambulance personnel.
- A locally approved leaflet should be adopted for handing to bereaved relatives.
- Any consideration for organ donation should not influence resuscitation attempt decision making:
  - If there is no ROSC, it is unlikely organ donation will occur.
  - If there is ROSC but the patient is not suitable for critical care, they are unlikely to be admitted solely for donation purposes.
  - A long downtime usually makes organs unsuitable for donation.
  - Tissue donation occurs the next day in the mortuary, not in the hospital, so transport to hospital does not change the chance of tissue donation.

8. Supporting Bystanders Witnessing Cardiac Arrest

- In many cases of out-of-hospital cardiac arrest (OHCA), a close relative or friend may have performed CPR before ambulance service help arrives; it is important to provide reassurance about the actions they have taken and their resuscitation efforts.

Termination of Resuscitation and Verification of Death in Adults

- Relatives may find it more distressing to be separated from their family member during the resuscitation attempt, and there may be advantages to them being present.
- However, it is also important to acknowledge that these are distressing events, and so there can be disadvantages to the relative being present.
- There are a number of key principles, actions and safeguards that ambulance clinicians should be aware of, and adopt, to support relatives through the witnessing of a resuscitation attempt and its termination when appropriate:
  - Always acknowledge the difficulty of the situation.
  - When possible, try to ensure that one member of the team is with the relative at all times. This can be challenging to achieve with limited numbers of people on scene, but will ensure the relative is supported as much as possible during the event.
  - Ensure the bystander understands they have a choice of whether or not to be present.
  - Ensure that introductions are made and names known.
  - Give clear, simple and honest explanations of what is happening.
  - Ask the relative, in a sensitive manner, not to interfere with the resuscitation process, but allow them to touch the patient when it is safe to do so should they so wish (assuming that there are no issues in relation to a possible crime scene).
  - Answer what questions they have and explain the procedures in simple terms.
  - When it becomes clear that the resuscitation attempt is unlikely to have a successful outcome, take time to prepare relatives by keeping them updated, using sensitive warnings. Examples include, 'despite all we are doing there has been no change', 'it is unlikely their heart is going to restart' or 'they are not responding to the drugs we are giving'.
  - When the decision has been made to terminate the resuscitation attempt, explain that you will be stopping CPR and ask if the relative would like to be present when this happens.
  - When the patient has died, explain that there will be a period where actions will need to be taken, for example that equipment will need to be removed. Depending on the situation, explain that some medical devices will need to be left in situ.
  - Allow relatives time to say goodbye; advise that it is ok to talk to the deceased or to touch them if they wish and this is appropriate to the situation.
- Best attempts should be made to ensure that any member of the public who has delivered CPR is supported at the scene and given welfare advice. Bystanders should be signposted to their GP in the first instance.

8.1 Breaking Bad News

- Breaking bad news is best done with a well-prepared, honest and simple approach.
- Relatives will often not remember the details of what was said, but they will remember how they were made to feel.
- Ambulance clinicians should try to:
  - Take time to prepare personal appearance; check and tidy uniform/clothing, remove gloves and, if necessary, wash hands.
  - Confirm the name of the deceased before speaking to the relatives, establish their relationship and confirm the correct relatives where there are multiple patients.
  - Adopt a position at the same level as the relative.
  - Use simple language and avoid medical jargon.
  - Avoid long preamble such as asking about the patient's pre-morbid health.
  - Ensure the word 'dead' or 'died' is introduced early in the conversation.
  - Allow periods of silence to enable the relatives to absorb and process what they are being told.
  - Check if they have understood what you have told them: you may need to repeat the information
- Remember to anticipate the types of reaction or emotional response to the bad news and be ready to support the relatives as much as possible.

8.2 Children and Young People Witnessing Cardiac Arrest

- Children and young people that witness and are present at a cardiac arrest, particularly of a close relative, may need additional support.
- They may have questions about what they have witnessed. Always talk to them with a family member or someone who knows them. Try to ascertain their understanding; their awareness of death and reaction will depend on their age and stage of development. Follow the child's lead, be open and honest, use simple terms and avoid long explanations which may cause confusion.
- Before leaving the scene, consider making a referral to their GP.
- Consider signposting parents/carers to organisations that provide specific support for bereaved children, as per local procedures.

Termination of Resuscitation and Verification of Death in Adults

KEY POINTS!

Termination of Resuscitation and Verification of Death in Adults

- Paramedics are increasingly being called upon to diagnose death and initiate the appropriate clinical response.
- After cardiac arrest, resuscitation efforts including ALS must be made whenever there is a chance of survival, unless the person has made an ADRT refusing CPR in these circumstances.
- Some conditions are incompatible with recovery and, in these cases, resuscitation should not be attempted.
- In some situations, once the facts of the patient and situation are known, resuscitation efforts can be discontinued.
- Patients can and do make anticipatory decisions NOT to be resuscitated. An ADRT must be respected and a DNACPR recommendation should be used to guide decision making on whether or not to attempt CPR.
- These guidelines should be read in conjunction with local policies and procedures.

Bibliography

1. Soar J, Bottiger BW, Carli P, Couper K, Deakin CD, Djavf T, Lott C, Olasveengen T, Paal P, Pellis T, D. Perkins GD, Sandroni C, Nolan JP. European Resuscitation Council Guidelines 2021: adult advanced life support. *Resuscitation* 2021, 161: 115–151. Available from: https://www.resuscitationjournal.com/article/S0300-9572(15)00328-7/pdf.

2. Resuscitation Council (UK). Resuscitation Guidelines 2021. *Prevention of Cardiac Arrest and Decisions about CPR*. 2021. Available from: https://resus.org.uk/resuscitation-guidelines/prevention-of-cardiac-arrest-and-decisions-about-cpr/.

3. British Medical Association, Resuscitation Council (UK), Royal College of Nursing. *Decisions Relating to Cardiopulmonary Resuscitation*. 3rd end. 2016. Available from: https://www.resus.org.uk/sites/default/files/2020-05/20160123%20Decisions%20Relating%20to%20CPR%20-%202016.pdfhttps://resus.org.uk/EasySiteWeb/GatewayLink.aspx?alId=16643.

4. Ambitions Partnership. *Universal Principles for Advance Care Planning (ACP)*. NHS England and NHS Improvement. 2022. Available from: https://www.england.nhs.uk/publication/universal-principles-for-advance-care-planning/.

5. British Medical Association. *2020/21 General Medical Services (GMS) Contract Quality and Outcomes Framework (QOF)*. London: NHS England and NHS Improvement, 2021. Available from: https://www.england.nhs.uk/coronavirus/wp-content/uploads/sites/52/2020/03/C0713-202021-General-Medical-Services-GMS-contract-Quality-and-Outcomes-Framework-QOF-Guidance.pdf

6. UK Government Office of the Public Guardian. *Mental Capacity Act 2005 Code of Practice*. London: The Stationary Office Ltd, 2007. Available from: https://assets.publishing.service.gov.uk/government/uploads/system/uploads/attachment_data/file/921428/Mental-capacity-act-code-of-practice.pdf

7. Mentzelopoulos, SD et al. European Resuscitation Council Guidelines 2021: thics of resuscitation and end of life decisions. *Resuscitation* 2021, 161: 408–432. Available from: https://www.resuscitationjournal.com/article/S0300-9572(21)00070-8/pdf

8. Department of Health (NI). *Review of the Law Relating to Advance Decisions to Refuse Treatment Mental Capacity Act (NI) 2016 section 284*. 2019. Available from: Mental Capacity Act (NI) 2016 Advance Decision to Refuse Treatment and Mental Health Paper – Review (health-ni.gov.uk).

9. Hospice UK. *Special Edition of Care After Death: Registered Nurse Verification of Expected Adult Death (RNVoEAD) Guidance*. 2020. Available from: https://professionals.hospiceuk.org/docs/default-source/What-We-Offer/Care-Support-Programmes/Care-after-death/rnvoead-special-covid-19-edition-final_2.pdf?sfvrsn=2H.

10. Resuscitation Council (UK). *ReSPECT Recommended Summary Plan for Emergency Care and Treatment*. 2017. Available from: https://www.resus.org.uk/respect/.

11. Ridley D. *Regulation 28 Report to Prevent Future Deaths. Mary Johnson*. 2020. Available from: Mary Johnson, Courts and Tribunals Judiciary.

12. Scottish Government. *Adults with Incapacity (Scotland) Act 2000. Proposals for Reform*. 2018. Available from: Adults with Incapacity (Scotland) Act 2000: Proposals for Reform (www.gov.scot).

13. Yoshikazu G. Relationship between the duration of cardiopulmonary resuscitation and favorable neurological outcomes after out-of-hospital cardiac arrest: a prospective, nationwide, population-based cohort study. *Journal of the American Heart Association* 2016, 5(3).

Termination of Resuscitation and Verification of Death in Children

1. Introduction

- Being called to a death of an infant, child or adolescent is one of the most difficult experiences to encounter. Paramedics are usually the first professionals to arrive at the scene, and, at the same time as making difficult judgements about resuscitation, they have to deal with the devastating initial shock of the parents/carers.

- Despite the recent fall in incidence, sudden unexpected death in infancy (SUDI) remains the largest single cause of death in infants aged 1 month to 1 year. SUDI can also occasionally occur in children older than one year of age. The 1991 national 'Reduce the Risk' campaign advocating that infants sleep on their backs produced a dramatic reduction (70%) in sudden infant deaths.

- In 50% of SUDIs, a specific cause for the death is found. The vast majority of SUDIs occur from natural causes. SUDIs can result from child prompting a joint paediatric and police investigation. When informed of a SUDI, ambulance control should immediately notify the police to initiate this process.

- This section draws on national experience and follows the Kennedy Report's (2016) recommendations.

2. Considerations for Paediatric Cardiac Arrest/Death

Resuscitation should always be attempted unless there is a condition unequivocally associated with death or the child has an advanced and irreversible condition and their Advance Care Plan recommends that CPR is not appropriate.

- The immediate consideration(s) when called to a paediatric cardiac arrest/child death include:

  1) **Resuscitation** This must be attempted in **ALL** cases, unless there is a condition unequivocally associated with death or the child has a life-limiting condition AND the child has an Advance Care Plan that states that CPR is not appropriate (refer to **Basic Life Support in Children** and **Advanced Life Support**).

  2) **Verification of death and termination of resuscitation** As in adult practice, asystole should be confirmed by ECG when determining death. (Pulse checks are particularly unreliable in sick children. Similarly, sick infants may demonstrate marked peripheral cyanosis and cold extremities prior to death (refer to **Medical Emergencies in Children – Overview** and **Trauma Emergencies in Children – Overview**).

- Unlike for adults, resuscitation of children should almost always be undertaken and continued (unless an Advance Care Plan recommends otherwise) while rapidly conveying the child to the nearest suitable Emergency Department, continuing resuscitation en route (even in circumstances where resuscitation appears futile and death inevitable).

- Parents/carers need to be assured that resuscitation was attempted (even if unsuccessful), rather than forever questioning whether their child was denied potentially life-saving treatment(s).

- An initial presumption in favour of performing CPR should be made when a child does not have an Advance Care Plan and there is no documented advance decision about attempting resuscitation.

- Every effort should be made to identify children with an Advance Care Plan, Recommended Summary Plan for Emergency Care and Treatment (ReSPECT) form or Treatment Escalation Plan that includes recommendations for resuscitation.

- On rare occasions, it may be appropriate to continue CPR when a child has a condition unequivocally associated with death until patient privacy and dignity can be assured before stopping the resuscitation attempt.

2.1 Conditions Unequivocally Associated with Death in Children

- **Decapitation.**
- **Massive cranial and cerebral destruction.**
- **Hemicorporectomy** (or similar massive injury).
- **Decomposition/putrefaction** – where tissue damage indicates that the patient has been dead for some hours, days or longer.
- **Incineration** – full-thickness burns and charring of greater than 95% of the body surface.
- **Hypostasis** – pooling of blood in congested vessels in the dependent parts of the body, in the position in which it lies after death. In very sick children, mottling of the skin may mimic hypostasis so hypostasis alone should not be used as the only factor to withhold paediatric resuscitation.
- **Rigor mortis** – stiffness occurring after death as a result of the enzymic muscle fibres breakdown. This can occur rapidly in children but sometimes does not occur at all, so resuscitation should be attempted unless there is another condition unequivocally associated with death.
- **Foetal maceration in a newborn** – children delivered with severe abnormalities incompatible with life. A stillborn child that died more than a day before birth may have skin loosening and sloughing off when touched.

Note: Do not withhold or terminate resuscitation:

(i) where these criteria have not been met or

(ii) where CPR appears futile or inappropriate, until senior clinical advice has been sought.

If access to the patient is restricted and it is believed that one of the conditions above may exist, then a

Termination of Resuscitation and Verification of Death in Children

multi-agency decision (Fire, Police, Coastguard etc.) should be made on whether ongoing rescue should continue or the incident becomes that of body recovery, applying JESIP principles and considering the risks posed to the rescue team.

Other conditions where resuscitation may be withheld or discontinued

In addition to the conditions above, other criteria can be applied to confirm death, and can be used when considering whether resuscitation need not be attempted or should be discontinued:

a. The child has a life-limiting condition, an Advance Care Plan, a ReSPECT form or Treatment Escalation Plan that advises resuscitation is not attempted.

b. Submersion (refer to **Drowning**).

> **Care Plans for Children and Young People**
>
> - Children and young people with complex illnesses are likely to have a detailed Advance Care Plan in place.
> - This is likely to be documented within the nationally recognised Child and Young Persons Advance Care Plan (CYPACP), although localised forms may also be used.
> - The CYPACP may or may not include a ReSPECT form.
> - Children and young people who have reached an age where they have an understanding and competence should be involved in decision making around their care. Parents should also be involved in this joint decision making process.
> - For additional support and guidance when using a care plan for children and young people, their specialist care team should be contacted.

2.2 Expected Deaths

- It is uncommon for ambulance paramedics to be called to attend to an expected death of a child.
- When a child has a life-threatening or life-limiting condition and is nearing death, the child's clinical team will have made plans, in conjunction with the child's parents (and the child if appropriate). These can include discussions about care after death, and written Advance Care Planning documentation will be prepared to guide ambulance paramedics.
- It is important to remember that even though the family may have been caring for the child for many years and anticipated their death, when the death occurs they are likely to experience overwhelming grief at their loss.
- Parents may have made decisions in advance about their child's care but can change their mind; be guided by them and contact the child's clinical team for advice and support.
- Following verification of death, family members may want time alone with the child but may be reassured by and benefit from your continuing presence; be guided by their needs. If transporting the child, ask if they have a favourite blanket or toy to take with them and pre-alert the receiving hospital so they can prepare for the child's arrival.
- Remember the needs of wider family members who may be with the child (particularly siblings), who will need support and sensitive communication.

3. Care of the Family

- Families are profoundly affected by the initial response and care that professionals offer their child in these circumstances. Not only is your role essential for immediate practical reasons but it also has a great influence on how the family deals with the death in the future.
- Communication and empathy are essential, and the family must be treated with compassion and sensitivity throughout. The Foundation for the Study of Infant Deaths found that parents/carers regard the actions and attitudes of those who tend to them as extremely important and typically speak very highly of the way both themselves and their child were treated.
- Explain what you are doing at every stage.
- Parents/carers exhibit a variety of reactions (e.g. overwhelming grief, anger, confusion, disbelief or guilt). Be prepared to deal with any of these feelings with empathy and sensitivity, remembering some reactions may be directed towards the attending ambulance paramedics as a manifestation of their distress.
- Avoid any criticism of the parents/carers, either direct or implied.
- Think before you speak. Chance remarks may cause offence and may be remembered indefinitely (e.g. 'I'm sorry; he looks so awful').
- Ask the child's name and use it when referring to them (do not refer to the child as 'it').

Termination of Resuscitation and Verification of Death in Children

- Allow the parents/carers to hold the child if they so wish (unless there are obvious indications of trauma or obvious suspicious circumstances that result in the police declaring a crime scene), as long as it does not interfere with clinical care.
- If possible, do not put children in body bags. It is known that relatives do not perceive very traumatic events in the way that unrelated onlookers might, and it is important they can see, touch and hold their loved one.
- Ensure the family is aware of where you are taking their infant/child. The parents/carers may wish to accompany you when you take the child to hospital. If appropriate, offer to take one or both in the ambulance. Alternatively, ensure that they have other means of transport, and that they know where to go.
- If they have no telephone, offer to help in contacting a relative or friend who can give immediate support, such as looking after other children or making sure the premises are secure.
- Explain sensitively that it is routine practice to involve both the coroner and the police in unexpected child deaths and that they may wish to attend the scene and/or speak to the carers.

4. Document

- Collect information pertaining to:
  - The situation in which you find the child (e.g. position in cot, bedding, proximity to others, room temperature etc.).
  - A history of the last 24–48 hours' events, including a brief description from the parents/carers of the events that led up to them finding the deceased child (e.g. when last seen alive, health at that time, position when found etc.). The police and the paediatrician will go through these events in greater detail, but the parent/carer's initial statement to you may be particularly valuable in the investigation.
  - Any significant past medical history.
- Write all this information down as soon as you have the opportunity, recording times and other details as accurately as possible.

5. Multi-agency Approach

The Kennedy Report requires a multi-agency approach to the management of SUDI, in which all the professionals involved keep each other informed and collaborate. Follow agreed protocols with regards to inter-agency communication and informing the police.

5.1 Communication with Other Agencies

- After you have arrived at the house and confirmed that the infant is deceased, the police Child Abuse Investigation Team (CAIT) must be informed (refer to locally agreed procedure). In unexpected deaths, the police will attend the scene and they can offer further advice regarding the Coroner's Officer's investigation.
- Share the information you have collected with the police and with relevant health professionals.

6. Transferring the Child

- The child should be taken to the nearest appropriate emergency department, not direct to a mortuary, even when the child has clearly been dead for some time and a death has been medically confirmed at home (there will be occasions where it is necessary to remind a doctor that taking the child to a hospital is now the preferred procedure, as recommended by Kennedy).
- Pre-alert the emergency department of your arrival, asking them to be ready to take over resuscitation if this is ongoing. Inform them if the parent(s)/carer(s) are accompanying the child.
- In hospital, an immediate examination will be made by a paediatrician, bodily samples (blood, urine, CSF) can be taken for analysis, parents/carers can talk with the paediatricians and support services can be contacted.

7. Support

- A child death is one of the most emotionally traumatic and challenging events to encounter and is very distressing for all involved.
- Opportunities for debriefing or counselling for ambulance staff should be available.
- Follow local procedures for post-critical incident debriefing local guidelines/processes.
- Some people will feel ongoing distress. This is normal and should be recognised: other forms of therapy, from informal support from colleagues to formal counselling, may be required.
- As part of the ambulance service safeguarding processes, information from local paediatricians and ambulance service safeguarding leads will be available if required for further discussion.
- Unsuccessful attempts at resuscitating children weigh heavily on individuals despite recognised poor outcomes following paediatric out-of-hospital cardiac arrest (OHCA). The vast majority of children having a cardiac arrest outside of hospital die, irrespective of response times, personnel or intervention/availability of advanced life support – less than 10% of paediatric OHCAs survive, despite those attempting resuscitation having done everything possible to help that child.

Termination of Resuscitation and Verification of Death in Children

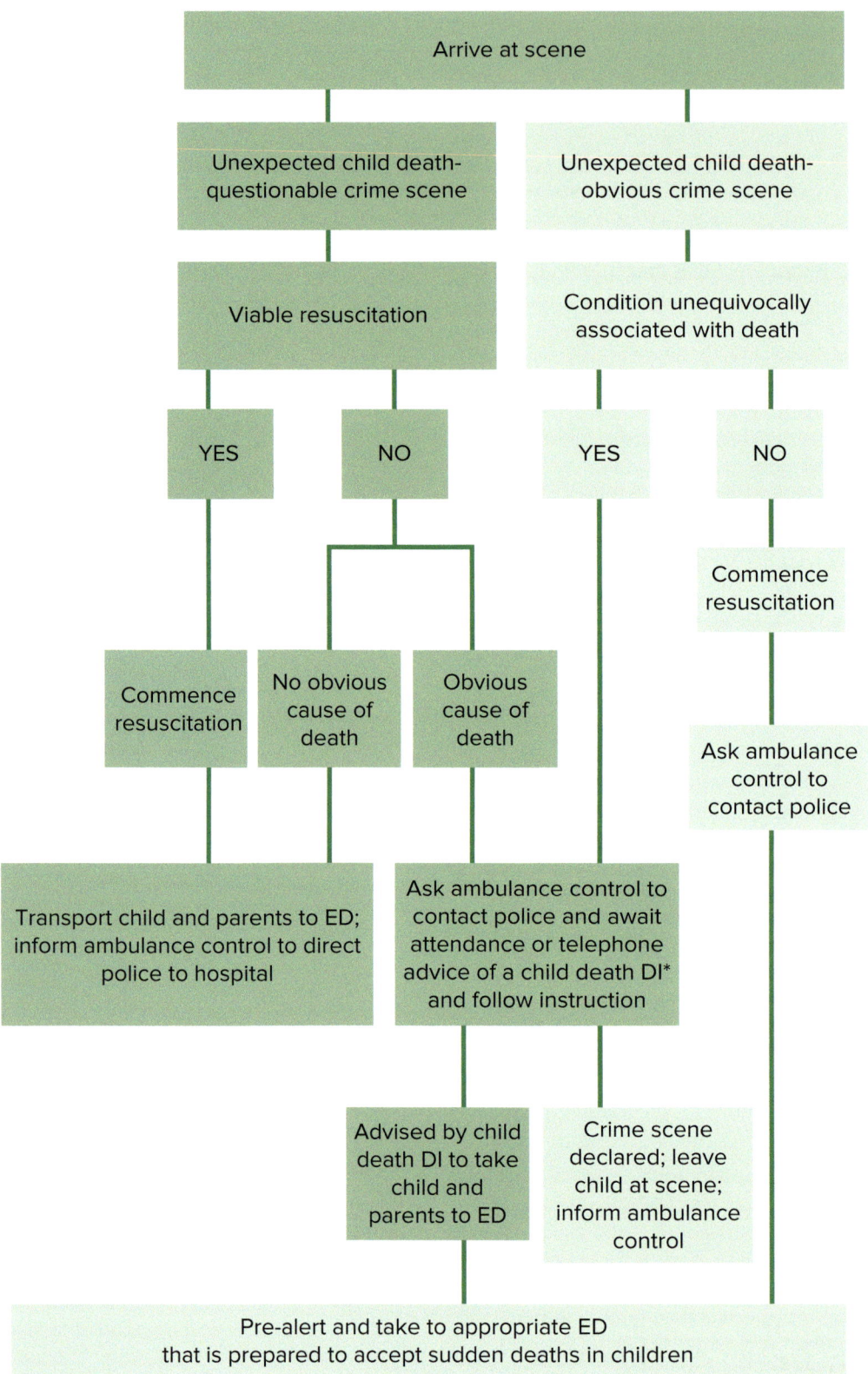

*Child Death Detective Inspector (child death DI) – A Detective Inspector who is trained in the management of child death; oversees the multiagency investigation and collection of evidence.

Figure 2.20 – Death of a child, including sudden unexpected death in infancy, children and adolescents (SUDICA).

Termination of Resuscitation and Verification of Death in Children

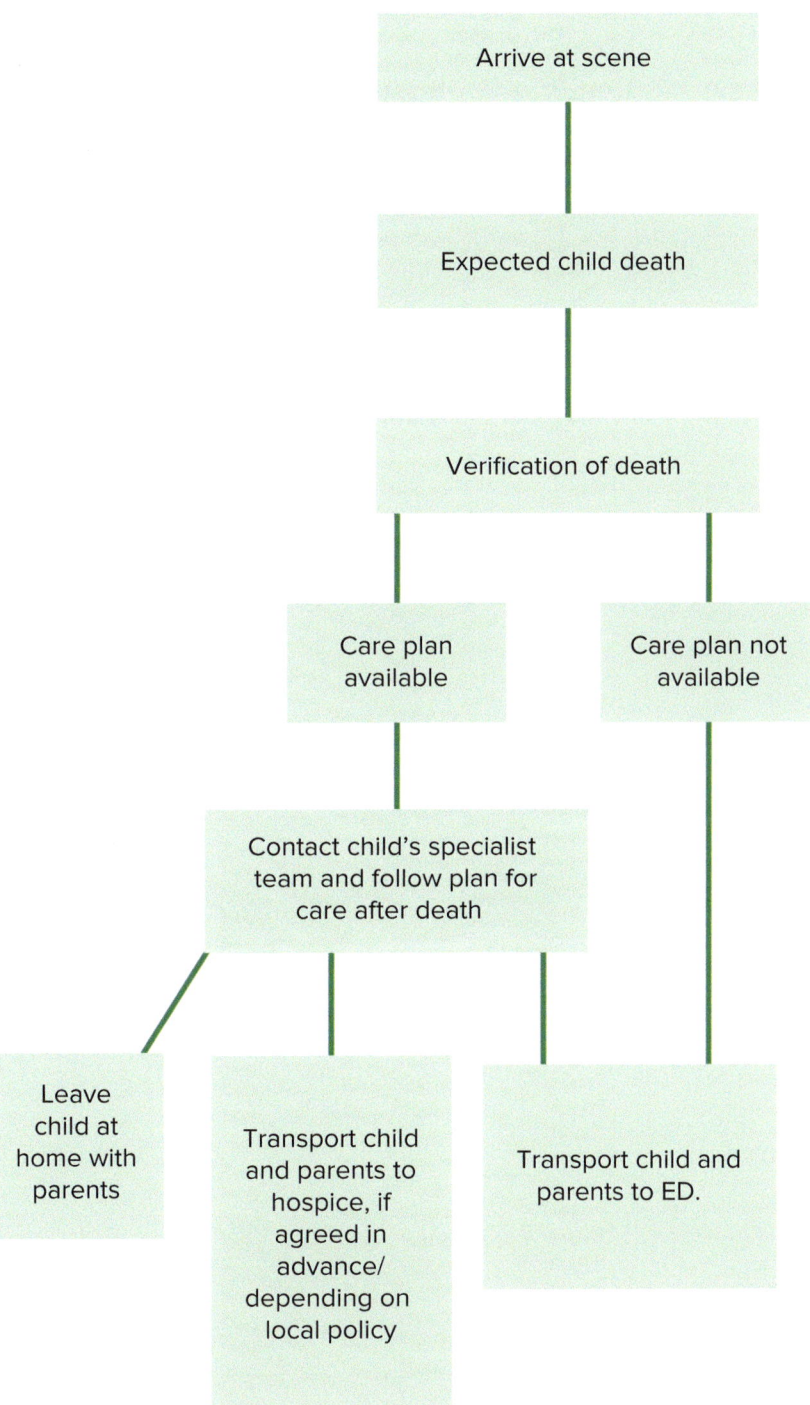

Figure 2.21 – Expected child death.

Termination of Resuscitation and Verification of Death in Children

> **KEY POINTS!**
>
> **Termination of Resuscitation and Verification of Death in Children**
> - A child death is one of the most emotionally traumatic and challenging events to encounter.
> - Resuscitation should always be attempted unless there is a condition unequivocally associated with death or a valid advance decision.
> - Communication and empathy are essential, and the family must be treated with compassion and sensitivity throughout. Parents/carers regard the actions and attitudes of those who tend to them as extremely important and speak very highly of the way both they and their child were treated.
> - Your role is not only essential for immediate practical reasons but also has a great influence on how the family deals with the death, long after the initial crisis is over.
> - Ensure the family is aware of where you are taking their infant/child.
> - Collect information pertaining to the situation in which you find the child, a history of events and any significant past medical history.
> - Follow agreed protocols with regards to inter-agency communication and informing the police.
> - In unexpected deaths, explain to the family that the death will be reported to the Coroner and that they will be interviewed by the Coroner's Officer and the police in due course.

Bibliography

1. Resuscitation Council (UK). *Resuscitation Guidelines 2015. Prevention of Cardiac Arrest and Decisions About CPR.* London: Resuscitation Council, 2015. Available from: https://resus.org.uk/resuscitation-guidelines/prevention-of-cardiac-arrest-and-decisions-about-cpr/.

2. British Medical Association, Resuscitation Council (UK), Royal College of Nursing. *Decisions Relating to Cardiopulmonary Resuscitation.* 3rd edn. London: British Medical Association, 2016. Available from: https://www.resus.org.uk/library/publications/publication-decisions-relating-cardiopulmonary.

3. Kennedy H. Royal College of Pathologists, Royal College of Paediatrics. *Sudden Unexpected Death in Infancy and Childhood.* London: Royal College of Pathologists, 2016. Available from: https://child-protection.rcpch.ac.uk/resources/sudden-unexpected-death-in-infancy-and-childhood-multi-agency-guidelines-for-care-and-investigation/.

4. Together for Shorter Lives. *Caring for a Child at End of Life.* 2nd edn. Together for Shorter Lives, 2019. Available from: https://www.togetherforshortlives.org.uk/app/uploads/2019/11/TfSL-Caring-for-a-child-at-end-of-life-Professionals.pdf.

3

Medical Emergencies

Medical Emergencies in Adults – Overview

1. Introduction

Although the care of a wide range of medical conditions will be quite specific to the presenting condition, there are general principles of care that apply to most medical cases, regardless of underlying condition(s).

2. Patient Assessment

- In order to gather as much relevant information as possible, without delaying care, the accepted format of history-taking is as follows:
    - Presenting complaint – why the patient or carer called for help at this time
    - The history of presenting complaint – details of when the problem started, exacerbating factors and previous similar episodes. **NB** The patient history can provide valuable insight into the cause of the current condition
    - Direct questioning about associated symptoms, by system. Ask about all appropriate systems. Refer to Table 3.1
    - Past medical history, including current medication
    - Family history
    - Social history.

- Combined with a good physical examination (primary and secondary survey), this format of history-taking should ensure that you correctly identify those patients who are time-critical, urgent or routine. The history taken must be fully documented. In many cases, a well-taken history will point to the diagnosis.

- The presence of MedicAlert®-type jewellery (bracelets or necklets), or emergency card (steroids, oxygen), can provide information on the patient's pre-existing health risk (e.g. diabetes, anaphylaxis, Addison's disease, COPD etc.) that may be relevant to the current medical emergency.

- Consider scoring a patient's level of frailty. Refer to Figure 3.1.[2]
    - The Rockwood Clinical Frailty Scale (CFS) is a judgement-based frailty assessment tool. It is not validated for people under the age of 65 years or those with long-term disabilities. Frailty must be sensed, described and measured: not guessed. If the patient you are assessing is acutely unwell and over 65 years, consider using the CFS, as per local pathways.
    - The score is based on the patient's baseline, so use the tool to score how the patient was 2 weeks ago (prior to deterioration) or their

CLINICAL FRAILTY SCALE

	1	VERY FIT	People who are robust, active, energetic and motivated. They tend to exercise regularly and are among the fittest for their age.
	2	FIT	People who have **no active disease symptoms** but are less fit than category 1. Often, they exercise or are very **active occasionally**, e.g., seasonally.
	3	MANAGING WELL	People whose **medical problems are well controlled**, even if occasionally symptomatic, but often **are not regularly active** beyond routine walking.
	4	LIVING WITH VERY MILD FRAILTY	Previously "vulnerable," this category marks early transition from complete independence. While **not dependent** on others for daily help, often **symptoms limit activities**. A common complaint is being "slowed up" and/or being tired during the day.
	5	LIVING WITH MILD FRAILTY	People who often have **more evident slowing**, and need help with **high order instrumental activities of daily living** (finances, transportation, heavy housework). Typically, mild frailty progressively impairs shopping and walking outside alone, meal preparation, medications and begins to restrict light housework.
	6	LIVING WITH MODERATE FRAILTY	People who need help with **all outside activities** and with **keeping house**. Inside, they often have problems with stairs and need **help with bathing** and might need minimal assistance (cuing, standby) with dressing.
	7	LIVING WITH SEVERE FRAILTY	**Completely dependent for personal care**, from whatever cause (physical or cognitive). Even so, they seem stable and not at high risk of dying (within ~6 months).
	8	LIVING WITH VERY SEVERE FRAILTY	Completely dependent for personal care and approaching end of life. Typically, they could not recover even from a minor illness.
	9	TERMINALLY ILL	Approaching the end of life. This category applies to people with a **life expectancy <6 months**, who are **not otherwise living with severe frailty**. (Many terminally ill people can still exercise until very close to death.)

SCORING FRAILTY IN PEOPLE WITH DEMENTIA

The degree of frailty generally corresponds to the degree of dementia. Common **symptoms in mild dementia** include forgetting the details of a recent event, though still remembering the event itself, repeating the same question/story and social withdrawal.

In **moderate dementia**, recent memory is very impaired, even though they seemingly can remember their past life events well. They can do personal care with prompting.

In **severe dementia**, they cannot do personal care without help.

In **very severe dementia** they are often bedfast. Many are virtually mute.

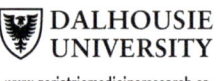
www.geriatricmedicineresearch.ca

Clinical Frailty Scale ©2005–2020 Rockwood, Version 2.0 (EN). All rights reserved. For permission: www.geriatricmedicineresearch.ca
Rockwood K et al. A global clinical measure of fitness and frailty in elderly people. CMAJ 2005;173:489–495.

Figure 3.1 – Clinical Frailty Scale. Used with permission from Dr. Rockwood and the Geriatric Medicine Research Unit.

Medical Emergencies in Adults – Overview

usual level of functioning when well, rather than how they present today. If possible, cross-reference what the patient describes to you with a description from relatives/carers.
- Do NOT compare the patient to the pictures (e.g. person using walking aids) alone to make a judgement on the level of frailty.

2.1 Primary Survey

- The primary survey should take 60–90 seconds for assessment and follow the approach set out in Table 3.1. This rapid assessment should quickly identify patients with actual or potential life-threatening conditions or symptoms.
- Assessment and management should proceed in a 'stepwise' manner and abnormalities should be managed as they are encountered; that is, do not move onto breathing and circulation until the airway is managed. Every time an intervention has been carried out, re-assess the patient.
- If haemorrhage cannot be controlled or airway and breathing cannot be corrected, evacuate immediately, continuing resuscitation as appropriate en route.

TABLE 3.1 – ASSESSMENT and MANAGEMENT of: Medical Emergencies

Assess <C>ABCDE

All stages should be considered, but some more detailed elements may be omitted if not considered appropriate.

At each stage, consider the need for **early senior clinical support**.

- Start correcting any **<C>ABCDE** problems as below.
- Undertake a **TIME-CRITICAL** transfer to nearest appropriate receiving hospital.
- Provide an ATMIST information call.

Catastrophic Haemorrhage

- Look for evidence of external catastrophic haemorrhage.
- Consider whether occult catastrophic haemorrhage could be occurring. For example, following trauma or as a result of an aneurysm rupture.

Stem external bleeding.

- Apply a tourniquet and/or apply direct pressure to the site.
- Dress the site with appropriate haemorrhage/trauma dressing.
- Elevate the site if possible.

Airway

- Assess the airway (refer to **Airway and Breathing Management**).
- **Look for** obvious obstructions, e.g. teeth/dentures, foreign bodies, vomit, blood (refer to **Foreign Body Airway Obstruction**).
- **Listen for** noisy airflow, e.g. snoring, gurgling or no airflow (refer to **Dyspnoea**).
- **Feel for** air movement.
- Airway constriction is a life-threatening condition and can result from an immune response to an allergen (refer to **Allergic Reactions including Anaphylaxis**).
- Correct any airway problems immediately by:
  - Positioning – head tilt, chin lift, jaw thrust.
  - Suction (if available and appropriate).
  - Oropharyngeal airway.
  - Nasopharyngeal airway.
  - Supraglottic mask airway (SGA) (if appropriate).
  - Endotracheal intubation (if appropriate, appropriately trained and only if waveform capnography is available).
  - Needle cricothyroidotomy.

(continued)

Medical Emergencies in Adults – Overview

TABLE 3.1 – ASSESSMENT and MANAGEMENT of: Medical Emergencies *(continued)*

Breathing

- Expose the chest and assess (refer to **Airway and Breathing Management**).

Inspect:

- Respiratory rate (<10 or >30).
- Adequacy and depth of chest movements.
- Symmetry of chest movement.
- Effectiveness of ventilation.
- Cyanosis (which may appear pale grey/blue), anaemia or pallor is more difficult to detect in people with dark skin tones. Look for central cyanosis around the lips, inside the mouth and in the oral mucous membranes (buccal or sublingual). Peripheral cyanosis is usually seen in the hands or feet, and may occur with or without central cyanosis.
- In anaemia the conjunctiva may appear to be pale pink or white, regardless of the patient's skin tone. In patients with dark skin tones there may be reduced darkness in the palmar creases, although this sign cannot be used on its own. The patient's palms can be compared to that of a family member with the same skin tone.
- Position of trachea in suprasternal notch

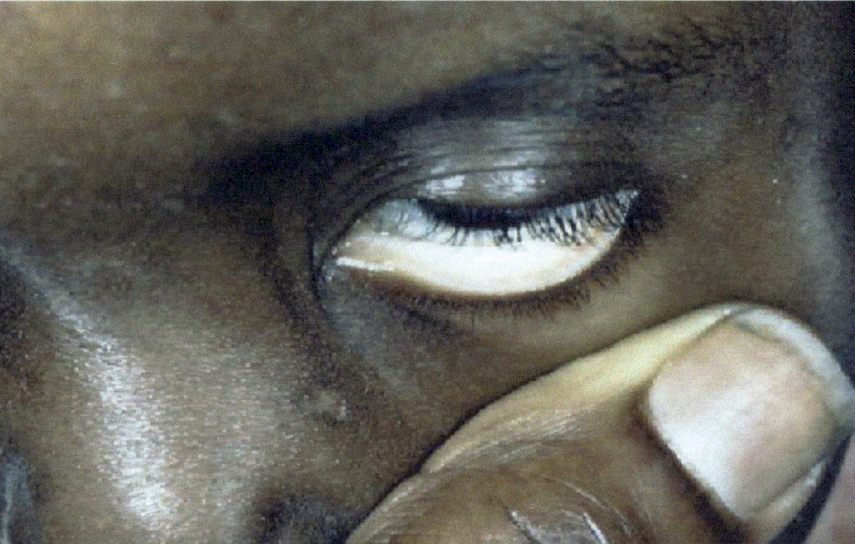

Figure 3.2 – Conjuctival pallor in a patient with severe anaemia. Reproduced with permission. Available from: https://www.hst.org.za/publications/NonHST%20Publications/malaria_36.pdf.

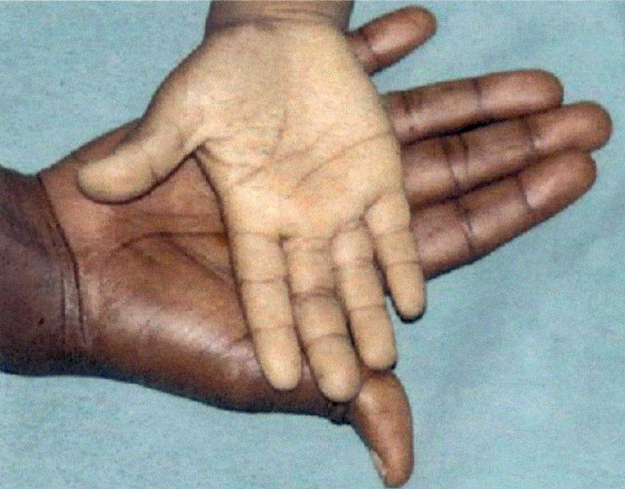

Figure 3.3 – Pallor of a child's palm, with the mother's for comparison. Republished with permission. Available from: https://pubmed.ncbi.nlm.nih.gov/20417858/.

Medical Emergencies in Adults – Overview

TABLE 3.1 – ASSESSMENT and MANAGEMENT of: Medical Emergencies *(continued)*

Palpate:
- Any instability of chest wall and note any areas of tenderness.
- Note depth and equality of chest movement.

Percuss for:
- Dullness or hyperresonance.

Auscultate:
- Altered breathing patterns with a stethoscope – ask the patient to take deep breaths in and out briskly through their mouth if possible – listen on both sides of the chest:
  - above the nipples in the mid-clavicular line
  - laterally in the mid-axillary line
  - below the shoulder blade (front and back).
- Auscultate to assess air entry and compare sides. Equality of air entry.
- Crepitations at the rear of the chest (crackles, heard low down in the lung fields at the rear – may indicate fluid in the lung in heart failure).
- Wheezing, noisy respiration on inspiration or expiration.
- Stridor (higher-pitched noise on inspiration), suggestive of upper respiratory obstruction.

Additional crackles and wheeze on inspiration may be associated with inhalation of blood or vomit.

- Correct any breathing problems immediately.
- Consider patient positioning (e.g. sitting upright for respiratory problems).
- If breathing is absent, refer to appropriate **Resuscitation** guidelines.
- If the breathing is inadequate, refer to **Airway and Breathing Management**.
- Treat underlying cause of unilateral chest movement if tension pneumothorax.

Monitor the patient's SpO_2; administer oxygen to achieve saturations of >94% if the patient presents as hypoxaemic on air; refer to **Oxygen**.

NB This is except for patients with COPD or other risk factors for hypercapnia (refer to **Oxygen**).

In patients with a decreased level of consciousness (Glasgow Coma Scale (GCS) <15), administer the initial supplemental oxygen dose until the vital signs are normal, then reduce the oxygen dose and aim for a target saturation (SpO_2) of >94%. Refer to **Altered Level of Consciousness**.

In patients with sickle cell crisis, administer supplemental oxygen via an appropriate mask/nasal cannula until a reliable SpO_2 measurement is available; then adjust the oxygen flow to aim for target saturation within the range of 94–98%. Refer to **Sickle Cell Disease**.

Consider assisted ventilation at a rate of 12–20 respirations per minute if any of the following are present:
- Oxygen saturation (SpO_2) <90% on levels of supplemental oxygen.
- Respiratory rate <10 or >30 bpm.
- Inadequate chest expansion.

NB Restraint (positional) asphyxia – If the patient is required to be physically restrained (e.g. by police officers) in order to prevent them injuring themselves or others, or for the purpose of being detained under the Mental Health Act, then it is paramount that the method of restraint allows both for a patent airway and adequate respiratory volume.

- **Under these circumstances, it is essential to ensure that the patient's airway and breathing are adequate at all times.**

(continued)

Medical Emergencies in Adults – Overview

> **TABLE 3.1** – ASSESSMENT and MANAGEMENT of: Medical Emergencies *(continued)*
>
> ### Circulation
>
> - Assess for evidence of external haemorrhage (e.g. epistaxis, haemoptysis, haematemesis, melaena). For suspected gastrointestinal bleeding, refer to **Gastrointestinal Bleeding**.
> - Assess skin colour and temperature.
> - Palpate for a radial pulse – if absent, feel for a carotid pulse. **NB** The estimation of blood pressure by pulse is inaccurate and unreliable; however, the presence of a radial pulse suggests adequate perfusion of major organs. The presence of a femoral pulse suggests perfusion of the kidneys, while a carotid pulse and coherent mental state suggests adequate perfusion of the brain.
> - Assess pulse rate, volume and rhythm.
> - Check capillary refill time centrally (forehead or sternum – normal <2 seconds).
> - Arrest external haemorrhage.
> - In cases of internal or uncontrolled haemorrhage, undertake a **TIME-CRITICAL** transfer to further care; provide an alert/information call.
> - Patients with acute adrenal insufficiency (adrenal crisis) and/or sepsis will usually benefit from early fluid therapy and an appropriate hospital alert/information call. Adrenal insufficiency patients with hypotension and hypovolaemia must be given IV fluids and injected hydrocortisone prior to transportation to minimise the risk of circulatory collapse. See **Adrenal Insufficiency Patients** and **Sepsis**.
>
> Consider hypovolaemic shock and be aware of its early signs:
>
> - Pallor.
> - Cool peripheries.
> - Anxiety, abnormal behaviour.
> - Increased respiratory rate.
> - Tachycardia.
>
> ### Recognition of Shock
>
> Shock is difficult to diagnose. In certain groups of patients the signs of shock may appear late (e.g. patients with acute adrenal insufficiency (adrenal crisis), pregnant women, patients on medication such as beta-blockers, and the physically fit).
>
> Blood loss of 750–1000 ml will produce little evidence of shock; blood loss of 1000–1500 ml is required before more classical signs of shock appear. **NB** This loss is from the circulation NOT necessarily visible externally.
>
> ### Fluid Therapy
>
> - If fluid replacement is indicated refer to **Intravascular Fluid Therapy in Adults**.
>
> Rapid fluid replacement into the vascular compartment can overload the cardiovascular system particularly where there is pre-existing cardiovascular disease and in older people. Gradual rehydration over many hours rather than minutes may be indicated for rehydration. **NB** Monitor fluid replacement closely in these cases.
>
> ### Disability
>
> - Note the initial level of responsiveness on the AVPU scale and the time of assessment.
> - **A** – Alert.
> - **V** – Responds to voice.
> - **P** – Responds to painful stimulus.
> - **U** – Unresponsive.
> - Detail how to check pain.
> - Assess and note pupil size, equality and response to light.
> - **NB** In patients with fixed pinpoint pupils, suspect opiate use.
> - Check for purposeful movement in all four limbs.
> - Check sensory function.
> - Assess blood glucose levels in all patients with diabetes, impaired consciousness, convulsions, collapse, or alcohol consumption, a history of Addison's disease or an other form of adrenal insufficiency.
> - Check blood glucose level to rule out hypo/hyperglycaemia as the cause (refer to **Glycaemic Emergencies in Adults and Children**).

Medical Emergencies in Adults – Overview

TABLE 3.1 – ASSESSMENT and MANAGEMENT of: Medical Emergencies *(continued)*

- Also check blood glucose levels in all patients with a history of diabetes, impaired consciousness, seizures, collapse or alcohol/drug consumption.
- Consider adrenal crisis as a cause and provide drug therapy as required; refer to appropriate drug guidelines. In adrenal crisis, refer to **Hydrocortisone** and **Adrenal Insufficiency Patients**.
- If the level of consciousness deteriorates or respiratory depression develops in cases where an overdose with opiate-type drugs may be a possibility, consider administering naloxone; refer to **Naloxone Hydrochloride**.
- For patients with decreased consciousness and active seizure, refer to **Seizures in Adults**.

Vital Signs and NEWS2

NB Complete a full set of observations for all patients; repeat after intervention or when any value is outside normal parameters.

Respiratory Rate
- Measure and record respiratory rate.

Pulse
- Measure and record pulse.

Oxygen Saturation
- Monitor the patient's SpO_2; administer oxygen to achieve saturations of >94% if the patient presents as hypoxaemic on air; refer to **Oxygen**.

Blood Pressure and Fluids
- Measure and record blood pressure. If required, administer fluids; refer to **Intravascular Fluid Therapy in Adults**.

Blood Glucose
- If appropriate, measure and record blood glucose for hypo/hyperglycaemia; refer to **Glycaemic Emergencies in Adults and Children**.

Temperature
- Measure and record temperature.

NEWS2
For cancer patients, consider UKONS Tool (see **End of Life Care**, 3. Management – Patients Who Are Not Expected to Die Within 72 Hours).

These observations will enable you to calculate a NEWS2 score.

ECG
- If required, monitor and record 12-lead ECG. Assess for abnormality; refer to **Cardiac Arrhythmia and Sudden Cardiac Death**.

Assess the Patient's Pain
- Where present, assess the SOCRATES of pain and record initial and subsequent pain scores.
- Consider analgesia if appropriate (refer to **Pain Management in Adults and Children**).

Documentation
- Complete documentation to include all clinical findings, advice from other clinicians, onward referral and worsening advice given.

2.2 Secondary Survey

- A secondary survey should only commence after the primary survey has been completed and an assessment of the patient's critical status has been made.
- The secondary survey is a more thorough 'head-to-toe' assessment of the patient, including their past medical history (refer to Table 3.2). It is important to monitor the patient's vital signs during the survey.
- A complete and thorough secondary survey may not be possible in some patients with **TIME-CRITICAL** conditions.
- Follow additional medical guidelines as indicated by the patient's condition (e.g. cardiac arrhythmia and sudden cardiac death).

Medical Emergencies in Adults – Overview

TABLE 3.2 – Clinical Assessment

- Continually re-assess <C>ABCDE throughout clinical assessment.
- Assess all patients holistically considering the implications of any of the following:
  - Congenital defects/malformations – kyphosis/scoliosis – causing compression.
  - Dentition – this may indicate level of nutrition.
  - Jugular vein distension – cardiac history.
  - Oedema (ankles/orbital) – failure or kidney disease.
  - Central cyanosis.
  - Finger clubbing/splinter haemorrhage – respiratory or cardiac history.
  - Bruising – injury (consider non-accidental injury in vulnerable patient groups).
  - Surgical scars – previous procedures.

Respiratory

- Inspect, palpate, percuss and auscultate the chest, examining for signs which could indicate a respiratory cause for the presenting condition:
  - Accessory muscles/recession/nasal flaring.
  - Chest shape and symmetry.
  - Palpate for tactile fremitus which may indicate mucus plug or pneumonia.
  - Central trachea.
- Assess for pneumothorax – in small pneumothorax no clinical signs may be detected. A pneumothorax causes breathlessness, reduced air entry and chest movement on the affected side. If this is a tension pneumothorax, then the patient will have increasing respiratory distress; distended neck veins, and tracheal deviation (late sign) away from affected side may also be present.

Cardiac

- Auscultate and palpate, examining for signs which could indicate a cardiac cause for the presenting condition.
- Assess skin colour and temperature.
- Record pulse oximeter reading including heart rate.
- Assess heart sounds and bruits.
- Palpate bilateral pulses for equality.
- Obtain a blood pressure reading, using a sphygmomanometer; consider bilateral and standing and sitting blood pressures – consider postural drop.

Neurological

- Establish Glasgow Coma Scale (refer to **Altered Level of Consciousness**).
- Assess cranial nerves.
- Consider gait.
- Asses tone, strength and sensation to separate limbs and dermatomes.
- Consider assessing reflexes.
- **NB** Patients on long-term steroids or who have adrenal insufficiency may deteriorate rapidly because of steroid insufficiency. If significantly unwell, the patient should be given hydrocortisone and fluids if required, refer to **Adrenal Insufficiency Patients**.
- Some patients, especially those with spinal cord injury above T6, are particularly susceptible to the potentially life-threatening condition autonomic dysreflexia, which is characterised by a rapid rise in blood pressure, bradycardia, tachycardia, arrhythmia, headache or sweating due to unregulated sympathetic hyperactivity. This can cause cerebral haemorrhage and death.
- A small number of patients who have had a severe stroke or who have severe forms of Parkinson's disease, multiple sclerosis, cerebral palsy or spina bifida may also be susceptible to autonomic dysreflexia.
  - Patients with spinal cord injury or neurological conditions may have neurogenic bowel dysfunction. They may depend on routine interventional bowel care, including manual removal of faeces. Autonomic dysreflexia can be caused by non-adherence to a patient's usual bowel routine or during or following interventional bowel care.
- Patients that present to ambulance services may have difficulty when their normal bowel routine does not occur, for example due to illness or injury. The condition autonomic dysreflexia should always be considered.

Medical Emergencies in Adults – Overview

TABLE 3.2 – Clinical Assessment *(continued)*
Gastrointestinal
• Auscultate, percuss and palpate, examining for signs which could indicate a gastrointestinal cause for the presenting condition.
• Auscultate for bowel sounds and bruits.
Percuss for hypo/hyper resonance (e.g. dull = solid, high pitch = gas, shifting dullness = fluid)
• Feel for tenderness and guarding in all four quadrants.
Musculoskeletal/Skin
• Check for MSC in four limbs: – Test for movement and power.   – Apply light touch to evaluate sensation.   – Assess pulse and skin temperature.
• Assess for rashes, localised inflammation, bruising, swelling, erythema or other abnormalities.
• Assess for jaundice.

ADDITIONAL INFORMATION

The following may assist in determining the diagnosis:

- Relatives, carers or friends with knowledge of the patient's history.
- Packets or containers of medication (including domiciliary oxygen) or evidence of administration devices (e.g. nebuliser machines).
- Warning stickers, often placed by the front door or the telephone, directing the health professional to a source of detailed information (one current scheme involves storing the patient details in a container in the fridge, as this is relatively easy to find in the house).
- Patient-held warning cards denoting previous thrombolysis, at-risk COPD patients or those taking monoamine oxidase inhibitor (MAOI) medication.
- Patients' individualised treatment plans.

Appendix

TABLE 3.3 – GLASGOW COMA SCALE		
Item	**Element**	**Score**
Eyes Opening:		
	Spontaneously	4
	To speech	3
	To pain	2
	None	1
Verbal Response:		
	Orientated	5
	Confused	4
	Inappropriate words	3
	Incomprehensible sounds	2
	No verbal response	1
Motor Response:		
	Obeys commands	6
	Localised pain	5
	Withdraws from pain	4
	Abnormal flexion	3
	Extensor response	2
	No response to pain	1

Medical Emergencies in Adults – Overview

> **KEY POINTS!**
>
> **Medical Emergencies in Adults – Overview**
> - Detect TIME-CRITICAL problems early.
> - Minimise time on scene.
> - Continuously re-assess <C>ABCDE.
> - Initiate treatments en route if the patient is deteriorating.
> - Provide an ATMIST information call for TIME-CRITICAL patients.

Bibliography

1. Sharif H, Hou S. Autonomic dysreflexia: a cardiovascular disorder following spinal cord injury. *Neural Regen Res* 2017,12(9): 1390–1400.

2. Rockwood, K et al. (2005) A global clinical measure of fitness and frailty in elderly people. *Canadian Medical Association Journal 2005* 173(5): 489–95: available from: https://pubmed.ncbi.nlm.nih.gov/16129869/.

Medical Emergencies in Children – Overview

1. Introduction

- A problem-based approach to paediatric emergencies is to be encouraged. Identifying the features of possible serious illnesses (and addressing them) is more important than identifying the child's underlying diagnosis.
- Assessment priorities include the detection of respiratory distress, circulatory impairment or decreased consciousness.
- Good patient assessment will allow potentially life-threatening illnesses or injuries to be recognised sooner. This should allow treatments and interventions to be given at the earliest opportunity, including rapid hospital transfer for urgent assessment and further treatments when needed.

2. History

- In most cases, a well-taken history will point to the diagnosis. When combined with the findings of your physical examination, this format of history-taking should allow **TIME-CRITICAL** patients, urgent patients and routine patients to be correctly identified.
- History-taking should adhere to the following format and be fully documented:
  - **Presenting complaint** — why did the patient or carer call for help?
  - The **history** of the presenting complaint — details of when the problem started, exacerbating factors and previous similar episodes.
  - Direct questioning about associated **symptoms**, by system. Ask about all appropriate systems.
  - **Past medical history**, including current medication.
  - **Family history**.
  - **Social history**.
- The following should also be considered:
  - **Previous** treatment/contact with healthcare services or episodes of a similar nature.
  - **Feeding and appetite** — note how the child is typically fed: bottle/breast/solids. Button battery ingestion may need to be considered (refer to **Overdose and Poisoning in Adults and Children**).
  - **Activity/Apathy** — does the child act and respond appropriately?
  - **Urine and Faeces** — is this more or less than usual? Wet/dry nappies can be used as a measure of hydration/dehydration.
  - **Growth** — is the child's growth following expected and previously measured centiles?
  - **Sleeping** — is this normal for the child?
  - **Pregnancy** — maternal illness or drug ingestion during pregnancy may have affected the child.
  - **Birth** — antenatal complications, premature labour and birth complications may impact a child's weight and development.
  - **Immunisation and Health Screening**.
  - **Development** — is the child meeting their expected developmental milestones, e.g. hearing, speech or motor ability? Have there been any backward steps/developmental regression? The child's *Red Book* or other documentation may provide useful supporting information.
- Remember that the history of the child and parent provides invaluable insights into the cause of the current condition.
- In making an assessment, make use of the following sources of additional information:
  - Relatives, carers or friends
  - Packets or containers of medication
  - Administration devices, e.g. inhalers, spacers etc.
  - MedicAlert®-type jewellery, e.g. bracelets, or emergency cards (steroids, oxygen), detailing underlying health issues (diabetes, anaphylaxis, drug allergy etc.), as well as a 24-hour telephone number to obtain a more detailed patient history
  - Child protection concerns may become apparent during the initial medical assessment and should be appropriately dealt with (refer to **Safeguarding Children**).
- Having called the emergency services, it is also important to address parental ideas, concerns and expectations regarding their child's current health.

Medical Emergencies in Children – Overview

3. Assessment and Management

TABLE 3.4 – ASSESSMENT and MANAGEMENT of: Medical Emergencies in Children

Assess <C>ABCDE

All stages should be considered but some more detailed elements may be omitted when not clinically appropriate.

- At each stage, consider the need for early senior clinical support.
- Start correcting any <C> **ABCDE** problems.
- Undertake a **TIME-CRITICAL** transfer to nearest appropriate receiving hospital.
- Continue patient management en route.
- Provide an ATMIST information call.

Catastrophic Haemorrhage

- Look for evidence of significant external haemorrhage.
- Consider occult sources of internal bleeding, especially following trauma.

Arrest external bleeding

- Apply a tourniquet and/or apply direct pressure to the site.
- Dress the site with an appropriate haemorrhage or trauma dressing.
- Elevate the site if possible.

Airway

- Manage the child's airway in a stepwise manner.
- Exercise extreme caution when managing epiglottitis (refer to **Respiratory Illness in Children**).

Position the head to open the airway.

Abnormal upper airway sounds

- **Look for** physical obstructions, e.g. teeth, foreign bodies, vomit or blood (refer to **Foreign Body Airway Obstruction**).
- **Listen for** noisy airflow, e.g. snoring, gurgling or no airflow (refer to **Dyspnoea**).
  - Inspiratory noises (stridor) suggest an airway obstruction near the larynx.
  - A snoring noise (stertorous breathing) may be present when there is obstruction in the pharynx, e.g. enlarged tonsils.
- **Feel for** air movement:
  - Airway constriction is a life-threatening condition and can result from an immune response to an allergen (refer to **Allergic Reactions including Anaphylaxis**).

Manual extension manoeuvres, head tilt, chin lift or jaw thrust

- The younger the child, the less neck extension will be required. A newborn's head should be placed in the neutral position, while an older child should be extended into a 'sniffing the morning air' position.
- Do not place pressure on the soft tissues under the chin or in front of the neck – this can obstruct the airway.

Aspiration, foreign body removal

- Blind finger sweeps must be avoided as they may push material further down the airway or damage the soft palate.
- Refer to **Foreign Body Airway Obstruction**.

Oropharyngeal airway (OPA)

- Ensure the OPA is of the appropriate size (refer to Page for Age) and inserted using the correct technique. Discontinue insertion or remove if the child gags (refer to **Paediatric Resuscitation**).

Medical Emergencies in Children – Overview

TABLE 3.4 – ASSESSMENT and MANAGEMENT of: Medical Emergencies in Children *(continued)*

Nasopharyngeal airway
- Correct sizing is essential.
- In small children, a size smaller than estimated may be required.
- Care should be taken not to damage tonsillar or adenoidal tissues.

Endotracheal intubation
- The hazards associated with intubation in children are considerable and usually outweigh the advantages. It should only be attempted where other more basic methods of ventilation have failed and only when capnography is available (ETT sizes are listed on Page for Age).
- Only attempt paediatric intubation if authorised to do so and follow local protocols.

Needle cricothyroidotomy
- Needle cricothyroidotomy is considered a method of last resort.
- Surgical airways should not be performed on children under the age of 12 years.
- The initial oxygen (O_2) flow rate in litres per minute should be set to equal the child's age in years and gradually increased (in 1 litre min^{-1} increments) until adequate chest wall movements are seen.
- Allow ~4 sec for exhalation.

Breathing

Measure the respiratory rate (see Page for Age).
- Tachypnoea, a rapid respiratory rate, in a child at rest indicates a need for increased ventilation and suggests:
  - an airway problem
  - a lung problem
  - a circulatory problem or
  - a metabolic problem.

Recession (indrawing, retraction)
- Intercostal recession (indrawing of the space between the ribs) and subcostal recession (along the costal margins at the point of diaphragmatic attachment) are seen when respiratory effort is high, due to the pliable nature of children's rib cages. In infants, the sternum itself may even be drawn in (sternal recession), but as children get older the rib cage becomes less pliable and other signs of accessory muscle use (other than recession) are seen (see below). If recession is seen in older children, it suggests severe respiratory difficulty.

Accessory muscle use
- As in adult life, when the work of breathing is increased, the sternocleidomastoid muscle may be used as an accessory respiratory muscle. This can cause head-bobbing (the head bobs up and down with each breath) in infants.

Flaring of the nostrils
- This is a subtle sign that is easily missed. It indicates significant respiratory distress.

Inspiratory or expiratory noises
- Wheezing indicates lower airway narrowing and is most commonly heard on expiration. The volume of the wheeze is **NOT** an indicator of severity – it may diminish with increasing respiratory distress because less air is being moved.

Inspiratory noises (stridor)
- This suggests an imminent danger to the airway due to reduction in airway circumference to approximately 10% of normal. Again, the volume of stridor does **NOT** reflect severity and may also diminish with increasing respiratory distress as less air is moved.

Grunting
- This is produced by exhalation against a partially closed laryngeal opening (glottis). This is more likely to be seen in infants and is a sign of severe respiratory distress.

Effectiveness of breathing — chest expansion and breath sounds
- Note the degree of expansion on both sides of the chest and whether it is equal.

(continued)

Medical Emergencies in Children – Overview

TABLE 3.4 – ASSESSMENT and MANAGEMENT of: Medical Emergencies in Children *(continued)*

Auscultate the chest with a stethoscope

- A silent chest is a pre-terminal sign, as it indicates that very little air is moving in or out of the chest.

Pulse oximetry

- This can be used at all ages to measure oxygen saturation (readings are less reliable in the presence of shock, hypothermia and other conditions such as carbon monoxide poisoning and severe anaemia).
- For additional signs of breathing compromise, refer to Table 3.5.
- All sick children require adequate oxygenation.
- Administer high levels of supplemental oxygen (O_2) via a non-rebreathing mask.
- If the child finds the face mask distressing, ask the parent to help by holding the mask as close to the child's face as possible. If this still produces distress, wafting O_2 across the face directly from the tubing, with the face mask detached from the tubing, is better than nothing.
- In children with sickle cell disease or cardiac disease, high levels of O_2 should be administered routinely, whatever their oxygen saturation.
- Consider assisted ventilation at a rate equivalent to the normal respiratory rate for the age of the child (refer to paediatric resuscitation charts for normal values) if:
  - The child is hypoxic (SpO_2 <90%) and remains so after being placed on high flows and concentration O_2.
  - Respiratory rate is <50% normal or >3 times normal.
  - Expansion is inadequate.
- Use an appropriately sized mask to ensure a good seal.
- Try to avoid hyperventilation to minimise the risks of gastric insufflation or barotrauma. The bag-valve-mask should have a pressure release valve as an added safety measure. If this is not available, extreme care must be taken not to over-expand the lungs. No bag smaller than 500 ml volume should be used for bag-valve-mask ventilation unless the child is <2.5 kg, i.e. preterm baby size.

Wheezing

- The management of asthma is discussed elsewhere (refer to **Asthma in Adults and Children**).
- See **Respiratory Illness in Children** for further guidance on childhood respiratory illnesses.

Circulation

Assessment and recognition of potential circulatory failure (shock)

- Circulatory assessments in children are difficult, as each physical sign may have a number of confounding variables.
- When assessing whether a child is shocked, it is important to assess and evaluate each of the signs below:

Heart rate: (see Page for Age)

- **Tachycardia** results from loss of circulatory volume. Heart rates, particularly in infants, can be very high (up to 220 beats per minute). (Heart rates greater than 220 bpm are seen in supraventricular tachycardia).
- An abnormally slow pulse, or **bradycardia**, is defined as less than 60 bpm or a rapidly falling heart rate associated with poor systemic circulation. Bradycardia is a pre-terminal sign and becomes apparent before cardiac arrest (see above).

Pulse volume

- Peripheral pulses become weak and then absent as shock advances.
- Children peripherally vasoconstrict their extremities as shock progresses, initially cooling skin distally and then more proximally as shock advances.
- There is no validated relationship between the presence of certain peripheral pulses and the systemic blood pressure in children.

Capillary refill

- This should be measured on the forehead or sternum.
- A capillary refill time of >2 seconds indicates poor perfusion, although this is influenced by a number of factors, including cold and poor lighting conditions.

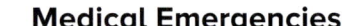

Medical Emergencies in Children – Overview

TABLE 3.4 – ASSESSMENT and MANAGEMENT of: Medical Emergencies in Children *(continued)*

Blood pressure:
- Varies with age
- Is difficult to reliably measure, increasing on-scene times, and therefore is not routinely measured in pre-hospital practice
- Hypotension is a very late (and pre-terminal sign) in shocked children and so other signs of circulatory inadequacy will manifest (and should have been recognised) long before hypotension occurs.
- For other signs of circulatory compromise, refer to Table 3.6.

Arrest external haemorrhage
- Do not attempt to gain intravenous (IV) or intraosseous (IO) access at the scene. Obtain access en route unless delay is unavoidable.

Cannulation
- Attempt cannulation with the widest bore cannula that can be confidently placed. The vehicle can be stopped briefly to allow for venepuncture and disposal of the sharp, with transport being recommenced before applying the IV dressing.
- The IO route may be required where venous access has failed on two occasions or no suitable vein is apparent within a reasonable timeframe. The IO route is the preferred route for vascular access in all cases of cardiac arrest in young children.
- Blood glucose level should be measured in (i) all children in whom vascular access is being obtained and (ii) any child with decreased conscious level (refer to **Altered Level of Consciousness**).

Fluid administration
- Use sodium chloride 0.9% to treat shock.
- Fluids should be measured in millilitres and documented as volume administered — not as the volume of fluid chosen.
- Fluids should be administered as boluses rather than 'run in'.
- Handover at the receiving unit must include details of volume and type of fluid administered.

Fluid volumes
- 10 ml/kg boluses of 0.9% Sodium Chloride are used to resuscitate medically ill children with shock from circulatory failure, to restore vital signs to normal.
- No more than two boluses should be given except on medical advice (refer to **Intravascular Fluid Therapy in Children** and **Sodium Chloride 0.9%**).

Exceptions
- In diabetic ketoacidosis, fluids are administered more cautiously to reduce the risk of cerebral oedema (refer to **Glycaemic Emergencies in Adults and Children**).
- In diabetic ketoacidosis, fluid should be withheld unless severe shock is present, in which case 10 ml/kg should be administered over 10–15 minutes (refer to **Glycaemic Emergencies in Adults and Children**).
- If a child has heart failure or renal failure, give a 5 ml/kg bolus but stop if the patient deteriorates. Transfer to hospital as a priority.
- Seek medical advice when exceptional circumstances are present, such as a long transfer time.

Disability

Recognition of potential neurological failure
- Note the initial level of responsiveness on the AVPU scale, and time of assessment:
    - **A** — Alert.
    - **V** — Responds to voice.
    - **P** — Responds to painful stimulus.
    - **U** — Unresponsive.

Response to a painful stimulus
- Pinch a digit or pull frontal hair. A child who is unconscious or who only responds to pain has a significant degree of coma (refer to Glasgow Coma Scale — Appendix 1. **NB** the 'adult' GCS should be used in children over 4 years of age).

(continued)

Medical Emergencies in Children – Overview

TABLE 3.4 – ASSESSMENT and MANAGEMENT of: Medical Emergencies in Children *(continued)*

Posture: observe the child's posture

- Children may:
  - be floppy (hypotonic) – recent floppiness in a child suggests a serious illness
  - be stiff (hypertonic) or
  - have back arching (opisthotonus).
- New onset stiffness suggests severe cerebral disturbance.
- Decerebrate or decorticate postures suggest a serious underlying cerebral abnormality.

Pupils

- Test pupil size and reaction.
- Pupils should be equal, of normal size and react briskly to light.
- Any abnormality or change in pupil size or reaction may be significant.
- For additional signs of neurological compromise, refer to Table 3.7.
- **NB** The whole assessment should take less than 2 minutes unless intervention is required.
- Re-assessment of <C>ABCD is necessary to assess the response to treatment or to detect deterioration. (Blood glucose levels should be measured in any seriously ill child.)
- The aim of management of any child with a cerebral insult is to minimise further insult by optimising their circumstances. This usually concerns management strategies designed to:
  - prevent hypoxia (see above)
  - normalise circulation without causing fluid overload
  - identify and treat hypoglycaemia (refer to **Glycaemic Emergencies in Adults and Children**).
- Other conditions that can be treated out of hospital and are discussed elsewhere include:
  - convulsions (refer to **Seizures in Children**)
  - opiate poisoning (refer to **Overdose and Poisoning in Adults and Children**)
  - meningococcal septicaemia (refer to **Meningococcal Meningitis and Septicaemia**).

Vital Signs

NB Complete a full set of observations for all patients, and repeat after intervention or when any value is outside normal parameters.

Respiratory rate

- Measure and record respiratory rate.

Pulse

- Measure and record pulse.

Oxygen saturation

- Monitor the patient's SpO$_2$; administer oxygen to achieve saturations of >94% if the patient is hypoxic in air (refer to **Oxygen**).

Blood pressure

- Measure and record blood pressure.
- **NB** This is difficult to reliably measure, increasing on-scene times, and as a result is not routinely measured in out-of-hospital practice.

Fluids

- If required, administer fluids (refer to **Intravascular Fluid Therapy in Children**).

Neurology

- Assess AVPU, GCS, pupils and posture.

Blood glucose

If appropriate, measure and record blood glucose for hypo/hyperglycaemia (refer to **Glycaemic Emergencies in Adults and Children**).

Temperature

- Measure and record temperature.

Medical Emergencies in Children – Overview

TABLE 3.4 – ASSESSMENT and MANAGEMENT of: Medical Emergencies in Children *(continued)*

Traffic lights
- Refer to specific guidelines to perform a NICE (National Institute for Health and Care Excellence) '**traffic light**' assessment, prioritising children into three groups according to the presence of certain symptoms and signs:
    - '**Green**' – low risk.
    - '**Amber**' – intermediate risk.
    - '**Red**' – high risk.
- Refer to **Febrile Illness in Children**, Table 3.53.

ECG
- If required, monitor and record 12-lead ECG. Assess for abnormality (refer to **Cardiac Arrhythmia and Sudden Cardiac Death**).

Pain assessment
- Use the **SOCRATES** pain mnemonic and record initial (and subsequent) pain scores.
- Offer analgesia where appropriate (refer to **Pain Management in Adults and Children**).

Documentation
- Complete documentation to include all clinical findings, advice from other clinicians, onward referral and worsening advice given.

TABLE 3.5 – Additional Signs of Compromised Breathing

Heart rate
- Tachycardia, or eventually bradycardia, may result from hypoxia and acidosis.
- Bradycardia in a sick child is a pre-terminal sign.

Skin colour
- Flushing of the skin (vasodilation) is seen in early respiratory distress due to elevated carbon dioxide levels.
- Hypoxia causes vasoconstriction and skin pallor.
- Cyanosis is a pre-terminal sign of hypoxia.

Mental status
- Hypoxia makes children agitated and drowsy.
- Agitation may be difficult to recognise due to the child's distress. Use parents to help make this assessment.
- Drowsiness gradually progresses, leading to unconsciousness.

TABLE 3.6 – Additional Signs of Circulatory Compromise

Respiratory rate
- The combination of both rapid respiratory rate and no recession may indicate circulatory insufficiency.
- Tachypnoea occurs as the body tries to correct metabolic derangements.

Skin
- Mottled, cold, reduction in skin colour (paler) reflects poor perfusion. Mottling may be difficult to detect in dark skin tones.

Mental status
- Agitation is seen in early shock, progressing to drowsiness as shock advances.
- Poor cerebral perfusion may ultimately result in loss of consciousness.

Medical Emergencies in Children – Overview

TABLE 3.7 – Additional Signs of Neurological Compromise

Respiratory system
- Brain insults produce abnormal breathing patterns, e.g. hyperventilation, Cheyne–Stokes breathing or apnoea.

Circulatory system
- Bradycardia may be a result of dangerously raised intracranial pressure.

Summary

- The primary assessment of the child should establish whether they are seriously ill.
- Immediate correction of any problems must be undertaken without delay at the scene.
- Continually monitor and reassess the child en route to hospital.
- Children who are found to be seriously ill must be considered to have a **TIME-CRITICAL** condition and be taken to the nearest suitable receiving hospital without delay.
- A hospital **ATMIST** call should be made whenever a seriously ill child is transported.
- Paediatric drug dosages are calculated as 'mg per kilogram' (refer to Page for Age and specific medicine guidelines for dosages and information).
- Drug doses **MUST** be checked before **ANY** drug administration, no matter how confident the practitioner may be.

Appendix

TABLE 3.8 – Modified Glasgow Coma Scale for Children Under 4-Years of Age

Item	Element	Score
Eyes Opening:		
	Spontaneously	4
	To speech	3
	To pain	2
	None	1
Verbal Response:		
	Orientated (appropriate words or social smiles, and fixes on and follows objects)	5
	Confused (cries, but is consolable)	4
	Inappropriate words (persistently irritable)	3
	Incomprehensible sounds (restless, agitated)	2
	No verbal response (silent)	1
Motor Response:		
	Obeys commands	6
	Localised pain	5
	Withdraws from pain	4
	Abnormal flexion	3
	Extensor response	2
	No response to pain	1

Medical Emergencies in Children – Overview

> **KEY POINTS!**
>
> **Medical Emergencies in Children – Overview**
> - The child and parent's history will provide a valuable insight into the cause of the child's current condition.
> - Hypoxia and hypovolaemia need urgent correction.
> - Emergency airway management rarely requires intubation.
> - Check the blood glucose in all seriously ill children and those with a decreased level of consciousness.
> - <C>ABCDE problems should be corrected and managed en route to further care. Do not delay on scene.
> - It is important to address ideas, concerns and expectations, especially of the parents who are often concerned, hence the call to emergency services.

Further Resources

1 **Spotting the Sick Child**. Available from: https://spottingthesickchild.com/**SSC** is an interactive tool commissioned by the Department of Health and Health Education England to support health professionals in the assessment of the acutely sick child.

Abdominal Pain

1. Introduction

- Abdominal pain is a common presenting symptom to ambulance services. The specific cause can be difficult to identify in pre-hospital care and a definitive diagnosis may require in-hospital investigations.
- The nature, location and pattern of the pain, together with associated symptoms, may indicate a possible cause (refer to Table 3.10). Many of the causes for abdominal pain can be self-limiting. However, it is important to recognise the risk associated with those conditions that need further input, as well as those that need more urgent life saving interventions.
- Abdominal pain in older people, patients who are immunocompromised, those with alcohol dependence and pregnant women often present atypically, which can lead to delayed diagnosis of life-threatening abdominal pathology.
- This guideline covers adults, infants and children. In this guideline, the term 'child' includes infants, unless specified otherwise.
- Abdominal pain can arise from both acute conditions and exacerbations of chronic abdominal conditions:
  - **Acute conditions:** e.g. appendicitis, cholecystitis, intestinal obstruction, ureteric colic, gastritis, perforated peptic ulcer, gastroenteritis, pancreatitis, diverticular disease, leaking or ruptured abdominal aortic aneurysms and gynaecological disorders.
  - **Chronic conditions:** e.g. irritable bowel syndrome (IBS), inflammatory bowel syndromes (ulcerative colitis and Crohn's disease), gastric and duodenal ulcers and intra-abdominal malignancy.

2. Severity and Outcome

- The most common diagnosis of patients presenting to ED with abdominal pain is non-specific abdominal pain, followed by renal colic.
- Many cases are relatively minor in nature (e.g. constipation, UTI); however, 25% of patients contacting the ambulance service with abdominal pain have serious underlying conditions.
- In patients >65 years there is a 6–8 times higher mortality rate often with atypical clinical presentations and the presence of co-morbidities.

3. Pathophysiology

Abdominal pain can be localised and referred, due to overlapping innervations of the organs contained in the abdomen (e.g. small and large intestines).

4. Causes and Symptoms

For possible causes and symptoms of abdominal pain, refer to Table 3.9 and Table 3.10.

Abdominal Pain

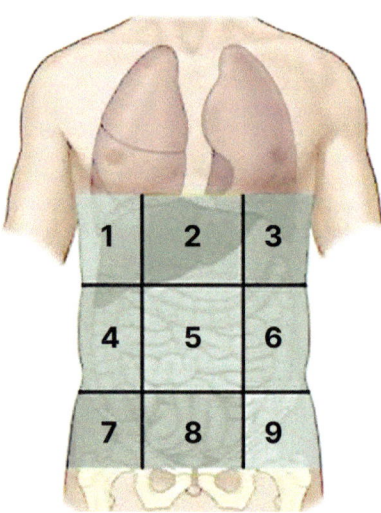

1	Right Hypochondrium Region • Liver • Gallbladder • Right kidney	2	Epigastric Region • Stomach • Liver • Pancreas • Right and left kidneys	3	Left Hypochondrium Region • Stomach • Liver (tip) • Left kidney • Spleen
4	Right Lumbar Region • Liver (tip) • Small intestines • Ascending colon • Right kidney	5	Umbilical Region • Stomach • Pancreas • Small intestines • Transverse colon	6	Left Lumbar Region • Small intestines • Descending colon • Left kidney
7	Right Iliac Region • Small intestines • Appendix • Cecum and ascending colon	8	Hypogastric Region • Small intestines • Sigmoid colon • Bladder	9	Left iliac region • Small intestines • Descending colon • Sigmoid colon

Figure 3.4 – Abdominal regions.

Abdominal Pain

TABLE 3.9 – Common Causes of Abdominal Pain in Children

< 2 Years	2 to 12 Years	12 to 16 Years
• Gastroenteritis. • Constipation. • Intussusception. • Infantile colic. • UTI. • Incarcerated inguinal hernia. • Trauma. • Pneumonia. • Diabetes.	• Gastroenteritis. • Mesenteric adenitis (inflammatory condition of lymph nodes in lower right abdomen). • Acute appendicitis. • Constipation. • UTI. • Onset of menstruation. • Psychogenic. • Testicular torsion. • Trauma. • Pneumonia. • Diabetes. • Tonsillitis, Otitis media	• Mesenteric adenitis. • Acute appendicitis. • Menstruation. • Mittelschmerz (ovulation pain). • Ovarian cyst torsion. • UTI. • Miscarriage. • Ectopic pregnancy. • Testicular torsion. • Psychogenic. • Trauma. • Pneumonia. • Diabetes.

TABLE 3.10 – Causes and Symptoms of Abdominal Pain in Adults and Children

CONDITION	CHARACTERISTICS OF PAIN	ASSOCIATED SYMPTOMS
Torsion of the testis **NB** This is a surgical emergency and if suspected the patient should be admitted to the nearest appropriate ED immediately.	• Sudden onset of severe pain in lower abdominal region or in the scrotum. • Pain may have subsided in case of torsion-detorsion. If history of severe self-limiting scrotal/testicular pain treat as torsion.	• Acute swelling of the scrotum (swelling is not *always* present). • Nausea and vomiting often occur. **NB** These symptoms indicate torsion of the testis until proven otherwise.
Leaking or ruptured abdominal aortic aneurysms (AAAs) Consider AAA in patients >50 years who present with the symptoms listed. Most deaths occur in older people. Refer to **Vascular Emergencies**	• Sudden severe abdominal pain or backache. • Renal colic-type pain – a new diagnosis of renal colic in a patient over 50 years of age raises the concern of AAA even in the absence of a palpable mass. **NB** Given that <25% of all AAA patients present with classic signs and symptoms, there is a risk of misdiagnosis.	• Collapse. • Hypotension. • Bilateral lower limb ischaemia or mottling (a late sign). • History of smoking. • History of hypertension and hypercholesterolaemia.

(continued)

Abdominal Pain

TABLE 3.10 – Causes and Symptoms of Abdominal Pain in Adults and Children *(continued)*

CONDITION	CHARACTERISTICS OF PAIN	ASSOCIATED SYMPTOMS
Appendicitis Frequently misdiagnosed. Approximately one-third of women of childbearing age with appendicitis are considered as having pelvic inflammatory disease or urinary tract infection (UTI). Appendicitis accounts for more than 40,000 hospital admissions in England each year (more common in children aged 12–16).	• An initially colicky then constant pain, increasing in intensity, often starting in the peri-umbilical area. • The pain may settle in the right lower quadrant, but the location may vary in the early stages. • Tenderness on palpation/percussion, guarding (muscular rigidity). The site of maximal tenderness is often said to be over McBurney's point, which is two-thirds of the way along a line drawn from the umbilicus to the anterior superior iliac spine. • There may be rebound tenderness in the right iliac fossa and coughing and walking may exacerbate the pain. • Older patients may present with generalised pain, distension and decreased bowel sounds. • In children, if asked to hop, the child will refuse as this causes pain. • Rovsing's sign – palpation of the left lower quadrant increases the pain felt in the right lower quadrant. • Psoas sign – extending the right thigh with the person in the left lateral position elicits pain in the right lower quadrant. • Obturator sign – internal rotation of the flexed right thigh elicits pain in the right lower quadrant.	• Nausea. • Vomiting (profuse vomiting may indicate development of peritonitis). • Loss of appetite. • Constipation. • Increased low grade temperature >37.5°C. • Diarrhoea. • Facial flushing, dry tongue, halitosis. • Tachycardia. **NB** Assess for potential complications: • Tachycardia and sudden easing of pain may be signs of a perforated appendix. • Palpable abdominal mass and swinging pyrexia may be signs of an appendix abscess. • High fever (more than 40°C), severe abdominal tenderness and absent bowel sounds may be signs of peritonitis.
Ectopic pregnancy Pregnancy not implanted in the uterus. It affects 1 pregnancy in 80 and accounts for 13% of all pregnancy-related deaths. Refer to **Vaginal Bleeding during Pregnancy up to 20 Weeks Gestation**	• Pain in the lower abdomen, pelvic area or back. **NB** Patients may present atypically but pain is almost always present.	• PV bleeding • Syncope or orthostatic hypotension • Nausea. • Missed last menstrual period (though can occur before this). • History of pelvic inflammatory disease. • Previous ectopic pregnancy. If the pregnancy ruptures, patients may report: • Severe lower abdominal pain. • Shoulder tip pain. • Feeling faint/collapse.

Abdominal Pain

TABLE 3.10 – Causes and Symptoms of Abdominal Pain in Adults and Children *(continued)*

CONDITION	CHARACTERISTICS OF PAIN	ASSOCIATED SYMPTOMS
Intestinal obstruction A partial or complete obstruction of the small or large intestine. Intussusception (bowel obstruction caused by a segment of intestine sliding inside another part of the intestines). Most commonly found in infants; another peak in incidence occurs at six years of age. Volvulus (a loop of intestine twisting around itself, resulting in obstruction).	• Abdominal pain that is cramping in nature. • Intermittent colicky pain associated with bouts of screaming and drawing up legs.	• Abdominal distension. • Nausea and vomiting. • Absolute constipation (late stage). • 'Currant jelly stool' – blood and mucus. • Faeculant vomiting. • Bile-stained vomiting. • Absence of passing flatus/wind. • Increased bowel sounds. • Visible distended loops of bowel. • Visible peristalsis. • Scars. • Swellings at the site of hernial orifices and of the external genitalia.
Ischaemic bowel Ischaemic bowel is a group of conditions that are associated with reduced blood flow and potential infarction of the intestines. This can occur within both the small intestine and the large intestine. This is a medical emergency, with mortality rates up to 90% in missed recognition or delayed diagnosis and treatment. The main contributing cause is a thrombus, and specific risk factors include AF, particularly where patient is not medicated, mitral stenosis, and strangulated hernias.	• Moderate to severe colic type or constant and poorly localised pain.	• Physical findings and observations that are out of proportion to the degree of pain reported. • Gastrointestinal symptoms such as nausea and vomiting, PR bleeds and bowel problems may also be present. • In early presentation, the abdominal examination may not show any significant findings, but later stages may include signs of peritonitis.
Peritonitis Inflammation of the lining of the abdominal cavity and abdominal organs. Requires urgent assessment and treatment	• Refusal or inability to walk. • Slow walk or stooped forward. • Pain on coughing or jolting.	• Lying motionless. • Decreased/absent abdominal wall movements with respiration. • Abdominal distension. • Abdominal tenderness – localised/generalised. • Abdominal guarding/rigidity. • Percussion tenderness. • Palpable abdominal mass. • Bowel sounds – absent/decreased (peritonitis). • Associated non-specific signs – tachycardia, fever.

(continued)

Abdominal Pain

TABLE 3.10 – Causes and Symptoms of Abdominal Pain in Adults and Children *(continued)*

CONDITION	CHARACTERISTICS OF PAIN	ASSOCIATED SYMPTOMS
Acute cholecystitis/ Biliary colic A common cause of patients attending ED for acute abdominal pain.	• Sudden onset sharp pain in the right upper quadrant of the abdomen. • Typically lasts several hours. • Pain may radiate through to the back • May experience right shoulder-tip pain. • Murphy's sign positive (unable to take a deep breath due to pain when palpating right subcostal area).	• Nausea and vomiting. • Increased temperature >38°C. • History of fat intolerance.
Acute pancreatitis Inflammation of the pancreas.	• Constant pain in the epigastrium • The pain may radiate to the patient's back.	• Abdominal tenderness. • Hypotension. • Nausea and vomiting. • Dehydration. • Shock. • History of alcohol misuse or gallstones.
Constipation Constipation is generally defined as passage of stools less frequently than their normal pattern.	• Abdominal tenderness.	• Infrequent bowel activity (less than 3 times per week or less than normal). • Foul-smelling wind and stools. • Excessive flatulence. • Irregular stool texture. • Passing occasional enormous stools or frequent small pellets. • Withholding or straining to stop passage of stools. • Soiling or overflow. • Abdominal distension. • Poor appetite. • Lack of energy. • Unhappy, angry or irritable mood and general malaise.
Gastritis An inflammation of the gastric lining can be caused by medication (aspirin, non-steroidal anti-inflammatory drugs), alcohol, *Helicobacter pylori* or stress.	• Upper abdominal pain. • Lower/central chest pain/ epigastric pain.	• Nausea and vomiting. • Loss of appetite. • Haematemesis.
Infective diarrhoea	• Intermittent generalised abdominal pain.	• Blood mixed with stools – ask about travel history and recent antibiotic therapy.

Abdominal Pain

TABLE 3.10 – Causes and Symptoms of Abdominal Pain in Adults and Children *(continued)*

CONDITION	CHARACTERISTICS OF PAIN	ASSOCIATED SYMPTOMS
Urinary tract pathology Infection arising from the kidneys, ureters, bladder and/or urethra. Urinary tract obstruction. Renal (ureteric) colic	• Pain in the lower abdomen and/or back. • Ureteric colic – colicky loin pain, pacing up and down.	• Pain/burning sensation when urinating. • Urinary frequency and nocturia. • Offensive urine. • Nausea and vomiting. • Cloudy/bloody urine with a malodour. • Lethargy. • Irritability. • Poor feeding/appetite • Fever. • If the infection involves the kidneys, the patient may have increased temperature >38°C, and fatigue. • Rigors may be present.
Abdominal migraine	• Presents typically as recurrent bouts of generalised abdominal pain.	• Nausea and vomiting. • No headache, followed by sleep and recovery.
Diverticular disease Inflammation of diverticula in the large intestine.	• Abdominal pain in the lower left quadrant.	• Nausea and vomiting. • Altered bowel habit. • Bloating. • Increased temperature >38°C.
Hepatitis	• Abdominal pain. • Jaundice	• This is due to liver inflammation and swelling.
Inflammatory bowel disease	• Increased frequency of defaecation and loose motions.	• Blood in stools.
Lower lobe pneumonia (children)	• Abdominal pain.	• Fever. • Cough. • Tachypnoea. • Desaturation.
Pelvic inflammatory disease A common cause of abdominal pain in females but rarely presents as an acute collapse.	• Pain in the lower abdomen, pelvic area or back. Usually bilateral pain. • Abdominal tenderness.	• Abnormal vaginal bleeding • Vaginal discharge. • Nausea. • Fever. • History of sexually transmitted infections and pelvic inflammatory disease.
Peptic ulcer An erosion of the lining of the stomach or small intestine, forming an ulcer.	• Central burning abdominal pain. • Back pain. • Perforation may lead to abrupt onset epigastric pain.	• Nausea and vomiting – haematemesis. • Fatigue. • Weight loss.

Abdominal Pain

5. Assessment and Management

For the assessment and management of abdominal pain, refer to Table 3.11.

TABLE 3.11 – ASSESSMENT and MANAGEMENT of: Abdominal Pain

Assess <C>ABCDE

If any of the following **TIME-CRITICAL** features present:

- major **<C>ABCDE** problems (refer to **Medical Emergencies in Adults – Overview** and **Medical Emergencies in Children – Overview**).
- suspected leaking or ruptured aortic aneurysm
- torsion of the testis
- ectopic pregnancy
- sepsis resulting from perforation
- traumatic disruption of abdominal organs, e.g. liver, spleen, then:
  – Start correcting any **<C>ABCDE** problems.
  – Undertake a **TIME-CRITICAL** transfer to nearest appropriate receiving hospital – for patients with suspected leaking or ruptured aortic aneurysm, follow local vascular care pathway.
  – Continue patient management en route.
  – Provide an ATMIST information call.

Differential Diagnoses

- If no immediately life-threatening signs are identified during the primary survey, then continue to a secondary survey to understand causes of pain and form differential diagnoses. Refer to Table 3.10.

NB For indigestion-type pain, have a high index of suspicion that it may be cardiac in origin.

Examination

- Assess the patient's abdomen, where possible in a supine position. Flexing the knees to 90 degrees relaxes the abdominal wall. The physical abdominal examination should include:
  – Inspection for distention, scars, bruising, temperature, etc.
  – Auscultating the abdomen for bowel sounds and their frequency.
  – Palpating for tenderness, rebound tenderness and guarding.
  – Consideration for special tests where relevant, e.g. Murphy's Sign, McBurney point tenderness.

NB Hyperactive bowel sounds in children commonly stem from gastroenteritis; however, consider bowel obstructions or gastro-intestinal (GI) haemorrhage/infection as a risk when completing the assessment.

History

- During history-taking, ask about gastrointestinal symptoms and genitourinary symptoms as the systems are interlinked.
- Ask about sexual history.
- Be aware of bowel obstructions caused by conditions such as intussusception (bowel obstruction caused by a segment of intestine sliding inside another part of the intestines) or volvulus (a loop of intestine twisting around itself resulting in obstruction), which are surgical emergencies and need to be conveyed to an ED within an hour of presentation.

Associated Symptoms/Conditions

- Altered bowel habit or flatulence.
- Nausea and vomiting – haematemesis/malaena may indicate gastrointestinal pathology – refer to **Gastrointestinal Bleeding**.
- Vaginal bleeding/pregnancy/previous ectopic pregnancy – refer to relevant Maternity Care guidelines.
- Burning on urination.
- Females: Menstrual history in females of childbearing age (is there any possibility of pregnancy?).

NB For details of signs and symptoms of specific conditions, refer to Table 3.10.

NB Bites, stings and poisons: ask about the possibility of bites, stings or ingestion of poisons. Adder envenomation can result in abdominal pain and vomiting.

Abdominal Pain

TABLE 3.11 – ASSESSMENT and MANAGEMENT of: Abdominal Pain *(continued)*
If Patient Is Female and of Childbearing Age, Consider Additional Causes
• Where available consider a pregnancy test.
• Consider ectopic pregnancy, pelvic inflammatory disease or other STD.
• Other gynaecological problems.
• Mittelschmerz (one-sided lower abdominal pain associated with ovulation).
• Torsion of the ovary.
• Pelvic inflammatory disease.
Known Congenital or Pre-existing Condition
• Previous abdominal surgery (adhesions).
• Nephrotic syndrome (primary peritonitis).
• Mediterranean background (familial Mediterranean fever).
• Hereditary spherocytosis (cholelithiasis).
• Cystic fibrosis (meconium ileus equivalent).
• Cystinuria.
• Porphyria.
• Current drug treatment if any.
• Recent travel.
• Presence of similar symptoms in others.
Red Flags
The following red flags require a discussion with a senior healthcare professional where not being conveyed.

• Suspected time-critical conditions:
   – suspected leaking or ruptured aortic aneurysm
   – torsion of the testis
   – ectopic pregnancy
   – sepsis resulting from perforation

• Severe pain, especially with a rigid abdomen.
• Persistent vomiting.
• Distended abdomen associated with absolute constipation.
• Unintentional weight loss.
• Blood in stool.
• Sudden change in bowel habit.
Respiratory Rate
• Measure and record respiratory rate.
Pulse
• Measure and record pulse.
Oxygen Saturation
• Monitor the patient's SpO$_2$, administer oxygen to achieve saturations of >94% if the patient presents as hypoxaemic on air (refer to **Oxygen**).
Blood Pressure and Fluids
• Measure and record blood pressure. If required, administer fluids (refer to **Intravascular Fluid Therapy in Adults** and **Intravascular Fluid Therapy in Children**).

(continued)

Abdominal Pain

TABLE 3.11 – ASSESSMENT and MANAGEMENT of: Abdominal Pain *(continued)*

Blood Glucose and Ketones
- If appropriate, measure and record blood glucose for hypo/hyperglycaemia (refer to **Glycaemic Emergencies in Adults and Children**).
- If appropriate, measure and record blood ketones (refer to **Glycaemic Emergencies in Adults and Children**).

Temperature
- Measure and record temperature.

NEWS2
- These observations will enable you to calculate a NEWS2 Score (refer to **Sepsis**).

ECG
- If appropriate, monitor and record 12-lead ECG. Assess for abnormality (refer to **Cardiac Arrhythmia and Sudden Cardiac Death**).

Assess the Patient's Pain
- Where present, assess the SOCRATES of pain and record initial and subsequent pain scores.
- Consider analgesia if appropriate (refer to **Pain Management in Adults and Children**).

Documentation
- Complete documentation to include all clinical findings, advice from other clinicians, onward referral and worsening advice given.

Transfer to Further Care
- Where conveyance is required transfer to further care (consider most appropriate centre). This may be Same Day Emergency Care (SDEC), Surgical Assessment Unit (SAU) or Emergency Department depending upon pathways at local hospital.
- Transfer all children with bile-stained (green) vomit.
- A new diagnosis of renal colic in a patient over 50 years of age raises the concern of AAA even in the absence of a expansile palpable mass.

5.1 Community Management

- Where the working diagnosis is of a minor illness, e.g. gastroenteritis or a single episode of self-limiting abdominal pain, discharge in the community may be appropriate. These patients do not routinely require discussion with a senior healthcare professional unless the clinician needs further advice.
- Discussion with a senior healthcare professional should be considered prior to leaving scene where:
  – Further management, input or advice is needed to continue this episode of care (e.g. medications, antibiotics).
  – Relevant surgical or past medical history are identified.
  – Recent involvement with another healthcare professional for the same or related condition in the past 72 hours.
  – A need for further GP assessment or urgent outpatient referral has been identified on assessment/ history taking (e.g. unintentional weight loss, recent change in bowel habit, blood in motions).

Follow local Trust procedures for accessing this advice.

- Should the patient be discharged on scene, provide the following advice to the patient/parent/carer:
  – Reassure the patient and encourage them to rest.
  – If they are not vomiting, advise regular paracetamol for pain relief.
  – Encourage the patient to drink plenty of clear fluids (e.g. cooled boiled water).
  – Do not push the patient to eat if they feel unwell.
  – If the patient is hungry, encourage them to eat bland food (e.g. crackers, rice, bananas or toast).
  – Many patients with abdominal pain get better without intervention over a few hours or days. However, if problems persist, encourage them to seek further medical advice.

Abdominal Pain

> **KEY POINTS!**
>
> **Abdominal Pain**
>
> - The most important diagnoses to consider are those that are life-threatening, as the result of either internal haemorrhage or perforation of a viscus and sepsis.
> - For indigestion-type pain, have a high index of suspicion that it may be cardiac in origin. In the absence of a specific working diagnosis obtain a 12-lead ECG for older patients and patients with cardiac risks presenting with upper abdominal pain.
> - If a patient is in pain, adequate analgesia should be given.
> - A precise diagnosis of the cause of abdominal pain is often not possible without access to tests and investigations in hospital or via primary care.
> - Patients presenting with recent onset of symptoms which require further GP/Outpatient assessment need to receive clearly documented advice on this and the clinical record sent to the GP practice.

Acknowledgements

We would like to gratefully acknowledge the contribution of the South Western Ambulance Service to this JRCALC guideline.

Bibliography

1. Clinical Knowledge Summaries, 2024. *Appendicitis*. Available from: https://cks.nice.org.uk/appendicitis.
2. Clinical Knowledge Summaries, 2024. *Scrotal Pain*. Available from: https://cks.nice.org.uk/topics/scrotal-pain-swelling/management/testicular-torsion/
3. Clinical Knowledge Summaries, 2021. *Acute Cholecystitis*. Available from: https://cks.nice.org.uk/topics/cholecystitis-acute/
4. Clinical Knowledge Summaries, 2024. *Constipation*. Available from: https://cks.nice.org.uk/topics/constipation/
5. Clinical Knowledge Summaries, 2024. *PID*. Available from: https://cks.nice.org.uk/topics/pelvic-inflammatory-disease/
6. Kavanagh S. The acute abdomen: assessment, diagnosis and pitfalls. *UK MPS Casebook* 2004, 12(1): 11–18.
7. Manterola C, Vial M, Moraga J, Astudillo P. Analgesia in patients with acute abdominal pain. *Cochrane Database of Systematic Reviews* 2011, 1. Available from: http://www.mrw.interscience.wiley.com/cochrane/clsysrev/articles/CD005660/frame.html: doi 10.1002/14651858.CD005660.pub3.
8. Agarwal T, Butt MA. Small bowel obstruction. *Emergency Medicine Journal* 2007, 24(5): 368.
9. Amoli HA, Golozar A, Keshavarzi S, Tavakoli H, Yaghoobi A. Morphine analgesia in patients with acute appendicitis: a randomised double-blind clinical trial. *Emergency Medicine Journal* 2008, 25(9): 586–589.
10. Beck J, Jang TB. Short answer question case series: controversies in the diagnosis and management of diverticulitis. *Emergency Medicine Journal* 2012, 29(6): 517–518.
11. Beck J, Jang TB. Short answer question case series: diagnosis of acute cholecystitis. *Emergency Medicine Journal* 2012, 29(5): 430–431.
12. Beckingham IJ, Bornman PC. Acute pancreatitis. *British Medical Journal* 2001, 322(7286): 595–598.
13. Car J. Urinary tract infections in women: diagnosis and management in primary care. *British Medical Journal* 2006, 332(7533): 94–97.
14. Cartwright SL, Knudson MP. Evaluation of acute abdominal pain in adults. *American Family Physician* 2008, 77(7): 971–978.
15. Chan SSW, Ng KC, Lyon DJ, Cheung WL, Cheng AFB, Rainer TH. Acute bacterial gastroenteritis: a study of adult patients with positive stool cultures treated in the emergency department. *Emergency Medicine Journal* 2003, 20(4): 335–338.
16. Chong CF, Wang TL, Chen CC, Ma HP, Chang H. Pre-consultation use of analgesics on adults presenting to the emergency department with acute appendicitis. *Emergency Medicine Journal* 2004, 21(1): 41–43.
17. Gray J, Wardrope J, Fothergill DJ. The ABC of community emergency care: 7 Abdominal pain: abdominal pain in women, complications of pregnancy and labour. *Emergency Medicine Journal* 2004, 21(5): 606–613.
18. Hall J, Driscoll P. The ABC of community emergency care: 10 Nausea, vomiting and fever. *Emergency Medicine Journal* 2005, 22(3): 200–204.
19. Humes DJ, Simpson J. Acute appendicitis. *British Medical Journal* 2006, 333(7567): 530–534.
20. Kingsnorth A, O'Reilly D. Acute pancreatitis. *British Medical Journal* 2006, 332(7549): 1072–1076.
21. Lehnert T, Sorge I, Till H, Rolle U. Intussusception in children: clinical presentation, diagnosis and management. *International Journal of Colorectal Disease* 2009, 24(10): 1187–1192.
22. Lewis SRR, Mahony PJ, Simpson J. Appendicitis. *British Medical Journal* 2011, 343: d5976.
23. Little P, Merriman R, Turner S, Rumsby K, Warner G, Lowes JA, et al. Presentation, pattern, and natural course of severe symptoms, and role of antibiotics and antibiotic resistance among patients presenting with suspected uncomplicated urinary tract infection

Abdominal Pain

in primary care: observational study. *British Medical Journal* 2010, 340: b5633.

24. Lynch RM. Accuracy of abdominal examination in the diagnosis of non-ruptured abdominal aortic aneurysm. *Accident and Emergency Nursing* 2004, 12(2): 99–107.

25. Metcalfe D, Holt PJE, Thompson MM. The management of abdominal aortic aneurysms. *British Medical Journal* 2011, 342: d1384.

26. Ranji SR, Goldman L, Simel DL, Shojania KG. Do opiates affect the clinical evaluation of patients with acute abdominal pain? *Journal of the American Medical Association* 2006, 296(14): 764–774.

27. Royal College of Obstetricians and Gynaecologists. *Management of Acute Pelvic Inflammatory Disease* (Green-top Guideline 32). London: RCOG, 2008. Available from: https://www.rcog.org.uk/en/guidelines-research-services/guidelines/gtg32/.

28. Sakalihasan N, Limet R, Defawe OD. Abdominal aortic aneurysm. *The Lancet* 2005, 365(9470): 1577–1589.

29. Touzios JG, Dozois EJ. Diverticulosis and acute diverticulitis. *Gastroenterology Clinics of North America* 2009, 38(3): 513–525.

30. Trowbridge RL, Rutkowski NK, Shojania KG. Does this patient have acute cholecystitis? *Journal of the American Medical Association* 2003, 289(1): 80–86.

31. National Collaborating Centre for Women's and Children's Health. *Urinary Tract Infection in Children: Diagnosis, treatment and long-term management* (CG54). London: Royal College of Obstetricians and Gynaecologists, 2007. Available from: http://www.nice.org.uk/nicemedia/pdf/CG54fullguideline.pdf.

32. National Institute for Health and Clinical Excellence. *Diarrhoea and Vomiting in Children: Diarrhoea and vomiting caused by gastroenteritis: diagnosis, assessment and management in children younger than 5 years* (CG84). 2009. Available from: https://www.nice.org.uk/guidance/cg84.

33. Scottish Intercollegiate Guidelines Network. *Management of Acute Upper and Lower Gastrointestinal Bleeding* (Guideline 105). Edinburgh: SIGN, 2008.

34. Gloucestershire Clinical Commissioning Group. 2015. *The Big 6*.

35. Bickley, LS., *Bates' Guide to Physical Examination and History Taking*. Philadelphia: Lippincott Williams & Wilkins, 2013.

Acute Behavioural Disturbance (ABD)

1. Introduction

This guideline must be considered in conjunction with the **Agitated Patients** and **Delirium** guidelines.

- This guideline covers caring for patients aged 12 years and over with severe agitation and delirium thought to be due to acute behavioural disturbance (ABD), when the level of agitation is posing a risk to the safety of the patient or others.
- Seek clinical advice if the patient is aged less than 12 years.
- Do **NOT** use this guidance if the patient has agitation without delirium or has delirium without agitation.

1.1 Definition

- ABD has been defined as 'a state of extreme mental and physiological excitement, characterised by extreme agitation, delirium, hyperthermia, hostility, exceptional strength and endurance without apparent fatigue' (refer to Figure 3.5).
- To have agitation, a patient must have an abnormal increase in motor activity or restlessness, e.g. trying to climb off the ambulance stretcher, trolley or cot, or actively resisting assessment, treatment or transport, or some combination of these. Anxiety or signs of mental distress or both are not enough by themselves to define the patient as being agitated.
- To have delirium, a patient must have recently (i.e. in the last few hours or days) developed signs of an abnormal state of mind, e.g. confusion, delusions or significantly abnormal behaviour.
- Clinicians must assess the patient's mental capacity to make decisions about their care and treatment. The presence of ABD signs or symptoms does not automatically mean a patient lacks capacity.

1.2 Terminology

- ABD is not a formal diagnosis. It is the 'umbrella' term for the clinical presentation of a number of possible conditions.
- ABD may also be known as:
  - acute behavioural disorder
  - acute severe behavioural disturbance
  - agitated delirium
  - excited delirium
  - excited delirium syndrome (ExD)
  - severe agitated delirium.
- Many of these terms are used interchangeably but they are not interchangeable terms. The term 'acute behavioural disorder' is widely used by the police but it is not a recognised medical condition.
- Most clinical professionals prefer the term ABD, as it describes behaviour that can have a number of causes without implying a discrete and defined condition.
- 'Excited delirium' is not a generally recognised medical condition, although it has been used in some health guidance, as well as by witnesses in UK Coroners' Courts, and it is a somewhat controversial concept. It is applied to a number of different conditions that have in common some or all of the following:
  - a state of high psychological and mental arousal

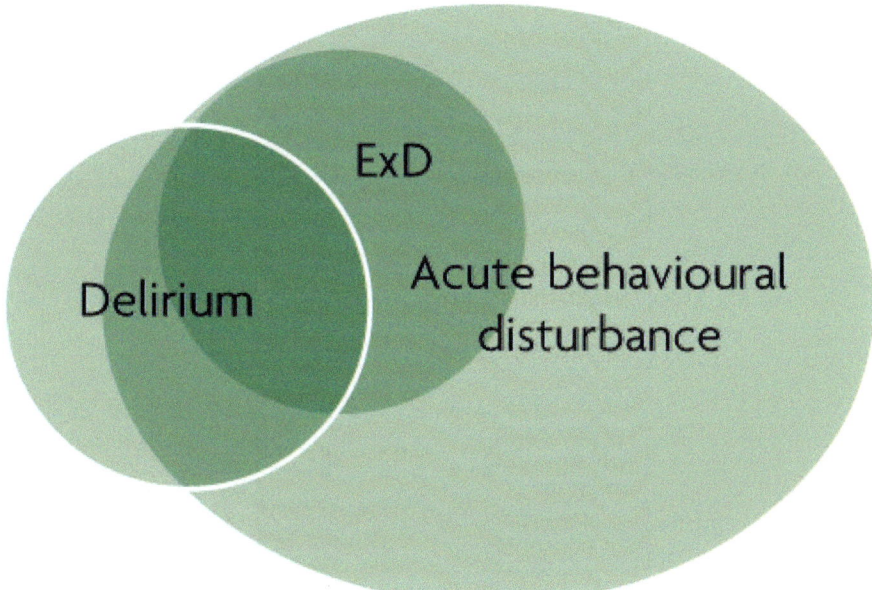

Figure 3.5 – Acute behavioural disturbance. Republished with kind permission of Professor Keith Rix. Available from: https://napicu.org.uk/wp-content/uploads/2019/04/K-Rix-Acute-Behavioural-Disburbance-20-March-14.05-14.30.pdf.

Acute Behavioural Disturbance (ABD)

- agitation
- tactile warmth or 'warm to touch'
- hyperthermia, which is abnormally elevated temperature, sweating
- violence, aggression and hostility with insensitivity to pain.

- Regardless of this terminological controversy, the significance of this group of signs and symptoms is that it constitutes a potentially fatal medical emergency.

2. Incidence, Severity and Outcome

- The incidence of life-threatening ABD in the UK is unknown, partly as there are a number of potential causes of similar presenting features, but there have been a number of deaths attributed to this condition. Its presentation has been associated with sudden death in approximately 10% of cases in some countries. The majority of patients who have died have deteriorated within an hour of the first contact with emergency services. However, it is important to realise that the patient may have been experiencing symptoms for some hours prior to first contact. Patients with ABD may come into contact with the police first as they are usually called to attend due to a person's sudden onset of bizarre or violent behaviour. The presenting behaviours can range from mildly erratic to a state of extreme agitation and physical exertion. ABD may be associated with fatality even when appropriately treated, the risk extending for as long as 24–48 hours after treatment, but the likelihood of successful treatment is increased with immediate appropriate clinical interventions.

- Some high-profile deaths of individuals displaying features of ABD have occurred whilst they have been in police custody. This has attracted much media coverage and ABD has become a controversial condition, with significant distress for the families involved. The early recognition, intervention and proactive treatment of ABD, with a collaborative response between the police and NHS Ambulance Services, may improve outcomes.

3. Pathophysiology

- ABD is most commonly associated with the use of illegal recreational drugs.
- ABD may be caused by drugs, infection; metabolic disorders (e.g. hypoglycaemia, hyponatraemia); liver failure; mental health disorders; dementia; drug or alcohol withdrawal.
- The most common cause internationally is recreational drug ingestion, particularly of methamphetamines, cocaine, legal- or illegal-high drugs or synthetic cannabinoids or novel psychoactive substance, as a toxidrome.

- ABD may be associated with serious mental illness, especially if antipsychotic medicine is stopped abruptly.
- The presentation may be also due to a physical illness. It is thought some individuals may have a genetic predisposition to developing ABD. It is essential to consider a range of differential diagnoses.
- The topic of ABD is controversial for a number of reasons, not least because it describes clinical presentations rather than a single disease.
- Patients have physiological signs of autonomic dysfunction, including significant tachycardia, tachypnoea, hyperthermia and sweating – these may be associated with multi-organ failure and death.
- The mechanism of ABD-related pathophysiological changes is unclear and there are a number of different theories. One current theory is that in some patients, ABD may be related to their dopamine levels, dopamine being a neurotransmitter in the brain. This is especially so in those cases involving novel psychoactive substances, particularly cocaine, illegal- and legal-high drugs or similar stimulants, or where patients on antipsychotic mediations have suddenly stopped taking them. Another theory is related to serotonin pathways, particularly when MDMA has been taken. There is also a theory related to genetic susceptibility, particularly in cocaine use, where some patients have fatal outcomes with lower doses of cocaine use than those who survive. Extreme agitation depletes the patient's oxygen and glucose reserves, producing CO_2 and water. CO_2 dissociates into hydrogen ions and bicarbonate, increasing any metabolic lactic acidosis. CO_2 is removed acutely via an increase in respiratory rate; if respiration is restricted or inadequate, the body cannot correct the resultant acidosis, leading to arrythmia risk and further metabolic disturbances. Patients are also at risk of dehydration, rhabdomyolysis producing acute renal failure from myoglobinaemia and hyperkalaemia, which may provoke life-threatening arrhythmias. It is important to try to minimise physical restraint to less than 10 minutes and to avoid airway or respiratory compromise.
- Many factors have been proposed as contributory to sudden death in ABD, such as positional asphyxia secondary to restraint, drug toxicity itself or underlying cardiac disease resulting in cardiac arrhythmias.
- Severe metabolic acidosis associated with life-threatening ABD is now thought to be the most significant factor in cardiovascular collapse and sudden death. Ambulance clinicians must be able to recognise that the presenting signs and symptoms of possible ABD represent an **emergency condition**.

Acute Behavioural Disturbance (ABD)

4. Assessment

- The identification of life-threatening ABD can be difficult clinically as the spectrum of behaviours and signs (refer to Table 3.12) overlap with many other disease presentations (refer to Table 3.13).

There is no definitive diagnostic test for the condition.

- Once potentially life-threatening ABD is suspected, attending ambulance clinicians should consider the need for additional clinical support and request this as per local procedures.

TABLE 3.12 – Possible Signs and Symptoms of ABD

- Acute psychosis with fear of impending doom or paranoia
- Constant or near-constant physical activity without fatigue
- 'Hot to touch' or tactile hyperthermia, profuse sweating or inappropriate state of undress
- Insensitivity to pain, including that caused by irritant sprays
- Extreme aggression or violent behaviour against inanimate objects or people when restraint is attempted
- Excessive strength or continued struggle in restraint to the point of collapse
- Attraction to glass
- Rapid breathing
- Lack of response to or engagement with others
- Lack of fear, e.g. running into the path of a moving vehicle or standing on a roof.

TABLE 3.13 – Differential Diagnoses of ABD

- Common conditions which may have similar presentations:
  - sepsis
  - hypoxia
  - hypoglycaemia
  - substance intoxication or withdrawal
  - meningitis or encephalitis
  - head injury
  - seizure, in the post-ictal phase
  - subarachnoid haemorrhage
  - psychiatric disorder.

- Rare conditions which may have similar presentations:
  - heat stroke
  - thyrotoxic storm or hyperthyroid crisis
  - neuroleptic malignant syndrome, which is a rare, severe, idiosyncratic adverse reaction to antipsychotics
  - serotonin syndrome, which is SSRI antidepressant toxicity
  - akathisia, which is an adverse effect of antipsychotic drugs, characterised by restlessness and mental unease, both of which can be intense.

- Although trauma is rarely the cause of death in ABD cases, many patients sustain trauma as part of the condition. It is recognised that this is due to:
  - lack of fear or risky behaviour by the patient
  - accidental injury in agitated state, especially where patients exhibit glass attraction
  - reduced pain perception
  - injury during restraint.
- Other potential pitfalls include:
  - assuming a medical cause or drug-related condition without considering the possibility of significant trauma
  - symptoms of trauma may be masked by the signs of ABD
  - misinterpretation of physiological observations.
- ABD may make the clinical assessment of possible major trauma more difficult. Physiological observations will be difficult to take, symptoms may be masked and a full account of the history is unlikely to be available.
- Information from bystanders and the police can be helpful and signs of minor trauma may be significant as they may indicate underlying major trauma.

Acute Behavioural Disturbance (ABD)

5. Management

- The Royal College of Emergency Medicine, UK, published an ABD Guideline in 2016 regarding the management of ABD in the Emergency Department. They and others have recommended joint guidelines between all those involved in the management of ABD from scene to hospital.
- This guideline provides the NHS ambulance services with clinical guidance to link the out-of-hospital phase to the emergency department phase for these patients.

5.1 Verbal Calming and De-escalation

- Verbal de-escalation is often under-utilised. Provided there is not an immediate risk to life, verbal de-escalation should be attempted before restraint or pharmacological agents are used.
- The key aspects to successful verbal and non-verbal de-escalation are:
  - Allow sufficient time to attempt verbal de-escalation.
  - Maintain a safe distance between you and the patient.
  - Have only one person verbally engage with the patient.
  - Introduce yourself; state that you are there to help and provide reassurance.
  - Use a calm voice and adopt a non-threatening stance.
  - Use short sentences and keep messages simple. Repetition is essential as the patient will usually have a short attention span.
  - Minimise the number of people in the immediate vicinity to those required for the safety of the patient and staff on scene.
  - Limit unnecessary noise and distractions, e.g. radio noise, blue lights, sirens, etc.
  - Minimise any painful stimuli for the patient.
  - Actively listen to the patient and try to gain an understanding of their concerns.
  - Try to establish rapport and offer choices; if appropriate, allow them to have a drink or a cigarette.
  - Avoid provocative statements, e.g. do not say 'If you don't calm down, we will have to sedate you'.
  - Once rapport has been established, continue clinical care.
- Patients with ABD are often highly agitated, with altered mental status or lacking mental capacity, making their response to de-escalation techniques unpredictable.
- In close liaison with police and/or other relevant healthcare professionals on scene, attempts at verbal calming by one person and other de-escalation techniques should be considered as the first-line intervention in attempting to manage individuals displaying possible ABD. Consider removal of any causes of the presenting symptoms where appropriate. Where patients present in the context of custodial settings, it is essential to establish if any pharmacological therapy has already been commenced, as this may affect decisions on further clinical care. A mental capacity assessment must also be undertaken in accordance with relevant legislation and their associated codes of practice (refer to **Mental Capacity Act 2005**).
- NICE recommend all health organisations provide their staff with training in de-escalation for:
  - recognising the early signs of agitation, irritation, anger and aggression
  - understanding the likely causes of aggression or violence
  - using techniques for distraction and calming, and ways to encourage relaxation
  - recognising the importance of personal space
  - responding to a patient's anger in an appropriate, measured and reasonable way to avoid provocation.
- Friends, family members or both may be helpful but ask them to desist if they are making the situation worse.
- In a 2-year audit by the London Ambulance Service for cases where appropriately trained critical care paramedics responded to assess ABD, 62% of patients were managed using only verbal de-escalation followed by standard care.
- Where de-escalation interventions are unsuccessful after a short period, attending ambulance clinicians should consider the need for additional clinical or police support or both and request this via the emergency operations centre if not already done.

5.2 Physical Restraint

- Physical restraint in ABD may be considered as part of patient management and planned by the police in conjunction with ambulance clinicians where possible before being applied.
- Clinicians should request senior support at the earliest opportunity, especially non-registered ambulance clinicians and newly qualified paramedics (NQPs).
- Clinicians on-scene are responsible for the clinical safety of the patient at all times and should immediately inform any other personnel on-scene if they believe the patient's clinical condition is at risk of deteriorating, particularly if there is any restriction to the patient's airway or breathing.
- The first healthcare professional on scene should be specifically responsible for monitoring and treating the patient. Any other healthcare professionals or ambulance staff in attendance should closely liaise with the designated police safety officer.

Acute Behavioural Disturbance (ABD)

- Assistance from police should be requested if:
  - There is significant risk of injury to the patient, personnel or bystanders.
  - The patient has agitation causing a severe to immediate life-threatening risk to safety.
- Physical restraint by the police can form part of patient care. It should be kept to a minimum, using a level of force that is justifiable, reasonable and proportional to the individual case, with close monitoring of the patient clinically. During restraint, clinicians should be prepared for a rapid deterioration in the patient's condition, including cardiovascular collapse.
- If any patient needs physical restraint, the ambulance clinician should actively monitor the patient's vital signs where possible and observe for any deterioration in the patient's condition.
- Police officers must be alerted to any concerns regarding the patient's welfare or clinical deterioration during restraint.
- The police have the legal authority to restrain a patient if:
  - There is an immediate need for care and control of the patient in their best interests under the Mental Capacity Act (MCA).
  - It is needed for the protection of the public.
  - It is needed to remove the patient to a place of safety (s136 MHA).
  - The patient is considered to be 'disturbing the peace'.
  - The police have other grounds in relation to their powers as police officers.
- Where legally possible to do so, consideration must be given by the police to using section 136 (s136) under the Mental Health Act (MHA) to detain the patient, to allow for mental health assessment after clinical management of the initial emergency.
- Section 136 can be used by the police in suspected ABD, **unless** the situation occurs in a private dwelling where s136 cannot legally be used. In those cases, if there is thought to be a potentially life-threatening emergency, the police would assist the ambulance clinician by considering the use of the MCA if the patient lacks capacity, and then acting in the best interests of the patient.
- Before ambulance clinicians use physical restraint they must, if the circumstances permit, consider the patient's mental capacity, their care and treatment. That assessment and the reasons for restraint must be documented after its use.
- Prolonged physical restraint must be, wherever practicable, avoided due to the associated risk of injuries to patients, as well as it being a potentially contributing factor in clinical deterioration. Care must be taken to ensure that the patient's airway or respiratory function is not compromised – this is particularly likely if the patient is kept in a prone position with pressure applied on their head, neck, chest or shoulder region. The use of the prone position should be avoided wherever possible or used for a very short period of time only, with the patient placed on their side and hand restraints moved to the patient's front. Handcuffs restraining the arms to the rear of the body are more likely to cause respiratory compromise than arms placed to the front of the body.
- Particular care should be taken where patients are thought to be obese, critically ill or injured, have a disability or are pregnant.
- When considering the use of restraint under the MCA it is necessary to evidence that the intervention is in the best interests of the patient, necessary in order to prevent the patient from coming to harm and proportionate in terms of the likelihood of the harm occurring and the severity of that harm. Clinicians must achieve a fair and reasonable balance between the risks associated with a particular form of restraint and the aim of the restraint. There are well-evidenced risks associated with any form of restraint (physical, mechanical or pharmacological) that must be considered and mitigated against as far as reasonably possible. The clinician must believe that the use of restraint is the least restrictive available to achieve safe and effective patient care. There must be a genuine belief that restraint is necessary.
- A 'proportionate response' means the least intrusive type and minimum amount of restraint to achieve a specific outcome in the best interests of the patient who lacks capacity.
- On the occasions when the use of force may be necessary, carers and healthcare and social care staff should use the minimum amount of force for the shortest possible time (MCA Code of Practice).
- Clinicians must not place themselves or others in danger. In some rare circumstances, ambulance clinicians may consider it appropriate to restrain a patient because of the risk of harm the patient potentially poses to the public in the absence of police support. Where appropriate, common law, criminal law and mental health law can be relied upon to justify such action, even though it may not be directly in the patient's best interests.
- Significant physiological derangements, such as acidosis, electrolyte abnormalities, rhabdomyolysis, cardiac arrhythmias, etc., can occur due to the underlying condition or as a result of resisting restraint. These may be exacerbated by other clinical factors, e.g. cardiac disease, obesity or taking medications or illicit substances.
- Physiological monitoring and clinical observations must be undertaken as soon as possible; **the patient may have to be clinically monitored from a distance**.

Acute Behavioural Disturbance (ABD)

- Attempts must be made to monitor the patient's respiratory rate, level of consciousness and skin colour, e.g. pallor or other change in colour, during restraint. A NEWS2 score should be measured and documented as soon as possible. If there is new confusion, this scores 3 points in NEWS2.

- If there is **any** evidence of possible trauma, complete a primary survey, extricate rapidly, provide an ATMIST pre-alert (refer to Trauma guidelines) and be prepared for sudden cardiovascular collapse.

- There is limited research on the effects of Tasers or conducted energy devices (CEDs) in ABD. A risk assessment will be completed and a decision made on the use of a Taser or CED by the police if other methods of de-escalation have failed. In rare circumstances where an immediate threat to life exists, it may be appropriate for a Taser or CED to be used by police, before or after ambulance clinician arrival, to gain initial control, so that restraint and possibly pharmacological agents can be safely used.

- In patients with ABD, the risks of deploying a Taser or CED predominantly relate to the risk of injury associated with the fall.

TABLE 3.14 – ASSESSMENT and MANAGEMENT of: Acute Behavioural Disturbance

Assessment of the Level of Risk to Safety

- The risk to consider is the likelihood of harm occurring and the severity of that harm. The level of risk may range from mild to immediately life-threatening. Determining the level of risk to safety requires clinical judgement that takes into account the risk to the patient, to emergency services and to others on scene.

Mild to Moderate Risk to Safety

- Signs include but are not limited to:
  - verbal aggression
  - actions not involving immediate risk of serious harm to personnel, e.g. pushing or grabbing
  - pulling at equipment
  - trying to climb off the stretcher
  - agitation preventing control of moderate external bleeding.
- Attempt verbal de-escalation and move sequentially through the steps below if the level of agitation continues to pose a risk to safety. Consider calling for police assistance.
- Provide restraint if safe to do so without additional assistance.
- Gain IV access if it is feasible and safe to do so.
- If the patient has a reduced level of consciousness:
  - Position the patient on their side.
  - Provide restraint as required.
  - Administer oxygen and continually monitor the patient's airway, breathing, SpO$_2$, end-tidal CO$_2$ and level of consciousness.
  - Monitor heart rate, blood pressure and capillary refill time, particularly in restrained limbs, if possible.

Severe to Immediate Life-threatening Risk to Safety

- Signs include but are not limited to:
  - dangerous physical aggression
  - wielding a weapon
  - actions involving immediate risk of serious harm to personnel, e.g. punching or kicking
  - destruction of physical surroundings
  - trying to get out of a moving ambulance
  - agitation preventing control of severe or life-threatening external bleeding.
- Call for urgent police assistance, clinical advice and additional clinical support in line with local procedures.
- Consider moving to create a safe distance between yourself and the patient.
- Attempt verbal de-escalation or provide restraint or both only if it is safe to do so.
- Once patient control has been obtained:
  - Position the patient on their side or allow them to sit up if cooperative and clinically appropriate.
  - Administer oxygen and continually monitor the patient's airway, breathing, SpO$_2$, end-tidal CO$_2$ and level of consciousness.

Acute Behavioural Disturbance (ABD)

TABLE 3.14 – ASSESSMENT and MANAGEMENT of: Acute Behavioural Disturbance *(continued)*

	– Monitor heart rate, blood pressure and capillary refill time, particularly in restrained limbs, if possible. – Gain IV access if not already achieved. – Consider IV fluids (refer to **Intravascular Fluid Therapy in Adults**). – Undertake a TIME-CRITICAL transfer and hospital pre-alert. The police must travel with the patient.
Assess <C>ABCDE	• If any of the following TIME-CRITICAL features are present: – Major <C>ABCDE problems (refer to **Medical Emergencies in Adults – Overview**), then: – Start correcting any <C>ABCDE problems. – Undertake a TIME-CRITICAL transfer to nearest appropriate receiving hospital. – Continue patient management en route. – Provide an ATMIST information call.
Respiratory Rate	• Measure and record respiratory rate.
Pulse	• Measure and record pulse.
Oxygen Saturation	• Monitor the patient's SpO_2; administer oxygen to achieve saturations of >94% if the patient presents as hypoxaemic on air (refer to **Oxygen**).
Blood Pressure	• Measure and record blood pressure.
Blood Glucose	• If appropriate, measure and record blood glucose for hypoglycaemia and hyperglycaemia (refer to **Glycaemic Emergencies in Adults and Children**).
Temperature	• Record temperature. If it has increased, allow passive cooling.
NEWS2	• These observations will enable you to calculate a NEWS2 Score (refer to **Sepsis**).
ECG	• Monitor the ECG and if possible and appropriate record a 12-lead ECG (refer to **Cardiac Arrhythmia and Sudden Cardiac Death**).
Assess the Patient's Pain	• Where present, assess the SOCRATES of pain and record initial and subsequent pain scores. • Consider analgesia if appropriate (refer to **Pain Management in Adults and Children**).
Documentation	• Complete documentation to include all clinical findings, advice from other clinicians, onward referral and details of the use of any physical restraint or use of rapid tranquilisation.

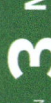

5.3 Rapid Tranquillisation (RT)

- Although verbal de-escalation and joint management with the police have been found to be effective in the majority of possible cases of ABD, in a small proportion of cases rapid tranquilisation (RT) may be an option.

- In some ABD cases, appropriately qualified clinicians may use medicines parenterally to calm the patient sufficiently to allow clinical care to be provided or the use of out-of-hospital anaesthesia. Clinicians must follow local trust guidelines and the situation must be otherwise unmanageable.

- The National Institute for Health and Care Excellence (NICE) uses the term 'rapid tranquillisation' to define using medicines parenterally to reduce the risk of harm and minimise agitation and violence. Ideally, these would have a very rapid onset of action with a high safety profile. No medicines are ideal for use in these extremely physiologically compromised patients; only a few medicines have been

Acute Behavioural Disturbance (ABD)

- used and these should only be administered by advanced clinicians approved by each ambulance trust, as per local guidelines.

- There are currently three types of medicines used internationally for rapid out of hospital tranquilisation in ABD: benzodiazepines, antipsychotics and dissociative agents. Currently, there is a lack of high-quality evidence in the medical literature to determine the most suitable single agent or combination of agents.

- There are significant risks during and after RT as usually there is limited access to information on the patient's past medical history or medication and drug history, and the environment is much less controlled. This makes this a high-risk clinical intervention given the already potentially seriously compromised physiology of patients with ABD. People with mental health problems are at increased risk of coronary heart disease, cerebrovascular disease, diabetes, epilepsy and respiratory disease, all of which can be exacerbated by the effects of rapid tranquillisation.

- The rapid control and calming of a patient displaying the extreme physical exertion associated with ABD may prevent further deterioration of their metabolic status. Ideally, medicines should be administered via the intravenous route; however, this route is unlikely to be immediately available, and the intra-nasal route is likely to present a risk to the clinician, so the intra-muscular route is generally the most suitable.

- The aim of RT is to reduce the level of agitation, making the patient calmer or more 'tranquil' **without** reducing their level of consciousness, although the latter may occur inadvertently if the patient is already physiologically seriously compromised.

- The clinician providing the RT must be accompanied by an appropriate second clinician who is able to provide clinical management of the patient's respiratory and cardiovascular systems. Clinicians should ensure that appropriate equipment is immediately available to manage a patient's airway, breathing and circulation.

- Clinicians must ensure that appropriately trained and equipped personnel accompany the patient during ambulance transfer to the ED. This will normally be the clinician who administers RT.

After Rapid Tranquilisation (RT)

- After RT the patient should be quickly and safely moved into a supine, lateral or reclined position where possible, depending on the risk assessment, then moved onto the ambulance and rapidly transferred to an ED. A police presence in the back of the ambulance will provide ongoing support, including altering any restraints such as handcuffs to reposition the patient.

- Physiological monitoring **must** be undertaken immediately post-RT and continued until ED clinicians take over care of the patient.

- A brief primary survey should be undertaken, looking for any potentially life-threatening injuries or conditions requiring immediate clinical treatment.

- An **early** pre-alert to include an SBAR summary and an ATMIST, if there may have been trauma, should be passed to the receiving ED.

- As well as having received agents that might depress respiration, many of these patients will be hypoxic or have a high oxygen demand due to their hyper-metabolic state. Oxygen should be given as soon as possible to achieve a target saturation of 94–98%.

- Hypovolaemia is common in ABD, attributable to the excess physical activity or hyperthermia or both. Where possible, patients should receive IV crystalloid. IV fluid will help correct metabolic acidosis and reduce end organ damage; aim to give 1 litre IV crystalloid stat on the way to hospital. Clinicians must monitor the patient's response to fluids and consider additional IV fluids.

- Hyperthermia is common in individuals presenting with ABD. This is due to a combination of the individual's state of constant physical exertion, which itself will generate heat, and hyperthermia due to dopamine dysfunction. 'Hot-to-touch' ABD patients need to be cooled to, but not below, normal body temperature. This can usually be achieved out of hospital with basic cooling methods such as the removal of clothing, where practical, if not already removed.

- After handover at the ED, detailed information regarding the clinical presentation, clinical risk assessments, clinical decision making, clinical findings and clinical care must be documented. These cases are also likely to be subject to internal and external reviews.

- Episodes of physical restraint must be documented for monitoring purposes; this must be managed in accordance with individual ambulance trust policy.

5.4 ABD in Custody Suites and Police Stations

- In 2019 the Faculty of Forensic and Legal Medicine (FFLM) in the UK issued guidance to healthcare professionals working in and on-call for police custody suites.

- The FFLM advised healthcare professionals (HCPs) covering custody suites, who may or may not have personally assessed the patient, that if anyone exhibits any of the following, they are to call or advise the custody staff that an ambulance should be called to transfer the patient to an ED: tactile hyperthermia or 'hot to touch'; constant or near-constant physical activity; extreme agitation or aggression. They have also advised the police that any individual with any of these presenting features is to be taken to an ED, not to a custody suite.

Acute Behavioural Disturbance (ABD)

- The custody suite HCP may have assessed the patient and given pre-rapid tranquillisation (pre-RT) using oral lorazepam (benzodiazepine) up to a maximum of 4 mg in 24 hours. The effect of pre-RT medication must be taken into consideration when assessing any patient clinically.

> **KEY POINTS!**
>
> **Acute Behavioural Disturbance (ABD)**
> - The majority of acutely disturbed or delirious patients can be managed using de-escalation techniques.
> - ABD is a clinical emergency – the patient may suffer sudden cardiovascular collapse or cardiac arrest or both with little or no warning.
> - Once ABD is identified, additional clinical support must be requested.
> - Dynamic risk assessments and non-clinical management of ABD cases should be conducted jointly with the police.
> - The clinician must take all reasonable actions to clinically monitor the patient throughout restraint where possible.
> - Patient restraint time must be kept to an absolute minimum – the degree of restraint used must be justifiable, reasonable and applied for the minimum time necessary and proportional to the situation.
> - The risks associated with the selected method of restraint must be considered and mitigated against as far as reasonably possible.
> - Early management of hyperthermia, hypovolaemia and acidosis should be instituted with IV fluids and oxygen.
> - Undertake a time-critical transfer and hospital pre-alert.

Acknowledgements

We gratefully thank the New Zealand Ambulance Service for sharing their guidelines and the many individuals who have provided invaluable advice and comments on this new guideline.

Bibliography

1. American College of Emergency Physicians. *White Paper Report on Excited Delirium Syndrome*, 2009.
2. NICE. *Violence and Aggression: Short-term management in mental health, health and community settings NICE guideline [NG10]*. 2015. Available from: https://www.nice.org.uk/guidance/ng10/chapter/1-Recommendations.
3. Hick JL, Smith S, Lynch MT. Metabolic acidosis in restraint-associated cardiac arrest: a case series. *Academic Emergency Medicine* 1999, 6(3): 239–243.
4. Rt. Hon. Dame Elish Angiolini DBE QC. Report of the Independent Review of Deaths and Serious Incidents in Police Custody. 2017. Available from: https://assets.publishing.service.gov.uk/government/uploads/system/uploads/attachment_data/file/655401/Report_of_Angiolini_Review_ISBN_Accessible.pdf.
5. The Royal College of Emergency Medicine. *Guidelines for the Management of Excited Delirium/Acute Behavioural Disturbance (ABD)*. 2016. Available from: https://www.rcem.ac.uk/docs/College%20Guidelines/5p.%20RCEM%20guidelines%20for%20management%20of%20Acute%20Behavioural%20Disturbance%20(May%202016).pdf.
6. UK Public General Acts. *Mental Health Act*. 1983, c. 20. Available from: http://www.legislation.gov.uk/ukpga/1983/20/contents.
7. UK Public General Acts. *Mental Capacity Act*. Available from: http://www.legislation.gov.uk/ukpga/2005/9/contents, 2005, c. 9.
8. NICE. *Violence and Aggression: Short-term management in mental health, health and community settings NICE guideline [NG10]*. 2015. Available from: https://www.nice.org.uk/guidance/ng10.
9. Green SM, Roback MG, Kennedy RM, Krauss B. Clinical practice guideline for emergency department ketamine dissociative sedation: 2011 update. *Annals of Emergency Medicine* 2011, 57(5): 449–461.
10. FFLM. *ABD 2019 Guidance*. 2019. Available from: https://fflm.ac.uk/resources/publications/guidelines-for-the-management-of-acute-behavioural-disturbance/.
11. Academy of Medical Royal Colleges. *Safe Sedation Practice for Healthcare Procedures*. 2013. Available from: https://www.rcoa.ac.uk/system/files/PUB-SafeSedPrac2013.pdf.
12. Baldwin S, Hall C, Bennell C et al. Distinguishing features of Excited Delirium Syndrome in non-fatal use of force encounters. *Journal of Forensic and Legal Medicine* 2016, 41: 21–27.
13. Wetli CV, Fishbain DA. Cocaine-induced psychosis and sudden death in recreational cocaine users. *Journal of Forensic Sciences* 1985, 30(3), 873–880.
14. Mash D. Excited delirium and sudden death: a syndromal disorder at the extreme end of the neuropsychiatric continuum. *Front Physiol* 2016, 7: 435.
15. Gonin P, Excited *delirium: a systematic review. Acad Emerg Med* 2018, 25(5): 552–565.
16. NICE. *Violent and Aggressive Behaviours in People with Mental Health Problems, Quality standard [QS154]*. 2017. Available from: https://www.nice.org.uk/guidance/qs154.

Acute Coronary Syndrome

1. Introduction

- The term "acute coronary syndromes" (ACS) encompasses a range of conditions including unstable angina, non-ST-segment-elevation myocardial infarction (NSTEMI) and ST-segment-elevation myocardial infarction (STEMI). The majority of these are due to a sudden reduction of blood flow to the heart muscle, usually caused by the rupture or erosion of an atherosclerotic plaque within the wall of a coronary artery leading to the formation of a blood clot within the artery.

- The most common symptom of acute coronary syndromes is severe pain in the chest and/or in other areas (for example, the arms, back or jaw), which can last for several hours. Other symptoms include sweating, nausea and vomiting, breathlessness and feeling faint.

- People with acute coronary syndromes may have a poor prognosis without prompt and accurate diagnosis. Treatments are available to help ease the pain, improve the blood flow and to prevent any future complications.

- The highest priority in managing STEMI is to restore an adequate coronary blood flow as quickly as possible by revascularisation. This applies to all people with STEMI, including those who have been resuscitated after cardiac arrest. The time taken to restore coronary blood flow is very important because heart muscle starts to be lost as soon as the coronary artery is blocked.

- In people with NSTEMI and unstable angina, the aim of treatment is to alleviate pain and anxiety and prevent recurrence of ischaemia. For people with unstable angina, treatment also aims to prevent or limit progression to acute myocardial infarction. The type of treatment is determined by the person's individual risk of future adverse cardiovascular events (heart attack and stroke, repeat treatment or death).[1]

- For patients with STEMI, time is of the essence, as delays in receiving reperfusion treatment (predominantly percutaneous coronary intervention, PCI) can increase chances of death, complications or significant long-term morbidity with heart failure. Longer prehospital delays, particularly those resulting from patients having haemodynamic complications on scene, are associated with worse outcomes.[1] Every effort must be made to expedite transfer to a hospital capable of providing primary percutaneous coronary intervention (PPCI) (sometimes called a 'Heart Attack Centre' or HAC) once STEMI is suspected from clinical and ECG findings.

2. Incidence

- Between 1st April 2020 and 31st March 2021, 82,471 cases of suspected heart attack hospital admissions were submitted to the Myocardial Ischaemic National Audit Project (MINAP)[2], of which 73,867 were confirmed as MI (either STEMI or NSTEMI). This represented a 14.8% reduction on the previous year, possibly due to patient help-seeking behaviour changing due to the COVID-19 pandemic. The reduction in the number of patients presenting with MI was greatest in those with NSTEMI, of which there were more than 10,000 fewer cases, an 18% year-on-year reduction. STEMI cases fell by 9% over the period.

3. Health Inequalities

Racial Differences

- The literature on racial differences in patients presenting with ACS is extensive but mostly drawn from the USA which, unlike the UK, does not have universal healthcare. But disparities in healthcare delivery and outcomes still exist in the UK.[3] Racial differences in management and outcome of acute myocardial infarction in the UK were further underlined during the COVID-19 pandemic, where, compared with white people, those from black, Asian and minority ethnic (BAME) communities had proportionally higher hospitalisation rates with AMI, less frequently received guideline indicated care (e.g. angiography), had longer delays to reperfusion (for STEMI) and had higher early mortality compared with the pre-COVID era.[4]

- In another recent UK study, compared with White British, BAME patients tended to be younger at time of presentation, and to have higher rates of diabetes, hypertension and chronic renal failure.[5] And there is some evidence from the UK that BAME patients experiencing ACS symptoms were less likely to use the ambulance service than white patients.[6]

Women

- The British Heart Foundation state that ACS 'kills twice as many women as breast cancer each year', and that it is a common misconception that men and women have different symptoms of a heart attack. Women with ACS do have different symptoms at presentation than men with ACS, but there is also considerable overlap. Although most sexes present with chest pain, women with ACS have higher odds of presenting with pain between the shoulders, nausea or vomiting or shortness of breath. Women are more likely to dismiss the idea that they may be having a heart attack and delay seeking medical attention. It's important to recognise the symptoms of a heart attack, take them seriously and act quickly to prevent damaging the heart muscle.[7]

- There is extensive literature showing that women have higher mortality after STEMI than men. This might be explained by what researchers have called 'unfavourable risk profile' (e.g. women tend to be older, and have more diabetes and hypertension when presenting with STEMI) and experience longer delays to reperfusion.[8]

Acute Coronary Syndrome

There is some evidence that women take longer to call emergency services when experiencing symptoms of ACS and have longer delays to first ECG recording. Bystanders appear to act more promptly when a man becomes ill with symptoms of ACS compared to women.[9]

- UK evidence shows that women are less likely to receive guideline-recommended care for a STEMI, including having a 12 lead ECG recorded by ambulance crews.[6,10]

4. Severity and Outcome

- Mortality rates for acute admissions with MI during 2020–21 were unchanged from pre-pandemic times (STEMI 7%, NSTEMI 3.3%).[2]
- The risk of cardiac arrest from ventricular fibrillation (VF) or other arrhythmias is highest in the first few hours after symptom onset. VF can occur without warning. For some patients, cardiac arrest is the first presentation of an acute coronary syndrome.

5. Assessment and Management

- NICE state: Immediately assess eligibility (irrespective of age, ethnicity or sex) for coronary reperfusion therapy (primary percutaneous coronary intervention [PCI]) or fibrinolysis in people with acute ST-segment elevation myocardial infarction (STEMI).[11]
- Do not use level of consciousness after cardiac arrest caused by suspected acute STEMI to determine whether a person is eligible for coronary angiography (with follow-on primary PCI if indicated). (Refer to **Return of Spontaneous Circulation**).
- The diagnosis of STEMI is dependent on rapid clinical assessment and recording of a 12 lead ECG. International guidelines recommend 12 lead ECG recording and interpretation as soon as possible from 'first medical contact', with a maximum delay target of 10 minutes.[12]
- Clinical risk factors should be considered together when assessing the likelihood of myocardial ischaemia, prompting rapid recording of the 12 lead ECG. Such factors include smoking, high cholesterol, higher age, family history of coronary disease, prior history of ischaemic heart disease and peripheral vascular disease, diabetes and chronic kidney disease. High risk features include:
  - Worsening angina
  - Prolonged pain (>20 minutes)
  - Pulmonary oedema
  - Hypotension
  - Arrhythmias.
- ECG rhythm monitoring with defibrillator availability is indicated as soon as possible in all patients with suspected ACS. This monitoring should continue until handover at hospital.

- Undertake a risk benefit analysis regarding the most appropriate method of transferring the patient to the ambulance with the aim of limiting patient movement and walking to reduce stress on the myocardium.

The 12-lead ECG

- Criteria for referral to a heart attack centre (HAC) may differ across the country, it is therefore recommended that locally agreed pathways are followed.
- Patients with bundle branch block of any type who have ongoing ischaemic symptoms should prompt discussion with the heart attack centre as per local pathways.
- If facilities exist, transmit 12 lead ECG for expert review in cases of uncertainty about interpretation, or seek senior clinician support using ambulance services local pathways. Automated ECG interpretation is widely available and is a useful support tool.
- The pre-hospital 12 lead ECG (PHECG) is the principal component of decision making regarding where the patient should be taken. If STEMI is suspected based on PHECG findings, immediate contact with the nearest 'heart attack centre' should be made according to locally agreed pathways. Conveyance to hospital, under emergency conditions, must be the main priority where STEMI is suspected (see below).
- There is evidence that recording PHECG is associated with short term mortality benefit for both STEMI and NSTEMI patients. However, one third of eligible patients did not receive a PHECG recording. Women, older people and those with comorbidities were less likely to have a PHECG recorded.[6]
- Some patients do not have 'classical' presentations (especially older people, and those with diabetes). This group have a high mortality due to delayed diagnosis and treatment, therefore paramedics should have a low threshold for recording a 12 lead ECG in unwell patients without chest pain.
- The diagnostic criteria for STEMI set out by the European Society of Cardiology are as follows:

ST-segment elevation (measured at the J-point): at least two contiguous leads with ST-segment elevation:
- 2.5 mm in men aged under 40 years,
- 2 mm in men aged over 40 years,
- 1.5 mm in women.

in leads V2 AND V3

and/or

In the inferior and/or lateral leads:
- 1 mm in two or more contiguous leads (in the absence of left ventricular hypertrophy or left bundle branch block (LBBB).

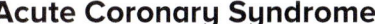

Acute Coronary Syndrome

- The presence of a Q-wave on the ECG should not necessarily change the reperfusion strategy in patients presenting within 12 hours of onset of their symptoms.
- ST-segment depression in leads V1–V3 suggests myocardial ischaemia, especially when the terminal T-wave is positive (ST-segment elevation equivalent), and confirmation by detecting concomitant ST-segment elevation > 0.5 mm recorded in leads V7–V9 should be considered as a means to identify posterior MI.
- Use of additional right precordial leads (V3R and V4R) should be considered in patients with inferior MI (ST elevation in leads II, III and aVF) to identify concomitant right ventricular infarction.
- In the presence of left bundle branch block (LBBB), the ECG diagnosis of AMI is challenging, but may be possible if there are superimposed marked ST-segment abnormalities consistent with STEMI. There are a number of algorithms available to support ECG diagnosis of STEMI in the presence of LBBB but none provide diagnostic certainty. Presence of concordant ST-segment elevation (i.e., in leads with positive QRS deflections) may indicate ongoing AMI. Patients with a clinical suspicion of ACS and LBBB should be managed in a way similar to STEMI patients, regardless of whether the LBBB is previously known. The presence of a (presumed) new LBBB does not necessarily indicate an AMI.
- Patients with MI and right bundle branch block (RBBB) have a poor prognosis. The ESC 12 suggests a PPCI strategy (emergency coronary angiography and PCI if indicated) should be considered when ongoing ischaemic symptoms occur in the presence of RBBB.

TABLE 3.15 – ASSESSMENT and MANAGEMENT of: STEMI

Assess <C>ABCDE

- 12 lead ECG showing STEMI – TIME-CRITICAL TRANSFER to heart attack centre.
- Administer aspirin as soon as possible (refer to **Aspirin**).
- Administer a $P2Y_{12}$ inhibitor or other antiplatelet in line with local policies.

TABLE 3.16 – ASSESSMENT and MANAGEMENT of: Acute Coronary Syndrome

NB A defibrillator must always be taken at the earliest opportunity to patients with symptoms suggestive of ACS and remain with the patient until handover to hospital staff.

Assess <C>ABCDE

- If any of the following TIME-CRITICAL features are present:
  - major **<C>ABCD** problems (refer to **Medical Emergencies in Adults –Overview**).
  - 12-lead ECG shows STEMI or bundle branch block (BBB) with other clinical features suggestive of ACS
  - suspected ACS with haemodynamic instability, then:
- Start correcting any **<C>ABCDE** problems.
- Undertake a **TIME-CRITICAL TRANSFER** to the nearest appropriate receiving hospital.

For patients with STEMI, undertake a direct admission to a PPCI-capable hospital ('Heart Attack Centre') according to local network pathways.

- Minimise delay to reperfusion by continuing management en route:
  - If facilities exist, transmit 12-lead ECG for expert review where possible in cases of uncertainty about interpretation. Where the initial ECG does not indicate STEMI, repeat ECGs at least every 10 minutes and be prepared to change planned destination or seek further advice if STEMI develops.
  - In comparison with placebo, aspirin halves the rate of vascular events (cardiovascular death, non-fatal MI and non-fatal stroke) in patients with unstable angina and reduces it by nearly a third in those with acute MI. Administer aspirin as soon as possible (refer to **Aspirin**).
  - Follow local policies guidelines for $P2Y_{12}$ inhibitor antiplatelet agents (e.g., ticagrelor, prasugrel).
  - Administer sublingual glyceryl trinitrate (GTN) for patients with ongoing ischaemic discomfort unless the patient is hypotensive or otherwise contraindicated (refer to **Glyceryl Trinitrate**). A recent (2022) meta-analysis concluded that there is no statistically significant difference in the rate of adverse events when nitrates are administered to patients with right ventricular MI (RVMI) compared to other infarct regions. Adverse events in the included studies were minor and transient.[13]
  - Provide an ATMIST pre-alert information call.

Acute Coronary Syndrome

TABLE 3.16 – ASSESSMENT and MANAGEMENT of: Acute Coronary Syndrome *(continued)*

NB A defibrillator must always be taken at the earliest opportunity to patients with symptoms suggestive of ACS and remain with the patient until handover to hospital staff.

Respiratory Rate
- Measure and record respiratory rate.

Pulse
- Measure and record pulse.

Blood Pressure
- Measure and record blood pressure.

Blood Glucose
- If appropriate, measure and record blood glucose for hypo/hyperglycaemia (refer to **Glycaemic Emergencies in Adults and Children**). Ideally, do this en route to hospital to avoid delay to reperfusion.

Assess Whether the Chest Pain May Be Cardiac
- Pain typically comes on over seconds and minutes rather than starting abruptly. If truly sudden onset, consider other diagnoses, such as aortic dissection, and seek advice (refer to **Non-Traumatic Chest Pain/Discomfort**). Refer to **Vascular Emergencies** 'Think Aorta'

NB Many patients do not have 'classical presentation' and some people, especially women, older people and those with diabetes, may not experience pain as their chief complaint. This group has a high mortality. Have a low threshold for recording 12-lead ECG.

A normal ECG does NOT exclude ACS and must not be used in isolation to determine patient disposition. Transient ST elevation should be taken seriously, seek senior clinical advice.

Assess for Accompanying Features
- Nausea and vomiting.
- Marked sweating.
- Breathlessness.
- Pallor.
- Combination of chest pain associated with haemodynamic instability.
- Feelings of impending doom.
- Skin that is clammy and cold to the touch.

NB These may not always be present.

ECG
- Aim to record 12 lead ECG within 10 minutes of first patient contact.[12]
- A normal 12-lead ECG alone must not be used to exclude ACS.
- Repeat the 12-lead ECG if there is diagnostic uncertainty (e.g. the initial ECG does not show ST elevation) or a change in the clinical status of the patient.
- Automated ECG interpretation can be a useful support tool.

Assess Oxygen Saturation
- There is no high-quality evidence that routine use of supplementary oxygen in normoxic patients with AMI is either helpful or harmful, nor that it reduces ischaemic chest pain. There is some evidence suggesting that hyperoxia may be harmful in patients with AMI.
- Monitor the patient's SpO_2 but do not administer oxygen unless the patient is hypoxaemic on air (SpO_2 <94%) (refer to **Oxygen**).

Undertake Further Assessment and Management in the Order Appropriate to the Circumstances
- Continuous cardiac monitoring is essential to detect arrhythmias and should continue until handover at the hospital.
- Obtain intravenous access if clinically indicated, but do not delay transfer to hospital.
- Monitor vital signs.
- Repeat dose of GTN if chest discomfort persists.
- 12-lead ECG (as above).

(continued)

Acute Coronary Syndrome

TABLE 3.16 – ASSESSMENT and MANAGEMENT of: Acute Coronary Syndrome *(continued)*

NB A defibrillator must always be taken at the earliest opportunity to patients with symptoms suggestive of ACS and remain with the patient until handover to hospital staff.

Assess Patient's Pain

- Where present, assess the **SOCRATES** of pain and record initial and subsequent pain scores.
- Consider analgesia if appropriate (refer to **Pain Management in Adults and Children**).
- While there are suggestions that morphine is associated with worse outcomes in STEMI patients, the evidence is of low quality, contradictory and thus uncertain.[15]
- Morphine often delays the onset of action of $P2Y_{12}$ inhibitors.
- Morphine remains the analgesia of choice in moderate/**severe pain** associated with STEMI.
- IV paracetamol or Entonox are acceptable alternatives for moderate pain where morphine is contraindicated.

Documentation

- Complete documentation to include all clinical findings, advice from other clinicians and onward referral.

Additional Information

- National and international standards and guidelines for ACS care consistently emphasise the importance of rapid access to defibrillation and reperfusion, and specialist cardiological care.
- Pre-alerting the hospital can speed up appropriate treatment of STEMI patients.
- National data suggest 'call to balloon' times are increasing year on year in patients receiving PPCI, with ambulance delays a significant factor.[2]
- **Make every effort to reduce on-scene time.**
- Pre-hospital thrombolysis is rarely given by UK ambulance services to treat STEMI. PPCI is the preferred reperfusion strategy. Refer to local policies.[16]
- Patients post ROSC with ST elevation should be taken to a PPCI-capable hospital.
- The role of emergency angiography (and PCI if indicated) in patients resuscitated from cardiac arrest but without ST-segment elevation on the pre-hospital 12-lead ECG is uncertain. Such patients should be treated according to locally agreed pathways of care. It is important to establish a history of the events prior to the cardiac arrest and whether the patient suffered chest pain. (Refer to **Advanced Life Support** guideline).
- The diagnosis of NSTEMI cannot be made pre-hospital as it requires use of biomarkers. Point of care (POC) troponin assays are insufficiently sensitive to 'rule out' ACS in the pre-hospital environment and are not recommended at this time.[17]

KEY POINTS!

Acute Coronary Syndrome

- **Make every effort to reduce on-scene time.**[1,2]
- **Obtain a 12 lead ECG as soon as possible, ideally within 10 minutes of arrival on scene.**[1]
- **Once STEMI has been identified, the priority is to get the patient to the heart attack centre as per local pathways.**
- **Risk of VF is high in the early stages of ACS. Always take a defibrillator to the patient.**
- **Patients with a presentation suggestive of ACS but without ST elevation should be considered at high risk and treated as a medical emergency.**
- **A normal ECG does not exclude ACS.**
- **Consider repeating the 12 lead ECG at regular intervals if the first recording is not indicative of STEMI, or the patient's condition changes, and be prepared to change destination hospital if STEMI develops. Automated ECG interpretation is widely available and a useful support tool.**

Acute Coronary Syndrome

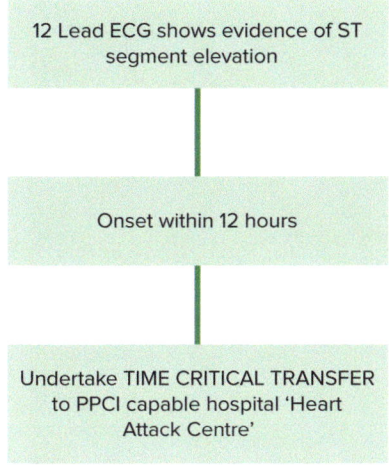

Figure 3.6 – ACS Algorithm.

Further Reading

Wrightington, Wigan and Leigh NHS Foundation Trust. *Performing a 12 lead ECG* (video) 2015. Available at https://www.youtube.com/watch?v=LlmtCDl0DuQ

CPDme. *A beginner's guide to basic ECG interpretation* (video). 2021. Available at https://www.youtube.com/watch?v=wH2SS8Jk41k

Till C. *Clinical ECGs in Paramedic Practice*. 2021. Class Publishing.

Master S. *Understanding right ventricular infarction in prehospital care*. 2021. Available at https://www.paramedicpractice.com/features/article/understanding-right-ventricular-myocardial-infarction-in-prehospital-care

Roos E. M. van Oosterhout, BSc, Annemarijn R. de Boer, MD, Angela H. E. M. et al. *Differences in Symptom Presentation in Acute Coronary Syndromes: A Systematic Review and Meta Analysis*. Journal of the American Heart Association. 2020. Available at https://www.ahajournals.org/doi/epdf/10.1161/JAHA.119.014733

Gorog D, Price S, Sibbing D, et al. *Antithrombotic therapy in patients with acute coronary syndrome complicated by cardiogenic shock or out-of-hospital cardiac arrest: a joint position paper from the European Society of Cardiology (ESC) Working Group on Thrombosis, in association with the Acute Cardiovascular Care Association (ACCA) and European Association of Percutaneous Cardiovascular Interventions* (EAPCI). Eur Heart J Cardiovasc Pharmacother. 2021, Mar 15;7(2):125–140. Available at https://pubmed.ncbi.nlm.nih.gov/32049278/

Nakashima T, Hashiba K, Kikuchi M et al. *Impact of Prehospital 12-Lead Electrocardiography and Destination Hospital Notification on Mortality in Patients With Chest Pain – A Systematic Review*. Circ Rep. 2022,15;4:187–193. Available at https://www.jstage.jst.go.jp/article/circrep/4/5/4_CR-22-0003/_article

Tanaka A, Matsuo K, Kikuchi M et al. *Systematic Review and Meta-Analysis of Diagnostic Accuracy to Identify ST-Segment Elevation Myocardial Infarction on Interpretations of Prehospital Electrocardiograms*. Circ Rep. 2022,4:289–297 Available at https://www.jstage.jst.go.jp/article/circrep/4/7/4_CR-22-0002/_article

JRCALC do not formally endorse these resources, but recognise they are useful sources of information.

Acute Coronary Syndrome

Bibliography

1. Alrawashdeh A, Nehme Z, Williams B, et al. *Impact of emergency medical service delays on time to reperfusion and mortality in STEMI Open Heart*, 2021 May;8(1):e001654. Available at https://openheart.bmj.com/content/8/1/e001654.long

2. National Cardiac Audit Programme. *Myocardial Ischaemia national audit project (MINAP).* 2022 Summary Report (2020/21 data). Available at https://www.nicor.org.uk/wp-content/uploads/2022/06/NICOR-MINAP_2022-FINAL.pdf

3. Cader A, Yancy C, Banerjee S. To be, or not to be BAME, in the time of COVID-19: does it matter? *Heart* 2021, 107(9): 692–693. Available at https://heart.bmj.com/content/107/9/692.long.

4. Rashid M, Timmis A, Kinnaird T, et al. Racial differences in management and outcomes of acute myocardial infarction during COVID-19 pandemic. *Heart* 2021;107(9): 734–740. Available at https://heart.bmj.com/content/107/9/734.long

5. Moledina S, Shoaib A, Weston C, et al. Ethnic disparities in care and outcomes of non-ST-segment elevation myocardial infarction: a nationwide cohort study. *Eur Heart J Qual Care Clin Outcomes* 2021, Apr 21; qcab030. doi: 10.1093/ehjqcco/qcab030.

6. Quinn T, Johnsen S, Gale CP et al. Effects of prehospital 12-lead ECG on processes of care and mortality in acute coronary syndrome: a linked cohort study from the Myocardial Ischaemia National Audit Project. *Heart* 2014, 100(12): 944–50. Available at https://heart.bmj.com/content/100/12/944.long

7. British Heart Foundation. *Heart Attack Symptoms.* Available at https://www.bhf.org.uk/informationsupport/conditions/heart-attack/symptoms

8. van der Mee M, Nathoe H, van der Graaf Y et al. Worse outcome in women with STEMI: a systematic review of prognostic studies. *European Journal of Clinical Investigation* 2015, 45(2): 226–235. Available at https://onlinelibrary.wiley.com/doi/10.1111/eci.12399

9. Lawesson S, Isaksson R, Ericsson M et al. Gender disparities in first medical contact and delay in ST-elevation myocardial infarction: a prospective multicentre Swedish survey study. *BMJ Open* 2018; 8:e020211. doi: 10.1136/bmjopen-2017-020211. Available at https://bmjopen.bmj.com/content/8/5/e020211

10. Wilkinson C, Bebb O, Dondo T et al. Sex differences in quality indicator attainment for myocardial infarction: a nationwide cohort study. *Heart* 2019, 105(7): 516–523. Available at https://heart.bmj.com/content/105/7/516.long

11. NICE. *[NG185] Acute coronary syndromes.* 2020. Available at https://www.nice.org.uk/guidance/ng185

12. Ibanez B, James S, Agewell S et al. 2017 ESC Guidelines for the management of acute myocardial infarction in patients presenting with ST-segment elevation: The Task Force for the management of acute myocardial infarction in patients presenting with ST-segment elevation of the European Society of Cardiology (ESC). *Eur Heart J* 2018, 39(2): 119–177. Available at https://academic.oup.com/eurheartj/article/39/2/119/4095042

13. Wilkinson-Stokes M, Betson J, Sawyer S. Adverse events from nitrate administration during right ventricular myocardial infarction: a systematic review and meta-analysis. *Emerg Med J.* 2022, Sep 30. Available at https://emj.bmj.com/content/early/2022/09/29/emermed-2021-212294

14. Sepehrvand N, James SK, Stub D, et al. Effects of supplemental oxygen therapy in patients with suspected acute myocardial infarction: a meta-analysis of randomised clinical trials. *Heart*, 2018 Oct;104(20):1691–1698. Available at https://heart.bmj.com/content/104/20/1691.long

15. Duarte GS, Nunes-Ferreira A, Rodrigues FB, et al. Morphine in acute coronary syndrome: systematic review and meta-analysis. *BMJ Open*, 2019 Mar 15;9(3):e025232. Available at https://bmjopen.bmj.com/content/9/3/e025232.long

16. Association of Ambulance Chief Executives. *NASMeD position statement, The use of pre-hospital thrombolysis for ST elevation myocardial infarction.* 2021. Available at https://aace.org.uk/wp-content/uploads/2021/07/AACE-NASMeD-pre-hospital-thrombolysis-position-statement-July-2021-FINAL.pdf

17. Cooper J, Ferguson J, Donaldson L et al. The Ambulance Cardiac Chest Pain Evaluation in Scotland Study (ACCESS): A Prospective Cohort Study. *Ann Emerg Med.* 2021 Jun;77(6): 575–588. Available at https://www.annemergmed.com/article/S0196-0644(21)00060-3/fulltext

18. https://www.ahajournals.org/doi/10.1161/JAHA.119.014733

Adrenal Insufficiency Patients

1. Introduction

- While there are many types of steroids, the two most encountered in the pre-hospital setting are corticosteroids and anabolic-androgenic steroids.

1.1 Corticosteroids

- Corticosteroids are a naturally occurring group of hormones produced by the adrenal glands, which are located just above both kidneys. They help to manage stress, blood pressure and blood glucose, immune function and anti-inflammatory processes. The pituitary gland produces adrenocorticotropic hormone (ACTH) which stimulates the adrenal glands to produce cortisol.
- Synthetic pharmaceutical corticosteroids are commonly prescribed to reduce inflammation and the activity of the immune system throughout the body, or to replace endogenous corticosteroids where the adrenal glands do not produce sufficient by themselves.
- Common conditions treated with corticosteroids include:
  - Rheumatoid arthritis
  - Asthma
  - Chronic obstructive pulmonary disorder (COPD)
  - Lupus and other autoimmune disorders
  - Multiple sclerosis
  - Inflammatory bowel diseases, e.g. Crohn's disease
  - Rashes and skin conditions, e.g. eczema
  - Endocrine conditions, e.g. adrenal insufficiency and pituitary disorders.
- Synthetic pharmaceutical corticosteroids come in many different forms and are used to treat a wide range of conditions. Common examples of corticosteroids can be found in Table 3.17.

TABLE 3.17 – Common Examples of Corticosteroids

ROUTE	FORM	COMMON EXAMPLES
Oral	Tablets, syrups, liquids	Prednisolone, Dexamethasone, Hydrocortisone, Betamethasone
Inhaled	Inhalers, nasal spray	Beclomethasone, Fluticasone
Injected	Injections (given into joints, muscles or blood vessels)	Methylprednisolone, Hydrocortisone, Triamcinolone
Topical absorption	Creams, lotions, eye drops, gels	Hydrocortisone skin cream, Beclomethasone dipropionate

1.2 Anabolic Steroids

- Anabolic steroids are manufactured drugs that mimic the effects of the male hormone testosterone.
- They may be legitimately prescribed to treat several conditions such as delayed puberty, and growth and weight gain in those with cachexia (secondary to conditions such as cancer and Advanced HIV disease), and to support in producing masculine characteristics in transgender men.
- However, more commonly, anabolic steroids are misused to gain muscle mass and improve athletic performance; misused anabolic steroids may come in tablet or injectable form. Common slang terms for anabolic steroids include 'roids', 'gear' and 'juice'.
- Although physical effects from sudden withdrawal of anabolic steroids are unpleasant, they are rarely dangerous. Withdrawal symptoms may include depression, aggressive behaviour, headache, anxiety, insomnia, nausea, vomiting, abdominal pain and hypotension.
- Symptoms should resolve once the body can restore its normal production of testosterone.

2. Incidence

- Primary adrenal insufficiency (when the adrenal glands cannot produce cortisol) affects around 3,400 people in the UK, and 1 in 20,000 people in western Europe.
- Secondary adrenal insufficiency (when the pituitary gland cannot produce ACTH, and therefore cannot stimulate the adrenal gland to produce cortisol) is more common, with 150–280 people per million affected. It is more common in women than men. The peak age of onset is between 50 and 60 years.
- The incidence of tertiary adrenal insufficiency (when the adrenal glands are supressed by a long course of exogenous corticosteroids) is unknown as it is commonly unreported.

3. Pathophysiology

3.1 Glucocorticoid Steroid-dependent Patients

- The cause of steroid dependency can be broken down into three types: primary, secondary and tertiary.

Adrenal Insufficiency Patients

- Regardless of type, those with adrenal insufficiency are at risk of adrenal crisis which can be life-threatening.
- Primary adrenal insufficiency occurs in patients who have direct impairment of the adrenal glands such as those with Addison's disease (autoimmune endocrine condition where the adrenal glands cease to function), congenital adrenal hyperplasia (genetic condition) or surgery or trauma to the adrenal glands.
- Secondary adrenal insufficiency is caused by pituitary disease, hypothalamic or pituitary tumours and their treatment (surgery and radiotherapy) or brain injury.
- Tertiary adrenal insufficiency may occur in patients who have taken high doses or multiple courses of steroids, or who have taken steroids for prolonged periods of time or via multiple routes. Prolonged use may lead to a reduction or cessation of naturally occurring cortisol production by the adrenal glands.
- Patients may be taking a maintenance dose (for example of prednisolone) and may be at risk after only 3 or 4 weeks of treatment.

3.2 Adrenal Crisis

- Adrenal crisis, also termed acute adrenal insufficiency, is a **life-threatening endocrine emergency** due to a lack of production of the adrenal hormone cortisol.
- Adrenal crisis can also occur if existing cortisol replacement does not meet the body's increased need for cortisol due to illness such as fever, persistent vomiting or diarrhoea or trauma.
- Equally, sudden cessation of corticosteroid medication for conditions listed above will risk adrenal crisis in those with adrenal insufficiency.
- Identifying patients at risk and prompt management can save lives.
- National guidance promotes a patient-held Steroid Emergency Card (see Figure 3.7) to help healthcare staff identify patients with adrenal insufficiency and provide information on emergency treatment if the patient is acutely ill or experiences trauma, surgery or other major stressors.

Figure 3.7 – NHS Steroid Emergency Card (Adult).

Adrenal Insufficiency Patients

4. Assessment and Management

TABLE 3.18 – ASSESSMENT and MANAGEMENT of: Steroid-Dependent Patients/Patients at Risk of Adrenal Insufficiency

Assess <C>ABCDE

- If any of the following **TIME-CRITICAL** features present:
  - Major **<C>ABCDE** problems (refer to **Medical Emergencies in Adults – Overview** and **Medical Emergencies in Children – Overview**).
- Start correcting **<C>ABCDE** problems.
- Give IM or IV Hydrocortisone before moving patient.
- Consider giving fluids prior to moving patient (refer to **Sodium Chloride 0.9%**).
- Undertake a **TIME-CRITICAL** transfer to nearest receiving hospital.
- Continue patient management en route.
- Provide an ATMIST information call.

Symptoms and Signs

- Symptoms and signs of adrenal insufficiency include:
  - Severe fatigue, lethargy, drowsiness, confusion, coma
  - Low blood pressure, postural dizziness and hypotension (≥20 mmHg drop in BP from supine to standing position), dizziness, collapse and hypovolaemic shock in severe cases
  - Abdominal pain, tenderness and guarding, anorexia, nausea, vomiting (in particular in primary adrenal insufficiency), diarrhoea
  - Fever
  - Patients may have a history of weight loss and increasing skin pigmentation over weeks to months (primary adrenal insufficiency).
- Assess patient for underlying acute conditions that may have precipitated the adrenal crisis and treat that condition too.
- Follow guidance in **Medical Emergencies in Adults – Overview** and **Medical Emergencies in Children – Overview** in addition to the specific management detailed below.

Pulse

- Measure and record pulse rate.

Respiratory Rate

- Measure and record respiratory rate.

Oxygen

- Measure oxygen saturations.

Blood Glucose and Ketones

- Measure and record blood glucose for hypoglycaemia.
- Check ketones.
- Treat hypoglycaemia (refer to **Glycaemic Emergencies in Adults and Children**).

Temperature

- Measure and record temperature.

NEWS2

- These observations, along with a blood pressure, will enable you to calculate a NEWS2 score (refer to **Sepsis**).

ECG

- If required, monitor and record 12-lead ECG and assess for abnormality (refer to **Cardiac Arrhythmia and Sudden Cardiac Death**).

(continued)

Adrenal Insufficiency Patients

TABLE 3.18 – ASSESSMENT and MANAGEMENT of: Steroid-Dependent Patients/Patients at Risk of Adrenal Insufficiency *(continued)*

Blood Pressure and Fluids

- Measure and record blood pressure.
- Give 1 litre of 0.9% sodium chloride intravenous infusion over 30 minutes if having an adrenal crisis (refer to **Intravascular Fluid Therapy in Adults** and **Sodium Chloride 0.9%**).
- Patients with adrenal crisis may be hypotensive or have postural hypotension. Assess for postural hypotension if normotensive when lying/sitting.
- There may be a profound postural drop in blood pressure when the patient is moved from the lying position to the semi-recumbent or sitting position. It may be necessary to give IV fluids prior to moving the patient if extrication requires a head-up posture.

Administer Hydrocortisone

- Administer hydrocortisone to:
  - Patients in an established adrenal crisis (IV or IM administration). Ensure parenteral hydrocortisone is given prior to transportation.
  - Patients with suspected adrenal insufficiency or on long-term steroid therapy who have become unwell or have suffered trauma, to prevent them having an adrenal crisis.
- If in doubt about adrenal insufficiency, hydrocortisone should be administered.
- Pregnant women who have Addison's disease who are established in labour should receive hydrocortisone.
- Refer to **Hydrocortisone**.

Conveyance to Hospital

- Convey patients who are in adrenal crisis, have required intravenous fluids or management of hypoglycaemia.
- Convey patients if the underlying condition precipitating the adrenal crisis needs hospital assessment/management.
- Convey patients if the underlying condition prevents them taking their prescribed steroids (e.g. diarrhoea and vomiting).

Consider Management in the Community or Referral to Other Services

- Patients with mild illness/injury where they have followed their treatment plan to increase steroid dose and have normal physiological parameters.

Appropriate Advice

- Patients on replacement steroids (e.g. Addison's disease or hypopituitarism) may have a treatment plan to increase their maintenance steroids in the event of illness/injury. This should be followed but they may require monitoring and higher doses for more significant illness/injury.
- Check that patients on replacement steroids have sufficient doses, access to an emergency kit if they are to remain at home.

Documentation

- Complete documentation to include all clinical findings, advice from other clinicians, onward referral and worsening advice given.

Adrenal Insufficiency Patients

> **KEY POINTS!**
>
> **Adrenal Insufficiency Patients**
> - Adrenal crisis is a medical emergency requiring prompt treatment with hydrocortisone and IV fluids.
> - Steroid-dependent patients can have an adrenal crisis triggered when the body's requirement for corticosteroids increases, such as due to infection or trauma, as the body is unable to increase its own production.
> - If extrication requires a head-up posture, IV fluids may be required before moving the patient, to prevent profound postural hypotension.
> - Look for an underlying cause that may have triggered the episode and treat that condition too.
> - If in doubt about adrenal insufficiency, hydrocortisone should be administered.

Acknowledgements

We would like to gratefully acknowledge the Addison's Disease Self-Help Group and The Pituitary Foundation for their contributions, comments and input to this JRCALC guideline.

Bibliography

1. NHS. *Steroids*. 2020. Available from: https://www.nhs.uk/conditions/steroids/.
2. Addison's Disease Self-help Group. *What Is Addison's Disease?* n.d. Available from: https://www.addisonsdisease.org.uk/what-is-addisons-disease.
3. Society for Endocrinology. *Adrenal Crisis Information*. n.d. Available from: https://www.endocrinology.org/adrenal-crisis.
4. NICE. Adrenal insufficiency: identification and management, NICE guideline [NG243]. Available from: https://www.nice.org.uk/guidance/NG243

Agitated Patients

1. Introduction

- This guideline must be considered in conjunction with the **Acute Behavioural Disturbance (ABD)** and **Delirium** guidelines.
- The clinical management of an agitated patient can be one of the most challenging presentations for any pre-hospital clinician. Agitation itself is not a diagnosis, it is a presentation seen in many different conditions.
- Agitation can be related to a physical and/or mental health condition. It is also worth noting that agitation presents as a spectrum; at one end the cooperative but distressed patient, and at the other a patient with a potentially life-threatening condition referred to as Acute Behavioural Disturbance (ABD) (Refer to **Acute Behavioural Disturbance (ABD)**) who, due to their severe nature of agitation, may have been or are actively being physically restrained before a clinician arrives on scene.

2. Causes

There are multiple causes of agitation in the pre-hospital patient (list not exhaustive):

TABLE 3.19 – Possible Causes of Agitation
Pain
Hypoxia
Head injury
Hypoglycaemia
Hypo or Hyperthermia
Meningitis/Encephalitis
Sepsis
Cerebral space-occupying lesion (brain tumour)
Dementia
Toxicological including substance misuse
Some strokes
Medication-related
Patients who are post seizure
Alcohol intoxication or alcohol withdrawal
Thyrotoxicosis
Some mental health presentations
A full bladder
Substance withdrawal
Patients receiving End of life Care

- The focus should be on identifying and treating, or arranging to treat the underlying cause.
- For a number of these conditions, it will be possible to form an impression of what may be contributing to the patient's agitated pre-hospital presentation, but in many cases it will not. For a number of patients, this may be an "acute on chronic" level of increased agitation. This can be seen in patients living with dementia where they are unsettled and distressed daily but the reason for their presentation to the ambulance service can be an acute worsening in their agitation. This might be due to a worsening or decline in their dementia but if the change is acute could more likely be due to another cause, such as infection or a recent unknown head injury.
- It is worth considering that a clinician should work on the assumption that forming a differential impression that a patient's agitation is due to their mental health should be by exclusion of other possible causes. Clinical assessments should be focussed on exploring these other clinical causes, prior to coming to a conclusion that the cause of the altered behaviour is due to a mental health presentation.

3. Bias

- All clinicians need to be aware that labelling a patient's presentation may lead to either a conscious or unconscious bias. Where a clinician refers to patient as "being ABD" or as agitated, this has the potential to influence their onward care. Clinicians should adopt an approach of using neutral terminology and aiming to describe the exact behaviour exhibited rather than broad-brush terminology, noting that terms such as ABD have a place when requesting prompt enhanced clinical assistance and support. Every patient contact should be based upon a holistic assessment of the patient, undertaken by the clinician and be based on that direct assessment as opposed to what any other individuals or agencies have reported.

4. Assessment

Assess the level of agitation

- Remember to consider the safety of yourself and others on scene when managing the agitated patient. For many patients it is obvious how severe a patient's agitation is, but it is important to formally assess and document this. The system in Table 3.20 shows a helpful way of assessing the level of agitation.

TABLE 3.20 – Agitation Level Descriptors	
Descriptor	Description
Mild	Agitated but cooperative
Moderate	Disruptive without danger
Severe	Dangerous to self and/or staff

- Consider requesting additional support if the patient has severe agitation, particularly if the patient is a danger to themselves or others.

Agitated Patients

- There are many scales which could be used to further describe a patient's level of agitation.
- The Brøset Checklist provides a helpful evidence-based methodology for assessing the agitated patient and helps describes the patient's presentation to others as well as recording it within the clinical notes.
  - Confused – Appears obviously confused and disorientated. May be unaware of time, place or person.
  - Irritable – Easily annoyed or angered. Unable to tolerate the presence of others.
  - Boisterous – Behaviour is overtly "loud" or noisy. For example, slams doors, shouts out when speaking etc.
  - Physically threatening – Where there is a definite intent to physically threaten another person. For example the taking of an aggressive stance; the grabbing of another person's clothing; the raising of an arm, leg, making of a fist or modelling of a head-butt directed at another.
  - Verbally threatening – A verbal outburst which is more than just a raised voice; and where there is a definite intent to intimidate or threaten another person. For example, verbal attacks, abuse, name calling, verbally neutral comments uttered in a snarling aggressive manner.
  - Attacking objects – An attack directed at an object and not an individual. For example the indiscriminate throwing of an object; banging or smashing windows; kicking, banging or head-butting an object; or the smashing of furniture.

Gathering information and communication with the patient

An initial stage of patient assessment is to gather information, from family and friends, carers and other agencies on scene (or remotely). Useful information may also be available from the patient care records if accessible.

- Take into account previous violent or aggressive episodes because these are associated with an increased risk of future violence and aggression but these should not overtly bias your assessment on this occasion.
- Do not make negative assumptions based on culture, religion or ethnicity.
- Recognise that unfamiliar cultural practices and customs could be misinterpreted as being aggressive.
- Ensure that your dynamic risk assessment is objective and take into account the degree to which the perceived risk can be verified.

Assess the mental capacity of the patient

While communicating with the patient, assess the capacity of the patient using the two-structured approach laid down in the Mental Capacity Act (2005) (refer to **Mental Capacity Act (2005)**):

1. Does the person have an impairment of their mind or brain, whether as a result of an illness, or external factors such as alcohol or drug use?
2. Does the impairment mean the person is unable to make a specific decision when they need to?

- Remember that in patients presenting with agitation, some will maintain capacity to make decisions while others may not. Where a patient lacks capacity we are legally mandated to act in the best interest of the patient. We are also required to act in a way that is less restrictive of the person's rights and freedom. In essence we must choose the option which is in the best interests of the patient but also the option that is least restrictive.
- Where a patient has mental capacity, the patient must consent to any intervention.

5. Consider Potentially Modifiable or Reversible Pathology

- There will be cases where attempts to modify or reverse the cause of the agitation on scene may resolve the agitation.
- Consider if there are other factors causing the patient's agitation:
  - Hypoxia – a patient who is profoundly hypoxic can become extremely agitated.
  - Hypoglycaemia – consider a low blood glucose early in the agitated patient remembering that although commonly associated with diabetes mellitus, a reduced blood glucose can be seen in other conditions.
  - Pain – consider if the patient is in pain and is struggling to express their pain. Also consider if the patients position is causing pain; are they lying on an item of equipment?
  - Is the patient's bladder full? Are they in retention of urine?
  - Post-ictal patients – allow them an appropriate period of time to recover following a seizure.
  - Other medical conditions – think about what may be causing the altered behaviour.
- A dynamic assessment needs to be conducted and consideration given as to the time a patient needs to safely recover. If agitation remains after management of reversible conditions, we need to consider other causes, which may need further in-hospital assessment. The patient who is agitated post-seizure may require some time to recover but if the agitation persists and/or the cause of the seizure is not known the patient is likely to require transfer to hospital.

Agitated Patients

6. Management

Non-pharmacological management

- Consideration should always be given to non-pharmacological management initially, using verbal de-escalation. Verbal de-escalation is often under-utilised and friends or family members may be helpful (but ask them to desist if their intervention is making the situation worse). For mild and moderate agitation presentations, the use of verbal de-escalation is often effective, but requires a calm and deliberate approach. Provided there is not an immediate risk to life, verbal de-escalation should be attempted before restraint or pharmacological agents are considered.
- It is important to consider both your body language and the tone, pitch and speed of verbal communications. Try and ensure the following:
  – One person delegated to lead the communication – this can change but having multiple clinicians and others talking to the patient at the same time may worsen distress and agitation
  – Ensure a quiet environment – turn radios/TVs down
  – Monitor your own emotional and physiologic response – try to remain calm
  – Use simple and compassionate language that does not appear to judge the patient or their behaviour
- The SAVE mnemonic can provide a useful starting point for communication:
  – Support – "Let's work together…"
  – Acknowledge – "I see this has been hard for you."
  – Validate – "I'd probably be reacting the same way if I was in your shoes."
  – Emotion naming – "You seem upset."
- Attempt a process of de-escalation:
  – Use calming techniques and distraction.
  – Offer the patient the opportunity to move away from the situation in which the agitation is occurring where possible, for example to a quiet room or area.
  – Aim to build emotional bridges and maintain a therapeutic relationship.
- The key aspects of successful verbal and non-verbal de-escalation are:
  – Allow sufficient time to attempt verbal de-escalation.
  – Maintain a safe distance between you and the patient.
  – Have only one person verbally engage with the patient.
  – Introduce yourself; state you are there to help and provide reassurance.
  – Use a calm voice and adopt a non-threatening stance.
  – Use short sentences and keep messages simple. Repetition is essential as the patient will usually have a short attention span.
  – Minimise the number of people in the immediate vicinity to those required for the safety of the patient and staff on scene.
  – Limit unnecessary noise and distractions, e.g. radio noise, blue lights, sirens, etc.
  – Minimise any painful stimuli for the patient.
  – Actively listen to the patient and try to gain an understanding of their concerns.
  – Try to establish rapport and offer choices; if appropriate, allow them to have a drink or a cigarette.
  – Avoid provocative statements, e.g. do not say "If you don't calm down, we will have to…".
  – Once rapport has been established, continue clinical care.
- If verbal de-escalation is unsuccessful consider the need for additional support or seek senior clinical advice as per local procedures.

Pharmacological management

- There will be times where the patient may benefit from a pharmacological intervention to aid in their clinical management. It is worth noting that some of these interventions will take time to reach a therapeutic threshold and the benefit may not be seen until the patient is handed over; but there will be a benefit as part of the patient's continuing care.
- Always consider that an intervention should only be undertaken in the best interests of the patient and should be the least restrictive intervention.
- If a decision has been reached that the patient will need further assessment and clinical management in hospital, pre-hospital clinicians may need to wait an appropriate period to see if a pharmacological intervention (if available) calms the agitation, before transfer to definitive care. Where a patient's agitation is such that (outside of end-of-life care), they require pharmacological intervention, the patient will need hospital face-to-face assessment. All patients given medication to reduce agitation where this is not to reverse a specific clinical condition, should be conveyed, even if a care pathway is being arranged in the community too.
- Rapid parenteral (IM or IV) pharmacological tranquilisation of a patient with extreme agitation, described as presenting with ABD, is clinically challenging and requires Advanced Practice pre-hospital clinicians with specific experience and education/training in this area, which is not currently within the scope of practice of most ambulance clinicians.

Oral tranquilisation

- Patients may benefit from low dose oral tranquilisation agents such as lorazepam

Agitated Patients

(administered by Trust approved clinicians, or it may have been given by custody suite clinicians). For this to be administered the patient must be fully conscious and able to safely swallow. No attempt should ever be made to force a patient to take oral medication. The patient must be willing to take the medication themselves. The patient must be fully informed and consent to taking the medication or, if they lack mental capacity to make such a decision, any actions taken by the treating clinicians must be the least restrictive option which is within the best interests of the patient.

- Consideration should be given to the fact that such medication is designed to moderate the agitation displayed and this may impact on the ability of other clinicians to assess the patient. Wherever possible the plan should be to avoid the need to medicate and to use other methods such as reassurance to manage behaviour. There is a difference between distress, pain and agitation and a careful clinical assessment should be conducted to determine what is causing the altered behaviour. The use of an oral tranquilisation agent in an ambulance setting will mean the patient must be conveyed for further assessment (unless the patient is an End-of-Life patient with a community plan to support their care at home), as the effects of any sedative may be shorter than the cause of the agitation.

- Consideration should always be given to other medicines the patient may have taken, either prescribed medicines or recreational depressant drugs or alcohol. In these cases, a risk assessment should be made and oral *tranquilisation may not be administered to some patients*.

- Where a patient is unable to swallow the medication due to their agitation and is unable to be safely transferred to hospital, this should prompt escalation to enhanced care practitioners/teams.

7. Ongoing Care and Management

Most patients who present with new acute agitation, wherever they are on an agitation spectrum, will require assessment in hospital or by an appropriate community team to investigate the causes and for further treatment. Prior to referring a patient for solely clinical management in the community, consideration should be given to the events which have caused the ambulance service to be contacted. Where a patient's agitation has increased over a period of time the ambulance service often becomes involved when family/carers are at a point of crisis. This needs to be taken into account when considering a care plan, as often support structures will already be exhausted and at crisis point.

- Agitation itself is not a diagnosis, it is a presentation seen in many different conditions.

- There are multiple causes of agitation, the focus should be on identifying and treating the underlying cause.

- Consideration should always be given to non-pharmacological management initially, including using verbal de-escalation.

- If verbal de-escalation is unsuccessful consider the need for additional support or seek senior clinical advice as per local procedures.

- Most patients who present with new acute agitation will require assessment in hospital or by an appropriate community team to investigate the causes and for further treatment.

References

1 Abderhalden C, Needham I, Dassen T, Halfens R, Haug H, Fischer J. Predicting inpatient violence using an extended version of the Brøset-Violence-Checklist: Instrument development and clinical application. *BMC Psychiatry.* 2006; 6: 9–17.

2 Alexander J, Tharyan P, Adams C, John T, Mol C, Philip J. Rapid tranquillization of violent or agitated patients in a psychiatric emergency setting: pragmatic randomised trial of intramuscular lorazepam v. haloperidol plus promethazine. *The British Journal of Psychiatry.* 2004; 185: 63–69.

3 Ashcraft L, Anthony W. Eliminating seclusion and restraint in recovery-oriented crisis services. *Psychiatric Services.* 2008; 59: 1198–202.

4 Baldaçara L, Sanches M, Cordeiro DC, Jackoswski AP. Rapid tranquilization for agitated patients in emergency psychiatric rooms: a randomized trial of olanzapine, ziprasidone, haloperidol plus promethazine, haloperidol plus midazolam and haloperidol alone. *Revista Brasileira de Psiquiatria.* 2011; 33: 30–39.

5 Barzman DH, Brackenbury L, Sonnier L, Schnell B, Cassedy A, Salisbury S, et al. Brief Rating of Aggression by Children and Adolescents (BRACHA): Development of a tool for assessing risk of inpatients' aggressive behavior. *Journal of the American Academy of Psychiatry and the Law Online.* 2011; 39: 170–79.

6 Bourn J, Maxfield A, Terry A, Taylor K. *A Safer Place to Work: Protecting NHS Hospital and Ambulance Staff from Violence and Aggression.* London 2003.

7 Chang JC, Lee CS. Risk factors for aggressive behavior among psychiatric inpatients. *Psychiatric Services.* 2004; 55: 1305–07.

8 Department of Health. Mental Health Act 1983: Code of Practice. London 2015.

9 Gerdtz MF, Daniel C, Dearie V, Prematunga R, Bamert M, Duxbury J. The outcome of a rapid training program on nurses' attitudes regarding the prevention of aggression in

Agitated Patients

emergency departments: a multi-site evaluation. *International Journal of Nursing Studies.* 2013; 50: 1434–45.

10 HM Government. Mental Health Crisis Care Concordant: Improving outcomes for people experiencing mental health crisis. 18 February. London: Department of Health; 2014.

11 James A, Madeley R, Dove A. Violence and aggression in the emergency department. Emergency Medicine Journal. 2006; 23: 431–34. Jansen G, Dassen T, Moorer P. The perception of aggression. *Scandinavian Journal of Caring Sciences.* 1997; 11: 51–55.

12 NICE Violence and Aggression Short-term management in mental health, health and community settings Updated edition NICE Guideline NG10 2015.

13 Swift RH, Harrigan EP, Cappelleri JC, Kramer D, Chandler LP. Validation of the behavioural activity rating scale (BARS): a novel measure of activity in agitated patients. *J Psychiatr Res.* 2002 Mar-Apr; 36(2): 87–95.

Alcohol-use Disorders

1. Introduction

- In 2017 in the UK, 7,697 people died from alcohol-specific conditions. This was equivalent to 12.2 deaths per 100,000 population. The latest figure is the highest rate since 2008, when the rate was recorded as 12.7 alcohol-specific deaths per 100,000.[1] Alcohol-use disorders are a common and increasing reason for a request for an emergency ambulance response.[2]
- Assessment, diagnosis and effective management of patients with alcohol-use disorders improve patient safety by reducing the acute and chronic complications caused by alcohol intoxication and acute withdrawal.[3] Remember that the use of other substances as well as alcohol may enhance the effect of each individual substance.
- Alcohol is associated with an increased chance of avoidable deaths from cancer, trauma and communicable diseases.[3] Whenever the opportunity arises, appropriate advice on consumption should be provided to the patient, and then they should be referred to specialist alcohol liaison services where available or through primary care, in line with Making Every Contact Count (MECC) guidance.
- Co-morbid mental health disorders commonly include depression, anxiety disorders and drug misuse. Physical co-morbidities are common, including gastrointestinal (GI) disorders, in particular liver disease, and GI haemorrhage; neurological and cardiovascular diseases are also common. In some people, these co-morbidities may remit with abstinence or reduced alcohol consumption, but many experience long-term consequences of alcohol-use disorders that may significantly shorten their life expectancy.
- Alcohol-use disorders are also associated with increased safeguarding risks affecting patients, other vulnerable adults around them or children in affected families. There should be a low threshold for safeguarding referrals.

2. Categorisation

2.1 Hazardous Drinking

- Hazardous drinking, or increasing-risk drinking, is categorised by the World Health Organization as 'a pattern of alcohol consumption that increases someone's risk of harm'.[3]
- Consumption, measured as units per week:
  – drinking more than 14 units a week, but less than 35 units a week, for women
  – drinking more than 14 units a week, but less than 50 units, for men.
- Some would limit this definition to the physical or mental health consequences (directly harmful use); others would include the wider social consequences. The term is currently used to describe this pattern of alcohol consumption; it is not a diagnostic term.

2.2 Harmful Drinking

- Harmful drinking (high-risk drinking) is categorised as 'a pattern of alcohol consumption that is causing mental or physical damage'.[3]
- Consumption, measured as units per week:
  – drinking 35 units a week or more for women
  – drinking 50 units a week or more for men.[3]

3. Conditions

3.1 Wernicke-Korsakoff Syndrome

- Wernicke-Korsakoff syndrome is caused by a lack of Vitamin B1 (also known as Thiamine). Thiamine cannot be produced by the body and is absorbed from foods. In chronic alcohol dependency, there is reduced absorption of thiamine as well as impaired utilisation of thiamine by cells, especially those in the cardiac and nervous systems. The condition causes lesions within the brain that disrupt neurological function; this can lead to irreversible neurological changes. Any patient who presents with loss of balance, tremor, confusion, agitation, visual disturbance or loss of muscle control may have an alcohol use disorder and should be considered at high risk of Wernicke-Korsakoff syndrome and be conveyed to hospital.[4]
- Emergency management for this condition may be needed urgently, with an intravenous administration of B vitamins in an Emergency Department.
- People with suspected Wernicke-Korsakoff syndrome are at higher risk if they are malnourished, at risk of malnourishment or have decompensated liver disease.

3.2 Alcohol-related Pancreatitis

- Alcohol-related pancreatitis is a potentially fatal condition, where alcohol even in small amounts may trigger a major inflammatory response. Patients presenting with abdominal pain, nausea and vomiting should be treated and transported to an Emergency Department for further investigation and management. The risk of developing pancreatitis grows with increased acute or chronic consumption of alcohol.

3.3 Alcoholic Ketoacidosis

- Alcoholic ketoacidosis can occur when a person who is alcohol dependant or has had a prolonged alcohol binge, abruptly stops drinking and at the same time stops eating. The alcohol will have reduced the body's ability to make glucose that can be used by cells so fatty acids are metabolised to create energy and this results in ketoacidosis. The glucose level is usually normal. Symptoms include vomiting and

Alcohol-use Disorders

abdominal pain. In the early stages the conscious level is normal. Diagnosis requires laboratory tests to calculate the anion gap and to exclude other diagnoses such as acute pancreatitis, so ED attendance is required. Treatment of Alcoholic ketoacidosis differs from the treatment of Diabetic ketoacidosis as large volumes of sodium chloride 0.9% alone can be detrimental. The requirement is for 5% dextrose.

3.4 Delirium

- Alcohol intoxication and withdrawal are frequently associated with delirium. Delirium is an acute, fluctuating change in mental status, with inattention, disorganised thinking and altered levels of consciousness.[5] There is a correlation between recent binge drinking and alcoholic ketoacidosis, which can lead to delirium.
- Delirium Tremens (DTs) is the most severe form of alcohol withdrawal, manifested by altered mental status (global confusion) and sympathetic overdrive (autonomic hyperactivity), which can progress to cardiovascular collapse.

3.5 Gastrointestinal Bleeding

- Patients may have acute or chronic GI haemorrhage; these are a major cause of alcohol-related morbidity and mortality.
- Mallory-Weiss syndrome is a common cause of upper GI haemorrhage in patients with recurrent and active drinking abuse. Alcohol has a reported association with Mallory-Weiss tear in 40% to 80% of patients.[6] Oesophageal or gastric varices (dilated veins) can be a cause of potentially life-threatening upper GI haemorrhage.

3.6 Hepatic Encephalopathy

- This condition can occur in acute or chronic liver failure. Increases in serum ammonia levels cause cerebral oedema. Initially, the signs may be very vague with general malaise, progressing to a flapping tremor of the limbs and then unconsciousness.

4. Assessment

- Multiple factors can affect the diagnosis in a patient with chronic alcohol use and there are several differential diagnoses that cannot be formally excluded within the pre-hospital environment.
- Remember that many of these signs (refer to Tables 3.21 and 3.22) can also be present in patients with head injuries, and any history of recent trauma should raise suspicion of an intracranial head injury (refer to **Trauma Emergencies in Adults – Overview** or **Trauma Emergencies in Children – Overview**).
- Consider mixed intentional or unintentional overdose in addition to alcohol use (refer to **Overdose and Poisoning in Adults and Children**).

TABLE 3.21 – Signs and Symptoms of Alcohol Intoxication[4]

- Impairment of tasks requiring skill.
- Increased talkativeness.
- Relaxation.
- Ataxia.
- Hyperreflexia.
- Reduced levels of capacity.
- Lack of coordination.
- Loss of inhibition, change in mood, excitability, aggression.
- Prolonged reaction times.
- Slurred speech.
- Amnesia.
- Diplopia.
- Dysarthria.
- Hypothermia.
- Nausea and vomiting.
- Respiratory depression.
- Reduced consciousness.

TABLE 3.22 – Signs and Symptoms of Acute Alcohol Withdrawal

- Confusion.
- Uncontrollable shaking.
- Nausea or vomiting.
- Paroxysmal sweats.
- Agitation.
- Hallucinations.
- Headaches.
- Convulsions.
- Depression.
- Tremor.
- Anxiety.
- Tactile disturbances.
- Visual disturbances.
- Disorientation.

Alcohol-use Disorders

5. Management

- Refer to Table 3.23 for the assessment and management of alcohol-use disorders.

5.1 Safety

- The management of patients experiencing alcohol-use disorders must always start with an assurance of the safety of the clinicians, the patient and any bystanders. Acute alcohol use can be associated with a sudden change in behaviour that may result in aggressive or violent outbursts.

5.2 Mental Capacity

- Careful assessment of the patient's mental capacity should be undertaken and the least restrictive methods of clinical management used, to ensure patient and clinician safety. Refer to **Safeguarding Adults at Risk** and **Mental Capacity Act 2005**.

5.3 Admission to Hospital

- Patients with signs of acute alcohol withdrawal should attend an Emergency Department or be seen by another healthcare professional. They are at high risk of developing alcohol withdrawal seizures or delirium tremens.
- Have a lower threshold for admission for vulnerable patients. For example, those who are frail or cognitively impaired; those who have multiple co-morbidities, a lack of social support or learning difficulties; and those who are children under 18 years old or pregnant women. These patients often need further physical, psychosocial and safeguarding support.
- Patients without time-critical **<C>ABCDE** issues but with signs of acute alcohol withdrawal **should not** be discouraged from the ingestion of alcohol prior to leaving the scene of the incident.[6]

TABLE 3.23 – ASSESSMENT and MANAGEMENT of: Alcohol-Use Disorders

Assess <C>ABCDE:

- If any of the following **TIME-CRITICAL** features are present:
  - major **<C>ABCDE** problems (refer to **Medical Emergencies in Adults – Overview**)
  - convulsions (relatively common in alcohol withdrawal; refer to **Seizures in Adults** or **Seizures in Children**).
- Start correcting any **<C>ABCDE** problems.
- Undertake a **TIME-CRITICAL** transfer to nearest appropriate receiving hospital.
- Continue patient management en route.
- Provide an ATMIST information call.

Respiratory Rate

- Measure and record respiratory rate.

Pulse

- Measure and record pulse

Oxygen Saturation

- Measure and record the patient's SpO$_2$, and administer oxygen to achieve saturations of >94% if the patient presents as hypoxaemic on air (refer to **Oxygen**).

Blood Pressure

- Measure and record blood pressure.

Blood Glucose

- Measure and record blood glucose for hypo/hyperglycaemia (refer to **Glycaemic Emergencies in Adults and Children**).
- Unless the patient refuses, this assessment should always be undertaken because acute alcohol intoxication and hypoglycaemia share many signs and symptoms.
- Glycogen stores can be very low and rebound hypoglycaemia may occur following pre-hospital glucose administration.
- Have a low threshold for transfer to hospital.

Temperature

- Measure and record temperature.

(continued)

Alcohol-use Disorders

TABLE 3.23 – ASSESSMENT and MANAGEMENT of: Alcohol-Use Disorders *(continued)*

NEWS2
- Calculate NEWS2 score (refer to **Sepsis**).

ECG
- If required, monitor and record 12-lead ECG. Assess for abnormality (refer to **Cardiac Arrhythmia and Sudden Cardiac Death**).

Assess the Patient's Pain
- Where present, assess the **SOCRATES** of pain, and record initial and subsequent pain scores.
- Consider analgesia if appropriate (refer to **Pain Management in Adults and Children**).

Documentation
- Complete documentation to include all clinical findings, advice from other clinicians, onward referral and worsening advice given.
- If the patient is not conveyed to hospital, they must not be advised to suddenly reduce their alcohol intake.
- If convulsions occur, refer to **Seizures in Adults** or **Seizures in Children**.

6. Making Every Contact Count

- Ambulance clinicians have a role to play in having conversations with people who are drinking harmful amounts of alcohol. The evidence-based MECC approach can be applied, or other locally agreed methods of ensuring health prevention messages can be given. An MECC interaction takes a matter of minutes and should be part of the clinical conversation with the patient if appropriate.
- Men should drink no more alcohol than 3–4 units each day and women no more than 2–3 units each day, with at least two alcohol-free days every week. A unit is half a pint of (3.5% ABV) beer, cider or lager, a small (125ml) glass of 8% wine or a single (25ml) measure of spirits.
- Most patients express the view that they expect to be asked about lifestyle behaviours by health professionals. Most people want to make changes to their unhealthy behaviours. They do, however, need some support to change. MECC is a great way to deliver consistent lifestyle advice messages.
- Consider referring or signposting the patient to primary care, local pathways or alcohol-use disorder services. Consider leaving an appropriate leaflet with the patient about local services for alcohol-use disorder.
- Discussing conditions associated with long-term alcohol use such as Wernicke-Korsakoff syndrome with patients and relatives helps to warn them about red flag symptoms and their causes.

KEY POINTS!

Alcohol-use Disorders
- **Rates of alcohol-use disorders are on the rise.**
- **Chronic alcohol use is associated with several serious conditions.**
- **People with chronic alcohol dependency must never be advised to stop drinking without clinically managed withdrawal by a specialist alcohol service.**
- **There is an increased risk of intracranial haemorrhage with heavy alcohol consumption.**
- **Paramedics should be aware of the pharmacological interactions that alcohol has, which reduce or increase the effects of some medicines.**

Further Reading

Further important information and evidence in support of this guideline can be found in the Bibliography.[7,8,9,10,11,12]

Alcohol-use Disorders

Bibliography

1. ONS. *Alcohol-specific Deaths in the UK*. 2017. Available from: https://www.ons.gov.uk/peoplepopulationandcommunity/healthandsocialcare/causesofdeath/bulletins/alcoholrelateddeathsintheunitedkingdom/registeredin2017.

2. NAO. *NHS Ambulance Services*. 2017. Available from: https://www.nao.org.uk/wp-content/uploads/2017/01/NHS-Ambulance-Services.pdf.

3. NICE. *Alcohol-use Disorders: Diagnosis and management of physical complications*. 2017. Available from: https://www.nice.org.uk/guidance/cg100/chapter/Recommendations#acute-alcohol-withdrawal.

4. NICE. *Alcohol-use Disorders: Diagnosis, assessment and management of harmful drinking (high-risk drinking) and alcohol dependence*. 2011. Available from: https://www.nice.org.uk/guidance/cg115.

5. Inouye SK, Schlesinger MJ, Lydon TJ. Delirium: a symptom of how hospital care is failing older persons and a window to improve quality of hospital care. *Am J Med* 1999, 106(5): 565–573.

6. Kortas DY, Haas LS, Simpson WG, Nickl NJ, Gates LK. Mallory-Weiss tear: predisposing factors and predictors of a complicated course. *Am. J. Gastroenterol* 2001, 96(10): 2863–2865.

7. Martin RP, Singleton CK, Hiller–Sturmhöfel S. The role of thiamine deficiency in alcoholic brain disease. *Alcohol Research & Health* 2003, 27(2): 134–142. Available from: https://pubs.niaaa.nih.gov/publications/arh27-2/134-142.htm.

8. Vonghia L. Acute alcohol intoxication. 2007. Available from: https://doi.org/10.1016/j.ejim.2007.06.033.

9. Griswold MG, Fullman N, Hawley C, Arian N, Zimsen SR, Tymeson HD, Venkateswaran V, Tapp AD, Forouzanfar MH, Salama JS, Abate KH 2018. Alcohol use and burden for 195 countries and territories, 1990–2016: a systematic analysis for the Global Burden of Disease Study. *The Lancet* 2016, 392(10152): 1015–1035.

10. NICE. *Alcohol-Use Disorders – NICE Pathways*. 2020. Available from: https://pathways.nice.org.uk/pathways/alcohol-use-disorders#path=view%3A/pathways/alcohol-use-disorders/acute-alcohol-withdrawal.xml&content=view-node%3Anodes-information-and-support.

11. NICE. *Alcohol-use Disorders: Diagnosis and management of physical complications*. 2017. Available from: https://www.nice.org.uk/guidance/cg100.

12. Alcohol Change UK. *Unit Calculator*. 2020. Available from: https://alcoholchange.org.uk/alcohol-facts/interactive-tools/unit-calculator.

Allergic Reactions including Anaphylaxis

1. Introduction

- The incidence of allergic reactions continues to rise. It is estimated that allergic reactions affect 30% of adults and 40% of children, while anaphylaxis affects up to 2% of the population.
- The most common triggers are food, drugs/medicines and venom but in 30% of cases the trigger is unknown.
- Anaphylaxis is defined as a severe, life-threatening, generalised or systemic hypersensitivity reaction. This is characterised by rapidly developing life-threatening airway and/or breathing and/or circulation problems, usually associated with skin and mucosal changes.
- Injected allergens can result in cardiovascular compromise, with hypotension and shock predominating. Inhaled and ingested allergens typically cause rashes, vomiting, facial swelling, upper airway swelling and wheeze. Slow release drugs/medicines prolong absorption and exposure to the allergen, meaning the action onset can be delayed.

2. Severity and Outcome

- The severity of symptoms varies from a localised urticaria to life-threatening respiratory and/or cardiovascular compromise – anaphylaxis.
- Some patients relapse after an apparent recovery (biphasic response); therefore, patients who have experienced an anaphylactic reaction should be transferred to hospital for further evaluation. The risk of an individual suffering a recurrent anaphylactic reaction is estimated to be approximately 1:12 per year.
- Patients with other allergic conditions, such as asthma or atopic eczema, are more at risk of developing anaphylaxis, and risk of death is increased in those with pre-existing asthma, particularly if the asthma is poorly controlled.
- Patients who have experienced previous episodes of anaphylaxis may wear a 'Medic Alert' bracelet or necklace and carry an adrenaline auto-injector (e.g. Anapen®, EpiPen®). It is now advised that all patients who have previously experienced an anaphylactic reaction are prescribed two auto-injectors that should be carried at all times.
- The mortality associated with anaphylaxis is estimated to be <1%.

3. Triggers

- Allergic reaction and anaphylaxis can be caused by a broad range of triggers, including food, drugs and insect stings. Food is a common trigger in children, while drugs/medicines are a more common trigger in older people. Virtually any food or class of drug can be implicated, although the classes of foods and drugs responsible for the majority of reactions are well described. For common triggers, refer to Table 3.24.
- The time it takes for the symptoms of anaphylaxis to develop depends on how the trigger enters the body. Death can occur quickly after contact with the trigger or allergen, with approximately 50% of fatalities due to circulatory collapse (shock) and the rest due to respiratory failure (asphyxia).

4. Assessment of Allergic Reactions and Anaphylaxis

- Anaphylaxis is likely when all of the following criteria are met:
  1. Sudden onset and rapid progression of symptoms.
  2. Life-threatening Airway and/or Breathing and/or Circulation problems.
  3. Skin and/or mucosal changes (flushing, urticaria, angioedema). Heightened skin colour (flushing) relating to increased blood flow may not be detected in dark skin tones. Assess for local skin temperature changes.
- The diagnosis is supported if a patient has been exposed to an allergen known to affect them.

TABLE 3.24 – Common Triggers of Allergic Reactions

1 – Foods

Nuts (e.g. peanuts, walnuts, almonds, Brazil nuts and hazel nuts), pulses, sesame seeds, milk, eggs and fish/shellfish.

2 – Venom – insect stings/bites

Insect stings and bites (e.g. wasps and bees).

NB Bees may leave a venom sac, which should be scraped off (not squeezed).

3 – Drugs

Antibiotics (e.g. penicillin, cephalosporin, ciprofloxacin and vancomycin), non-steroidal anti-inflammatory drugs, angiotensin-converting enzyme inhibitors, gelatins, protamine, vitamin K, amphotericin, etoposide, acetazolamide, pethidine, local anaesthetic, diamorphine and streptokinase.

4 – Other causes

Latex, hair dye, semen and hydatid.

Allergic Reactions including Anaphylaxis

- The skin and/or mucosal changes that occur in allergic reactions and anaphylaxis include:
  - Erythema (superficial reddening of the skin, caused by dilatation of the capillaries).
    - If erythema is identified, it may be pink, purple or red, or the skin may become darker than the surrounding area.
    - Assess for skin changes closely using natural light if possible (or non-fluorescent light to avoid a blue tinge).
    - Palpate the skin gently for a raised rash and/or changes in temperature.
    - Consider moistening the skin (if unbroken) to enhance the visibility of skin changes.
  - Urticaria (a raised itchy rash (also known as hives), nettle rash, weals or welts)
  - Angioedema (swelling in the dermis, subcutaneous and submucosal tissues).
- Isolated skin or mucosal changes without life-threatening airway, breathing or circulatory problems do not signify an anaphylactic reaction. Skin and mucosal changes can be subtle or absent in up to 20% of anaphylactic patients.
- Angioedema most commonly occurs with urticaria, but may occur in isolation. It can occur anywhere on the body, but most often involves the eye, lips, hands and feet. Less commonly, submucosal swelling affects the airway. Angioedema may be considered part of the continuum of anaphylaxis, but in isolation, without respiratory difficulty or circulatory collapse, is not anaphylaxis.
- The mechanism for angioedema and anaphylaxis is the same, in that both histamine and bradykinin are involved. However, in anaphylaxis the reaction is more marked, resulting in an increase in vascular permeability and circulatory collapse.
- Anaphylaxis can occur despite a long history of previously safe exposure to a potential trigger. Reactions can be rapid, slow or biphasic.
- For a list of signs and symptoms which may occur during an allergic reaction or anaphylaxis, refer to Table 3.25.
- For the assessment and management of anaphylaxis and allergic reactions, refer to Table 3.26.

TABLE 3.25 – Signs and Symptoms of Allergic Reactions or Anaphylaxis

Airway problems	- Throat and tongue swelling (laryngeal/pharyngeal oedema) - Difficulty in breathing and swallowing - Hoarse voice - Stridor (high-pitched inspiratory noise caused by upper airway obstruction).
Breathing problems	- Bronchospasm - Tachypnoea/dyspnoea - Wheeze/stridor - Fatigue - Confusion caused by hypoxia - Cyanosis (usually a late feature) - SpO_2 <92% - Respiratory arrest.
Circulatory problems	- Hypotension - Tachycardia - Pallor with clammy skin - Dizziness - Decreased conscious level - Myocardial ischaemia - Bradycardia (usually a late feature) - Cardiac arrest.
Other	- Skin/mucosal changes (urticarial/hives) - Diarrhoea and/or vomiting - Abdominal pain - Anxiety.

Allergic Reactions including Anaphylaxis

5. Management of Allergic Reactions and Anaphylaxis

5.1 Immediate Management (Figure 3.8)

- Adrenaline is the first-line treatment for anaphylaxis and immediate administration is a priority. Follow the algorithm for initial treatment of anaphylaxis (Figure 3.8).
  - Give intramuscular (IM) adrenaline early (in the anterolateral thigh) for Airway/Breathing/Circulation problems.
  - A single dose of IM adrenaline is well tolerated and poses minimal risk to an individual having an allergic reaction. If in doubt, give IM adrenaline.
  - Repeat IM adrenaline after 5 minutes if Airway/Breathing/Circulation problems persist.
- Self-administration of IM adrenaline (via an EpiPen® or similar) is not always reliable. Do not assume that any self-administered adrenaline has been delivered effectively.
- Lie the patient flat (elevate legs if hypotensive). A sitting position is acceptable if that makes breathing easier for the patient. If patient is pregnant, lie her on left side. Avoid any sudden change in posture.
- Treat life-threatening features using the Airway, Breathing, Circulation, Disability, Exposure (ABCDE) approach.
- Rapid conveyance to hospital is indicated in patients whose respiratory and/or cardiovascular problems persist despite two doses of IM adrenaline.

5.2 Management of Refractory Anaphylaxis (Figure 3.9)

- Patients who fail to respond to a second IM dose of adrenaline have refractory anaphylaxis. If further treatment is indicated, first ensure that all steps recommended in 'Immediate Management' have been undertaken.
- Continue to administer the appropriate dose of IM adrenaline at 5-minute intervals until the patient begins to improve or is handed over to emergency department (ED) clinicians.
- Histamine release during an anaphylactic reaction leads to increased vascular permeability, causing large volumes of fluid to leak from the patient's circulation. If haemodynamically compromised, refer to **Intravascular Fluid Therapy in Adults** and **Intravascular Fluid Therapy in Children**.
  - Adult: 500–1000 mL per bolus
  - Child: 10 mL/kg per bolus.

NB Large volumes may be required (e.g. 3–5 L in adults).

- Consider nebulised Salbutamol and Ipratropium Bromide for bronchospasm (refer to **Salbutamol** and **Ipratroprium Bromide**); refer to Page for Age for children's doses.

5.3 Management of Cardiac Arrest due to Anaphylaxis

- Start chest compressions early.
- Use IV or IO **Adrenaline 1 milligram in 10 ml (1 in 10,000)** bolus (cardiac arrest protocol).
- Aggressive fluid resuscitation.
- Consider prolonged resuscitation/extracorporeal CPR.

Allergic Reactions including Anaphylaxis

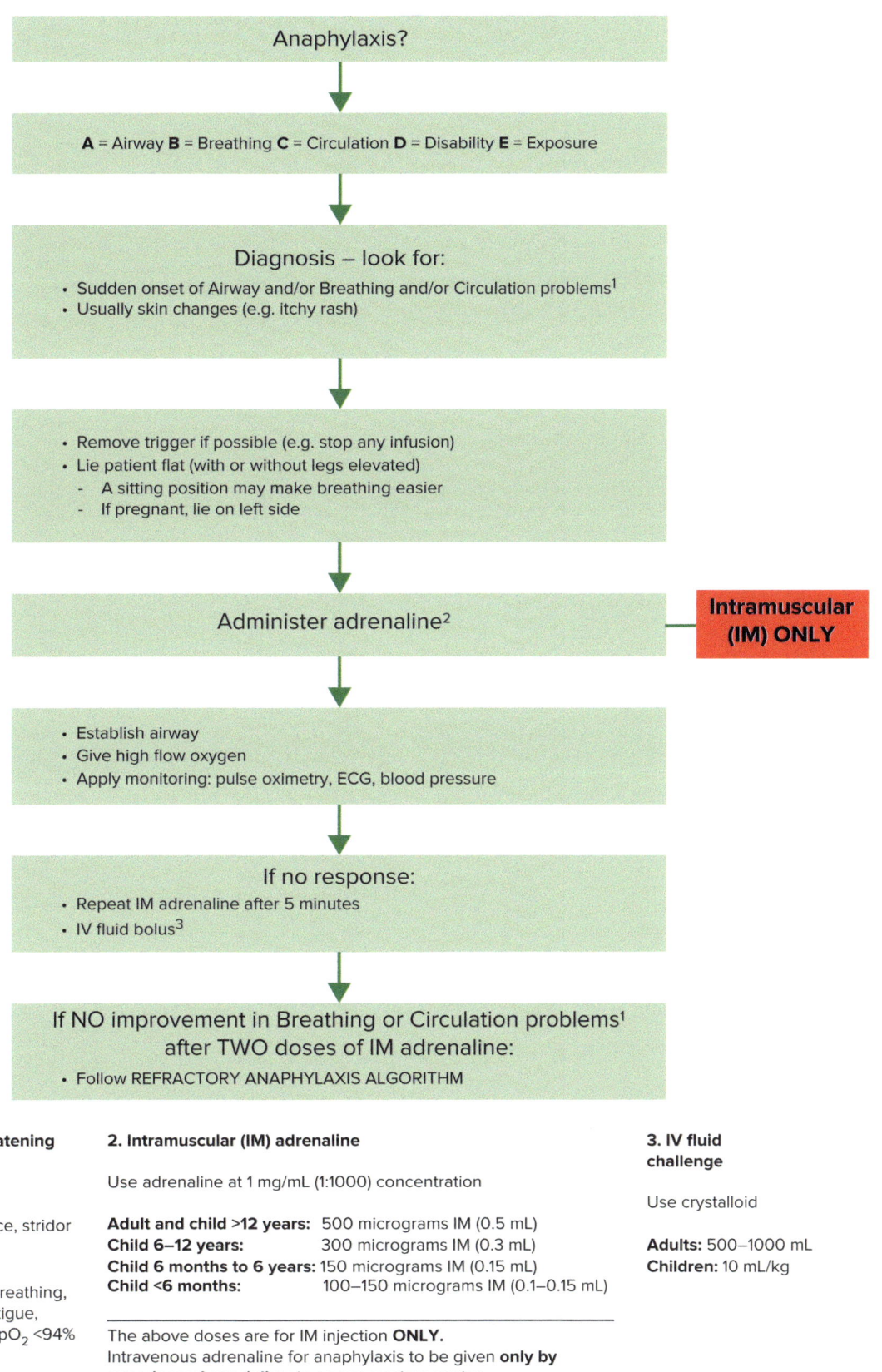

Figure 3.8 – Immediate management of anaphylaxis.

Allergic Reactions including Anaphylaxis

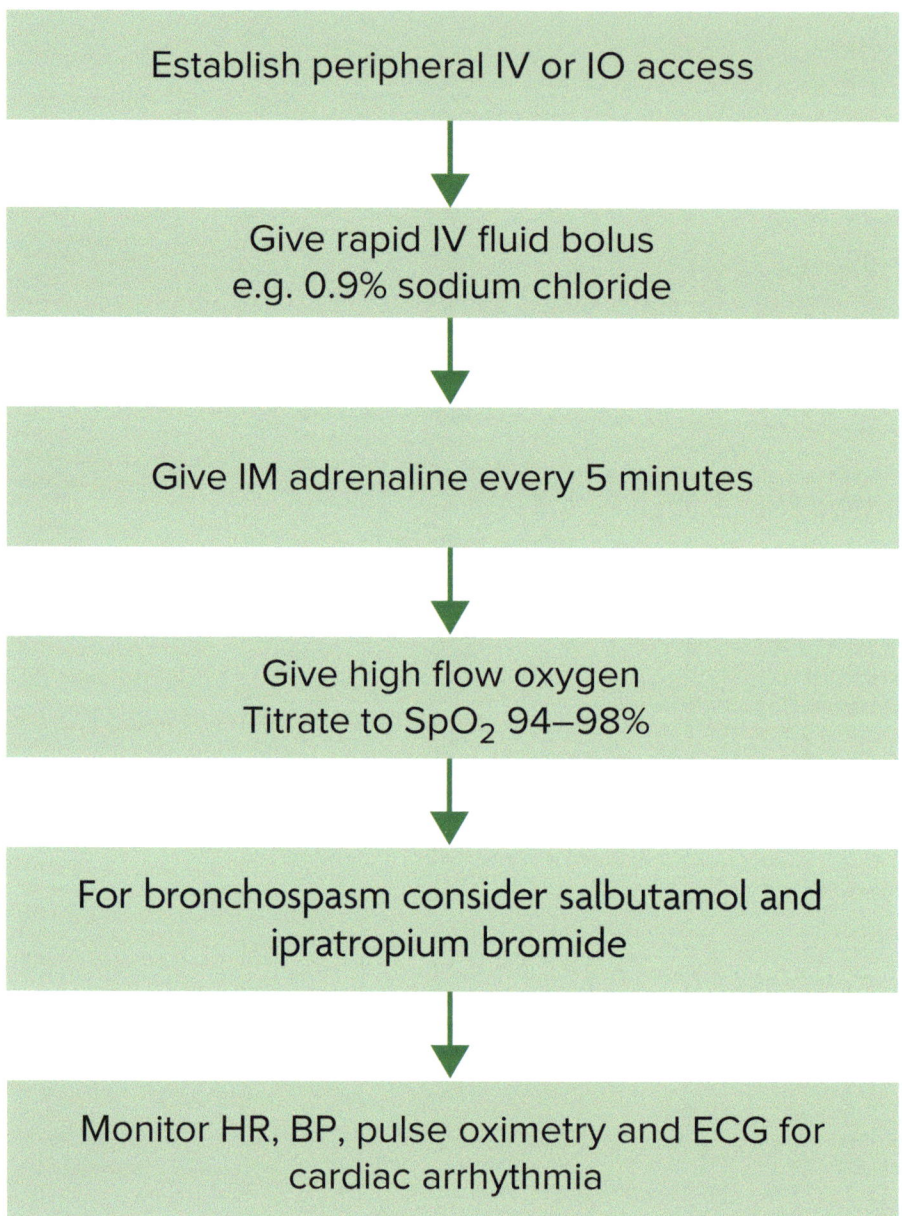

Figure 3.9 – Management of refractory anaphylaxis.

Allergic Reactions including Anaphylaxis

TABLE 3.26 – ASSESSMENT and MANAGEMENT of: Allergic Reactions and Anaphylaxis

Trigger
- Quickly remove the patient from the trigger. Do not delay definitive treatment if this is not possible or where the trigger is unknown.
- Where an insect sting is the trigger, early removal is more important than the method of removal. If the trigger has been ingested, attempts to make the patient vomit are not recommended.

For Anaphylaxis
- Administer Adrenaline **SAFETY NOTE 1:1,000 IM ONLY**. Intramuscular adrenaline is the most important drug for the treatment of anaphylactic reactions (refer to **Adrenaline 1 milligram in 1 ml (1 in 1,000)**); refer to **Page for Age** for children's doses.
- **NB** Drug check **MUST** be completed before administration, including clarification of route to be used **(IM ONLY)**.

Assess <C>ABCDE
- If any of the following **TIME-CRITICAL** features are present:
  - Major **<C>ABCDE** problems (refer to **Medical Emergencies in Adults – Overview** and **Medical Emergencies in Children – Overview**).
  - Administer high levels of supplementary oxygen to achieve saturations of >94% if the patient presents as hypoxemic on air (refer to **Oxygen**).
- Start correcting any **<C>ABCDE** problems.
- Undertake a **TIME-CRITICAL** transfer to nearest appropriate receiving hospital.
- Continue patient management en route.
- Provide an ATMIST information call.

Mild or Moderate Allergic Reaction
- Consider a mild/moderate allergic reaction if the onset of the presentation has progressed over minutes to hours, and there are skin and/or mucosal changes in the absence of life-threatening features. In this scenario, adrenaline is not appropriate.
  - For mild and moderate allergic reactions, oral antihistamine is the treatment of choice.
  - For a mild reaction, consider the appropriateness of advising the patient to purchase their own over-the-counter antihistamine. If this is not possible, consider referral for oral antihistamine supply.

FOR ALL PATIENTS WITH SYMPTOMS OF ANAPHYLAXIS OR ALLERGY

Respiratory Rate
- Measure and record respiratory rate.

Pulse
- Measure and record pulse.

Oxygen Saturation
- Monitor the patient's SpO_2, administer oxygen to achieve saturations of >94% if the patient presents as hypoxemic on air (refer to **Oxygen**).

Blood Pressure and Fluids
- Measure and record blood pressure; if required, administer fluids (refer to **Intravascular Fluid Therapy in Adults** and **Intravascular Fluid Therapy in Children**).

Blood Glucose
- If appropriate, measure and record blood glucose for hypo/hyperglycaemia (refer to **Glycaemic Emergencies in Adults and Children**).

Temperature
- Measure and record temperature.

NEWS2
- These observations will enable you to calculate a NEWS2.

(continued)

Allergic Reactions including Anaphylaxis

TABLE 3.26 – ASSESSMENT and MANAGEMENT of: Allergic Reactions and Anaphylaxis *(continued)*

ECG
- If required, monitor and record 12-lead ECG. Assess for abnormality (refer to **Cardiac Arrhythmia and Sudden Cardiac Death**).

Assess the Patient's Pain
- Where present, assess the **SOCRATES** of pain and record initial and subsequent pain scores.
- Consider analgesia if appropriate (refer to **Pain Management in Adults and Children**).

Transfer to Further Care
- Convey all patients who have experienced an anaphylactic reaction to the Emergency Department as some patients may relapse hours after an apparent recovery from anaphylaxis (biphasic response).
- Patients who have experienced an allergic reaction and do not require attendance at the Emergency Department should be advised to see their GP for consideration of oral steroids (where not already prescribed) if their symptoms are persistent. For first presentations of an allergic reaction, consider informing the patient's GP.

Documentation
- Complete documentation to include all clinical findings, advice from other clinicians, onward referral and worsening advice given.

KEY POINTS!

Allergic Reactions including Anaphylaxis
- **Remove from trigger if possible.**
- **Anaphylaxis can occur despite a long history of previously safe exposure to a potential trigger.**
- **Consider anaphylaxis in the presence of acute cutaneous symptoms, bronchospasm or cardiovascular compromise.**
- **Anaphylaxis may be rapid, slow or biphasic.**
- **Immediate administration of adrenaline is key in managing anaphylaxis. Repeat every 5 minutes until symptoms show signs of improving.**
- **Large volumes of intravenous fluids may be needed to support the circulation.**
- **For mild and moderate allergic reactions, oral antihistamine is the treatment of choice.**

Acknowledgements

We would like to gratefully acknowledge the contribution of the Resuscitation Council UK to the JRCALC guideline.

Bibliography

1. Lott C, Truhlar A, Alfonzo A, et al. European Resuscitation Council Guidelines 2021: Cardiac arrest in special circumstances. *Resuscitation* 2021, 161: 152–219.

2. Deakin CD, Soar J, Davies R, et al. (2021) *Resuscitation Guidelines: Special Circumstances Guidelines*. Resuscitation Council UK, 2021. Available from: https://www.resus.org.uk/library/2021-resuscitation-guidelines/special-circumstances-guidelines.

3. National Institute for Health and Clinical Excellence. *Anaphylaxis: Assessment to Confirm an Anaphylactic Episode and the Decision to Refer after Emergency Treatment for a Suspected Anaphylactic Episode (CG134)*. 2011. Last updated 2020. Available from: https://www.nice.org.uk/guidance/cg134.

Altered Level of Consciousness

1. Introduction

- Pre-hospital presentation of altered level of consciousness (ALoC) can be a major challenge.
- In patients with ALoC it is important to undertake a rapid assessment for **TIME-CRITICAL** conditions.
- It is important to understand, where possible, the cause of altered consciousness which can range from diabetic collapse, to factitious illness (refer to Table 3.27).
- The patient history may provide valuable insight into the cause of the current condition. Gaining information from all appropriate sources can be key to a future diagnosis. The patient, family, carers, bystanders and reviewing any video recording of the event (if appropriate) can all aid in forming the history. Consider the following in formulating your diagnosis.
- Ask the patient, relatives or bystanders if there is:
  - any history of recent illness or pre-existing chronic illness (e.g. diabetes, steroid-dependent adrenal insufficiency, epilepsy, or cardiac abnormality)
  - any past history of mental health problems
  - any preceding symptoms such as headache, fits, confusion
  - any history of trauma
  - any history of similar events
  - any chance of being pregnant.

NB Remember, an acute condition may be an exacerbation of a chronic condition or a 'new' illness superimposed on top of a pre-existing problem, such as adrenal crisis triggered by infective gastroenteritis.

- However, often there is little available information – in these circumstances the scene may provide clues to assist in formulating a diagnosis:
  - Environmental factors (e.g. extreme cold, possible carbon monoxide sources).
  - Evidence of tablets, ampoules, pill boxes, syringes, including domiciliary oxygen (O_2), or administration devices (e.g. nebuliser machines). Review end of life medication charts to consider accidental or intentional overdoses.
  - Evidence of alcohol or medication abuse.

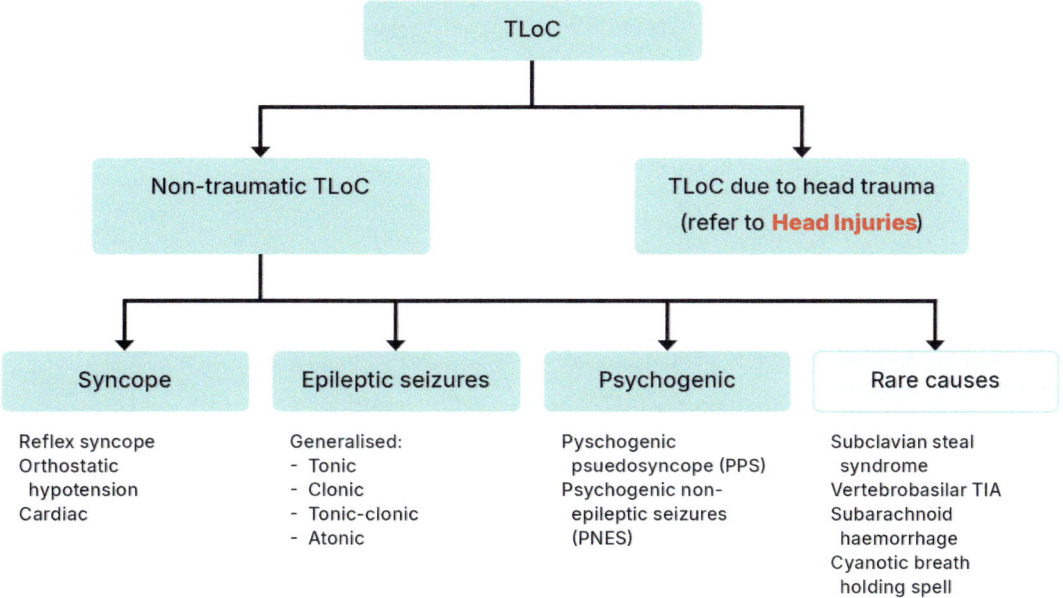

Figure 3.10 – The two main groups of TLoC.
Source: European Society of Cardiology

Altered Level of Consciousness

TABLE 3.27 – Conditions That May Result in ALoC (Altered Level of Consciousness)

Alterations in pO_2 (hypoxia) and/or pCO_2 (hyper/hypocapnia)

Inadequate airway.

Inadequate ventilation or depressed respiratory drive.

Persistent hyperventilation.

Inadequate perfusion

Cardiac arrhythmias (refer to **Cardiac Arrhythmia and Sudden Cardiac Death**).

Distributive shock.

Hypovolaemia.

Neurogenic shock.

Raised intracranial pressure.

Altered metabolic states

Hypoglycaemia and hyperglycaemia (refer to **Glycaemic Emergencies in Adults and Children**).

Acidosis.

Intoxication or poisoning

Alcohol intoxication.

Carbon monoxide poisoning.

Drug overdose (intentional or accidental) (refer to **Overdose and Poisoning in Adults and Children**).

Medical conditions

Adrenal crisis (risk of adrenal crisis with hypoglycaemia) (refer to **Hydrocortisone** and **Adrenal Insufficiency Patients**).

Epilepsy (refer to **Seizures in Adults** and **Seizures in Children**).

Hypo/hyperthermia.

Infection (especially in the young and elderly).

Meningitis.

Psychogenic non epileptic seizures (PNES).

Sepsis (refer to **Sepsis**).

Stroke (refer to **Stroke/Transient Ischaemic Attack**).

Subarachnoid haemorrhage (refer to **Headache**).

Trauma

Refer to **Trauma Emergencies in Adults–Overview** and **Trauma Emergencies in Children–Overview**.

Head injury (refer to **Head Injury**).

This guideline contains guidance for managing patients with transient loss of consciousness (TLoC) (section 2) and reduced level of consciousness (section 3).

2. Transient Loss of Consciousness (TLoC)

- Transient loss of consciousness (TLoC) may be defined as spontaneous loss of consciousness with complete recovery, i.e. full recovery of consciousness without any residual neurological deficit.
- An episode of TLoC is often described as a 'blackout' or a 'collapse'. There are various causes of TLoC, including:
  - cardiovascular disorders (which are the most common)
  - neurological conditions such as epilepsy, and psychogenic attacks.
- The diagnosis of the underlying cause of TLoC is often inaccurate and delayed. Some people have expensive and inappropriate tests or referrals; others with potentially dangerous conditions may not receive appropriate assessment, diagnosis and treatment. This is why a full and comprehensive history taking and all environmental factors need to be considered and documented as appropriate.

2.1 Assessment and Management

For the assessment and management of TLoC, refer to Table 3.28.

Altered Level of Consciousness

TABLE 3.28 – ASSESSMENT and MANAGEMENT of: Transient Loss of Consciousness

Assess <C>ABCDE
- If any of the following **TIME-CRITICAL** features are present:
  - major **<C>ABCDE** problems
  - unexpected OR persistent loss of consciousness, ECG abnormalities, TLoC during exertion, new, unexplained breathlessness, then:
- Start correcting any **<C>ABCDE** problems.
- Undertake a **TIME-CRITICAL** transfer to nearest appropriate receiving hospital.
- Continue patient management en route.
- Provide an ATMIST information call.

Ascertain from the Patient or Witnesses What Happened Before, During and After the Event

Record details about:
- Circumstances of the event.
- The patient's posture immediately before loss of consciousness.
- Prodromal symptoms (such as sweating or feeling warm/hot).
- Appearance (whether eyes were open or shut) and colour of the patient during the event.
- Presence or absence of movement during the event (limb-jerking and its duration).
- Any tongue-biting (record whether the side or the tip of the tongue was bitten).
- Injury occurring during the event (record site and severity). Refer to relevant guideline.
- Duration of the event (onset to regaining consciousness).
- Presence or absence of confusion during the recovery period.
- Weakness down one side during the recovery period.
- Details of any previous TLoC, including number and frequency.
- The patient medical history and any family history of cardiac disease (personal history of heart disease or family history of sudden cardiac death).
- Current medication that may have contributed to TLoC (diuretics).
- Other cardiovascular and neurological signs.

Assess Vital Signs
- Pulse rate, respiratory rate and temperature. Calculate NEWS2 score and if pregnant refer to the **Prehospital Maternity Decision Tool**.

Blood Pressure
- Lying and standing blood pressure if clinically appropriate.

ECG
- Monitor and record 12-lead ECG.
- Assess for abnormality (refer to **Cardiac Arrhythmia and Sudden Cardiac Death**).

The following ECG abnormalities are considered red flags and in these cases the patient must be conveyed to the Emergency Department for assessment:
- New conduction abnormalities (complete right or left bundle branch block or any degree of heart block).
- Evidence or prolonged (>440 ms for males or >460 ms for females) or shortened QTc intervals (<350 ms for both).
- Any ST segment or T-wave abnormalities (e.g. brugada syndrome, abnormal T-wave inversion).
- Pathological Q waves.
- Paced rhythm.
- Inappropriate persistent bradycardia.
- Ventricular arrhythmia.

(continued)

Altered Level of Consciousness

> **TABLE 3.28** – ASSESSMENT and MANAGEMENT of: Transient Loss of Consciousness *(continued)*
>
> - Ventricular pre-excitation (e.g. Wolff-Parkinson-White syndrome).
> - Sustained atrial arrhythmias.
> - Left or right ventricular hypertrophy.
>
> **If an Underlying Cause Is Suspected**
>
> - Undertake relevant examinations and investigations; for example, check blood glucose levels if hypoglycaemia is suspected – refer to relevant guideline.
> - Epilepsy (refer to **Seizures in Adults** and **Seizures in Children**).
>
> **Assess for Uncomplicated Faint and Situational Syncope**
>
> Diagnose uncomplicated faint (uncomplicated vasovagal syncope) on the basis of the initial assessment when:
>
> - There are no features that suggest an alternative diagnosis (**NB** brief seizure activity can occur during uncomplicated faints and is not necessarily diagnostic of epilepsy).
>
> **AND**
>
> - There are features suggestive of uncomplicated faint (the 3 'P's) such as:
>   - **posture** – prolonged standing, or similar episodes that have been prevented by lying down
>   - **provoking** factors (such as pain or a medical procedure)
>   - **prodromal** symptoms (such as sweating or feeling warm/hot before TLoC).
>
> Diagnose situational syncope on the basis of the initial assessment when:
>
> - There are no features from the initial assessment that suggest an alternative diagnosis.
>
> **AND**
>
> - Syncope is clearly and consistently provoked by straining during micturition (usually while standing) or by coughing or swallowing.
> - Distinguish whether the syncope occurred during exercise (when a cardiac arrhythmic cause is probable) from those whose syncope occurred shortly after stopping exercise (when a vasovagal cause is more likely).
>
> **Care Pathway**
>
> **Red Flags**
>
> The presence of any of the following during physical examination should be considered a red flag, resulting in conveyance to the Emergency Department:
>
> - New ECG abnormalities (listed below).
> - Physical signs of heart failure.
> - TLoC during exertion.
> - Family history of sudden cardiac death in people aged younger than 40 years and/or an inherited cardiac condition (see section 4).
> - New or unexplained breathlessness.
> - A heart murmur, not previously diagnosed.
>
> Conveyance should be considered for anyone older than 65 years of age who has experienced a TLoC without prodromal symptoms. Where not conveyed, these patients must be discussed directly with a senior clinician as per local pathways.
>
> **Alternative care pathway**
>
> - If a diagnosis of uncomplicated faint or situational syncope is made, there is nothing in the initial assessment to raise clinical or social concern and there are no red flags present then only patients with a GCS 15, with normal blood glucose and responsible adult supervision present may be left at scene.
> - **Advise the patient to take a copy of the clinical record and the ECG record to their GP and follow local protocols to safely hand over clinical responsibility.** Take the opportunity, if appropriate, to discuss and record any lifestyle factors which may influence the cause of any TLoC episode. Making Every Contact Count can prevent future reoccurrence.

Altered Level of Consciousness

TABLE 3.28 – ASSESSMENT and MANAGEMENT of: Transient Loss of Consciousness *(continued)*

Driving

- Road traffic collisions resulting from blackouts are two or three times more common than those resulting from seizures. The DVLA has specific and legal regulations regarding causes of lost/altered consciousness.
- It is a legal requirement for drivers to inform the DVLA themselves if they have a medical condition that could affect driving.
- **All licence holders or applicants should be informed that they must notify DVLA if TLoC occurs while sitting.**
- **All licence holders or applicants should be informed that they must notify DVLA if TLoC occurs following cough syncope.**
- There are differences in requirements to report to the DVLA between Group 1 (cars and motorbikes) and Group 2 (bus or lorry) drivers. Further information is available from the DVLA.

Please note. Group 2 drivers (bus or lorry) must notify the DVLA of ANY TLoC.

- When it is appropriate, particularly when discharging a patient who is a driver and not conveying them to a healthcare facility, ambulance clinicians should:
  - advise the patient on the possible impact of their medical condition for safe driving ability.
  - advise the patient on their legal requirement to notify the DVLA about TLoC.
  - document any of the above if it is discussed with the patient.
  - note that the patient could be fined up to £1,000 if they do not tell the DVLA about a medical condition that affects their driving, and they could be prosecuted if they are involved in an accident as a result.
  - If an ambulance clinician is concerned that the patient cannot or will not notify the DVLA themselves, it would be appropriate to liaise with the patient's GP and to document these actions.

3. Reduced Level of Consciousness

3.1 Introduction

- Any patient presenting with a decreased level of consciousness (GCS <15) mandates further assessment and, possibly, treatment.
- There are a number of causes of reduced level of consciousness; refer to Table 3.27.

3.2 Assessment and management

For the assessment and management of reduced level of consciousness, refer to Table 3.29.

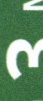

TABLE 3.29 – ASSESSMENT and MANAGEMENT of: Reduced Level of Consciousness

Assess <C>ABCDE

- Start correcting any **<C>ABCDE** problems.
- Undertake a **TIME-CRITICAL** transfer to the nearest appropriate receiving hospital.
- Consider an early call for Specialist or Advanced Care to scene. Consider time to hospital for definitive care against time to scene for these resources.
- Continue patient management en route.
- Provide an ATMIST information call.

Oxygen

- Administer high levels of supplementary oxygen and aim for a target saturation within the range of 94–98% (refer to **Oxygen**).

Assess for Hypoxia

- Apply pulse oximetry.
- Obtain IV access if appropriate.

Assess Heart Rhythm for Arrhythmias

- Undertake a 12-lead ECG.

(continued)

Altered Level of Consciousness

TABLE 3.29 – ASSESSMENT and MANAGEMENT of: Reduced Level of Consciousness *(continued)*

Assess Level of Consciousness

- Assess using the AVPU scale or Glasgow Coma Scale (GCS) (refer to Appendix):

A – Alert

V – Responds to voice

P – Responds to painful stimulus

U – Unresponsive.

- Assess and note pupil size, equality and response to light.
- Check for purposeful movement in all four limbs and note sensory function.
- Do not delay on scene attempting to calculate a GCS if red flags present. Use the AVPU scale initially and complete a full detailed GCS score after red flags have been corrected and/or en route to hospital.

Assess Blood Glucose Level

- If hypoglycaemic (<4.0 mmol/l) or suspected, refer to **Glycaemic Emergencies in Adults and Children**.

Assess Vital Signs

- Pulse rate, respiratory rate and temperature. Calculate NEWS2 score and if pregnant refer to the **Prehospital Maternity Decision Tool**.

Blood Pressure

- Measure blood pressure.
- Correct blood pressure with fluid administration if required (refer to **Sodium Chloride 0.9%**).

Assess for Significant Injury Especially to the Head

- If trauma is detected or suspected, refer to **Spinal Injury and Spinal Cord Injury**.

Assess for Other Causes

- Breath for ketones, alcohol and solvents.
- Evidence of needle tracks/marks.
- MedicAlert® -type jewellery (bracelets or necklets), or emergency card (steroids, oxygen), which detail the patient's primary health risk (e.g. diabetes, anaphylaxis, Addison's disease, COPD etc.) – also list a 24-hour telephone number to obtain a more detailed patient history. If appropriate, consider mobile phone devices for emergency health information.
- Warning stickers, often placed by the front door or the telephone, directing the health professional to a source of detailed information (one current scheme involves storing the patient details in a container in the fridge, as this is relatively easy to find in the house).
- Patient-held warning cards, for example for those taking monoamine oxidase inhibitor (MAOI) medication.
- Social carers notes often hold valuable medical information about the patient – consider when in home environment.
- End of life patients conscious level can reduce, consider the whole history and ensure shared decision making as per local policies. Refer to **End of Life Care**.
- **For management, refer to relevant guideline(s).**

Assess for Respiratory Depression

- In cases of severe respiratory depressions, refer to **Airway and Breathing Management**.
- If the level of consciousness deteriorates or respiratory depression develops in cases where an overdose with opiate-type drugs may be a possibility, consider naloxone (refer to **Naloxone Hydrochloride**).
- In a patient with fixed pinpoint pupils, suspect opiate use/overdose.

NB Any patient with a decreased level of consciousness may have a compromised airway.

Altered Level of Consciousness

> **TABLE 3.29** – ASSESSMENT and MANAGEMENT of: Reduced Level of Consciousness *(continued)*
>
> **Re-assess <C>ABCDE**
> - Document any changes/note trends in:
>   - GCS
>   - altered neurological function
>   - base-line observations.

4. Sudden Cardiac Death

- This is defined by the European Society of Cardiology as cardiac arrest presumed to be of cardiac cause, within one hour of onset of symptoms in witnessed cases, and within 24 hours of last being seen alive in unwitnessed cases. About one third of cases are unwitnessed. Incidence increases markedly with age, with the majority of cases over the age of 60. Causes vary, with electrical and structural abnormalities, myocarditis and cardiomyopathies accounting for most young deaths gradually changing to predominantly coronary artery disease during the 5th decade. Coronary artery disease accounts for 75-80% of cases.
- There are a few cardiac conditions which heighten the risk for sudden cardiac death. Some are not identifiable on an ECG, so careful history taking is important.

History 'red flags' for possible cardiac risk in younger people

- Syncope (especially during exercise, while supine or without 'prodrome').
- Dizziness, breathlessness or chest pain, especially during exercise or heightened emotional states.
- Family history of sudden death (particularly under the age of 40) or Sudden Infant Death Syndrome (SIDS).
- Family history of heart conditions (e.g. need for a pacemaker at <50 years of age).
- Palpitations.
- Previous cardiac arrest.

APPENDIX

GLASGOW COMA SCALE		
Item	**Element**	**Score**
Eyes Opening:		
	Spontaneously	4
	To speech	3
	To pain	2
	None	1
Verbal Response:		
	Orientated	5
	Confused	4
	Inappropriate words	3
	Incomprehensible sounds	2
	No verbal response	1
Motor Response:		
	Obeys commands	6
	Localised pain	5
	Withdraws from pain	4
	Abnormal flexion	3
	Extensor response	2
	No response to pain	1

Altered Level of Consciousness

> **KEY POINTS!**
>
> **Altered Level of Consciousness**
> - The cause of altered consciousness can be difficult to ascertain.
> - Ensure a comprehensive history is gained and documented.
> - Identify red flags.
> - Patients over 65 years are known to have more serious underlying causes of TLoC.
> - Manage treatable causes.
> - Consider specialist support/senior clinician inout and shared decision making e.g. for conveyance decisions.
> - For patients at end of life, consider causes and appropriate management (refer to care plans).

Bibliography

1. National Collaborating Centre for Acute Care. *Head Injury: Triage, assessment, investigation and early management of head injury in infants, children and adults* (CG56). London: National Collaborating Centre for Acute Care at The Royal College of Surgeons of England, 2007. Available from: https://www.nice.org.uk/guidance/cg176.

2. National Institute for Health and Clinical Excellence. *Stroke: The diagnosis and initial management of acute stroke and transient ischaemic attack* (CG68). London: NICE, 2008.

3. National Institute for Health and Clinical Excellence. *The Epilepsies: The diagnosis and management of the epilepsies in adults and children in primary and secondary care* (CG137). London: NICE, 2012. Available from: https://nice.org.uk/guidance/CG137.

4. National Institute for Health and Clinical Excellence. *Transient Loss of Consciousness in Adults and Young People* (CG109). London: NICE, 20 23. Available from: https://www.nice.org.uk/guidance/cg109https://www.nice.org.uk/guidance/qs71.

5. Task Force for the Diagnosis and Management of Syncope, European Society of Cardiology, European Heart Rhythm Association, Heart Failure Association, Heart Rhythm Society, Moya A, Sutton R, Ammirati F, Blanc JJ, Brignole M, Dahm JB, et al. Guidelines for the diagnosis and management of syncope (version 2009). *European Heart Journal* 2009, 30(21): 2631–2671.

6. Michele Brignole, Angel Moya, Frederik J de Lange, Jean-Claude Deharo, Perry M Elliott, Alessandra Fanciulli, Artur Fedorowski, Raffaello Furlan, Rose Anne Kenny, Alfonso Martín, Vincent Probst, Matthew J Reed, Ciara P Rice, Richard Sutton, Andrea Ungar, J Gert van Dijk, 2018 ESC Guidelines for the diagnosis and management of syncope. *European Heart Journal* 2018, 39(21)1: 1883–1948. https://doi.org/10.1093/eurheartj/ehy037.

7. Driver & Vehicle Licensing Agency. *Assessing fitness to drive – a guide for medical professionals.* May 2022. Available from: http://www.gov.uk/dvla/fitnesstodrive.

8. Health Education England. Making Every Contact Count. Available from: http://www.makingeverycontactcount.co.uk/.

Asthma in Adults and Children

1. Introduction

- Asthma has varying levels of severity and patients usually present to the ambulance service with one of four presentations: mild/moderate, severe, life-threatening or near-fatal (refer to Table 3.30).
- This guideline covers asthma in adults and children. A child is defined as between one year and puberty.
- Typically in patients requiring hospital admission the symptoms will have developed gradually over a number of hours (>6 hours).
- There may be a history of increasing wheeze or breathlessness which is often worse at night or early in the morning. Respiratory infections, allergy, cold weather and physical exertion are common triggers.
- Known asthmatics may be on regular medication, taking inhalers ('preventers' and/or 'relievers') and sometimes oral medications such as Montelukast (Singulair®) or theophyllines.
- Some patients with asthma will have an individualised treatment plan with detailed information regarding their daily symptom control as well as what to do in an acute exacerbation. They may have their own antibiotics and steroids to start when they get an exacerbation.
- **Consider anaphylaxis** where there is a sudden onset or in a patient without a history of asthma that has severe wheezing.
- **Inhaled foreign body:** Consider an inhaled foreign body in a child experiencing their first wheezy episode, or if there is a history of playing with small toys and the wheeze was of sudden onset, particularly if the wheeze is unilateral. These children must be transferred for medical assessment. If they are unwell during transport, bronchodilators may provide some clinical benefit.
- Patients over 50 years of age who are long-term smokers with a history of exertional breathlessness and no other known cause of breathlessness should be treated as having COPD (refer to **Chronic Obstructive Pulmonary Disease**).

2. Incidence

- Asthma is rare in the older population and practitioners should be aware that many people will describe a range of other respiratory conditions as 'asthma', and therefore other causes of breathlessness need to be considered.
- In adults, asthma may often be complicated and mixed in with a degree of bronchitis, especially in smokers. This can make the condition much more difficult to treat, both routinely and in emergencies. The majority of asthmatic patients take regular 'preventer' and 'reliever' inhalers.
- Asthma is rare in very young children (under one year), and other causes of wheeze (such as bronchiolitis or viral induced wheeze) should be considered.

3. Severity and Outcome

- Severe asthma is a **TIME-CRITICAL** emergency – in the UK some 2,000 people a year die as a result of asthma. Patients with severe asthma and one or more risk factor(s) (refer to Table 3.30) are at greater risk of death.
- In patients ≤40 years, asthma deaths peak in the summer (July/August), whereas deaths peak in the winter (December/January) for asthmatics aged >40 years.

TABLE 3.30 – Risk Factors for Developing Near-Fatal Asthma

Medical

- Previous near-fatal asthma (e.g. previous ventilation or respiratory acidosis).
- Previous admission requiring intensive care.
- Previous hospital admission for asthma especially if using three or more classes of asthma medication in the last year.
- Anaphylaxis.
- High β2 agonist requirements, especially with little or no response.
- Repeated asthma-related ED attendances, particularly in the last 12 months.
- Brittle asthma.

Psychological/behavioural

- Non-compliance with treatment or monitoring.
- Failure to attend appointments.
- Fewer GP contacts.
- Frequent home visits.
- Self-discharge from hospital.
- Psychosis, depression, other psychiatric illness or deliberate self-harm.
- Current or recent major tranquilliser use.
- Denial.
- Alcohol or drug abuse.
- Obesity.
- Smoking.
- Learning difficulties.
- Employment problems.
- Income problems.
- Social isolation.
- Childhood abuse.
- Severe domestic, marital or legal stress.

Asthma in Adults and Children

TABLE 3.31 – Features of Severity

Life-threatening asthma	Any one of the following in a patient with severe asthma: • Altered conscious level. • Exhaustion. • Cyanosis. • Silent chest. • Poor respiratory effort. • PEF <33% best or predicted. • SpO_2 <92%. • Arrhythmia. • Hypotension.

Acute severe asthma	Any one of:
	• PEF 33–50% best or predicted.
	• Inability to complete sentences in one breath.
	• Pulse:
	  – >110/minute in adults
	  – >125/minute in children >5 years
	  – >140/minute in children 1–5 years.
	• Respiration:
	  – >25/minute in adults
	  – >30/minute in children >5 years
	  – >40/minute in children 1–5 years.

Moderate asthma exacerbation	• Moderate asthma exacerbation.
	• Able to speak in sentences.
	• Increasing symptoms.
	• PEF >50–75% best or predicted.
	• No features of acute severe asthma.
	• Heart rate:
	  – ≤140/min in children aged 1–5 years
	  – ≤125/min in children >5 years.
	• Respiratory rate:
	  – ≤40/min in children aged 1–5 years
	  – ≤30/min in children >5 years.

Mild asthma	• Below best level of functioning due to wheeze. • PEFR >75% best or predicted. • No features of moderate or acute severe asthma.

4. Pathophysiology

- Asthma is caused by inflammation of the bronchi, making them narrower. The muscles around the bronchi become irritated and contract, causing sudden worsening of the symptoms. The inflammation can also cause the mucus glands to produce excessive sputum, which further blocks the air passages.

- Small airway obstruction and narrowing is caused by three factors:
  a bronchial mucosal swelling
  b bronchial muscle spasm and constriction
  c increased bronchial mucus and secretions.

- Since inspiration is an active process involving the muscles of respiration, the obstruction of the airways is overcome on breathing in. Expiration occurs with muscle relaxation and is severely delayed by the narrowing of the airways in asthma, producing the characteristic expiratory wheeze.

- Asthma is managed with a variety of inhaled and tablet medications. Inhalers are divided into two broad categories: preventer and reliever.

1 The preventer inhalers are normally anti-inflammatory drugs and these include steroids and other milder anti-inflammatories and long-acting beta agonists such as salmeterol or formoterol. The common steroid inhalers are beclometasone (Clenil, Qvar), budesonide (Pulmicort), fluticasone (Flixotide) and tiotropium (Spiriva). These drugs act on the lung over a period of time to reduce the inflammatory reaction that causes the asthma. Regular use of these inhalers often eradicates all symptoms of asthma and allows for a normal lifestyle. A combination of maintenance and reliever inhaler therapy (MART) may be given as a single inhaler (AirFluSal, Flutiform, Relvar Ellipta).

2 The short-acting beta agonist reliever inhalers include salbutamol (Ventolin) and terbutaline (Bricanyl); the inhaled muscarinics include ipratropium bromide (Atrovent). These inhalers work rapidly on the lung to relax the smooth muscle spasm when the patient feels wheezy or tight-chested. They are used in conjunction with preventer inhalers. Inhalers are commonly given through a spacer device, such as a Volumatic® or an Aerochamber®, improving drug administration. In mild and moderate asthma attacks, some patients may be treated with high doses of 'relievers' through a spacer device. This has been shown to be as effective as nebulisation.

5. Assessment

- Assess <C>ABCDE (refer to **Medical Emergencies in Adults – Overview** and **Medical Emergencies in Children – Overview**), but specifically assess for the severity of the asthma attack (refer to asthma algorithm – Figure 3.12 and Table 3.31).

Asthma in Adults and Children

6. Management

- Refer to the asthma algorithm (Figure 3.12 and Table 3.33) for the management of mild/moderate, severe, life-threatening and near-fatal.
- Always ask if the patient has an individualised asthma treatment plan and follow it, unless clinical circumstances dictate otherwise.

6.1 For less severe attacks

- Where possible, the patient's own β2 agonist should be given (ideally using a spacer) as first-line treatment.
  - Short acting beta-agonist (e.g. salbutamol, terbutaline) – Increase the dose by two puffs every 2 minutes according to response, up to ten puffs according to response
  - Long acting beta-agonist (e.g. formoterol, salmeterol) – One puff every minute up to six puffs according to response
- If symptoms are not controlled by maximum inhaler use, then start nebulised salbutamol whilst transferring to the emergency department (ED).

NB Children aged under two years old who do not appear to be responding to salbutamol (administered with adequate technique) and/or ipratropium may not be having an asthma attack; alternative diagnosis and treatments should be considered (refer to **Respiratory Illness in Children**).

- Patients (or friends/bystanders) who have previously experienced a severe asthma attack may be more likely to call for help early in the development of an attack, and the symptoms may appear mild on arrival of the ambulance.
- Some patients may be appropriate for alternative care pathways, for example early referral to primary or urgent care. However, apparently minor symptoms should not preclude onward referral, especially where an alternative pathway is not readily accessible. Local care pathways should be followed where patients are considered for non-conveyance. However, caution should be exercised in known severe asthmatics and robust safety-netting of patients must be in place.
- Worsening advice should be given to seek further advice if there is further deterioration, which includes increasing breathlessness, decrease in peak expiratory flow rate (PEFR) and exhaustion.

6.2 Peak expiratory flow rate (PEFR)

- Peak flow is a rapid measurement of the degree of obstruction in the patient's lungs. It measures the maximum flow on breathing out, or expiring, and therefore can reflect the amount of airway obstruction. Whenever possible, peak flow should be performed before and after nebulised treatment. Many patients now have their own meter at home and know what their normal peak flow is. Clearly, when control is good, their peak flow will be equivalent to a normal patient's measurement, but during an attack it may drop markedly (refer to Figure 3.11).
- There is no place for PEFR measurements in pre-school children, as developmentally they do not have the technical ability to reliably perform this task.
- PEFR should be attempted where possible before and after nebulised therapy in mild to moderate asthma. However, care should be taken in severe life-threatening attacks as it could exacerbate the attack and the patient may deteriorate. Predicted PEFR is shown in Figure 3.11.

TABLE 3.32 – Peak Expiratory Flow Rates in Children

Height (m)	Height (ft)	Predicted EU PEFR (L/min)
1.25	4'1"	192
1.30	4'3"	212
1.35	4'5"	233
1.40	4'7"	254
1.45	4'9"	276
1.50	4'11"	299
1.55	5'1"	323
1.60	5'3"	346
1.65	5'5"	370
1.70	5'7"	393

Asthma in Adults and Children

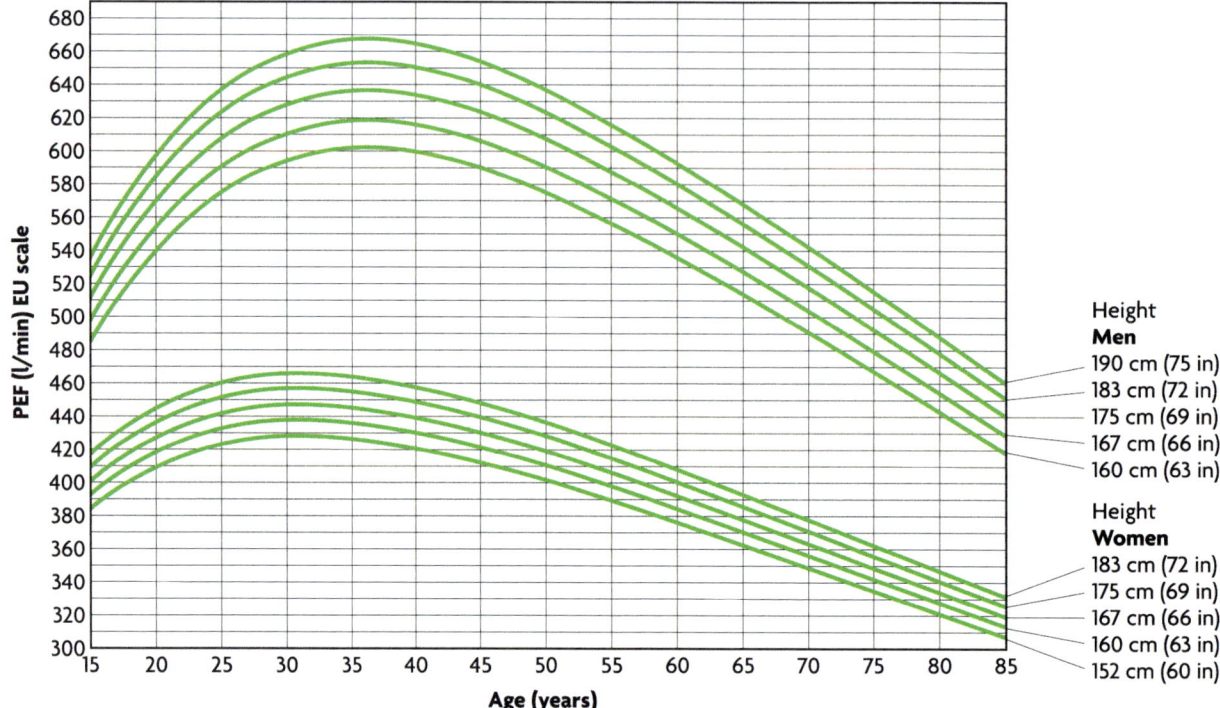

Figure 3.11 – Peak flow charts – Peak expiratory flow rate – normal values. For use with EU/EN13826 scale PEF meters only.

Adapted by Clement Clarke for use with EN13826/EU scale peak flow meters from Nunn AJ Gregg I, Br Med J 1989:298;1068–70.

TABLE 3.33 – ASSESSMENT and MANAGEMENT of: Asthma

Assess <C>ABCDE

- If any of the following **TIME-CRITICAL** features present:
  - major <C>ABCDE problems (refer to **Medical Emergencies in Adults – Overview** and **Medical Emergencies in Children – Overview**).
  - extreme difficulty in breathing or requirement for assisted ventilations. **NB** Asthma is predominantly a disease of exhalation; therefore care should be taken not to over-ventilate. Adequate expiration must be achieved.
  - exhaustion
  - cyanosis (may be more difficult to detect in patients with dark skin. Examine fingertips using additional non-fluorescent light. Look at the palms, mucous membranes and tongue for pallor)
  - silent chest
  - SpO_2 <92%
  - PEF <33% best or predicted.
- Start correcting any <C>ABCDE problems.
- Undertake a TIME-CRITICAL transfer to nearest appropriate receiving hospital.
- Continue patient management en route.
- Provide an ATMIST information call.

Respiratory Rate

- Measure and record respiratory rate.

Pulse

- Measure and record pulse.

Oxygen Saturation

- Monitor the patient's SpO_2, administer oxygen to achieve saturations of 94–98% if the patient presents as hypoxemic on air (refer to **Oxygen**).

Asthma in Adults and Children

TABLE 3.33 – ASSESSMENT and MANAGEMENT of: Asthma *(continued)*

Specifically Assess for the Severity of the Asthma Attack (refer to Figure 3.12 and Table 3.31)

- Move to a calm, quiet environment.
- Encourage use of own inhaler, using a spacer if available. Ensure correct technique is used (refer to Figure 3.12).

NB In children under two who have a poor response to salbutamol, consider an alternative cause (refer to **Respiratory Illness in Children**).

- If unresponsive:
  – Administer high levels of supplementary oxygen.
- Administer nebulised salbutamol (refer to **Salbutamol**; refer to Page for Age for children's doses).

Mild Asthma

- For cases of mild asthma that respond to treatment, consider alternative care pathway where appropriate. **NB** Exercise caution in known severe asthmatics.

Moderate Asthma

- For moderate asthma, administer Prednisolone. Refer to **Prednisolone**.

Severe Asthma

- Administer high levels of supplementary oxygen.
- Administer nebulised salbutamol (refer to **Salbutamol**; refer to Page for Age for children's doses).
- If no improvement, administer ipratropium bromide (refer to **Ipratropium Bromide**; refer to Page for Age for children's doses).
- Administer steroids (refer to **Prednisolone/Hydrocortisone**; refer to Page for Age for children's doses).
- Continuous salbutamol nebulisation may be administered unless clinically significant side effects occur (refer to **Salbutamol**; refer to Page for Age for children's doses).

Life-threatening Asthma

- Give early consideration and low threshold to activate enhanced care support.
- Continuous salbutamol nebulisation may be administered unless clinically significant side effects occur (refer to **Salbutamol**; refer to Page for Age for children's doses).
- If there is no improvement, administer ipratropium bromide (refer to **Ipratropium Bromide**; refer to Page for Age for children's doses).
- If there is no improvement, administer a single dose of intravenous magnesium (refer to **Magnesium Sulfate**; refer to Page for Age for children's doses).
- If the patient continues to deteriorate, administer adrenaline. **SAFETY NOTE: 1:1000 IM ONLY** (refer to **Adrenaline 1 milligram in 1 ml (1 in 1,000)**; refer to Page for Age for children's doses).

NB: Drug check MUST be completed before administration, including clarification of route to be used (IM ONLY).

- Administer steroids (refer to **Prednisolone/Hydrocortisone**; refer to Page for Age for children's doses).
- Assess for bilateral tension pneumothorax.
- Transfer rapidly to nearest receiving hospital.
- Provide an ATMIST information call.
- Continue patient management en route.

Blood Pressure and Fluids

- Measure and record blood pressure; if required administer fluids (refer to **Intravascular Fluid Therapy in Adults** and **Intravascular Fluid Therapy in Children**).

Blood Glucose

- If appropriate, measure and record blood glucose for hypo/hyperglycaemia (refer to **Glycaemic Emergencies in Adults and Children**).

(continued)

Asthma in Adults and Children

TABLE 3.33 – ASSESSMENT and MANAGEMENT of: Asthma *(continued)*

Temperature
- Measure and record temperature.

NEWS2
- These observations will enable you to calculate a NEWS2 Score.

ECG
- If required, monitor and record 12-lead ECG. Assess for abnormality (refer to **Cardiac Arrhythmia and Sudden Cardiac Death**).

Documentation
- Complete documentation to include all clinical findings, advice from other clinicians, onward referral and worsening advice given.

KEY POINTS!

Asthma in Adults and Children
- Asthma is a common life-threatening condition.
- Its severity is often not recognised.
- Accurate documentation is essential.
- A silent chest is a pre-terminal sign.
- Bronchodilators are the mainstay of treatment.
- Ipatropium bromide should be considered in severe cases.
- Clinical assessment should determine the severity of the asthma attack.
- Consider magnesium in life-threatening asthma not improving with continuous nebulised Salbutamol.
- Consider adrenaline for life-threatening asthma continuing to deteriorate with continuous nebulised Salbutamol.
- Asthma is rare in very young children (under one year) and other causes of wheeze (such as bronchiolitis or viral-induced wheeze) should be considered.

Bibliography

1. Soar J, Perkins GD, Abbas G, Alfonzo A, Barelli A, Bierens JJLM, et al. European Resuscitation Council Guidelines for Resuscitation 2010 Section 8: Cardiac arrest in special circumstances: electrolyte abnormalities, poisoning, drowning, accidental hypothermia, hyperthermia, asthma, anaphylaxis, cardiac surgery, trauma, pregnancy, electrocution. *Resuscitation* 2010, 81(10): 1400–1433.

2. Health Improvement Scotland, British Thoracic Society, *SIGN 158 British Guideline on the Management of Asthma*. Revised July 2019.

3. Rubin BK, Dhand R, Ruppel GL, Branson RD, Hess DR. Respiratory care year in review 2010. Part 1: asthma, COPD, pulmonary function testing, ventilator-associated pneumonia. *Respiratory Care* 2011, 56(4): 488–502.

4. Nunn AJ, Gregg I. New regression equations for predicting peak expiratory flow in adults. *British Medical Journal* 1989, 298(6680): 1068–1070.

Asthma in Adults and Children

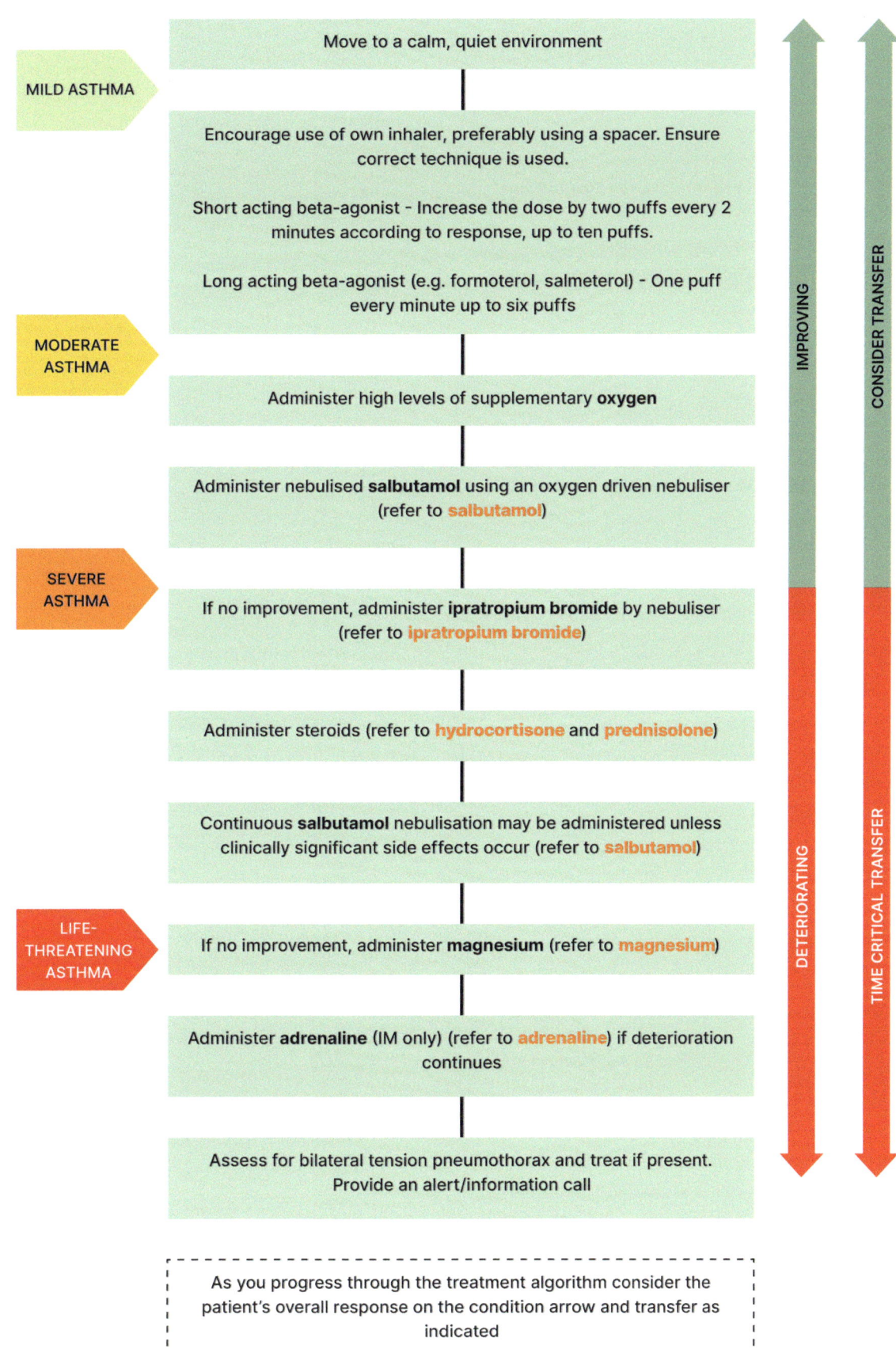

Figure 3.12 – Asthma assessment and management algorithm.

Behavioural Emergencies

1. Introduction

There are many physiological and psychological causes of an acute change in a person's behaviour. The primary aim is to maintain the safety of yourself, other responders, carers, the patient and the wider public.

Behavioural disturbances, agitation or aggression are an increasingly more common presentation encountered by pre-hospital clinicians. When assessing any patient with an acute behavioural change it is important to assess and manage the patient safely and systematically, without biases, and only reach decisions that the behaviour might be deliberate if organic or acute mental health causes can be ruled out (which may not be possible out of hospital).

These are challenging patients with a potential for risks to yourself or others. They often involve the attendance of the police either before your arrival or at your request due to a perceived level of risk.

These patients have higher morbidity and mortality rates than other people, they present an even higher medico-legal risk from their behaviour, injuries they may have sustained, or from an underlying illness that may be causing their adverse behaviour.

There are specific legal and clinical conditions to consider when using this guideline, and other JRCALC guidelines to consider include:

- **Mental Capacity act 2005**
- **Mental Health presentations**
- **Agitated Patients**
- **Acute Behavioural Disturbance**
- **Delirium**
- **Duty of care**

Behavioural changes present challenges in assessing the patient and reaching a specific diagnosis. Consideration and where possible exclusion of life-threatening conditions including, but not limited to:

- Hypoxia and or hypercapnia
- Hypo/hyperthermia
- Hypo/hyperglycaemia
- Intracranial haemorrhage
- Infection e.g. bacterial meningococcal meningitis, sepsis
- Toxins – legally prescribed or illegal substances
- Shock/hypoperfusion

Considering the reversibility of specific conditions can help in developing a management plan.

2. Pre-dispatch Information

Consider any information from the pre-dispatch information. Consider other agencies in the response to incidents and any in-service teams that may have additional information regarding the patient. If possible and where appropriate, review the NHS care record of the patient at an early stage.

3. Dynamic Risk Assessments

Ensure that a dynamic risk assessment is undertaken to mitigate the risk to yourself and others attending the scene and the patient (refer to **Major, Complex and High-Risk Incidents**). Remember – dynamic risk assessment is a continuous approach and should involve the environment, scenario and time. Consider if it is safe to approach the patient or remain at a safe distance. Consider exit routes.

Acute behavioural changes introduce a level of unpredictability to the situation; continued assessment and a flexible approach should be used.

In some cases, it may not be possible to be in physical contact with the patient due to a perceived or actual risk. Police involvement should be considered and where required they should be requested to attend. A strategy must be developed using the joint decision model this may include:

- Extraction/withdrawal from the scene
- De-escalation
- Isolation
- Restrictive interventions – direct and indirect
- Rapid tranquilisation (or escalation for consideration of this)

Restrictive interventions should be considered only when it is safe and appropriate to do so and where staff have had the training to do this.

4. Assessment

Physiological monitoring and clinical observations must be undertaken as soon as possible; the patient may have to be clinically monitored from a distance.

Due to the risks discussed it may be appropriate initially to make an assessment without direct physical contact considering Table 3.34.

Behavioural Emergencies

TABLE 3.34 – Initial Patient Assessment	
Appearance	Jaundice – suspect hepatic encephalitis
	Anaemia – shock, hypoperfusion
	Cyanosis – hypoxia
	Apparent pain – grimace, guarding
	Skin tone – pale, flushed, sweating
	Breathing – rate, pattern and effort
	Pupils – dilated, pin-point, unequal
	Limb movement – controlled, weakness/palsy
	Gait – steady, staggering
Behaviour	General behaviour (intoxicated, anxious, hyperactive)
	Irritability
	Hostility, anger
	Impulsivity
	Restlessness, pacing
	Agitation
	Suspiciousness/fear
	Property damage
	Rage (especially children)
	Intimidating physical behaviour (clenched fist, "shaping up")
Communication	Alert and orientated to time, place, people?
	Delirium – static or fluctuating
	Threats
	Reports of weapons
	Expressed thoughts
	Reports drug or alcohol use
	Reports hallucinations

Once contact can safely occur, the assessment and management of the patient can be undertaken according to Table 3.35.

TABLE 3.35 – ASSESSMENT and MANAGEMENT of: Behavioural Emergencies
NOTE – Consider referring to other relevant clinical guidelines:
• **Mental Capacity Act 2005**
• **Mental Health Presentations**
• **Agitated Patients**
• **Acute Behavioural Disturbance**
• **Delirium**
• **Duty of Care**

(continued)

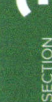

Behavioural Emergencies

TABLE 3.35 – ASSESSMENT and MANAGEMENT of: Behavioural Emergencies *(continued)*

Assess C<ABCDE>

If any of the following **TIME CRITICAL** features are present:
- Major problems (refer to **Medical Emergencies Overview**).
- List other relevant problems to that condition.

Start correcting any **C<ABCDE>** problems.

Undertake a **TIME CRITICAL** transfer to nearest appropriate receiving hospital.

Continue patient management en route.

Provide an ATMIST information call.

Mental Capacity

- Assess the mental capacity of the patient. Refer to **Mental Capacity Act 2005**. Adults with incapacity (Scotland) Act 2000.

Respiratory Rate

Measure and record respiratory rate.

Pulse

Measure and record pulse.

Oxygen Saturation

Monitor the patient's SpO2, administer oxygen to achieve saturations of >94% if the patient presents as hypoxaemic on air (refer to **Oxygen**).

Blood Pressure

Measure and record blood pressure.

Consider measuring lying and standing blood pressures.

Blood Glucose and Ketones

Measure and record blood glucose for hypo/hyperglycaemia (refer to **Glycaemic Emergencies in Adults and Children**).

Check ketones

Temperature

Measure and record temperature.

NEWS2

Calculate a NEWS2 Score.

Fluids

Assess hydration status and encourage oral fluid intake.

Always consider if the patient may have had an unwitnessed seizure and/or has a history/diagnosis of epilepsy. They may be in the post-ictal stage.

Always consider if the patient may be under the influence of drugs or alcohol.

As part of history taking, ask close friends/relatives/neighbours if new or worsening confusion and/or alteration in behaviour is worse than normal.

Behavioural changes and agitation can be challenging and difficult to manage and there are a number of options, including safe holding techniques or the use of appropriate medications. Advanced/specialist paramedics may have received additional training in this area. Refer to local procedures.

Clinicians on scene are responsible for the clinical safety of the patient at all times and should immediately inform any other personnel on scene if they believe the patient's clinical condition is at risk of deteriorating, particularly if there is any restriction to the patient's airway or breathing.

ECG

If appropriate, monitor the rhythm and record a 12-Lead ECG. Assess for abnormality (refer to **Cardiac Arrhythmia and Sudden Cardiac Death** and **Acute Coronary Syndrome**).

Behavioural Emergencies

TABLE 3.35 – ASSESSMENT and MANAGEMENT of: Behavioural Emergencies *(continued)*
Assess the Patient's Pain
Where present, assess the **SOCRATES** of pain and record initial and subsequent pain scores.
Consider using Abbey Pain Score (refer to **Pain Management in Adults and Children**)
Consider analgesia if appropriate (refer to **Pain Management in Adults and Children**).
Differential Diagnosis
Reaching an absolute diagnosis can be difficult in this patient group.
Review each relevant clinical guideline within the suite of behavioural emergencies.
Where possible treat identified reversible causes.
Seek senior clinical advice.
Referral Decision Making
Not all patients with behavioural changes need to attend an emergency department.
Consider advanced care and treatment escalation plans.
Consider the safety of the patients, carers and others when making a referral.
Utilise specialist community services and teams where appropriate.
Where police are involved in the continuing care of the patient, ensure use of JESIP principles in making referral decisions.
Documentation
Complete documentation to include all clinical findings, advice from other clinicians, onward referral and worsening advice given.

KEY POINTS!

Behavioural Emergencies

- Behavioural emergencies are complex, requiring consideration of medical, trauma, toxicological, mental health or deliberate causes.
- Safety of the responders, the patient and bystanders is pivotal and should be assessed and managed using dynamic and joint decision-making.
- An initial hands-off approach to the assessment of the patient requires consideration for remote assessment techniques.
- Specific guidelines are available for specific conditions and advice and direct support should be sought from senior clinicians and multiagency commanders where required.

References

1. Burnett AM, Peterson BK, Stellpflug SJ, Engebretsen KM, Glasrud KJ, Marks J and Frascone RJ. The association between ketamine given for prehospital chemical restraint with intubation and hospital admission. *The American Journal of Emergency Medicine* 2015, 33(1): 76–79. doi: https://doi.org/10.1016/j.ajem.2014.10.016.
2. Dunn T, Dempsey C, Zeller S, Nordstrom K and Wilson M, 2017. Agitation in field settings: emergency medical services providers and law enforcement. *The Diagnosis and Management of Agitation* 2017, 156.
3. Karch SB. The problem of police-related cardiac arrest. *Journal of Forensic and Legal Medicine* 2016, 41: 36–41.

Cardiac Arrhythmia and Sudden Cardiac Death

1. Introduction

Cardiac arrhythmia and sudden cardiac death is a common finding in the pre-hospital environment, particularly in older people, where it is more prevalent. The most common arrhythmias are atrial fibrillation, bradyarrhythmia and rhythm disturbance caused by conduction system disease.

- Cardiac arrhythmia is a common complication of acute myocardial ischaemia or infarction and may precede cardiac arrest or complicate the early post-resuscitation period. Arrhythmias are also commonly found in those with chronic cardiovascular disease.
- The diagnosis and management of disorders of cardiac rhythm is a specialised subject, often requiring detailed investigation and management strategies that are not available outside hospital.
- In the pre-hospital environment, safe care consists of high risk arrhythmia identification, treatment (if indicated) and conveyance to appropriate care. For lower risk arrhythmias, signposting or referring for follow-up, with safety netting, may be sufficient.
- Cardiac monitors used by UK Ambulance Services use algorithms which can provide automated interpretation of arrhythmias. However, poor electrode placement will seriously undermine algorithm accuracy. It is therefore important to place electrodes accurately.[5]

2. Principles of Treatment

- Management is determined by the condition of the patient as well as the nature of the rhythm. Use the standard <C>ABCDE approach.
- In all cases follow the **Oxygen** guideline and administer oxygen if indicated.
- Establish and maintain cardiac rhythm monitoring as soon as possible. This should be done with a 12-lead ECG whenever possible. Many arrhythmias (e.g. AV nodal heart blocks) can be more easily identified via a printed rhythm strip over several seconds.
- Identify life-threatening signs or symptoms:
  - Evidence of low cardiac output: pallor, sweating, cold clammy extremities, impaired consciousness or hypotension (SBP <90 mmHg), recent syncope
  - Severe heart failure
  - Ischaemic chest pain.

Some arrhythmias may be high risk but can present without overt symptoms. If unsure, seek senior clinical advice or convey to hospital for further assessment.

- Gain venous access if indicated, e.g. if there is a high risk arrhythmia, or life-threatening signs or symptoms.
- Provide a named ECG recording for the hospital, and, if possible, archive the record electronically so that further copies can be available at a later time if needed. Consider also giving the patient a named copy of the ECG.
- Repeat the recording if the rhythm changes at any time, during any intervention (e.g. vagal procedures or the administration of drugs) and during transfer. Ambulance clinicians may greatly assist the subsequent diagnosis and management of patients by obtaining good-quality 12 lead ECG recordings. Record the patients name on all ECGs to ensure the ECG stays with the correct patient record.
- Some arrhythmias may put the patient at a higher risk of stroke, due to increased incidence of blood clots, the most common of which is atrial fibrillation which increases this risk by a factor of five. Many of these patients will need to be on anticoagulant medication in order to reduce this stroke risk. Patients with arrhythmias that are not conveyed to hospital, which have not previously been diagnosed, should be sign-posted to primary care for follow-up.

3. Bradycardia

3.1 Introduction

- Bradycardia is defined as a ventricular rate of less than 60 beats per minute. However, some people have low heart rates normally and are asymptomatic (for example, athletes or people with bradycardia as a normal variant). Others have bradycardia as a result of medications such as beta-blockers or sedatives, and may or may not be symptomatic. It is therefore important to be able to recognise, ascertain the cause (if possible) and treat bradycardia if there are life-threatening signs or symptoms.

3.2 Assessment and Management

For the assessment and management of high risk bradycardia, refer to Table 3.36 and Figure 3.13.

TABLE 3.36 – ASSESSMENT and MANAGEMENT of: Bradycardia

Assess to Determine If One or More Life-Threatening Signs or Symptoms Are Present

- Shock (systolic blood pressure <90 mmHg), syncope (including recent) or reduced consciousness
- Ventricular rate of less than 40 beats per minute and symptomatic
- Severe heart failure

Cardiac Arrhythmia and Sudden Cardiac Death

TABLE 3.36 – ASSESSMENT and MANAGEMENT of: Bradycardia *(continued)*

- Myocardial ischaemia (including STEMI)
- Recent asystole
- Mobitz II AV block
- Complete heart block
- Ventricular pauses for greater than 3 seconds.

Management:

- Follow the **Oxygen** guideline and administer oxygen if indicated.
- Undertake a 12 lead ECG, with a 3 lead 'rhythm strip' as necessary.
- Gain IV access if indicated (life-threatening signs or symptoms).
- Consider atropine (refer to **Atropine Sulfate**), check for response and repeat after 3–5 minutes if indicated.
- If patient is **not** responsive to atropine (improvement in heart rate and blood pressure) consider 50 micrograms (0.5 mL) of Adrenaline 1:10,000 (refer to **adrenaline 1:10,000**)
- Consider transcutaneous pacing (if available from specialists or within your scope of practice):
  - if there is no response to atropine and adrenaline
  - if the patient is severely symptomatic, particularly when high risk AV block is present.
- Transfer to further care with a pre-alert if appropriate.
- Continuous ECG monitoring should be undertaken during transfer.
- For patients with no life-threatening signs or symptoms, and where a likely cause is known (for example, new beta-blockers or where there has been recent weight loss causing the need for a medication adjustment) consider referral or signposting to local pathways of care according to local policies. Provide worsening care advice and safety netting. If cause is unknown, convey for further assessment.

4. Tachycardia

4.1 Introduction

- **These guidelines are intended for the treatment of patients who maintain a cardiac output in the presence of tachycardia where there is no clear normal physiological cause.**
- **Pulseless ventricular tachycardia is treated according to the cardiac arrest algorithm for the treatment of pulseless VT/VF.**
- Tachycardia is defined as a heart rate greater than 100 beats per minute. Tachycardia may be a normal physiological response to another condition (for example, anxiety, infection, hypoxia, hypovolaemia or exercise) in which case, the underlying cause should be identified and treated if indicated. Anti-arrhythmic manoeuvres (e.g. Valsalva) are not indicated in these circumstances.
- Supra-ventricular tachycardia (SVT) is a generic term encompassing most tachycardias arising from the HIS bundle or above. It also includes some rhythms arising from re-entry circuits between the atria and ventricles or nodal areas. It may not be possible (or necessary) to identify the exact type of arrhythmia in the pre-hospital environment. If the rhythm has a narrow QRS, has a regular R-R interval and is tachycardic without a normal physiological cause, it can be treated as an SVT. All three of these criteria must be present.
- As with bradycardia, the primary aim is to identify life-threatening signs and symptoms, treat if indicated, and convey for further care.
- In some cases the patient will have a management plan and consideration may be given to discharge on scene or non-ED pathways according to local policies.

4.2 Assessment and Management

For the assessment and management of tachycardia, broad complex tachycardia and narrow complex tachycardia, refer to Table 3.37.

Cardiac Arrhythmia and Sudden Cardiac Death

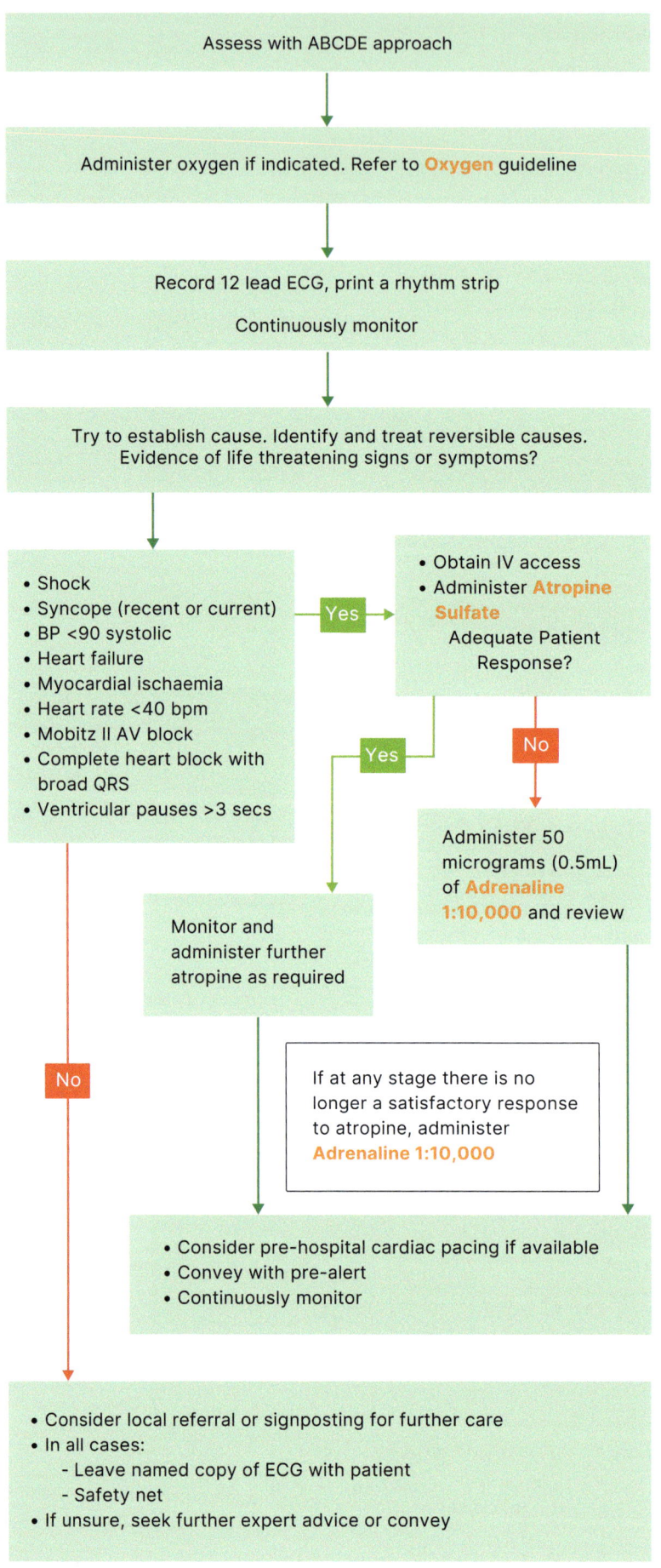

Figure 3.13 – Management of bradycardia.

Cardiac Arrhythmia and Sudden Cardiac Death

> **TABLE 3.37** – ASSESSMENT and MANAGEMENT of: Tachycardia
>
> - These guidelines are intended for the treatment of patients who maintain a cardiac output in the presence of tachycardia where there is no clear physiological cause.
> - **Pulseless ventricular tachycardia** is treated with immediate attempts at defibrillation following the algorithm for the treatment of pulseless VT/VF.
>
> **Assess to Determine If One or More Life-threatening Signs or Symptoms Are Present**
>
> - Shock (systolic blood pressure <90 mmHg), syncope or reduced consciousness
> - Severe heart failure
> - Myocardial Ischaemia (**NB** it may be impossible to identify STEMI with tachycardia. Most heart attack centres request the patient is taken to ED to slow the rate before accepting).
>
> **Management**
>
> - Follow the **Oxygen** guideline and administer oxygen if indicated.
> - Undertake a 12 lead ECG, with a 3 lead 'rhythm strip' as necessary.
>
> If one or more life-threatening signs or symptoms are present:
>
> - Gain IV access.
> - Consider pre-hospital cardioversion if available from specialists or within your scope of practice.
>
> **For SVT** without life-threatening signs or symptoms, consider vagal manoeuvres if trained and unless contraindicated (see **Figure 3.14**). The Modified Valsalva Manoeuvre has been shown to be very effective for SVT. Perform continuous ECG rhythm recording as you undertake any manoeuvre. The response to treatment can provide important additional information about the arrhythmia.
>
> **For broad complex tachycardia (regular or irregular),** treat as VT until proved otherwise. It can be difficult in the pre-hospital environment to identify whether the rhythm is a true VT, or tachycardia with aberrant conduction (e.g. bundle branch block with tachycardia). In VT, there is a risk of deterioration into VF or pulseless VT so it is important to continuously monitor for this.
>
> **It is not necessary to identify which type of broad complex tachycardia is present – in all cases assess for and treat life-threatening signs and symptoms, and transfer to definitive care for follow-up.**

5. Sudden Cardiac Death

- This is defined by the European Society of Cardiology as cardiac arrest presumed to be of cardiac cause, within one hour of onset of symptoms in witnessed cases, and within 24 hours of last being seen alive in unwitnessed cases.[2] About one third of cases are unwitnessed. Incidence increases markedly with age, with the majority of cases over the age of 60. Causes vary, with electrical and structural abnormalities, myocarditis and cardiomyopathies accounting for most young deaths gradually changing to predominantly coronary artery disease during the 5th decade. Coronary artery disease accounts for 75–80% of cases.

- There are a few cardiac conditions which heighten the risk for sudden cardiac death. Some are not identifiable on an ECG, so careful history taking is important (see **Altered Level of Consciousness**).

History 'red flags' for possible cardiac risk

🚩 Syncope (especially during exercise, while supine or without 'prodrome').

🚩 Dizziness, breathlessness or chest pain, especially during exercise or heightened emotional states.

🚩 Family history of sudden death (particularly under the age of 40) or Sudden Infant Death Syndrome (SIDS).

🚩 Family history of heart conditions (e.g. need for a pacemaker at <50 years of age).

🚩 Palpitations.

🚩 Previous cardiac arrest.

5.1 Assessment

There are several abnormal ECG findings which may support a higher risk of sudden cardiac death, and a comprehensive list is beyond the scope of these guidelines.

If an abnormal ECG is found or is indicated on the auto interpretation, seek senior clinical advice before dis-charging the patient, or convey to hospital. The following are some more well-known arrhythmias.

- **Brugada syndrome.** This is more common in males than females, and those of Asian ancestry (particularly Japan and SE Asia). Diagnosis consists of ECG findings plus clinical criteria. If Brugada-type ECGs are found incidentally or with other findings (see history above) the patient should be conveyed for further assessment. Most 12-lead ECG auto-interpretation software will recognise some forms of Brugada ECG patterns and will state it on the ECG recording.

- **Long QT syndrome.** The QT interval on an ECG is measured from the start of the QRS complex to the end of the T wave. As heart rates vary, the corrected QT interval (the 'QTc') is an estimate

Cardiac Arrhythmia and Sudden Cardiac Death

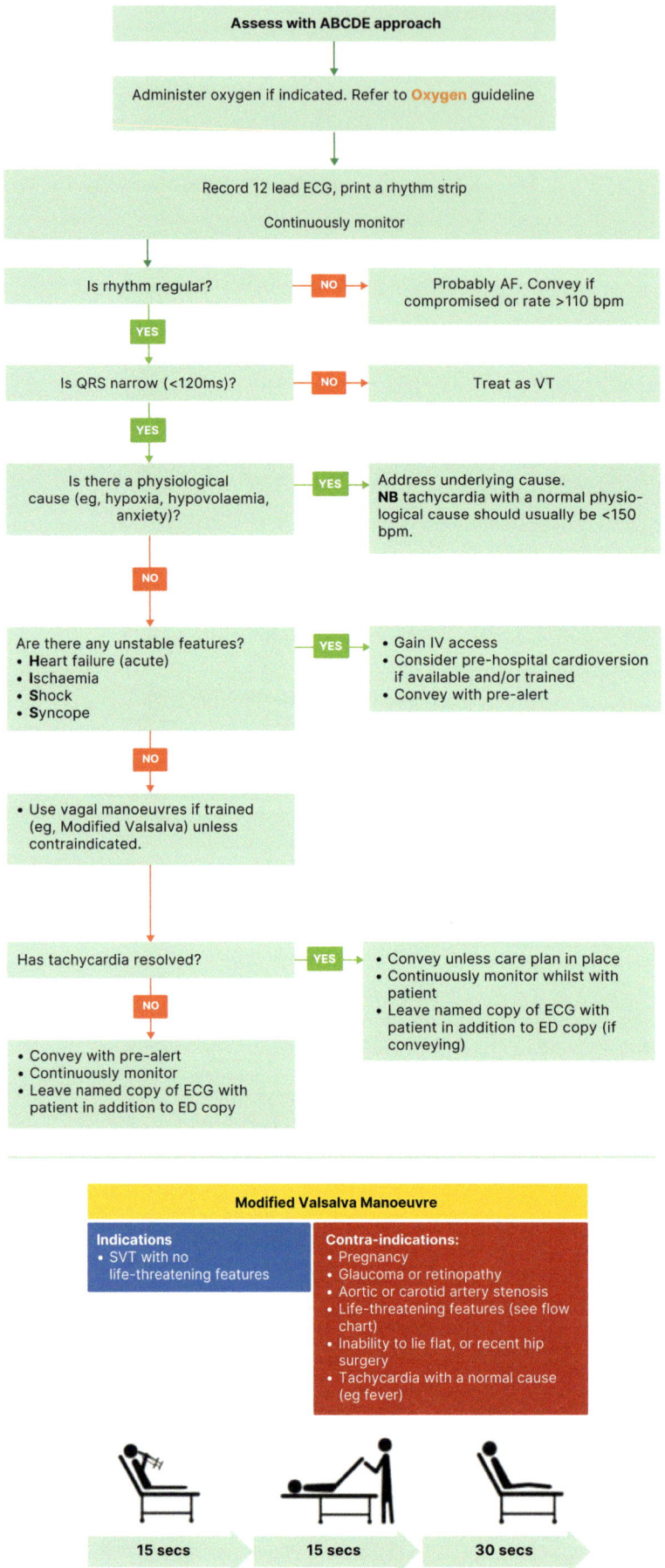

Figure 3.14 – Management of tachycardia.

Cardiac Arrhythmia and Sudden Cardiac Death

of the QT interval at a heart rate of 60 bpm and can be found as a data reading on the ECG. Normal QTc for women is 360–460ms; normal QTc for men is 350–450ms. An excessively long QT puts patients at risk of arrhythmias such as VF and Torsades de Pointes. There are many acquired causes of long QT, including electrolyte disturbances, cardiac ischaemia, hypothermia and many medications. Long QT syndrome is genetically acquired, and can put the patient at higher risk of sudden cardiac death, depending on the extent of the prolongation. A careful history of red flags should be taken and if long QT is suspected, the patient should be conveyed for further investigation. Regardless of history, a QTc of >500 for either sex is considered high risk.

- **Cardiomyopathies.** There are several types of cardiomyopathies. ECG abnormalities are common. A careful history should be taken, and the patient conveyed if the history suggests a cardiac abnormality or sudden unexplained unconsciousness (refer to **Altered Level of Consciousness**).

APPENDIX

Common Cardiac Arrhythmias and Treatment Pathways: Arrhythmias Table

(**NB** It is beyond the scope of these guidelines to describe all possible arrhythmias. If unsure, seek senior clinical advice or convey the patient)

	Look for	Risk/Signs and symptoms	Pre-hospital care	ECG examples
ATRIAL				
Sinus bradycardia	Regular rate <60bpm. P waves before each QRS. QRS can be normal or wide (for example if BBB).	Usually asymptomatic. Dizziness, syncope, fatigue, shortness of breath in more severe cases. Mild symptoms in less severe cases. Can be normal in athletes or a normal variant.	Look for cause. Mild symptoms may be suitable for referral/signposting (for example if due to beta-blockers). If unsure of cause and/or more severely symptomatic, convey. Consider O2. Consider atropine sulphate.	
Atrial fibrillation	No P waves, irregular R-R intervals. Ventricular rate unlikely to exceed 160bpm. Lead V1 can look like atrial flutter.	Stroke; dizziness, fatigue, shortness of breath, syncope if rate is fast. May be asymptomatic if rate <110bpm.	Symptomatic or >110bpm: convey. Asymptomatic and <110bpm: routine referral or signposting for anti-coagulation if not already in place.	
Atrial flutter	Flutter waves, particularly in inferior leads. QRS interval will usually be around 150 or 75, or vary between both.	Stroke; dizziness, fatigue, shortness of breath, syncope if R-R rate is fast. May be asymptomatic if rate <100bpm.	Convey for further assessment unless care plan and anti-coagulation in place. If not anti-coagulated, refer/signpost for meds follow-up.	

(continued)

Cardiac Arrhythmia and Sudden Cardiac Death

SUPRA-VENTRICULAR TACHYCARDIA (SVT)				
SVT	R-R Rate >100; regular; narrow QRS (<120ms). May be unifocal atrial tachycardia, AVNRT, AVRT, tachycardic atrial flutter or junctional tachycardia. **It is not important (or always possible) to distinguish type.**	Range between mild symptoms (for example palpitations) to severe (for example syncope, dizziness, shortness of breath) depending on cardiac co-morbidities and rate. Can be sudden onset and may self-terminate.	Convey unless rate has resolved, asymptomatic and care plan in place. Consider O2. Consider modified Valsalva manoeuvre (unless contraindicated – **see SVT flow-chart**).	
AV NODE OR JUNCTION				
1st degree AV nodal block	Long PR interval (>200ms).	Usually incidental finding. Very long ('marked') first degree AV block can cause heart failure in the longer term.	No action needed unless marked first degree or symptomatic. If PR interval >300ms refer/signpost for routine follow-up.	Source: ECG reproduced with kind permission from Charles L. Till. *Clinical ECGs in Paramedic Practice*. 2021. Class Professional Publishing.
2nd degree AV block Mobitz type I	Increasingly long PR interval then missed beat (2nd degree will always have missed beats).	Usually incidental finding. Can be the result of high vagal tone.	Only convey if symptomatic (for example fatigue or breathlessness). If symptomatic and bradycardic, consider atropine sulphate. If cardiac disease, refer/signpost for routine follow-up.	Source: ECG reproduced with kind permission from Charles L. Till. *Clinical ECGs in Paramedic Practice*. 2021. Class Professional Publishing.
2nd degree AV block Mobitz type II	Constant P-P interval but 'dropped' QRSs.	Indicates heart disease. Higher risk due to unreliability of junctional or ventricular escape beats. Risk of total heart block or sinus arrest.	Convey even if asymptomatic. If bradycardic, consider O2. Consider atropine sulphate.	Source: ECG reproduced with kind permission from Charles L. Till. *Clinical ECGs in Paramedic Practice*. 2021. Class Professional Publishing.

Cardiac Arrhythmia and Sudden Cardiac Death

3rd degree (total) AV block	Constant P-P interval, constant R-R interval, but no relationship between the two. P-P interval will be faster than the R-R interval.	Indicates heart disease. High risk due to unreliability of escape rhythm. May be bradycardic. Risk of cardiac arrest.	Convey even if asymptomatic. Consider atropine sulphate if bradycardic.	Source: ECG reproduced with kind permission from Charles L. Till. *Clinical ECGs in Paramedic Practice*. 2021. Class Professional Publishing.
VENTRICULAR				
Right bundle branch block	QRS 120ms or slightly longer, rSR pattern in V1, V2 or V3, 'slurred' S wave in V5 and V6.	Often incidental finding. Can be a normal variant in younger people. Often seen in the context of pulmonary infection or pressure (eg, COPD).	No action needed if asymptomatic. If symptomatic, treat for primary cause (for example, chest pain, pulmonary symptoms).	
Left bundle branch block	QRS >120ms deep S waves in V1 – V3, wide R wave in V5 and V6. ST elevation in anterior leads is a normal finding in LBBB.	Always a result of heart disease. May be known if long standing, or as a result of a newer event. Can be result or cause of heart failure.	Seek advice on appropriate acute pathway in the context of possible cardiac symptoms (eg appropriate ACS pathways). Refer for routine follow-up if no cardiac symptoms.	
Premature ventricular complex (PVC)	Wide complex QRS occurring too soon after previous normal QRS and before the next expected P wave.	Very common in healthy people. Sensation of palpitations. Where frequent (>5 in a minute, or runs of PVCs) there is a risk of progression to VT or longer term heart failure. May be fatigue, shortness of breath if frequent.	If runs of 3 or more in a row, >5 a minute, or a history of heart disease, convey or seek advice regarding urgent follow-up. If infrequent, otherwise healthy and no shortness of breath or chest pain, reassurance only.	

(continued)

Cardiac Arrhythmia and Sudden Cardiac Death

Monomorphic Ventricular Tachycardia (VT)	3 or more identical ventricular escapes or PVCs in a row. Wide complex QRS, regular R-R interval, rate >100. Can be difficult to distinguish from BBB with tachycardia, in which case, treat as VT.	Dizziness, syncope, shortness of breath. Can progress to VF arrest.	Convey even if resolved or asymptomatic unless care plan in place. Treat all wide complex QRS tachycardia as VT until proven otherwise. Consider O2. Be prepared for cardiac arrest.	
Polymorphic VT, including Torsade De Pointes	3 or more wide QRSs in a row of varying morphologies, varying R-R interval, rate >100.	Dizziness, syncope, shortness of breath. High risk of progression to VF arrest.	Convey even if resolved or asymptomatic. Consider O2. Be prepared for cardiac arrest.	

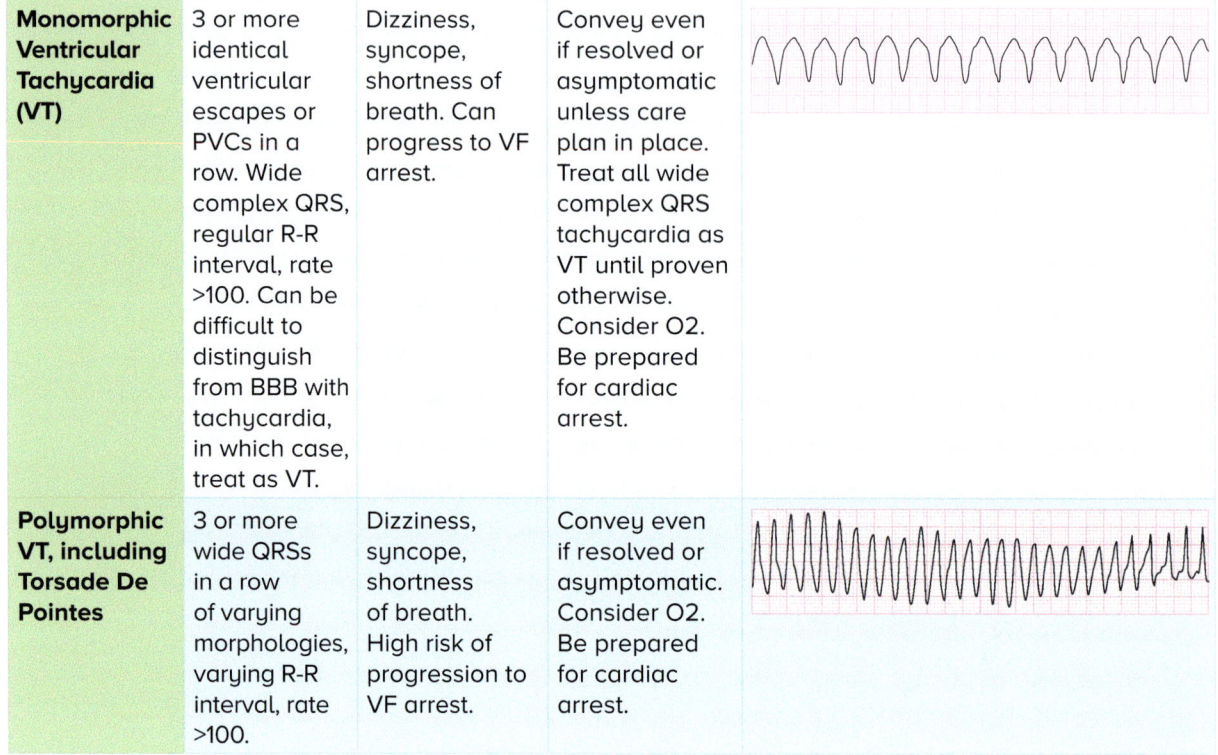

Source: Table reproduced with kind permission from Claire Hall, St George's, University of London.

KEY POINTS!

Cardiac Arrhythmia and Sudden Cardiac Death

- Continuous monitoring should be used for all patients with arrhythmias.
- Longer rhythm strips are invaluable for identifying and recording many arrhythmias.
- Assess for life-threatening signs and symptoms, and convey if unsure.
- Seek senior advice if you are in doubt about the type of arrhythmia or care pathway.
- Record the ECG rhythm during any intervention. Ensure all ECGs are named and safely handed over to receiving staff, so further copies can be retrieved if necessary.

Acknowledgments

We would like to gratefully acknowledge the contribution of Charlie Till for the ECG images, and Claire Hall for the aide-memoire table in this JRCALC guideline.

Further Resources

Modified Valsalv Manoeuvre: https://youtu.be/8DIRiOA_OsA

Bibliography

1. European Resuscitation Council Guidelines. 2021. Available from: European Resuscitation Council guidelines 2021
2. Katja Zeppenfeld, Jacob Tfelt-Hansen, Marta de Riva et al. ESC Guidelines for the management of patients with ventricular arrhythmias and the prevention of sudden cardiac death: Developed by the task force for the management of patients with ventricular arrhythmias and the prevention of sudden cardiac death of the European Society of Cardiology (ESC) Endorsed by the Association for European Paediatric and Congenital Cardiology (AEPC). *European Heart Journal 2022*, 43(40): 3997–4126, https://doi.org/10.1093/eurheartj/ehac262
3. British Heart Foundation. Arrhythmias – Abnormal heart rhythms – BHF
4. Arrhythmia Alliance UK. Home – Arrhythmia Alliance – UK
5. Clinical Guidelines by Consensus. Recording a Standard 12-Lead Electrocardiogram. An approved method by The Professional Body for Cardiac Scientists (SCST). 2024. Available from: https://scst.org.uk/wp-content/uploads/2024/09/2024_ECG_Recording_Guidelines_26-09-2024_V5_FINAL.pdf
6. Till CL. 2021. *Clinical ECGs in Paramedic Practice*. Class Professional Publishing.

Chronic Obstructive Pulmonary Disease

1. Introduction

- Chronic obstructive pulmonary disease (COPD) is a chronic progressive disorder characterised by airflow obstruction.
- A diagnosis of COPD is usually made in the presence of airflow obstruction in people >35 years of age, who are or were previously smokers and may have one or more risk factors (refer to Table 3.38).
- Patients over 50 years of age who are long-term smokers with a history of exertional breathlessness and no other known cause of breathlessness should be treated as having COPD.

TABLE 3.38 – Signs/Symptoms of COPD

Signs/symptoms

- Exertional breathlessness.
- Chronic cough.
- Regular sputum production.
- Frequent winter 'bronchitis'.
- Wheeze.

- Patients with COPD usually present to the ambulance service with an acute exacerbation of the underlying illness. COPD is a concomitant/secondary illness in many incidents with other chief complaints.
- Some patients with COPD are at increased risk of hypercapnic respiratory failure (Type 2) and respiratory acidosis due to carbon dioxide retention. It is vital for any patient who has a history of this to know their baseline oxygen saturation levels (when well), to have an oximeter (where possible) and to be issued an 'alert card' by their specialist so that respiratory failure is not worsened by high levels of oxygen administration. Ambulance clinicians should be aware of the British Thoracic Society and **Oxygen** guidelines; however, these patients may require a tailored approach.
- Excessive oxygen administration in these patients can lead to:
  - Worsened ventilation-perfusion matching due to attenuation of hypoxic pulmonary vasoconstriction
  - Decreased binding affinity of haemoglobin for carbon dioxide
  - Decreased minute ventilation.

2. Incidence

- It is estimated that approximately 3 million people have COPD, affecting 2–4% of the population over 45 years of age. However, only 1.5% of the population are diagnosed with the condition.
- In the UK, COPD is the fifth leading cause of death and it is estimated that by 2020 it will be the third leading cause of death worldwide.

3. Severity and Outcome

- COPD results in disability and impaired quality of life, leading to 30,000 deaths per annum in the UK.
- COPD is the second leading cause of emergency admission in the UK, with 130,000 cases per annum and direct costs estimated at £800 million and indirect costs of £24 million.

4. Pathophysiology

- Airflow obstruction is the result of airway and parenchymal damage due to chronic inflammation.
- COPD increases the risk of co-morbidities such as lung cancer and cardiovascular disease.
- An acute exacerbation refers to a worsening of the patient's symptoms (refer to Table 3.39). There is no single feature that defines an exacerbation, although there are a number of known causes (refer to Table 3.41); however, in 30% of cases the cause is unknown.
- COPD patients generally have lower than normal SpO_2 levels, and British Thoracic Society oxygen guidelines should be followed to maintain a target saturation of 88–92% SpO_2.
- Some exacerbations are mild and self-limiting whilst others are more severe, potentially life-threatening and require intervention – not all features will be present (refer to Table 3.39).
- Some conditions may present with symptoms similar to an exacerbation of COPD – consider these when diagnosing an exacerbation of COPD (refer to Table 3.40).

TABLE 3.39 – Features of an Acute Exacerbation of COPD

Features

- Increased dyspnoea – particularly on exertion.
- Increased sputum volume/purulence.
- Increased cough.
- Upper airway symptoms (e.g. colds and sore throats).
- Increased wheeze.
- Chest tightness.
- Reduced exercise tolerance.
- Fluid retention.
- Increased fatigue.
- Acute confusion.
- Worsening of a previously stable condition.

(continued)

Chronic Obstructive Pulmonary Disease

TABLE 3.39 – Features of an Acute Exacerbation of COPD *(continued)*

Severe features
- Marked dyspnoea.
- Tachypnoea.
- Pursed-lips breathing.
- Use of accessory respiratory muscles (sternomastoid and abdominal) at rest.
- Acute confusion.
- New-onset cyanosis.
- New-onset peripheral oedema.
- Marked reduction in activities of daily living.

TABLE 3.40 – Conditions with Similar Features to an Acute Exacerbation of COPD

Features
- Asthma.
- Pneumonia.
- Pneumothorax.
- Left ventricular failure/pulmonary oedema.
- Pulmonary embolus.
- Lung cancer.
- Upper airway obstruction.
- Pleural effusion.
- Recurrent aspiration.

TABLE 3.41 – Causes of Exacerbation of COPD

Infections
- Rhinoviruses (common cold).
- Influenza.
- Parainfluenza.
- Coronavirus.
- Adenovirus.
- Respiratory syncytial virus.
- *C. pneumoniae*.
- *H. influenzae*.
- *S. pneumoniae*.
- *M. catarrhalis*.
- *S. aureus*.
- *P. aeruginosa*.

Pollutants
- Nitrogen dioxide.
- Particulates.
- Sulphur dioxide.
- Ozone.

5. Assessment and Management

For assessment and management of chronic obstructive pulmonary disease, refer to Table 3.42 and Figure 3.15.

TABLE 3.42 – ASSESSMENT and MANAGEMENT of: Chronic Obstructive Pulmonary Disease

Assess <C>ABCDE
- If any of the following **TIME-CRITICAL** features present:
  - major <C> **ABCDE** problems
  - extreme breathing difficulty (by reference to patient's usual condition)
  - cyanosis (although peripheral cyanosis may be 'normal' in some patients)
  - exhaustion
  - hypoxia (oxygen saturation <88%) unresponsive to oxygen (O_2) – some COPD patients normally have a lower than normal oxygen saturation (SpO_2) at baseline. It is important to ask if patients know what their baseline levels are, and if they have had problems with oxygen treatment previously.
- Start correcting any **<C> ABCDE** problems.
- Undertake a **TIME-CRITICAL** transfer to nearest appropriate receiving hospital.
- Continue patient management en route.
- Provide an ATMIST information call.

Position
- Position the patient for comfort and ease of respiration, often sitting forwards, but be aware of potential hypotension.

Ventilation
- Consider non-invasive ventilation if not responding to treatment.

Chronic Obstructive Pulmonary Disease

TABLE 3.42 – ASSESSMENT and MANAGEMENT of: Chronic Obstructive Pulmonary Disease
(continued)

Ask the Patient if They Have an Individualised Treatment Plan

- Follow the individualised treatment plan or alert card if available.
- The patient will often be able to guide their care.
- Alert cards outline emergency treatment, with specific target oxygen saturation as decided by the specialist, according to most recent investigations. As part of general history-taking and scene survey, ambulance clinicians should be mindful of the need to find out if such a card exists. Many patients may also have a special message passed from the GP surgery to the Ambulance Clinical Hub.
- A typical card will be similar to the one shown below, as recommended by the British Thoracic Society (BTS, 2017).

OXYGEN ALERT CARD

Name: _____

I have a chronic respiratory condition and I am at risk of having a raised carbon dioxide level in my blood during flare-ups of my condition (exacerbations)

Please use my _____% Venturi mask to achieve an oxygen saturation of

_____% to _____% during exacerbations of my condition

Use compressed air to drive nebulisers (with nasal oxygen a 2 l/min)
If compressed air is not available, limit oxygen-driven nebulisers to 6 minutes

---

Republished with kind permission of the British Thoracic Society. BTS Guideline for oxygen use in adults in healthcare and emergency settings 2017. Thorax Vol 72, Suppl 1.

- Patients with COPD can easily become anxious, making it feel harder to breathe. They may have received advice about using specific breathing control techniques to help reduce breathlessness; one example is pursed-lips breathing. Encourage the patient to use these techniques if appropriate and if the patient has found them helpful previously.

Specifically assess:

Diagnosis
- Assess whether this is an acute exacerbation of COPD (refer to Table 3.39 for the features of COPD).
- Or another condition (refer to Table 3.40 and **Dyspnoea** for conditions with similar features to an acute exacerbation of COPD).

NB Chest pain and fever are uncommon symptoms of COPD – therefore consider other possible causes.

Airway
- Maintain airway patency.

NB Noises (e.g. 'bubbling' or wheeze) associated with breathing, indicating respiratory distress.

Bronchodilators
- Administer nebulised salbutamol (refer to **Salbutamol**).
- In severe cases, administer ipratropium bromide (refer to **Ipratropium Bromide**).
- If inadequate response after 5 minutes, a further dose of nebulised salbutamol may be administered.
- Ipratropium can only be administered ONCE; salbutamol may be repeated at regular intervals unless the side effects of the drug become significant.

NB Limit oxygen-driven nebulisation to 6 minutes. If journey time is significant, consider a further 6 minutes of nebulisation therapy ONLY if clinically indicated, but aim for a target saturation within the range of 88–92%.

(continued)

Chronic Obstructive Pulmonary Disease

TABLE 3.42– ASSESSMENT and MANAGEMENT of: Chronic Obstructive Pulmonary Disease *(continued)*

Steroids
- Administer Prednisolone (refer to **Prednisolone**) or Hydrocortisone (refer to **Hydrocortisone**).

Respiratory Rate
- Measure and record respiratory rate.

Oxygen

If the primary illness in a patient with COPD requires high-concentration oxygen (refer to **Oxygen**), then this should **NOT BE WITHHELD**. The patient should be continually monitored closely for changes in respiratory rate and depth and the inspired concentration adjusted accordingly. In the short time that a patient is in ambulance care, hypoxia presents a much greater risk than hypercapnia in most cases.

- Measure oxygen saturation. Pulse oximetry, whilst important in COPD patients, will not indicate carbon dioxide (CO_2) levels which are assessed by capnography or, more commonly, blood gas analysis in hospital.
- Administer supplemental oxygen; aim for a target saturation within the range of 88–92% or the prespecified range – refer to the patient's individualised treatment plan or alert card if available.

NB The aim of oxygen therapy is to prevent life-threatening hypoxia – administer cautiously, as a proportion of COPD sufferers are chronically hypoxic and when given oxygen may develop increasing drowsiness and loss of respiratory drive. If this occurs, reduce oxygen concentration and support ventilation if required.

Pulse
- Measure and record pulse.

Blood Pressure and Fluids
- Measure and record blood pressure; if required, administer fluids (refer to **Intravascular Fluid Therapy in Adults** and **Intravascular Fluid Therapy in Children**).

Blood Glucose
- If appropriate, measure and record blood glucose for hypo/hyperglycaemia (refer to **Glycaemic Emergencies in Adults and Children**).

Temperature
- Measure and record temperature.

NEWS2
- These observations will enable you to calculate a NEWS2 Score (refer to **Sepsis**).

ECG
- If required, monitor and record 12-Lead ECG. Assess for abnormality (refer to **Cardiac Arrhythmia and Sudden Cardiac Death**).

Assess the Patient's Pain
- Where present, assess the **SOCRATES** of pain and record initial and subsequent pain scores.
- Consider analgesia if appropriate (refer to **Pain Management in Adults and Children**).

Documentation
- Complete documentation to include all clinical findings, advice from other clinicians, onward referral and worsening advice given.

Transfer
- Consider alternative care pathway where appropriate (refer to Table 3.43).
- Arrange a follow-up, such as visiting a nurse, a GP review or referral to other support before discharge.

Chronic Obstructive Pulmonary Disease

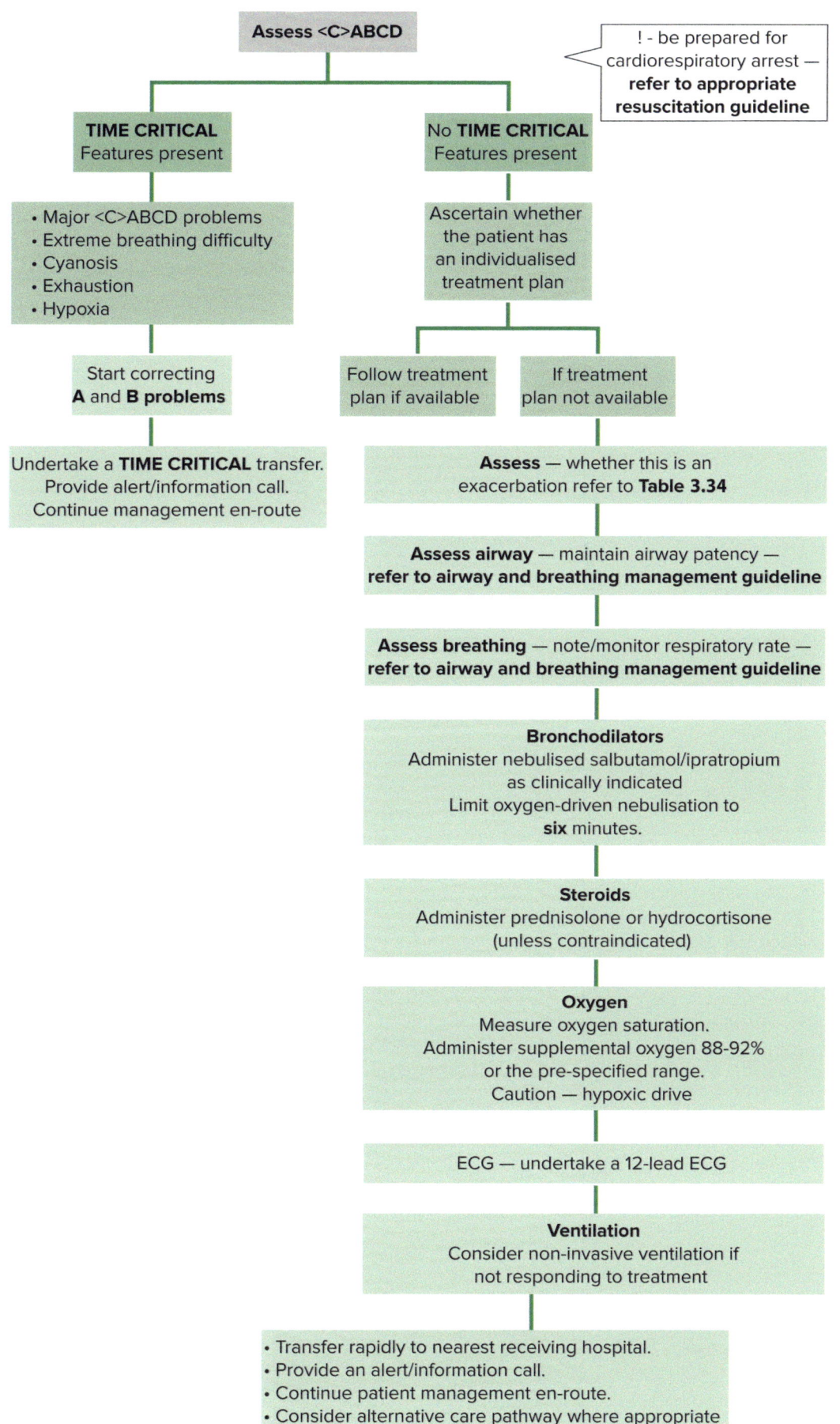

Figure 3.15 – Assessment and management of chronic obstructive pulmonary disease algorithm.

Chronic Obstructive Pulmonary Disease

TABLE 3.43 – Factors to Consider When Deciding Where to Treat a Person with COPD

Factor	Treat at home	Treat in hospital
Able to cope at home	Yes	No
Breathlessness	Mild	Severe
General condition	Good	Poor/deteriorating
Level of activity	Good	Poor/confined to bed
Cyanosis	No	Yes
Worsening peripheral oedema	No	Yes
Level of consciousness	Normal	Impaired
Already receiving long-term oxygen therapy	No	Yes
Social circumstances	Good	Living alone/not coping
Acute confusion	No	Yes
Rapid rate of onset	No	Yes
Significant comorbidity (particularly cardiac disease and insulin-dependent diabetes)	No	Yes
SpO_2 <90%	No	Yes

KEY POINTS!

Chronic Obstructive Pulmonary Disease

- Early respiratory assessment (including oxygen saturation) is vital.
- If in doubt, provide oxygen therapy, titrating en route, aiming for oxygen saturation of 88–92%.
- Provide nebulisation with salbutamol and assess response.

Bibliography

1. National Institute for Health and Clinical Excellence. *Chronic Obstructive Pulmonary Disease in over 16s: diagnosis and management*. London: NICE, 2018. Available from: https://www.nice.org.uk/guidance/ng115/chapter/Recommendations#managing-exacerbations-of-copd

2. British Thoracic Society Emergency Oxygen Guideline Development Group. BTS Guideline for Oxygen Use in Adults in Healthcare and Emergency Settings. *Thorax: An International Journal of Respiratory Medicine*. 2017, 72: 1. Available from: https://www.brit-thoracic.org.uk/quality-improvement/guidelines/emergency-oxygen/.

3. Rubin BK, Dhand R, Ruppel GL, Branson RD, Hess DR. Respiratory care year in review 2010. Part 1: Asthma, COPD, pulmonary function testing, ventilator-associated pneumonia. *Respiratory Care* 2011, 56(4): 488–502.

4. Austin MA, Wills KE, Blizzard L, Walters EH, Wood-Baker R. Effect of high flow oxygen on mortality in chronic obstructive pulmonary disease patients in pre-hospital setting: randomised controlled trial. *British Medical Journal* 2010, 341: c5462.

5. Austin MA, Wood-Baker R. Oxygen therapy in the pre-hospital setting for acute exacerbations of chronic obstructive pulmonary disease. *Cochrane Database of Systematic Reviews* 2006, 3. DOI:10.1002/14651858.CD005534.pub2. Available from: https://pubmed.ncbi.nlm.nih.gov/31934729/

6. National Institute for Health and Clinical Excellence. *Chronic Obstructive Pulmonary Disease: Management of chronic obstructive pulmonary disease in adults in primary and secondary care (partial update)* (CG101). London: NICE, 2010. Available from: http://www.nice.org.uk/nicemedia/live/13029/49397/49397.pdf.

7. NHS Evidence. *COPD*. 2012. Available from: http://www.evidence.nhs.uk/topic/chronic-obstructive-pulmonarydisease?q=copd.

8. Ram FSF, Picot J, Lightowler J, Wedzicha JA. Non-invasive positive pressure ventilation for treatment of respiratory failure due to exacerbations of chronic obstructive pulmonary disease. *Cochrane Database of Systematic Reviews* 2004, 3. DOI:10.1002/14651858.CD004104.pub3.

9. Schmidbauer W, Ahlers O, Spies C, Dreyer A, Mager G, Kerner T. Early pre-hospital use of non-invasive ventilation improves acute respiratory failure in acute exacerbation of chronic obstructive pulmonary disease. *Emergency Medicine Journal* 2011, 28(7): 626–627.

10. The Global Initiative for Chronic Obstructive Lung Disease. *Global Strategy for Diagnosis, Management, and Prevention of COPD*. 2011. Available from: http://goldcopd.org/gold-2017-global-strategy-diagnosis-management-prevention-copd/.

11. Uronis H, McCrory DC, Samsa G, Currow D, Abernethy A. Symptomatic oxygen for non-hypoxaemic chronic obstructive pulmonary disease. *Cochrane Database of Systematic Reviews* 2011, 6. DOI:10.1002/14651858.CD006429.pub2. Available from: https://www.cochranelibrary.com/cdsr/doi/10.1002/14651858.CD006429.pub2/full

12. O'Driscoll BR, Howard LS, Davison AG, on behalf of the British Thoracic Society. BTS guideline for emergency oxygen use in adult patients. *Thorax* 2008, 63(suppl. 6): vi1–vi68.

13. Healthcare Commission. *Clearing the Air: A national study of chronic obstructive pulmonary disease*. London: Healthcare Commission, 2006.

Delirium

1. Introduction

This guideline must be considered in conjunction with the **Acute Behavioural Disturbance (ABD)** and **Agitated Patients** guidelines.

- Delirium is an acute deterioration in mental status that can develop over hours or days and can last for days to weeks. Although people of any age are at risk of delirium, it is most common in older adults due to aging and aging-related brain changes.[7] Delirium is 10 times more common in persons with dementia.[5]

- Delirium can be triggered by numerous causes including acute medical illness, a drug side-effect or withdrawal, trauma, or surgery.[21] A serious clinical syndrome and a common medical emergency, delirium is characterised by an acute change in attention, cognition, level of awareness.[1]

- Delirium is often unrecognised in routine clinical care and is associated with significant distress in patients and caregivers and can sometimes be the only symptom of serious underlying disease.[13] In some people the risk of a future diagnosis of dementia is increased after an episode of delirium[8] and it is known to worsen cognitive decline.[9] Zazzara et al., (2020) found in community-based patients, that there was higher prevalence of possible delirium in the frail and older adult with COVID-19.[23]

- Lack of detection of delirium is associated with poor outcomes (National Institute of Health and Care Excellence (NICE). These include increased mortality, increased length of hospital stay, increased risk of readmission and higher rates of institutionalisation.[22]

- There are three subtypes of delirium recognised: hypoactive (drowsy), hyperactive (agitated) and mixed delirium where a patient can exhibit features of both. It can occur acutely or subacutely and symptoms often fluctuate. The most common form of delirium is hypoactive, especially in older adults, and many of these patients subsequently do not return to their cognitive baseline.[1]

- Patients may appear confused or 'not with it' when talking to them. Alternatively, it may be their family or carer who may notice a change in the patient. Delirium should be distinguished from dementia and depression as these conditions share some features (see chart, Moore 2019).[15]

- Delirium can be prevented in many cases (up to one third), and the lack of awareness of delirium is leading to a large amount of morbidity and mortality and a burden to families and friends, carers, Social Care, and the NHS.

- When assessing a patient with suspected delirium it is important to undertake a comprehensive history and examination. Consideration should be given to previous and current medical history, recent surgery, acute social and environmental changes (e.g. loss of or changes to family and carers) and medications can all cause delirium. In addition, there may be factors that for ambulance clinicians, may need special consideration such as a delayed emergency response to the patient that may have resulted in the patient being at risk of a long lie (refer to **Falls in Older Adults**).

- Delirium detection should be undertaken at the earliest opportunity with lack of detection associated with poor outcomes and increased mortality. Screening tools, such as the four 'A's Test (4AT), have been developed to improve early identification of possible delirium which can prompt a more accurate diagnosis and consideration of underlying causes.[12] Ambulance clinicians are in the unique position to be able to undertake early assessment for delirium, often in the patient's own environment, prior to a hospital admission which, in itself, is a risk factor of delirium.[20]

2. Incidence

- The incidence and prevalence of delirium can vary depending on several factors, the diagnostic criteria being used, and the population and setting being studied (NICE, 2012). Within the community setting, prevalence is thought to be 1–2%, but higher in people aged 85 years and over. Those living in long-term care facilities aged 65 years and older being as high as 10–40%. Within the emergency department setting delirium can occur in 30% of those aged 65 years and older.

- There are multiple predisposing factors that increase the risk of developing delirium. These include:
  - Aged 65 years and older
  - Cognitive impairment and/or dementia
  - Previous diagnosis of delirium
  - Living with frailty or multiple co-morbidities
  - Multiple medications
  - Severe illness
  - Current hip fracture
  - Visual or hearing impairment
  - Recent surgery
  - Terminal illness.

3. Severity and Outcome

- Delirium is persistently associated with nearly a three-fold increase in one-year mortality. This is independent of age, gender, morbidity, functional status, and dementia. Delirium is also independently linked with poor outcomes including medical complications, increased

Delirium

length of hospital stays (2–3 fold), new institutionalisation as well as admission and readmission to hospital.[11] Older persons, frailty, hypoactive delirium and the duration and severity of the delirium can worsen the outcomes.

4. Signs and Symptoms

The table below provides information on how delirium, dementia and depression differ, to assist with making the correct diagnosis.

TABLE 3.44 – Table of 3 D's – Delirium, dementia and depression

	Delirium	Dementia	Depression
Onset	Sudden (hours/days)	Usually gradual and progressive (months and years)	Gradual (weeks/months)
Duration	Usually less than a month	Years to decades	Months, can be chronic
Course	Reversible, when causes identified	Not reversible, progressive deterioration	Recovers within months, can relapse
Alertness, levels of consciousness	Fluctuates (sleepy/agitated) known as hyper or hypo types	Generally normal or slowed	Generally normal
Attention	Flucutates, difficulty concentrating, easily distracts	Generally normal	May have difficulty concentrating
Sleep	Change in pattern, often awake through the night and more confused	Can be disturbed/nighttime wandering and confusion possible as disease progresses	May experience early morning wakening, or difficulty in getting off to sleep
Thinking	Disorganised, jumping from one idea to another	Abstract thought problems, poor judgement, sometimes problems word finding	Slower, preoccupied with negative thoughts e.g. hopelessness/helplessness/self-depreciation
Perception	Illusions, delusions and hallucinations common	Generally normal in early stages	Generally normal

Hyperactive Delirium

- Less aware of what is going on around them.
- Unsure about where they are or what they are doing there.
- Unable to follow a conversation or to speak clearly.
- Have vivid dreams, which are often frightening and may be agitated or confused when they wake up.
- Hearing noises or voices when there is nothing or no one to cause them.
- Seeing people or objects which are not there.
- Worry that other people are trying to harm them.
- Be very agitated or restless, unable to sit still and wandering about.
- Have moods that change quickly; frightened, anxious.
- Depressed or irritable, aggressive, biting.
- Fluctuations in behaviour being more confused at some times than at others – often in the evening or at night.

Hypoactive Delirium

Hypoactive delirium can be easily missed and difficult to diagnose, therefore have a high index of suspicion. The patient may present with:

- Less aware of what is going on around them with reduced attention.
- Reduced alertness.
- Unsure about where they are or what they are doing there.
- Unable to follow a conversation or to speak clearly.
- Be slow or sleepy.
- Sleep during the day but wake up at night.
- Appears low in mood, frightened, anxious.
- Depressed.
- Fluctuations in behaviour be more confused at some times than at others – often in the evening or at night.
- Not eating and drinking.

Delirium

Always consider an alternative diagnoses such as depression, other mental health conditions or other medical causes, and whether the cause is likely to be reversible and treatable.

Mixed Delirium

Very often the person experiencing delirium can have symptoms of both hypoactive and hyperactive delirium, this is known as mixed delirium. The patient's symptoms may vary throughout the day and night.

5. Causes

In older people the cause of delirium is usually multifactorial. Some of the more common causes of delirium can be remembered using the mnemonic PINCH ME:

TABLE 3.45 – PINCH ME	
Pain	This can be difficult to detect in delirium but should always be an early consideration especially in hyperactive delirium. Look for non-verbal signs of pain, particularly those with communications difficulties. Consider use of abbey pain scale score for the assessment of pain. Consider silent MI. Refer to **Pain Management in Adults and Children**.
Infection **I**ntracerebral	Does the patient have clinical signs that could indicate an infection? *Look for possible sources of infection. Alternative sources of infection and causes of delirium other than urinary tract (UTI) infection must be excluded before a working diagnosis of UTI is made.* (NICE, 2022)
(mal) **N**utrition	*Malnutrition is a state in which a deficiency of nutrients such as energy, protein, vitamins, and minerals causes measurable adverse effects on body composition, function, or clinical outcome. Malnutrition is both a cause and a consequence of ill health. It is common and increases a patient's vulnerability to disease.* (NICE, 2017). Some patients with delirium may not eat as much as usual which can lead to poor nutrition. Consider has there been any changes in nutritional intake or any recent weight loss. Consider ill-fitting dentures or poor mouth care which can lead to pain.
Constipation	Many older patients with delirium, if they do not have an adequate fluid intake or nutrition, may become constipated. Constipation can cause pain and discomfort and if not correctly managed can lead to other complications.
(de) **H**ydration **H**ypoxia **H**ypoglycaemia	Many patients with delirium are dehydrated. Consider this in people with a long lie who have not been able to access fluids. Refer to **Intravascular Fluid Therapy in Adults**, **Sodium Chloride 0.9%** and **Glycaemic Emergencies**. Consider urine output, urine retention and urine concentration (be aware of other factors that affect the colour of urine e.g. medication, diet, haematuria).
Medications **M**etabolic	Many medications can directly or indirectly change a person's cognitive function. Consider have there been any recent changes in medication, have any medications been stopped or started. Typical offending medications include: • Tricyclic antidepressants e.g. amitriptyline • Antimuscarinics e.g. oxybutynin • Antihistamines e.g. cetirizine, loratadine hydroxyzine • H2 receptor antagonists e.g. ranitidine • Opioids e.g. codeine • Benzodiazepines e.g. lorazepam • Gabapentin, pregabalin • Theophylline • Hyoscine. Many longstanding medications may also play a role in development of delirium. Consider if patient has taken or had access to other medicines, this could be accidental or deliberate. Patients with pre-existing cognitive impairment are at higher risk of accidental ingestion of medications and mis-dosing.

(continued)

Delirium

TABLE 3.45 – PINCH ME *(continued)*	
	Also consider over-the-counter medications and complementary/alternative medications may have been taken.
	When did the patient last have a medication review?
	Also consider alcohol intoxication or drug/alcohol withdrawal (BGS, 2019).
Environment	Consider any recent changes in a person's environment or being moved to an unfamiliar environment. Disturbed sleep, sensory deficits, recent major surgery, falls, over or under simulation etc. can all increase the risk of developing delirium. Have there been changes in social care circumstances such as a partner who normally cares for the person being admitted to hospital or the lack of suitable health and social care package in place?

6. Pathophysiology

- It is not known why some patients may become hypoactive or hyperactive.
- Hypoactive delirium can be easily missed.
- Mechanisms are not fully understood but may involve:
  – Reversible impairment of cerebral oxidative metabolism.
  – Multiple neurotransmitter abnormalities, especially cholinergic deficiency.
  – Generation of inflammatory markers, including C-reactive protein, interleukin-1 beta and 6, and tumour necrosis factor–alpha.
- Stress of any kind upregulates sympathetic tone and downregulates parasympathetic tone, impairing cholinergic function and thus contributing to delirium. Older people are particularly vulnerable to reduced cholinergic transmission, increasing their risk of delirium.
- Regardless of the cause, the cerebral hemispheres or arousal mechanisms of the thalamus and brain stem reticular activating system become impaired.

7. Assessment and Management

Assess the patient for risk factors for delirium, consider age 65 years and older, cognitive impairment, falls and if present use the 4AT screening tool.

TABLE 3.46 – 4AT Screening tool		
[1] ALERTNESS	*This includes patients who may be markedly drowsy (e.g., difficult to rouse and/or obviously sleepy during assessment) or agitated/hyperactive. Observe the patient. If asleep, attempt to wake with speech or gentle touch on shoulder. Ask the patient to state their name and address to assist rating.*	
	Normal (fully alert, but not agitated, throughout assessment)	0
	Mild sleepiness for <10 seconds after waking, then normal	0
	Clearly abnormal	4
[2] Abbreviated Mental Test 4	*Age, date of birth, place (name of hospital or building), current year*	
	No mistakes	0
	1 mistake	1
	2 or more mistakes/untestable	2
[3] ATTENTION	*Ask the patient: "Please tell me the months of the year in backwards order, starting at December." To assist initial understanding one prompt of "what is the month before December?" is permitted.*	
Months of the year backwards	Achieves 7 months or more correctly	0
	Starts but scores <7 months/refuses to start	1
	Untestable (cannot start because unwell, drowsy, inattentive)	2
[4] ACUTE CHANGE OR FLUCTUATING COURSE	*Evidence of significant change or fluctuation in: alertness, cognition, other mental function (e.g., paranoia, hallucinations) arising over the last 2 weeks and still evident in last 24 hrs*	

Delirium

TABLE 3.46 – 4AT Screening tool *(continued)*		
	No	0
	Yes	4
		4AT SCORE:
	4 or above: possible delirium +/- cognitive impairment	
	1–3: possible cognitive impairment	
	0: delirium or severe cognitive impairment unlikely (but delirium still possible if [4] information incomplete)	

Reproduced with permission from https://www.the4at.com/.

TABLE 3.47 – ASSESSMENT and MANAGEMENT of: Delirium
Assess C<ABCDE>
If any of the following **TIME CRITICAL** features are present:
• Major **C-ABCDE** problems (refer to **Medical Emergencies Overview Guideline**).
• list other relevant problems to that condition.
Start correcting any **C<ABCDE>** problems.
Undertake a **TIME CRITICAL** transfer to nearest appropriate receiving hospital.
Continue patient management en route.
Provide an ATMIST information call.
Respiratory Rate
Measure and record respiratory rate.
Pulse
Measure and record pulse.
Oxygen Saturation
Monitor the patient's SpO$_2$, administer oxygen to achieve saturations of >94% if the patient presents as hypoxaemic on air (refer to **Oxygen** guideline).
Blood Pressure
Measure and record blood pressure.
Consider measuring lying and standing blood pressures.
Blood Glucose
Measure and record blood glucose for hypo/hyperglycaemia (refer to **Glycaemic Emergencies in Adults and Children).**
Temperature
Measure and record temperature.
NEWS2
Calculate a NEWS2 Score.
Frailty
The level of frailty of the patient should be assessed. The score is based on the patients baseline so use the tool to score how the patient was two weeks ago (prior to deterioration), or their usual level of functioning when well rather than how they present today. Refer to JRCALC **Clinical Frailty Score in Falls in Older Adults**.
Fluids
Assess hydration status and encourage oral fluid intake.

(continued)

Delirium

TABLE 3.47 – ASSESSMENT and MANAGEMENT of: Delirium *(continued)*

Always consider if the patient may have had an unwitnessed seizure and has a history/diagnosis of epilepsy. They may be in the post-ictal stage.

Always consider the patient may be under the influence of drugs or alcohol.

As part of history taking, ask close friends/relatives/neighbours if new or worsening confusion and/or alteration in behaviour is worse than normal.

Assess using a screening tool such as the 4AT (see Table 3.46).

Mental Capacity
Assess the mental capacity of the patient. Refer to **Mental Capacity Act 2005**. Adults with incapacity (Scotland) Act 2000.

ECG
If appropriate, monitor and record a 12-Lead ECG. Assess for abnormality (refer to **Cardiac Arrhythmia and Sudden Cardiac Death** and **Acute Coronary Syndrome**).

Assess the Patient's Pain
Where present, assess the **SOCRATES** of pain and record initial and subsequent pain scores.

Consider using Abbey Pain Score (refer to **Pain Management in Adults and Children**)

Consider analgesia if appropriate (refer to **Pain Management in Adults and Children**).

Documentation
Complete documentation to include all clinical findings, advice from other clinicians, onward referral and worsening advice given.

- To treat delirium, you need to identify and manage the cause or combination of causes. Refer to PINCH ME, Table 3.45.
- For patients that are difficult to manage due to their delirium and if agitated, refer to **Agitated Patients** guideline. Always consider the use of non-pharmacological interventions first. Verbal de-escalation is effective but often under-utilised, and friends or family members may be helpful (but ask them to desist if their intervention is making the situation worse).
- Pharmacological intervention would be considered but is likely to be outside the routine scope of a paramedic not in a specialist or advanced role; refer to local guidelines.
- Rapid parenteral (IM or IV) pharmacological tranquilisation of a patient with extreme agitation caused by delirium is clinically challenging and requires a senior clinician with specific experience and education/training in this area.
- Patients may benefit from low dose oral tranquilisation agents such as lorazepam (administered by Trust approved clinicians). Refer to **Acute Behavioural Disturbance (ABD)** and **Agitated Patients** guidelines.
- You can help someone with delirium feel calmer and more in control if you:
  - Stay calm and provide reassurance.
  - Remind them of where they are, who they are and what your role is.
  - Explain what is happening and how they are doing.
  - Involve those who are familiar with the patient in the assessment.
  - Talk to the person in short, simple sentences.
  - Check understanding – repeat things if necessary.
  - Try not to agree with any unusual or incorrect ideas, but tactfully disagree or change the subject.
  - Talk to the person to reorientate them of the time and date.
  - Make sure they can see a clock or a calendar.
  - Try to make sure that someone they know well is with them. This is often most important during the evening when confusion often gets worse.
  - If they are going to hospital, take some familiar objects from home.
  - Make sure they have their glasses, hearing aids and dentures.
  - Support them to eat and drink.
  - Have a light on at night so that they can see where they are if they wake up.
  - Consider playing music and use dementia friendly ambulance if available.
  - Keep warm.

Delirium

8. Referral and Decision Making

- Not all patients who have been assessed as having a potential delirium will require conveyance to the emergency department (ED). Decisions around conveyance or community management will depend on whether the cause or combination of causes of the delirium has been identified and if the patient can be managed in the community, as per local pathways.

- Careful consideration must be given to whether to convey the patient direct to an ED or other hospital receiving areas such as a frailty unit, same day emergency care (SDEC), medical assessment unit, as per local pathways. The ED route may lead to worsening of the delirium due to the environment and other factors relating to a busy ED. Follow Trust guidelines or seek senior clinical advice regarding appropriate destination.

- Depending on the underlying cause of the delirium, management in the community can be considered with direct referral to urgent community response teams (UCR), primary care or other appropriate community team for rapid community review and management based on local pathways.

- Always consider if the patient has an advanced care plan or ReSPECT plan to aid decisions about management and conveyance. Consider that this may be an end-of-life event causing signs and symptoms of delirium.

- Decisions around home management and community-based care must consider whether the patient can undertake activities of daily living, manage their personal care-hygiene/toilet, nutrition, and hydration.

- Consider if the patient is within their normal baseline, asking relatives and carers can be helpful.

- Consider if the patient lives alone and what support they have available, including care packages and other forms of home and family/friend's support.

- Ensure, where possible, personal items such as glasses, dentures, hearing aids etc. are transported with the patient as not having these items can increase the risk of delirium if an inpatient stay is required.

- For patients discharged at scene/referred for onward community assessment consider signposting to delirium resources which give key information on how family and carers can support someone with delirium.

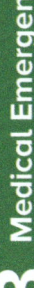

KEY POINTS!

Delirium

- **Consider if the patient needs hospital admission or if a community referral is appropriate.**
- **Consider delirium early in the assessment of the patient.**
- **Delirium is an acute deterioration in mental status that can develop over hours or days and can last for days to weeks.**
- **Delirium can be triggered by numerous causes.**
- **Delirium is often not recognised and is associated with poor outcomes.**

References

1. Anand A & MacLullich AMJ. Delirium in older adults. *Medicine* 2020, 49(1). doi: https://doi.org/10.1016/j.mpmed.2020.10.002.

2. Agar RM. Age and Ageing 2020, 49(3): 337–340. https://doi.org/10.1093/ageing/afz171

3. Alagiakrishnan K, Wiens CA. An approach to drug induced delirium in the elderly. Postgraduate Medical Journal 2004, 80: 388–393.

4. Bourne RS et al. Drug treatment of delirium: Past, present, and future. Journal of Psychosomatic Research 2008, 65: 273–282.

5. British Geriatrics Society (2020). End of Life Care in Frailty: Delirium. Available at: https://www.bgs.org.uk/resources/end-of-life-care-in-frailty-delirium.

6. Brown B & Boyle M. Delirium. In: ABC of Psychological Medicine, 2003. BMJ Books.

7. Bugiani O. Why is delirium more frequent in the elderly? *Neurol Sci.* 2021, 42(8): 3491–3503. doi: 10.1007/s10072-021-05339-3. Epub 2021 May 24. PMID: 34031797; PMCID: PMC8143064.

8. Davis DH, Muniz Terrera G, Keage H, et al. Delirium is a strong risk factor for dementia in the oldest-old: a population-based cohort study. *Brain* 2012, 135(9): 2809–2816.

9. Davis DH, Muniz-Terrera G, Keage HA, et al. Association of delirium with cognitive decline in late life: a neuropathologic study of 3 population-based cohort studies. *JAMA psychiatry* 2017, 74(3): 244–251.

10. de Lange E, Verhaak PFM and van der Meer K. Prevalence, presentation and prognosis of delirium in older people in the population, at home and in long term care: a review. *International Journal of Geriatric Psychiatry*

Delirium

10. 2012, 28(2): 127–134. doi: https://doi.org/10.1002/gps.3814.

11. SIGN (2019). Risk reduction and management of delirium A national clinical guideline. Available at: https://www.sign.ac.uk/media/1423/sign157.pdf.

12. Maclullich, A. (2019). 4AT – RAPID CLINICAL TEST FOR DELIRIUM. Available at: https://www.the4at.com/

13. Manning W et al (2013) Delirium. (2nd ed.) Stirling: University of Stirling/Hammond Press.

14. Marcantonio ER. Clinical management and prevention of delirium. *Psychiatry* 2008, 7: 42–48

15. Moore A (2019) Delirium and dementia. In Harrison Dening K (Ed) Evidence-Based Practice in Dementia for Nurses and Nursing Students. Jessica Kingsley Publishers, London, 237–248.

16. MSD Manual, Professional Version. https://www.msdmanuals.com/en-gb/professional/neurologic-disorders/delirium-and-dementia/delirium#:~:text=Pathophysiology%20of%20Delirium&text=Stress%20of%20any%20kind%20upregulates,increasing%20their%20risk%20of%20delirium.

17. NICE 2019. Nutrition support for adults: oral nutrition support, enteral tube feeding and parental nutrition. London: NICE, 2019. Available from: https://www.nice.org.uk/guidance/cg32/resources/nutrition-support-for-adults-oral-nutrition-support-enteral-tube-feeding-and-parenteral-nutrition-pdf-975383198917

18. NICE 2017. Recognising and prevention delirium: A quick guide for care home managers | Quick guides to social care topics | Social care | NICE Communities | About. Available at: https://www.nice.org.uk/about/nice-communities/social-care/quick-guides/recognising-and-preventing-delirium#:~:text=Hypoactive%20delirium[Accessed 5 Jan. 2023].

19. O'Malley G et al. The delirium experience: a review. *Journal of Psychosomatic Research* 2008, 65: 223–228.

20. Richardson, S. J. (2020). The DECIDE Study: Delirium and Cognitive Impact in Dementia (Doctoral dissertation, Newcastle University).

21. Wilson JE, Mart MF, Cunningham, C et al. Delirium. *Nat Rev Dis Primers* 2020, 6:90. https://doi.org/10.1038/s41572-020-00223-4

22. Witlox J, Eurelings LS, de Jonghe JF, et al. Delirium in elderly patients and the risk of postdischarge mortality, institutionalization, and dementia: a meta-analysis. *Jama* 2010, 304(4): 443–451.

23. Zazzara et al. Probable delirium is a presenting symptom of COVID-19 in frail, older adults: a cohort study of 322 hospitalised and 535 community-based older adults. *Age and Ageing* 2020, 50(1): 40–48. doi: https://doi.org/10.1093/ageing/afaa223.

Further Information

European Delirium Association https://www.europeandeliriumassociation.org/

Greater Manchester Hospital Delirium Toolkit https://dementia-united.org.uk/greater-manchester-hospital-delirium-toolkit/

Royal College of Physicians The prevention, diagnosis, and management of delirium in older people – national guidelines.

Royal College of Physicians. Guidelines for health professionals working with people with delirium.

Royal College of Psychiatrists Delirium https://www.rcpsych.ac.uk/mental-health/problems-disorders/delirium

The British Geriatrics Society Delirium Hub https://www.bgs.org.uk/resources/delirium-hub-introduction

Training Resources

Dementia United. Resources: https://dementia-united.org.uk/resources/

Health Education England. Raising awareness of delirium http://portal.e-lfh.org.uk/Component/Details/664998 https://www.nice.org.uk/about/nice-communities/social-care/quick-guides/recognising-and-preventing-delirium

The British Geriatrics Society Delirium Hub: Education and training https://www.bgs.org.uk/resources/delirium-hub-education-and-training

West Yorkshire and Healthcare Partnership. Raising awareness and training of delirium. https://www.wypartnership.co.uk/our-priorities/mental-health/mental-health/dementia/raising-awareness-and-training-delirium

Dyspnoea

1. Introduction

- Dyspnoea (pronounced *duhsp-nee-uh*) is a subjective feeling of breathlessness that is felt by patients when there is an underlying acute or chronic pathology and is one of the most common presentation faced by ambulance clinicians.
- Dyspnoea is a common but important clinical symptom present in up to half of patients admitted to acute hospitals, increasing significantly during winter months.
- Dyspnoea may indicate underlying pathology for a large range of conditions (refer to Table 3.48), particularly those affecting the respiratory and cardiac systems.
- The most common causes of acute dyspnoea are asthma, chronic obstructive pulmonary disease (COPD), heart failure and infection (often pneumonia).
- Many people living with long-term respiratory or cardiac conditions have poor quality of life due to chronic dyspnoea, fatigue and other symptoms.
- Some patients with respiratory conditions will have their own pulse oximeter to monitor their saturations and may contact the ambulance service should their oxygen saturations drop below their target.
- Patients may describe the sensation as:
  - Sensation of work or effort
  - Tightness
  - Air hunger/unsatisfied inspiration (BMJ).
- Acute episodes of dyspnoea often have a pulmonary or cardiac cause. Asthma, cardiogenic pulmonary oedema, COPD, pneumonia, cardiac ischaemia, and interstitial lung disease are common causes and account for approximately 85% of all ED cases of dyspnoea. In 15% of cases dyspnoea is unexplained.
- Breathlessness can be classified by speed of onset:
  - **Acute** — when it develops suddenly or in a matter of minutes.
  - **Subacute** — when it develops over hours or days.
  - **Chronic** — when it develops over weeks or months.
- An acute/subacute worsening of dyspnoea in a patient with a known cardiovascular, pulmonary, or neuromuscular condition may represent a deterioration of the underlying condition or the appearance of a new problem. Rapid treatment and conveyance to an appropriate hospital should be undertaken unless an advance care plan states otherwise.
- Dyspnoea may also present in patients towards the terminal stage of illness or actively dying (refer to **End of Life Care**).
- Many cases of dyspnoea can be managed by community teams, and person-centred, holistic management is paramount. Depending on the underlying cause, alternatives to ED and management in the community can be considered with direct referral to Same Day Emergency Care (SDEC), urgent community response teams (UCR), primary care specialist or advanced paramedics or other appropriate community team for rapid community review and management based on local pathways.

2. Severity and Outcome

- Dyspnoea is an important clinical symptom which in some circumstances can be severe or life-threatening. Dyspnoea varies in intensity and can be a distressing symptom, especially for patients at the end of life.
- Not all patients presenting with dyspnoea are life threatening, and some patients may experience dyspnoea as part of their normal disease pattern, such as those living with COPD or heart failure.
- Time course:
  - Acute dyspnoea appears over **minutes to hours**. Many presentations of this nature may be life-threatening, such as pulmonary embolism, myocardial infarction, anaphylaxis, foreign body aspiration or cardiogenic shock.
  - Sub-acute dyspnoea appears over **hours to days**. Acute exacerbations of long-term conditions such as asthma, COPD, infection or heart failure may present this way, as well as sub-acute pulmonary emboli. Less common causes include cardiac tamponade, myocarditis or superior vena cava syndrome.
  - Chronic dyspnoea appears over **weeks to months**. This is patients living with chronic or long-term conditions experiencing dyspnoea as their baseline, but varying day to day. Such diagnoses include COPD, pulmonary fibrosis, heart failure, valvular heart disease or chronic anaemia.
  - Dyspnoea that comes and goes may indicate a transient problem, such as paroxysmal tachycardia or intermittent heart blocks.
- Many patients experiencing dyspnoea, especially those with long-term conditions, may be suitable for community treatment. Depending on the underlying cause, alternatives to ED and management in the community can be considered with direct referral to urgent community response teams (UCR), Same Day Emergency Care (SDEC), primary care specialist or advanced paramedics or other appropriate community team for rapid community review and management based on local pathways.
- These patients may have an advance care plan, such as a ReSPECT form, which will guide your treatment and conveyance decisions. Where

Dyspnoea

available, seek joint decision making with a senior clinician.

- Dyspnoea from any cause can manifest in anxiety, however a diagnosis of anxiety is a **diagnosis of exclusion**, and all other differentials should be ruled out before discharge.
- **For details of the severity and outcome for specific conditions refer to the individual guidelines.**

3. Pathophysiology

- Dyspnoea is a multi-dimensional process involving physiological and psychological systems. There are many causes of dyspnoea which should be explored during history taking. Table 3.48 details these.
- The respiratory system is designed to match alveolar ventilation with metabolic demand. Disruption of this process may lead to the conscious awareness of breathing and dyspnoea. Dyspnoea is an uncomfortable sensation and may include chest tightness, air hunger, effortful breathing, the urge to cough and a sense of suffocation.
- Some patients living with long term conditions such as COPD or heart failure may have normally abnormal clinical signs and symptoms, such as lower oxygen saturations. Patients tend to know what is normal for them, and they are often documented in their care plans. These should routinely be asked as part of history taking.
- It must be noted that dyspnoea does not always mean the patient is hypoxemic, and similarly those living with chronic hypoxaemia may not present with dyspnoea.
- Dyspnoea in pregnancy should always be treated with a high degree of suspicion, as pregnant patients are more susceptible to DVT and pulmonary embolism.
- Increases of patients presenting with dyspnoea has been shown to be linked with health inequalities, social and environmental factors. Air pollution, social-economic deprivation, and internal mould have all been linked to worsening of chronic conditions and increased 999 calls for dyspnoea, or exacerbation of long-term conditions. This is particularly pertinent for the very young, or patients living with frailty. As ambulance staff, we are privileged to experience patient's environments, and must act on any reversible environmental factors we see. Usually, this will be in the form of a safeguarding referral.
- During extremes of temperature, there may be more patients presenting with dyspnoea due to exacerbated long term conditions and seasonal infections. These are more prevalent in patients over age 65 and under fives. Consider carbon monoxide poisoning particularly during winter months and consider making safeguarding or fire home safety referrals as per local pathways. Refer to **Overdose and Poisoning in Adults and Children**.

TABLE 3.48 – Causes of Dyspnoea

Pulmonary causes	Cardiac causes	Other causes
Acute exacerbation of asthma.	Aortic aneurysm.	Anaphylaxis.
Bronchiectasis.	Aortic dissection.	Carbon monoxide exposure.
COPD including acute exacerbation.	Cardiac arrhythmia.	Chemicals/poisons.
Cystic fibrosis.	Cardiac tamponade.	Diabetic ketoacidosis.
Flail chest.	Heart failure including acute exacerbation.	Diaphragmatic splinting – obesity ascites.
Interstitial lung disease.	Ischaemic heart disease.	Pregnancy due to physiological changes.
Lung/lobar collapse.	Myocardial infarction (consider atypical presentations without chest pain).	End of life.
Massive haemothorax.		Epiglottitis.
Pleural effusion.	Pericarditis.	Hyperventilation/Anxiety.
Pneumonia/Lower respiratory tract infection.	Superior vena cava syndrome.	Medication – Short-term opioid or sedative use (in patients with long term respiratory conditions).
Pneumothorax.	Valvular dysfunction.	Metabolic causes.
Pulmonary embolism.		Neuromuscular disorders (Guillan-Barre Syndrome, Myasthenia Gravis).
Upper airway obstruction.		Pain.
Viral respiratory infections.		Sepsis.
		Severe hypovolaemia.
		Severe anaemia.
		Thyrotoxicosis.

Dyspnoea

4. Assessment and Management

- Diagnosis of the underlying cause of the patient's presenting illness can be difficult and may require in-hospital investigations. Assessment must include a detailed history and a thorough physical examination. For the assessment and management of patients with dyspnoea refer to Table 3.50.
- For patients living with chronic conditions or frailty, hospital conveyance may not be in their best interest or be the patient's preferred place of care, and community or primary care teams may be better placed to assess and treat a dyspnoea. Consider SDEC, UCR, primary care, specialist or advanced paramedic, or other community referral.
- Clinical decisions around non-conveyance and treatment must be guided by the patient's wishes, any advance care plans, and in all cases be in the patient's best interest. Senior clinical support should be sought for joint decision making. Consider if the patient is already known to community services for their condition.

TABLE 3.49 – Differential Diagnosis for Common Conditions

Condition	Symptoms	Signs	Auscultation or audible sounds	History
Acute exacerbation of asthma Refer to **Asthma in Adults and Children**	Dyspnoea Cough Unable to complete sentences	Wheeze Tachypnoea Tachycardia Pulsus paradoxus Hyperresonant chest Accessory muscle use	Decreased or absent breath sounds if severe Wheeze	Previous asthma Recent increase in inhaler use Allergen exposure Concurrent LRTI
Acute Coronary Syndrome, for example, STEMI or NSTEMI Refer to **Acute Coronary Syndrome**	Central chest pain for >15 minutes, constricting or crushing that radiates to arm/neck (chest pain may be absent in female patients, advanced age or diabetic patients) Dyspnoea	Tachycardia Arrhythmia Pallor/Reduction in normal skin colour Diaphoretic	Wheeze Crepitations	Symptoms suggestive of ischaemic heart disease (IHD) or previous investigations for chest pain
Acute Heart Failure Refer to **Heart Failure**	Dyspnoea especially on exertion Orthopnoea/paroxysmal nocturnal dyspnoea Cough producing frothy, white or pink phlegm	Peripheral oedema Tachycardia Raised JVP Pleural effusion	Heart murmur Crepitations	Angina Hypertension History of heart failure, for example, left ventricular failure, right ventricular failure or cor pulmonale Valvular dysfunction or congenital heart problems

(continued)

Dyspnoea

TABLE 3.49 – Differential Diagnosis for Common Conditions *(continued)*

Condition	Symptoms	Signs	Auscultation or audible sounds	History
Anaphylaxis Refer to **Allergic Reactions including Anaphylaxis**	Dyspnoea Dysphagia Chest tightness Confusion Hypoxia/Cyanosis Circulatory collapse	Tachycardia Tachypnoea Erythema Urticaria Angioedema Pharyngeal or laryngeal oedema Pallor/Reduction in normal skin colour	Decreased breath sounds Wheeze Stridor	Allergen exposure
Chronic Obstructive Pulmonary Disease (COPD) Refer to **Chronic Obstructive Pulmonary Disease**	Progressive dyspnoea Chest tightness Cough – increase in sputum volume or colour Confusion Ankle swelling	New-onset cyanosis Peripheral oedema Accessory muscle use Pursed lip breathing Decreased oxygen saturations (more than normal)	Course crepitations Wheeze	Smoking >35 years of age
End of life dyspnoea Refer to **End of Life Care**	Dyspnoea	Tachypnoea	Decreased breath sounds	Long term respiratory conditions such as COPD or heart failure
Foreign Body Airway Obstruction (FBAO) Refer to **Foreign Body Airway Obstruction**	Dyspnoea Inability to speak Cough	Clutching at neck Sudden onset Cyanosis	Stridor Wheeze	Eating – especially fish, meat, or poultry Illicit drug ingestion or substance misuse
Hyperventilation Refer to **Hyperventilation Syndrome**	Dyspnoea Acute agitation and anxiety Chest pain which may resemble angina pectoris Palpitations	Sudden dyspnoea Hyperpnoea Tachypnoea Numbness and tingling in the limbs and around the mouth	Clear chest	**NB** ensure other more serious conditions are excluded before considering this diagnosis
Pneumonia/LRTI Refer to **Medical Emergencies in Adults – Overview** and **Medical Emergencies in Children – Overview**	Dyspnoea Fever Cough	Tachycardia Decreased oxygen saturations CRB-65 score	Coarse or fine crepitations Dull percussion	Smoking Ischaemic heart disease (IHD) Mould exposure

Dyspnoea

TABLE 3.49 – Differential Diagnosis for Common Conditions *(continued)*

Condition	Symptoms	Signs	Auscultation or audible sounds	History
Pneumothorax Refer to **Thoracic Trauma**	Dyspnoea Sudden onset pleuritic chest pain	Dyspnoea	Decreased breath sounds Hyper-resonant percussion	Trauma Previous pneumothorax COPD Asthma Smoking Tall, thin stature
Pulmonary Embolism Refer to **Pulmonary Embolism**	Dyspnoea Pleuritic chest pain Cough or haemoptysis Possible DVT Leg oedema Syncope Fever	Tachycardia Tachypnoea Fever ECG: Non-specific ST wave changes Hypotension	Focal crepitations	Prolonged immobilisation Recent surgery Thrombotic disease Active cancer Pregnancy DVT Previous history of DVT or PE Smoking Obesity Oral contraceptive pill use
Pleural Effusion	Localised chest pain Progressive dyspnoea	Dull percussion Reduced chest wall movements on affected side	Decreased or absent breath sounds Pleural 'rub'	May be associated with pneumonia or heart failure
Epiglottitis	Rapidly progressing sore throat Fever Dyspnoea Dysphagia	Drooling Stridor Unwell looking Tripod position Irritable		Can occur **in all age groups and is becoming more prevalent due to decreased uptake of Hib Vaccine** 2–3 days of worsening symptoms followed by acute airway obstruction

Dyspnoea

TABLE 3.50 – ASSESSMENT and MANAGEMENT of: Dyspnoea

NB Take a defibrillator at the earliest opportunity and keep this with the patient until handover/discharge.

Assess <C>ABCDE

- If any of the following **TIME-CRITICAL** features present:
  - major **<C>ABCDE** problems, refer to **Medical Emergencies in Adults – Overview** and **Medical Emergencies in Children – Overview**
  - extreme airway/breathing difficulty or cyanosis
  - features of life-threatening asthma, refer to **Asthma in Adults and Children**
  - features of tension pneumothorax or major chest trauma, refer to **Thoracic Trauma**
  - acute myocardial infarction, refer to **Acute Coronary Syndrome**
  - anaphylaxis, refer to **Allergic Reactions including Anaphylaxis**
  - foreign body airway obstruction, refer to **Foreign Body Airway Obstruction**
  - reduced level of consciousness, refer to **Altered Level of Consciousness**, then:
- Start correcting **<C>ABCDE** problems
- Undertake a **TIME-CRITICAL** transfer to the nearest receiving hospital.
- Continue patient management en route.
- Consider a hospital pre-alert call.

Position

- Position the patient for comfort, usually sitting upright.

Ask the Patient If They Have an Individualised Treatment Plan

- Be aware that the patient may have a treatment plan or an advance care plan – consider discussion with a senior clinician.
- Patients with long term conditions will often be able to guide their care and have an advance care plan, ReSPECT form or DNACPR form in place.
- Hospital conveyance may not be in their best interest or be the patient's preferred place of care, and community or primary care teams may be better placed to assess and treat a dyspnoea. Consider SDEC, UCR, primary care, specialist or advanced paramedic, or other community referral.
- Patients may also be known to a named community team. Consider contacting these providers prior to conveyance.

If the patient is not time-critical

- Obtain a thorough history to help identify the cause of dyspnoea.

Specifically assess:

- Effort and effectiveness of ventilation – rate and depth.
- Level of consciousness.
- Skin – cyanosis/diaphoresis/pallor/capillary refill time.
- Duration of difficulty breathing – acute, sub-acute, chronic or intermittent?
- Pain associated with breathing – any pattern of breathing/depth of respiration?
- Associated syncope? Chest pain? Fever? Palpitations?
- Signs of DVT? Consider PE.
- 12-Lead ECG.
- Advanced age, male sex, multiple co-morbidities, cancer, chronic renal disease, low systolic blood pressure and abnormal temperature are associated with increased mortality when dyspnoea is the presenting complaint.
- Do certain positions exacerbate breathing (e.g. unable to lie down, must sit upright, sleeping with more pillows)?
- Does the patient have a cough?

Dyspnoea

TABLE 3.50 – ASSESSMENT and MANAGEMENT of: Dyspnoea *(continued)*
NB Take a defibrillator at the earliest opportunity and keep this with the patient until handover/discharge.

- If yes, is the cough productive:
  - **sputum or bubbling**: consider infection or heart failure
  - **frothy white/pink sputum**: consider acute heart failure
  - **yellow/green sputum**: consider chest infection
  - **haemoptysis**: consider PE, chest infection or carcinoma of the lung.
- Has the patient increased their use of respiratory medications/inhalers recently?
- Signs of anaphylaxis:
  - urticarial rash
  - facial swelling
  - circulatory collapse.
- Is the patient on long term oxygen therapy (LTOT) and have they had to increase their oxygen lately?
- Impact on activities of daily living, and managing at home – walking, dressing etc. (exercise tolerance).
- Rockwood Clinical Frailty Score (refer to **Medical Emergencies in Adults – Overview**).
- Calculate CRB-65 for community acquired pneumonia? (See Table 3.51)
- Sore throat and drooling – consider Epiglottitis.
- Smoking/vaping history.
- Recent travel history.
- Close contact with anyone else unwell.

Percuss the Chest

To determine if there are collections of air (pneumothorax) or fluid (pneumonia, pleural effusion, haemothorax) in the lungs.

Auscultate the Chest

To determine adequacy of air entry on both sides of the chest.

To determine chest sounds:
- audible wheeze on expiration – consider asthma, ACS, anaphylaxis, COPD or heart failure (especially in older patients with no history of asthma).
- audible stridor (upper airway narrowing) – consider anaphylaxis, or foreign body airway obstruction.
- crepitations (fine crackling in lung bases) – ACS, heart failure.
- rhonchi (harsher, rattling sound) indicating collections of fluid in larger airways – pneumonia.
- rales (clicking, rattling or crackling noises) – heart failure, COPD, pulmonary embolism.

Consider Possible Causes

- Refer to Table 3.48 and Table 3.49.

Known cause

- If the cause of dyspnoea is known follow relevant guideline, as per Table 3.49.
- Exacerbations of chronic conditions can often be managed in the community by referral to UCR, primary care, or other community teams – if in the patient's best interest contact these teams prior to conveyance.

Unknown cause

- If cause of dyspnoea unknown refer to **Medical Emergencies in Adults – Overview** and **Medical Emergencies in Children – Overview** and follow management below.
- Have a low threshold for conveying a patient with unexplained dyspnoea to ED in order to rule out serious diagnosis.
- Anxiety is a diagnosis of exclusion, and all other pathologies should be ruled out before discharging the patient.
- Dyspnoea as a symptom will cause a patient to feel anxious.

(continued)

Dyspnoea

TABLE 3.50 – ASSESSMENT and MANAGEMENT of: Dyspnoea *(continued)*

NB Take a defibrillator at the earliest opportunity and keep this with the patient until handover/discharge.

Ventilation

Consider assisted ventilation at a rate of 12–20 breaths per minute if:

- SpO_2 is <90% on high concentration O_2, or
- Expansion is inadequate, refer to **Airway and Breathing Management**.

If the patient has a diagnosis of COPD or other respiratory conditions, they may know their own target oxygen saturations and have an oxygen alert card – manage accordingly (refer to **Chronic Obstructive Pulmonary Disease**).

Fluid

- Administer fluid as required, refer to **Intravascular Fluid Therapy in Adults** and **Intravascular Fluid Therapy in Children**.

Pain Management

- Administer pain relief if indicated, refer to **Pain Management in Adults and Children**.
- Have a low threshold for administration of morphine for those patients at end of life presenting with dyspnoea (refer to **End of Life Care**).

Transfer or Referral to Further Care

- Patients with an unexplained cause of dyspnoea.
- Where the cause is known refer to the relevant guideline for care pathway.
- For pregnant patients presenting with dyspnoea, a low threshold for conveyance should be adopted, even if they look well – all pregnant patients should be discussed with a senior clinician prior to discharge.
- If a community referral pathway exists for the identified presentation, seek to refer where the patient meets the criteria.
- Hospital conveyance may not be in their best interest or be the patient's preferred place of care, and community or primary care teams may be better placed to assess and treat a dyspnoea. Consider SDEC, UCR, primary care, specialist or advanced paramedic, or other community referral.

TABLE 3.51 – CRB-65 Score for Community Acquired Pneumonia

Confusion	+ 1 point
Respiratory rate ≥30	+ 1 point
Blood Pressure <90 mmHg or Diastolic BP ≤60 mmHg	+ 1 point
Age ≥65	+ 1 point
Score	Total/4
Low Risk Group: 0 Points: 0.6% 30-Day mortality. Consider community referral.	
Low Risk Group: 1 Point: 2.7% 30-Day mortality. Consider community referral.	
Moderate Risk Group: 2 Points: 6.8% 30-day mortality. Consider inpatient treatment of community referral.	
Severe Risk Group: 3 Points: 14% 30-Day mortality. Consider Inpatient admission/ITU involvement.	
Highest Risk Group: 4 Points: 27.8% 30-Day mortality. Consider Inpatient admission/ITU involvement	

Reference: Lim et al. (2003); Metley at al. (2019)

Dyspnoea

> **KEY POINTS!**
>
> **Dyspnoea**
> - Is dyspnoea a result of respiratory, cardiac, both or other causes?
> - Consider time-critical causes.
> - Dyspnoea can be acute, sub-acute, chronic, or intermittent.
> - Consider possible causes and refer to relevant guidelines for assessment and management.
> - Dyspnoea may be experienced by those at end of life or actively dying.
> - Consider environmental causes and refer to safeguarding where appropriate.
> - Anxiety is a diagnosis of exclusion, and dyspnoea itself can cause anxiety.
> - Many presentations of dyspnoea are suitable for community treatment and referral.

Bibliography

1. Parshall MB, Schwartzstein RM, Adams L, Banzett RB, Manning HL, Bourbeau J, et al. An official American Thoracic Society statement: update on the mechanisms, assessment, and management of dyspnea. *American Journal of Respiratory and Critical Care Medicine* 2012, 185(4): 435–452.

2. Kemp S and Hopkin J. 2020. *The clinical presentation of respiratory disease*. In: Firth J, Conlon C and Cox T (Eds.). Oxford Textbook of Medicine, 6th edition. Oxford: Oxford University Press.

3. Karras DJ, Sammon ME, Terregino CA, Lopez BL, Griswold SK, Arnold GK. Clinically meaningful changes in quantitative measures of asthma severity. *Academic Emergency Medicine* 2000, 7(4): 327–334.

4. British Medical Journal Best Practice. *Epiglottitis*. 2023. Available from: https://bestpractice.bmj.com/topics/en-gb/452.

5. Hale ZE, Singhal A, Hsia RY. Causes of Shortness of Breath in the Acute Patient: A National Study. *Acad Emerg Med*. 2018. 25(11): 1227–234.

6. British Medical Journal Best Practice. Assessment of *Dyspnoea*. 2023. Available from: https://bestpractice.bmj.com/topics/en-gb/862.

7. National Institute for Health and Care Excellence. *Angio-oedema and Anaphylaxis*. Clinical Knowledge Summaries. 2022. Available from: https://cks.nice.org.uk/topics/angio-oedema-anaphylaxis/diagnosis/diagnosis-of-anaphylaxis/.

8. National Institute for Health and Care Excellence. *Chronic Obstructive Pulmonary Disease*. Clinical Knowledge Summaries. 2023. Available from: https://cks.nice.org.uk/topics/chronic-obstructive-pulmonary-disease/diagnosis/diagnosis-acute-exacerbation/.

9. National Institute for Health and Care Excellence. *Pulmonary Embolism*. Clinical Knowledge Summaries. 2023. Available from: https://cks.nice.org.uk/topics/pulmonary-embolism/.

10. National Institute for Health and Care Excellence. *Breathlessness*. Clinical Knowledge Summaries. 2022. Available from: https://cks.nice.org.uk/topics/breathlessness/.

11. National Institute for Health and Care Excellence. *Pneumonia in adults*. Quality Standard [QS110]. 2016. Available from: https://www.nice.org.uk/guidance/qs110/chapter/quality-statement-1-mortality-risk-assessment-in-primary-care-using-crb65-score

12. National Institute for Health and Clinical Excellence. *Chest Pain – Pulmonary Causes*. Clinical Knowledge Summaries. 2022. Available from: https://cks.nice.org.uk/topics/chest-pain/diagnosis/pulmonary-causes/.

13. British Geriatric Society. *Information for healthcare professionals caring for older people during cold weather*. 2023. Available from: https://www.bgs.org.uk/coldweather.

14. Metlay JP, Waterer GW, Long AC, Anzueto A, Brozek J, Crothers K, Cooley LA, Dean NC, Fine MJ, Flanders SA, Griffin MR, Metersky ML, Musher DM, Restrepo MI, Whitney CG. Diagnosis and Treatment of Adults with Community-acquired Pneumonia. An Official Clinical Practice Guideline of the American Thoracic Society and Infectious Diseases Society of America. *Am J Respir Crit Care Med*. 2019, Oct 1;200(7): e45–e67. doi: 10.1164/rccm.201908–1581ST.

15. Lim WS, van der Eerden MM, Laing R, Boersma WG, Karalus N, Town GI, Lewis SA, Macfarlane JT. Defining community acquired pneumonia severity on presentation to hospital: an international derivation and validation study. *Thorax* 2003, May;58(5): 377–82. doi: 10.1136/thorax.58.5.377. PMID: 12728155; PMCID: PMC1746657.

16. Balen F, et al. Predictive factors for early requirement of respiratory support through phone call to Emergency Medical Call Centre for dyspnoea: a retrospective cohort study. *European journal of emergency medicine: official journal of the European Society for Emergency Medicine* 2023, 30(6): 432–437.

17. Booth S and MJ Johnson. Improving the quality of life of people with advanced respiratory disease and severe breathlessness. *Breathe* 2019, 15(3): 198–215.

18. Christiaens H, et al. Winter virus season impact on acute dyspnoea in the emergency department. *The clinical respiratory journal* 2019, 13(11): 722–727.

19. Kauppi W, et al. Pre-hospital predictors of an adverse outcome among patients with dyspnoea as the main symptom assessed by pre-hospital emergency nurses – a retrospective observational study. *BMC emergency medicine* 2020, 20(1): 89.

20. Le TT, et al. Respiratory events associated with concomitant opioid and sedative use among Medicare beneficiaries with chronic obstructive pulmonary disease. *BMJ open respiratory research* 2020, 7(1).

21. Zhou J, et al. Epidemiology, outcomes and predictors of mortality in patients transported by ambulance for dyspnoea: A population-based cohort study. *Emergency medicine Australasia: EMA* 2023, 35(1): 48–55.

22. Regulation 28 Report to Prevent Future Deaths: Leonard King. (2023). Available from: https://www.judiciary.uk/wp-content/uploads/2023/09/Leonard-King-Prevention-of-future-deaths-report-2023–0294_Published.pdf. Accessed March 2024.

Febrile Illness in Children

1. Introduction

- There are many important differences between children and adults in their anatomy, their physiology and their immunity, as well as differences in the types of illnesses they encounter and the ways these conditions present, develop and progress.
- The assessment and management of children poses many potential pitfalls for the unwary and inexperienced, and presents healthcare providers with significant challenges, whatever the setting.
- Children may struggle to verbalise and communicate their condition to you, adding to the challenges faced when assessing and caring for them.

1.1 'Major' and 'Minor' Childhood Illnesses

- Sick children are notoriously difficult to assess, except when they are obviously very ill or injured, with grossly deranged vital signs. The younger the child, the more difficult the assessment.
- Before considering 'minor' illnesses in children, it is crucial to both appreciate and understand that 'major' childhood illnesses (including life-threatening conditions such as meningococcal disease and sepsis) do not commonly present in extremis, but typically present with relatively innocent features that can easily be mistaken for minor illnesses.
- Children's vital signs may well be deranged when their illness (or injury) is advanced (significant), and these abnormalities should be readily detected. However, earlier in the same illness, these same children may appear relatively well and exhibit 'normal' physiology. There is a risk that the significance of these children's illnesses may not be appreciated if assessed early in the course of their illness.
- In critically ill children, temperature is not routinely recorded as part of the 'ABC' assessment as it delays treatment without altering management.
- Temperature should however be measured in the less-ill child, where it forms part of the picture of their illness and is an essential sign that informs clinical decision making.
- Staff should be familiar with NICE's *Feverish Illness in Children* guidance (on which this guideline is based).

1.2 Fever

- Normal body temperature is 37°C. A temperature of 38°C and above is likely to be significant.
- Fever is part of the immune system's response to infection and is not thought to be harmful (although lay people often assume that it is).
- It can herald a significant underlying infection, hence the importance of identifying its cause.
- Throughout most of childhood, the height of the fever bears little relationship to the gravity of the illness, although in babies aged under 6 months a high temperature is much more likely to be significant.
- When facing serious infections, small babies often have unstable body temperatures and may paradoxically present with a low body temperature.
- Febrile illnesses in children aged between 6 months and 5 years can produce a seizure – a febrile convulsion – following a rapid rise in body temperature (refer to **Seizures in Children**).
- A child with a fever is a very common presentation. Such children may have a self-limiting viral condition or else another obvious cause, such as an ear infection or upper respiratory tract infection. However, for some febrile children no obvious cause will be found and a small number of these will have a serious illness.
- Ambulance clinicians have an important role to play in the reduction of the mortality rate for children with feverish illness, which remains higher in the UK than in many other European countries. The main priorities are to:
  – Identify any immediately life-threatening features.
  – Assess whether the child has (i) a serious illness requiring intervention or (ii) a self-limiting illness, without necessarily diagnosing a specific condition.
  – Determine a likely source of the illness to direct specific treatment.
  – Make appropriate management decisions based upon the results of the assessment.
- NICE defines a fever as 'an elevation of body temperature above the normal daily variation'. It recognises that this is often hard to define, as normal temperature varies depending on the individual, the body site where temperature is measured and the time of day.

2. Incidence

- Febrile illness is the most common medical problem in childhood. Younger children are the most vulnerable due to the immaturity of their immune systems. By the age of 18 months, an otherwise healthy child would be expected to have had around eight acute febrile illnesses.

3. Severity and Outcome

- Infectious diseases are a major cause of childhood mortality and morbidity.
- Most febrile illnesses are due to self-limiting viral infections requiring little or no intervention. However, fever is a common presenting feature of serious bacterial infections (SBI) such as meningitis, septicaemia, urinary tract infections and

Febrile Illness in Children

pneumonia, and distinguishing between a simple viral infection and a more serious bacterial infection is a real diagnostic challenge. 1% of the UK's under-5 population will have an SBI each year.

4. Assessment

4.1 Febrile Child Assessment

Carry out a primary survey immediately on any ill child to exclude any evidence of life-threatening illness. For the assessment and management of a febrile child, refer to Table 3.52.

- Use the traffic light system shown in Table 3.53 to support the assessment and management of the child.
- When assessing children with learning disabilities, take the individual child's learning disability into account when interpreting the traffic light table.

TABLE 3.52 – ASSESSMENT and MANAGEMENT of: a Febrile Child

Assess <C>ABCDE
- If any of the following **TIME-CRITICAL** features are present:
  - Major **<C>ABCDE** problems (refer to **Medical Emergencies in Children – Overview**).
  - Active seizure (refer to **Seizures in Children**).
- Start correcting any **<C>ABCDE** problems.
- Undertake a **TIME-CRITICAL** transfer to nearest appropriate receiving hospital.
- Continue patient management en route.
- Provide an ATMIST information call.

Respiratory Rate
- Measure and record respiratory rate. For specific ranges, refer to Table 3.55.

Pulse
- Measure and record pulse. For specific ranges, refer to Table 3.55.

Oxygen Saturation
- Monitor the patient's SpO_2; administer oxygen to achieve saturations of >92% if the patient presents as hypoxemic on air (refer to **Oxygen**).

Blood Pressure and Fluids
- Measure and record blood pressure; if required, administer fluids (refer to **Intravascular Fluid Therapy in Children**).

Blood Glucose
- If appropriate, measure and record blood glucose for hypo/hyperglycaemia (refer to **Glycaemic Emergencies in Adults and Children**).

Overall Assessment
- AVPU.
- Consider the overall impression of the child (e.g. playful, lively, disinterested, miserable, floppy etc.).
- Capillary refill.

Temperature
- Measure and record temperature.

Take and Record a Full History
- Length of illness.
- Other symptoms besides fever, specifically asking about:
  - urinary symptoms
  - abdominal pain
  - abnormal skin colour, cold hands and feet, muscle pains
  - headache, photophobia, neck stiffness
  - other complaints, such as a painful joints, sore throat, ear pain etc.

(continued)

Febrile Illness in Children

TABLE 3.52 – ASSESSMENT and MANAGEMENT of: a Febrile Child *(continued)*
- Is fluid intake adequate? A febrile child needs extra fluids to prevent dehydration. - If they are vomiting, they may become dehydrated and be unable to absorb medication. - Diarrhoea also increases fluid losses, increasing the risk of dehydration. - Underlying (chronic) medical problems, including advice that the parent may have been given by specialists regarding actions to be taken if their child develops a fever. (This should include whether the child is under current investigation or management by a doctor.) - Medications, antibiotics or steroids (or other drugs reducing immunity). To assess a child properly, you will need to be aware of the action of any drug they are taking as this may be relevant. If in doubt, this must be checked. - Any other illness in the family, the nursery or school etc.? - Recent foreign travel – consider malaria or other tropical illness.
ECG
- If required, monitor and record 12-lead ECG. Assess for abnormality (refer to **Cardiac Arrhythmia and Sudden Cardiac Death**).
Assess the Patient's Pain
- Where present, assess the SOCRATES of pain and record initial and subsequent pain scores. - Consider analgesia if appropriate (refer to **Pain Management in Adults and Children**).
Documentation
- Complete documentation to include all clinical findings, advice from other clinicians, onward referral and worsening advice given.

TABLE 3.53 – Traffic Light System for Assessing Paediatric Fever

	Green – Low Risk	Amber – Intermediate Risk	Red – High Risk
Colour (of skin, lips or tongue)	- Normal colour	- Pallor reported by parent/carer	- Pallor/cyanotic/a reduction in normal skin colour. Mottling may be difficult to detect in dark skin
Activity	- Responds normally to social cues - Content/smiles - Stays awake or awakens quickly - Strong normal cry/not crying	- Not responding normally to social cues - No smile - Wakes only with prolonged stimulation - Decreased activity	- No response to social cues - Appears ill to a healthcare professional - Does not wake or if roused does not stay awake - Weak, high-pitched or continuous cry

Respiratory		- Nasal flaring
		- Tachypnoea: respiratory rate
		  – >50 breaths/minute, age 6–12 months
		  – >40 breaths/minute, age >12 months
		- Oxygen saturation ≤95% in air
		- Crackles in the chest
			- Grunting
			- Tachypnoea: respiratory rate >60 breaths/minute
			- Moderate or severe chest indrawing

Febrile Illness in Children

TABLE 3.53 – Traffic Light System for Assessing Paediatric Fever *(continued)*

Circulation and hydration	• Normal skin and eyes
	• Moist mucous membranes
		• Tachycardia:
		  – >160 beats/minute, age <12 months
		  – >150 beats/minute, age 12–24 months
		  – >140 beats/minute, age 2–5 years
		• Capillary refill time ≥3 seconds
		• Dry mucous membranes
		• Poor feeding in infants
		• Reduced urine output
			• Reduced skin turgor

Other	• None of the amber or red symptoms or signs	• Age 3–6 months, temperature ≥39°C • Fever for ≥5 days • Rigors • Swelling of a limb or joint • Non-weight-bearing limb/not using an extremity	• Age <3 months, temperature ≥38°C* • Assess closely for a non-blanching rash using natural light if possible (or non-fluorescent light to avoid a blue tinge) • Consider moistening the skin (if unbroken) to enhance the visibility of skin changes • Bulging fontanelle • Neck stiffness • Status epilepticus • Focal neurological signs • Focal seizures

*Some vaccinations have been found to induce fever in children aged under 3 months.

© NICE 2013 *Table 1 Traffic light system for identifying risk of serious illness.* Available from: www.nice.org.uk/guidance/cg160. All rights reserved. Subject to Notice of rights.

NICE guidance is prepared for the National Health Service in England. All NICE guidance is subject to regular review and may be updated or withdrawn. NICE accepts no responsibility for the use of its content in this product/publication.

Note: The traffic light system does not seek to make a specific diagnosis but simply identifies which symptoms and signs should receive the highest priority, guiding subsequent management.

4.2 Temperature Measurement

- Any reported parental perception of a fever should be considered valid and taken seriously.
- Do not take temperatures orally in the under 5s. Even in older children, it may be easier to avoid using the oral method.
- In order to obtain an accurate temperature, an appropriate thermometer must be used:
  - In children **under** 4 weeks of age, use an electronic thermometer placed in the child's axilla. **NB** The thermometer must be left in place for at least the minimum recommended time, otherwise it may under-record.
  - In children **over** 4 weeks of age, use either an electronic thermometer or a tympanic thermometer.
- Earlier treatment with antipyretics (e.g. paracetamol, ibuprofen) must be considered, as it may mask the child's fever.
- Chemically sensitive strips placed on the forehead are inaccurate and should not be used.
- Mercury-containing, glass thermometers are no longer used, for safety reasons.

4.2.1 Important clinical points

Tachycardia frequently accompanies a fever and is suggestive of an underlying infection, while **tachypnoea** suggests an underlying respiratory illness.

A child's resting heart rate increases 10 bpm for every 1°C rise in body temperature.

Febrile Illness in Children

A **disproportionate tachycardia** – i.e. above the accepted normal range (refer to Table 3.55) having taken account of the fever – is seen in early sepsis and meningococcal disease. Such children must receive further medical assessment.

Other features suggesting sepsis include cold hands and feet, abnormal skin colour and muscle pains in the legs.

Infants and small children with meningococcal disease rarely exhibit 'classical' textbook signs (**neck stiffness, photophobia** and **non-blanching rash**), but more commonly present with features that might suggest a non-specific viral illness such as an upper respiratory tract infection (URTI) or gastroenteritis.

In such circumstances, seek (and document) evidence to rule out the possibility of meningococcal disease.

- Conduct an assessment of dehydration (refer to **Paediatric Gastroenteritis**).
- Examine all other systems (including skin) to determine the source of the fever and estimate the disease severity.
- A positive sign must be 'seen' rather than assumed (e.g. otitis media cannot be diagnosed on a history of 'ear ache' alone). Direct visualisation of the tympanic membrane using an auroscope is required to diagnose otitis media.
- **NB It is possible for a child to have a common infection as well as a more serious underlying one; a child with coryza and runny nose could still have meningitis.**

4.3 Specific Febrile Illnesses

The following potential diagnoses must each be specifically considered; some typical signs and symptoms are shown in Table 3.54:

- **Meningococcal septicaemia** – often the child does not present as acutely as tradition would have it.
- **Meningitis** (pre-school children rarely have neck stiffness).
- **Urinary tract infection (UTI)** – UTIs are particularly common in babies and young children and can cause permanent kidney damage. UTIs can also progress to life-threatening septicaemia. Symptoms can again be very non-specific and include: poor feeding, lethargy and abdominal pains. In hospital practice, clean catch urine samples are collected on every febrile child to exclude UTIs.
- **Pneumonia** – typical chest signs may be absent.
- **Herpes simplex encephalitis** – classical pointers include focal neurological signs and focal seizures.
- **Septic arthritis/osteomyelitis** – fever plus very tender swollen joint(s)/bone(s), with a refusal to weight-bear.
- **Kawasaki's disease** – a collection of signs including: fever for >5 days; cervical lymphadenopathy; mucosal changes in the upper respiratory tract (e.g. redness and cracked lips); peripheral limb changes (e.g. oedema, peeling skin); a non-specific, blanching 'measles-like' rash; and bilateral conjunctival redness.

5. Management

(Using the **Traffic Light System for Assessing Paediatric Fever** as shown in Table 3.53).

5.1 Red Traffic Light Features

Children with any of the NICE Red Traffic Light features or Red Flags must be conveyed to an ED with appropriate paediatric services for further specialist assessment.

Provide an ATMIST pre-alert and convey under emergency driving conditions where required. Consider sepsis or meningitis as possible causes and provide care en route according to Trust/JRCALC guidelines.

TABLE 3.54 – Symptoms and Signs Suggestive of Specific Diseases

Diagnosis to be considered	Symptoms and signs in conjunction with fever
Meningococcal disease	Non-blanching rash, particularly with one or more of the following: - an ill-looking child - lesions larger than 2 mm in diameter (purpura) - capillary refill time ≥3 seconds - neck stiffness
Bacterial meningitis	Neck stiffness Bulging fontanelle Decreased level of consciousness Convulsive status epilepticus

Febrile Illness in Children

TABLE 3.54 – Symptoms and Signs Suggestive of Specific *(continued)*

Herpes simplex encephalitis	Focal neurological signs
	Focal seizures
	Decreased level of consciousness
Pneumonia	Tachypnoea (respiratory rate >60 breaths/min, age 0–5 months; >50 breaths/min, age 6–12 months; >40 breaths/minute, age >12 months)
	Crackles in the chest
	Nasal flaring
	Chest indrawing
	Cyanosis
	Oxygen saturation ≤95%
Urinary tract infection	Vomiting
	Poor feeding
	Lethargy
	Irritability
	Abdominal pain and tenderness
	Urinary frequency or dysuria
Septic arthritis	Swelling of a limb or joint
	Not using an extremity
	Non-weight-bearing
Kawasaki disease	Fever for more than 5 days and at least four of the following: • bilateral conjunctival infection • change in mucous membranes • change in extremities • polymorphous rash • cervical lymphadenopathy

© NICE 2013 Table 2 *Summary table for symptoms and signs suggestive of specific diseases*. Available from: www.nice.org.uk/guidance/cg160. All rights reserved. Subject to Notice of rights.

NICE guidance is prepared for the National Health Service in England. All NICE guidance is subject to regular review and may be updated or withdrawn. NICE accepts no responsibility for the use of its content in this product/publication.

5.2 Amber Traffic Light Features

Children with amber traffic light features may be considered for an alternative treatment pathway. Children presenting with multiple amber features must be considered for hospital assessment.

Note: If a child has amber traffic light features and a decision is made **not** to transport the child OR a child has green traffic light features but a cause for the fever has not been found, the following 'safety nets' **MUST** be put in place:

- The patient MUST be discussed with a GP or paediatric healthcare professional, following local protocols, for urgent follow-up arrangements giving a specified time and place (e.g. for the child to be seen within the next 2–6 hours, exact timing to be decided by the attending staff).

- Direct verbal handover to the doctor is important but may not always be possible.

- The arrangements must be made by the attending ambulance staff.

- **It is not adequate to tell the parents to make their own arrangements to see the GP.**

5.3 Green Traffic Light Features

Children who have only green traffic light features may be managed at home. Record that the child has been assessed as having only green features on the patient clinical record and ensure that negative findings are noted to demonstrate the absence of amber or red features, e.g. no nasal flaring.

Ensure that parents/carers are provided with a patient information leaflet if one is available. They should receive specific, written worsening advice, including expectations on length of illness. Ensure that they are aware of the following:

- Suitable antipyretic interventions available.

Febrile Illness in Children

- The importance of offering the child regular fluids (if breastfeeding, then continue as normal).
- How to identify a non-blanching rash.
- Checking the child during the night.
- Keeping the child away from nursery/school while the fever persists and to notify the nursery/school of the illness.
- The common signs of dehydration:
  - sunken fontanelle
  - dry mouth
  - sunken eyes
  - absence of tears
  - poor overall appearance.

Advise parents/carers to seek further advice if:

- The child has a fit.
- The child develops a non-blanching rash.
- They are worried that the child is becoming dehydrated.
- Nappies are becoming drier or changed much less frequently.
- They feel that the child's health is getting worse.
- They are more worried than when they last received advice.
- The fever lasts longer than 5 days.
- They are distressed or concerned that they are unable to look after their child.

TABLE 3.55 – 'Normal' Paediatric Physiological Values

Age	Respiratory rate (bpm)	Heart rate (bpm)
<1 year	40–60	110–160
1–2 yrs	25–35	110–150
2–5 yrs	25–30	95–140
5–12 yrs	20–25	80–120
Over 12 yrs	15–20	60–100

🚩 TABLE 3.56 – Red Flags

Febrile children fulfilling the following red flag criteria **must** be transported to hospital:

- Any febrile baby <1 month old (irrespective of the absolute temperature).
- Any febrile child <3 months old without an obvious cause (as a minimum, an urgent urine sample will be required).
- Any febrile child <3 years without an obvious cause, if a urine sample cannot be arranged at the time through the GP.
- Those with any signs of serious illness (refer to **Medical Emergencies in Children – Overview**).

🚩 TABLE 3.56 – Red Flags (continued)

- Any child with a significant fever but no localising symptoms or signs, who has received antibiotics within the last 48 hours (signs of meningitis can be masked by antibiotic use; so-called 'partially treated' meningitis).
- Any child on steroids or other medication known to suppress the immune system.
- Any child, regardless of age, where there is any doubt that they could be seriously ill.
- Any child where the social or psychological environment suggests that they may not receive adequate supervision or care if left at home.
- Those with a medical protocol saying that transport is necessary.

Use local referral pathways to inform the child's GP as required. Arrange for infants and children presenting with unexplained fever of 38°C or higher to have a urine sample tested after 24 hours at the latest.

Important clinical points – antipyretics and antibiotics

- Tepid sponging is not recommended. Do not over- or under-dress a child with fever.
- Giving an **antipyretic** such as paracetamol or ibuprofen purely to treat the fever is not necessary, but parental sensitivities should be observed.
- An analgesic/antipyretic may help relieve misery and other unpleasant symptoms that often accompany febrile illnesses (e.g. aches, pains and other symptoms which the child is often unable to fully describe).
- Antipyretics do not protect against febrile convulsions. Giving antipyretics to a child who either has just had a seizure or is thought to be at risk of having a seizure has not been shown to be beneficial.
- Note: Antipyretics are effective, even in children with SBI. It would therefore be wrong to assume that a clinical improvement seen following an antipyretic excludes a serious underlying infection.
- Combinations of paracetamol and ibuprofen should not be given. Only consider alternating these agents if the distress persists or recurs before the next dose is due.
- Paracetamol is normally given every 6 hours and ibuprofen every 8 hours; care needs to be taken not to exceed the maximum dose of each drug in a 24-hour period. A treatment diary may be useful if the parents or carers find it difficult to remember which was the last drug given and at what time.
- **Antibiotics** should not be given to a febrile child where the diagnosis is not known. This can delay the subsequent diagnosis of a serious infection such as meningitis.

Febrile Illness in Children

5.4 Febrile convulsions

Febrile convulsions commonly occur in children who are aged between 6 months and 3 years and who have a temperature greater than 38°C. Most febrile convulsions occur in those aged approximately 18 months, although children up to 5 years of age can be affected.

Ambulance clinicians must not apply the diagnosis of febrile convulsion to patients aged over 5 years; older children require a paediatrician to rule out other causes of the convulsion first.

For the management of active febrile convulsions, refer to **Seizures in Children**.

KEY POINTS!

Febrile Illness in Children

- Febrile illness is the most common paediatric presentation and suggests underlying infection.
- Always seek the underlying cause of the fever.
- All febrile children must be assessed with a full history and examination.
- Physiological parameters must be measured, documented and compared against age-specific, 'normal' values.
- Significant tachycardia suggests sepsis.
- Use the NICE 'traffic light' system.
- The early features of serious infections are often non-specific (e.g. meningococcal disease often mimics URTIs and gastroenteritis).
- Small children rarely exhibit the 'classical' meningococcal signs – neck stiffness, photophobia or non-blanching rash; these features are more likely in older children and teenagers. In all age groups, important early features include fever, cold hands and feet, abnormal skin colour and muscle pains or confusion.
- Improvement following antipyretics does not rule out a serious underlying infection.
- Antibiotics should not be blindly given to a febrile child where the diagnosis is not known.
- Where a justifiable clinical reason not to transport a child to hospital has been found and a decision made to stay at home, these decisions must be carefully documented.
- Provide a 'safety net', with written information, to any febrile child not transferred to hospital.
- If uncertain, seek advice from either their GP or out-of-hours doctor.
- The GP should be routinely informed of any consultation.

Bibliography

1. National Collaborating Centre for Women's and Children's Health. *Urinary Tract Infection in Children: Diagnosis, treatment and long-term management* (CG54). London: Royal College of Obstetricians and Gynaecologists, 2007. Available from: http://www.nice.org.uk/nicemedia/pdf/CG54fullguideline.pdf.

2. Hanna CM, Greenes DS. How much tachycardia in infants can be attributed to fever? *Annals of Emergency Medicine* 2004, 43(6): 699–705.

3. Hay AD, Costelloe C, Redmond NM, Montgomery AA, Fletcher M, Hollinghurst S, et al. Paracetamol plus ibuprofen for the treatment of fever in children (PITCH): randomised controlled trial. *British Medical Journal* 2008, 337: a1302.

4. National Collaborating Centre for Women's and Children's Health. *Feverish Illness in Children: Assessment and initial management in children younger than 5 years* (CG47). London: National Institute for Health and Clinical Excellence, 2007.

5. National Collaborating Centre for Women's and Children's Health. *Patient's Information Sheet.* London: National Institute for Health and Clinical Excellence, 2007.

6. National Collaborating Centre for Women's and Children's Health. *Bacterial Meningitis and Meningococcal Septicaemia: Management of bacterial meningitis and meningococcal septicaemia in children and young people younger than 16 years in primary and secondary care* (CG102). London: National Institute for Health and Clinical Excellence, 2010. Available from: https://www.nice.org.uk/guidance/cg102.

7. Woollard M, Pitt K. Antipyretic pre-hospital therapy for febrile convulsions: does the treatment fit? A literature review. *Health Education* 2003, 62(1): 23–28.

8. Sharp A. Management of febrile convulsions within the pre-hospital environment. *Journal of Paramedic Practice* 2016, 8(9): 447–451.

9. National Institute for Health and Clinical Excellence. *Febrile Convulsions.* NICE Clinical Knowledge Summaries. NICE, 2013. Available from: https://cks.nice.org.uk.

10. National Institute for Health and Clinical Excellence. *Feverish Illness in Children: Assessment and Initial Management in children younger than five years.* NICE, 2013. Available from: https://www.nice.org.uk/guidance/cg160/resources/fever-in-children-younger-than-5-years-pdf-246224941765.

11. National Institute for Health and Care Excellence. *Fever in Under 5s: Assessment and initial management* [CG160]. London: NICE, 2017. Available from: https://www.nice.org.uk/guidance/cg160.

Gastrointestinal Bleeding

1. Introduction

Gastrointestinal (GI) bleeding is a common medical emergency accounting for 7,000 admissions per year in Scotland alone.

Gastrointestinal haemorrhage is commonly divided into:

- Upper gastrointestinal haemorrhage.
- Lower gastrointestinal haemorrhage.

2. Incidence

- Upper GI bleeding is more common than lower GI bleeding and is more prevalent in socioeconomically deprived areas.
- Upper GI bleeding accounts for up to 85% of gastrointestinal bleeding events.

3. Severity and Outcome

- The severity of gastrointestinal bleeding can range from clinically insignificant blood loss to significant life-threatening haemorrhage.
- Death is uncommon in patients less than 40 years of age; it is estimated that the overall mortality rate in the UK for patients admitted with acute GI bleeding is approximately 7%. The majority of deaths occur in older people, particularly those with comorbidities. There are many factors that are associated with a poor outcome, including liver disease, acute haemodynamic disturbance, clotting abnormalities, continued bleeding, haematemesis, haematochezia and elevated blood urea.
- Upper GI bleeding tends to be more severe and in extreme circumstances can rapidly lead to hypovolaemic shock.

4. Pathophysiology

- The upper gastrointestinal tract comprises the oesophagus, stomach and duodenum. For common causes of bleeding, refer to Table 3.57.
- The lower gastrointestinal tract comprises the lower part of the small intestine, the colon, rectum and anus. Common causes of bleeding include diverticular disease, inflammatory bowel disease, haemorrhoids and tumour.

4.1 ACUTE UPPER GI BLEEDING

- More than 50% of cases are due to peptic ulcers which, together with oesophagitis and gastritis, account for up to 90% of all upper GI bleeding in older people. Eighty-five percent of deaths associated with upper GI bleeding occur in persons older than 65 years.
- Patients presenting with upper GI bleeding may have a history of aspirin or non-steroidal anti-inflammatory drug (NSAID) use.
- Only 50% of patients present with haematemesis alone, 30% with melaena and 20% with haematemesis and melaena
- Patients with haematemesis tend to have greater blood loss than those with melaena alone. Patients older than 60 years account for up to 45% of all cases (60% of these are women).

TABLE 3.57 – Common Causes of Upper Gastrointestinal Bleeding

Common causes

- Peptic ulcers:
  - Duodenal ulcers
  - Gastric ulcers
- Oesophageal varices
- Gastritis
- Oesophagitis
- Mallory–Weiss tears
- Caustic poison
- Tumour

Peptic Ulcers

- Peptic ulcers are commonly associated with the use of aspirin, non-steroidal anti-inflammatory drugs, corticosteroids, anticoagulants, alcohol and cigarettes.

Oesophageal Varices

- It is estimated that variceal bleeding is the cause of 10% of cases. These patients can bleed severely, with up to 8% dying within 48 hours from uncontrolled haemorrhage. It is commonly associated with alcoholic cirrhosis and increased portal pressure (causing progressive dilation of the veins and protrusion of the formed varices into the lumen of the oesophagus). Spontaneous rupture of the varices will cause the patient to become haemodynamically unstable within a very short period of time due to large volumes of blood loss.

Mallory–Weiss Tears

- Approximately 10% are caused by oesophageal tears, which are more common in the young. Predisposing factors include hiatal hernia and alcoholism. Initiating factors are persistent coughing or severe retching and vomiting, often after an alcoholic binge; haematemesis presents after several episodes of non-bloody emesis. Bleeding can be mild to moderate.

Gastritis

- Drugs, infections, illnesses and injuries can cause inflammation of the lining of the stomach and lead to bleeding.

Gastrointestinal Bleeding

Oesophagitis
- Gastroesophageal reflux disease or alcohol can lead to inflammation and ulcers in the lining of the oesophagus which may lead to bleeding.

Tumour
- A tumour in the oesophagus, stomach or duodenum can cause bleeding.

4.2 ACUTE LOWER GI BLEEDING

Patients with a lower GI bleed commonly present with bright-red/dark blood with clots per rectum (PR); bright-red blood PR in isolation excludes upper GI bleeding in over 98% of cases (unless the patient appears hypovolaemic). Lower GI bleeding is less likely to present with signs of haemodynamic compromise, is more prevalent in men and also has a common history of aspirin or NSAID use. The mean age for lower GI bleeding is 63–77 years, with mortality around 4% (even serious cases have rarely resulted in death). Common causes include:

Diverticular disease
- Diverticular bleeding accounts for up to 55% of cases. Patients commonly present with an abrupt but painless PR bleed. The incidence of diverticular bleeding increases with age.

Inflammatory Bowel Disease
- Major bleeding from ulcerative colitis and Crohn's disease is rare. Inflammatory bowel disease accounts for less than 10% of cases.

Haemorrhoids
- Haemorrhoids account for less than 10% of cases. Bleeding is bright red and usually noticed on wiping or in the toilet bowl. The incidence is high in pregnancy, a result of straining associated with constipation and hormonal changes. Further evaluation may be needed if the patient complains of an alteration of bowel habit and blood mixed with the stool.

Tumour
- Tumour in the large bowel can cause bleeding.

Differential diagnosis
- Post-rectal bleeding can cause significant embarrassment for the patient and care must be taken when assessing female patients that per vaginum (PV) bleeding is excluded.

5. Assessment and Management

For the assessment and management of gastrointestinal bleeding, refer to Table 3.58.

TABLE 3.58 – ASSESSMENT and MANAGEMENT of: Gastrointestinal Bleeding

Assess <C>ABCDE
- If any of the following **TIME-CRITICAL** features present:
  – major **<C>ABCDE** problems (refer to **Medical Emergencies in Adults – Overview** and **Medical Emergencies in Children – Overview**).
  – haematemesis – large volume of bright-red blood
  – haemodynamic compromise
  – decreased level of consciousness.
- Start correcting any **<C>ABCDE** problems.
- Undertake a **TIME-CRITICAL** transfer to nearest appropriate receiving hospital.
- Continue patient management en route.
- Provide an ATMIST information call.

Assess Blood Loss

Where does the bleeding originate – upper or lower GI tract?

- **Haematemesis** – vomited fresh/dark red/brown/black or 'coffee ground' blood (depending on how long it has been in the stomach). Did this occur after an increase in intra-abdominal pressure (e.g. retching or coughing).
- Ascertain how many episodes of non-bloody emesis.
- **Melaena** – malodorous, liquid, black stool or bright-red/dark blood with clots PR. It can be difficult to estimate blood loss when mixed with faeces.
- Estimate blood loss – if not visible, ask the patient or relatives/carers to estimate colour/volume – PR blood loss is difficult to estimate. (**NB** The blood acts as a laxative, but repeated blood-liquid stool, or just blood, is associated with more severe blood loss than maroon/black solid stool.)
- If the patient has suffered unexplained syncope, this may indicate concealed GI bleeding. Ensure PV bleeding is excluded in females.

(continued)

Gastrointestinal Bleeding

TABLE 3.58 – ASSESSMENT and MANAGEMENT of: Gastrointestinal Bleeding *(continued)*

History
- **When did the bleeding begin?**
- Is/has the patient:
  - currently taking or recently taken aspirin or NSAID?
  - currently taking iron tablets?
  - consumed food or drink containing red dye(s)?
  - currently taking beta-blockers or calcium-channel blockers – may mask tachycardia in the shocked patient?
  - currently taking or recently taken anticoagulatory or antiplatelet therapy?
- **Is there a history of:**
  - bleeding disorders?
  - liver disease?
  - abdominal surgery, in particular, abdominal aortic surgery?
  - alcohol abuse?
  - syncope?

Oxygen Saturation
- Monitor the patient's SpO_2; administer oxygen to achieve saturations of >94% if the patient presents as hypoxaemic on air; refer to **Oxygen**.

Respiratory Rate
- Measure and record respiratory rate.

Pulse
- Measure and record pulse.

ECG
- If required, monitor and record 12-lead ECG. Assess for abnormality (refer to **Cardiac Arrhythmia and Sudden Cardiac Death**).

Assess the Patient's Pain
- GI bleeding is not generally associated with pain.
- Where present, assess the SOCRATES of pain and record initial and subsequent pain scores.
- Consider analgesia if appropriate (refer to **Pain Management in Adults and Children**).

Fluid
- Measure and record blood pressure; if required, administer fluids (refer to **Intravascular Fluid Therapy in Adults** and **Intravascular Fluid Therapy in Children**).
- Tranexamic acid is not indicated in GI haemorrhage due to a lack of current evidence for benefit.

Blood Glucose
- If appropriate, measure and record blood glucose for hypo/hyperglycaemia (refer to **Glycaemic Emergencies in Adults and Children**).

Temperature
- Measure and record temperature.

NEWS2
- These observations will enable you to calculate a NEWS2 score (refer to **Sepsis**).

Transfer to Further Care
- Continue patient management en route.
- Provide an alert/information call.

Documentation
- Complete documentation to include all clinical findings, advice from other clinicians, onward referral and worsening advice given.

Gastrointestinal Bleeding

> **KEY POINTS!**
>
> **Gastrointestinal Bleeding**
> - Haematemesis or melaena indicates an upper GI source.
> - Bright-red or dark blood with clots per rectum indicates a lower GI source.
> - Almost all deaths from GI bleeds occur in older people.
> - Approximately 80% of all GI bleeds stop spontaneously or respond to conservative management.
> - Tranexamic acid is not indicated in GI haemorrhage due to a lack of current evidence for benefit.

Bibliography

1. Bennett C, Klingenberg SL, Langholz E, Gluud LL. *Tranexamic acid for upper gastrointestinal bleeding (Review)*. London: Cochrane Library and Wiley, 2014. Available from: https://www.cochranelibrary.com/cdsr/doi/10.1002/14651858.CD006640.pub3/epdf/standard.

2. Scottish Intercollegiate Guidelines Network. *Management of Acute Upper and Lower Gastrointestinal Bleeding* (Guideline 105). Edinburgh: SIGN, 2008.

3. Cappell MS, Friedel D. Initial management of acute upper gastrointestinal bleeding: from initial evaluation up to gastrointestinal endoscopy. *Medical Clinics of North America* 2008, 92: 491–509.

4. Edwards AJ, Maskell GF. Acute lower gastrointestinal haemorrhage. *British Medical Journal* 2009, 339: b4156.

5. Michels SL, Collins J, Reynolds MW, Abramsky S, Paredes-Diaz A, McCarberg B. Over-the-counter ibuprofen and risk of gastrointestinal bleeding complications: a systematic literature review. *Current Medical Research and Opinion* 2012, 28(1): 89–99.

6. Palmer K. Acute upper gastrointestinal haemorrhage. *British Medical Bulletin* 2007, 83(1): 307–324.

7. Szajerka T, Jablecki J. Upper gastrointestinal bleeding in a young female with AIDS: a case report. *International Journal of STD & AIDS* 2012, 23(3): e33–34.

8. van Leerdam ME. Epidemiology of acute upper gastro-intestinal bleeding. *Best Practice & Research in Clinical Gastroenterology* 2008, 22(2): 209–224.

9. Alkhatib AA, Elkhatib FA, Maldonado A, Abubakr SM, Adler DG. Acute upper gastrointestinal bleeding in elderly people: presentations, endoscopic findings, and outcomes. *Journal of the American Geriatrics Society* 2010, 58(1): 182–185.

10. Kent AJ, O'Beirne J, Negus R. The patient with haematemesis and melaena. *Acute Medicine* 2011, 10(1): 45–49.

Glycaemic Emergencies in Adults and Children

1. Introduction

- A person who does not have diabetes normally maintains their blood glucose level within a narrow range.
- This is achieved by a balance between glucose entering the blood stream (from the gastrointestinal tract or from the breakdown of stored energy sources) and glucose leaving the circulation through the action of insulin.
- The prevalence of type 1 diabetes (previously known as juvenile diabetes) is increasing in the adult population. Diagnosis of type 2 diabetes in children is also occurring. It is important to note that type 2 diabetes is not always associated with obesity.

2. Considerations for Patients with Diabetes

2.1 Blood Glucose Monitors

- Prior to testing capillary blood glucose or ketones, the patient's fingers must be cleaned using a non-alcohol based wipe, or gauze with sterile water or sodium chloride, and dried thoroughly with a gauze swab. This prevents contamination of blood glucose results from residual deposits on the skin. Alcohol-based wipes should not routinely be used as research suggests their use may adversely affect blood glucose and ketone readings if the test is taken prior to the alcohol evaporating. Rinsing hands thoroughly in tap water and drying thoroughly is an acceptable alternative.[1,2]
- Blood glucose and ketone meters should be routinely checked for accuracy using control solutions provided by the manufacturer. Patients with type 1 diabetes should have their own meters, and ambulance clinicians may encounter a wide variety of different devices, which may not be regularly checked. It is recommended that clinicians only use service-issue meters.
- Patients with type 2 diabetes may not have their own blood glucose meter, and their blood glucose levels may only be tested sporadically at their GP's surgery. A person with type 2 diabetes and prescribed insulin will normally have been issued with a blood glucose meter by their diabetes team.

2.2 Continuous Glucose Monitors (CGMs) and Flash Glucose Monitoring

- These devices are now very common.[23] These are subcutaneous devices that read interstitial fluid glucose levels at approximately 5-minute intervals.
- These CGM monitors cannot be relied on by ambulance clinicians in lieu of capillary blood glucose testing, as interstitial glucose changes lag behind that of capillary blood glucose and should not be used to influence treatment decisions.

2.3 Blood Ketone Meters

- Most patients with type 1 diabetes will have a blood ketone meter issued to them. These are operated in the same way as blood glucose meters. When available, blood ketone meters can assist the ambulance clinician in determining the risk of diabetic ketoacidosis (DKA).
- When to consider testing for ketones:
  - Any systemically unwell patient with diabetes.
  - Unexplained hyperglycaemia (blood glucose >11 mmol/L).
  - Recent history of starvation and or high alcohol intake (this may be chronic or acute).
  - Clinician concern (e.g. no obvious cause for acute illness).
- Ketone testing should only be performed when indicated (i.e. it is not a standard observation).
- Pregnant women with type 1 diabetes are more prone to ketosis and thus ketoacidosis, even when glucose levels may be relatively normal (i.e. euglycaemia). If there is any doubt they should be referred or conveyed for further assessment either in a maternity assessment unit or an emergency department.
- Ketoacidosis can occur in patients with type 2 diabetes during acute illness.[3,4] DKA has also been observed in those type 2 patients who take a "... flozin " tablet to control their diabetes (dapagliflozin, canagliflozin, empagliflozin, ertugliflozin). It is not uncommon for blood glucose levels to be relatively normal in this situation ('euglycaemic ketoacidosis'). While this is a rare complication of " flozin " treatment, consider ketoacidosis if the patient appears unwell or has symptoms suggestive of DKA.
- Alcoholic ketoacidosis can occur when a person who has alcohol-dependency or prolonged/excessive alcohol use, abruptly stops drinking and also stops eating. The alcohol use reduces the body's ability to generate glucose that can be used by cells, so fatty acids are metabolised instead to create energy and this results in ketoacidosis. The glucose level is usually normal. Refer to **Alcohol-use Disorders**.

Glycaemic Emergencies in Adults and Children

TABLE 3.59 – Blood Ketones and DKA risk levels

DKA Risk Level	Blood Ketone Level	Considerations
Minimal	< 0.6 mmol/L	**Ketonaemia not present** Ketoacidosis unlikely If there is significant hyperglycaemia consider Hyperosmolar Hyperglycaemic State (HHS) Hospital assessment is not required based on ketone level alone but may be required if the patient is systemically unwell and has high blood glucose levels, or for other reasons.
Elevated	0.6 – 2.9 mmol/L	**Ketonaemia present** Ketoacidosis possible Consider conveyance to hospital in the presence of illness and/or vomiting, or where clinical concern is associated with an elevated ketone reading. For non-conveyed patients, follow **Sick-day Rules** principles and refer them to primary care or their diabetes team. The patient should be able to reliably eat and drink, administer additional doses of rapid-acting insulin (as per 'Sick-Day Rules'), retest their glucose and ketones every 2 hours, and know how to access their diabetes team. If there is significant hyperglycaemia (>=30 mmol/L), consider HHS. Children under 1 should always be conveyed to hospital. For children over 1, specialist diabetes teams should always be contacted for ongoing care advice and the child either conveyed to hospital or referred to primary care.
High	>=3.0 mmol/L	**Excessive ketonaemia present** High Risk Ketoacidosis Commence fluid therapy Convey to hospital with pre-alert

2.4 Sick-day Rules

- Illness generally raises blood glucose levels and increases the risk of ketone body production. This can result in DKA if adequate insulin and hydration are not maintained.[5]

- Increased levels of stress hormones during illness may also contribute to high blood glucose levels. Diarrhoea and vomiting may reduce blood glucose levels, with a possibility of hypoglycaemia rather than hyperglycaemia. However, ketones (known as starvation ketones) may still be produced in significant quantities.

- NICE guidelines recommend that people with type 1 diabetes mellitus should be provided with clear guidance for the management of diabetes during periods of illness and many patients with type 1 diabetes will be able to competently manage transient episodes of hyperglycaemia at home. Timely and appropriate sick-day management may prevent progression to DKA and consequent admission to hospital.

General Sick-day Rule Principles

- Never stop the insulin.
- Insulin dosages may need to be increased or decreased depending on blood glucose or ketone levels following advice from their specialist team. Most patients (or parents of paediatric patients) will be aware of the relevant correction dosages. Patients should have access to their specialist team for further advice and support.
- Encourage oral fluids (non-sugar based) to prevent dehydration.
- Increase the frequency of monitoring of blood glucose levels. A minimum of one test every 2 hours is generally suggested.

Glycaemic Emergencies in Adults and Children

- When available, blood ketone levels should also be closely monitored. Urinalysis for ketones can be used, but is less reliable as ketones take longer to be detected and normalised. However, in the absence of a blood ketone meter, urinary ketones may still be used to guide patients on additional insulin doses.

2.5 Insulin Pumps

- Increasing numbers of patients with type 1 diabetes, especially children, now wear insulin pumps. These deliver a continuous flow of rapid-acting insulin via a subcutaneous cannula, combined with manual bolus deliveries for correction doses and at mealtimes to cover the carbohydrate content of the meal.
- At no time should these devices be removed or altered by ambulance clinicians.
- After episodes of hypoglycaemia, patients using insulin pump therapy will generally not need to consume a slow-release carbohydrate, such as a biscuit or toast once blood glucose levels have returned to normal. This is due to being solely on rapid-acting insulin. Patients should be advised to monitor their glucose levels more closely following a hypoglycaemic episode. If in doubt, consult the patient or the child's caregivers.
- Patients using insulin pumps are at a high risk of developing DKA in cases of cannula blockage or pump failure, due to only rapid-acting insulin being infused. If needing to transfer a patient with type 1 diabetes on insulin pump therapy, encourage the patient to bring a supply of pump consumables with them. Hospitals do not routinely stock insulin pump consumables, potentially risking an interruption in insulin delivery for the patient, which may lead to ketosis and DKA. Also advise the patient to take their long-acting and rapid-acting insulin pens with them and, if possible, label them with their name, or ask receiving staff to do so.

Hybrid-closed loop insulin pumps

- Patients with type 1 diabetes may use a hybrid closed-loop insulin pump system which combines the benefits of a CGM device with an insulin pump. The CGM device communicates with the insulin pump which, according to an algorithm in the pump, aims to deliver the correct amount of insulin to achieve a steady glucose level in the target range. These systems are approved and are becomingly increasingly common in type 1 diabetes treatment.
- The hybrid closed-loop system should help protect the person with type 1 diabetes from developing hypoglycaemia as the delivery of insulin ceases/reduces if the patient's glucose level is falling towards the hypoglycaemia range.
- Whilst a hybrid closed-loop system controls the delivery of basal insulin, the person with diabetes is still required to instruct the pump to deliver a bolus dose when eating carbohydrates according to their 'insulin to carb' ratio, e.g. 1 unit insulin for 10 grams carbohydrate.
- There are a variety of combinations of pumps and CGM devices many of which are available with an app on a smart phone, examples include Tandem T-slim pump with DEXCOM G6 sensor, Medtronic 780G with Guardian 4 CGM sensor, YpsoPump with DEXCOM G6 sensor.
- Occasionally, if glucose levels are rising quickly, the pump will discontinue the 'loop' and the system reverts to 'manual' mode with pre-set delivery of hourly basal rates – requiring the user to input manual correction doses.
- A minority of patients with type 1 diabetes will use 'DIY' looping. This term refers to a system set-up by the patient using a CGM device and a pump (which may or may not be in warranty); in this case the algorithm has been developed in an app by the patient. 'DIY' looping is unapproved and whilst these systems have been shown to work successfully, they have not been subject to rigorous clinical trials. Patients who use such systems do so at their own risk.
- Leave all insulin devices and pumps in-situ for hospital teams to manage. **Do not remove devices.**

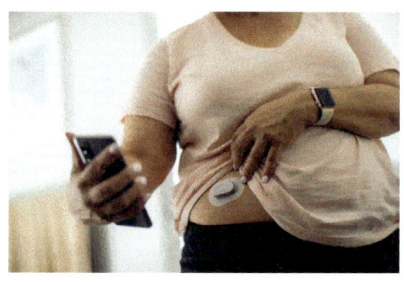

Dexcom G6

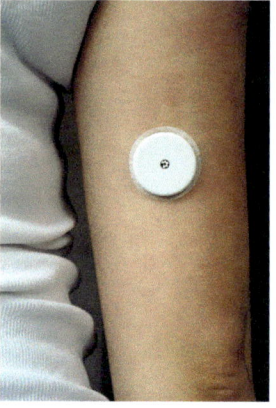

Freestyle Libre

Glycaemic Emergencies in Adults and Children

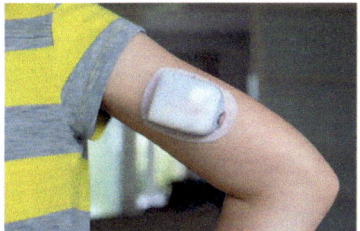

Omnipod

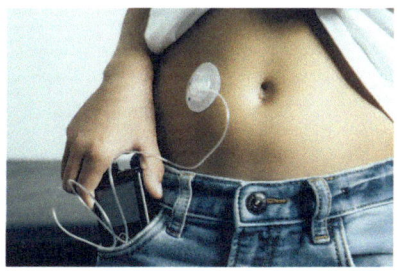

Medtronic Insulin Pump

2.6 Driving

- It is a legal requirement for drivers to inform the DVLA if their diabetes is treated by insulin injections. Diabetes treated by non-insulin injections or tablets may need to be reported to the DVLA. Further information is available from the DVLA.[6, 7, 20]

- When it is appropriate – particularly when discharging a patient who is a driver after a hypoglycaemic episode and not conveying them to a healthcare facility – ambulance clinicians should:
  - advise the patient on the impact of their medical condition for safe driving ability
  - advise the patient on their legal requirement to notify the DVLA of the episode
  - document any of the above if it is discussed with the patient.

Note that the patient could be fined up to £1,000 if they do not tell the DVLA about a medical condition that affects their driving, and they could be prosecuted if they are involved in an accident as a result.[7]

- There are differences in requirements to report to the DVLA between Group 1 (cars and motorbikes) and Group 2 (bus or lorry) drivers
  - Group 1 drivers (car and motorcycle) need to tell the DVLA if:
    - they have had more than one episode of severe hypoglycaemic while awake (needing the assistance of another person within the last 12 months)
    - they develop impaired awareness of hypoglycaemia (difficulty in recognising the warning symptoms of low blood sugar)
  - Group 2 drivers (bus and lorry) must stop driving group 2 vehicles and tell the DVLA if:
    - they have a single episode of hypoglycaemia requiring the assistance of another person, even if this happened during sleep
    - they have any degree of impaired awareness of hypoglycaemia (difficulting in recognising the warning signs and symptoms of low blood sugar)
  - All drivers (Group 1 and Group 2) must tell DVLA if:
    - They suffer severe hypoglycaemia while driving
    - they or their medical team feel they are at high risk of developing hypoglycaemia
    - an existing medical condition gets worse or they develop any other condition that may affect their ability to drive safely.

- Appropriate glucose monitoring systems for driving:
  - Group 1 drivers may not use finger prick glucose testing and continuous glucose monitoring systems (flash glucose and CGM) for the purposes of driving.
  - Group 2 drivers must continue to use finger prick testing for the purposes of driving. CGM and flash glucose monitoring systems are not legally permitted for the purposes of Group 2 driving.

- If an ambulance clinician is concerned that a patient cannot or will not notify the DVLA themselves after recurrent episodes of hypoglycaemia requiring assistance, it would be appropriate to liaise with the patient's GP and again, document these actions

3. Hypoglycaemia

- Hypoglycaemia is the term used to describe low blood glucose levels.[8] For patients with type 1 diabetes, hypoglycaemia is due to a relative excess of insulin over available glucose, resulting in a disturbance of glucose metabolism. There are both medical and lifestyle risk factors for hypoglycaemia (refer to Table 3.60).

- The definition of hypoglycaemia is a blood glucose of <4.0 mmol/L for patients with diabetes.[8] This should not be confused with the lower minimum level of <3.0–3.9 mmol/L used for patients without diabetes who are symptomatic.

- Correction of hypoglycaemia is a medical emergency. If left untreated, hypoglycaemia may lead to the patient suffering permanent brain damage and may even prove fatal.

Glycaemic Emergencies in Adults and Children

- There are three classes of hypoglycaemia: mild, moderate and severe (see Figure 3.16). In mild cases, the person can treat themselves, whereas in severe cases, third-party assistance will be required.
- Some patients can detect the early symptoms for themselves, but others may be too young or deteriorate rapidly and without apparent warning.
- Any person with a reduced level of consciousness, who is having a convulsion, is seriously ill or is traumatised should have hypoglycaemia excluded.
- Abnormal neurological features may occur, for example unilateral weakness, similar to a stroke. Patients with symptoms indicative of a stroke should have an immediate blood glucose test to exclude hypoglycaemia.
- Signs and symptoms for hypoglycaemia can vary from person to person. Symptoms may be masked due to medication or other injuries, for example with beta-blocker medicines (refer to Table 3.61).
- It should be noted that classical symptoms of hypoglycaemia may **NOT** always be present, and children may have a variety of unusual symptoms with low blood glucose (refer to Table 3.61).

TABLE 3.60 – Risk Factors for Hypoglycaemia

Medical risk factors[10]	Lifestyle risk factors
- Insulin or other hypoglycaemic drug treatments. - Tight glycaemic control. - Previous history of severe hypoglycaemia. - Undetected nocturnal hypoglycaemia. - Long duration of type 1 diabetes. - Duration of insulin therapy in type 2 diabetes. - Lipohypertrophy at injection sites. - Impaired awareness of hypoglycaemia. - Overcorrections of hyperglycaemia. - Preceding hypoglycaemia (<3.5 mmol/L). - Severe hepatic dysfunction. - Renal dialysis therapy. - Impaired renal function. - Sudden cessation of peritoneal dialysis. - Inadequate treatment of previous hypoglycaemia. - Terminal illness. - Sepsis. - Endocrine illness (including Addisonian crisis; refer to **Adrenal Insufficiency Patients**). - Hypothermia (especially in very young babies). - Sudden cessation of tube or IV feeding. - Very sick or traumatised children. - Very young babies (especially preterm). - Ketotic hypoglycaemia of infancy.	- Drug ingestion, e.g. oral hypoglycaemic drugs, beta-blockers, alcohol. - Inadequate carbohydrate intake. - Increased exercise (relative to usual)/ excessive physical activity. - Irregular lifestyle (or supervision if the patient is a child). - Increasing age. - Excessive or chronic alcohol intake. - Early pregnancy. - Breastfeeding. - No or inadequate blood glucose monitoring.

Glycaemic Emergencies in Adults and Children

TABLE 3.61 – Signs and Symptoms of Hypoglycaemia

• **Autonomic**	• Sweating
	• Trembling/shaking
	• Palpitations/pounding heart
	• Hunger
• **General malaise**	• Headache
	• Nausea
• **Neuroglycopenic**	• Incoordination
	• Confusion
	• Speech difficulty
	• Drowsiness
	• Odd behaviour
	• Aggression/combative behaviour
	• Fitting
	• Unconsciousness

3.1 Hypoglycaemia in the Absence of Diabetes

Occasionally, hypoglycaemia will be experienced by patients who do not have a diagnosis of diabetes.[10] Hyperinsulinaemia, extreme diet restriction, severe illness (especially in children) and long periods of sustained intense exercise can result in hypoglycaemia.

This can generally be divided into two broad categories:

- **Reactive hypoglycaemia** – may be the result of gastrointestinal surgery or enzyme deficiency and may occasionally be found in patients with pre-diabetes as the body struggles to regulate insulin production.

- **Fasting hypoglycaemia** – may occur as a result of medications such as salicylates e.g. aspirin, certain antibiotics, pentamidine or quinine; with excessive alcohol intake, especially binge drinking; serious illnesses, especially those affecting the liver, heart or kidneys; hormonal abnormalities; or the presence of certain types of tumours, particularly those in the pancreas.

Note that hypoglycaemia in the absence of diabetes could be considered if blood glucose is between 3.0 and 3.9 mmol/L and the patient is also symptomatic.

3.2 Impaired Awareness of Hypoglycaemia

- Impaired awareness (IA) arises in patients whose perception of hypoglycaemia is reduced or absent, and the possibility of severe hypoglycaemic events is increased. IA is more commonly associated with insulin therapy and may be induced by recurrent hypoglycaemic episodes and/or strict glycaemic control, which cause a dampening of the sympathetic response.[11] The condition can be objectively identified using a number of validated tools and is reversible for many through strict avoidance of hypoglycaemia for a period of weeks or months.

- In patients with type 1 diabetes, the prevalence of IA varies: 25–40% has been reported. Recent evidence suggests the prevalence may be significantly higher (53–57%) in hypoglycaemic patients attended by the ambulance services.[12.]

- NICE Guidelines recommend the use of CGM/Flash Glucose Systems for patients with diabetes and prescribed insulin with Impaired Awareness of Hypoglycaemia. For patients not currently using a CGM, discuss its use with them and consider referral to appropriate primary/secondary care services, with the recommendation of CGM prescription, as per local pathways.

3.3 Assessment and Management of Hypoglycaemia

For the assessment and management of hypoglycaemia, refer to Tables 3.62 and 3.63 and Figure 3.16. The principles of assessment and management are essentially the same in adults and children both with and without diabetes.
NB Note that the lower blood glucose level for hypoglycaemia in the patient without diabetes is 3.0–3.9 mmol/L who is also symptomatic.

TABLE 3.62 – ASSESSMENT and MANAGEMENT of: Hypoglycaemia

Assess <C>ABCDE

- Start correcting <C>ABCDE problems (refer to **Medical Emergencies in Adults – Overview** and **Medical Emergencies in Children – Overview**).
- Consider and look for medical alert/information signs (alert bracelets, chains and cards).

Assess Blood Glucose Level

- Measure and record blood glucose level (pre-treatment measure).
- Clean the patient's fingers prior to testing blood glucose levels as they may have been in contact with sugary substances (e.g. sweets). It is vital that fingers are cleaned using a non-alcohol based wipe, or gauze with sterile water or sodium chloride, and dried thoroughly with a gauze swab prior to obtaining a blood glucose reading. Do NOT use alcohol-based wipes as these may give a false high reading.

(continued)

Glycaemic Emergencies in Adults and Children

TABLE 3.62 – ASSESSMENT and MANAGEMENT of: Hypoglycaemia *(continued)*

Severe

Patient unconscious (GCS ≤8), convulsing or very agitated, or aggressive.

- Check <C>ABCDE and correct as necessary.
- Administer IV glucose 10% (refer to **Glucose 10%** for dosages).
- Only administer IM glucagon if IV glucose 10% is not possible. **NB** IM glucagon to be given ONCE ONLY.
- The onset time for glucagon is 10 minutes (but it can take up to 15 minutes to take effect). Glucagon requires the patient to have adequate glycogen stores so may be ineffective if they have been exhausted through frequent episodes of hypoglycaemia, alcohol use or low carbohydrate diet. Also, it is less effective in patients who take a sulphonylurea medicine (e.g. gliclazide, glipizide, tolbutamide, glimepiride), are chronically malnourished or take excess alcohol, so IV glucose 10% is preferred in these groups.
- Keep nil by mouth as there is an increased risk of aspiration/choking.
- Titrate further doses of IV Glucose 10% to effect – an improvement in clinical state and glucose level should be observed rapidly.
- Re assess blood glucose level after 5 minutes. If <4.0 mmol/L, administer a further dose of IV glucose 10%.
- Re assess blood glucose level after a further 15 minutes.
- Consider rapid transfer to the nearest suitable receiving hospital if no improvement.
- Monitor vital signs and conscious level en route. Check glucose again if patient deteriorates, or half-hourly.
- Provide a pre-alert/information call if necessary.

Mild to Moderate

Patient conscious, orientated, able to swallow.

- If capable, cooperative and deemed to have a safe swallow, administer 15–20 grams of quick-acting carbohydrate, such as one of the following:
  – 5–7 Dextrosol® tablets (or 4–5 Glucotabs®) or
  – 1 bottle (60 ml) Glucojuice® or
  – 150–200 ml pure fruit juice, e.g. orange (avoid pure fruit juice if a renal dialysis patient because of potassium content) or
  – 1–2 tubes of 40% glucose gel or
  – 3–4 heaped teaspoons of sugar dissolved in water (**NB** this is not an effective treatment for patients taking acarbose as it prevents the breakdown of sucrose to glucose).
- Do not give chocolate, as it is slower acting.
- If **NOT** capable and cooperative, but able to swallow, administer 1–2 tubes of 40% glucose gel to the buccal mucosa or give IV glucose 10% or IM glucagon (refer to **Glucagon**) if IV access is not possible. **NB** IM glucagon to be given **ONCE ONLY**.
- Re-assess blood glucose level after 10–15 minutes and ensure blood glucose level has improved to at least 4.0 mmol/L in addition to an improvement in level of consciousness.
- If no improvement, repeat oral treatment up to three times in total.
- If no improvement after three treatments or 30–45 minutes, give IV glucose 10% (refer to **Glucose 10%**).
- For ongoing care refer to Table 3.63.
- Once blood glucose is >4 mmol/L, give a starchy snack, e.g. two biscuits, one slice of bread/toast, 200–300 ml glass of milk (not soya) or a normal meal if due (must contain carbohydrate).
- **NB** Patients given glucagon require a larger portion of long-acting carbohydrate to replenish glycogen stores (double the suggested amount above).
- **NB** Patients who self-manage their insulin pumps (CSII) may not need a long-acting carbohydrate. (See **Section 2.5**)
- Transfer to the nearest suitable receiving hospital if the patient requires further treatment, otherwise the patient can usually be safely left at home. If the patient is a child, ensure they are left with a responsible adult.

Glycaemic Emergencies in Adults and Children

TABLE 3.63 – Care Pathway

Patients who do not need conveyance to hospital

- The following patients may not need conveyance to hospital:
  - patients whose episode was mild or moderate and who are now fully recovered after treatment
  - patients with a sustained blood glucose level of >4.0 mmol/L
  - patients who have been able to eat/drink a glucose- and carbohydrate-containing food where relevant.
- If the patient is a child, they must be in the care of a responsible adult.
- Advise patients/carers to call for help if any symptoms of hypoglycaemia recur.
- Ambulance services must arrange for a message to be forwarded to a primary healthcare team or diabetes team as per local pathways. All patients with hypoglycaemia who require third-party assistance should be referred to a specialist diabetes team as per local procedure. Where these pathways do not exist, the patient's GP must be informed. For all patients who use insulin and are not currently using CGM/Flash Glucose systems, consider recommending the patient contacts their diabetes team to discuss these, as they are proven to reduce severe hypoglycaemic episodes.
- Patient consent is not required in order to make a referral, although the patient should be informed that a referral is being made.
- Consider giving the patient and carers a hypoglycaemia patient information leaflet where available.
- Consider advising the patient about their responsibilities in relation to driving.

Patients who require further care

Consider conveying to hospital patients that are older, frail, have a low BMI, live alone or are on multiple medications.

- The following patients should be transferred to further care, with continuing patient management en route:
  - patients who have had recurrent treatment for hypoglycaemia within the previous 48 hours
  - patients whose episode was severe and who had a very slow response and recovery after treatment
  - patients taking **sulphonylureas** (glibenclamide, glipizide, gliclazide, tolbutamide, glimepiride). **These can be longer acting and result in a prolonged or recurrent hypoglycaemic event. Be aware that these patients may need to be monitored for a longer time period and therefore consider conveying or discuss with primary care/specialist team.**
  - patients with no previous history of diabetes who have suffered their first hypoglycaemic episode
  - patients with a blood glucose level of ≤4.0 mmol/L after treatment
  - patients who have not returned to normal mental status within 10 minutes of treatment
  - patients with any additional disorders or other complicating factors (e.g. renal dialysis, chest pain, cardiac arrhythmias, Addison's disease, alcohol consumption, dyspnoea, seizures or focal neurological signs/symptoms, active cancer treatment)
  - patients with signs of infection (e.g. urinary tract infection, upper respiratory tract infection) and/or who are unwell ('flu-like symptoms).

4. Hyperglycaemia

- Hyperglycaemia is the term used to describe elevated blood glucose levels (capillary blood glucose greater than 11 mmol/L). Symptoms associated with high blood glucose levels include unusual thirst (polydipsia), urinary frequency (polyuria), tiredness, weight loss, thrush (candidiasis) or recurrent infections. They are usually of slower onset in comparison to those of hypoglycaemia but can develop relatively quickly (days to weeks) in those with newly presenting type 1 diabetes.
- Patients with diabetes (types 1 and 2) may develop raised blood glucose in response to infection and follow '**Sick-day Rules- section 2.4**' to manage their glucose levels (and blood ketones, if appropriate).
- Hyperglycaemia can occur transiently in patients who are severely physically stressed (e.g. during a convulsion).
- Higher glucose levels may be acceptable in some patients according to their care plan e.g. End of life.
- The underlying reason for raised blood glucose should be determined as it may be an emergency in its own right.

High blood sugars in patients that are not known to have diabetes

- A high blood sugar can be an important incidental finding. If adult patients have no

Glycaemic Emergencies in Adults and Children

MILD	MODERATE	SEVERE
The patient is conscious, orientated and able to swallow.	The patient is conscious and able to swallow, but may be confused, disoriented and/or combative.	The patient is unconscious/fitting or combative or where there is increased risk of aspiration/choking.

MILD
- Give 15–20 g quick acting carbohydrate, such as:
  - 4–5 Glucotabs or
  - 1 bottle (60 ml) Glucojuice® or
  - 1–2 tubes 40% glucose gel or
  - 3–4 heaped teaspoons of sugar dissolved in water or
  - 150–200 ml pure fruit juice.
- Re-test blood glucose after 15 mins.
- If blood glucose remains <4 mmol/l, repeat above treatment up to twice more at 15-minute intervals until a blood glucose of >4 mmol/l is obtained.
- If blood glucose fails to rise >4 mmol/l AFTER 3 cycles of oral treatment (i.e. 45 mins), consider IV 10% glucose or IM glucagon.

MODERATE
If capable and cooperative:
- Give 15–20 g quick acting carbohydrate, such as:
  - 4–5 Glucotabs or
  - 1 bottle (60 ml) Glucojuice® or
  - 1–2 tubes 40% glucose gel or
  - 3–4 heaped teaspoons of sugar dissolved in water or
  - 150–200 ml pure fruit juice.

If **NOT** capable and cooperative, but able to swallow:
- Administer 1–2 tubes of glucose gel 40% to the buccal mucosa or give 1 mg glucagon IM (refer to **Glucagon**).
- Re-test blood glucose after 15 mins. If <4 mmol/l, repeat administration of 40% glucose gel. NB IM glucagon cannot be repeated.
- If 40% glucose gel cannot be administered due to patient disposition, consider IV 10% glucose (refer to **Glucose 10%**).
- If blood glucose remains <4 mmol/l, repeat above treatment up to twice more at 15-minute intervals until a blood glucose of >4 mmol/l is obtained.

SEVERE
- Check ABC and correct as necessary.
- Administer IV glucose 10% (refer to **Glucose 10%** for dosages).
- If IV not possible administer IM glucagon (may take up to 15 minutes to work and IM glucagon ONCE ONLY).
- Re-assess blood glucose level after 10 minutes.
- If blood glucose remains <4.0 mmol/l, administer a further dose of IV 10% glucose.
- Repeat treatment until a blood glucose of >4 mmol/l is obtained.
- If no improvement, convey to nearest suitable receiving hospital.
- Check glucose again if patient deteriorates.
- Provide a pre-alert/information call if necessary.

Blood glucose level should now be 4 mmol/l or above.
- Once a blood glucose of >4 mmol/l is achieved, give a starchy snack, e.g. two biscuits; one slice of bread/toast; 200–300 ml glass of milk (not soya); a normal meal if due (must contain carbohydrate).
- **NB** Patients given glucagon require a larger portion of long-acting carbohydrate to replenish glycogen stores (double the suggested amount above).
- **NB** Patients who self-manage their insulin pumps (CSII) may not need a long-acting carbohydrate.
- In most cases patients who have fully recovered and maintain glucose levels >4 mmol/l will not require admission to ED.

If blood glucose is now >4 mmol/l, follow up treatment as described on the left.

Glucagon may take up to 15 minutes to work and can be ineffective in the very young, older people, undernourished patients or those with hepatic disease.
In patients with renal/cardiac disease, use IV fluids with caution.
Avoid fruit juice in renal failure. **Note:** the carbohydrate content of some commercially available glucose-containing drinks varies – individual product labels should be checked. Diet drinks may not contain sugar.

Figure 3.16 – Hypoglycaemic emergencies algorithm.
Source: http://www.diabetologists-abcd.org.uk/JBDS/JBDS_HypoGuideline_FINAL_280218.pdf.

Glycaemic Emergencies in Adults and Children

symptoms of diabetes but have a capillary blood glucose of >11.0 mmol/L, they should be advised to contact their GP for a risk assessment to determine their risk of type 2 diabetes.[13] Further information can be found at the NHS Know Your Risk Score website: www.riskscore.diabetes.org.uk

- A blood glucose measurement of more than 7.8 mmol/L but less than 11.1 mmol/L may indicate: a risk of type 2 diabetes; non-diabetic hyperglycaemia (raised blood glucose levels but not in the diabetic range, also known as 'impaired glucose regulation') or 'stress hyperglycaemia' (transient rise in blood glucose levels due to acute illness); or medication that causes a rise in blood glucose, e.g. steroids, antiretrovirals.

Patient Management (Adult)

- If an adult has a high blood glucose and is symptomatic (e.g. have shortness of breath, tachycardia, hypotension, temperature, dehydration, thirst, polyuria, generally unwell), convey them to hospital.

- If their blood glucose is high and they have no other symptoms i.e. no ketones or/and signs of acidosis (i.e. deep, sighing respirations – Kussmaul breathing), contact their GP/primary care/OOH to discuss the clinical findings and agree a care plan. Keep the patient (and carer, as appropriate) involved in this process.

Patient Management (Paediatric)

- The majority of children who develop diabetes have type 1 diabetes. DKA is the principal cause of death in children with diabetes, so recognition and treatment are a medical emergency. Clinicians should maintain a high index of suspicion when presented with any generally ill child with a blood glucose >11 mmol/L and convey immediately to ED/Paediatric Assessment Unit (PAU). Diabetes or hyperglycaemia due to illness should be considered if their blood glucose is 7–10.9 mmol/L. Contact their GP/Primary care to discuss ongoing care plans.

- Type 1 diabetes can occur in infants. These children may have blood glucose levels that are particularly difficult to control.

5. Diabetic Ketoacidosis (DKA)

- A relative lack of circulating insulin means that cells cannot take up glucose from the blood and use it to provide energy. This forces the cells to provide energy for metabolism from other sources, such as fatty acids. Ketones are produced as a by-product of fatty acid metabolism in the liver. They are acidic chemicals whose accumulation leads to the development of a metabolic acidosis. Ketone production ceases with insulin therapy, which allows the body to convert from fat to its preferred fuel substrate, glucose.

- Blood ketone measurement is used in the diagnosis of DKA, and patients with **capillary blood ketones of 3.0 mmol/L or more are considered to be at high-risk of DKA**. Urinary ketone measurements can also be used but note that urine ketostix tests can remain positive even after DKA has resolved.

- For a confirmed diagnosis of DKA, the following must be present: capillary blood glucose above 11 mmol/L; capillary ketones above 3 mmol/L or urine ketones ++ or more; and venous pH less than 7.3 and/or bicarbonate less than 15 mmol/L.[14]

- Risk factors for DKA are summarised in Table 3.65. DKA can complicate intercurrent illness in a person with diabetes. Infections, myocardial infarction (which may be silent) or a stroke may precipitate DKA.

- Patients with DKA may present with one or more signs and symptoms and this should alert the ambulance clinicians to the possibility of DKA (refer to Table 3.64).

- Un diagnosed patients with type 1 diabetes may present with DKA due to early symptoms being missed. When assessing unwell patients, remember the 4 T's – Thirsty, Tiredness, Thinner and Toilet (increased urination).[15] When these symptoms are present with hyperglycaemia, consider undiagnosed diabetes.

- DKA may occur relatively rapidly in children, sometimes without a long history of the classical symptoms. The absolute blood glucose level is not a good indicator of the presence of DKA – some children with blood glucose levels in the >20 range may appear quite well and not have DKA.

Fluid Management (Adult)

- Adults at high-risk of DKA (**capillary blood ketones of 3.0 mmol/L or more**) should receive IV fluid resuscitation in line with intravascular fluid therapy guidelines (Intravascular Fluid Therapy in Adults). Note that rapid fluid replacement into the vascular compartment can compromise the cardiovascular system, particularly where there is pre-existing cardiovascular disease and in the elderly. Gradual rehydration over hours rather than minutes is indicated.

- Patients may present with significant dehydration, resulting in reduced fluid in both the vascular and tissue compartments. Often this has taken time to develop and will take time to correct.

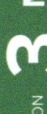

Glycaemic Emergencies in Adults and Children

Fluid Management (Paediatric)
- Children and young adults with DKA may also present with significant dehydration (refer to **Intravascular Fluid Therapy in Children**).
  - If **SHOCKED**, establish IV/IO access and commence fluids en route to hospital giving an initial fluid bolus of 10ml/kg (over **15** minutes) and pre-alerting the ED. Further fluid may be required, using smaller volumes, but only after discussion with a senior clinician as per local procedure.
  - If **NON-SHOCKED** patients with DKA showing early signs of dehydration, an inital 10 ml/kg bolus should be given (over **30** minutes).
- Do not try to give oral fluids to children with DKA – they have a very high risk of aspiration.

TABLE 3.64 – Signs and Symptoms of Hyperglycaemia and DKA

Hyperglycaemia	Diabetic ketoacidosis
The symptoms of hyperglycaemia include: - polyuria - polydipsia - weight loss - lethargy - recurrent infections especially thrush - blurred vision	A patient presenting with DKA may have: - vomiting - abdominal pain - rapid breathing/hyperventilation or Kussmaul breathing - evidence of ketones: fruity odour on the breath (resembling nail varnish remover) **NB** Not everyone can detect this odour - evidence of ketones: presence of ketones in capillary blood (3.0 mmol/L or more) and/or urine (urinary ketones: ++ or more) - dehydration, dry mouth and possible circulatory failure due to hypovolaemia - confusion/reduced level of consciousness - weight loss - other autoimmune conditions that are more common in type 1 diabetes, e.g. Addison's disease which can predispose to DKA - evidence of diabetes complications, e.g. previous toe/foot amputation or foot ulceration - consider pregnancy in women of child-bearing age – the fetus is very sensitive to ketosis.

TABLE 3.65 – Risk factors for DKA[18]

- Inadequate or inappropriate insulin therapy
- Infection
- Myocardial infarction
- Pancreatitis
- Stroke
- Acromegaly
- Hyperthyroidism
- Certain drugs, including corticosteroids, thiazides, pentamidine, sympathomimetics, antipsychotics, cocaine, certain immunotherapy medications and SGLT2 inhibitors (the 'flozins': e.g. dapagliflozin, canagliflozin, empagliflozin, ertugliflozin)
- Cushing's syndrome
- Hispanic or black ancestry
- Bariatric surgery
- Undiagnosed type 1 Diabetes

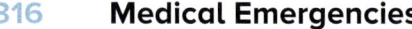

Glycaemic Emergencies in Adults and Children

TABLE 3.66 – ASSESSMENT and MANAGEMENT of: DKA in Adults and Children

Assess <C>ABCDE

- Start correcting ABC problems (refer to **Medical Emergencies in Adults – Overview** and **Medical Emergencies in Children – Overview**). Correct life-threatening conditions, airway and breathing on scene.
- For high-risk DKA patients (capillary blood ketone level of 3.0 mmol/L or more) administer IV fluids in accordance to **Intravascular Fluid Therapy in Adults** and **Intravascular Fluid Therapy in Children** and/or **Sodium Chloride 0.9%**.
- **DO NOT** delay at scene for fluid replacement.
- Transfer to nearest suitable receiving hospital, with a pre-alert/information call. Include term 'high-risk DKA' and ketone value when known.
- These patients have a potentially life-threatening condition – they require urgent hospital treatment including insulin and fluid/electrolyte therapy.
- Consider and look for medical alert/information signs (alert bracelets, chains, tattoos and cards).

Assess Blood Glucose and Ketone Levels

- Measure and record blood glucose level.
- Where ketone meters are available, measure and record blood ketone level. Patients with a **capillary blood ketone level** of **3.0 mmol/L or more** are **considered to be at high-risk of DKA**.
- If the patient has records of their blood glucose and ketone levels, ensure these accompany the patient.
- Always use water or water-based wipes when cleaning fingers prior to blood testing.

Assess for Signs of Dehydration

- Signs may include:
  - The skin of the forearm remains tented following a gentle pinch, only returning to its normal position slowly.
  - Dry mouth.
- In severe cases this may lead to hypovolaemic shock. Patients who are shocked, have poor capillary refill, tachycardia, reduced Glasgow Coma Score (GCS) and hypotension should receive fluids in accordance with **Intravascular Fluid Therapy in Adults** and **Intravascular Fluid Therapy in Children.**
- **DO NOT** delay at scene for fluid replacement – DKA is a time critical emergency.

Assess Heart Rhythm

- Undertake ECG.

Measure Oxygen Saturation (SpO$_2$)

- Administer supplemental oxygen if the patient is hypoxaemic, SpO$_2$ <94%.
- Refer to **Oxygen**.

6. Hyperosmolar Hyperglycaemic State (HHS)

- Hyperosmolar Hyperglycaemic State (HHS) usually affects those with pre-existing type 2 diabetes but may sometimes be the first presentation of this condition.[19]
- HHS characteristics include high blood glucose (hyperglycaemia >=30 mmol/L), absence of hyperketonaemia (ketones <=3.0 mmol/L), marked hypovolaemia and hyperosmolality.
- Typically, HHS occurs in those aged over 45 years old, but it can affect younger adults and teenagers.
- It often develops over several days, and consequently the dehydration and metabolic disturbances are more extreme. HHS has a high mortality, as such, it is a medical emergency and requires prompt recognition, treatment and urgent transfer to definitive care.
- The predominant cause of HHS is usually a respiratory or urinary tract infection.
- HHS used to be known as HONK (Hyperglycaemic Hyperosmotic Non-Ketotic coma), however, the majority of patients presenting with this condition are not comatose but may still be seriously ill.

Glycaemic Emergencies in Adults and Children

TABLE 3.67 – Characteristics of and Risk Factors for HHS

Characteristics:	Risk factors:
• Type 2 diabetes • Hypovolaemia • Marked hyperglycaemia (>30 mmol/L) without significant ketosis (<=3.0 mmol/L) • Severely dehydrated and unwell	• Undiagnosed type 2 diabetes • Infection • Certain medications, in particular recent use of steroids, such as Prednisolone or Dexamethasone • Co-existing disease • Persistent hyperglycaemia in type 2 diabetes • Substance misuse

6.1 Management

- Patients should undergo urgent transfer to definitive care.
- Patients should be encouraged to drink fluids, if able to tolerate without nausea.
- Administer IV 0.9% sodium chloride in line with intravascular fluid therapy guidelines to restore circulating volume and commence rehydration (refer to **Intravascular Fluid Therapy in Adults** and **Intravascular Fluid Therapy in Children**). Care should be taken to prevent fluid overload, and risk of cerebral oedema must be considered.

7. Diabetes and Mental Health

- In recent years, more has been understood about the psychological impact of living with and managing diabetes. Increased incidents of depression, anxiety and eating disorders are now clinically recognised consequences of managing this lifelong, challenging and frustrating disease.
- Clinicians may see evidence of this in their interactions with patients and should be able to signpost patients to seek support and advice as appropriate; this may be from their specialist diabetes team, primary care experts or mental health services.
- Clinicians should be mindful of their use of language when dealing with patients living with diabetes, avoiding terms which imply blame such as 'non-compliant' or 'poor management'.[21]

7.1 Diabulimia

- This is a recently recognised eating disorder affecting the type 1 diabetes patient population.[22]
- Insulin-treated patients will often withhold insulin with the intent to lose weight. This will happen rapidly as the patient puts themselves into a state of moderate DKA. Carbohydrate food intake is then not absorbed by the normal digestive process but is expelled from the body by increased micturition. These patients can be secretive and difficult to manage as their desire to lose weight may often take precedence over their physical health.
- Clinicians may observe repeated episodes of DKA, extreme weight loss and a reluctance to attend hospital.
- Suspicion of diabulimia should be shared with receiving clinicians or referred to GP or diabetes services.

KEY POINTS!

Glycaemic Emergencies in Adults and Children

- Clean and thoroughly dry the patient's fingers prior to obtaining a capillary blood sample using a non-alcohol based wipe, or gauze with sterile water or sodium chloride, and dried thoroughly with a gauze swab – rinsing hands thoroughly in tap water is an acceptable alternative.
- Patients not conveyed to hospital should be referred to primary healthcare or diabetes team as per local pathways.
- Glucagon may be used intramuscularly to treat hypoglycaemia if treatment with oral or IV glucose is not possible.
- Patients whose hypoglycaemia is not due to diabetes may not respond well to glucagon.
- If GCS ≤13, consider IV 10% glucose (first line) or IM glucagon, refer to **Glucose 10%** and review patient's condition, titrate to effect.
- Do not remove wearable pumps/devices from the patient.
- High-Risk DKA patients (capillary blood ketones >=3.0 mmol/L) should receive IV fluids.
- DKA is a time critical emergency – and time on scene should be minimised where possible.

Glycaemic Emergencies in Adults and Children

Bibliography

1. Hirose T, Mita T, Fujitani Y, Kawamari R, Watada H. Glucose monitoring after fruit peeling: pseudohyperglycemia when neglecting hand washing before fingertip blood sampling. *Journal of Diabetes Care* 2011, 34: 596–597.

2. Ferretti DO, Martin KD. Isopropyl alcohol left on the skin falsely lowers capillary glucose values. *Journal of Clinical Outcomes Management* 2008, 15: 179–181.

3. Rosenstock J, Ferrannini E. Euglycemic diabetic ketoacidosis: a predictable, detectable, and preventable safety concern with SGLT2 inhibitors. *Diabetes Care* 2015, 38(9): 1638–1642.

4. Umpierrez GE, Smiley D, Kitabchi AE. Narrative review: ketosis-prone type 2 diabetes mellitus. *Annals of Internal Medicine* 2006, 144: 350–357.

5. Ng SM, Soni A, Agwu JC, Edge JA, Drew JH et al. *Sick Day Rules*. ACDC Clinical Guideline, version 3, 2015.

6. Driver and Vehicle Licensing Agency. *Diabetes and driving*. Available from: https://www.gov.uk/diabetes-driving.

7. Driver and Vehicle Licensing Agency (2019) INF294: A guide to insulin treated diabetes and driving. Available from: https://assets.publishing.service.gov.uk/government/uploads/system/uploads/attachment_data/file/834451/inf294-a-guide-to-insulin-treated-diabetes-and-driving.pdf.

8. Joint British Diabetes Societies for inpatient care (2023). The Hospital Management of Hypoglycaemia in Adults with Diabetes Mellitus. Available from: https://abcd.care/sites/abcd.care/files/site_uploads/JBDS_Guidelines_Current/JBDS_01_Hypo_Guideline_with_QR_code_January_2023.pdf.

9. Deary IJ, Hepburn DA, MacLeod KM, Frier BM. Partitioning the symptoms of hypoglycaemia using multi-sample confirmatory factor analysis. Diabetologia 1993, 36(8): 771–7.

10. Kabadi U (2021) BMJ Best Practice: Non-diabetic hypoglycaemia. Available from: https://bestpractice.bmj.com/topics/en-gb/509/pdf/509/Non-diabetic%20hypoglycaemia.pdf

11. Lin YK, Fisher SJ and Pop-Busui, R. Hypoglycemia unawareness and autonomic dysfunction in diabetes: Lessons learned and roles of diabetes technologies. *J Diabetes Investig*. 2020, 11(6), 1388–1402

12. Duncan EAS, Fitzpatrick D, Ikegwuonu T et al. Role and prevalence of impaired awareness of hypoglycaemia in ambulance service attendances to people who have had a severe hypoglycaemic emergency: a mixed-methods study. *BMJ Open* 2018, 8: e019522.

13. NICE (2017) Type 2 diabetes: prevention in people at high risk: Encouraging people to have a risk assessment. Available from: https://www.nice.org.uk/guidance/ph38/chapter/recommendations#encouraging-people-to-have-a-risk-assessment

14. Joint British Diabetes Societies Inpatient Care Group (2021). The Management of Diabetic Ketoacidosis in Adults. Available from: https://diabetes-resources-production.s3.eu-west-1.amazonaws.com/resources-s3/public/2021-06/JBDS%2002%20DKA%20Guideline%20amended%20v2.pdf

15. Diabetes UK. What are the signs and symptoms of diabetes? Available from: https://www.diabetes.org.uk/diabetes-the-basics/diabetes-symptoms[Accessed 04/2023].

16. Glaser N, Kuppermann N. Fluid treatment for children with diabetic ketoacidosis. *Paediatric Diabetes* 2019, 20: 10–14.

17. British Society for Paediatric Endocrinology and Diabetes (2020). BSPED Interim Guideline for the Management of Children under the age of 18 years with Diabetic Ketoacidosis. Available from: https://www.bsped.org.uk/media/1745/bsped-dka-guidelines-no-dka-link.pdf.

18. Diabetic Ketoacidosis. BMJ Best Practice (2022) Diabetic ketoacidosis – Symptoms, diagnosis and treatment, BMJ Best Practice. Available from: https://bestpractice.bmj.com/topics/en-gb/3000097[Accessed 19/01/2023].

19. Joint British Diabetes Societies Inpatient Care Group (2022). The Management of the Hyperosmolar Hyperglycaemic State (HHS) in Adults. Available from: https://abcd.care/sites/abcd.care/files/site_uploads/JBDS_Guidelines_Current/JBDS_06_The_Management_of_Hyperosmolar_Hyperglycaemic_State_HHS_%20in_Adults_FINAL_0.pdf

20. Driver and Vehicle Licensing Agency (2019) INF188/2: Information for drivers with diabetes treated by non insulin medication, diet, or both. Available from: https://assets.publishing.service.gov.uk/government/uploads/system/uploads/attachment_data/file/795538/inf188x2-information-for-drivers-with-diabetes-treated-by-non-insulin.pdf

21. Diabetes UK (2018) Language Matters: Language and diabetes. Available from: language-matters_language and diabetes.pdf language-matters_language and diabe-tes.pdf

22. Diabetes UK. Diabulimia and Diabetes. Available from: Diabulimia and diabetes | Diabetes UK

23. NICE (2022) Resource impact report for continuous glucose monitoring recommendations in: Type 1 diabetes in adults: diagnosis and management (NG17) Type 2 diabetes in adults: management (NG28) Diabetes (type 1 and type 2) in children and young people: diagnosis and management (NG18). Available from: https://www.nice.org.uk/guidance/ng18/resources/resource-impact-report-type-1-and-type-2-diabetes-and-continuous-glucose-monitoring-pdf-11020390813

Headache

1. Introduction

- Headache disorders are among the most common disorders of the nervous system and are a feature of both minor and major illness, which can prove challenging for a clinician.
- Most headaches are simple and not serious, but care must be taken to ensure that **TIME-CRITICAL** conditions are not missed.
- A detailed history is vital when dealing with headache, as the aetiology may go back hours, days, months or even years in relation to family history or childhood illness, e.g. tumours.

2. Incidence

- More than 10 million people in the UK suffer from headaches. Most headaches are not serious and can be treated with over-the-counter medicines and lifestyle changes such as getting more rest and drinking enough fluids. However, there are red flags in both history and examination that may indicate more concerning causes.
- The severity of headaches varies from patient to patient in terms of the pain the patient experiences. Although the pain may be the primary concern of the patient, it may not be associated with the severity of the underlying cause.
- The outcome for a patient presenting to ambulance services for headache will be as varied as the cause of the headache: the clinical significance of the headache and the progression are all dependent on the presenting factors.

3. Types of Headache

- Headaches can be broadly defined as primary or secondary:
  - **Primary headaches** are those which occur spontaneously (simple headaches); occur in response to a lifelong condition (e.g. migraines); are 'tension-type' headaches (various aetiologies); or are severe, short-lasting headaches (cluster headaches). These should not be considered as being pathophysiological as that is normal for the patient.
  - **Secondary headaches** are secondary to illness or injury and are pathological in origin, for instance head trauma (skull fracture); infective origin (i.e. meningitis); intracranial haemorrhage (i.e. spontaneous subarachnoid bleed or subdural bleed following trauma); or vascular (i.e. temporal arteritis).
- It is difficult to accurately differentiate between a simple headache, which requires no treatment, and a potentially more serious condition. Table 3.68 lists **'red flag'** symptoms that require the patient to undergo hospital assessment. **NB** This does not mean that any patient presenting without these symptoms is safe to be left at home.
- Consideration should be given to transferring all first presentations of severe headache to the emergency department for further investigation.

TABLE 3.68 – Red Flag Signs and Symptoms

🚩 Headache localised to the vertex, i.e. top of the head.

🚩 Escalating headache of an unusual nature.

🚩 Changed visual acuity.

🚩 Meningeal irritation, i.e. neck stiffness and photophobia.

🚩 Cranial nerve palsy.

🚩 Worsening headache with fever.

🚩 Sudden-onset or thunderclap headache reaching maximum intensity within 5 minutes.

🚩 New-onset neurological deficit, i.e. loss of function or altered sensation.

🚩 New-onset cognitive dysfunction.

🚩 Change in personality.

🚩 Impaired level of consciousness.

🚩 Recent head trauma, typically within the past three months.

🚩 Headache triggered by cough, Valsalva (trying to breathe out with nose and mouth blocked) or sneeze.

🚩 Headache triggered by exercise.

🚩 Orthostatic headache, i.e. a headache that changes with posture.

🚩 Symptoms suggestive of giant cell arteritis, which could include pain and tenderness over the temples, jaw pain while eating or talking and vision problems.

🚩 Symptoms and signs of acute narrow-angle glaucoma, i.e. red eye.

🚩 A substantial change in the characteristics of the headache.

🚩 Vomiting without other obvious cause.

🚩 Newly presenting ataxia, i.e. a neurological sign consisting of a lack of voluntary coordination of muscle movements.

🚩 Any evidence of a rash.

3.1 Migraine

- A migraine is a severe headache felt as a throbbing pain that is usually unilateral and frontal, often accompanied by nausea and vomiting. Some people also have other symptoms, such as sensitivity to light. Migraine is a common health condition, affecting about 15% of adults in the UK.

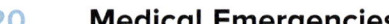

Headache

- There are several types of migraine, including:
  - **Migraine with aura**: this has the presence of a warning sign, known as an aura, before the migraine begins. About a third of people with a migraine have this. Warning signs may include visual problems such as flashing lights; stiffness in the neck, shoulders or limbs; or occasionally limb weakness or altered limb sensations. The migraine with aura may appear like a transient ischaemic attack (TIA) or stroke — great care is needed to differentiate between the two diagnoses; if there is any doubt, treat this as a TIA/stroke.
  - **Migraine without aura**: this is a headache without the signs and symptoms of an aura listed above.
  - **Migraine without headache**: also known as a silent migraine, this is when an aura or other migraine symptoms are experienced in the absence of a headache. Particular attention should be paid to this condition, as the symptoms can clearly mimic those of other conditions such as a TIA. If in any doubt, treat as a TIA/stroke.
- Migraines affect 1 in 4 women and 1 in 12 men in the UK. Some women find that migraine attacks are more frequent around the time of their menstruation, although this association has not been proven. Migraines usually begin in young adults. About 9 in 10 have their first migraine before they are 40 years old, although it is possible for migraines to begin later in life.
- Everyone will experience migraines differently. Some people have attacks frequently, up to several times a week. Other people only have a migraine occasionally and it is possible for years to pass between migraine attacks. Sometimes migraine attacks are associated with certain triggers, such as stress and certain foods.

3.2 Tension-type Headaches

- Tension-type headaches are the most common type of headache and the ones we think of as normal, everyday headaches. Most people are likely to have experienced them at some point. Up to 70% of the whole population will experience a tension headache during their lifetime; however, they are most prevalent up to the age of 30.
- Tension-type headaches may feel like a constant ache that affects both sides of the head and is often frontal. Patients may also complain of their neck muscles tightening and a feeling of pressure behind the eyes. The headaches usually last for 1 to 6 hours, but some people may have more persistent headaches that last for several days.
- Tension-type or chronic daily headaches can be caused by medication overuse or withdrawal. These should be considered to be secondary headaches.
- A tension-type headache is the most common symptom of mild carbon monoxide poisoning. Refer to **Overdose and Poisoning in Adults and Children**.

3.2.1 Medication-overuse Headaches

- Be alert to the possibility of medication-overuse headache in people whose headache developed or worsened while they were taking the following drugs for 3 months or more:
  - Triptans, opioids, ergots or combination analgesic medications on 10 days per month or more.
  - Paracetamol, aspirin or an NSAID, either alone or in any combination, on 15 days per month or more.
- The body gets used to the painkillers that are being taken. A rebound headache develops, particularly if patients have not taken a painkiller within a day or so of the last dose. Patients assume that they are suffering from a further tension headache or migraine and take a further dose of painkiller. When the effect of the painkiller wears off, another rebound headache develops and the cycle continues. Patients may start to take painkillers every day as a prophylactic measure to prevent headaches, which can further compound the problem.

3.3 Cluster Headaches

- Cluster headaches are excruciating attacks of pain in one side of the head, often felt behind the eye. Sufferers often call them 'suicidal headaches' because they are so severe. Cluster headaches begin unexpectedly and they are much more painful than migraines or any other type of headache.
- They are called cluster headaches because sufferers usually get one to three of the attacks every day, for several weeks or months, before they subside. A pain-free period will follow, which sometimes lasts months or years, before the headache attacks start again.
- Each cluster headache lasts between 15 minutes and 3 hours, but often less than 1 hour. They may start in the early hours of the morning and wake the person from sleep. Because of the intensity of the pain, some people will pace the room, rock or may even bang their head against the wall out of frustration, restlessness and despair.
- There are two types of cluster headaches:
  - **Episodic headache clusters** are separated by headache-free periods of 1 month or more.
  - **Chronic headache clusters** are separated by headache-free periods of less than 1 month, or are not separated at all. About 10% of cluster headache cases are chronic.
- Cluster headaches are rare and affect around 1 in 1,000 people. Anyone can be affected, but

Headache

approximately 80% of sufferers are male and most are smokers. It is not known what causes cluster headaches, but they are more common in autumn and spring. In some people, an attack can be triggered by drinking alcohol or an extreme increase in temperature, such as from exercising in hot weather.

3.4 Subarachnoid Haemorrhage

- Subarachnoid haemorrhage (SAH) is usually the result of bleeding from an aneurysm. It was previously thought to be mostly congenital but the cause is now considered to vary from genetic malformations of the elastic lamina to stressors such as hypertension and atherosclerosis.
- SAH affects 6–12 people per 100,000 of the population per year and constitutes about 6% of first strokes. Although SAH represents a small proportion of strokes, it tends to affect younger people, of whom about half die due to the episode.
- Risk factors include hypertension, smoking and excessive alcohol; however, the bigger the aneurysm, the more likely it is to bleed.
- The most characteristic feature is a sudden headache. This may last a few seconds or even a fraction of a second. Patients may even look round and accuse someone of hitting them on the back of the head.
- SAH should be considered in any patients presenting with sudden-onset, severe and unusual headache with or without any associated alteration in consciousness:
  – The headache is often diffuse.
  – The dominant feature is the severity, rather than the suddenness, of the headache, often being described as the most severe ever experienced.
  – It may last a week or 2.
  – Vomiting may occur; however, this does not distinguish it from other causes of headache.
  – Seizures occur in only about 7% of patients but, when they do, they are highly suggestive of a haemorrhage.

4. Assessment and Management

- For the assessment and management of headaches, refer to Table 3.69.

TABLE 3.69 – ASSESSMENT and MANAGEMENT of: Headache

Assess <C>ABCDE

- Start correcting any <C>ABCDE problems (refer to **Medical Emergencies in Adults – Overview** and **Medical Emergencies in Children – Overview**).
- Exclude the following or refer to the specific guidelines for:
  – **Stroke/Transient Ischaemic Attack**
  – **Head Injury**
  – **Glycaemic Emergencies in Adults and Children**.
- Consider carbon monoxide poisoning (refer to **Overdose and Poisoning in Adults and Children**).

Levels of Consciousness

- Assess AVPU:
  – **A** — Alert
  – **V** — Responds to voice
  – **P** — Responds to painful stimulus
  – **U** — Unresponsive.
- **NB** The only normal GCS is 15.

Respiratory Rate

- Measure and record respiratory rate.

Pulse

- Measure and record pulse.

Oxygen Saturation

- Monitor the patient's SpO_2; administer oxygen to achieve saturations of >94% if the patient presents as hypoxemic on air; refer to **Oxygen**.

Blood Pressure and Fluids

- Measure and record blood pressure; if required, administer fluids (refer to **Intravascular Fluid Therapy in Adults** and **Intravascular Fluid Therapy in Children**).

Headache

TABLE 3.69 – ASSESSMENT and MANAGEMENT of: Headache (continued)

Blood Glucose
- If appropriate, measure and record blood glucose for hypo/hyperglycaemia (refer to **Glycaemic Emergencies in Adults and Children**).

Temperature
- Measure and record temperature.

NEWS2
- These observations will enable you to calculate a NEWS2 score (refer to **Sepsis**).

Record Pain Score
- Assess the **SOCRATES** of the pain:
  - **S**ite — where exactly is the pain?
  - **O**nset — what was the patient doing when the pain came on?
  - **C**haracter — what does the pain feel like?
  - **R**adiates — where does the pain spread to?
  - **A**ssociated symptoms — e.g. nausea, dizziness.
  - **T**iming — how long has the patient had pain?
  - **E**xacerbating/relieving factors — what makes it better or worse?
  - **S**everity — obtain an initial pain score.
- Offer symptomatic pain relief for clinically benign headaches, using appropriate pain management drug therapy and taking into account the patient's preference, comorbidities and risk of adverse events.
- Consideration should therefore be given to initial management with NSAID and/or paracetamol, combined with onward referral for consideration of additional therapies, such as anti-emetics and triptans, EXCEPT in cluster headaches where paracetamol, NSAIDs, opioids, ergots or oral triptans should NOT be offered for the acute treatment. In this instance, the patient should be referred to their GP for onward management. Beware of making the diagnosis of cluster headaches, as it is very rare and other serious conditions may present in this way.
- Where medication overuse is the cause, advise the patient to stop taking all overused acute headache medication and to see their GP. It is best to stop abruptly rather than gradually. It is important to note that headache symptoms are likely to get worse in the short term before they improve and that there may be associated withdrawal symptoms.

Key Questions for a Patient with Headache
- Is this the worst headache ever?
- Is it different from your usual headache?
- Is this a new headache?

Assess for Red Flag Symptoms (refer to Table 3.68)
- Multiple red flags significantly increase the risk of serious pathology.
- Undertake a TIME-CRITICAL transfer to the nearest suitable receiving hospital.
- Provide an alert or information call.

Documentation
- Complete documentation to include all clinical findings, advice from other clinicians, onward referral and worsening advice given.

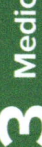

- Patients may deteriorate rapidly if they have a space-occupying condition, e.g. a haemorrhage resulting in a mass effect.
- Clinicians must ensure that patients receive the safest pathway of care. It is always better to be cautious, especially in children and those patients who are on their own.

- **NB** Where patients are not conveyed, follow-up care **MUST** be arranged. Always liaise with the patient's GP (or out-of-hours doctor) to discuss onward care. Ensure that, where practicable, patients are not left alone while awaiting follow-up.

Headache

> **KEY POINTS!**
>
> **Headache**
> - It is preferable to be cautious when dealing with patients with headaches, as diagnosis can be challenging.
> - Headaches with different or unusual characteristics are significant.
> - Sufferers of migraines are at risk of serious intracranial events.
> - With headache, blood pressure must be checked.
> - Any headache is significant if it is persistent or if it is associated with altered conscious levels or unusual behaviour.
> - Sinister headaches may or may not be accompanied by neurology. Do not exclude simply based on physical examination — **HISTORY IS KEY**.
> - A tension-type headache is the most common symptom of mild carbon monoxide poisoning.

Bibliography

1. NHS Evidence. *Headache Assessment/Management: How Should I Assess Someone Presenting with a Headache?* Clinical Knowledge Summaries. London: NHS Evidence, 2010.

2. Scottish Intercollegiate Guidelines Network. *Diagnosis and Management of Headache in Adults* (Guideline 107). Edinburgh: SIGN, 2008. Available from: http://www.sign.ac.uk/assets/sign107.pdf.

3. The Headache Classification Subcommittee of the International Headache Society. *The International Classification of Headache Disorders*. 2nd edn. (ICHD-II). 1st revision. The International Headache Society, 2005.

4. World Health Organization. *Headache Disorders* (Fact sheet 277). Available from: http://www.who.int/mediacentre/factsheets/fs277/en, 2004.

Heart Failure

1. Introduction

- Heart failure is not a specific disease entity; rather, it is a clinical syndrome characterised by several clinical signs, symptoms and diagnostic findings. Heart failure is caused by a structural or functional cardiac abnormality, resulting in a reduced cardiac output and/or increased intra-cardiac pressures. The most common cause of heart failure in the UK is coronary artery disease, and many patients have had a myocardial infarction in their past medical history. Heart failure can also be caused by abnormalities of the valves, pericardium, endocardium, heart rhythm and conduction system.[1]

- It is important to recognise that heart failure is a long-term condition and many people live in the community with **chronic heart failure**, which is a generic term that means they have already been diagnosed with heart failure and are receiving treatment. People may develop **acute on chronic heart failure** (decompensated) if they already have a diagnosis of heart failure but develop worsening symptoms quite quickly, despite treatment.

- **Acute heart failure** may therefore represent a decompensation of stable chronic heart failure or may be the patient's first presentation of symptoms. As part of clinical history-taking, you may find the patient has had some preceding dyspnoea; they may also have chest pain and acute coronary syndrome or/and arrhythmias such as atrial fibrillation (refer to **Acute Coronary Syndrome**).

- Acute heart failure can present in three major forms:
  - **Acute pulmonary oedema**. This is the sudden development of interstitial oedema in the lungs with severe dyspnoea, with or without peripheral oedema. It may come on very suddenly or patients may have had some dyspnoea for weeks or days that suddenly worsens.
  - **Predominant peripheral oedema with or without pulmonary oedema**. The patient may have significant fluid-loading, with swollen legs, abdomen and scrotum, as well as elevated jugular venous pressure (JVP) and pleural effusions.
  - **Cardiogenic shock**. This is rare and occurs in 5–8% of cases of acute heart failure. The commonest cause in a new presentation of heart failure is STEMI, but this may be a decompensation of advanced chronic heart failure. These cases require rapid treatment.

- Patients with an existing diagnosis of heart failure may be known to or be currently under the care of a specialist multidisciplinary heart failure team. The team may include services such as rehabilitation, tertiary care, palliative care and community nursing care. Patients may have a personal, anticipatory care plan that details what should happen if their condition deteriorates.

- Heart failure patients in the palliative phase of their illness may develop decompensated heart failure, and it is important to refer to any palliative plans or pathways in place, including any DNACPR or ReSPECT forms. This is to ensure the patient's and/or their family's and carers' wishes are adhered to in an emergency.

- Acute heart failure is a life-threatening medical condition, so for all new cases and all chronic cases, unless there is an advance care plan/palliative management in place, a TIME-CRITICAL transfer to hospital is required for urgent assessment and treatment, ideally at a hospital that has a coronary care unit.

1.1 Terminology

- There are many different terms and acronyms related to heart failure and some of them mean the same thing. Some terms are older and tend not to be referred to as often, but you may still see or hear them used.

- Some important terms are:
  - **Ejection fraction (EF):** The percentage of blood ejected by the ventricles relative to its filled volume.
  - **HFrEF:** Heart failure with reduced ejection fraction which is also referred to as LVSD – left ventricular systolic dysfunction. This is heart failure with an ejection fraction of <40%. There is reduced contractility of the left ventricle, so the heart is not able to pump blood around the body efficiently. Diagnosis is via an echocardiogram.
  - **LVSD:** Left ventricular systolic dysfunction, see also HFrEF above. This can be mild, moderate or severely impaired and is diagnosed usually on echocardiogram or MRI.
  - **HFpEF:** Heart failure with preserved ejection fraction, previously known as diastolic dysfunction. This is where on echocardiography the left ventricle is pumping well but it may have a problem relaxing and filling up with blood. The ejection fraction is ≥50%.
  - **HFmrEF:** Heart failure with a mid-ranged ejection fraction of 40–49%. This group of patients is in a 'grey area' and has elements of systolic and diastolic dysfunction.
  - **CCF:** Congestive cardiac failure. This is now an old-fashioned term and relates to people with both pulmonary and peripheral oedema. It involves the left and right ventricle.
  - **LVF:** Left ventricular failure. These patients tend to be breathless on exertion and may have signs of pulmonary oedema, including bi-basal crepitations on chest auscultation.

Heart Failure

They may also have signs of right-sided heart failure.
- **RVF:** Right ventricular failure. These cases have symptoms such as significant peripheral oedema, ascites, elevated JVP and pleural effusions. The lungs are often clear to auscultation.
- **De novo heart failure:** A term for the first presentation of heart failure. There has been no previous history or diagnosis of heart failure.
- **Cor pulmonale:** These cases have symptoms and signs of predominantly right heart failure but are primarily caused by chronic lung disease.

2. Incidence

Around 900,000 people in the UK have heart failure. It is estimated that there is also a similar number of patients with impaired heart function that have not yet been diagnosed with heart failure. Both the incidence and prevalence of heart failure increase steeply with age, with the average age at first diagnosis being 76 years. The prevalence of heart failure is expected to rise in the future as a result of an ageing population, improved survival of people with ischaemic heart disease and more effective treatments for heart failure.[2,3]

3. Severity and Outcome

- Acute heart failure carries an inpatient mortality of around 10%. In the long term, 27% of community heart failure patients are alive after 10 years.

4. Pathophysiology

- In HFrEF, reduced ejection fraction increases preload and results in left ventricular dilation to maintain stroke volume. This mechanism cannot be sustained, and ventricular remodelling occurs, reducing cardiac output.
- The signs and symptoms generated can be grouped together depending on whether the left or right side of the heart is involved. Left ventricular failure is the most common and most frequently caused by a previous myocardial infarction. Poor ventricular contraction occurs, and blood backs up into the lungs. This increases pulmonary vein hydrostatic pressure and subsequently causes fluid to enter the alveoli, seen as pulmonary oedema. The presence of this fluid causes a reduction in gas exchange (refer to Figure 3.17).
- Right heart failure is primarily caused by left heart failure but can also be caused in isolation by lung disease, such as COPD or pulmonary embolism as well as valvular disease. An increase in pressure in the pulmonary vasculature causes an increase in right ventricular afterload, resulting in ventricular hypertrophy, and subsequently leads to progressive dilation and eventual failure.
- This mechanism gives rise to the common signs and symptoms seen in a right-sided pathology – raised JVP, hepatomegaly, ascites and significant peripheral oedema.

4.1 Factors Triggering Acute Heart Failure

- An identifiable trigger/s causing the acute decompensation of heart failure can be found in two-thirds of cases. This is relevant as you may need to address two or more acute conditions at once. Some triggers, such as ischaemia and pneumonia, are associated with increased mortality risk. The commonest triggers are:
  - myocardial infarction
  - acute coronary syndrome
  - tachyarrhythmia, e.g. atrial fibrillation or ventricular tachycardia
  - infection, e.g. pneumonia, infective endocarditis or sepsis
  - excessive rise in blood pressure
  - non-adherence to medications
  - bradyarrhythmia
  - toxic substances, e.g. alcohol or recreational drugs
  - drugs, e.g. NSAIDs, corticosteroids, negative inotropic substances or cardiotoxic chemotherapeutics
  - exacerbation of chronic obstructive pulmonary disease
  - pulmonary embolism.
- Chest trauma, cardiac intervention, acute native or prosthetic valve incompetence secondary to endocarditis, aortic dissection or thrombosis are also causes.

5. Assessment and Management

- It can be difficult to differentiate heart failure from other causes of breathlessness, such as exacerbation of COPD, pulmonary embolism or pneumonia. Acute heart failure is frequently mistaken for sepsis as both can present with collapse and hypotension. If the patient has a history of heart failure or valve disease, STOP and THINK before administering intravenous fluids, as these can be harmful, especially if given quickly and in large amounts. A thorough history and physical examination of the patient is required. Assessment should focus on signs and symptoms associated with heart failure.
- Red flag indicators for heart failure are:
  - **Orthopnoea:** increased breathlessness on lying down. The patient may have slept in the chair on preceding nights.
  - **Paroxysmal nocturnal dyspnoea (PND):** waking up at night short of breath and relieved by sitting up.
  - **New dyspnoea** with a past history of myocardial infarction/hypertension/angina.

Heart Failure

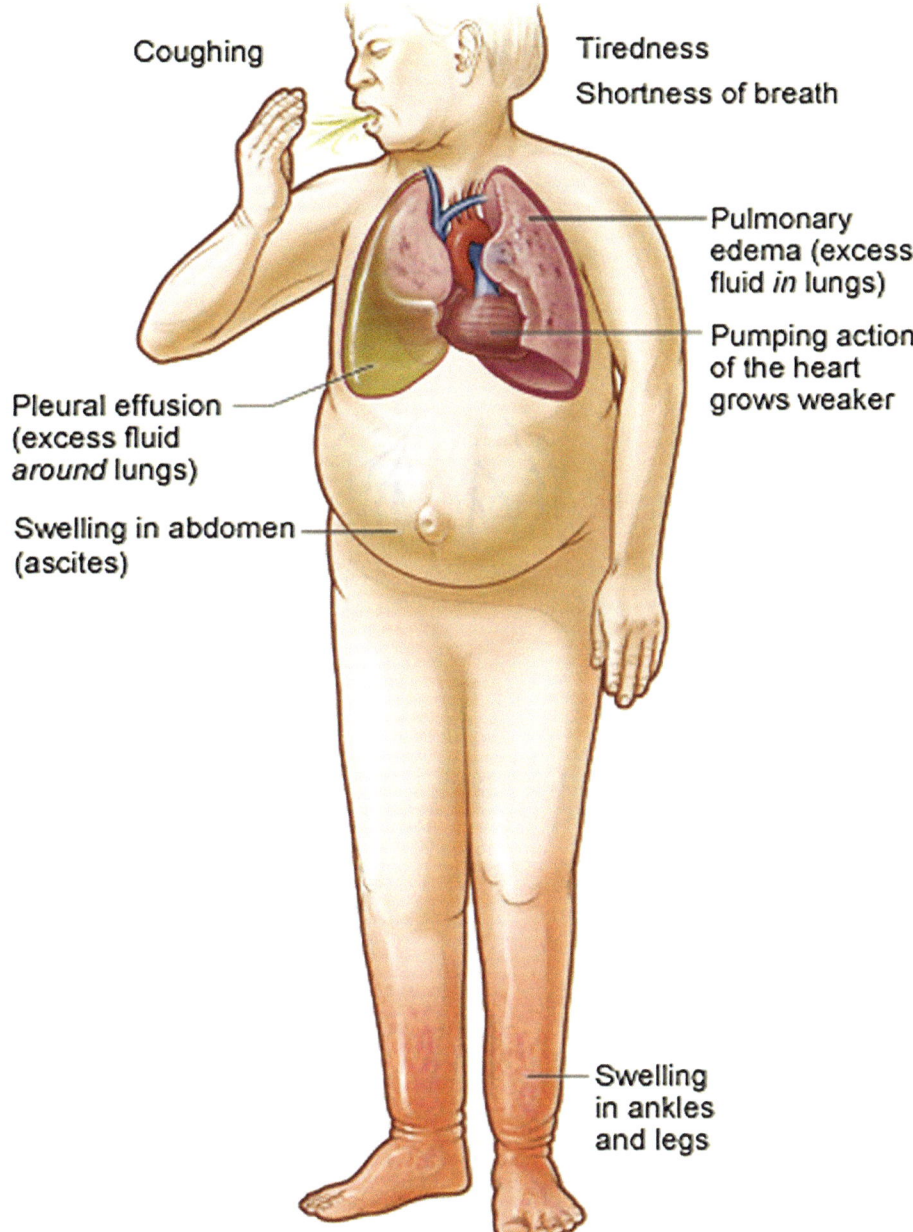

Figure 3.17 – Signs and symptoms of heart failure. Source: National Heart, Lung, and Blood Institute; National Institutes of Health; U.S. Department of Health and Human Services. Available from: https://www.nhlbi.nih.gov/health-topics/heart-failure.

- **New peripheral oedema**, accompanied by dyspnoea.
- **Coughing up pink frothy sputum**.

• Patients with an existing diagnosis of chronic heart failure may be known to or be currently under the care of a specialist multidisciplinary heart failure team. These teams often know the patients well and can offer advice on treatment. If the patient is sufficiently stable and there is time to do so, contact the team for advice. Not all chronic heart failure patients are palliative, and the majority should still be managed actively and conveyed to hospital. Good care plans, if available, should help decisions around need for conveyance to hospital.

• Patients with advanced disease may have a personal or anticipatory care plan/end of life plan in place. This may be available by contacting a locally agreed directory of service or may be accessible electronically. For these patients, try to follow the care plan or contact the team for advice before admission. Following the care plan may involve assisting or instructing patients to take prescribed anticipatory medications such as extra oral diuretics, i.e. furosemide, bumetanide, bendroflumethiazide or metolazone, or taking the

Heart Failure

- next dose early, in conjunction with a care plan/contact with the community team.
- Currently, many more heart failure patients who are palliative or at the end of their life are cared for at home in their final days with the express wish to remain at home. Consider end of life plans and refer to **End of Life Care**.
- Some patients with advanced heart failure may have a left ventricular assist device (LVAD), a mechanical pump that is implanted inside a person's chest to augment the weakened heart (refer to **Management and Resuscitation of Patients with Left Ventricular Assist Devices (LVADs)**).
- Assessment and management of acute heart failure should focus on identifying the underlying cause, stabilisation and transport to the most appropriate facility (refer to Table 3.70 and Figure 3.18).
- If conveyance to hospital is necessary, the patient should be conveyed rapidly to the most appropriate receiving hospital as per local pathways, preferably to a site with a cardiology department and/or CCU/ICU. Recent data suggest that acute heart failure might have a 'time-to-therapy' concept. Accordingly, pre-hospital management is considered a critical component of care. Many patients with acute heart failure have normal or high blood pressure at presentation and are admitted with symptoms and/or signs of congestion. This is quite unlike cardiogenic shock where low cardiac output leads to symptomatic hypotension and signs/symptoms of hypoperfusion, a circumstance that is relatively rare and associated with a particularly poor outcome. Therefore, it is important to note that appropriate therapy requires appropriate identification of the specific acute heart failure presentation. Caution must be noted regarding giving IV fluids for heart failure.
- It is accepted that the diagnosis of acute heart failure is difficult, especially in the pre-hospital setting, and it is recognised that where doubt exists as to whether the condition is exacerbation of COPD rather than acute heart failure, administration of salbutamol may be considered (refer to **Dyspnoea** and **Medical Emergencies in Adults – Overview**).

TABLE 3.70 – ASSESSMENT and MANAGEMENT of: Acute Heart Failure

Assess <C>ABCDE

- Start correcting <C>ABCDE problems (refer to **Medical Emergencies in Adults – Overview**).
- If the patient is **TIME-CRITICAL**:
  – Correct life-threatening conditions, airway and breathing on scene.
  – Then commence transfer to the nearest suitable receiving hospital.
  – If the patient is in the palliative care stage, refer to their end of life pathway or anticipatory care plans and medicines. Be aware that a number of heart failure patients will have community DNACPR forms. Ask if the patient has an active DNACPR form.
  – If the patient is stable and known to community heart failure services, consider contacting them for advice.

History

- Document history and review any existing care plans for:
  – HF diagnosis
  – SOB/SOBOE
  – chest pain
  – COPD/asthma
  – orthopnoea
  – paroxysmal nocturnal dyspnoea.

Examination

- Examine:
  – heart rate
  – blood pressure
  – respiratory rate
  – SpO_2
  – oedema
  – auscultation.

Heart Failure

TABLE 3.70 – ASSESSMENT and MANAGEMENT of: Acute Heart Failure *(continued)*

- Non-invasive monitoring, including pulse oximetry, blood pressure, respiratory rate and a continuous ECG, should be instituted within minutes of patient contact and continued during transport to hospital.

Clinical Indicators of Potential Heart Failure

- Symptoms include dyspnoea, worsening cough, waking at night gasping for breath, breathlessness on lying down and anxiousness/restlessness.
- Fine crackling sounds (rales) are suggestive of pulmonary oedema, commonly heard in the lung bases, but may be heard over other lung fields as well. These crackles are often accompanied by expiratory wheeze.
- Coughing up of frothy sputum, white or pink (blood stained) in colour in decompensated heart failure.
- Although peripheral oedema is a common sign of heart failure, it is not specific to heart failure and may be a consequence of numerous pathologies. Peripheral oedema starts at the feet and extends up the body as the condition progresses. The patient may also have abdominal ascites and pleural effusion. People with venous insufficiency, obesity or lymphoedema may have chronic oedema.
- JVP provides an estimation of right atrial filling pressure as there are no valves between the right atrium and the internal jugular vein. It is accepted that assessment of JVP can be challenging, particularly in the pre-hospital environment. Assessment of JVP may be undertaken but should not delay treatment.

Oxygen

- Oxygen therapy is recommended for patients with acute heart failure.
- Target saturations 94–98%.
- Administer the initial oxygen dose until a reliable SpO_2 measurement is available, then adjust oxygen flow to aim for a target saturation within the range of 94–98% (refer to **Oxygen**).
- For all patients, sit the patient fully upright immediately. Doing so lowers left atrial pressure, the driving pressure for pulmonary oedema. Sitting the patient fully upright also reduces the abdominal pressure on the bases of the lungs by lowering the diaphragm and enables the patient to use accessory muscles fully. The importance of positioning cannot be overstated. The patient may be nearing exhaustion and will slump quickly so may need repositioning repeatedly during transfer to hospital.

ECG

- Record a 12-lead ECG.
- It is rare for patients with heart failure to have a normal ECG. Where no ECG abnormalities are identified, clinicians should consider the possibility of an alternative diagnosis.
- Where the ECG indicates that heart failure may be due to acute coronary syndrome, refer to **Acute Coronary Syndrome**.

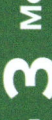

Heart Failure

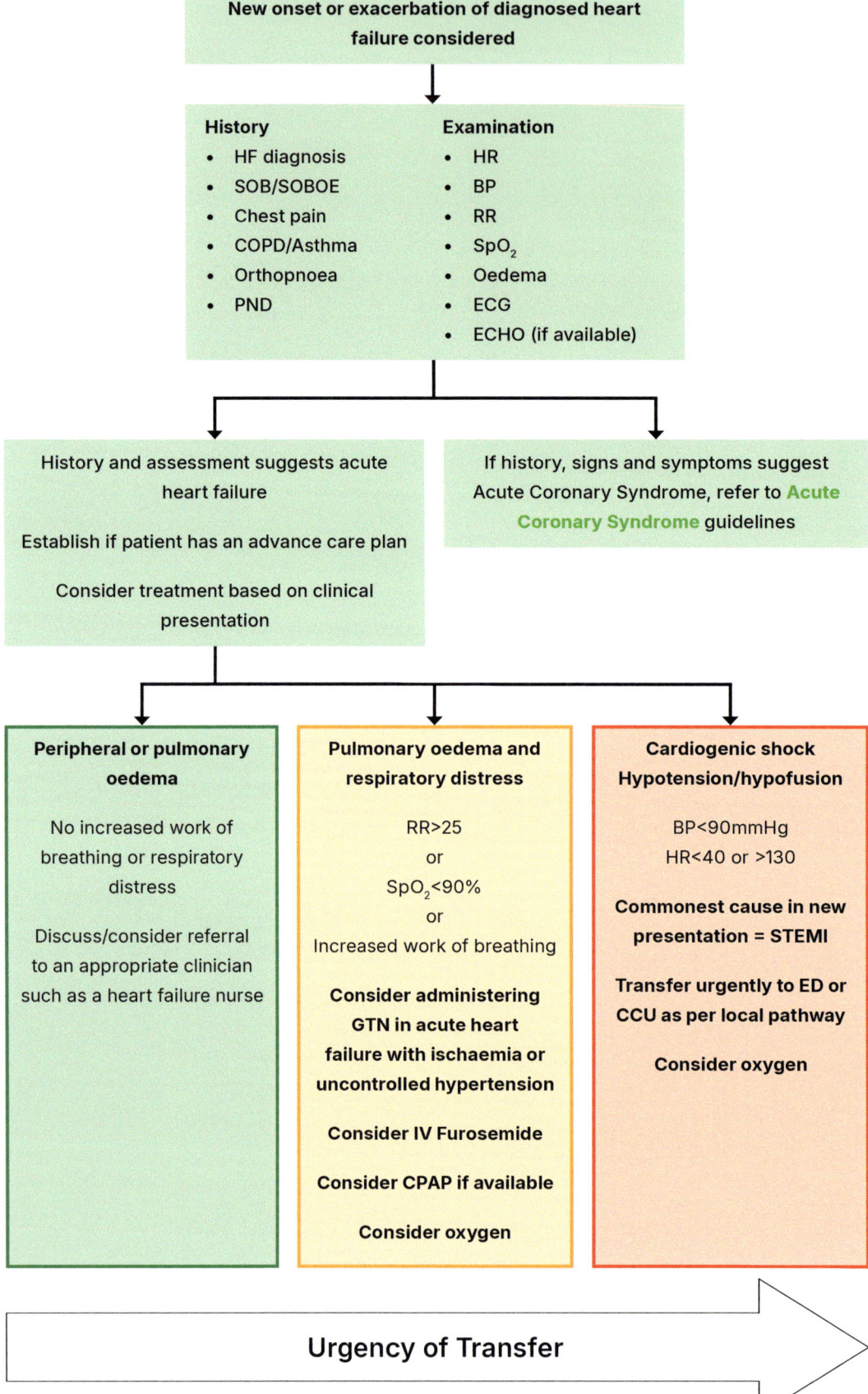

Figure 3.18 – Heart failure algorithm.

Heart Failure

6. Therapies in Heart Failure

6.1 GTN

- Vasodilators are frequently used in heart failure for symptomatic relief; however, there is no robust evidence confirming their beneficial effects. They have dual theoretical benefit by decreasing venous tone (to optimise preload) and arterial tone (to decrease afterload). Consequently, they may also increase stroke volume. Vasodilators are especially useful in patients with hypertensive acute heart failure, whereas in patients with systolic BP <110 mmHg (or with symptomatic hypotension) they should be avoided. Vasodilators should be used with caution in patients with significant aortic stenosis.

6.2 Furosemide

- Furosemide has been the cornerstone of treatment of patients with both acute heart failure and chronic heart failure and signs of fluid overload and congestion for many years. Although there is little high-level evidence for or against its use to improve long-term mortality, it is required for symptomatic benefit. Diuretics increase renal salt and water excretion and have some vasodilatory effect. Initially, 40 milligrams of intravenous furosemide can be considered in acute heart failure patients, excluding cardiogenic shock. If the patient has chronic heart failure, consider reviewing the patient's care plan or contacting the local team/pathway. If the patient requires active management, do not delay conveyance to hospital. Depending on the severity of symptoms, the care plan may advise giving a short-term increase in oral diuretic therapy, particularly if not conveying to hospital.

6.3 Morphine

- Analysis of large heart failure registries suggests that the use of opiates in heart failure increases mortality. Therefore, opiates should not routinely be used but should be considered if the patient is complaining of chest pain. Patients with advanced heart failure under the care of a palliative care team may also have morphine listed as part of their routine care plan (refer to **End of Life Care**).

6.4 Continuous Positive Pressure Ventilation

- Continuous positive pressure ventilation (CPAP), if available, should be considered in patients with respiratory distress (respiratory rate >25 breaths/min, SpO_2 <90%) and started as soon as possible to decrease respiratory distress and reduce the rate of mechanical endotracheal intubation. With CPAP therapy, pressure remains constant through the inspiratory and expiratory phases.

- Prospective randomised controlled trials have demonstrated that CPAP improves survival to hospital discharge and decreases intubation rates.

- A systematic review of eight pre-hospital randomised trials of CPAP and BiPAP suggested that CPAP is the most effective treatment in terms of mortality and intubation rate compared to standard care. The effect of BiPAP on mortality and intubation rate was uncertain.

- The objective of non-invasive positive pressure ventilation (CPAP) is two-fold. The first is to 'splint' open collapsing alveoli and increase intra-alveolar pressure. The increase in pressure helps shift fluid present in the alveoli back into the pulmonary capillaries, thereby reducing pulmonary oedema. The second is to raise intrathoracic pressure throughout the respiratory cycle. This increase in intrathoracic pressure increases pressure in the vena cavae, and consequently serves to reduce filling pressures. Combined, these two actions reduce congestion.

Heart Failure

> **KEY POINTS!**
>
> **Heart Failure**
> - Acute heart failure is a life-threatening medical condition. For all new cases and all chronic cases, unless there is an advance care plan or palliative management in place, a TIME-CRITICAL transfer to hospital is required for urgent assessment and treatment, ideally at a hospital that has a coronary care unit.
> - If the patient has a history of heart failure or valve disease, STOP and THINK before administering intravenous fluids, as these can be harmful, especially if given quickly and in large amounts.
> - Consider administering IV furosemide.
> - Consider administering GTN in Acute Heart Failure with ischaemia or uncontrolled hypertension.
> - In patients with systolic BP <110 mmHg, or with symptomatic hypotension, GTN/nitrates should be avoided.
> - CPAP should be utilised where equipment and suitably trained clinicians are available.
> - Pulmonary oedema can be difficult to differentiate from other causes of breathlessness, such as exacerbation of COPD, pulmonary embolism or pneumonia; therefore, a thorough history and physical examination are needed.
> - Establish if the patient has a personal care plan or end of life plan and if they are being managed by a specialist heart failure team. Follow plans or liaise with other healthcare professionals to manage the patient appropriately.
> - Initial management depends on the clinical presentation: acute pulmonary oedema, peripheral oedema, respiratory distress or cardiogenic shock.

Further Reading

Further important information and evidence in support of this guideline can be found in the Bibliography.[4,5,6,7,8,9]

Bibliography

1. Ponikowski P, Voors AA, Anker SD et al. 2016 ESC Guidelines for the diagnosis and treatment of acute and chronic heart failure: the Task Force for the diagnosis and treatment of acute and chronic heart failure of the European Society of Cardiology (ESC). *European Heart Journal* 2016, 37(27): 2129–2200.

2. National Institute for Health and Care Excellence. *Acute Heart Failure: Diagnosis and management* [CG187]. Manchester: NICE, 2014. Available from: https://www.nice.org.uk/guidance/cg187.

3. National Institute for Health and Care Excellence. *Chronic Heart Failure in Adults: Management* [CG108]. Manchester: NICE, 2010. Available from: https://www.nice.org.uk/guidance/cg108.

4. British Medical Association and the Royal Pharmaceutical Society. *British National Formulary 75 (BNF) March – September 2018*. London: The Pharmaceutical Press.

5. Goodacre S, Stevens JW, Pandor A et al. Prehospital noninvasive ventilation for acute respiratory failure: systematic review, network meta-analysis, and individual patient data meta-analysis. *Academic Emergency Medicine* 2014, 21: 960–970.

6. Vital FMR, Saconato H, Ladeira MT, Sen A, Hawkes CA et al. Non-invasive positive pressure ventilation (CPAP or bilevel NPPV) for cardiogenic pulmonary edema (Review). *Cochrane Database Systematic Review* 2013, CD005351.

7. Wakai A, McCabe A, Kidney R et al. Nitrates for acute heart failure syndromes. *Cochrane Database Systematic Review* 2013, CD005151.

8. Peacock WF, Emerman C, Costanzo MR et al. Early vasoactive drugs improve heart failure outcomes. *Congest Heart Fail.* 2009, 15: 256–264.

9. Vaswani A, Khaw HJ, Dougherty S et al. *Cardiology in a Heartbeat*. Banbury: Scion Publishing, 2016.

Heat Related Illness

1. Introduction

- Heat related illnesses are relatively uncommon presenting condition to ambulance services in the United Kingdom but they can be life-threatening.
- Heat related illness can be **exogenous** caused by environmental factors, e.g. the sun and/or **endogenous**, e.g. increased metabolic workload.
- Heat related illness refers to a continuum of conditions (refer to Figure 3.19).

The clinical management of heat related illnesses focusses on the rapid reduction of core temperature and ongoing supportive care, refer to Table 3.75.

Heat stress

- Heat stress occurs when thermal homeostasis begins to fail. This can be due to excessive internal or external heat generation, or dysregulation of normal compensatory mechanisms.

Signs and symptoms of heat stress (Table 3.71) are a warning of impending heat exhaustion if left untreated.

TABLE 3.71 – Features of Heat Stress (European Resuscitation Council Guidelines)

Heat stress
- Heat cramps: sodium depletion causing cramps.
- Heat oedema: swelling of feet and ankles.
- Heat syncope: vasodilation and dehydration causing hypotension.
- Normal or mild temperature elevation.

Heat exhaustion

- Heat exhaustion is a mild form of Heat Related Illness.
- Core temperature may be moderately elevated along with any on the features from Table 3.72.
- If not managed appropriately it can progress to heat stroke.

TABLE 3.72 – Features of Heat Exhaustion

Heat exhaustion
- Core temperature >37°C and <40°C.
- Haemoconcentration.
- Headache, dizziness, nausea, vomiting, tachycardia.
- Hyponatraemia or hypernatraemia.
- Hypotension, sweating, muscle pain, weakness and cramps.
- May progress rapidly to heat stroke.

Heat stroke

- Heat stroke is a life-threatening heat related illness.
- It is defined as a core body temperature (above 40°C) with central nervous system dysfunction such as delirium, convulsions or coma, and systemic organ damage.[3]

There are two types of heat stroke:

1. **Non-exertional heat stroke (or classic heat stroke)** due to very high external temperatures with or without associated high humidity. It is more common in hot climates but also occurs during heatwaves.[3] It tends to occur in the:
   - very young
   - elderly
   - those with chronic illness or frailty.

2. **Exertional heat stroke** is due to excess heat production with impaired ability to dissipate this thermal load, either due to rapid heat production, insulating clothing or warm environs.[3] This tends to occur in:
   - athletes
   - manual workers
   - firefighters
   - military recruits.[5,6]

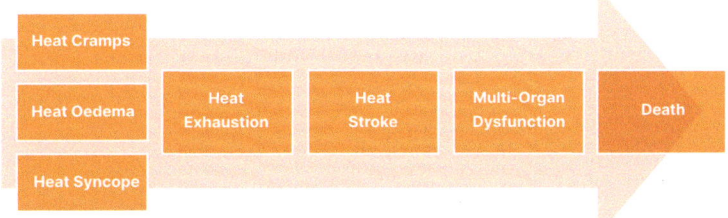

Figure 3.19 – Continuum of heat related illness.

Heat Related Illness

TABLE 3.73 – Features of Heat Stroke

Heat stroke

- Cardiovascular dysfunction including arrhythmias and hypotension.
- Central nervous system dysfunction including seizures and coma.
- Coagulopathy.
- Core temperature ≥40°C.
- Early signs and symptoms include extreme fatigue, headache, fainting, vomiting and diarrhoea, facial flushing (heightened skin colour (flushing) relating to increased blood flow may not be detected in dark skin tones. Assess for local skin temperature changes).
- Hot, dry skin (sweating is present in about 50% of cases of exertional heat stroke).
- Liver and renal failure.
- Respiratory dysfunction including acute respiratory distress syndrome (ARDS).
- Rhabdomyolysis.

2. Incidence

The exact incidence of heat stroke is unknown with many sufferers self-managing their condition. Incidence in the general population in the absence of a heat wave is relatively low.

A variety of medications may predispose to the development of heat illness, refer to Table 3.74.

In addition, individuals who use recreational drugs (e.g. cocaine, ecstasy, amphetamines) and then engage in vigorous or prolonged dancing in crowded "rave" settings may also develop heat illness.[8]

TABLE 3.74 – Medications Predisposing to Heat Related Illness[4]

- Alcohol
- Amphetamines
- Anticholinergics
- Antihistamines
- Antipsychotics
- Beta-Blockers
- Calcium Channel Blockers
- Desmopressin
- Diuretics
- SSRIs
- Theophylline
- Tricyclic antidepressants

3. Severity and Outcome

- Heat stroke is a life-threatening emergency that requires prompt appropriate treatment. Mortality for non-exertional heat stroke is between 10–60% and around 5–25% for exertional heat stroke, although this increases when patients present with concurrent hypotension.[1,3] Recovery from heat stroke even after appropriate treatment and rehabilitation may be incomplete and leave patients with persistent functional impairment.
- Outcome is best when rapid cooling has been provided at the earliest opportunity.[3] Cooling will ideally be undertaken within 30 minutes of patient presentation.[1,7]
- **Systemic effects** – Heat stroke can lead to a variety of life-threatening systemic conditions including: disseminated intravascular coagulation, renal failure, rhabdomyolysis, hepatic necrosis, metabolic acidosis, decreased tissue perfusion, in addition to cerebral and cerebellar damage.

4. Pathophysiology

- In heat related illnesses there is an imbalance in the metabolic production and subsequent loss of heat by the body. This increase in core body temperature has multiple undesirable effects on many body systems. Systemically this increased temperature leads to swelling and degeneration at both cellular and tissue levels.
- **Cellular changes** – At increased temperatures cellular organelles swell and stop functioning properly. Cell membranes become distorted leading to unwanted increased permeability and inappropriate movement of ions across, into and out of cells. Red blood cells also change shape at elevated temperatures and their capacity to carry oxygen is decreased. At high temperatures cells will undergo inappropriate apoptosis and die. Cellular damage correlates to the rise in temperature and the length of time that elevated core temperature is maintained before cooling.

Heat Related Illness

5. Assessment and Management

- For the assessment and management of heat exhaustion and heat stroke refer to Table 3.75.

TABLE 3.75 – ASSESSMENT and MANAGEMENT of: Heat Related Illness

Assess <C>ABCDE

- If any of the following **TIME-CRITICAL** features are present:
  - Major **ABC** problems
  - haemodynamic compromise
  - decreased level of consciousness, then:
- Start correcting **A** and **B** problems.
- Undertake a **TIME-CRITICAL** transfer to nearest appropriate receiving hospital.
- Provide an ATMIST information call.
- Continue patient management en route.

Assess

Undertake physical examination and assess for the presence of features of heat related illness (refer to Tables 3.69–3.71).

- Heat Stroke is potentially fatal and is a **TIME CRITICAL** diagnosis.
- Consider other potential causes for hyperthermia such as infection or side effects from medications or recreational drug use (e.g. amphetamines, cocaine, ecstasy).

Cooling

Initiate measures to cool the patient:

- Remove the patient from the hot environment or remove cause if possible[1]
- Manage in an air-conditioned cool vehicle where available
- Remove clothing[1]
- Apply ice packs to the patient's neck, axillae and groin (such cold packs must **NOT** be the only cooling method used)[9,10]
- Commence cooling with fanning, tepid sponging, water misting or with a wet sheet loosely over the patient's body[1]
- If cold or iced water is used, massaging of the skin may be needed to overcome cold induced vasoconstriction and ensure effective heat loss
- Transfer the patient with air conditioning turned on or with vehicle windows open.

NB Ice packs applied directly to the skin can cause frostbite, place a layer of material between the packs and the skin.

- **DO NOT** administer antipyretics (NSAIDs or paracetamol)[1]

NB Immersion in cold or ice water is highly effective at cooling[1] but usually not possible in the pre-hospital environment. Provision should be made for such an intervention at high-risk events.

Temperature

- Measure and record:
  - the patient's temperature.
  - record site and method of temperature measurement (i.e. tympanic, axillary, other).
  - if possible, and time allows, measure and record the environmental temperature.

NB The core temperature may or may not be elevated but patients may be tachycardic, hypotensive and/or sweating excessively.

Oxygen

- If the patient is hypoxaemic, administer high levels of supplemental oxygen and aim for a target saturation within the range 94–98%); refer to **Oxygen**.

(continued)

Heat Related Illness

TABLE 3.75 – ASSESSMENT and MANAGEMENT of: Heat Related Illness *(continued)*

Fluid Therapy

If fluid therapy is indicated refer to Intravascular Fluid Therapy guidelines. (**Intravascular Fluid Therapy for Adults** and **Intravasucular Fluid Therapy for Children**)

DO NOT administer warmed intravascular fluids.[11,12]

DO NOT delay on scene for fluid replacement; administer en route.

Blood Glucose

- Measure blood glucose; refer to **Glycaemic Emergencies in Adults and Children**.

Vital Signs

- Monitor vital signs.
- Monitor ECG.
- Assess AVPU and GCS.

Disposition

- Consider discharge on scene for patients with mild heat related illness who can: tolerate oral fluids, have rapid normalisation of physiology and become symptom free.
- For such patients, provide appropriate safety-netting
- Patients with Exertional Heat Illness should follow appropriate Return to Function guidelines after seeking specialist and personalised advice.[13]
- The guidance may include:
  – Restricted activities
  – Medical follow-up
  – Graded resumption of activity

Transfer

- Transfer patients with moderate or severe heat related illness to the nearest appropriate receiving hospital.
- Continue management en route.
- Complete documentation.

KEY POINTS!

Heat Related Illness

- Heat Related Illness occurs in three main settings; high external temperatures, as a result of excess heat production and with certain drugs.
- The higher the level of activity, the lower the environmental temperature required to produce heat stroke.
- Do not assume that collapse in an athlete is due to heat illness – check for other causes.
- In mild Heat Related Illness, the patient may present with flu-like symptoms, such as headache, nausea, dizziness, vomiting, and cramps; the core temperature may not be elevated.
- In severe Heat Related Illness, the patient will have neurological symptoms such as decreased level of consciousness, ataxia and convulsions, and core temperature will usually be elevated, typically >41°C.
- Remove the patient from the hot environment or remove cause, remove clothing and cool.

Heat Related Illness

Bibliography

1. Lipman GS, Gaudio FG, Eifling KP, Ellis MA, Otten EM, Grisson C (2019). Wilderness Medical Society Clinical Practice Guidelines for the Prevention and Treatment of Heat Illness: 2019 Update. Wilderness & Environmental Medicine. 30(4S): S33–S46

2. Heled Y, Rav-Acha M, Shani Y, Epstein Y, & Moran, DS (2004). The "golden hour" for heatstroke treatment. Military medicine, 169(3): 184–186.

3. Boucham A, Abuyassin B, Lehe C, Laitano, O, Jay O, O'Connor FG and Leon LR (2022). Classic and exertional heatstroke. Nature Reviews Disease Primers, 8(1): 8.

4. Dallimore J, Anderson SR, Imray C, Johnson, C., Moore, J. and Winser, S. (2023). Oxford Handbook of Expedition and Wilderness Medicine. 3rd Edition. Oxford University Press. Oxford.

5. Ogden HB, Rawcliffe AJ, Delves SK, & Roberts, A. (2022). Are young military personnel at a disproportional risk of heat illness?. BMJ Mil Health. 98–303.

6. Périard JD, DeGroot D, & Jay O (2022). Exertional heat stroke in sport and the military: epidemiology and mitigation. Experimental physiology, 107(10): 1111–1121.

7. Belval, Luke N, Douglas J. Casa, William M. Adams, George T. Chiampas, Jolie C. Holschen, Yuri Hosokawa, John Jardine et al. "Consensus statement-prehospital care of exertional heat stroke." Prehospital Emergency Care 22, no. 3 (2018): 392–397.

8. Yeo TP (2004). Heat stroke: a comprehensive review. AACN Advanced Critical Care, 15(2): 280–293.

9. Gaudio FG, & Grissom CK (2016). Cooling methods in heat stroke. The Journal of emergency medicine, 50(4): 607–616.

10. Kielblock AJ, Van Rensburg JP, & Franz RM (1986). Body cooling as a method for reducing hyperthermia. An evaluation of techniques. The South African Medical Journal. 69(6): 378–380.

11. Mok G, DeGroot D, Hathaway NE, Bigley DP, McGuire CS. Exertional heat injury: effects of adding cold (4 C) intravenous saline to prehospital protocol. Current sports medicine reports. 2017 Mar 1; 16(2): 103–8.

12. Morrison KE, Desai N, McGuigan C, Lennon M, Godek SF. Effects of Intravenous Cold Saline on Hyperthermic Athletes Representative of Large Football Players and Small Endurance Runners. Clinical Journal of Sport Medicine. 2018 Nov 1;28(6): 493–9.

13. O'Reilly M, Hu YWE, Gruber J, Jones DM, Daniel A, Marra J, & Fraser JJ (2022). Consistency and applicability of return to function guidelines in tactical-athletes with exertional heat illness. A systematic review. The Physician and Sports medicine, 1–10.

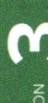

Hyperventilation Syndrome

1. Introduction

- Hyperventilation syndrome is defined as 'breathing in excess of metabolic requirements'.[1]
- It is characterised by an irregular and disorganised breathing pattern with an increased rate and depth of respirations, known as tachypnoea.[2]
- Hyperventilation has many causes, including a number of life-threatening conditions such as:
  - myocardial infarction
  - pulmonary embolism
  - diabetic ketoacidosis
  - asthma
  - sepsis.
- This guideline focuses on acute episodes of primary or idiopathic hyperventilation, which means there is no underlying cause.[3,4] This condition was initially termed Hyperventilation Syndrome (HVS), but more recently the term HVS has slowly disappeared in favour of:
  - Panic/anxiety attack
  - Panic/anxiety disorder
  - Dysfunctional breathing
  - Breathing pattern disorder.[5,6,7,8,9]

2. Incidence

- It is estimated that 6–10% of the general adult population may suffer from some form of HVS. The condition is more common in women.[6,7] Within UK ambulance services the prevalence of HVS is estimated to be 1%, which is comparable to estimates for emergency departments, which range from 0.3–6%.[10,11,3,12]
- HVS is rare in children, where the most likely cause is physical illness.
- Patients with HVS use a significant amount of hospital and emergency service resources because they frequently seek care in the emergency department or from paramedics due to fearing they are experiencing life-threatening emergencies.[11,13]

3. Severity and Outcome

- As per its definition, HVS has no organic cause and is self-limiting. No organic cause means that there is no underlying physical change to the patient's cells, tissues or organs which could account for the experienced symptoms. The signs and symptoms of HVS may be distressing for the patient but these will subside once a good respiratory pattern is established.
- Within the literature there are case study reports of apnoeic episodes following HVS, but these are rare.[14]
- **A diagnosis of HVS must be a diagnosis of exclusion of organic causes for hyperventilation.** This is due to the differential diagnoses of HVS including many life-threatening conditions with poor prognosis if the correct treatment is withheld. Potential differential diagnoses are listed in Table 3.76.

TABLE 3.76 – Differential Diagnoses of HVS by Body System[15,16,17,18]

BODY SYSTEM	DIFFERENTIAL DIAGNOSES	
Cardiovascular	- Angina - Aortic aneurysm - Coronary artery disease - Tachyarrhythmia	- Myocardial infarction - Pericarditis - Heart failure
Neurological	- Brain stem lesions - Encephalitis - Head trauma - Mèniére's disease	- Meningitis - Stroke - Vertigo
Respiratory	- Asthma - Chronic obstructive pulmonary disease - Cystic fibrosis - Interstitial lung disease	- Lung tumour - Pneumonia - Pneumothorax - Pulmonary embolism - Pleural effusion
Gastrointestinal	- Cholecystitis - Liver failure - Hiatus hernia	- Liver cirrhosis - Peptic ulcer

Hyperventilation Syndrome

TABLE 3.76 – Differential Diagnoses of HVS by Body System[15,16,17,18] *(continued)*

BODY SYSTEM	DIFFERENTIAL DIAGNOSES	
Endocrine	• Diabetic ketoacidosis • Pheochromocytoma	• Thyrotoxicosis
Renal	• Kidney failure	
Environmental	• Heat or altitude acclimatisation	• Carbon monoxide poisoning
Other	• Anaemia • Drug intoxication • Drugs or caffeine (withdrawal) • Pain	• Hypokalaemia • Sepsis • Serious aspirin overdoses • Pregnancy

4. Pathophysiology

- The basic rhythm of respiration is controlled subconsciously by the medullary respiratory centre.[19] The automatic control of respiration can be overridden by anxiety, which causes central stimulation of the medullary respiratory centre's inspiratory area, leading to an increased rate and depth of respiration.[20]

- An increased rate and depth of respiration results in faster elimination of carbon dioxide through exhalation, causing a decrease in alveolar and arterial carbon dioxide known as hypocapnia.[18] Hypocapnia reduces the formation of hydrogen ions and bicarbonate ions in the blood, causing a rise in pH levels known as respiratory alkalosis.[21]

- Hypocapnia also causes constriction of cerebral arteries, thereby increasing vascular resistance and reducing blood flow to the brain.[18] This diminished cerebral perfusion may explain some of the neurological symptoms associated with HVS.[22]

- The physiological mechanisms by which many of the other HVS symptoms occur are not entirely clear, but they must nonetheless be seen as genuine consequences of physiological imbalances rather than figments of patients' imagination.[23]

- Signs and symptoms of HVS are wide-ranging and vague and can vary between patients. Experiencing the frightening symptoms of HVS may exacerbate patients' anxiety which promotes further hyperventilation, resulting in HVS symptoms entering a vicious cycle.

TABLE 3.77 – Signs and Symptoms of HVS by Body System[2,4,20,22]

BODY SYSTEM	SIGNS AND SYMPTOMS
Cardiovascular	Palpitations, tachycardia, arrhythmias, chest pain, blotchy changes in skin colour
Neurological	Paraesthesia (numbness and tingling of the mouth/lips/extremities), dizziness/unsteadiness/light-headedness, syncope, headache, blurred or tunnel vision, impaired concentration and memory
Respiratory	Tachypnoea, shortness of breath, tightness in chest/throat, frequent sighing, yawning, feeling of suffocation/choking
Gastrointestinal	Globus, dysphagia, epigastric discomfort, excessive air-swallowing, dry mouth, belching, flatulence, nausea
Musculoskeletal	Aching of the muscles of the chest, tremors, weakness, tetany of hands or feet (e.g. carpopedal spasm)
Psychological	Tension, anxiety, panic, feelings of unreality or disorientation, fear of dying, fear of losing control or going crazy, hallucinations, phobias
General	Fatigue, exhaustion, sleep disturbance, sweating, weakness, chills or heat sensations

Hyperventilation Syndrome

5. Assessment and Management

For the assessment and management of hyperventilation syndrome, refer to Table 3.78 and Figure 3.20.

TABLE 3.78 – ASSESSMENT and MANAGEMENT of: Hyperventilation Syndrome

Assess <C>ABCDE

- If any of the following **TIME-CRITICAL** features present:
  - major **<C>ABCDE** problems
  - cyanosis
  - reduced level of consciousness (refer to **Altered Level of Consciousness**).
  - hypoxia (refer to **Oxygen**).
- Start correcting **<C>ABCDE** problems.
- Undertake a **TIME-CRITICAL** transfer to nearest receiving hospital.
- Continue patient management en route.
- Provide an alert/information call.

NB If any of the **TIME-CRITICAL** features listed above are present, it is unlikely to be due to hyperventilation syndrome and is more likely to be physiological hyperventilation, secondary to an underlying pathological process.

Individualised Treatment Plan

- Ask the patient if they have an individualised treatment plan, and follow the plan if available.
- The patient will often be able to guide their care.

History

⚠ **Always presume hyperventilation is secondary to hypoxia or another underlying respiratory or metabolic disorder until proven otherwise and such is a diagnosis of exclusion.**

- Cause of hyperventilation.
- Previous episodes of hyperventilation.
- Previous medical history.
- Features of hyperventilation syndrome (refer to Table 3.76).
- Did the patient's breathlessness occur at rest rather than exertion? This distinction points towards HVS.[24]

Differential Diagnosis

- Refer to Table 3.76.

Basic Observations

- Respiratory rate.
- Peripheral oxygen saturations (SpO_2): apply pulse oximeter. **DO NOT** administer supplemental oxygen unless hypoxaemic (SpO_2 <94%) (refer to **Oxygen**). **NB** Low SpO_2 is not a presenting feature of HVS and will indicate an underlying clinical condition.
- Heart rate.
- Blood pressure.
- Measure and record blood glucose for hypo/hyperglycaemia (refer to **Glycaemic Emergencies in Adults and Children**).
- If required, monitor and record a 12-lead ECG and assess for abnormality (refer to **Cardiac Arrhythmia and Sudden Cardiac Death**).
- Temperature.
- Respiratory rate and heart rate will likely be elevated in acute HVS patients alongside an abnormally high SpO_2 of 99%–100%.[25]

Hyperventilation Syndrome

TABLE 3.78 – ASSESSMENT and MANAGEMENT of: Hyperventilation Syndrome *(continued)*

Physical examination
- Auscultation of breath sounds to exclude physical causes of breathlessness as may be indicated by a wheeze or crackles.[24]
- Observation and palpation of the patient's chest may demonstrate paradoxical breathing associated with forced respiration, i.e. the abdomen retracts and upper chest expands on inhalation as supposed to normal abdominal protrusion and lower thorax expansion.[18]
- Refer to **Dyspnoea**.

Disease-specific Measurements
- Peak expiratory flow: readings should be compared with predicted values to exclude significant respiratory restriction.[18]
- ECG: temporary ECG changes can occur during acute episodes of HVS, and underlying cardiac conditions need to be excluded.[26]

Treatment
- Aim to restore a normal level of pCO_2 over a period of time by reassuring the patient and coaching them regarding their respirations.
- Practical ways to coach a patient's breathing include:
  - asking the patient to count to two between each breath
  - using distraction techniques
  - asking the patient to slowly breathe in through their nose and out through their mouth.
- Try to remove the source of the patient's anxiety – this is particularly important in the management of children.
- Promote a good patient–clinician relationship: communicate to patients that you believe they are suffering with HVS, as this may offer sufficient reassurance and relief of anxiety which in turn will reduce the severity and frequency of symptoms.[27]
- Paper bag rebreathing has not been recommended since 1990 due to the risk of hypoxia.[28]
- Refer to **Mental Health Presentations**.

Diagnosis
- There is a lack of agreement regarding specific HVS diagnostic criteria and no symptoms are absolutely diagnostic of HVS.[18]

Oxygen Saturation
- Apply pulse oximeter.
- **DO NOT** administer supplemental oxygen unless hypoxaemic (SpO_2 <94%) (refer to **Oxygen**).
- **NB** Low SpO_2 is not a presenting feature of HVS and will indicate an underlying clinical condition.

Breathing
- Consider auscultation of breath sounds during assessment of breathing.
- Aim to restore a normal level of pCO_2 over a period of time by reassuring the patient and coaching them regarding their respirations.
- Try to remove the source of the patient's anxiety – this is particularly important in the management of children.
- Refer to **Dyspnoea**.

Transfer
- Transfer to further care:
  - Patients experiencing their first episode.
  - Children aged <16 years.
  - Known HVS sufferers whose symptoms have not settled or which re-occur within 10 minutes.
  - Patients who have an individualised care plan and a responsible adult present may be considered for non-conveyance and managing at home according to local protocols.
  - Provide details of local care pathways if symptoms re-occur.

Hyperventilation Syndrome

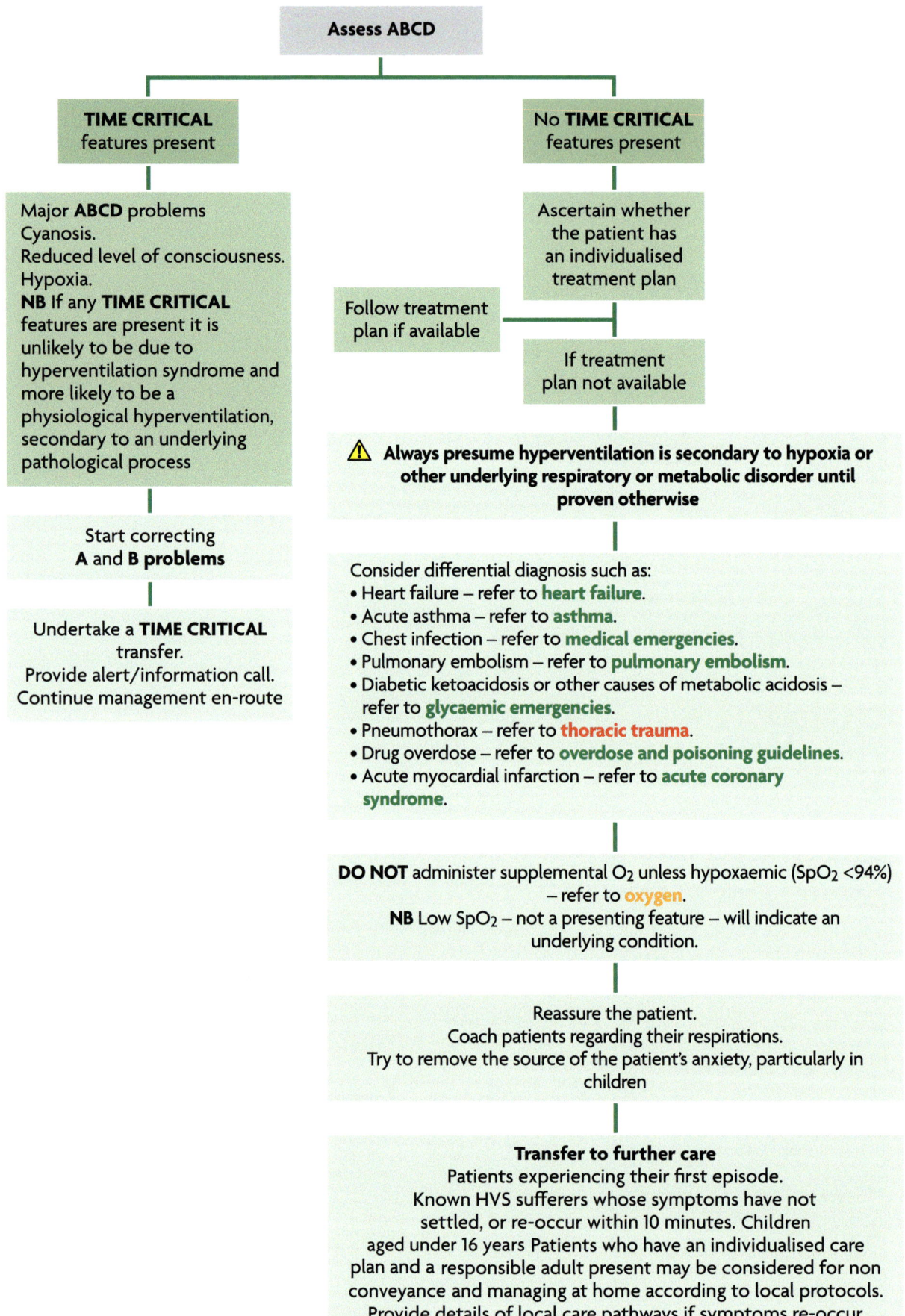

Figure 3.20 – Assessment and management of hyperventilation syndrome algorithm.

Hyperventilation Syndrome

> **KEY POINTS!**
>
> **Hyperventilation Syndrome**
> - HVS is a diagnosis of exclusion.
> - Differential diagnosis: many life-threatening medical conditions can cause hyperventilation.
> - In children a medical cause is more likely than anxiety.
> - Administer supplemental oxygen if hypoxaemic (SpO$_2$ <94%).
> - Reassure the patient and coach their breathing.

Further Reading

Further important information and evidence in support of this guideline can be found in the Bibliography.[29,30,31,32,33,34,35,36,37,38,39,40,41,42]

Bibliography

1. Gardner WN. Hyperventilation: a practical guide. *Medicine* 2003, 31(11): 7–8.
2. Caroline N. *Emergency Care in the Streets*. 7th edn. Burlington, MA: Jones and Bartlett, 2016.
3. Pfortmueller CA, Pauchard-Neuwerth SE, Leichtle AB, Fiedler GM, Exadaktylos AK, et al. Primary hyperventilation in the emergency department: a first overview. *PLOS ONE* 2015, 10(6).
4. Clarke V, Townsend P. Respiratory assessment. In Blaber AY, Harris G. *Assessment Skills for Paramedics*. 2nd edn. Maidenhead: Open University Press, 2016: 14–46.
5. Kerr WJ, Gliebe PA, Dalton JW. 1938. Physical phenomena associated with anxiety states: the hyperventilation syndrome. *Cal West Med* 1938, 48(1): 12–16.
6. Thomas M, McKinley RK, Freeman E, Foy C. Prevalence of dysfunctional breathing in patients treated for asthma in primary care. *BMJ* 2001, 322(7294): 1098–1100.
7. Thomas M, McKinley RK, Freeman E, Foy C, Price D. The prevalence of dysfunctional breathing in adults in the community with and without asthma. *Prim Care Respir J* 2005, 14(2): 78–82.
8. Warburton CJ, Jack S. Can you diagnose hyperventilation? *Chron Respir Dis* 2006, 3(3): 113–115.
9. Todd S, Walsted ES, Grillo L, Livingston R, Menzies-Gow A, Hull JH. Novel assessment tool to detect breathing pattern disorder in patients with refractory asthma. *Respirology* 2017, 23: 284–290.
10. Wilson C, Harley C, Steels S. PP09 Pre-hospital diagnostic accuracy for hyperventilation syndrome. *Emerg Med J* 2017: 34:e3.
11. Coley KC, Saul MI, Seybert AL. Economic burden of not recognizing panic disorder in the emergency department. *J Emerg Med* 2009, 36(1): 3–7.
12. Greenslade JH, Hawkins T, Parsonage W, Cullen L. Panic disorder in patients presenting to the emergency department with chest pain: prevalence and presenting symptoms. *Heart Lung Circ* 2017, 26(12): 1310–1316.
13. Katerndahl DA, Realini JP. Where do panic attack sufferers seek care? *J Fam Pract* 1995, 40(3): 237–243.
14. Munemoto T, Masuda A, Nagai N, Tanaka M, Yuji S. Prolonged post-hyperventilation apnea in two young adults with hyperventilation syndrome. *BioPsychoSocial Medicine* 2013, 7(1): 9.
15. Pfeffer JM. The aetiology of the hyperventilation syndrome. *Psychother Psychosom* 1978, 30(1): 47–55.
16. Ong JR, Hou SW, Shu HT, Chen HT, Chong CF. Diagnostic pitfall: carbon monoxide poisoning mimicking hyperventilation syndrome. *Am J Emerg Med* 2005, 23(7): 903–904.
17. Brashear RE. Hyperventilation syndrome. *Lung* 1983, 161(1): 257–273.
18. Pizzorno JE, Murray MT, Joiner-Bey H. *The Clinician's Handbook of Natural Medicine*. 3rd edn. St Louis: Elsevier, 2016.
19. Aehlert B. *Paramedic Practice Today: Above and beyond*. Burlington, MA: Jones and Bartlett, 2011.
20. Porth CM, Litwack K. Disorders of acid-base balance. In Porth CM, Matfin G. *Pathophysiology: Concepts of altered health states*. 8th edn. Philadelphia: Lippinkott Williams & Wilkins, 2009: 805–825.
21. Khurana I. *Medical Physiology for Undergraduate Students*. New Delhi: Elsevier, 2012.
22. Evans RW. Unilateral paresthesias due to hyperventilation syndrome. *Pract Neurol* 2005: 65–68.
23. Chapman S, Robinson G, Stradling J, West S. *Oxford Handbook of Respiratory Medicine*. Oxford: Oxford University Press, 2009.
24. National Institute for Health and Care Excellence. *Breathlessness*. Clinical Knowledge Summaries. 2017. Available from: https://cks.nice.org.uk/breathlessness.
25. O'Driscoll BR, Howard LS, Earis J on behalf of the British Thoracic Society Emergency Oxygen Guideline Group. BTS guideline for oxygen use in adults in healthcare and emergency settings. *Thorax* 2017, 72: ii1–ii90.
26. Michaelides AP, Liakos CI, Antoniades C, Tsiachris DL, Soulis D, Dilaveris PE, Tsioufis KP, Stefanadis CI. ST-segment depression in hyperventilation indicates a false positive exercise test in patients with mitral valve prolapse. *Cardiology Research and Practice*. 2015. Available from: https://www.hindawi.com/journals/crp/2010/541781.
27. Boulding R, Stacey R, Niven R, Fowler SJ. Dysfunctional breathing: a review of the literature and proposal for classification. *Eur Respir Rev* 2016 25(141): 287–294.
28. Kishikawa M. Re-evaluation of paper bag rebreathing for hyperventilation syndrome. *International Conference*

Hyperventilation Syndrome

and Exhibition on Lung Disorders & Therapeutics. 2015. Available from: http://lung.conferenceseries.com/abstract/2015/re-evaluation-of-paper-bag-rebreathing-for-hyperventilation-syndrome.

29. Wilson C. Hyperventilation syndrome: diagnosis and reassurance. *Journal of Paramedic Practice* 2018, 10(9): 370–375.

30. American Psychiatric Association. Diagnostic and Statistical Manual of Mental Disorders. 5th edn. 2013. Available from: https://dsm.psychiatryonline.org/doi/book/10.1176/appi.books.9780890425596.

31. Malmberg LP, Tamminen K, Sovijärvi ARA. Orthostatic increase of respiratory gas exchange in hyperventilation syndrome. *Thorax* 2000, 55(4): 295–301.

32. Maguire CA, Robson AG, Pentland J, McAllister D, Innes JA. Smoking status predicts benefit from breathing retraining for hyperventilation. *Thorax* 2010, 65(suppl. 4): A157.

33. Gardner W. Orthostatic increase of respiratory gas exchange in hyperventilation syndrome. *Thorax* 2000, 55(4): 257–259.

34. Bazin KA, Moosavi S, Murphy K, Perkins A, Hickson M, Howard LS. Carbon dioxide sensitivity in patients with hyperventilation syndrome. *Thorax* 2010, 65(suppl. 4): A134.

35. van den Hout MA, Boek C, van der Molen GM, Jansen A, Griez E. Rebreathing to cope with hyperventilation: experimental tests of the paper bag method. *Journal of Behavioral Medicine* 1988, 11(3): 303–310.

36. Tavel ME. Hyperventilation syndrome: hiding behind pseudonyms? *Chest* 1990, 97(6): 1285–1288.

37. Saisch SGN, Wessely S, Gardner WN. Patients with acute hyperventilation presenting to an inner-city emergency department. *Chest* 1996, 110(4): 952–957.

38. Hornsveld HK, Garssen B, Fiedeldij Dop MJC, van Spiegel PI, de Haes J. Double-blind placebo-controlled study of the hyperventilation provocation test and the validity of the hyperventilation syndrome. *The Lancet* 1996, 348(9021): 154–158.

39. Gardner WN. The pathophysiology of hyperventilation disorders. *Chest* 1996, 109(2): 516–534.

40. Folgering H. The pathophysiology of hyperventilation syndrome. *Monaldi Archives for Chest Disease* 1999, 54(4): 365–372.

41. Callaham M. Hypoxic hazards of traditional paper bag rebreathing in hyperventilating patients. *Annals of Emergency Medicine* 1989, 18(6): 622–628.

42. The British Thoracic Society, Scottish Intercollegiate Guidelines Network. *British Guideline on the Management of Asthma* (Guideline 101). London/Edinburgh: BTS and SIGN, 2008 (revised May 2012). Available from: https://www.brit-thoracic.org.uk/document-library/clinical-information/asthma/btssign-asthma-guideline-2014/.

Hypothermia

1. Introduction

- Hypothermia is defined as a core body temperature below 35°C (refer to Figure 3.21). It is a potentially life-threatening condition and a reversible cause of cardiac arrest.
- Primary hypothermia is due to environmental exposure, with no underlying medical condition causing disruption of temperature regulation.
- Secondary hypothermia results from a medical illness lowering the temperature set-point.
- The speed of onset of hypothermia can vary:
  i. **Acute hypothermia (immersion hypothermia)**
     – This occurs when a person loses heat very rapidly (e.g. by falling into cold water). It is associated with drowning. Acute hypothermia may also occur in a snow avalanche when it may be associated with asphyxia.
  ii. **Subacute hypothermia (exhaustion hypothermia)**
     – This typically occurs in a hill walker who is exercising in moderate cold who becomes exhausted and is unable to generate enough heat. Heat loss will occur more rapidly in windy conditions or if the patient is wet or inadequately clothed. It may be associated with injury, frostbite or non-freezing cold injury. Do not forget that if one person in a group of walkers is hypothermic, others in the party who are similarly dressed and who have been exposed to identical conditions may also be hypothermic.
  iii. **Chronic hypothermia**
     – In chronic hypothermia heat loss occurs slowly, often over days or longer. It most commonly occurs in the older person living in an inadequately heated house or the person who is sleeping rough. It can be associated with injury or illness (e.g. the patient who falls or has a stroke and who is on the floor overnight).
- Mixed forms of hypothermia may occur (e.g. the exhausted walker who collapses and falls into a stream).

1.1 Diagnosis

- In order to measure core body temperature accurately and make a diagnosis, a low-reading thermometer is required. However, most ambulance services do not carry low-reading thermometers. In the pre-hospital environment, measuring the patient's temperature using an oesophageal, bladder or rectal approach may not be practical. However, tympanic thermometry may not be reliable in cold environments (partly because the probe is not well insulated) or if the patient is in cardiac arrest, with no blood flow in the carotid artery.
- Because of the difficulty of diagnosing hypothermia in the pre-hospital environment, patients should be treated as having hypothermia if there is clinical suspicion of the diagnosis based on the risk factors in Table 3.79, the clinical history, examination and the presence of concurrent injuries or illness which may increase the likelihood of hypothermia.

TABLE 3.79 – Risk Factors for Hypothermia

Factors

- Older patients > 80 years due to impaired thermoregulation.
- Children due to their proportionately larger body surface area.
- Some medical conditions (e.g. hypothyroidism, stroke etc. due to impaired thermoregulation).
- Intoxicated patients (e.g. alcohol, recreational drugs).
- In association with drowning and in patients exposed to cold, wet and windy environments especially if inadequately dressed.
- Patients suffering from exhaustion.
- Injury and immobility.
- Decreased level of consciousness.

2. Incidence

- The true incidence is unknown but the ONS report fewer than 400 deaths per annum in England and Wales. However, it is suggested that hypothermia may be under-diagnosed in temperate climates such as the UK.
- Death from hypothermia is more common in those over the age of 70 and in males.

3. Pathophysiology

As the core body temperature falls, there may be:

- Progressive decrease in the level of consciousness (refer to **Altered Level of Consciousness**).
- Other brain dysfunction (e.g. slurring of speech, muscular incoordination).
- Slowing heart rate.
- Slowing respiratory rate.
- Development of cardiac arrhythmias, such as sinus bradycardia, atrial fibrillation, ventricular fibrillation and asystole.
- Cooling the body decreases oxygen demand and is protective for the brain and vital organs; therefore refer to the Hypothermia section within **Advanced Life Support** as good outcomes have resulted from prolonged resuscitation of hypothermic patients.

Hypothermia

4. Severity and Outcome

The severity of hypothermia can be classified as mild, moderate or severe depending on the patient's core body temperature (refer to Figure 3.21).

- However, in the pre-hospital environment, where appropriate thermometers and the skills to use them are often unavailable, it may be better to define the severity clinically (refer to Table 3.80).

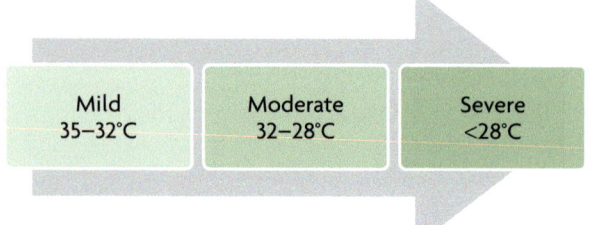

Figure 3.21 – Severity of hypothermia.

TABLE 3.80 – Clinical Stages of Hypothermia	
Stage	**Clinical Signs**
I	Conscious and shivering.
II	Reduced conscious level; may or may not be shivering.
III	Unconscious; vital signs present.
IV	Apparent death; vital signs absent.

5. Assessment and Management

For the assessment and management of hypothermia, refer to Table 3.81.

TABLE 3.81 – ASSESSMENT and MANAGEMENT of: Hypothermia
Assess <C>ABCDE

• If any of the following **TIME-CRITICAL** features are present:
  – major **<C>ABCDE** problems, refer to **Medical Emergencies in Adults – Overview** and **Medical Emergencies in Children – Overview**.
  – haemodynamic compromise.
  – decreased level of consciousness.
  – cardiac arrest, then:
• Start correcting any **<C>ABCDE** problems.
• Undertake a **TIME-CRITICAL** transfer to nearest appropriate receiving hospital or consider transfer to a hospital that provides extracorporeal life support (ECLS), as per local pathways.
• Continue patient management en route.
• Provide an ATMIST information call.

Assess
• Undertake physical examination and assess for the presence of features of hypothermia (refer to Table 3.80): symptoms are often non-specific and can include ataxia, slurred speech, apathy, irrational behaviour and decrease in the level of consciousness (refer to **Altered Level of Consciousness**), heart rate and rhythm and respiratory rate.
Temperature
• Measure and record the patient's core temperature. Temperature measurement in the field is difficult, therefore it is important to suspect and treat hypothermia from the history and circumstances of the situation. Shivering peaks around 34°C and is minimal or stopped by 31–32°C. Shivering is a very effective way of raising body temperature BUT there must be adequate energy stores to fuel it.

Hypothermia

TABLE 3.81 – ASSESSMENT and MANAGEMENT of: Hypothermia *(continued)*

Warming

PREVENT FURTHER HEAT LOSS, as in the mildly hypothermic patient, preventing further heat loss will enable the patient to warm up by their own metabolism.

- Place in vehicle.
- Consider using foil blankets. Foil blankets work by reflecting radiated heat so are only useful in mild hypothermia. In severe hypothermia, minimal heat is radiated.
- Some foil blankets may only have one reflective surface so must be placed the right way round.
- If the patient is conscious, provide a hot drink/food if available and appropriate.
- **DO NOT** rub the patient's skin as this causes vasodilatation and may increase heat loss.
- **DO NOT** give the patient alcohol as this causes vasodilatation and may increase heat loss.
- Manage co-existing trauma or medical conditions as they arise (refer to appropriate **trauma/medical** guidelines).

Resuscitation

BEWARE: Severely hypothermic patients may initially appear to be dead but frequently have a very slow and weak pulse, very slow and shallow respirations, fixed dilated pupils and increased muscle tone. Dilated pupils can be seen in hypothermia and therefore should not be used as a sign of death.

- Rough handling can invoke cardiac arrhythmias (including VF and pulseless VT), so handle patients carefully.
- Airway – clear the airway.
- Ventilation – if there are no signs of respiration, ventilate with high concentrations of oxygen, but do NOT hyperventilate. A respiratory rate and tidal volume appropriate in normothermia is inappropriate in hypothermia (refer to appropriate **Resuscitation** guidelines).
- Signs of life – look for signs of life (palpate central artery, ECG monitoring etc.) for up to 1 minute.
- Cardiac arrest – refer to appropriate **Resuscitation** guidelines and additional information below. Remember that the rules for normothermic arrest must not be extrapolated completely to hypothermic arrest.
- Cardiac arrythmias (except VF) will usually revert spontaneously with re-warming and do not need treatment unless they persist after re-warming.

Respiratory Rate

- Measure and record respiratory rate.

Pulse

- Measure and record pulse.

Oxygen

- It is unlikely that SpO_2 can be reliably measured using a finger probe in a hypothermic patient. Oxygen should be given in all cases, and particularly if the patient is shivering and has co-morbidities, as the metabolic demand of intense shivering puts an extra burden on the heart. Administer 15 litres per minute until a reliable SpO_2 measurement can be obtained and then adjust oxygen flow to aim for target saturation within the range of 94–98% (refer to **Oxygen**).

Blood Pressure and Fluids

- Measure and record blood pressure. If required, administer fluids (preferably warm fluids). (Refer to **Intravascular Fluid Therapy in Adults** and **Intravascular Fluid Therapy in Children**).

Blood Glucose

- Measure and record blood glucose for hypo/hyperglycaemia (refer to **Glycaemic Emergencies in Adults and Children**).

NEWS2

- These observations will enable you to calculate a NEWS2 Score (refer to **Sepsis**).

ECG

- Monitor and record 12-Lead ECG. Assess for abnormality (refer to **Cardiac Arrhythmia and Sudden Cardiac Death**).

(continued)

Hypothermia

TABLE 3.81 – ASSESSMENT and MANAGEMENT of: Hypothermia (continued)

Assess the Patient's Pain
- Where present, assess the **SOCRATES** of pain and record initial and subsequent pain scores.
- Consider analgesia if appropriate (refer to **Pain Management in Adults and Children**).

Transfer
- Transfer patients to the nearest appropriate receiving hospital. For patients with cardiac arrest, cardiovascular system instability (BP <90; irregular rhythm; ventricular arrhythmia), consider conveying to a hospital that provides ECLS, as per local pathways.
- In severe hypothermia with the presence of cardiac instability or arrest, the fastest way to re-warm patients is by extracorporeal warming – this may not be available in every hospital, so follow any local care pathways. Other patients can be re-warmed successfully by less invasive or non-invasive methods.
- Continue management en route.
- Complete documentation.

Additional Information for Cardiac Arrest in Hypothermia

While breathing continues, cardiac arrest has not occurred so do not start CPR.

Do not stop cardiac resuscitation in the field.

Follow the usual procedure (refer to appropriate **Resuscitation** guidelines) with the following minor changes:
- Hypothermia may cause chest wall stiffness, and ventilations and compressions may be more difficult.
- Drugs are less likely to be effective at low body temperatures: do not give ALS drugs if the core temperature is below 30°C.
- Defibrillation is less likely to be effective at low body temperatures: if VF persists after 3 shocks, delay further defibrillation until the core temperature is above 30°C.
- Hypothermia is protective and good outcomes have resulted from prolonged resuscitation of hypothermic patients.

Trauma (refer to appropriate **Trauma** guidelines) – hypothermia worsens the prognosis of trauma patients, so it is important that patients who are initially normothermic are not allowed to become hypothermic. This may occur for example during a prolonged extrication from a road traffic collision or from the cooling of burns.

Documentation
- Complete documentation to include all clinical findings, advice from other clinicians, onward referral and worsening advice given.

KEY POINTS!

Hypothermia
- **Do not stop cardiac resuscitation in the field.**
- **Hypothermia is defined as a core body temperature below 35°C.**
- **Prevent further heat loss; wrap the patient appropriately, do not rub the skin or give alcohol.**
- **If cardiac arrest occurs, ALS drugs may not be effective; prolonged (hours) CPR will be required.**

Bibliography

1. Gordon L, Paal P. Normothermic and hypothermic cardiac arrest – beware of Jekyll and Hyde. *Resuscitation* 2018, 129: e10–11.
2. Haverkamp FJC, Giesbrecht GG, Tan ECTH. The prehospital management of hypothermia – an up-to-date overview. *Injury* 2018, 49: 149–164.
3. Paal P, Gordon L, Strapazzon G, Brodmann Maeder M, Putzer G, Walpoth B, et al. Accidental hypothermia-an update: the content of this review is endorsed by the International Commission for Mountain Emergency Medicine (ICAR MEDCOM). *Scand J Trauma Resusc Emerg Med* 2016, 24: 111.
4. Truhlar A, Deakin CD, Soar J, Khalifa GE, Alfonzo A, Bierens JJ. European Resuscitation Council Guidelines

Hypothermia

for Resuscitation 2015. Section 8: cardiac arrest in special circumstances. *Resuscitation* 2015, 95: 148–201.

5. Caroselli C, Gabrieli A, Pisani A, Bruno G. Hypothermia: an under-estimated risk. *Internal and Emergency Medicine* 2009, 4(3): 227–230.

6. Strapazzon G, Procter E, Paal P, Brugger H. Pre-hospital core temperature measurement in accidental and therapeutic hypothermia. *High Alt Med Biol* 2014, 15(2): 104–111.

7. Ireland S, Endacott R, Cameron P, Fitzgerald M, Paul E. The incidence and significance of accidental hypothermia in major trauma—a prospective observational study. *Resuscitation* 2011, 82: 300–306.

8. Stroop R, Schone CH Grau Th. Incidence and strategies for preventing sustained hypothermia of crash victims during prolonged vehicle extrication. *Injury* 2019, 50: 308–317.

9. Waibel BH, Schlitzkus LL, Newell MA, et al. Impact of hypothermia (below 36°C) in the rural trauma patient. *J Am Coll Surg* 2009, 209: 580–588.

10. Shari S, Elliott AC, Gentilello L. Is hypothermia simply a marker of shock and injury severity or an independent risk factor for mortality in trauma patients? Analysis of a large national trauma registry. *J Trauma* 2005. 59: 1081–1085.

11. Eidstuen SC, Uleberg O, Vangberg G, Skogvoll E. When do trauma patients lose temperature – a prospective study. *Acta Aanes Scand* 2018, 62: 384–393.

12. Winkelmann M, Soechtig W, Macke C, et al. Accidental hypothermia as an independent risk factor or poor neurological outcome in older multiply injured patients with severe traumatic brain injury: a matched pair analysis. *Eur J Trauma Emerg Surg* 2019, 45: 255–261.

13. Trentzsche H, Huber-Wagner S, Hildebrand F, et al. Hypothermia for prediction of death in severely injured blunt trauma patients. *Shock* 2012, 37: 131–139.

14. Lapostolle F, Courvreur J, Koch FX, Savary D, et al. Hypothermia in trauma victims at first arrival of ambulance personnel: an observational study with assessment of risk factors. *Scand J Trauma Resus Emerg Med* 2017, 25: 43.

15. Khorsandi M, Dougherty S, Yound N, Kerslake D, Giordano V, Lendrum R, et al. Extracorporeal life support for refractory cardiac arrest from accidental hypothermia: a 1–year experience in Edinburgh. *J Emerg Med* 2016, 52: 160–168.

16. McCormack J, Percival D. HEMS advanced trauma team retrieval of a patient with accidental hypothermic cardiac arrest for ECMO therapy. *Resuscitation* 2016, 105: e23.

17. Ruttmann E, Dietl M, Kastenberger T, et al. Characteristics and outcome of patients with hypothermic out-of-hospital cardiac arrest: experience from a European trauma center. *Resuscitation* 2017, 120: 57–62.

18. Forti A, Brugnaro P, Crucitti M, Brugger H, Cipollotti G, Strapazzon G. Hypothermic cardiac arrest with full neurologic recovery after approximately nine hours of cardiopulmonary resuscitation: management and possible complications. *Ann Emerg Med* 2019, 73: 52–57.

Implantable Cardioverter Defibrillator

1. Introduction

- The implantable cardioverter defibrillator (ICD) has revolutionised the management of patients at risk of developing a life-threatening ventricular arrhythmia. Several clinical trials have testified to their effectiveness in reducing deaths from sudden cardiac arrest in selected patients, and the devices are implanted with increasing frequency.
- ICDs are used in both children and adults.
- ICD systems consist of a generator connected to an electrode or electrodes, usually placed transvenously into cardiac chambers (the ventricle, and sometimes the right atrium and/or the coronary sinus) (refer to Figure 3.22). The electrodes serve a dual function allowing the monitoring of cardiac rhythm and the administration of electrical pacing, defibrillation and cardioversion therapy. Modern ICDs are slightly larger than a pacemaker and are usually implanted in the left subclavicular area (refer to Figure 3.22). The ICD generator contains the battery and sophisticated electronic circuitry that monitors the cardiac rhythm, determines the need for electrical therapy, delivers treatment, monitors the response and determines the need for further therapy. Subcutaneous ICDs are usually placed in the left lateral chest wall, beneath the axilla, with a subcutaneous lead placed across the left precordium, and running up the edge of the sternum in a reverse "L" shape. Subcutaneous are more common in children and young adults, and avoid complications associated with long term intravascular hardware, but function in a similar way as the more frequently occurring subcutaneous system.
- The available therapies include:
  - Conventional programmable pacing for the treatment of bradycardia
  - Anti-tachycardia pacing (ATP) for ventricular tachycardia (VT) in trans-venous systems
  - Delivery of biphasic shocks for the treatment of ventricular tachycardia and ventricular fibrillation (VF)
  - Cardiac resynchronisation therapy (CRT) (biventricular pacing) for the treatment of heart failure.
- These treatment modalities and specifications are programmable and capable of considerable sophistication to suit the requirements of individual patients. The implantation and programming of devices is carried out in specialised centres. The patient should carry a card or documentation which identifies their ICD centre and may also have been given emergency instructions.
- The personnel caring for such patients in emergency situations are not usually experts in arrhythmia management or familiar with the details of the sophisticated treatment

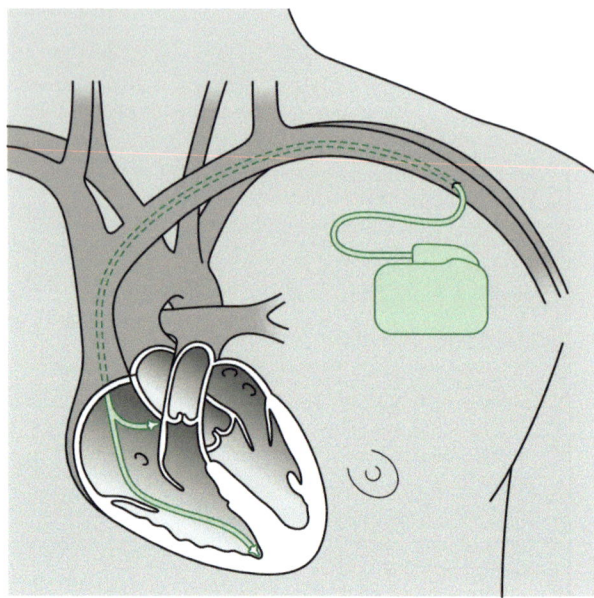

Figure 3.22 – Usual location of an ICD.

regimes offered by modern ICDs. Moreover, the technology is complex and evolving rapidly. In an emergency, patients will often present to the ambulance service or emergency department (ED) and the purpose of this guidance is to help those responsible for the initial management of these patients.

2. General Principles

Some important points should be made at the outset.

- The ICD has a simple algorithm to decide when to shock, first of all based on heart rate, and then by determining if the rate is regular or stable (i.e. not atrial fibrillation) and whether the QRS morphology is narrow or broad complex (e.g. SVT versus VT). However if in doubt the device will usually discharge, and so AF with rapid, aberrant QRS complexes may well prompt a so-called inappropriate shock.
- On detecting VF/VT, the ICD will usually discharge a maximum of eight times before shutting down. However, a new episode of VF/VT will result in the recommencing of its discharge sequence. A patient with a fractured ICD lead may suffer repeated internal defibrillation as the electrical noise is misinterpreted as a shockable rhythm, which is another cause of so-called inappropriate shock.
- These patients are likely to be conscious with a relatively normal ECG rate.
- When confronted with a patient in cardiac arrest, the usual management guidelines are still appropriate (refer to **cardiac arrest** and **arrhythmia** guidelines). If the ICD is not responding to VF or VT, or if shocks are ineffective, external defibrillation/cardioversion should be carried out. Avoid placing the

Implantable Cardioverter Defibrillator

defibrillator electrodes/pads/paddles close to or on top of the ICD; ensure a minimum distance of 8 cm between the edge of the defibrillator paddle pad/electrode and the ICD site. Most ICDs are implanted in the left sub-clavicular position (refer to Figure 3.22) and are usually readily apparent on examination; the conventional (apical/right subclavicular) electrode position will then be appropriate. The anterior/posterior position may also be used, particularly if the ICD is right sided.

- Whenever possible, record a 12-lead electrocardiogram (ECG) and record the patient's rhythm (with any shocks). Make sure this is printed out and stored electronically (where available) for future reference. Where an external defibrillator with an electronic memory is used (whether for monitoring or for therapy), ensure that the ECG report is printed and handed to appropriate staff. Again, whenever possible, ensure that the record is archived for future reference. Record the rhythm during any therapeutic measure (whether by drugs or electricity). All these records may provide vital information for the ICD centre that may greatly influence the patient's subsequent management.

- The energy levels of the shocks administered by ICDs (up to 40 Joules) are much lower than those delivered with external defibrillators (120–360 J). **Personnel in contact with the patient when an ICD discharges will not be harmed by the shock; often the reassurance of holding a patient's hand, or even a hug, can be beneficial to the patient. Leaping back from a patient suffering ICD shocks will often increase their stress and adrenaline levels, especially in the case of inappropriate shocks.** Chest compression and ventilation can be carried out as normal, and protective examination gloves should be worn as usual.

- Placing a ring magnet over the ICD generator can temporarily disable the shock capability of an ICD. The magnet does not disable the pacing capability for treating bradycardia. The magnet may be kept in position with adhesive tape if required. Removing the magnet returns the ICD to the status present before application. This is invaluable in the case of inappropriate shocks. The ECG rhythm should be monitored at all times when the device is disabled. An ICD should only be disabled when the rhythm for which shocks are being delivered has been recorded. If that rhythm is VT or VF, external cardioversion/defibrillation must be available. With some models, it is possible to programme the ICD so that a magnet does not disable the shock capabilities of the device. This is usually done only in exceptional circumstances, and consequently such patients are rare.

- The manufacturers of the ICDs also supply the ring magnets. Many implantation centres provide each patient with a ring magnet and stress that it should be readily available in case of emergency. With the increasing prevalence of ICDs in the community, it becomes increasingly important that emergency workers have this magnet available to them when attending these patients.

- Note that patients with an implantable cardioverter defibrillator may have a DNACPR form or ReSPECT plan. Follow these as appropriate. It is not expected that an ICD should be manually disabled with a magnet if the patient suffers a cardiac arrest. It may continue to fire until the patient enters a non-shockable rhythm.

- Many problems with ICDs can only be dealt with permanently by using the programmer available at the ICD centre.

- The guidelines should be read from the perspective of your position and role in the management of such patients. For example, the recommendation to 'arrange further assessment' will mean that the ambulance clinician should transport the patient to hospital. For ED staff, however, this might mean referral to the medical admitting team or local ICD centre.

- Coincident conditions that may contribute to the development of arrhythmia (e.g. acute ischaemia worsening heart failure) should be managed as appropriate according to usual practice.

- Maintain oxygen saturations above 94%.

- Receiving ICD therapy may be unpleasant 'like a firm kick in the chest', and psychological consequences may also arise. It is important to be aware of these, and help should be available from implantation centres. An emergency telephone helpline may be available.

- Recurrent ICD discharges can be harmful, and may indicate a "VT/VF Storm" – defined as >3 episodes in 24 hours, and will usually require admission; a single shock where the device has discharged appropriately and effectively will often not require admission, with the patient usually being asked to contact their implanting centre during office hours, in the absence of any other pathology that may have precipitated the attack.

3. Management

- The following should be read in conjunction with the treatment table (refer to Table 3.82) and algorithm (refer to Figure 3.23). Approach and assess the patient and perform basic life support according to current BLS guidelines.

Implantable Cardioverter Defibrillator

	Monitor the ECG
3.1	**If the patient is in cardiac arrest.**
3.1.1	Perform basic life support in accordance with current BLS guidelines. Standard airway management techniques and methods for gaining IV/IO access (as appropriate) should be established.
3.1.2	If a shockable rhythm is present (VF or pulseless VT) but the ICD is not detecting it, perform external defibrillation and other resuscitation procedures according to current resuscitation guidelines.
3.1.3	If the ICD is delivering therapy (whether by anti-tachycardia pacing or shocks) but is failing to convert the arrhythmia, then external defibrillation should be provided, as per current guidelines.
3.1.4	If a non-shockable rhythm is present, manage the patient according to current guidelines. If the rhythm is converted to a shockable one, assess the response of the ICD, performing external defibrillation as required.
3.1.5	If a shockable rhythm is converted to one associated with effective cardiac output (whether by the ICD or by external defibrillation), manage the patient as usual and arrange further treatment and assessment.
3.2	**If the patient is not in cardiac arrest.**
3.2.1	Determine whether an arrhythmia is present.
3.2.2	If no arrhythmia is present:
	If therapy from the ICD has been effective and the patient is in sinus rhythm or is paced, monitor the patient, give O_2 and arrange further assessment to investigate the possibility of new myocardial infarction (MI), heart failure, other acute illness or drug toxicity/electrolyte imbalance etc.
	An ICD may deliver inappropriate shocks (i.e. in the absence of arrhythmia) if there are problems with sensing the cardiac rhythm or with the leads. Record the rhythm (while shocks are delivered, if possible), disable the ICD with a magnet, monitor the patient and arrange further assessment with help from the ICD centre. Provide supportive treatment as required.
3.2.3	If an arrhythmia is present:
	If an arrhythmia is present and shocks are being delivered, record the arrhythmia (while ICD shocks are delivered if possible) on the ECG. Determine the nature of the arrhythmia. Transport rapidly to hospital in all cases.
TACHYCARDIA	
3.2.3.1	If the rhythm is a **supraventricular tachycardia** (i.e. sinus tachycardia, atrial flutter, atrial fibrillation, junctional tachycardia, etc.) and the patient is haemodynamically stable and is continuing to receive shocks, disable the ICD with a magnet. Consider possible causes, treat appropriately and arrange further assessment in hospital.
3.2.3.2	If the rhythm is **ventricular tachycardia**:
	• Pulseless VT should be treated as cardiac arrest (3.1.2 above).
	• If the patient is haemodynamically stable, monitor the patient and convey to the emergency department.
	• If the patient is haemodynamically unstable, and ICD shocks are ineffective, treat as per VT guideline.
	• An ICD will not deliver antitachycardia pacing (ATP) or shocks if the rate of the VT is below the programmed detection rate of the device (generally 150 beats/min). Conventional management may be undertaken according to the patient's haemodynamic status.
	• Recurring VT with appropriate shocks. Manage any underlying cause (acute ischaemia, heart failure etc.). Sedation may be of benefit.
INAPPROPRIATE/INEFFECTIVE ICD FIRING	
3.2.3.3	A ring magnet placed over the ICD box will stop the ICD from firing and may be considered in conscious patients where the ICD shocks are ineffective and the patient is distressed. In ICDs that have a dual pacing function, the magnet will also usually change the pacing function to deliver a paced output of 50 beats/min. Rarely, placing a magnet may trigger a fixed pacing mode from older devices – there is no harm from this, but it may look sudden and unusual on the monitor if not expected. This feature is rare nowadays and restricted to a minority of devices in usage within the UK.

Implantable Cardioverter Defibrillator

TABLE 3.82 – ASSESSMENT and MANAGEMENT of: Patients Fitted with an ICD

Patient in Cardiac Arrest:
- Assess the patient
  - Perform basic life support in accordance with current BLS guidelines.
  - Standard airway management techniques.
  - IV access (if required) should be used.
- Monitor the ECG.

Assess Rhythm:
- Shockable rhythm is present (VF or pulseless VT)
  - **BUT** the ICD is not detecting it, perform external defibrillation and other resuscitation procedures according to current resuscitation guidelines.
  - If the ICD is delivering therapy (whether by ATP or shocks) but is failing to convert the arrhythmia, then external defibrillation should be provided, as per current guidelines.
- Non-shockable rhythm
  - Manage the patient according to current guidelines. If the rhythm is converted to a shockable one, assess the response of the ICD, performing external defibrillation as required.
- If a shockable rhythm is converted to one associated with effective cardiac output (whether by the ICD or by external defibrillation)
  - Manage the patient as usual and arrange further treatment and assessment.

Patient NOT in Cardiac Arrest
- Determine whether an arrhythmia is present.

If no arrhythmia is present
- If therapy from the ICD has been effective, the patient is in sinus rhythm or is paced:
  - Monitor the patient.
  - Administer oxygen and aim for a saturation above 94% (refer to **Oxygen**).
  - Arrange further assessment to investigate possibility of new myocardial infarction (MI), heart failure, other acute illness or drug toxicity/electrolyte imbalance etc.
  - An ICD may deliver inappropriate shocks (i.e. in the absence of arrhythmia) if there are problems with sensing the cardiac rhythm or problems with the leads (e.g. a fractured lead may produce intermittent electrical noise that is mis-interpretated as VF by the device):
  - Record the rhythm (while ICD shocks are delivered, if possible).
  - Disable the ICD with a magnet (if available).
  - Monitor the patient.
  - Arrange further assessment with help from the ICD centre. Provide supportive treatment as required.
  - A ring magnet placed over the ICD box will stop the ICD from firing and may be considered in conscious patients where the ICD shocks are ineffective and the patient is distressed. In ICDs that have a dual pacing function, the magnet will also usually change the pacing function to deliver a constant paced output, dependent on the manufacturer.

If an arrhythmia is present
- If an arrhythmia is present and shocks are being delivered:
  - Record the arrhythmia (while ICD shocks are delivered, if possible) on the ECG.
  - Determine the nature of the arrhythmia.
  - Transport rapidly to hospital in all cases.

If the rhythm is **supraventricular** (i.e. sinus tachycardia, atrial flutter, atrial fibrillation, junctional tachycardia, etc.)
- If the patient is haemodynamically stable, and is continuing to receive shocks, disable the ICD with a magnet:
  - Consider possible causes, treat appropriately.
  - Arrange further assessment in hospital.

If the rhythm is **ventricular tachycardia**
- Pulseless VT should be treated as cardiac arrest (3.1.2 above).

(continued)

Implantable Cardioverter Defibrillator

TABLE 3.82 – ASSESSMENT and MANAGEMENT of: Patients Fitted with an ICD *(continued)*

If the patient is haemodynamically stable:
- Monitor the patient.
- Convey to the emergency department.

If the patient is haemodynamically unstable, and ICD shocks are ineffective, treat as per VT guideline.
- An ICD will not deliver ATP or shocks if the rate of the VT is below the programmed detection rate of the device. Conventional management may be undertaken according to the patient's haemodynamic status.
- For recurring VT with appropriate shocks, manage any underlying cause (acute ischaemia, heart failure etc.). Sedation may be of benefit.

KEY POINTS!

Implantable Cardioverter Defibrillators
- ICDs deliver therapy with bradycardia pacing, ATP and shocks for VT not responding to ATP or VF.
- ECG records, especially at the time that shocks are given, can be vital in subsequent patient management. A recording should always be made if circumstances allow.
- Cardiac arrest should be managed according to normal guidelines.
- Avoid placing the defibrillator electrode over or within 8 cm of the ICD box.
- A discharging ICD is unlikely to harm a rescuer touching the patient or performing CPR.
- An inappropriately discharging ICD can be temporarily disabled by placing a ring magnet directly over the ICD box.

Bibliography

1. Soar J, Bottinger BW, Carli P, Couper K, Deakin C, et al. European Resuscitation Council Guidelines 2021: adult advanced life support. *Resuscitation* 2021, 161: 115–151.
2. Perkins GD, Handley AJ, Koster RW, Ristagno G, Soar J, et al. European Resuscitation Council Guidelines 2015 Section 2: adult basic life sup-port and use of automated external defibrillators. *Resuscitation* 2015, 95: 81–99.
3. Perkins GD, Grasner JT, Semeraro F, Nolan JP, et al. European Resuscitation Council Guidelines 2021: executive summary. *Resuscitation* 2021, 161: 1–60.
4. Deakin CD, Nolan JP, Sunde K, Koster RW. European Resuscitation Council Guidelines for Resuscitation 2010 Section 3: electrical therapies: automated external defibrillators, defibrillation, cardioversion and pacing. *Resuscitation* 2010, 81(10): 1293–1304.
5. Deakin CD, Morrison LJ, Morley PT, Callaway CW, Kerber RE, Kronick SL, et al. Part 8: advanced life support: 2010 International Consensus on Cardiopulmonary Resuscitation and Emergency Cardiovascular Care Science with Treatment Recommendations. *Resuscitation* 2010, 81(1): e93–174.
6. Sunde K, Jacobs I, Deakin CD, Hazinski MF, Kerber RE, Koster RW, et al. Part 6: defibrillation: 2010 International Consensus on Cardiopulmonary Resuscitation and Emergency Cardiovascular Care Science with Treatment Recommendations. *Resuscitation* 2010, 81(1): e71–85.

Implantable Cardioverter Defibrillator

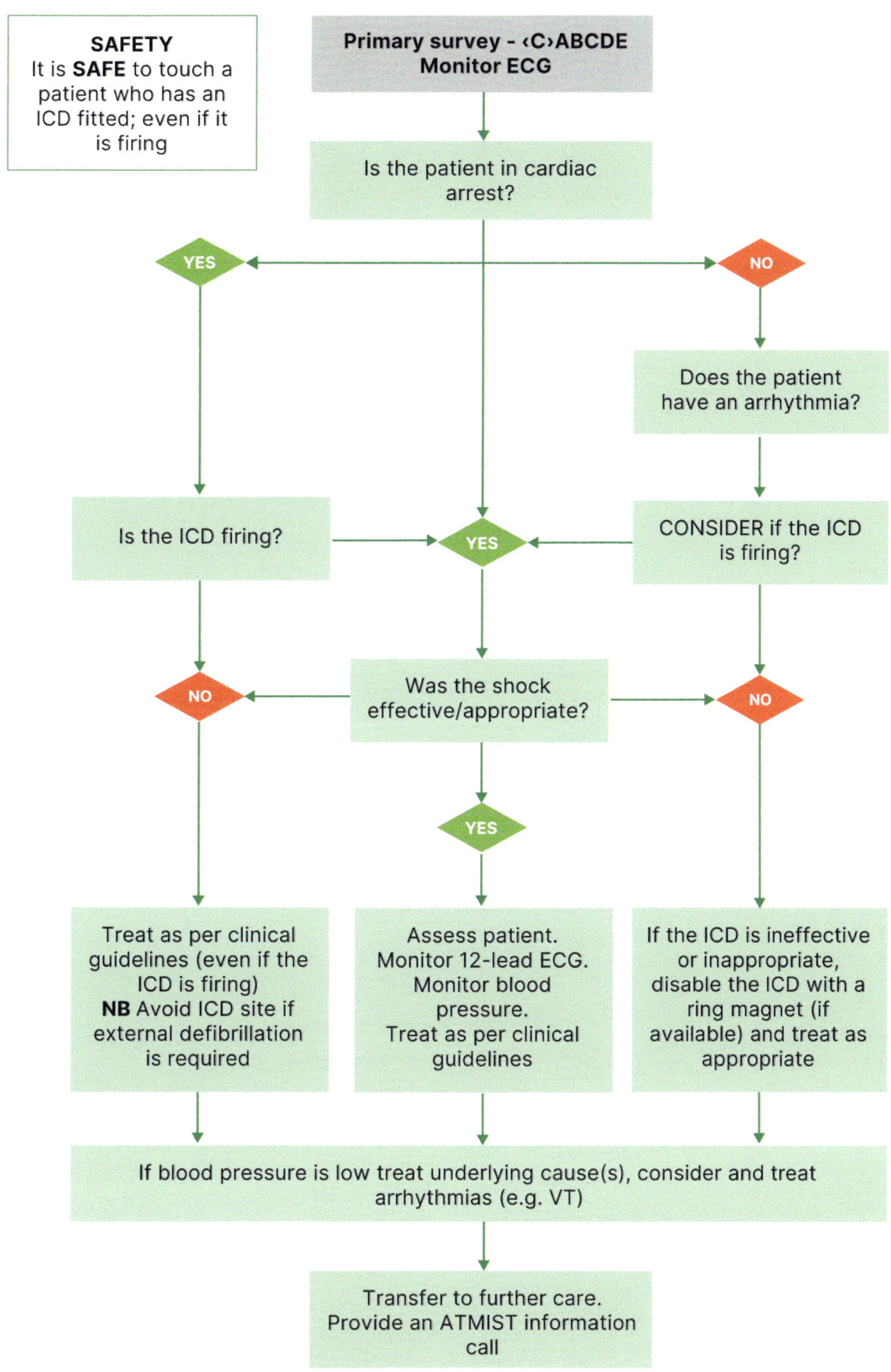

Figure 3.23 – Implantable cardioverter defibrillator algorithm.

Low Back Pain (Non-traumatic)

1. Introduction

- This guideline applies to adults over 18 years old. It does **not** apply to patients that have experienced recent trauma causing their low back pain (including axial-loading mechanisms to top of head through spine). In these instances, refer to **Trauma Emergencies in Adults – Overview** and **Spinal Injury and Spinal Chord Injury**.
- Many people experience back pain at some point in their adult life. Most often, symptoms resolve within 6 weeks with conservative management, including appropriate analgesia, exercise and lifestyle advice. Radiographs are not normally required for acute non-traumatic musculoskeletal back pain in healthy individuals with good bone health.
- Ambulance services are frequently called to patients experiencing severe and debilitating acute low back pain. Assistance is often required for these patients; however, the high severity of the symptoms may frequently exceed the severity of the underlying diagnosis, which will often be non-sinister musculoskeletal pain.
- The likelihood of serious pathology increases with age, and caution is advised in patients over 50 years of age. Alternative diagnoses should be considered in all patients, regardless of age, particularly where symptoms are new or have recently changed. Specific causes of lower back pain that should be considered include cancer, infection, fragility fractures, renal colic, inflammatory disease, abdominal aortic aneurysm, pancreatitis, aortic dissection and ectopic pregnancy. Lower back pain is commonly encountered in pregnancy and the same clinical assessment should be performed, making special consideration of pregnancy-associated emergencies (refer to **Maternity Care (including Obstetric Emergencies Overview)**).

2. Incidence

- Low back pain is a common cause of calls to ambulance services in the UK.[1]
- In the United Kingdom, over 2.5 million people consult their GP every year due to back pain. Up to 60% of the population will experience back pain at some point in their adult life, with over 28% of adults over 25 years experiencing low back pain each month.[2]
- Patients may present with new onset lower back pain, or with exacerbations of known chronic pain. Between 3% to 7% of adults are chronically disabled by lower back pain.[3]
- Low back pain is a leading cause of sickness absence from work in the European workforce.[4] However, data suggest that over 70% of people have returned to work at 1 month from onset, and over 93% at 1 year.[5]
- Chronic back pain is associated with mental health issues contributed to by ongoing pain and disability.

3. Severity and Outcome

- Low back pain is subdivided by time frame into:
  – Acute low back pain: less than 4 weeks' duration.
  – Subacute lower back pain: 4 to 12 weeks' duration.
  – Chronic low back pain: lasting more than 12 weeks.
- Most low back pain is musculoskeletal in origin and is defined as pain and/or stiffness in the lumbosacral area of the back, between the bottom of the ribs and the top of the legs.[6] The symptoms may arise from many anatomical structures of the lower back and surrounding area.
- Non-specific low back pain is a well-recognised clinical entity that is diagnosed when the pain cannot be attributed to a specific cause but may likely be related to muscular, ligamentous, intervertebral disc or joint-related origins.[3,7]
- While patients may complain of isolated pain in the lumbosacral region of the spine, they may also encounter radiation of pain unilaterally to the buttocks or thighs, and this may extend beyond the knee.

4. Differential Diagnosis

4.1 Key Differential Diagnoses

- While most low back pain is musculoskeletal in origin, other causes of back pain must always be considered. These include (but are not limited to):
  – renal colic
  – aortic aneurysm
  – aortic dissection
  – pancreatitis
  – ectopic pregnancy.
- Abdominal examination must form part of the examination of patients with low back pain, and must be performed prior to making a diagnosis of musculoskeletal back pain.

4.2 Red Flag Symptoms in Musculoskeletal Pain

- Serious pathology as a cause of musculoskeletal conditions is considered rare but must be managed as an emergency or as urgent depending on local pathways.
- The majority of serious pathology affecting the spine (such as vertebral fractures, cauda equina syndrome, malignant metastatic disease, infection) will most commonly present with back pain. Serious pathologies such as these can involve other body systems.

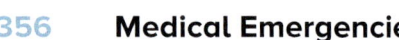

Low Back Pain (Non-traumatic)

- Consider serious pathology as a differential diagnosis to exclude where any of the following features are present:
  - escalating back pain and progressively worsening symptoms that have not responded to conservative management or analgesia
  - systemic illness (e.g. weight loss, fever)
  - night pain that prevents sleep, and/or difficulty in lying flat
  - saddle anaesthesia, disturbance of bladder or bowel function or bilateral sciatica
  - severe or progressive neurological deficit, motor weakness or paralysis.

5. Serious Pathologies (for Conveyance to Hospital)

5.1 Cauda Equina Syndrome (CES)

- Cauda equina syndrome (CES) is a rare but serious condition caused by compression to the nerve roots at the end of the spinal cord ('cauda equina' = 'horse's tail') typically at the levels from L2 to L5. It is a neurosurgical emergency requiring an urgent MRI scan to confirm or exclude the diagnosis. Where the diagnosis is confirmed, a neurosurgical strategy will typically involve emergency spinal decompressive surgery.
- CES should be suspected in people presenting with back pain. Specific symptoms to ask about include:
  - any changes in bladder or bowel function
  - bilateral sciatica (pain radiating down buttocks and thighs)
  - numbness or reduced sensation around or under the genitals, or around the anus
  - loss of anal tone (ability to squeeze anal muscles)
  - loss of sexual function.
- Care must be taken to enquire about these symptoms that may be embarrassing to patients, such as episodes of unexpected faecal incontinence or urinary retention, numbness affecting the perineum when they wipe themselves after going to the toilet or sensory disturbance affecting sexual function (including erectile dysfunction).

5.2 Metastatic Spinal Cord Compression (MSCC)

- Metastatic spinal cord compression (MSCC) occurs as a consequence of metastatic disease infiltrating the bones of the spine. It can lead to irreversible neurological damage.
- Symptoms can include:
  - banding pain (circulating around the torso)
  - rapidly escalating pain
  - disturbance of gait or coordination
  - pain that is worsened on lying flat
  - unremitting pain at night
  - systemic illness associated with advanced malignancy.
- Metastatic disease of the spine can originate from many different primary cancers, including lung, bowel, breast, prostate and blood cancers such as lymphoma. Bony infiltration of the metastatic cancer can lead to collapse of the vertebral bones due to loss of their structural integrity (leading to pain) and can also lead to neurological symptoms from invasion or compression at the spinal canal.

5.3 Infection

- Infections can occur within the spine, notably at the level of the intervertebral discs (discitis) or as collection of pus within the epidural space (abscess). These are uncommon infections in healthy individuals with an uncompromised immune system. However, it is important to consider infection as a cause of unexplained back pain, especially in immune-compromised patients such as those on medications or treatment that reduce their immunity. Intravenous drug users and patients with known active or suspected tuberculosis are also at particular risk of spinal infection.
- Infection should be suspected in patients with back pain, alongside systemic symptoms such as:
  - fever
  - weight loss
  - general malaise/lethargy
  - unexplained tachycardia (patients in severe pain may be tachycardic until this is controlled).

5.4 Vertebral Insufficiency Fracture(s)

- Patients may present with sudden onset of pain localised to the spine, usually in the thoraco-lumbar region. This may occur after low-impact trauma, and may be a sharp, severe pain that is exacerbated by movement.
- Risk factors that may be associated with vertebral insufficiency fractures include:
  - a history of other fragility fractures (such as neck of femur or distal radius fractures)
  - osteoporosis
  - long-term steriod use
  - renal disease.

5.5 Cervical Spondylotic Myelopathy (CSM)

- In rare cases, cervical spondylosis (age-related degeneration) can progress to this syndrome, which is characterised by worsening neck pain, incoordination (e.g. difficulty with simple motor tasks such as fastening buttons), heaviness or weakness in arms or legs, pins and needles in arms, difficulty walking and bowel or bladder disturbance.

Low Back Pain (Non-traumatic)

6. Urgent Conditions (May Be Appropriate for Community Management and/or Referral to Primary Care)

- In most instances, non-traumatic low back pain can be managed in the community with over-the-counter analgesic medications and simple exercises. Other conditions may be appropriate for management in the community but may nonetheless require investigation and support from primary care services. Ambulance clinicians should endeavour to contact a patient's own GP where possible (in-hours), and ensure that a copy of their assessment notes is available to the primary care services to access (as per local guidance and pathways).
- Patients should be provided with advice and guidance tailored to their needs and functional capabilities to empower them to provide self-care for their low back pain. This should include:
  - information relating to the nature of their back pain
  - encouragement to continue with normal activities and routines (where able).[8]

6.1 Rheumatological Conditions

- Osteoarthritis and rheumatoid arthritis may present with an acute flare or progression of symptoms affecting joints including the spine and sacro-iliac joints.

6.2 Known Primary or Secondary Cancers

- Red flag symptoms of MSCC or CES should be excluded (as previously described in section above); however, other patients with low back pain related to cancer may be appropriate for management in the community.

6.3 Acute Sciatica

- Sciatica is a painful syndrome caused by irritation or compression of the sciatic nerve that runs from the lower back to the feet. Sciatica is usually self-limiting within 4–6 weeks but may last longer. Symptoms may be exacerbated by movements such as bending, coughing or sneezing.
- Patients may complain of unilateral pain described as stabbing, burning or shooting in character, and may also encounter weakness, or tingling or numbness, to sensory areas of the buttock, back of leg, knee or foot.

7. Assessment and Management

- Taking a clear and thorough history is an essential part of the assessment in order to explore possible serious pathologies. This will require asking a range of questions, some of which may be intrusive or embarrassing, and so it should be explained to patients that these questions are important and relate to the symptoms of back pain.
- It may be helpful to explain that nerves supply all limbs and organs, and that the nerves at the lower part of the spine supply the bowel and bladder, as well as the patient's sexual function. It may be necessary to ask directly:
  - Have there been any episodes of incontinence (faeces or urine), or have they suffered urinary retention?
  - Have they been able to go to the toilet when they try to?
  - Have they been wet or soiled without knowing?
  - Does it feel different when they wipe themselves after going to the toilet?
- Ask how the patient is coping with the pain. This may be helpful in eliciting what they might be concerned about, and may also establish if the symptoms are exacerbating any chronic or acute mental health problems.
- Explain that medication and other substances can affect pain. Take a thorough social history, including a drug history of prescribed and non-prescribed drugs, alcohol and recreational substances. If necessary, refer to **Alcohol-use Disorders**.

TABLE 3.83 – ASSESSMENT and MANAGEMENT of: Low Back Pain

Assess <C>ABCDE

- If any of the following **TIME-CRITICAL** features are present:
  - Major **<C>ABCDE** problems (refer to **Medical Emergencies in Adults – Overview**).
- Start correcting any **<C>ABCDE** problems.
- Undertake a **TIME-CRITICAL** transfer to nearest appropriate receiving hospital.
- Continue patient management en route.
- Provide an ATMIST information call.

Respiratory Rate

- Measure and record respiratory rate.

Low Back Pain (Non-traumatic)

TABLE 3.83 – ASSESSMENT and MANAGEMENT of: Low Back Pain *(continued)*
Pulse
• Measure and record pulse and heart rate.
Oxygen Saturation
• Monitor the patient's SpO_2; administer oxygen to achieve saturations of >94% if the patient presents as hypoxaemic on air (refer to **Oxygen**).
Blood Pressure
• Measure and record blood pressure.
Blood Glucose
• If appropriate, measure and record blood glucose for hypo/hyperglycaemia (refer to **Glycaemic Emergencies**).
Temperature
• Measure and record temperature.
NEWS2
• These observations will enable you to calculate a NEWS2 score.
ECG
• If required, monitor and record 12-lead ECG. Assess for abnormality (refer to **Cardiac Arrhythmia and Sudden Cardiac Death**).
Assess the Patient's Pain
• Assessment of pain using SOCRATES and score pain using 0–10 rating (refer to **Pain Management in Adults and Children**).
Assess for Other Possible Emergency Medical Causes of the Back Pain
• Assess the abdomen.
• Consider dissecting thoracic or abdominal aortic aneurysm, pancreatitis, renal colic, aortic dissection and ectopic pregnancy.
Assess for Any Red Flags
• Chest pain radiating through to the back.
• Known or suspected underlying serious pathology.
• Bladder/bowels disturbance (new retention or incontinence).
• Bilateral leg pain/pins and needles/numbness.
• Saddle paraesthesia.
• Banding pain (circulating around the whole torso)/pins and needles/numbness.
• Sudden onset of thoracic pain.
• Upper limb incoordination/heaviness.
• Gait incoordination.
• Jaw pain.
• Signs or suspicion of fracture.
• Persistent headache.
• Dizziness.
• Drop attack/blackout/collapse.
• Visual disturbance.
• Any signs of infection.
• Systemically unwell.
• Unremitting night pain.
• Escalating and worsening pain.

(continued)

Low Back Pain (Non-traumatic)

TABLE 3.83 – ASSESSMENT and MANAGEMENT of: Low Back Pain *(continued)*

Inspect the Patient
- What position is the patient when found?
- Can the patient sit?
- Can the patient stand?
- Can the patient lie flat?
- Can the patient mobilise?
- Can the patient evenly bear weight?
- Does the patient's spine have normal curvature, or do they have a kyphosis (bent forwards) or scoliosis (curved sideways)?
- Is the patient experiencing any muscle spasm?
- Palpate the skin and assess closely for rashes, swelling and skin changes. Use natural light if possible (or non-fluorescent light to avoid a blue tinge).
- Does the patient have any fasciculation (muscle twitch/involuntary muscle contraction)?

Palpation
- Palpate the spine for any bony tenderness, crepitus or unnatural alignment of spinal processes.
- Palpate sacroiliac joint and paravertebral muscles for pain/tenderness/spasm/swelling.

Assess for Paraesthesia (Pins and Needles)
See Figure 3.24.
- Where does the patient feel paraesthesia?
- Does the patient feel this constantly or intermittently?

Functional Assessment
- Ask patient to perform a straight leg raise – if this is painful, it usually indicates sciatic nerve irritation due to intervertebral disc disease.
- Assess and document range of movement/strength. Can patient mobilise and manage to undertake basic personal care?

Other Social and Psychological Factors to Assess (Yellow Flags)
- Mental health problems (mood/stress/anxiety/depression).
- Misuse of alcohol or medication misuse (prescription and non-prescription).
- Is the pain affecting activities of daily living (ADLs)?

Functional levels of exercise and activity
- Weight loss or weight gain.
- A belief that pain and/or activity is harmful.
- Social withdrawal.
- Have they been unable to work due to the pain?
- Lack of support at home.

What are the patient's expectations for their care?
- It is not uncommon for patient's to seek diagnostic imaging in the hope that this will remedy their symptoms, and it may be appropriate to counsel patients that emergency MRI imaging is not generally indicated in the absence of red flag signs or symptoms.
- Medication history, including non-prescribed and over the counter medication – what's been tried, dosages etc.

Documentation
- Complete documentation to include all clinical findings, advice from other clinicians, onward referral and worsening safety-net advice provided.

Low Back Pain (Non-traumatic)

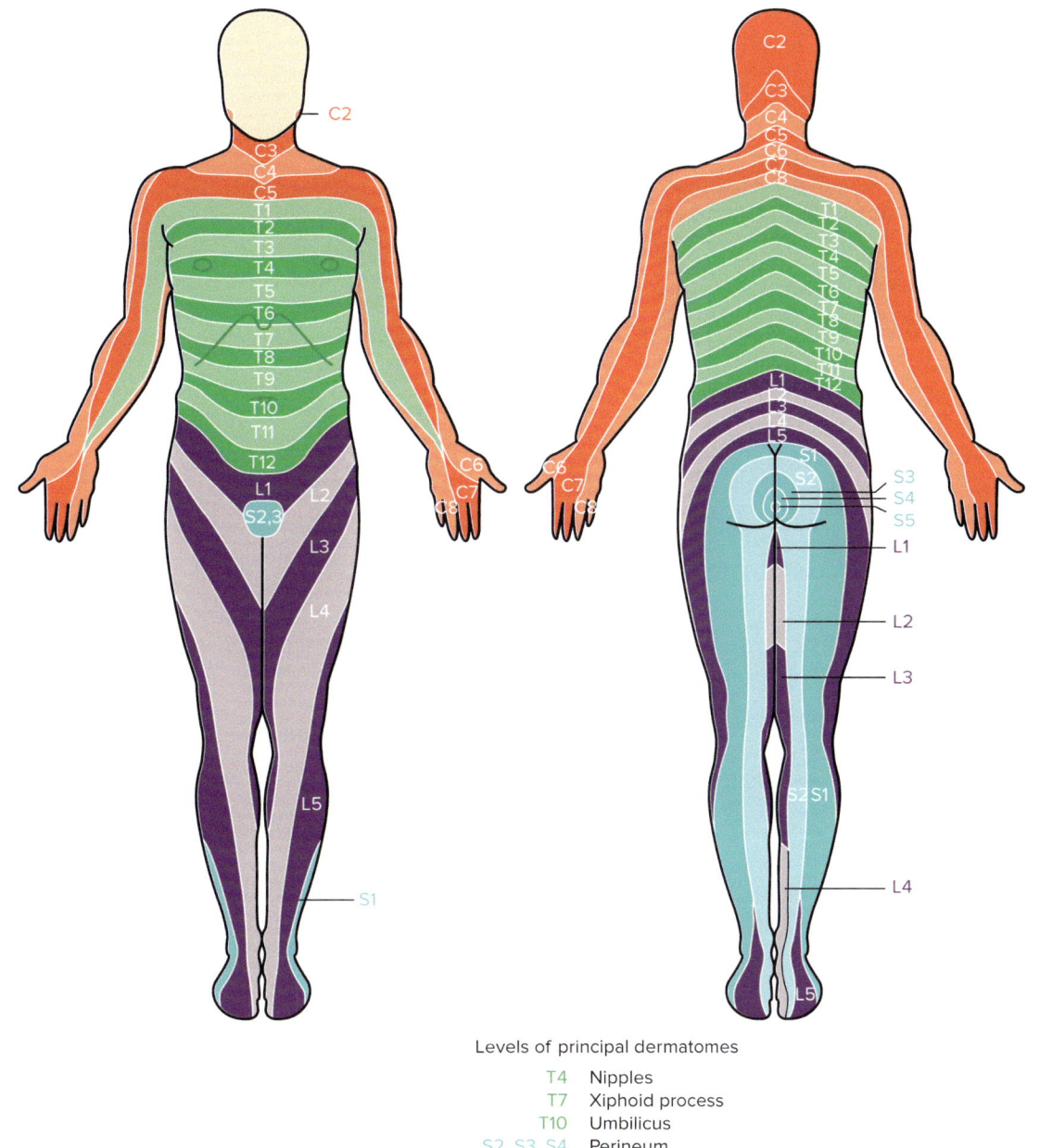

Levels of principal dermatomes
- T4 — Nipples
- T7 — Xiphoid process
- T10 — Umbilicus
- S2, S3, S4 — Perineum

Figure 3.24 – Dermatomes. Dermatomes show the distribution of pain that radiates from the spine at different levels.

8. Pain Management

Both pharmacological and non-pharmacological management options may be appropriate. As a general approach, the patient should be reminded that for simple low back pain their symptoms are likely to improve with a strategy of simple analgesia, gentle exercises and modification of lifestyle factors that may exacerbate the pain.

8.1 Pharmacological Management

- Refer to **Pain Management in Adults and Children**. If a patient already has a pain management plan, they should be advised to follow this and to seek advice from a pharmacist as required.

- Current guidance suggests offering a non-steroidal anti-inflammatory (NSAID) such as ibuprofen as first-line pharmacological treatment in low back pain. Instruction to take gastro-protective medication is recommended, as these reduce stomach acid secretion and mitigate the small risk of GI bleeding that is increased with NSAIDs. Both ibuprofen and proton-pump inhibitors such as omeprazole can be bought over the counter in large stores or pharmacies, where additional advice will also be available.

- Ibuprofen is indicated for mild to moderate pain and inflammation. Refer to **Ibuprofen** for doses, indications and contraindications. Ibuprofen works as an anti-inflammatory at higher (400–600 mg) doses, and effects are usually noted within 30 minutes.

Low Back Pain (Non-traumatic)

- Combined therapy with ibuprofen and paracetamol is a suitable initial strategy for the management of ongoing pain in most patients with low back pain. Patients should be counselled to take the medications regularly while experiencing the pain, rather than reactively if the pain is too severe. This will enable them to move and exercise more freely, a key component to recovery.
- If NSAIDs are contra-indicated or not tolerated, a weak opiate such as codeine is suggested, with or without paracetamol (co-codamol). Strong opiates such as morphine are not recommended for the treatment of acute non-traumatic low back pain.
- If pain is severe and uncontrolled, other analgesia may be necessary. However, in chronic or acute-on-chronic pain, additional analgesia may not be beneficial and can lead to increased dependency. Therefore, a cautious approach is advised for additional analgesics. When required, prescribing support may be required via a referral to the patient's GP, out-of-hours service, prescribing pharmacist or other local appropriate care pathway.
- Inhalational analgesia may be useful to help a person from the floor to a standing position to facilitate assessment and examination. Patients may require reassurance to overcome the apprehension of movement when in severe pain, and may feel 'trapped' on the floor or on low furniture. Once patients have been mobilised to a more comfortable position, they should be advised to remain on high-backed chairs or standing up while the pain remains very severe.

8.2 Non-pharmacological Management

- There is limited evidence of benefit for the use of warm or cold compresses, but some patients will seek to apply hot-water bottles or ice packs to their lower back.
- Patients should be advised that muscular relaxation is a key part of easing low back pain. Bed rest is not advised and will delay recovery, as it prevents them from moving freely and regularly. Patients should be encouraged to maintain their normal activities as much as they are able to tolerate, and should be reassured that it is highly unlikely that gentle activities would aggravate their pain or cause injury.
- Personalised care should be provided for patients with chronic pain, recognising new symptoms, understanding patients' concerns and perceptions regarding their pain and managing expectations around being conveyed to an emergency department and diagnostic imaging.
- It may be necessary to counsel the patient that they may remain in pain but that further pain relief may not be helpful, and that the goal is not to resolve the pain but to control it such that they are able to undertake activity.
- Patients may be advised to refer themselves for local physiotherapy (if this is available locally).
- If pain is not settling after 4–6 weeks, patients should seek further support from primary care services.

9. Simple Exercises – Advice

- Patients can be encouraged to perform regular, simple exercises to aid pain management and relieve stiffness and pain. Various NHS websites have a suite of exercises that be accessed for guidance, e.g. https://www.nhs.uk/conditions/back-pain/treatment/.
- Consider the appropriateness of different exercises for each patient. For instance, older patients may be advised to undertake exercises on the bed rather than on the floor.
- Simple exercises should be advised for patients with confirmed musculoskeletal (non-traumatic) low back pain that are not being conveyed to hospital. The exercises below should be done three times per day, consisting of two sets of five repetitions.

9.1 Simple Exercises

- Patients should be advised to try walking little and often and should remain as active as possible.

Knees to chest:

1. Lie on your back, with your knees bent and feet flat on the floor or bed.
2. Bring one knee up and use your hands to pull it gently towards your chest.
3. Hold the leg in position for 5 seconds, and then relax.
4. Repeat this exercise with the other knee.
5. Do the exercise five times on each side.

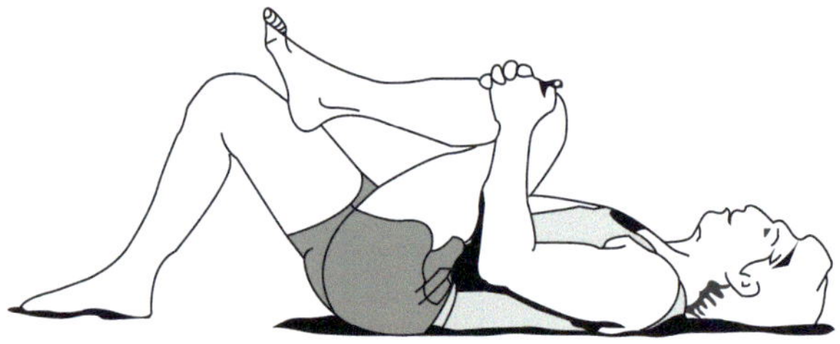

Figure 3.25 – Simple 'knees to chest' exercise.

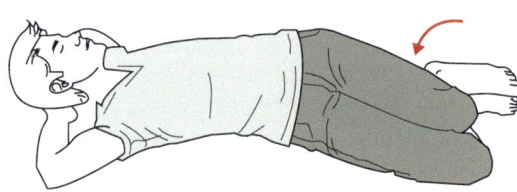

Figure 3.26 – Simple 'knee-rolling' exercise.

Low Back Pain (Non-traumatic)

Knee rolling:

1. Lie on your back, with your knees bent and your feet together.
2. Roll your knees to one side, keeping your shoulders flat on the bed or floor, and hold for 10 seconds.
3. Roll your knees back to the starting position, and then over to the other side and repeat.
4. Do this exercise three times on each side.

10. Safety-netting

- All safety-netting advice should be documented. The patient should be advised to contact their GP if pain is not settling within 4–6 weeks.
- Specific advice should be given to patients advising them to seek urgent help (i.e. attend an urgent treatment centre or emergency department) if they encounter any of the following symptoms:
  - New motor weakness affecting the lower limbs.
  - New onset of severe pain and/or new pins and needles/numbness affecting both legs.
  - Loss of sensation, numbness or pins and needles to inner thighs, genitals, anus or buttocks.
  - Altered sensation when wiping themselves after toileting.
  - New difficulty when trying to urinate, control urinary flow or new incontinence.
  - New loss of sensation when they pass urine.
  - New uncertainty regarding whether their bladder is full or empty.
  - Inability to control a bowel motion/faecal incontinence.
  - Loss of sensation when passing a bowel motion.
  - New change or inability to achieve an erection or ejaculate.
  - New altered sensation in genitals during sexual intercourse.

Further Reading

BMJ Best Practice. *Musculoskeletal Lower Back Pain*. 2020. Available from: https://bestpractice.bmj.com/topics/en-gb/778.

Booton P, Cooper C, Easton G, Harper M. *General Practice at a Glance*. Chichester: Wiley Blackwell, 2013.

Brotzman B, Manske R. *Clinical Orthopaedic Rehabilitation*. 3rd edn. Philadelphia: Mosby Elsevier, 2011.

Chartered Society of Physiotherapy. *Back Pain*. 2022. Available from: https://www.csp.org.uk/conditions/back-pain.

Dynamic Health. *Cauda Equina*. 2021. Available from: https://www.eoemskservice.nhs.uk/advice-and-leaflets/lower-back/cauda-equina.

Finucane LM, Downie A, Mercer C et al. International framework for red flags for potential serious spinal pathologies. *Journal of Orthopaedic & Sports Physical Therapy* 2020, 50(7): 350–371. Available from: https://www.jospt.org/doi/pdf/10.2519/jospt.2020.9971.

Henschke N, Maher CG, Refshauge KM et al. Prognosis in patients with recent onset low back pain in Australian primary care: inception cohort study. *BMJ* 2008, 337.

Hopcroft K, Forte V. *Symptom Sorter*, 6th Ed. Oxon: CRC Press, 2020.

NHS Mental Health. *Mental Health Services*, 2022. Available from: https://www.nhs.uk/mental-health/nhs-voluntary-charity-services/charity-and-voluntary-services/get-help-from-mental-health-helplines/.

RCGP. National Collaborating Centre for Primary Care (UK). *Low Back Pain: Early management of persistent non-specific low back pain*. London: Royal College of General Practitioners (UK), 2009. (NICE Clinical Guidelines, No. 88.) 2, Introduction. Available from: https://www.ncbi.nlm.nih.gov/books/NBK11709/.

Simon C, Everitt H, van Dorp F, Burkes M. *Oxford Handbook of General Practice*. 4th edn. Oxford: Oxford University Press, 2014. [p. 1288 of e-book]

The Christie NHS Foundation Trust. *MSCC Service Education Red Flag Card*. 2019. Available from: https://www.christie.nhs.uk/media/1125/legacymedia-1201-mscc-service_education_mscc-resources_red-flag-card.pdf.

Versus Arthritis. *Back Pain*. 2022. Available from: https://www.versusarthritis.org/about-arthritis/conditions/back-pain/.

Bibliography

1. Capsey M, Cormac R, Alexanders J, Martin D. Ambulance service use by patients with lower back pain: an observational study. *British Paramedic Journal* 2022, 6(4): 11–17. https://doi.org/10.29045/14784726.2022.03.6.4.11.
2. Macfarlane GJ, Beasley M, Jones EA, Prescott GJ, Docking R, Keeley P, McBeth J, Jones GT; MUSICIAN study team. The prevalence and management of low back pain across adulthood: results from a population-based cross-sectional study (the MUSICIAN study). *Pain* 2012, 153(1): 27–32. doi: 10.1016/j.pain.2011.08.005. Epub 2011 Oct 5. PMID: 21978663.

Low Back Pain (Non-traumatic)

3. National Institute for Health and Care Excellence (NICE). *Back Pain – Low (without radiculopathy).* 2022. Available from: https://cks.nice.org.uk/topics/back-pain-low-without-radiculopathy/.

4. Bevan S, Quadrello T, McGee R et al. *Fit for Work? Musculoskeletal Disorders in the European Workforce.* The Work Foundation Report, 2012.

5. Wynne-Jones G, Cowen J, Jordan JL et al. Absence from work and return to work in people with back pain: a systematic review and meta-analysis. *Occupational and Environmental Medicine* 2014, 71: 448–456.

6. Dionne CE, Dunn KM, Croft PR et al. A consensus approach toward the standardization of back pain definitions for use in prevalence studies. *Spine* 2008, 33(1): 95–103.

7. Deyo RA, Jarvik JG and Chou R. Low back pain in primary care. *BMJ* 2014, 349.

8. National Institute for Health and Care Excellence (NICE). *Low Back Pain and Sciatica in over 16s: Assessment and management* [NG59], 2016. Available from: https://www.nice.org.uk/guidance/ng59.

Management and Resuscitation of Patients with Left Ventricular Assist Devices (LVADs)

1. Introduction

- Left ventricular assist devices (LVADs) are implanted pumps used to replace or supplement cardiac function. The pump augments blood flow by draining blood from the left ventricle and ejecting it into the aorta. The pump is internally implanted but is powered by external batteries (or a mains transformer) and has an external controller, which is worn or carried by the patient (refer to Figure 3.27).

- Clinical trials have established the efficacy of LVAD therapy for advanced heart failure.[1,2,3,4] Ongoing technological improvements and a growing mismatch between the demand for donor hearts for transplantation and their supply have resulted in a progressive increase in the number of patients receiving LVAD support in the UK.[5,6] In

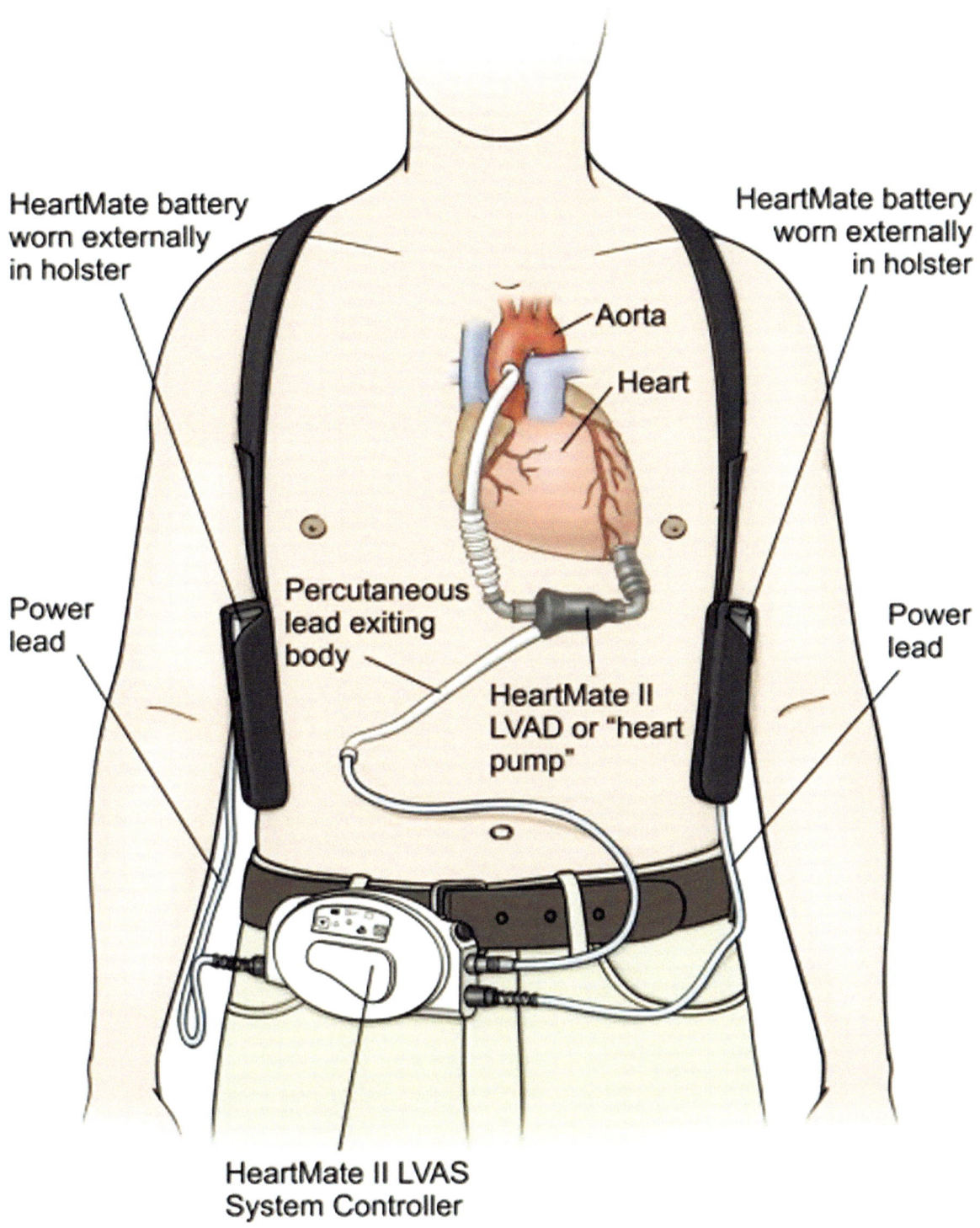

Figure 3.27 – Typical arrangement of the LVAD components.

Management and Resuscitation of Patients with Left Ventricular Assist Devices (LVADs)

January 2016, 207 adult patients were receiving LVAD therapy in the UK, 184 (89%) as outpatients. These numbers are predicted to increase. There are a number of children with LVADs, mostly teenagers.

- There is currently only one LVAD system, the Heartmate 3, which is implanted in the UK. However patients with four types of historical LVAD systems live in the UK. These devices are implanted by, and currently managed by, the six UK adult cardiac transplant centres.

- LVAD recipients are normally ambulatory adult outpatients who, despite subnormal exercise capacity,[7] may travel extensively within the UK. However, LVAD failure is a life-threatening emergency.[8,9,10,11,12] This dependency arises for two reasons:
  - If the LVAD does not operate, the already dysfunctional left ventricle may not be able to generate an adequate cardiac output to sustain life.
  - As the device contains no valves, if it fails there is retrograde blood flow through it during ventricular diastole, further limiting systemic perfusion.[13] Moreover, LVAD outpatients are vulnerable to other complications,[14,15] particularly stroke,[16] bleeding,[17,18] systemic infection and LVAD thrombosis.[19,20,21,22]

- Patients discharged with an LVAD device undergo an extensive package of familiarisation and training, which includes training of relatives/friends. It is fundamentally important where a trained family member or friend is on scene that they are involved in attempts to rectify the condition. They will be familiar with the exact device the patient has implanted. However, LVAD recipients are often unaccompanied in the community and therefore will not always be accompanied by a trained companion.

- On discharge, patients are presented with a patient-specific protocol (PSP). These are often shared with local ambulance services and may be flagged on control room systems. It should be noted that the patient could be mobile and may not be at their home address or that the PSP may not be readily accessible.

- Patients discharged with an LVAD will normally have spare batteries with them, along with a spare control unit. All LVAD equipment must be conveyed with the patient to hospital. Wherever possible, a family member/friend who is trained and familiar with the device should also accompany the patient to hospital.

2. Assessment

- The algorithms given in Figures 3.28–30 are intended only for use with LVAD recipients who have experienced sudden clinical deterioration. For clinically compromised LVAD recipients, where the LVAD has been non-functional for more than a few minutes, restarting the LVAD carries a theoretical risk of release of thrombus from the LVAD and embolic stroke. However, this risk may be offset by bidirectional blood flow through the non-functional LVAD13 and systemic anticoagulation. In a patient who is critically ill or in circulatory arrest, the balance of risk and benefit favours restarting a non-functioning LVAD. If LVAD non-function is suspected in a patient who is not severely compromised, immediate advice should be sought from the VAD centre (see Section 7 for contact details).

2.1 Assessment of Airway and Breathing

- The assessment starts with a rapid evaluation of the patient's responsiveness and breathing. In an unresponsive patient who is not breathing normally despite an open airway, that is, not breathing or giving only infrequent 'agonal' gasps (the features usually used to identify cardiac arrest),[23] ambulance clinicians should consider that a likely cause is that the LVAD has stopped and should proceed to the assessment of circulation. In the patient who is breathing normally, administration of oxygen and assessment to identify other respiratory conditions should follow standard guidelines.

2.2 Assessment of Circulation

- This part of the assessment starts by determining if the LVAD is running. Unresponsiveness and absence of normal breathing usually implies circulatory arrest.

- In an LVAD recipient, sudden failure of the LVAD is the cause most likely to be corrected by prompt, appropriate intervention.

- Sudden LVAD failure does not always cause circulatory arrest, so in an LVAD patient who is very ill but breathing, it is still important to check at this stage whether the LVAD is running.

- Clinicians should minimise delay by avoiding futile repeated attempts to palpate a pulse and record the arterial BP and oxygen saturation, as these may be difficult or impossible to detect in compromised LVAD recipients.

- A loud alarm coming from the controller is likely to indicate a stopped LVAD, unless its display shows another explanation.

- If no alarm is sounding, LVAD failure is still a possibility (due to alarm battery depletion or alarm failure), so a stethoscope should be placed over the apex of the heart to listen for a humming sound. Absence of a humming sound indicates that the LVAD is not working. If a loud alarm is sounding (with no other cause shown) or the pump is inaudible via stethoscope, the clinician is directed to Algorithm 2 (LVAD troubleshooting) (refer to Figure 3.29).

Management and Resuscitation of Patients with Left Ventricular Assist Devices (LVADs)

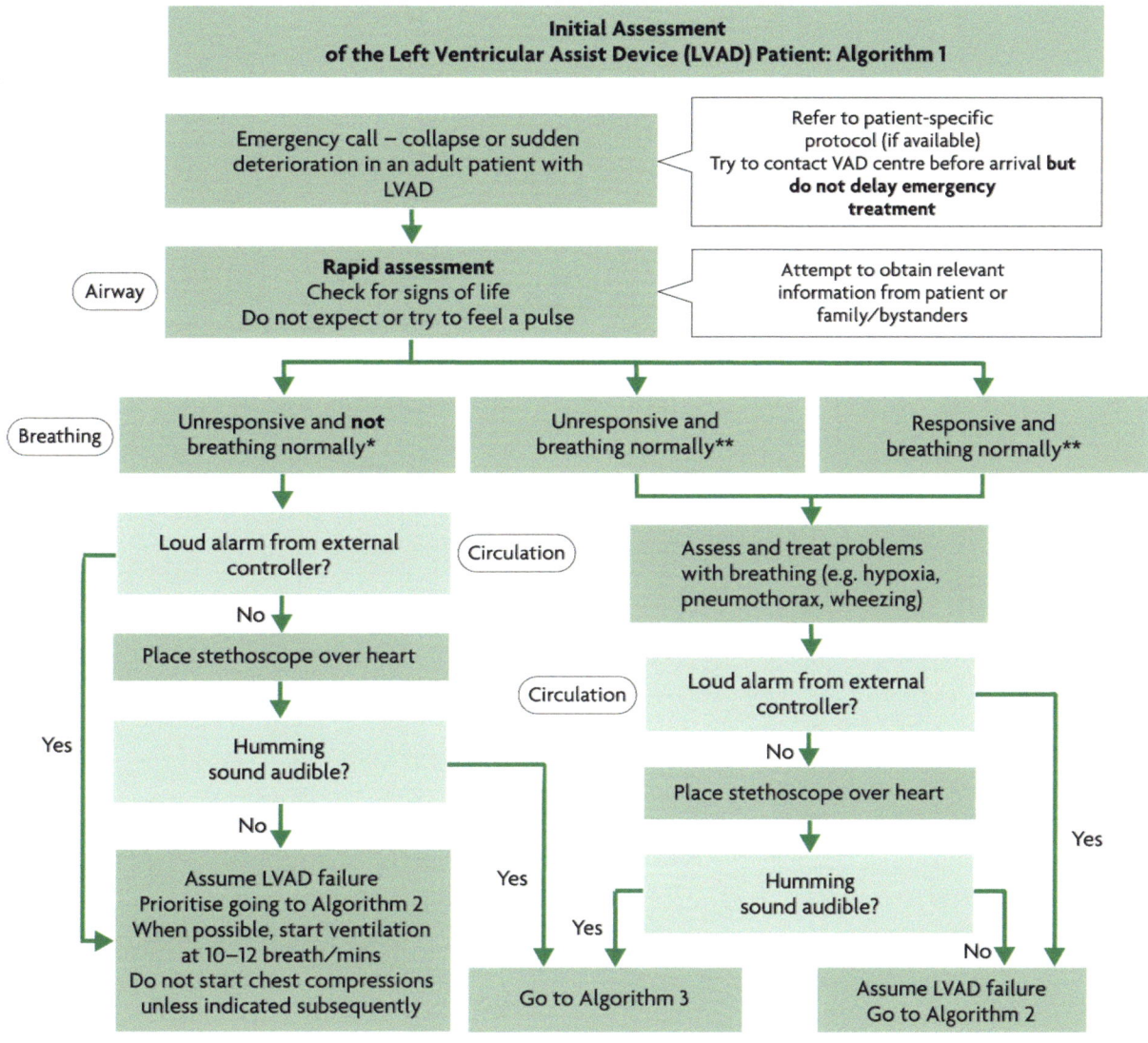

Figure 3.28 – Algorithm 1 – Initial assessment of the LVAD patient.

2.3 LVAD Troubleshooting

- If the LVAD has stopped, the most effective resuscitation manoeuvre is to restart it without delay. Operation of the LVAD is dependent on:

1. secure connection of an external controller to the percutaneous cable (driveline) of the implanted blood pump
   AND
2. the supply of power to the external controller, either via a rechargeable battery or via mains power.

- The percutaneous driveline usually exits the skin over the abdomen to the right of the umbilicus.
- All adult LVADs in use in the UK have two power connections to the controller, both of which are usually connected, although only a single working power source is needed for the LVAD to operate. This allows replacement of one power source without interrupting LVAD operation.
- The controller and batteries may be carried in a bag, contained within pockets of the patient's clothing or belt-mounted.
- If the LVAD is not running, first check the external components of the LVAD. The clinician should open the LVAD bag containing the controller and batteries to expose the contents, and check that all connections to the controller are fully engaged and secure.
- Next, check the battery charge by pressing a button on the battery that illuminates a display similar to a fuel gauge. If the battery charge level is low, the power source must be changed. Depleted batteries should be replaced with charged ones or with a mains power supply. If a mains power supply is in use and potentially defective, the device should be switched to a charged battery.
- If these measures fail to restart the LVAD, it is presumed that the controller is defective. The

Management and Resuscitation of Patients with Left Ventricular Assist Devices (LVADs)

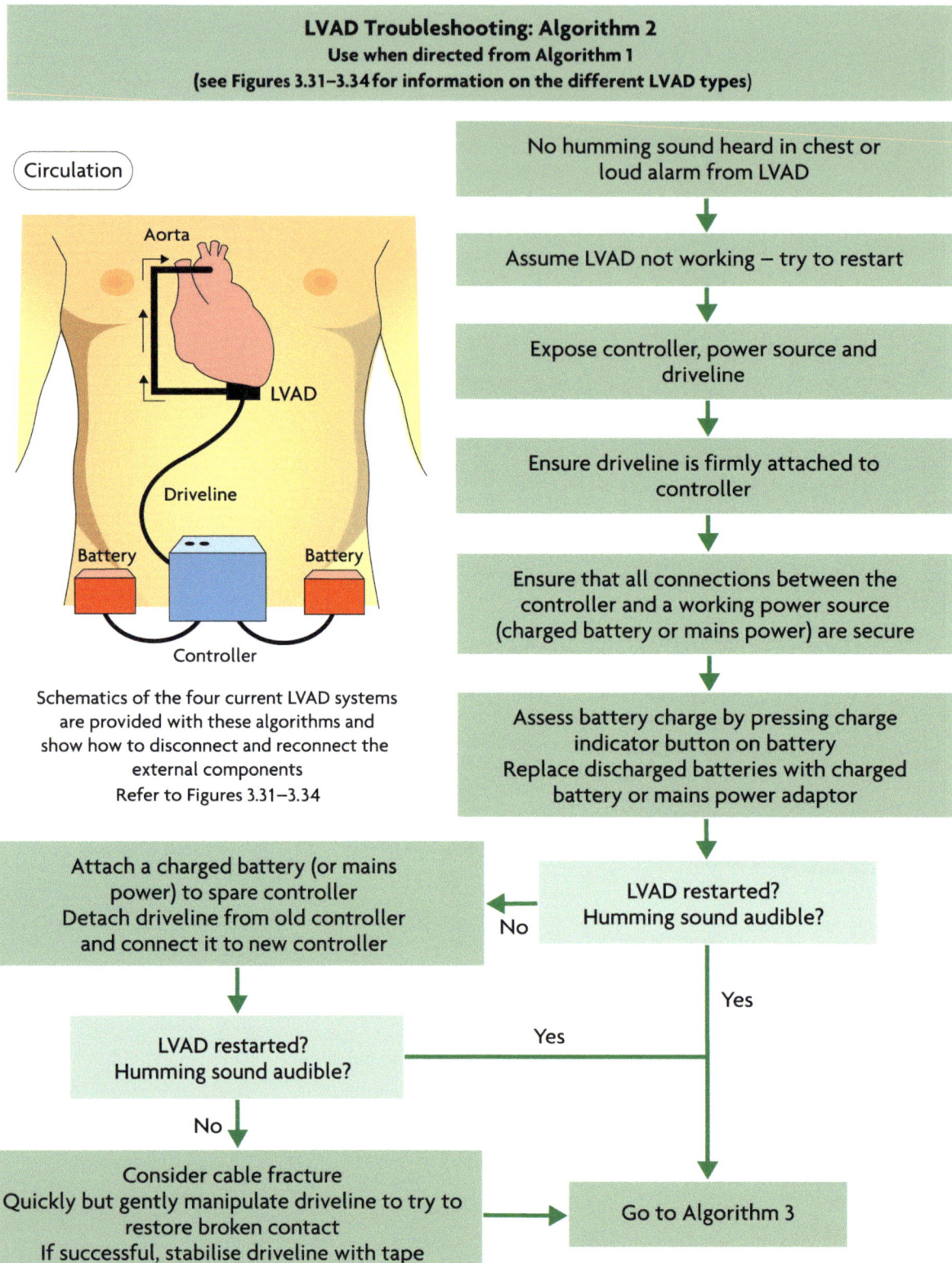

Figure 3.29 – Algorithm 2 – LVAD troubleshooting.

spare controller (carried by the patient at all times) should be connected to a charged battery (or mains power). Then, the driveline should be disconnected from the presumed-defective controller and connected to the replacement controller whereupon the LVAD should restart.

- If these actions do not restart the LVAD, the possibility of cable fracture within the driveline causing loss of electrical continuity should be considered. If this is suspected, gentle manipulation of the driveline may restore LVAD operation, in which case the driveline should be stabilised (using tape).

Management and Resuscitation of Patients with Left Ventricular Assist Devices (LVADs)

- If the LVAD cannot be restarted, or in the unlikely event that an LVAD patient is found in an unconscious state with a non-functioning LVAD that cannot be restarted and no spare equipment, the clinician should proceed to Algorithm 3 (Figure 3.30) and the VAD centre should be contacted using a telephone number located:
    - on an identification card or bracelet
    - on an Immediate Action Notice, in an envelope in the bag with the controller in use
    - on the LVAD controller itself
    - in an emergency bag carried separately by the patient.
- Where the specific VAD centre cannot be contacted, the ambulance crew should contact the operations centre and attempts can be made to contact the local VAD centre for further advice and support. **If the clinician cannot rapidly establish which VAD centre the patient is from, they should call the nearest VAD centre for further advice and support.**
- Active LVAD audible alarms are often accompanied by warning messages, which may be displayed on the controller screen. Such messages either indicate an LVAD fault, which may cause rapid clinical deterioration, or may be indicative of a clinical problem causing LVAD parameters to fall outside the normal operating range. Alarm messages thus facilitate diagnosis of LVAD-related or medical issues and should be reported to the VAD centre co-ordinator who can provide appropriate advice.

3. Ensuring Adequate Circulation

- Whether the LVAD was found to be running, or an attempt has been made to restart a non-functioning LVAD, Algorithm 3 (Figure 3.30) should always be followed irrespective of clinical status and aims to ensure an adequate circulation. This includes checking the underlying cardiac rhythm, looking for signs of adequate perfusion and treating if necessary. Subsequently, the patient should be assessed for disabilities (e.g. stroke, glucose, drugs) and examined for evidence of bleeding and infection. Finally, transfer arrangements are made in consultation with the VAD centre.

3.1 Cardiac Rhythm Management

- Many LVAD recipients also have a cardiac resynchronisation therapy (CRT) pacemaker and, in some, their device incorporates an implantable cardiac defibrillator (ICD). Some have an ICD without CRT. An ICD would be expected to deliver a shock in the event of ventricular fibrillation (VF) or rapid ventricular tachycardia (VT).
- If a patient is unresponsive, and has VF or VT (with ICD not present or ineffective), immediate defibrillation (VF) or cardioversion (VT) is indicated. If possible, anterior-posterior pad positioning would be preferable based on the LVAD position within the chest wall.
- Some LVAD recipients without ICDs may be temporarily tolerant of what would normally be considered to be life-threatening ventricular arrhythmia (VF or VT) because LVAD operation is ECG independent and passive blood flow through the right heart and pulmonary circulation may sustain enough venous return to the LVAD to maintain systemic blood flow and consciousness.[24] A responsive patient with VT or VF should be transported to hospital for urgent treatment. If the patient becomes unresponsive during an episode of VT or VF prior to arrival at hospital, they should receive immediate defibrillation or cardioversion.

3.2 Circulatory Assessment and Observations

- Ambulance clinicians should look for clinical signs of an adequate circulation (e.g. capillary refill time less than 2 seconds, absence of pallor/cyanosis). Emergency treatment must not be delayed while repeated attempts are made to measure arterial BP or pulse oximetry in LVAD patients; contemporary pumps produce continuous (non-pulsatile) blood flow, resulting in an attenuated arterial pulse pressure, which typically renders ineffective usual sphygmomanometry[25] and pulse oximetry.[26,27] If arterial BP can be recorded, hypotension is a normal finding in LVAD recipients; a mean arterial BP between 60 and 90 mmHg would be considered acceptable.

3.3 Chest Compressions

- There has been controversy as to whether chest compressions should be applied to LVAD recipients. The disagreement centres on safety, efficacy and when to start chest compressions.
- Evidence of compression efficacy in the presence of an LVAD is tenuous. Unsurprisingly, long periods of compressions were associated with poor outcomes. Short periods of compressions appeared to be associated with favourable outcomes, in keeping with a low risk of harm to an LVAD patient receiving CPR briefly, provided definitive treatment of the cause of circulatory arrest is not delayed.[28]
- It is reasonable to conclude that the balance of risks favours delivery of high-quality chest compressions by ambulance clinicians to LVAD recipients with out-of-hospital circulatory arrest either if attempts to restart an LVAD have failed or as a temporising measure until definitive intervention is possible, for example while searching for missing emergency LVAD equipment to restart an LVAD that is not running. Patients receiving CPR should have ECG monitoring in standard fashion; those with

Management and Resuscitation of Patients with Left Ventricular Assist Devices (LVADs)

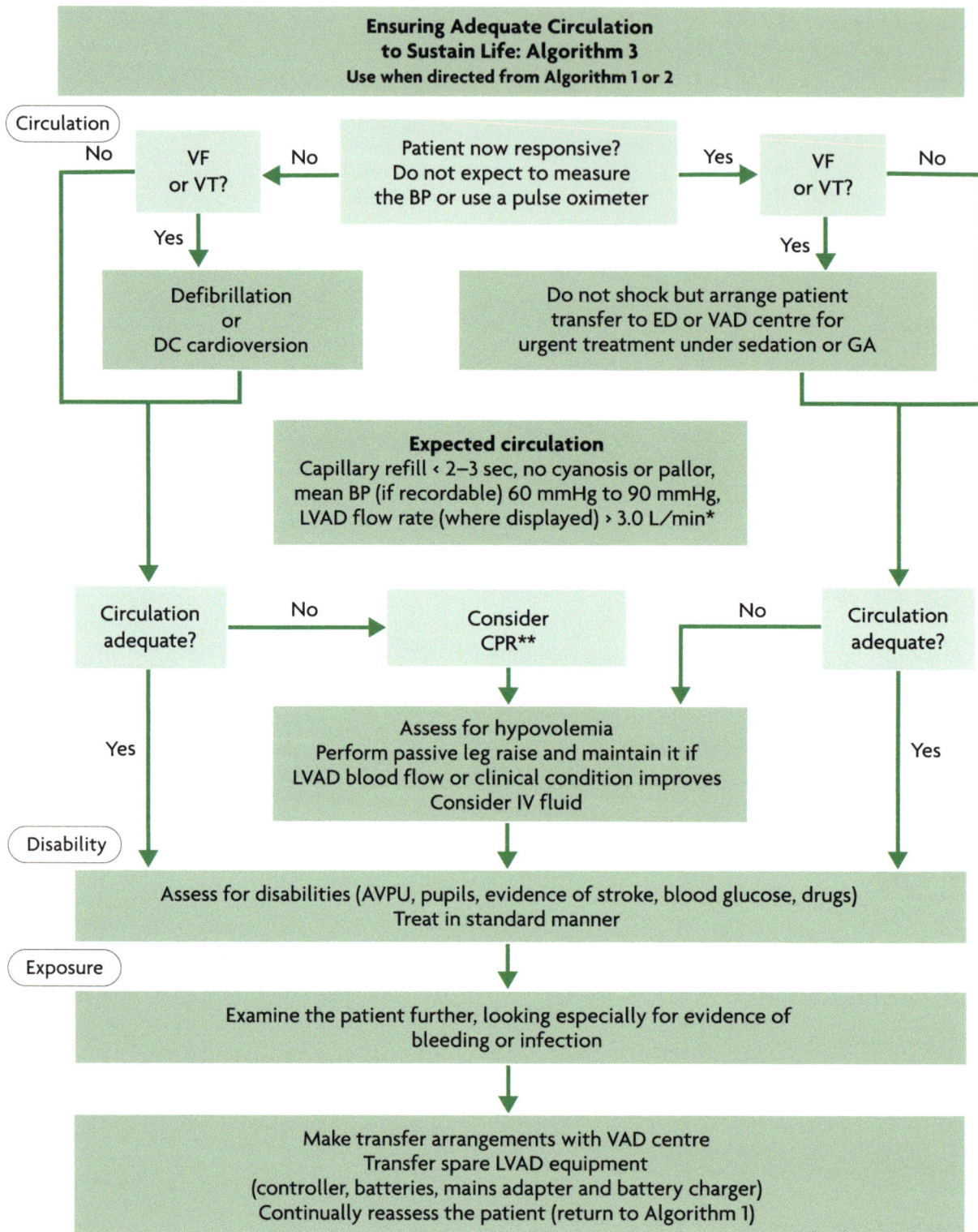

Figure 3.30 – Algorithm 3 – Ensuring adequate circulation.

recurrent VF or VT should receive immediate defibrillation. Adrenaline and amiodarone can be given during CPR according to standard ALS guidelines.

3.4 Consider Hypovolaemia

- Hypovolaemia can reduce LVAD flow to critical levels. If this is the case, chest compressions should be commenced prior to the assessment of hypovolaemia. Otherwise, hypovolaemia can be assessed and treated without CPR.

Management and Resuscitation of Patients with Left Ventricular Assist Devices (LVADs)

Hypovolaemia may be recognised by the display showing low LVAD flow (<3 L/min), with or without an audible alarm.

- Risk factors for hypovolaemia include a history of bleeding (notably gastrointestinal).
- When hypovolaemia is suspected, intravenous fluids should be given. Sustained passive elevation of the legs may provide a transient increase in venous return and help to maintain perfusion until the fluid has been administered.[26,29,30] If passive leg raising is followed by a transient increase in flow rate through the LVAD (sometimes for less than a minute), this supports the likely need for intravenous fluid.
- Positive responses to fluid administration include an increase in the displayed LVAD flow rate and clinical evidence of improved circulation. However, administration of excessive fluid can potentiate right heart failure; further advice can be provided by the VAD centre.

4. Transfer to Hospital

- Whether a patient should be transported to the local ED or to the VAD centre should be determined by dialogue with the VAD centre. This decision will depend on the patient's clinical condition and by logistical considerations. In cases of cardiac arrest, if the patient cannot be transported to a VAD centre within 45 minutes of CPR on-set then consideration should be made for any nearby Extracorporeal Membrane Oxygenation (ECMO) centres that can offer Extracorporeal CPR (ECPR).
- Appropriately trained caregivers should be encouraged to accompany the patient during ambulance transfer to hospital.
- It is of paramount importance that all emergency LVAD equipment (including the spare controller, rechargeable batteries, mains power adapter and battery charger) is transferred to hospital with the patient, as sustained LVAD function is dependent on the availability of these components.
- It is important to monitor the patient continuously during transfers, as clinical deterioration can be sudden.

5. Advance Decisions to Refuse Treatment and Do-Not-Attempt-CPR Decisions

- There is evidence of sporadic initiation of advance statements (living wills) or Advance Decisions to Refuse Treatment (England and Wales) (ADRTs) in UK LVAD outpatients. More frequently, do-not-attempt-CPR (DNACPR) decisions have been recorded by healthcare professionals for LVAD inpatients, typically with participation of the patient in the decision making process if they have the capacity, otherwise their family or authorised representative.[31] The increasing international use of LVADs for destination therapy in more elderly patients has focused debate on end-of life care planning, with more patients preferring to die in their home rather than in hospital.[32]
- It is recommended that the existence and location of advance statements, ADRTs and recommendations about CPR and/or other life-sustaining treatments should be recorded in the PSP. Unless there is a valid and applicable advance statement, ADRT or other recommendations warranting a different response in a community setting, the measures recommended in these guidelines may be assumed to be appropriate for any critically ill LVAD recipient.

6. Schematics of LVAD Types

Four different types of LVADs are implanted in the UK. Schematics of these different devices are included for reference purposes.

Management and Resuscitation of Patients with Left Ventricular Assist Devices (LVADs)

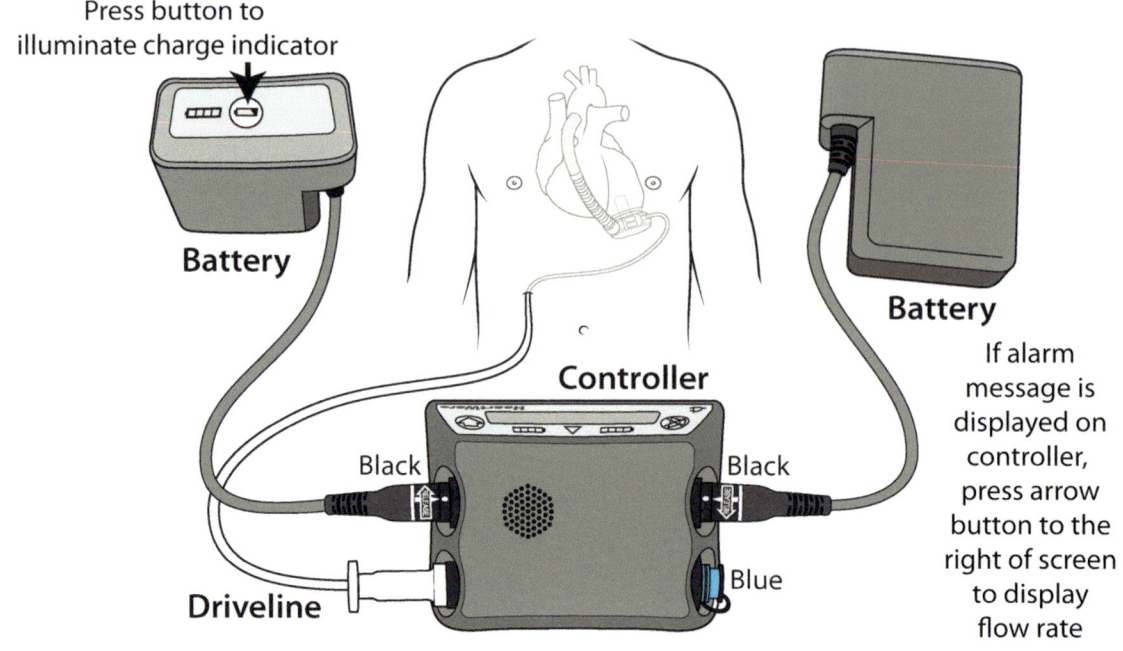

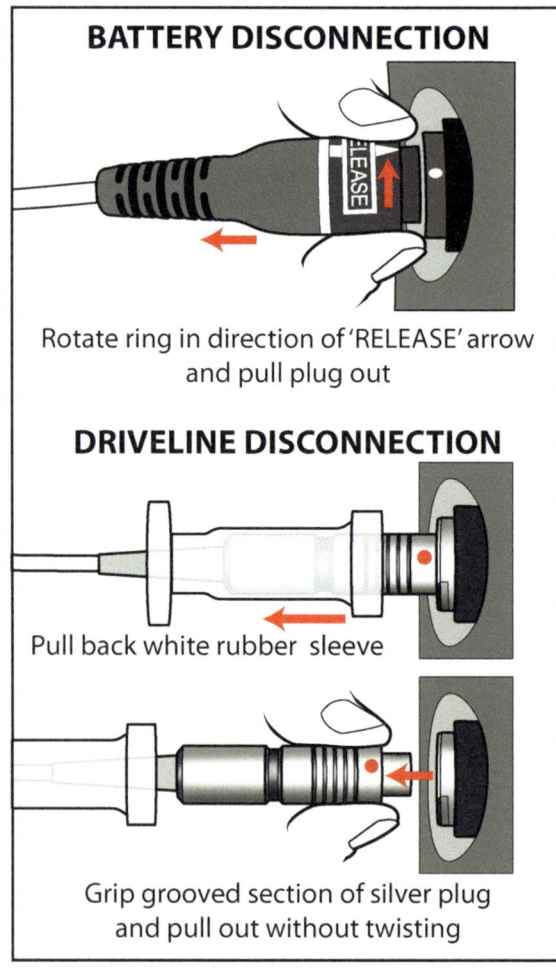

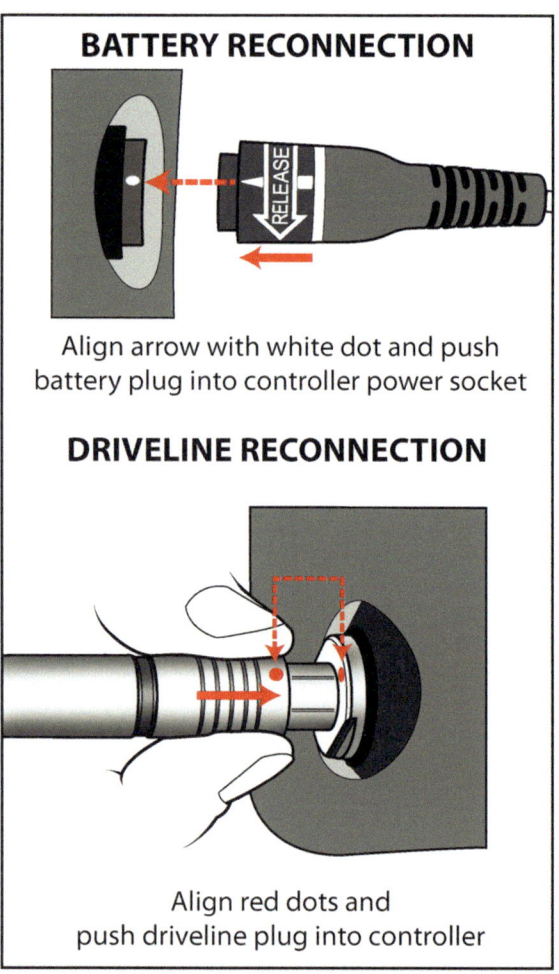

Figure 3.31 – Medtronic Inc. (formerly Heartware Inc.) HVAD.

Management and Resuscitation of Patients with Left Ventricular Assist Devices (LVADs)

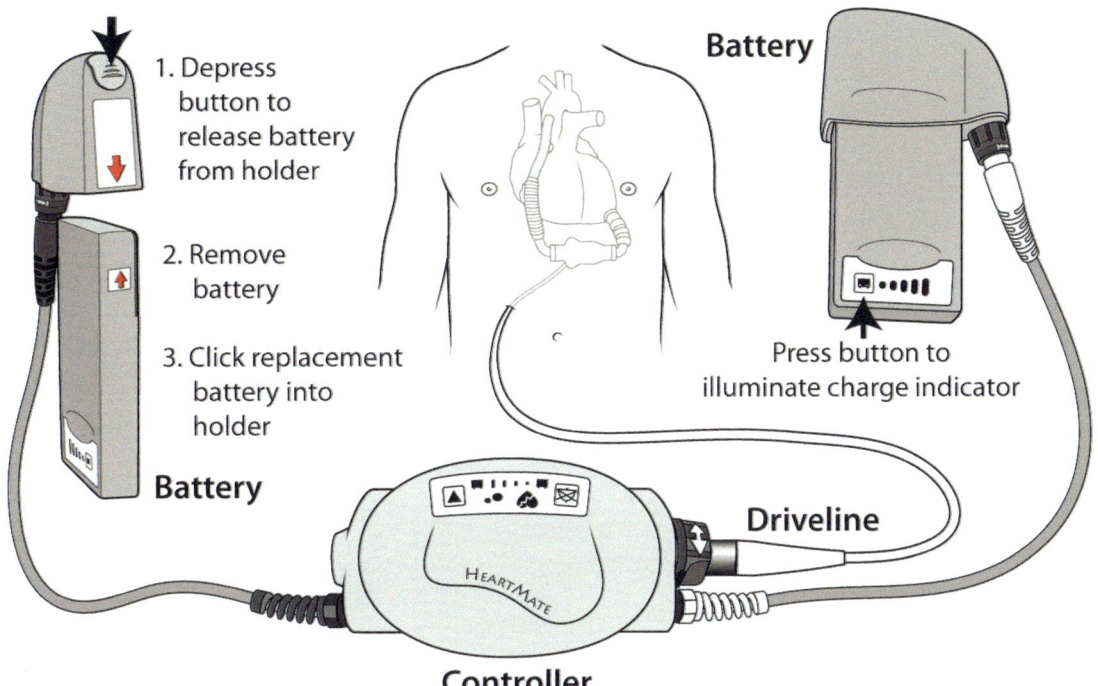
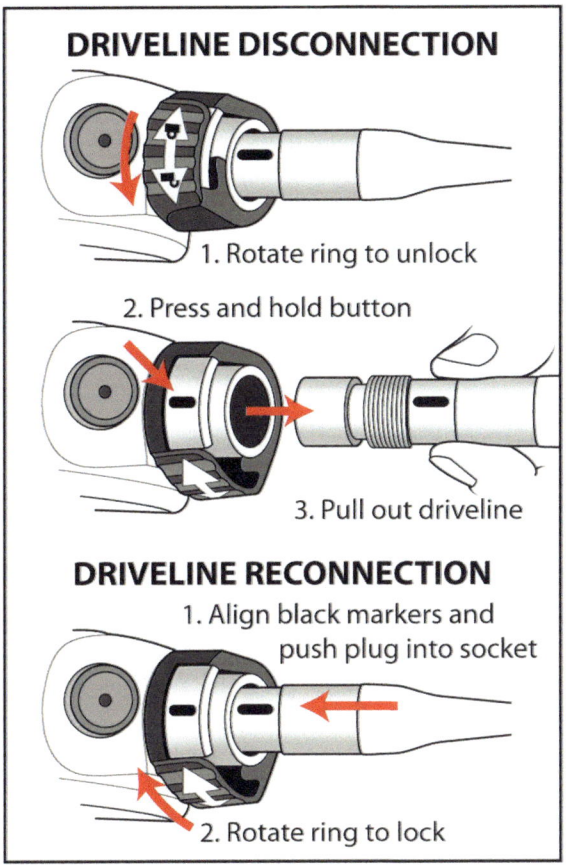
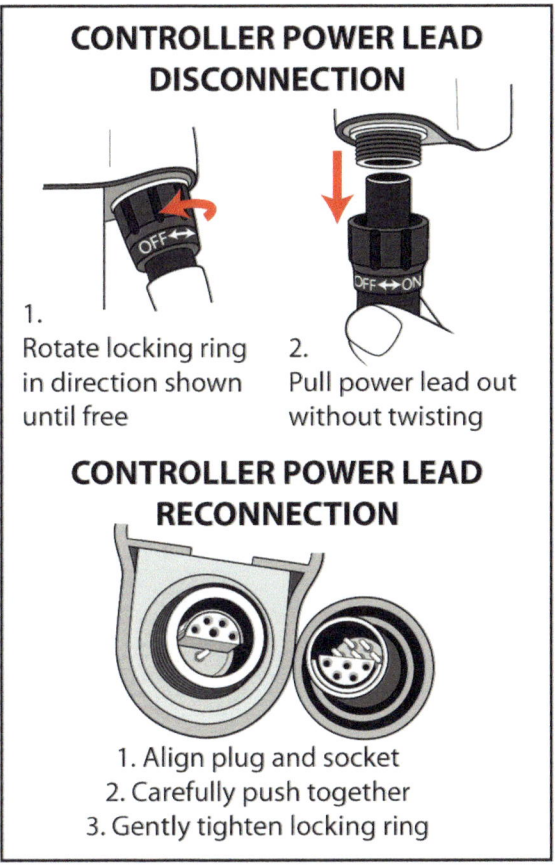

Figure 3.32 – LVAD type – Abbott Inc. (formerly Thoratec Inc.) HeartMate II, original version.

Management and Resuscitation of Patients with Left Ventricular Assist Devices (LVADs)

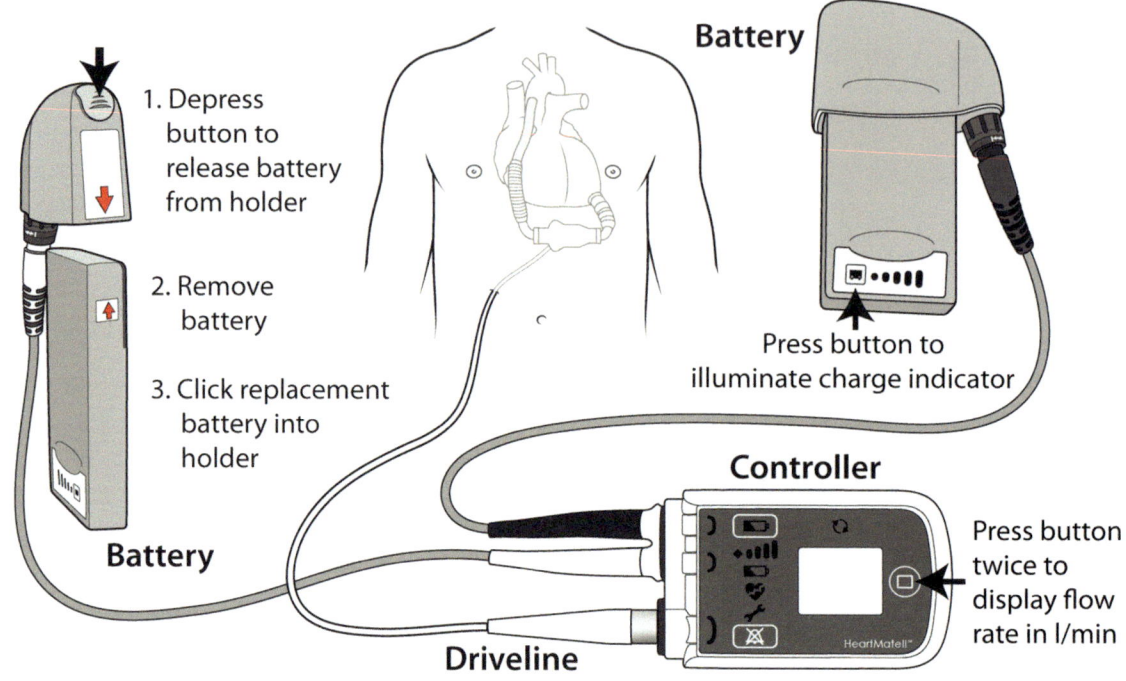

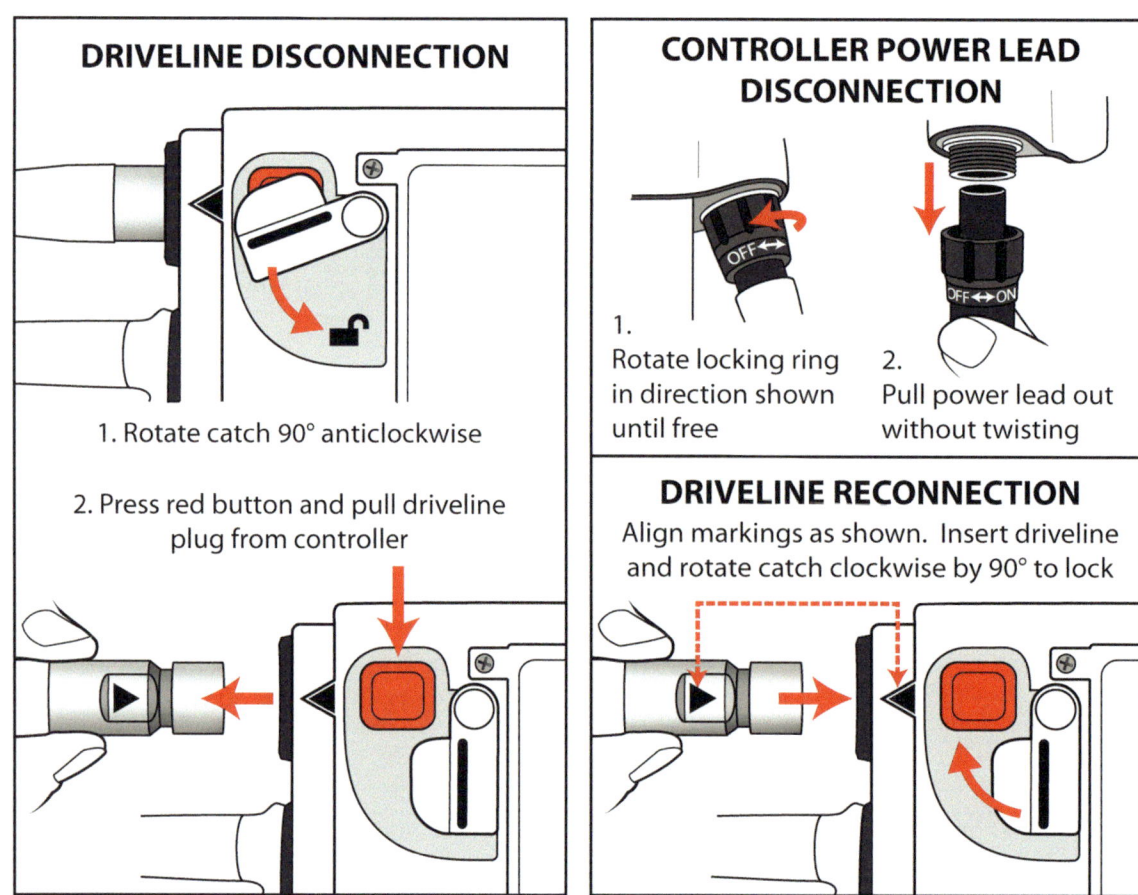

Figure 3.33 – LVAD type – Abbott Inc. (formerly Thoratec Inc.) HeartMate II, pocket controller version.

Management and Resuscitation of Patients with Left Ventricular Assist Devices (LVADs)

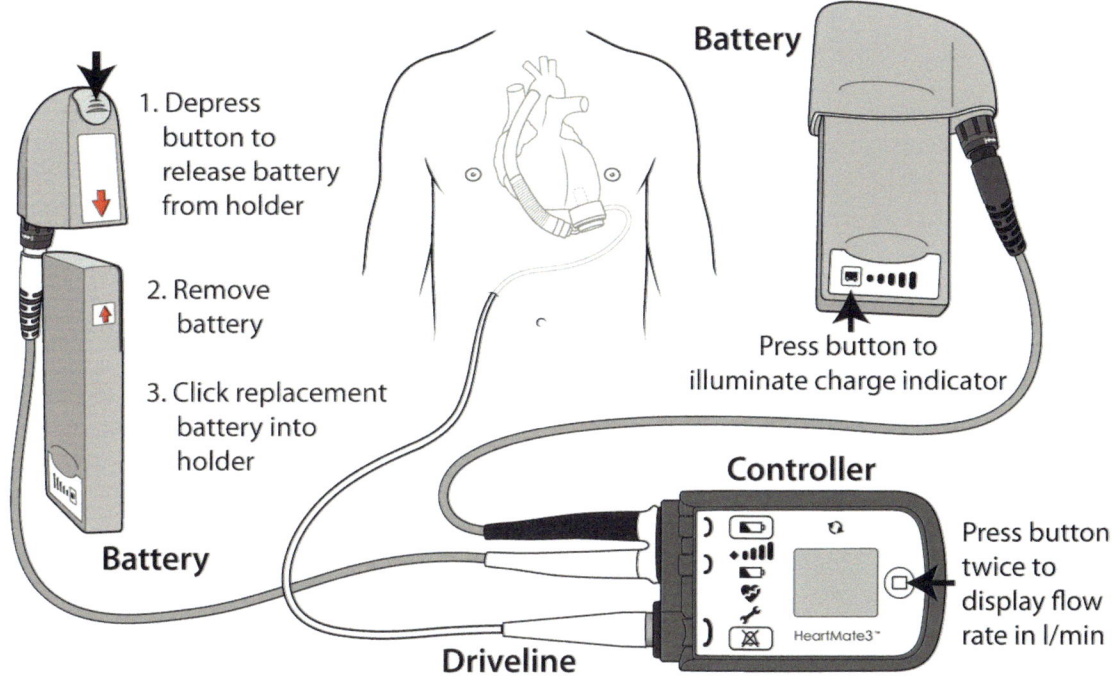

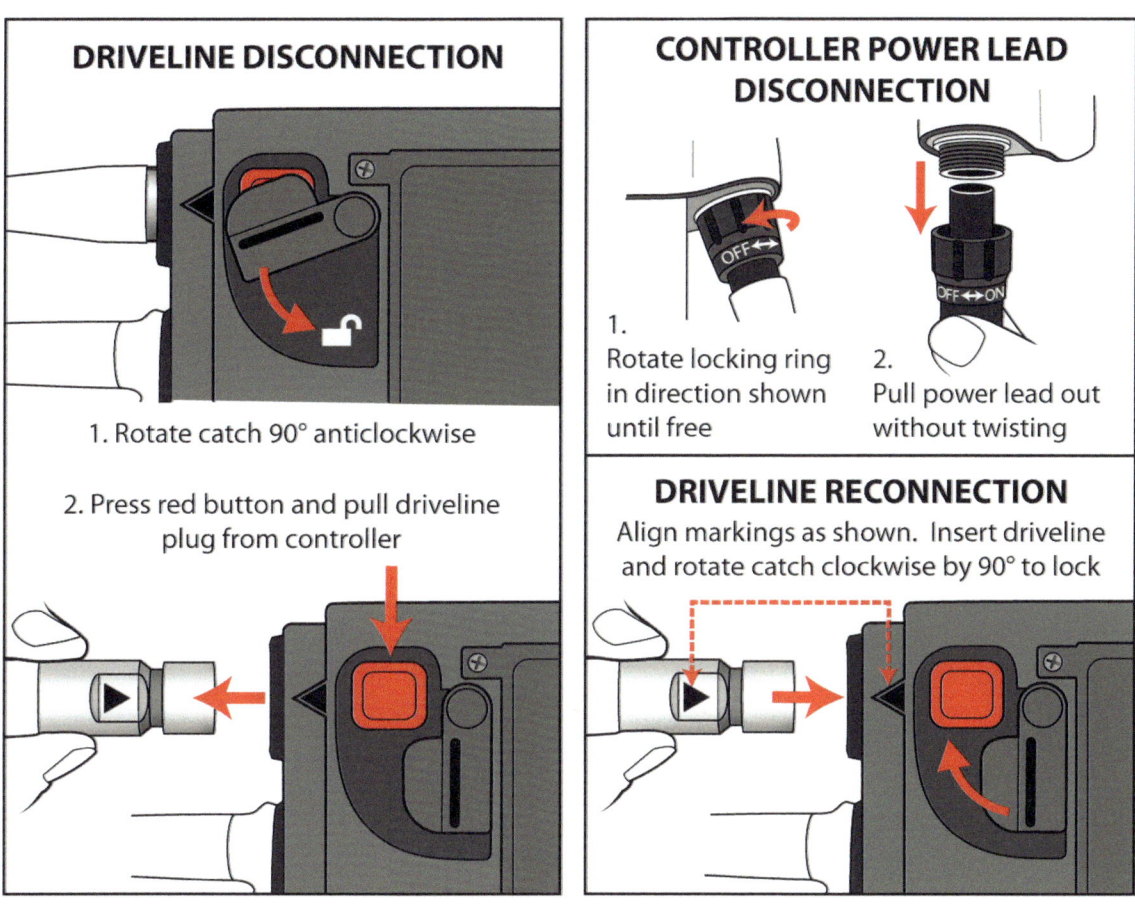

Figure 3.34 – LVAD type – Abbott Inc. (formerly Thoratec Inc.) HeartMate 3.

Management and Resuscitation of Patients with Left Ventricular Assist Devices (LVADs)

7. Contact Details for Ventricular Assist Device Implantation Centres

Centre	Service	Emergency Number	Hospital Switchboard
Birmingham, QEII	Adult	07920530026	0121 371 2000
Cambridge, Royal Papworth	Adult	01223 639300 Direct line for transplant coordinator	01223 638000
Glasgow, Golden Jubilee	Adult	0141 951 5784	0141 951 5000
London, Great Ormond Street	Paediatric	**Mon** to **Fri** 0800–1600 0207 405 9200 Ext. 5807 **Out of hours** Cardiology 0207 405 9200 Ext. 1632 **OR** bleep 0548	0207 405 9200
London, Harefield	Adult	07805768819	01895 823737
Manchester, Wythenshawe	Adult	0161 998 7070 **Ask for the VAD coordinator on call**	0161 998 7070
Newcastle, Freeman	Adult	0191 244 8444	0191 233 6161
	Paediatric	**Working hours:** 0191 244 8961 **Out of hours:** Ward 23, PICU 0191 213 7023 0191 213 7028	0191 233 6161

Ambulance services should use the emergency number in the first instance and, if there is no response, should ring the hospital switchboard and ask for the VAD coordinator, or alternative speciality, as detailed.

KEY POINTS!

Management and Resuscitation of Patients with LVADs

- The number of patients fitted with an LVAD is increasing and will continue to increase.
- LVADs are implanted by and currently managed by the six UK adult cardiac transplant centres.
- LVAD failure is a life-threatening emergency.
- A responsive patient with VT or VF should be transported to hospital for urgent treatment following discussion with the VAD centre.
- Measurement of BP and arterial saturation is challenging but hypotension is a normal finding in LVAD recipients. A mean arterial BP between 60 and 90 mmHg would be considered acceptable.
- Whether a patient should be transported to the local ED or to the VAD centre should be determined by dialogue with the VAD centre.
- All emergency LVAD equipment, including the spare controller, rechargeable batteries, mains power adapter and battery charger, must be transferred to hospital with the patient.

Management and Resuscitation of Patients with Left Ventricular Assist Devices (LVADs)

Acknowledgements

These algorithms were first published in the *Emergency Medicine Journal* and are republished with permission.

Bowles CT, Hards R, Wrightson N, Lincoln P, Kore S, Marley L, Dalzell JR, Raj B, Baker TA, Goodwin D, Carroll P, Pateman J, Black JJM, Katternhorn P, Faulkner M, Parameshwar J, Butcher C, Mason M, Rosenberg A, McGovern I, Weymann A, Gwinnutt C, Banner NR, Schueler S, Simon AR and Pitcher DW. Algorithms to guide ambulance clinicians in the management of emergencies in patients with implanted rotary left ventricular assist devices. *Emergency Medicine Journal* 2017, 34: 842–850.

We would like to gratefully acknowledge the contribution of John JM Black, Christopher T Bowles and Mark Faulkner to this JRCALC guideline.

Bibliography

1. Slaughter MS, Rogers JG, Milano CA et al. Advanced heart failure treated with continuous-flow left ventricular assist device. *N Engl J Med* 2009, 361: 2241–2251.

2. Aaronson KD, Slaughter MS, Miller LW et al. Use of an intrapericardial, continuous flow, centrifugal pump in patients awaiting heart transplantation. *Circulation* 2012, 125: 3191–3200.

3. Miller LW, Pagani FD, Russell SD et al. Use of a continuous-flow device in patients awaiting heart transplantation. *N Engl J Med* 2007, 357: 885–896.

4. Birks EJ, Tansley PD, Hardy J et al. Left ventricular assist device and drug therapy for the reversal of heart failure. *N Engl J Med* 2006, 355: 1873–1884.

5. Emin A, Rogers CA, Parameshwar J et al. Trends in long-term mechanical circulatory support for advanced heart failure in the UK. *Eur J Heart Fail* 2013, 15: 1185–1193.

6. National Health Service. *Annual Report on Ventricular Assist Devices*. London: National Health Service Blood and Transplant, 2015.

7. Jakovljevic DG, McDiarmid A, Hallsworth K et al. Effect of left ventricular assist device implantation and heart transplantation on habitual physical activity and quality of life. *Am J Cardiol* 2014, 114: 88–93.

8. Bischof D, Graves K, Genoni M et al. Fatal disconnection of a ventricular assist device in an out-of-hospital setting. *Emerg Med J* 2012, 29: 247–248.

9. Cubillo EI, Weis RA, Ramakrishna H. Emergent reconnection of a transected left ventricular assist device driveline. *J Emerg Med* 2014, 47: 546–551.

10. Schima H, Stoiber M, Schlöglhofer T et al. Repair of left ventricular assist device driveline damage directly at the transcutaneous exit site. *Artif Organs* 2014, 38: 422–425.

11. Man survives after LVAD battery almost fails. *J Emerg Med Serv* 2010. Available from: http://www.jems.com/articles/2010/08/man-survives-after-lvad-batter-0.html.

12. Tigges-Limmer K, Schönbrodt M, Roefe D et al. Suicide after ventricular assist device implantation. *J Heart Lung Transpl* 2010, 29: 692–694.

13. Noor MR, Ho CH, Parker KH et al. Investigation of the characteristics of Heartware HVAD and Thoratec Heartmate II under steady and pulsatile flow conditions. *Artif Organs* 2016, 40: 549–560.

14. MacGowan GA, Schueler S. Right heart failure after left ventricular assist device implantation: early and late. *Curr Opin Cardiol* 2012, 27: 296–300.

15. Patil NP, Sabashnikov A, Mohite PN et al. De novo aortic regurgitation after continuous-flow left ventricular assist device implantation. *Ann Thorac Surg* 2014, 98: 850–857.

16. Harvey L, Holley C, Roy SS et al. Stroke after left ventricular assist device implantation: outcomes in the continuous-flow era. *Ann Thorac Surg* 2015, 100: 535–541.

17. Islam S, Cevik C, Madonna R et al. Left ventricular assist devices and gastrointestinal bleeding: a narrative review of case reports and case series. *Clin Cardiol* 2013, 36: 190–200.

18. Bhat P, Nassif ME, Vader JM et al. Epistaxis in patients with left ventricular assist devices – incidence, risk factors, and implications. *J Heart Lung Transpl* 2014, 33: S246.

19. Stulak JM, Davis ME, Haglund N et al. Adverse events in contemporary continuous flow left ventricular assist devices: a multi-institutional comparison shows significant differences. *J Thorac Cardiovasc Surg* 2016, 151: 177–189.

20. Koval CE, Thuita L, Moazami N et al. Evolution and impact of drive-line infection in large cohort of continuous-flow ventricular assist device recipients. *J Heart Lung Transpl* 2014, 33: 1164–1172.

21. Starling RC, Moazami N, Silvestry SC et al. Unexpected abrupt increase in left ventricular assist device thrombosis. *N Engl J Med* 2014, 370: 33–40.

22. Najjar SS, Slaughter MS, Pagani FD et al. An analysis of pump thrombus events in patients in the HeartWare ADVANCE bridge to transplant and continued access protocol trial. *J Heart Lung Transpl* 2014, 33: 23–34.

23. Resuscitation Council. Resuscitation Guidelines 2015. *Adult Basic Life Support and Automated External Defibrillation*. Available from: https://www.resus.org.uk/resuscitation-guidelines/adult-basic-life-support-and-automated-external-defibrillation/.

24. Busch MC, Haap M, Kristen A et al. Asymptomatic sustained ventricular fibrillation in a patient with left ventricular assist device. *Ann Emerg Med* 2011, 57: 25–28.

25. Bennett MK, Roberts CA, Dordunoo D et al. Ideal methodology to assess systemic blood pressure in patients with continuous-flow left ventricular assist devices. *J Heart Lung Transpl* 2010, 29: 593–594.

26. Bramstedt KA, Simeon DJ. The challenges of responding to 'high-tech' cardiac implant patients in crisis. *Prehosp Emerg Care* 2002, 6: 425–432.

27. Moazami N. Patients with a ventricular assist device need special considerations. *J Emerg Med Serv* 2012. Available from: https://www.jems.com/articles/print/volume-37/issue-2/patient-care/patients-ventricular-assist-device-need.html.

28. Shinar Z, Bellezzo J, Stahovich M et al. Chest compressions may be safe in arresting patients with left ventricular assist devices (LVADs). *Resuscitation* 2014, 85: 702–704.

Management and Resuscitation of Patients with Left Ventricular Assist Devices (LVADs)

29. Powell KR, Flattery MP, Cei LF et al. Pre-hospital care for VAD patients: where are the gaps? *J Heart Lung Transpl* 2015, 34: S23.
30. Shah KB, Cei LF, Pinney SP et al. Emergency care for patients with continuous flow left ventricular assist devices. *J Heart Lung Transpl* 2014, 33: S220–221.
31. MacIver J, Ross HJ. Withdrawal of ventricular assist device support. *J Palliat Care* 2005, 21: 151–156.
32. Brush S, Budge D, Alharethi R et al. End-of-life decision making and implementation in recipients of a destination left ventricular assist device. *J Heart Lung Transpl* 2010, 29: 1337–1341.

Meningococcal Meningitis and Septicaemia

1. Introduction
- Meningococcal disease is the leading cause of death by infection in children and young adults and can kill a healthy person of any age within hours of their first symptoms.

2. Incidence
- In England and Wales, the incidence of meningococcal disease is falling, with around 750 cases being reported each year (decreased incidence attributed to the efficacy of Men C and Men B vaccines).

3. Pathophysiology
- Two clinical categories are described, although they often overlap:
1 meningitis.
2 septicaemia.
- In meningitis, the meninges covering the brain and spinal cord are infected by bacteria causing inflammation.
- In septicaemia, bacteria invade the bloodstream, releasing toxins and producing a clinical picture of shock and circulatory collapse. Deterioration can be rapid and may be irreversible, with treatment becoming less effective by the minute. Early recognition and prompt treatment improves clinical outcomes.
- A minority of patients will have pure septicaemia and it is these patients who carry the worse prognosis.

4. Severity and Outcome
- The mortality from septicaemia can be up to 40% but if recognised early, resuscitated aggressively and managed on ITU, mortalities of less than 5% can be achieved.

5. Assessment and Management
- These presentations should be managed in the same way as any other form of severe sepsis, with a <C>ABCDE approach and a **TIME-CRITICAL** transfer to hospital with an ATMIST pre-alert. Refer to **Sepsis**.

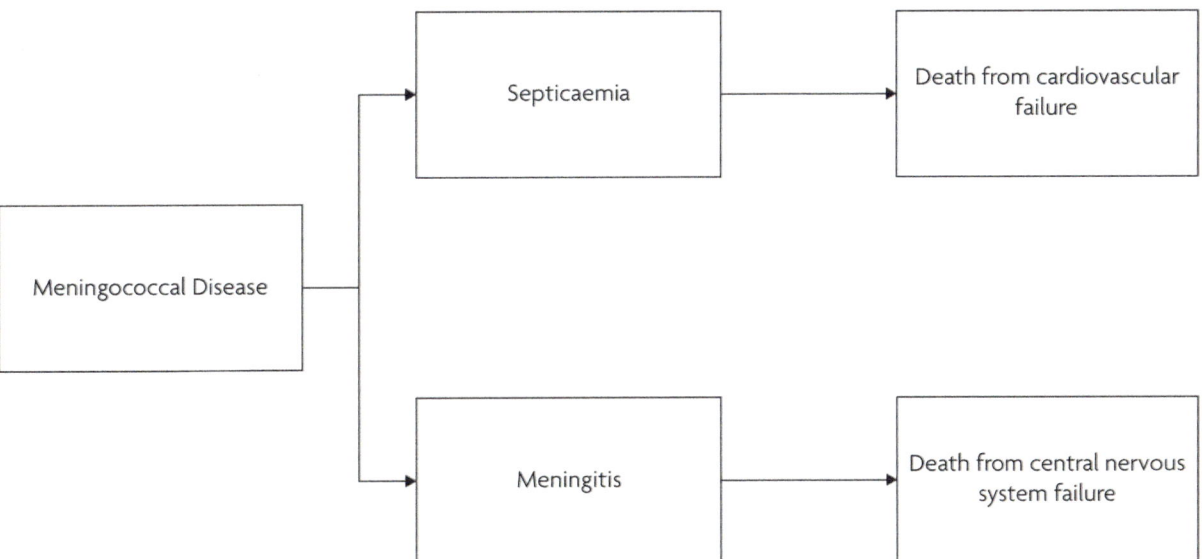

Figure 3.35 – Meningococcal meningitis and septicaemia.

Meningococcal Meningitis and Septicaemia

TABLE 3.84 – ASSESSMENT AND MANAGEMENT of: Meningococcal Meningitis and Septicaemia

Assess <C>ABCDE

- If any of the following **TIME-CRITICAL** features are present:
- Major **<C>ABCDE** problems (refer to Medical Emergencies in Adults – Overview and Medical Emergencies in Children – Overview).
    - Seizures.
    - Rash – progressive petechial rash becoming purpuric – like a bruise or blood blister. A purpuric rash may only be seen as an area of skin that is darker than its surroundings. It could alternatively be a purple/maroon colour. Use natural light if possible during a close examination (or a non-fluorescent light to avoid a blue tinge).
    - Start correcting any **<C>ABCDE** problems.
- Undertake a **TIME-CRITICAL** transfer to nearest appropriate receiving hospital.
- Continue patient management en route.
- Provide an ATMIST information call.

Clinical Findings

- The patient may have been previously unwell with non-specific symptoms, for example:
    - Irritability.
    - Pyrexia.
    - 'Flu-like' symptoms.
- The patient may be 'unwell' and deteriorate rapidly. In some individuals the meningococcal bacteria cross the blood – brain barrier, producing inflammation and swelling in the meninges and the brain tissue itself. This causes raised intracranial pressure, which can lead to neurological damage and death.
- The main symptoms of meningitis are due to central nervous system dysfunction. They may be very hard to assess and parents' anxieties about their child's condition must always be taken seriously.
- 'Classic' features (neck stiffness, photophobia and haemorrhagic rash) should be sought and can help you make the diagnosis when present. However, an absence of these signs should not be taken as evidence that meningococcal disease has been excluded. Do not be falsely reassured!
- Clinical features include:
    - Fever (may be masked by peripheral shutdown or antipyretics).
    - Cold, mottled skin (especially extremities). The skin may rarely be warm and flushed; features of 'warm shock'.
    - Raised respiratory rate and effort.
    - O$_2$ saturations – reduced or unrecordable (poor perfusion).
    - Raised heart rate.
    - Capillary refill time >2 seconds.
    - Pain in joints, muscles and limbs.
    - Rash – progressive petechial rash becoming purpuric – like a bruise or blood blister. A purpuric rash may only be seen as an area of skin that is darker than its surroundings. It could alternatively be a purple/maroon colour. Use natural light if possible during close examination (or a non-fluorescent light to avoid a blue tinge). **NB** These rashes are often not present at presentation.
    - Headache.
    - Vomiting, abdominal pain and diarrhoea.
    - Drowsiness/confusion.
    - Rigors.
    - Seizures.
    - Photophobia (less common in young children).
    - Neck stiffness (less common in young children).

Meningococcal Meningitis and Septicaemia

TABLE 3.84 – ASSESSMENT AND MANAGEMENT of: Meningococcal Meningitis and Septicaemia *(continued)*

The Rash
- The classic description of a haemorrhagic, non-blanching rash (may be petechial or purpuric) is only seen in approximately 40% of infected children.
- In pigmented skin it can be helpful to look at the conjunctiva under the lower eyelid.
- Early signs and symptoms are often subtle.
- Septicaemia: rashes do not necessarily develop at the same rate as the septicaemia.
- The rapidly evolving, haemorrhagic rash described in textbooks may be a very late sign – by the time this rash is present, resuscitative attempts may be too late.
- Up to 30% of cases start with a blanching rash, which fades with pressure, before becoming purpuric later. The rash may be pink, purple, maroon and may not be easily detectable without careful examination using natural light.
- The rash may be absent.

The 'glass' or 'tumbler' test
- A petechial or purpuric rash does not blanch/fade when pressed with a glass tumbler.
- **NB** If the 'glass' test is negative, do not assume that meningococcal disease has been excluded.

Specific Clinical Features
- Neck stiffness is rarely seen (but is more common in older children, teenagers and adults, being quite rare in pre-school children – the age group most at risk of infection). Small children often present with non-specific signs such as nausea, vomiting, loss of appetite, sore throat and coryzal symptoms – features that might otherwise suggest a diagnosis of viral illness.

Benzylpenicillin
- Where the patient meets the indication for administration of **Benzylpenicillin Sodium**, and where the clinician has a high index of suspicion of bacterial meningococcal septicaemia, even without the presence of a rash, benzylpenicillin should be administered.
- **NB** Meningococcal septicaemia can progress rapidly – early antibiotic administration is associated with better outcomes.
- Withhold benzylpenicillin only when there is a clear history of anaphylaxis after a previous dose; a history of a rash following penicillin is not a contraindication.
- In the unlikely event of an allergic reaction following administration of benzylpenicillin, manage according to **Allergic Reactions including Anaphylaxis**.
- Administer benzylpenicillin en route to further care.

Respiratory Rate
- Measure and record respiratory rate.

Pulse
- Measure and record pulse.

Oxygen Saturation
- Monitor the patient's SpO_2; administer oxygen to achieve saturations of >94% if the patient presents as hypoxemic on air; refer to **Oxygen**.

Blood Pressure and Fluids
- Measure and record blood pressure; if required, administer fluids, (refer to **Intravascular Fluid Therapy in Adults** and **Intravascular Fluid Therapy in Children**).
- Hypovolaemia complicating meningococcal septicaemia will require fluid resuscitation.
- **DO NOT** delay at scene for fluid replacement; cannulate and give fluid en route to hospital wherever possible.

Blood Glucose
- If appropriate, measure and record blood glucose for hypo/hyperglycaemia (refer to **Glycaemic Emergencies in Adults and Children**).

(continued)

Meningococcal Meningitis and Septicaemia

TABLE 3.84 – ASSESSMENT AND MANAGEMENT of: Meningococcal Meningitis and Septicaemia *(continued)*

Temperature
- Measure and record temperature.

NEWS2
- These observations will enable you to calculate a NEWS2 Score (refer to **Sepsis**). A National Paediatric Early Warning Score is still in development.

ECG
- If required, monitor and record 12-lead ECG. Assess for abnormality (refer to **Cardiac Arrhythmia and Sudden Cardiac Death**).

Assess the Patient's Pain
- Assess the **SOCRATES** of pain and record initial and subsequent pain scores.
- Consider analgesia if appropriate, (refer to **Pain Management in Adults and Children**).

Documentation
- Complete documentation to include all clinical findings, advice from other clinicians and onward referral.

6. Risk of Infection to Ambulance Personnel

- Meningococcal bacteria do not survive outside the nose and throat.
- Ambulance personnel directly exposed to large respiratory particles, droplets or secretions from patients with meningococcal disease should be offered preventative antibiotics. Such exposure is unlikely to occur unless working in very close proximity to the patient (e.g. inhaling droplets coughed or sneezed by the patient, or when undertaking airway management).
- Public Health will provide post-exposure antibiotics for meningococcal contacts who may otherwise be at increased risk of infection.

KEY POINTS!

Meningococcal Meningitis and Septicaemia

- Meningococcal disease is the leading cause of death from infection in children and young adults. It can kill a healthy person of any age within hours of their first symptoms.
- Two clinical categories are described – meningitis and septicaemia – although they often overlap.
- Non-specific symptoms, such as pyrexia or a 'flu-like' illness, may be the only clinical features at first presentation.
- A non-blanching rash should be sought, suggestive of meningococcal septicaemia (not universally present).
- A TIME-CRITICAL transfer should be undertaken whenever meningococcal disease is suspected (irrespective of the presence or absence of a rash).
- Administer benzylpenicillin if septicaemia is suspected. The illness progresses rapidly and early antibiotics can improve outcomes.

Meningococcal Meningitis and Septicaemia

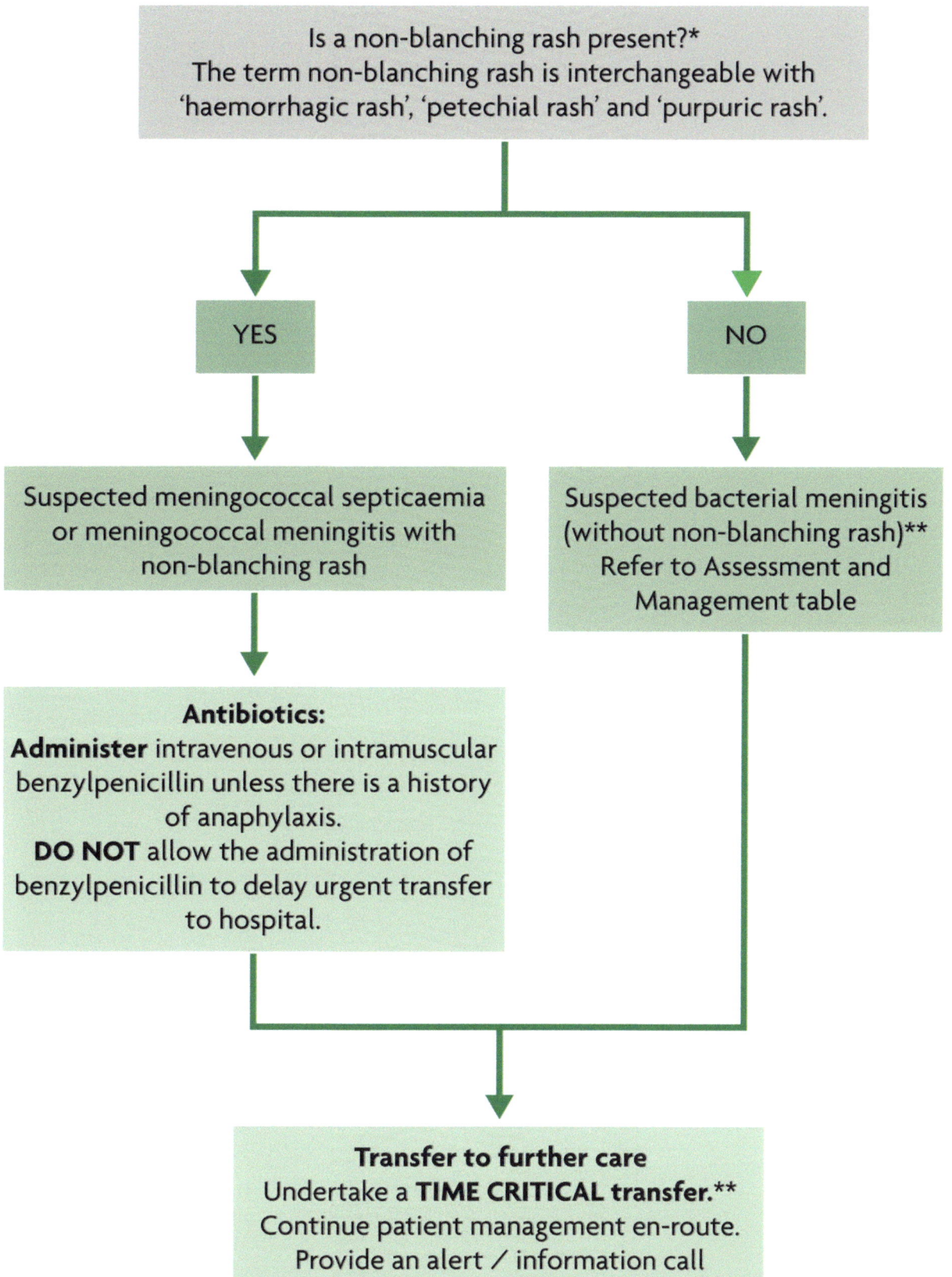

Figure 3.36 – Management algorithm for patients with suspected meningococcal disease.

* If bacterial meningitis is suspected and urgent transfer is not possible, administer antibiotics even in the absence of a non-blanching rash.

Meningococcal Meningitis and Septicaemia

Bibliography

1. National Institute for Health and Clinical Excellence. *Feverish Illness in Children: Assessment and Initial Management in children younger than five years.* NICE, 2013. Available from: https://www.nice.org.uk/guidance/cg160.

2. National Institute for Health and Clinical Excellence. *Meningitis – Bacterial meningitis and meningococcal disease.* London: NICE, 2019. Available from: https://cks.nice.org.uk/meningitis-bacterial-meningitis-and-meningococcal-disease.

3. Meningitis Research Foundation. *Lessons from Research for Doctors in Training: Recognition and early management of meningococcal disease in children and young people.* Bristol: MRF, 2004. Available from: https://www.meningitis.org/healthcare-professionals/resources.

4. National Collaborating Centre for Women's and Children's Health. *Bacterial Meningitis and Meningococcal Septicaemia: Management of bacterial meningitis and meningococcal septicaemia in children and young people younger than 16 years in primary and secondary care* (CG102). London: National Institute for Health and Clinical Excellence, 2010. Available from: https://www.nice.org.uk/guidance/cg102.

5. Thompson MJ, Ninis N, Perera R, Mayon-White R, Phillips C, Bailey L, et al. Clinical recognition of meningococcal disease in children and adolescents. *The Lancet* 2006, 367(9508): 397–403.

6. Strang JR, Pugh EJ. Meningococcal infections: reducing the case fatality rate by giving penicillin before admission to hospital. *British Medical Journal* 1992, 305(6846): 141–143.

7. Riordan FA, Thomson AP, Sills JA, Hart CA. Who spots the spots? Diagnosis and treatment of early meningococcal disease in children. *British Medical Journal* 1996, 313(7067): 1255–1256.

8. Scottish Intercollegiate Guidelines Network. *Management of Invasive Meningococcal Disease in Children and Young People* (Guideline 102). Edinburgh: SIGN, 2008.

9. Chief Medical Officer. *Meningococcal infection* (letter, PL/CMO/99/1). London: Department of Health, 1999.

10. Hart CA, Thomson AP. Meningococcal disease and its management in children. *British Medical Journal* 2006, 333(7570): 685–690.

11. Hahne SJ, Charlett A, Purcell B, Samuelsson S, Camaroni I, Ehrhard I, et al. Effectiveness of antibiotics given before admission in reducing mortality from meningococcal disease: systematic review. *British Medical Journal* 2006, 332(7553): 1299–1303.

12. Meningitis Research Foundation. *Meningococcal Septicaemia: Identification & management for ambulance personnel*, 2nd edition. Bristol/Edinburgh/Belfast: Meningitis Research Foundation, 2008.

13. Cartwright K, Reilly S, White D, Stuart J. Early treatment with parenteral penicillin in meningococcal disease. *British Medical Journal* 1992, 305(6846): 143–147.

14. Booy R, Habibi P, Nadel S, de Munter C, Britto J, Morrison A, et al. Reduction in case fatality rate from meningococcal disease associated with improved healthcare delivery. *Archives of Disease in Childhood* 2001, 85(5): 386–390.

15. Pollard AJ, Cloke A, Glennie L, Faust SN, Haines C, Heath PT, et al. *Management of Meningococcal Disease in Children and Young People.* 7th edition. Bristol/Edinburgh/Belfast: Meningitis Research Foundation, 2010. Incorporates NICE *Bacterial Meningitis and Meningococcal Septicaemia* (CG102). Distributed in partnership with NICE.

16. Health Protection Agency. *Meningococcal Reference Unit Isolates of Neisseria Meningitidis: England and Wales, by region, age group & epidemiological year, 2000–2001 to 2009–2010.* London: HPA, 2010.

17. Surtees SJ, Stockton MG, Gietzen TW. Allergy to penicillin: fable or fact? *British Medical Journal* 1991, 302(6784): 1051–2.

18. Carcillo JA, Davis AL, Zaritsky A. Role of early fluid resuscitation in pediatric septic shock. *Journal of the American Medical Association* 1991, 266(9): 1242–1245.

Mental Health Presentations

1. Introduction

- The World Health Organization (WHO) has defined mental health as 'a state of well-being in which every individual realises his or her own potential, can cope with the normal stresses of life, can work productively and fruitfully, and is able to contribute to her or his community.'
- Around 10–15% of presentations to ambulance services involve primary mental health needs, where a patient's mental state may be deteriorating or where there may be an established risk of harm to, or from a patient. This is in addition to co-morbid mental health needs which may exist alongside, or contribute to, both.
- It is known that often, mental health needs may be influenced by socioeconomic factors. Following the COVID pandemic and during/following periods of socioeconomic instability, it may be expected that there are substantial impacts on the mental wellbeing of the population.

Facts and Figures

- Each year in England, 1 in 4 people will be experiencing a diagnosed mental illness, and even more will be living with symptoms of an undiagnosed condition.
- In England, 1 in 6 people report a common mental health problem (e.g., depression/anxiety) in any given week.
- The most extreme outcome for some people experiencing mental distress is death by suicide. According to the most recent figures, there were 5,583 suicides registered in England and Wales in 2021 (10.7 per 100,000 population). In Scotland, the number of suicides per 100,000 population was slightly higher at 13.7.

Mental Health Services

- Statutory NHS services are most often provided in three distinct age groups (within community and inpatient settings):
  - Child and Adolescent Mental Health Services (CAMHS)
  - services for adults of working age
  - services for older people.
- Most people diagnosed with a common mental illness are treated in the community within primary care.
- However, there are many secondary care services available to support people diagnosed with a mental illness. These are provided by the NHS and private companies. Every region in England has a 24/7 freephone Urgent Mental Health Helpline which can be accessed by any person experiencing mental health needs.
- Some services offer a self-referral pathway however most secondary services are accessed following a referral by a healthcare professional (often the patient's GP) via a single point of access. There are also a range of specialist services.

Examples of secondary care services	Examples of specialist services
• Community Mental Health Teams	• Specialist eating disorder services
• Crisis Resolution Home Treatment Teams	• Personality disorder services
• Early Intervention Teams	• Rehabilitation services
• Assertive Outreach Teams	• Forensic services
• Acute Impact Wards	
• Psychiatric Intensive Care Units	

Broadly, treatment for mental ill health will fall into the domains of biological, psychological and social:

Biological

- Medication – based on symptoms and depending on need. The most prescribed are anxiolytics, antidepressants and antipsychotics.
- Electro-convulsive therapy (ECT) may benefit a small percentage of patients and is used in treatment resistive circumstances in long term illness where medications and talking therapies haven't been fully effective.

Psychological

- Talking therapy – there are a wide range of talking therapies, but common ones include counselling, Improving Access to Psychological Therapies (IAPT), cognitive behavioural therapy (CBT), dialectical behavioural therapy (DBT) and specialist counselling services (e.g., bereavement counselling). IAPT service can normally be accessed by self-referral – check local pathways.
- Relaxation/mindfulness.

Social

- Social Prescribing – helping to connect people with mental or physical health problems with non-medical services and activities near them.
- Social support via Social Care

Additional help and support can be accessed via several national and/or local charities and peer-support self-help groups. Increasingly these groups are becoming more formal parts of the pathways offered by statutory mental health providers to give a more holistic approach in the management of mental health needs.

Mental Health Presentations

2. Legal Framework

Mental Health Act

The Mental Health Act (1983) and subsequent amendments provide a framework to support and treat those experiencing significant mental health needs within England and Wales. Within Scotland the Mental Health (Care and Treatment) Act (2003) provides a similar framework, however there are some differences.

An Approved Mental Health Professional (AMHP) is a social worker, registered mental health nurse, occupational therapist or clinical psychologist who has undertaken a specific qualification and is warranted by their Local Authority. An AMHP cannot be a paramedic unless they are dual registered as one of the other professions detailed above. They lead in organising mental health act assessments, including co-ordinating the professionals required (such as doctors, police and ambulance staff). Following an assessment, they are responsible for the decision to make an application to detain the patient under the Mental Health Act 1983 and work within the guidance laid out within the Mental Health Act Code of Practice.

For a patient to be detained under the Mental Health Act, one or two doctors (depending on the circumstances) must make a medical recommendation. This recommendation forms the basis for an AMHP to make an application for detention. Such recommendations are based on the patient suffering from a mental disorder of a nature and severity that requires detention in hospital for either assessment of treatment, and, in the case of treatment, that appropriate therapeutic interventions are available. Where two doctors are involved in the assessment, at least one must be approved under section 12 of the Mental Health Act 1983.

Some of the key provisions of the Mental Health Act (1983) that may be encountered as part of pre-hospital mental health care are outlined in Table 3.85.

TABLE 3.85 – Mental Health Act Provisions

Section 2	Admission to hospital for a period of up to 28 days for assessment. Requires two recommendations from doctors (one of which must be approved under s12 MHA) and an application to be made by an AMHP.
Section 3	Admission to hospital for a period of up to 6 months (although this can be renewed) for treatment of a mental disorder. Requires two recommendations from doctors (one of which must be approved under s12 MHA) and an application to be made by an AMHP, or in rare cases, the nearest relative.
Section 4	Admission to hospital for a period of 72 hours in cases of urgent necessity. Requires a single recommendation from a s12 approved doctor and an application by either an AMHP or the patients nearest relative. Can be converted to a section 2 following a second recommendation.
Section 6	The power of the AMHP to convey (or delegate authority to convey i.e., to an ambulance clinician) a patient to hospital based on an application for admission. Where such authority is delegated, this conveys s137 powers upon the person(s) to which this is delegated to detain the patient.
Section 13	The duty upon the local authority to arrange for an AMHP to consider a patient's case where they have reason to think that an application for admission to hospital may need to be made.
Section 18	The power to return a patient to hospital who is absent without leave. This can be applied by AMHPs, an officer on the staff of the hospital, constable or any person authorised in writing by hospital managers. There is no specific power for ambulance staff and this would require a written authorisation from hospital managers.
Section 135(1)	A warrant, applied for by an AMHP, allowing a police officer to enter a property and remove a patient to a place of safety to make an application for admission under the Act.
Section 135(2)	A warrant that may be applied for by a police officer or any other person authorised by the Act, authorising a constable to enter a property to take a person into custody who is subject to detention or an application for detention under the Mental Health Act. Unlike Section 135(1), an AMHP is not lawfully mandated to be present when the warrant is executed.

Mental Health Presentations

TABLE 3.85 – Mental Health Act Provisions *(continued)*	
Section 136	The power of a police officer to detain a patient and take them to a place of safety for the purpose of an assessment under the Act where: • They are in a place other than a house, flat or room (or associated yard, garden, garage or outhouse) where they, or any other person is living. • They need immediate care or control; **and** • It is necessary in the best interests of the person or for the protection of others. Once enacted, a s136 can only be removed following an assessment by a doctor.
Section 137	The powers, authorities, protections and privileges conferred upon a police constable or any other authorised person (including ambulance staff) to detain and convey a patient to hospital. This includes the power to restrain patients.

Conveyance Under the Mental Health Act

Ambulance staff may be asked to convey a patient to hospital for several reasons. This may include both patients being admitted informally based on consent (under s131 MHA and only where the patient has the capacity to give consent under the Mental Capacity Act 2005), and those detained under the Act.

Ambulance staff must ensure that the patient is either accompanied by the relevant application paperwork, or the applicant has confirmed that the paperwork has been sent electronically to the receiving hospital. Staff should also ensure that authority to detain the patient under section 6 of the Act has been clearly delegated to them. This is not required in law to be completed in writing; however, it is best practice and provides clear, demonstrable evidence of the authority of ambulance staff to detain and convey the patient using powers and protections under s137. Where the applicant has left the patient in the care of another person or team (e.g. in the emergency department) it may not always be possible to obtain a specific delegation. As the applicant has the responsibility to arrange transport, in such circumstances, the fact that they have made an application and arranged transport is sufficient to demonstrate the intent to delegate authority to convey.

In the case of a section 136, the Mental Health Act code of practice states that patients should normally be transported by ambulance and that the police officer should remain with the patient during the journey.

For transfers between mental health facilities, an escort from the ward should normally be present. Section papers (or copies) should also be present.

3. Equality in Mental Health

The Equality Act 2010 outlines the obligation to ensure equality, particularly in relation to 9 protected characteristics. Racism, inequality, and stigma experienced by individuals can contribute to the circumstances that precipitate and perpetuate poor mental health.

The combination of increased psychosocial burden, exposure to direct and indirect inequalities and barriers in accessing care can impact on the risk to an individual in mental health. Such factors must be considered as part of a wider risk assessment approach to ensure a holistic approach to meeting the needs of all.

Specific groups of patients presenting with mental health needs may also be subject to further inequalities in care. It is important to ensure equality in the approach to all care needs. Particular consideration should be given to Children and Young People, Older Adults, LGBTQ+ patients and those from minority ethnic groups, to ensure that the impact and risk of symptoms is not minimised or discounted by virtue of their protected characteristics.

Government figures[16] identify that ethnic minority groups, particularly those from black African groups, have a significantly higher rate of detention under the Mental Health Act.

Individuals from some ethnic groups face disadvantages within society, with some being more likely to experience poverty or homelessness, do less well in education, be unemployed, have contact with the criminal justice system and face challenges in accessing services. In turn, each of these factors can increase the likelihood of an individual developing mental ill health.

The Mental Health Foundation[10] identify that black males are more likely to have experienced a psychiatric disorder in the last year than white males, that older south Asian women are a high-risk group for suicide and that refugees and asylum seekers may have higher incidences of mental ill health conditions such as PTSD, depression and anxiety when compared to the general population.

There are often many barriers to individuals from ethnic groups accessing care and support, including:

• The impact of cultural stigma on seeking access to mental healthcare

• The cultural appropriateness and relevance of mental health service provision

Mental Health Presentations

- The cultural competence of healthcare staff
- Being unaware of the available care and support
- Being seen by professionals who have no direct experience of racism or discrimination
- Language barriers
- Access to financial means to support private care, such as private counselling.

There is a well-recognised health inequality demonstrating that individuals living in areas of deprivation are more likely to experience mental health needs, alongside other health needs. This is impacted further in mental health presentations by social cohesion within communities which can also act as a determinant of mental health.

Mental health conditions are in themselves also considered as disabilities under the Equality Act, with many who experience mental ill health also facing discrimination, stigma and inequality directly as a result of their mental ill health.

In all cases, the experience of mental health needs is specific to the experience of the individual, including their symptoms, social circumstances, life experience and skills, cultural background, and ability to access care. No two patients presenting with mental health will have the same needs, nor respond equally to treatments and interventions from healthcare providers. Advocacy can be a helpful way to enable every individual to have their needs heard, gain access to available services, and facilitate the sharing and understanding of information relevant to decisions about care. Advocates could be friends, family members, charity organisations and in some cases, individuals may have a legal right to an advocate. In addition, clinicians should be diligent in taking a personalised approach to identifying, understanding and managing the needs of the individual.

4. Assessment

The assessment of patients with mental health needs is key to understanding the presentation of the patient, their needs and how ambulance service clinicians should manage those needs. When documenting an assessment, it is helpful to clearly record answers to subjective assessment questions using direct quotes from the patient, for example where the patient is expressing thoughts or emotions, in order to provide additional clarity.

An overview of the assessment of mental health patients considers History, Mental State Examination (MSE), Risk, Physical Assessment, Mental Capacity. Additional information is provided below to add further context.

History

Presenting complaint

A thorough history will help to shape your understanding of the patient's current presentation and needs. This is even more true as part of the assessment of an individual with mental health needs.

When considering the presenting complaint and history of presenting complaint, typical acronyms used for physical health presentations in pre-hospital practice may not always be the best fit for mental health needs. It is however important to consider, as a minimum:

- The nature, course, and severity of the patient's presentation
- What factors are making the presentation better or worse
- What has specifically led to the patient (or a third party) seeking support now
- How the presentation is impacting upon the patient's ability to undertake their normal activity
- What are the patient's expectations of the contact with professionals
- The patient's usual level of functioning
- The patient's usual mental state

Medical

As part of collecting relevant information about the patient's past medical history it is key to ensure that you identify any psychiatric history. This will include information about the patient's current and past engagement with mental health services, encompassing voluntary sector services, GPs and other primary care healthcare professionals, secondary care, and specialist services as well as any history of both inpatient admission under a Mental Health Act or as part of an informal voluntary admission.

As with any presentation, the medication history should include: prescribed, over the counter, herbal or illicit medications/substances. For mental health presentations this includes any psychiatric medications including Selective Serotonin Reuptake Inhibitors (SSRIs), Serotonin-Noradrenaline Reuptake Inhibitors (SNRIs), anxiolytics, mood stabilisers and anti-psychotic medications (including depot injections which provide a long term slow release dose of medication and are often administered monthly). This should also include timings of medication initiation (recent commencement of some anti-depressants may lead to increased suicidality for example), whether the patient is taking medication in line with their prescription and common side effects of psychiatric and physical health medications which may be contributing to the patient's presenting needs.

Family

Like many physical health conditions, some mental health conditions have a genetic component. As a result, it is important to consider the patient's family history of psychiatric illness. This also presents an opportunity to explore family support

Mental Health Presentations

and relationships which may be available and the impact of the presentation upon dependants as part of any subsequent safety or management plan.

Social

Given the social determinants of mental health conditions, a thorough social history is important as part of a holistic assessment of the patient's needs. This should include (where relevant):

- Drug and alcohol use, including any dependency or withdrawal
- Living circumstances
- Mobility
- Visual/auditory impairment
- Employment/occupation/ current education
- Finance
- Care arrangements, support mechanisms and social networks
- Adverse childhood experiences
- Sexuality
- Religious or cultural beliefs
- Forensic history (i.e., police involvement, imprisonment)
- Any other relevant social history.

Third-Party Information

Patients experiencing mental health needs may not always have full insight into their condition and others may have sought help on their behalf. The information provided by family, friends or bystanders can be important in generating as broad an understanding of the patient's circumstances as possible. Information from other healthcare professionals may also help guide the understanding of the individuals needs and how these can be most appropriately met. Confidentiality should be maintained appropriately (refer to **Patient Confidentiality**) and it is important to consider and document third party information as part of the assessment process, along with the context and intent with which it is shared.

Mental Capacity

See **Mental Capacity Act 2005** guideline.

Mental State Examination

The mental state examination (MSE) is a core component of a psychiatric assessment which builds upon the narrative created by the patient history to provide a snapshot of the patient's mental state at the time of the assessment. The MSE can help to support the identification of key symptoms and effects by considering a range of factors relevant to presentations of mental ill health. It is also particularly helpful when making referrals or discussing a patient with mental health professionals as it supports a common language which will help them to clearly understand the patient's presentation.

The MSE is an important element within the mental health assessment and should be documented within the patient record. An overview of the MSE is provided in Table 3.86. This is not an exhaustive, nor prescriptive, list of considerations and should be used to guide an approach to an assessment.

A range of tools and frameworks for the MSE exist, refer to local policy for specific guidance.

TABLE 3.86 – Mental State Examination Overview

Appearance Identify relevant information about the individual's appearance which may provide insight into their mental state	• General appearance and distinguishing features • State of dress (including whether appropriate to time, circumstance, weather etc.) • Personal hygiene • Evidence of self-harm or self-neglect
Behaviour Consider aspects of the individual's behaviour and mannerisms which may be linked to their mental state.	• General manner • Level of engagement • Rapport • Level of psychomotor activity • Level of eye contact • Gesticulation, facial expression, and involuntary movements
Speech Observe and record abnormalities of speech which may be indicative of altered mental state.	• Rate • Rhythm • Volume • Tone • Content

(continued)

Mental Health Presentations

TABLE 3.86 – Mental State Examination Overview *(continued)*

Mood/Affect
Consider both the subjectivity reported mood and observed affect.
	• Current expressed mood
	• Observed affect
	  – Observed emotion
	  – Nature, range and intensity of affect
	• Congruency of affect with expressed mood, thoughts, and other mental state findings

Thoughts
Consider the patient's thought process, content, and possession and how this might demonstrate underlying mental health needs.
Does the patient have any odd, unusual, or bizarre ideas? (delusions)
	• Process
	  – Are the patient's thoughts linear, tangential, circumstantial?
	  – Is the patient experiencing flight of ideas or thought block?
	• Content
	  – Is the patient experiencing intrusive thoughts of suicide, self-harm or harm to others?
	  – Is there evidence of obsessions, compulsions or over/under valued thoughts/ideas?
	• Possession
	  – Does the patient believe their thoughts are not their own or that they can be read by others?
	• Delusions
	  – Is the patient demonstrating a fixed belief that is not in line with objective evidence or the patients educational, cultural, or social background and circumstances?
	  – Is there evidence of persecutory delusion?

Perception
Consider whether the patient seems to be experiencing or responding to hallucinations.
	• Hallucinations
	  – Auditory
	  – Visual
	  – Tactile
	  – Olfactory (Smell)
	  – Gustatory (Taste)
	  – Command Hallucinations

Cognition
Consider the cognitive abilities of the patient as they apply to the patient mental state.
	• Orientation
	  – Is the patient oriented to time, place, and person?
	• Registration
	  – Is the patient able to understand and repeat new information?
	• Recall
	  – Is the patient able to recall information after a short time?
	• Concentration/Attention
	  – Is there any evidence of hypervigilance or a reduction in concentration/attention?

Insight Consider the patient's insight into their presentation, any required treatment or intervention and broader psychosocial circumstances.	• Does the patient understand the nature and severity of their illness? • Does the patient understand the available treatment and support for their illness?
Judgement Identify any impairment of judgement as part of the broader assessment of the patient's mental state.	• Is the patient's judgement impaired? • Is there evidence of impulsive/disproportionate/apathetic responses, or inaction when making decisions? • How might the patient respond to a common risk situation e.g. a fire alarm sounding?

Mental Health Presentations

Alongside this examination of mental state, it is important to consider the patient's sleep habits and appetite, as these are two areas very commonly affected by mental illness and can contribute significantly to worsening symptoms.

In respect of sleep, it is important to explore:

- Is the patient achieving an appropriate amount of sleep each night?
- Is sleep broken or of poor quality?
- Does the patient have difficulty in getting to sleep or waking?
- Does the patient have early morning wakening?
- Does the patient sleep during the day instead of overnight?

Advice can be provided to support sleep hygiene and establish routines for normal patterns of sleep, enabling appropriate rest and recovery.

When considering the patients appetite and food intake it is important to establish:

- Does the patient have a reduced or increased appetite and/or consumption?
- Is the patient binging eating food?
- Does the patient purge food (for example by vomiting or using laxatives)?
- Is the patient restricting their consumption?
- Is the patient only consuming fluids?
- Has there been any reduction or increase in weight in the last few weeks and months?

Risk Assessment

The purpose of a psychiatric risk assessment is to identify a range of risks, including:

- From the patient to themselves.
- From the patient to others.
- To the patient from others.
- Resulting from care provided to, or withheld from, the patient.

Both NICE guidelines and contemporary research into a range of psychiatric risk domains identify that risk assessment tools that stratify risk by score or category (e.g., high/medium/low) are often unable to predict adverse events and as a result are not recommended for use.

Structured professional judgement, through a combination of a structured assessment approach and professional clinical judgement, involves drawing together a range of information to facilitate an understanding of:

- The presenting risks.
- The likelihood, severity, and immediacy of the risk.
- How specific the risk is.
- Factors which may increase risk.
- Factors or interventions which may support an individual to mitigate risks as part of a care plan.

The process of assessing risk should form a collaborative approach in partnership with the patient, and not simply be an objective assessment of the patient. It will not always be possible to eliminate risk when supporting those experiencing mental health needs. Legal frameworks such as the Mental Health Act 1983 and Mental Capacity Act 2005 do exist to protect individuals where this is necessary, however there are clear ethical considerations to balance risk with the need to promote freedom, autonomy, and choice when supporting individuals with mental health needs. This is key to ensuring that individuals retain agency over their health to maximise their recovery.

TABLE 3.87 – General Risk Assessment Considerations

Presenting Risk	How is the patient presenting, what are their needs and what are the identified risks to and/or from the patient?
Predisposing Factors	What are the static risk factors which may place the individual at higher risk? These factors are often derived from population studies based upon elements of a person's biopsychosocial history which cannot be altered, and the presence, or absence, of these factors may not be predictive of risk in an individual. They should however be considered as part of a holistic assessment.
	Predisposing risk factors of suicide may include:
	• Previous self-harm/overdose suicide attempt
	• Previous psychiatric inpatient admission
	• Diagnosed mental disorder
	• Substance use disorder
	• Domestic violence
	• Chronic illness (especially pain)
	• Adverse childhood experiences

(continued)

Mental Health Presentations

TABLE 3.87 – General Risk Assessment Considerations *(continued)*

	- Family history/exposure to suicide
	- Age and gender
	  – Men are generally at higher risk
	  – The risk in both males and females is highest between age 45–49
	  – Females between 10–25 are also at increased risk.

Precipitating Factors	What are the factors, or triggers, which have contributed to the presentation and led a person to present in crisis? Consider particularly why this presentation has occurred now and any unmet needs the person may have.
Perpetuating Factors	What are the dynamic risk factors which may increase risk? These factors will depend on the circumstances of each case; however, examples of dynamic risk factors of suicide may include: - Ongoing thoughts, intent, or plan of suicide - Hopelessness, bereavement, or relationship breakdown - Active psychological/emotional distress - Non-adherence with treatment/disengagement with mental health services - Current substance use - Recent discharge from psychiatric hospital or community mental health services - Psycho-social stressors, including financial difficulties, homelessness, or risk to employment - Poor social/healthcare support mechanisms
Protective Factors	Consider specific opportunities to mitigate risk factors, particularly any preventable, precipitating or perpetuating factors (e.g., by removing/resolving the cause of the presentation, or by limiting exposure to perpetuating factors where possible). You should also consider the supportive mechanisms the individual has in place, including family/social support, GP, mental health teams, crisis lines, safety plan (see management section), distraction/coping strategies and available safety netting opportunities. It should be noted that protective factors are fluid and risk may increase if these mechanisms fail or become inaccessible.

TABLE 3.88 – Risk Specific Consideration

RISK TO SELF	
Suicide	Ideation - Frequency, severity, and intrusiveness of thoughts of suicide. Intent - The level of intent expressed by the patient in relation to making an attempt to end their life (for example does the patient have a specific intent to end their life or can they simply not see an alternative?) - The stated purpose of any intent to end their life. Plan - The method and potential lethality of any plan of suicide identified by the patient. - When and where the patient is planning to end their life. Preparation - Is the patient gathering means to carry out a plan? - Has the patient researched suicide methodology?

Mental Health Presentations

TABLE 3.88 – Risk Specific Consideration *(continued)*	
	• Has the patient made arrangements for after their death (e.g., funeral arrangements, wills, child/pet care)? Actions • Is the patient currently acting upon a plan to end their life? • Has the patient previously attempted to end their life? • When did the patient last attempt to end their life? • How does the patient feel about previous attempts?
Self-Harm	Intent • Why is the person considering/undertaking acts of self-harm? This might include, establishing a sense of control over circumstances, catharsis, self-punishment or management of psychological pain/distress and may not be an act of intended suicide. Severity • Consider the degree of harm and likely consequences, including complications such as infection. Method • How is the person harming themselves? Is there a risk of the person causing more harm than intended? Harm reduction • How does the patient usually manage thoughts to self-harm? • Has the patient considered using methods to minimise or reduce lasting harm, such as snapping elastic bands against their wrist (where this is age appropriate), or using ice as a sensory alternative?
Self-Neglect	Activities of daily life • Is the patient able to undertake normal activities of daily living? Evidence of self-neglect • Consider the patient's environment • Is the patient able to undertake activities of daily living? • Explore changes in physical condition (such as weight loss) • Consider if the patient is able to engage with recommended medical treatments (including taking medication as prescribed, counselling/therapy) • What support is available, has been previous offered or has been previously declined? Consider Safeguarding.
Substance Use	Including illicit drugs, alcohol, prescription medication or any other substance. Consider: • What substances are being used by the patient? • How much is the patient using? • How is the substance being used? • How often is the patient using the substance? • Does the patient depend on the substance to maintain their daily functioning? • Is the patient at risk of withdrawal?
Accidental Death/ Injury	Consider: • Is the patient demonstrating a pattern of behaviour that may place them at higher risk of accidental death or serious injury where this may not be their intent? • Are the factors which might increase the patient's impulsivity or reckless behaviour such as drug/alcohol use or severe emotional distress?

(continued)

Mental Health Presentations

TABLE 3.88 – Risk Specific Consideration *(continued)*

RISK TO OTHERS	
Agitation/Agression	Consider: • Does the patient have any physical or mental health illness or injury contributing to their agitation/aggression? • Is the aggression directed specifically at a specific individual? • Alcohol or drug intoxication • Could the agitation be caused by delirium? (See **Agitated Patients**) • Is this an Acute Behavioural Disturbance presentation? (See **Acute Behavioural Disturbance**)
RISK TO and/or FROM OTHERS	
Violence	Consider: • Identify any thoughts, plans or acts to harm or kill others, or animals. • Carefully explore any previous police engagement or imprisonment for violent offences.
Neglect	Consider: • Identify the needs of any dependants and the patient's ability to care for others, or for carers ability to support the patient. • Visually assess the patient and their surroundings for signs of neglect. • Where dependants are present, visually assess for signs of neglect. • Where possible, assess the home environment for signs of neglect. Refer to the Safeguarding guidelines – **Safeguarding Adults at Risk** and **Safeguarding Children**
RISK FROM OTHERS	
Abuse	Consider: • Any signs of abuse from or towards dependants, carers or domestic partners present at the time of assessment • Discuss the nature of the patient's close relationships Refer to the Safeguarding guidelines – **Safeguarding Adults at Risk** and **Safeguarding Children**
Exploitation	Explore circumstances/evidence which might suggest financial, emotional or sexual exploitation, forced labour, or any other form of exploitation. Refer to the Safeguarding guidelines – **Safeguarding Adults at Risk** and **Safeguarding Children**
Radicalisation	Consider PREVENT responsibilities: • Identify those at risk of radicalisation • Identify fantasies or idealisation of violence • Identify any recent history of altered behaviour, such as withdrawal, increased anger, or speaking from a script, which may indicate potential radicalisation Refer to the Safeguarding guidelines – **Safeguarding Adults at Risk** and **Safeguarding Children**
Victimisation	Consider: • Is the patient being victimised (or they might be) owing to their mentail ill health? • Is the patient at risk of becoming a victim of crime, such as harassment, theft or assault, owing to their mental health? Refer to the Safeguarding guidelines – **Safeguarding Adults at Risk** and **Safeguarding Children**
Iatrogenic Harm	Is there a risk of harm, or unintended consequences, arising from the patient's current or proposed treatment?

Mental Health Presentations

Physical Assessment

An assessment of the patient's physical health is a crucial part of the wider assessment of a mental health crisis presentation. This is covered in more detail in the physical health interface section of this guideline.

Mental Capacity

Where a patient presents with a mental disorder, it is important to consider the need to assess the patient's capacity. Mental health conditions can impact the ability of the patient to make a decision. Where the patient is found to lack capacity to make a decision, the Mental Capacity Act (2005) provides a framework for decisions to be made in the best interests of the patient. Remember that the presumption of capacity is not a substitute for an assessment of capacity where the patient's behaviour or circumstances cause doubt as to whether they have the capacity to make a decision. Where doubt exists, capacity must always be formally assessed and documented.

In particular, consider how mood, thoughts and perceptions may impact on the ability of the patient to weigh and use information in relation to specific decisions. Such factors render the individual unable to consider the merits of alternative courses of action. See **Mental Capacity Act 2005** for more information.

Children and Young People

In most mental health settings, the assessment and management of children and adolescents is conducted by staff specialised in delivering mental health care to this group. In the context of urgent and emergency presentations to the ambulance service, it is recognised that ambulance staff are not able to provide this level of specialist knowledge. The principles laid out in this guideline continue to apply, however, consider adapting communication styles and approaches to reflect the patient's needs.

Wherever possible it is highly advised to seek specialist advice from a CAMHS clinician or other suitably qualified or experienced mental health practitioner. Where this is not possible and there are concerns about the immediate safety of a child, consider conveyance to an appropriate mental health setting or to an emergency department.

Specific considerations that should be made in children and young people include:

- Adapting communication styles to be age appropriate.
- Considering additional factors relating to their engagement in education environments, including academic performance, truancy, bullying and developing social relationships.
- Exploring the relationship of the young person with their family members.
- Identifying any concerns which may give rise to a need to consider safeguarding the child or others within the household or family.

Where a child under the age of 16 is of an age and level of competence to be involved in making decisions around their care, make every effort to involve the child in that decision. Where this is not the case, or where care is refused by a child of such an age, clinicians should engage with those who hold parental responsibility for the child. Where appropriate care is refused by parents/guardians/caregivers, consider whether the Childrens' Act may apply in order to safeguard the child from a risk of harm. Refer to the Safeguarding guidelines – **Safeguarding Adults at Risk** and **Safeguarding Children**

Older Adults

Older adult mental health care is also often provided by mental health teams who specialise in the delivery of a more tailored approach to managing the needs of older people. As with children and young people, there is no expectation on ambulance staff to be able to offer specialist assessment and intervention in the context of emergency presentations. The general principles within this guideline should be used to support an assessment and understanding of the patient's needs. Wherever possible, seek advice from a specialist older adult mental health clinician, a specialist in geriatric medicine or the patient's GP.

Specific considerations which should be made for older adult patients presenting with mental health needs include:

- Always ascertain the patient's usual level of functioning. Age alone does not directly correlate with a person's day to day functioning. Are they usually self-caring, living independently, able to manage activities of daily living, mobile?
- Are they known to have any physical health problems, mental health conditions or dementia?
- If there is a rapid change to someone's level of functioning or they are more confused than usual, have a high index of suspicion of delirium. Delirium can be caused by pain, infection, constipation, dehydration, medication or environment factors (see **Agitated Patient**).
- Consideration of physical health needs which may be presenting as apparent mental health symptoms, including infection.
- What medications are they prescribed? Does it appear they have been taking these as prescribed? Have there been any new medications prescribed recently or any recent changes to doses of medication?
- Consideration of care and support needs arising as a result of any presenting illness.

Mental Health Presentations

5. Management

Therapeutic Approach

The approach taken by the health professional involved is fundamental to the management of any mental health incident. Often patients remember the warmth, empathy, compassion and concern of the healthcare professional who looked after them at a time of distress, rather than specific advice given. These aspects of care are particularly important when supporting patients with mental health concerns.

Staff who can establish rapport, manage distress, and provide reassurance, are more likely to elicit true expressions of feelings and worries from the patient, and this facilitates an effective assessment to formulate a safe outcome.

Ambulance clinicians are unlikely to be able to offer meaningful long-term interventions to support severe or enduring underlying mental health needs. However, the act of assessment in itself can be a cathartic process for patients that can help minimise the stigma of, and encourages future engagement with, assessment by healthcare services. Advocacy on behalf of our patients is also a key part of the role of ambulance services responding to mental health crisis. This ensures we amplify the voice of our patients and support them in accessing appropriate care and support.

Communication

Communication skills are a key component of completing an effective assessment of the patient, de-escalating distress, and working in partnership with the patient to establish a care plan.

Gaining an understanding of the patient's situation (and their perception of the situation) and developing a rapport with the patient is vital in eliciting their immediate needs and achieving an appropriate/safe outcome.

It is important to employ active listening as part of your engagement with the patient. This will allow the patient to express themselves and give confidence that they are being heard and understood. You can do this by:

- Maintaining concentration on what is being said and pay attention to how it is being said. Avoid being distracted by other tasks or preparing a response to what is being expressed.
- Demonstrating that you are listening and interested. Adopt an open body position and use body language, facial expressions, or gestures (such as nodding or smiling) to let the patient know you are engaged.
- Avoid interrupting the patient and allow them to finish before asking questions.
- Summarising what the patient has told you, and/or ask questions to clarify specific points to demonstrate that you have understood what has been communicated.
- Avoid minimising the experience of the patient.
- Remain calm, confident, sympathetic and non-judgemental throughout.
- Do not feel pressured to fill silence or space within the conversation. Do not rush – allow the patient to use this time to gather their thoughts or to add additional information.
- Apologise if you make a mistake in how you communicate.
- Demonstrate empathy.

Consider the following question types when communicating with the patient:

TABLE 3.89 – Type of Questions

• **Open questions** Leave the respondent free to answer as they wish. They are broad in nature, but are more time-consuming, and answers may contain irrelevant but valuable and unexpected information. They encourage the respondent to talk, leaving the questioner free to observe, listen and learn.	General 'open' questions • What's happened today to make your call for help? • How are you feeling? Specific 'open' questions • When did the increased anxiety/low mood/suicidal thoughts start? • What coping strategies have you used/tried?
• **Probing questions** Questions are designed to encourage the respondent to enlarge or expand on their initial responses. They are often the follow-up question to find out more about a certain aspect, or to clarify understanding	• Can you explain what you mean? • And then what happened? • What did you think would happen?
• **Closed questions** Place restrictions on the respondent. There is usually only one correct answer. They give the questioner control over the situation, and they provide focus.	• Have you taken any medication? • Have you called your CPN/Support worker?

Mental Health Presentations

De-escalation

De-escalation techniques are designed to support an individual in re-establishing control over their immediate situation and emotional state, or in responding to and mitigating the physiological effects of a mental health crisis presentation. This can be achieved in several ways:

- **Removing the stimulus**. Where something, or someone, is stimulating and exacerbating the patient's condition. For example, move to another room, or to the ambulance, where the patient is not directly being affected by the stimulus and may feel safer.
- **Reassurance**. Support patients to feel safe and listened to.
- **Acknowledge and validate** the patient's emotions and experience as being real. Do not minimise or dismiss the patient experience.
- **Providing the patient with space, and time**, to express and ventilate their emotion or experience can be a cathartic process which facilitates de-escalation. This can be a delicate balance and at times, consider the use of gentle challenge to ensure that such ventilation is productive and not escalating the patient's emotional state.
- **Distraction**. A powerful tool that helps patients to focus on something else for a short time, e.g. discussing something irrelevant to the patient's presentation (use environmental cues), or by specifically identifying and utilising useful distraction techniques in conjunction with the patient.
- **Using techniques such as controlled breathing techniques and mindfulness** to assist in the management of physiological symptoms arising as part of the autonomic response to mental health crisis, e.g. hyperventilation and tachycardia. This can help to make the patient feel more at ease and more able to engage in the assessment and management of their current needs.

Clinicians should also consider using any local conflict resolution, or de-escalation training.

Shared Decision Making

Working in partnership with both the patient, families, carers, and other professionals is fundamental to establishing a safe and effective care plan for patients.

Risk management is a statement of plans and allocation of responsibility (where appropriate) to support, contain or respond to the risk(s) identified.

Formulating and agreeing a plan of action provides challenges and opportunities for both the clinician and patient. Consent and collaboration need to be at the heart of the decision-making process.

The components of the plan of action should include:

- The immediacy and severity of the risk.
- Service options – what the ambulance service can provide. What mental health specific services are available in the area?
- What the patient wants.
- Duty of care – particularly with issues of confidentiality. Professionals have a duty of care to balance confidentiality with the need to know, particularly regarding colleagues from other agencies. The issue of confidentiality is further clouded by the duty of care you hold to others, to pass on information about a third party you know to be at risk.

In considering a plan to support an individual with mental health needs, it is important to explore a range of potential care and treatment options and demonstrate a rationale/justification for the decisions made.

Safety Planning

Safety plans are a powerful tool to empower an individual to utilise the resources and support available to them and identify new opportunities to maintain their safety. Safety plans should not be imposed upon patients – it is crucial that safety plans are established in partnership so that the patient can feel confident in it, and it accurately reflects the actions which are most likely to have a positive impact for them. Table 3.90 identifies a range of options which might be considered as part of a safety plan.

TABLE 3.90 – Considerations for Safety Planning

Existing Safety/Crisis Plans	If the patient is already known to local mental health services: • Ask to see a copy of their care plan and follow the recommendations/advice, as appropriate. • Contact their care co-ordinator (during normal office hours).
Improving Mood	In partnership with the patient, identify activities and circumstances where the patient's mood may be better, as well as where their mood may be worse. Consider how the patient might draw on this to respond to low mood/anxiety/stress.

(continued)

Mental Health Presentations

TABLE 3.90 – Considerations for Safety Planning *(continued)*

Improving Situation and Surroundings	Consider: • Is there something about the patient's current situation or surroundings which could be changed now? • Are there environments in which the patient feels more at ease?
Distraction	Are there any activities which the patient finds help distract them from negative thoughts? For example, this might include: • Going for a walk/exercising • Reading • Watching a film or TV programme • Drawing or painting
Support	What support does the patient have to maintain their safety and promote their recovery? Family and Friends • Does the patient have someone they are able to speak with about how they are feeling? • Does the patient have friends/family who might be able to spend time with them to offer a degree of reassurance and safety? GP • Is the patient currently engaging with their GP about their mental health? Mental Health Professionals • Is the patient currently receiving care under mental health services (including IAPT, primary care, voluntary or private services) VCSE and Community Services • Is the patient receiving support from charity or community groups?
Emergency Action Plan	How should the patient access care in an emergency where they are unable to keep themselves safe? 24/7 Crisis Line • Every area of the UK now has 24/7 freephone crisis lines able to support individuals experiencing a mental health crisis. Numbers for these crisis lines can be found on NHS. UK by searching for 'Urgent Mental Health Helplines' 111/999 • Where there is an immediate risk of harm, ask the patient and/or those close to them to contact 111/999

Referrals and Safety Netting

It is recommended that all providers of pre-hospital care have clear policies and procedures that set out the routes for onward referral to other agencies within their area. Examples of referral pathways are detailed below.

Direct consultation with a mental health professional – via an Ambulance Clinical Contact Centre (or equivalent), or locally agreed referral routes with statutory mental health service providers. This may include:

• Community mental health teams (usually during normal working hours)
• Crisis or other out-of-hours teams (24/7 or outside of normal working hours)
• Hospital mental health liaison services
• Locally agreed alternative care pathways – to avoid use of emergency departments where other clinical pathways would be more appropriate
• Using the Directory of Services Service Finder to identify appropriate local provision.

Wherever patients are referred to services and/or discharged by ambulance services without conveyance, it is imperative that consideration is given to safety-netting. This should include:

• Providing appropriate advice about the patient's presentation and the agreed next steps to access appropriate care.
• Identifying a safety plan.
• Giving clear advice about where to access help in an emergency.

Mental Health Presentations

- Wherever possible, identifying others who can support the individual and recontact mental health/emergency services if necessary.

Conveyance

In some circumstances, including where the patient may have concurrent physical health needs, it may be necessary to convey the patient to an emergency department.

It is recognised that conveyance to an emergency department can often be a sub-optimal pathway of care for patients with mental health needs. Wherever possible, clinicians should identify and consider alternative pathways which may better meet the needs of the patient where there is no clear requirement for emergency physical healthcare intervention.

Safeguarding

For most adults presenting with mental health needs, there will be no need to make a safeguarding referral – these patients should be conveyed/referred to mental health pathways as appropriate, unless there is a specific safeguarding risk identified.

The identification of mental health needs in children, or the exposure of a child to a serious mental health presentation within a domestic setting, should be a trigger to consider safeguarding risks. Where any such risks are identified, consider making a safeguarding referral.

Safeguarding referrals should be considered for:

- Adults at risk of abuse or neglect because of care or support needs.
- Children <18 who have taken an overdose or self-harmed.
- Children <18 who have witnessed acts of self-harm, suicide or been exposed to trauma because of a mental health presentation.
- Carers, families, or others at risk from the patient.

For further guidance refer to the JRCALC Safeguarding Guidelines: **Safeguarding Adults at Risk** and **Safeguarding Children**

Physical Interventions

Physical restraint techniques are potential interventions that should only be deployed when verbal de-escalation techniques have proved ineffective, and following formal consideration under the guidance of the Mental Capacity Act (MCA), Mental Health Act or any other legal framework.

It is beyond the scope of this guidance to recommend any specific training model for physical interventions, or to mandate the degree of training that each trust may adopt to safely discharge its duties to protect patients, staff and the public. This must be determined locally based on current national guidance, a training needs analysis and assessment of risk.

Physical interventions broadly fall into three areas:

1. **Disengagement techniques** often referred to as breakaway techniques which are skills designed to lead to physical disengagement or escape from an assailant.
2. **Physical restraint techniques**, which include manual holds and interventions to restrict the movement of an individual who may present a risk to themself or others. These techniques will require a minimum of two staff to intervene safely.
3. **Mechanical restraint**, which describes techniques to restrict movement, using devices designed for the purpose e.g. handcuffs.

Where a patient lacks capacity, ambulance staff are obliged under the MCA to act in the best interests of patients who lack capacity, even when the patient refuses treatment or is abusive, threatening, or violent.

The MCA also protects ambulance staff from liability when 'reasonable force' is required to ensure that a patient lacking capacity receives care that is in their best interests; or to protect the patient from harm. Section 6 of the Act defines restraint as the use, or threat, of force where an incapacitated person resists, and any restriction of liberty or movement whether or not the person resists. Refer to **Mental Capacity Act 2005** for more information.

6. Physical Health Interface

There are well established links between mental and physical health. The impact of a chronic health condition may lead to symptoms of mental illness, and those with mental ill health may be more likely to develop physical illness, or present with physical side-effects of common mental health treatments. Many medical conditions may present with symptoms consistent with mental ill health and patients with a diagnosed mental health condition may have concurrent physical health needs. These needs may be missed if a holistic approach to patient care and robust physical assessment is not undertaken. It is therefore important to always consider mental and physical health together to ensure a holistic approach to identifying and meeting the needs of the patient. Doing so establishes a parity between the consideration of mental and physical health concerns whilst enabling the clinician to ensure that assumptions about the patient's condition or needs do not lead to diagnostic overshadowing.

Physical assessment in mental health presentations should explore all presenting symptoms in light of both medical and psychiatric causes. Ensure appropriate physical examination and observations are completed to exclude acute medical or traumatic conditions.

Mental Health Presentations

There are a wide range of physical health conditions which should be considered when assessing a patient in mental health crisis, some of these are outlined in Table 3.91.

TABLE 3.91 – Physical Differentials for Psychiatric Presentations	
Respiratory	Pulmonary Embolism
	Asthma
	COPD
	Pneumothorax
Cardiac	Myocardial Infarction or other Acute Coronary Syndromes
	Arrhythmia (consider side-effects of psychiatric medications)
	Heart Failure
Neurological	Stroke/Transient Ischaemic Attack
	Head Injury
	Space Occupying Lesion
	Meningitis or encephalitis
Endocrine	Hypo/Hyperglycaemia
	Abnormal Electrolytes
	Hypo/hyperthyroidism
	Phaeochromocytoma
	Adrenal Insufficiency
	Hepatic Encephalopathy
Infection	Sepsis
	Pneumonia
	Endocarditis
	Meningitis
Substance Related	Intoxication
	Withdrawal
	Overdose
	Carbon monoxide poisoning
Other	Neuroleptic Malignant Syndrome
	Serotonin Syndrome
	Medication-induced psychosis
	Delirium (see **Agitated Patients**)
	Heat related illness

Red Flags requiring Physical Health Assessment

There are some conditions which, in all cases, will require assessment within a physical healthcare setting before an assessment of the patient's mental health needs might be considered by mental health services. These may include (but are not limited to):

- Overdose (including where a toxic dose of a single substance has been taken, or where multiple substances may have been taken)
- Self-harm requiring further assessment or wound closure
- Patients newly unable to weight bear
- Any Loss of Consciousness
- Head injury (refer to local head injury management policy)
- Ingested objects
- Physical abnormalities requiring further assessment e.g., NEWS2 > 3
- Prolonged physical restraint
- Taser/Incapacitant Spray Exposure (additional guidance relating to Controlled Energy Devices including Taser can be found in RCEM Best Practice Guidance, see Further Reading section)
- Completely incoherent patients e.g., acute intoxication, delirium, ABD

Mental Health Presentations

In such cases, these patients should be referred for assessment through the Emergency Department, Same Day Emergency Care, Frailty Unit or other appropriate destination from where a mental health assessment can be arranged if required.

Heat Illness in Mental Health

Evidence from North America has highlighted risks associated with heat illness in patients with mental health conditions. The effects of some psychiatric medications, including antipsychotics and some antidepressants may lead to patients having a reduced ability to thermoregulate. In addition, factors associated with mental ill health may put those with mental health needs in a disadvantaged position to adapt to, or mitigate for, extremes of heat. During periods of extreme heat, clinicians should be particularly vigilant for signs of heat related illness; refer to **Heat Related Illness**.

7. Self-Harm and Suicide

Self-Harm

Self-Harm is **NOT** classified as a specific mental disorder; however, a history of self-harm can be a strong predictor for repeated self-harm and completion of suicide. It is more commonly used as a way for a person to cope with life, rather than a failed attempt to end it; and there are many reasons why a person may self-harm. Some examples are listed below:

- Release or catharsis
- Making an emotional pain a 'real' physical pain
- Having control when feeling out of control
- As a self-punishment.

Self-harm describes a range of ways in which a person may cause themselves harm and may include by causing injury, intentionally neglecting their needs or sabotaging positive things (including for example relationships or employment).

A large part of the assessment by an ambulance clinician is likely to be centred on the physical nature of the self-harm. However, talking about the self-harm is vital as part of the assessment; it acknowledges what has happened and with this it communicates to the person that you are not rejecting them. This often helps reduce feelings of shame and stigma, which can help maintain self-harm.

When working with someone who has self-harmed it is important that these factors are addressed:

- What led up to it? (i.e. what was the trigger – interpersonal stressors and/or situational aspects?)
- What was the intent of the act?
- What was the motivation?
- Was it planned or impulsive?
- Are there practical protective factors in place to reduce the risk of harm occurring?

These questions may overlap somewhat with a suicide risk assessment; but ambulance clinicians should be aware to separate these two aspects and to treat each accordingly.

TABLE 3.92 – Tips of talking to someone about self-harm

Do ...	Don't ...
<ul><li>Actively listen.</li><li>Provide support and reassurance.</li><li>Encourage the use of any positive coping strategies.</li><li>Treat the patient with dignity and respect.</li></ul>	<ul><li>Minimise the person's feelings or problems.</li><li>Use statements that don't take the patient's pain seriously (such as "but you've got a great life" or "things aren't that bad").</li><li>Try to solve the patient's problems for them.</li><li>Touch (e.g., hug or hold the patient's hand/arm) without their permission.</li><li>Use terms such as 'self-harmer', 'self-mutilator', 'self-injurer' or 'cutter' to refer to the patient.</li><li>Accuse the patient of attention seeking.</li><li>Make the patient feel guilty about the effect their self-injuring is having on others.</li><li>Set goals or pacts.</li></ul>

Suicide

The act of suicide may be an act in isolation, or it may be after a lonely introspective mental journey, usually occurring gradually, progressing from suicidal thoughts, to planning, then attempting (or rehearsing) suicide, and finally dying. But, with the right help, many people who have been on a suicidal path do recover completely and go on to lead happy and fulfilling lives. However, some high lethality survivors do describe acting on impulse, often following acute loss or bereavement – partner, parent, child, job, freedom or when they have felt that they had a problem they couldn't solve any other way.

Mental Health Presentations

The clinical and risk assessments should therefore each time be specific to the individual in front of us in crisis. Debt, bereavement, guilt, shame, hopelessness, isolation and disconnection are the strongest predictors of suicidal risk, with ongoing clinical plans needed to reduce the risk for that individual. Following on from global experiences of isolation through COVID-19 measures and mental trauma associated with exposure to these measures, specific consideration may need to be given to issues surrounding this.

It is always appropriate to ask the question directly, in a compassionate way and at the right time – is the patient is considering taking their life? Appropriate questioning can open a window – possibly for the first time – on that journey and allow the individual to express their fears and accept support. It is therefore vital that ambulance clinicians can communicate effectively and identify key risks with a patient who is feeling suicidal.

- The key to assessing risk within any situation is to ask questions. These should be clear, unambiguous, and single. Do not use euphemisms. Adopting a sensitive but direct approach is usually best. For example:
  - Is life worth living?
  - Are you thinking about killing yourself? **OR**
  - Are you thinking about suicide? (Asking this question will **NOT** make somebody more likely to kill themselves.)
- If the patient denies any suicidal ideation (and this is consistent with the patient's presentation), the clinical assessment can continue without further risk assessment; but always advise the patient to seek further medical attention should this change.

Some strategies to help care for a suicidal patient are:

- Ask directly about suicide e.g., are you thinking about suicide – don't use euphemisms like 'harm yourself, or 'do something stupid'
- Your primary role at this stage is to listen intently – not to direct or to make plans for the person
- Ask the person to tell you their story. Listen carefully and without distraction – they will often talk about positives in their life as well as the crisis they are in today
- When someone mentions positive things e.g., relationships, pets, plans for tomorrow, reflect these things back, amplify these things and highlight that there are things or moments when they have been happy
- Ask the person if they would be prepared to think about how they could keep themselves safe for now – and what it would take to help them to keep safe
- Try to focus on the here and now
- Think about resources around the person – neighbours, friends, family, connections and supports that can help to keep the person safe
- Write the safety plan down with the person and ask them to keep adding ideas on how they might keep themselves safe. Explore with the patient what has helped in similar circumstances previously.
- Make the environment safe – people will often tell you about the means of suicide they are contemplating, and may be willing for you to remove the means from their home e.g., medications
- Work with the person to identify what helps to soothe them e.g., music, baths, walks, talking to others
- Identify people who might be able to offer immediate support and who can help to implement the safety plan.

Myth Busting – Common untrue assumptions about suicide

- People who talk about suicide won't really do it.
- Anyone who tries to kill themselves must be mentally ill.
- If someone is determined to kill themselves, there is nothing you can do.
- People who kill themselves were unwilling to seek help.
- Talking about suicide may give someone the idea.

8. Dementia

A diagnosis of dementia is made when a patient has impairment in more than one cognitive domain. The cognitive domains are memory, attention, reasoning, visuospatial, language, personality, and behaviour. Dementias are gradually progressive and impact on the patient's ability to function at work or in their usual activities. There are a wide spectrum of changes, and degrees of impairment, in dementia. Some patients will currently have only mild changes, whereas others will have more severe impairments. Dementia is common, 7% of over 65 year olds have dementia. It is also a growing issue in the UK with numbers of patients expected to be more than 1 million by 2025. The rate of 'young onset dementia' in those under the age of 65 is also increasing.

There are many causes of dementia. The most common causes in all age groups are Alzheimer's disease and vascular dementia. Other types of dementia include Lewy body dementia, Fronto-temporal lobe dementia, Creutzfeldt–Jakob disease, alcohol related dementia, HIV-related cognitive impairment, Parkinson's disease dementia.

Mental Health Presentations

Korsakoff's Syndrome or alcohol-related brain injury – Although sharing many common symptoms with dementia and often used in the same context, Korsakoff's is not a type of dementia. Brain damage can be caused by consistent alcohol misuse resulting in many of the symptoms of dementia.

If diagnosed early and abstinence is achieved, progression can sometimes be halted.

There are currently no cures for dementia; however, there are several medications that are used to alleviate symptoms and prolong the quality of the patient's life.

TABLE 3.93 – Common Medications for Dementia

• Treatment of mild-moderate cognitive symptoms	• Acetylcholinesterase inhibitors (or cholinesterase inhibitors) act to slow or reduce the progression of symptoms e.g. Donepezil hydrochloride, rivastigmine and galantamine.
• Treatment of moderate to severe cognitive symptoms	• NMDA receptor antagonists (N-methyl-D-aspartate receptor antagonist) e.g. Memantine hydrochloride.
• Treatment of behavioural symptoms in dementia (e.g., aggression, hallucinations, depression, agitation)	• Antipsychotic medications and benzodiazepines (used with caution due to side effects) e.g., Antidepressants, hypnotics.

Dementia and Mental Capacity

Patients with dementia generally experience a decline in their abilities over time. Therefore, the need to take into consideration a patient's capacity should not be underestimated (refer to **Mental Capacity Act 2005**).

A diagnosis of dementia does not mean that the patient lacks capacity, and all measures must be taken to ensure correct assessment and treatment. Check for the presence of an advance directive or living will, lasting power of attorney (for health and welfare), deputyship end of life plan, ReSPECT plan or check if the patient is currently subject to a section of the Mental Health Act or a deprivation of liberty order.

Any visit to hospital can be distressing and unpleasant, but in the case of a person with dementia, it can be significantly more distressing. Consider whether the patient needs to be conveyed to hospital and, if so, what specific issues and concerns they may have. Refer to local pathways, GPs, primary care and community care services when possible, to avoid hospital attendances.

When thinking about admission to hospital for a person living with severe dementia, carry out an assessment that balances their current medical needs with the additional harms they may face in hospital, for example:

- Disorientation
- A longer length of stay
- Increased mortality
- Increased morbidity on discharge
- Delirium
- The effects of being in an impersonal or institutional environment.

When thinking about admission to hospital for a person living with dementia, consider:

- Any RESPeCT, advance care and support plans
- The value of keeping them in a familiar environment.

Communication

Dementia causes damage to the areas of the brain that affect an individual's ability to communicate, retain information, make decisions or problem solve, eventually even on a very basic level. This can, and often does, lead to anxiety, frustration, and fear. Communicating effectively with someone who has dementia is a skill that, if used properly, can make a considerable difference to experience and outcome for patients.

Each patient with dementia must be treated as an individual with their own specific set of needs. Ensure patients are included, informed and consent is gained whenever possible to reduce their anxiety and fears.

Care home staff, family, carers, and friends should be asked to help provide a detailed history and can determine the changes in a patient from their normal state. Those who know the patient best should be asked to help you with assessing, moving, and handling, treating and helping a patient to understand what is happening.

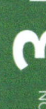

Mental Health Presentations

TABLE 3.94 – Tips for communicating with patients with Dementia

Do ...	Don't ...
• Consider the potential barriers to effective communication. Ensure only one person is talking/asking questions at a time. • Consider carefully what language and questions can be used to minimise confusion and worry. • Ask simple questions one at a time and wait for an answer. • Reduce distractions such as noise and activity. • Use non-verbal communication such as tone of voice, posture and body position making sure you appear approachable and non-threatening. • Using the person's name, make eye contact and appropriate touch. • Encourage the person to focus upon and communicate with you. Use environmental clues to build a rapport. • Take your time, try not to rush conversation. • Create a friendly and respectful rapport and environment. • Explore how the patient is feeling and avoid simply asking direct questions to test the patients recall. • Demonstrate empathy and empower the patient wherever possible to complete things that they are capable of.	• Do not finish their sentence or presume you know the answer. • Don't become frustrated.

9. Pregnancy and Mental Health

During pregnancy the mind changes as well as the body. It is important to consider that during and after pregnancy mothers may be particularly at risk of mental ill health. This includes mothers with pre-existing mental health problems, or those whose mental health illness is related to their pregnancy. Post-natal depression affects 10–15% of women who have recently given birth.

The MBRRACE-UK report in 2022[12] noted that "Deaths from mental health-related causes as a whole (suicide and substance abuse) account for nearly 40% of deaths occurring within a year after the end of pregnancy with maternal suicide remaining the leading cause of direct deaths in this period."

Women who present with any of the 'Red Flag' presentations described in Table 3.95 **MUST** be referred urgently to a specialist perinatal mental health team via mental health single points of access, 24/7 Urgent Mental Health Lines or in accordance with local protocol.

TABLE 3.95 – Pregnancy and Maternal Mental Health: Red Flag Signs and Risk Factors

Red Flags
- Recent significant change in mental state or emergence of new symptoms
- New thoughts or acts of violent harm to self or the infant
- New and persistent expressions of incompetency as a mother or estrangement from the infant.

Risk Factors
- Women with history of bipolar disorder, schizophrenia, severe depression, other psychotic disorder or previous inpatient/crisis care
- Women with a close family history of bipolar or psychosis
- Women presenting with uncharacteristic symptoms or behaviour and marked changes to normal functioning
- Partner, family or friends reporting significant change in presentation and acting out of character
- Older professional women with depression who appear to be functioning at a high level

Women presenting with anxiety or panic attacks or unusual/overvalued ideations which may appear out of context or extreme.

Mental Health Presentations

Refer to local pathways and consider the need for conveyance to ED or an alternative care facility. Consider safeguarding issues and referral (Refer to **Safeguarding Adults at Risk**).

Men can also experience major depressive episodes, with approximately 8–10% of fathers experiencing postpartum depression following the birth of a child. Many of the same red flag signs and risk factors will apply. Those predisposed to mental health conditions, regardless of gender, will be at a higher risk of developing symptoms and this may also be increased by marital discord, disrupted sleep, where the pregnancy was unintended and social deprivation.

10. Eating Disorders

There are several types of eating disorder, which can occur regardless of gender. The highest risk for development of eating disorders is between ages 13 and 17, however they can emerge at any age. Eating disorders are a particularly high risk form of mental illness, with Anorexia Nervosa being demonstrated to have the highest mortality rate of any psychiatric disorder.[22]

NICE Guidelines outline factors which should be taken into account when assessing a person with a potential eating disorder. These include:

- An unusually low or high body mass index (BMI) or body weight for their age
- Rapid weight loss
- Dieting or restrictive eating practices (e.g., dieting when they are underweight) that are worrying them, their family members or carers, or professionals
- Family members or carers report a change in eating behaviour
- Social withdrawal, particularly from situations that involve food
- Other mental health problems
- A disproportionate concern about their weight or shape (e.g., concerns about weight gain as a side effect of contraceptive medication)
- Problems managing a chronic illness that affects diet, such as diabetes or coeliac disease
- Menstrual or other endocrine disturbances, or unexplained gastrointestinal symptoms
- Physical signs of:
  - Malnutrition, including poor circulation, dizziness, palpitations, fainting or pallor
  - Compensatory behaviours, including laxative or diet pill misuse, vomiting or excessive exercise.
- Abdominal pain that is associated with vomiting or restrictions in diet, and that cannot be fully explained by a medical condition
- Unexplained electrolyte imbalance or hypoglycaemia
- Atypical dental wear (such as erosion)
- Whether they take part in activities associated with a high risk of eating disorders (for example, professional sport, fashion, dance, or modelling).

It is important to remember that patients with eating disorder may also present with a wide array of comorbid psychiatric illnesses, substance use disorders and physical illnesses including type 1 diabetes mellitus and other illnesses where symptoms or treatments may impact on body weight such as cystic fibrosis, thyroid abnormalities and inflammatory bowel disease.[22]

In the context of emergency presentations, it is important to always ensure a complete physical health assessment is undertaken. This should include a 12 lead ECG. Consideration should be given to nutritional, hydration and possible electrolyte imbalances.

Neither scoring tools, nor Body Mass Index should be used in isolation to determine whether a patient requires a referral in relation to an eating disorder. Wherever possible, given that eating disorders may be rooted in concerns over physical appearance, it may be beneficial to avoid a conversational focus during assessment upon physical appearance, but instead focusing on the factors outlined above. Those presenting with symptoms of an eating disorder should be referred to local mental health services in line with local policies/protocols. Where this is not possible locally, consideration should be given to engaging primary care or other professionals to support access to professional eating disorder support.

Clinicians should be aware of refeeding syndrome and the risks associated with advice to increase oral intake in this group of patients. Refeeding should be a closely monitored process led by specialists in eating disorders and advice to alter nutritional intake should be avoided by ambulance clinicians Symptoms of refeeding syndrome may include:

- Fatigue
- Weakness
- Confusion
- Difficulty breathing
- Abdominal pain
- Hypertension
- Seizures
- Arrhythmia
- Heart failure
- Liver failure.

Where clinicians identify a patient may be experiencing refeeding syndrome in the community, the patient should be conveyed for further assessment and management.

Mental Health Presentations

Mental Health Presentations Algorithm

EQUALITY IN MENTAL HEALTH

Ensure equality in the approach to all care needs. Particularly those in higher risk groups: Children and young people; older adults; LGBTQ+; ethnic minority groups.

No two patients will have the same needs, nor respond equally to treatments and interventions.

ASSESSMENT

Patient History
- History of Presenting Complaint
- Past Medical History
- Medications
- Social History
- Family History
- Drug/Alcohol Use

MSE (See Table 2)
- Appearance
- Behaviour
- Speech
- Mood
- Thought process
- Perception
- Cognition
- Insight
- Judgement

Risk (See Tables 3 & 4)
- Risk to self
- Risk to others
- Risks from others
- Vulnerability/safeguarding

Mental Capacity
- Refer to Mental Capacity Act 2005

Physical Assessment (See Table 7)
- Consider mental and physical health together. Many medical conditions may present with symptoms consistent with mental ill health and patients with a diagnosed mental health condition may have concurrent physical health needs.
- Undertake appropriate physical examination and observations to exclude acute medical or traumatic conditions.
- Red flag cases will always require assessment in a physical healthcare setting.

MANAGEMENT

Therapeutic
- Establish rapport
- Manage distress
- Provide reassurance

De-escalation
- Remove the stimulus
- Reassure patient
- Give patient space and time
- Distraction
- Breathing and mindfulness techniques

Shared decision making
- Work with patient, families, carers and other professionals
- Agree a plan of action
- Consent and collaboration

Safety Planning (See Table 6)
- Empower patient to use resources and support available to them
- Emergency action plan

Communication (See Table 5)
- Maintain concentration and avoid distractions
- Demonstrate you are listening and interested (body language, gestures)
- Don't interrupt. Wait before asking questions.
- Summarise what the patient has told you
- Remain calm and confident and non-judgemental
- Apologise if you make a mistake in how you communicated
- Demonstrate empathy

CONVEYANCE
- Where possible, consider alternative pathways for patient's best interests.

CONVEYANCE UNDER THE MENTAL HEALTH ACT
- Ensure staff have been delegated necessary authority to detain patient under section 6 of the Mental Health Act.
- Ensure all necessary paperwork has been completed to accompany patient, or has been sent ahead electronically to the receiving hospital.

Other considerations

SELF-HARM: More commonly a coping mechanism for life. Assess the physical injuries, and talk to the patient about it to acknowledge what has happened. It helps reduce feelings of shame and stigma. (See Table 8)

SUICIDE: Ask directly about suicide. Be compassionate and consider timing when asking questions. Listen. Reinforce positive things the patient mentions, e.g family, pets. Consider available resources; safety plans; environment.

DEMENTIA: Consider the patient's capacity. Conveyance may cause more distress. Refer to local pathways and consider alternatives where possible to avoid hospital attendance. Include patient during communication to reduce anxiety. (see Table 10)

PREGNANCY: Pregnant mothers presenting with Red Flags must be referred urgently to a specialist perinatal mental health team via local pathways. (See Table 11)

EATING ORDERS: Ensure a complete physical health assessment is undertaken, including a 12 lead ECG.

Figure 3.37 – Mental Health Presentations Algorithm

Mental Health Presentations

> **KEY POINTS!**
>
> **Mental Health Presentations**
> - Patients present frequently to ambulance services with mental health needs.
> - Clinicians should ensure a thorough and holistic assessment of need, including both physical and mental health needs, to inform clinical decision making, management and the utilisation of appropriate care pathways.
> - The management of patients experiencing mental health needs can be significantly improved through the use of appropriate communication approaches, de-escalation methods and offering an empathetic, non-judgemental approach.
> - The assessment of risk relating to mental health presentations, decision making relating to care pathways and safety planning should be undertaken collaboratively with the patient.
> - Clinicians should work to identify appropriate alternative care pathways where there is no clear necessity for conveyance to emergency departments.

12. Terminology

Caution should always be exercised in the use of acronyms in documentation, considering that some acronyms may have multiple meaning in different contexts. TCA for example may mean both Tricyclic antidepressants and traumatic cardiac arrest. The below acronyms are included purely for information and to support understanding.

Term	Explanation
AC	Approved Clinician
AMHP	Approved Mental Health Professional
AOT	Assertive Outreach Team
CAMHS	Child and Adolescent Mental Health Services
CBT	Cognitive Behavioural Therapy
CMHT	Community Mental Health Team
CPA	Care Programme Approach
CPN	Community Psychiatric Nurse
CRHT	Crisis Resolution Home Treatment
CTO	Community Treatment Order
CYP	Children and Younger People
DBT	Dialectical Behavioural Therapy
ECT	Electroconvulsive Therapy
GAU	General Admissions Unit
HTT	Home Treatment Team
IAPT	Improving Access to Psychological Therapies
LD	Learning Disability
LSU	Low Secure Unit
MCA	Mental Capacity Act (2005)
MHA	Mental Health Act 1983 (as amended by the Mental Health Act 2007)
MOAI	Monoamine Oxidase Inhibitors
MSE	Mental State Examination
MSU	Medium Secure Unit
PICU	Psychiatric Intensive Care Unit
RC	Responsible Clinician
RMN	Registered Mental Health Nurse

(continued)

Mental Health Presentations

Term	Explanation
SNRI	Serotonin Noradrenaline Reuptake Inhibitor
SOAD	Second Opinion Appointed Doctor
SSRI	Selective Serotonin Reuptake Inhibitor
TCA	Tri-cyclic Antidepressant

Bibliography

1. Bickley, L., Szilagyi, P. and Hoffman, R., 2017. Bates' guide to physical examination and history taking. 12th ed. Philadelphia: Wolters Kluwer.

2. McManus S, Meltzer H, Brugha TS, Bebbington PE, Jenkins R. Adult Psychiatric Morbidity in England, 2007: Results of a household survey. London: The NHS Information Centre for Health and Social Care, 2009.

3. McManus S, Bebbington P, Jenkins R, Brugha T (eds). Mental Health and Wellbeing in England: Adult psychiatric morbidity survey 2014. Leeds: NHS Digital, 2016.

4. Ministry of Justice. The Mental Capacity Act 2005 Code of Practice 2007. London: The Stationery Office, 2005. Available from: https://www.gov.uk/government/publications/mental-capacity-act-code-of-practice

5. Mental Health First Aid. Self-injury First Aid Guideline. Melbourne: MHFA, 2014.

6. Mental Health First Aid. Suicide First Aid Guideline. Melbourne: MHFA, 2014.

7. Alzheimers Research UK. Dementia Symptoms. Cambridge: Alzheimers Research UK, 2018. Available from: https://www.alzheimersresearchuk.org/about-dementia/types-of-dementia/frontotemporal-dementia/symptoms.

8. National Institute for Health and Care Excellence. Dementia: assessment, management and support for people living with dementia and their carers [NG97]. London: NICE, 2018.

9. Alzheimers Research UK. Frontotemporal Dementia. Cambridge: Alzheimer's Research UK, 2018. Available from: https://www.alzheimersresearchuk.org/about-dementia/types-of-dementia/frontotemporal-dementia/symptoms/.

10. Mental Health Foundation (2021) https://www.mentalhealth.org.uk/explore-mental-health/a-z-topics/black-asian-and-minority-ethnic-bame-communities.

11. Mothers and Babies: Reducing Risk through Audits and Confidential Enquiries across the UK (2015) Saving Lives, Improving Mothers' Care. https://maternalmentalhealthalliance.org/wp-content/uploads/MBRRACE-UK-Maternal-Report-2015-3.pdf.

12. Mothers and Babies: Reducing Risk through Audits and Confidential Enquiries across the UK (2022) Lessons learned to inform maternity care from the UK and Ireland Confidential Enquiries into Maternal Deaths and Morbidity 2018–20. https://www.npeu.ox.ac.uk/assets/downloads/mbrrace-uk/reports/maternal-report-2022/MBRRACE-UK_Maternal_MAIN_Report_2022_v10.pdf.

13. National Institute for Clinical Excellence (2017) Eating disorders: recognition and treatment. https://www.nice.org.uk/guidance/ng69.

14. National institute for Clinical Excellence (2022) Self-harm: assessment, management and preventing recurrence. https://www.nice.org.uk/guidance/NG225.

15. National Records of Scotland (2021) Probable Suicides 2021. https://www.nrscotland.gov.uk/files/statistics/probable-suicides/2021/suicides-21-report.pdf.

16. NHS Digital (2022) Detentions under the Mental Health Act. https://www.ethnicity-facts-figures.service.gov.uk/health/mental-health/detentions-under-the-mental-health-act/latest.

17. Office of the Chief Social Worker for Adults (2019) National Workforce Plan for Approved Mental Health Professionals (AMHPs). https://assets.publishing.service.gov.uk/government/uploads/system/uploads/attachment_data/file/843539/AMHP_Workforce_Plan_Oct19___3_.pdf

18. Parliament of the United Kingdom. The Mental Health Act 1983 (amended 2007). London: The Stationery Office, 2007.

19. Royal College of Emergency Medicine (2021) Management of Controlled Energy Device (Taser) Attendances. https://rcem.ac.uk/wp-content/uploads/2021/11/Management_of_Controlled_Energy_Device_Attendances_Taser_2021.pdf.

20. Royal College of Psychiatrists (2016). Assessing and Managing Risk of Patients causing harm. https://www.rcpsych.ac.uk/members/supporting-your-professional-development/assessing-and-managing-risk-of-patients-causing-harm.

21. Scarff J. R. (2019). Postpartum Depression in Men. Innovations in clinical neuroscience, 16(5–6), 11–14. https://www.ncbi.nlm.nih.gov/pmc/articles/PMC6659987/.

22. Scottish Intercollegiate Guidelines Network (2022) SIGN 164: Eating Disorders. https://www.sign.ac.uk/media/1987/sign-164-eating-disorders-v2.pdf.

23. Scowcroft E. Samaritans Suicide Statistics Report 2017. Surrey: Samaritans, 2017.

24. World Health Organization. Promoting Mental Health: Concepts, emerging evidence, practice (Summary Report). Geneva: WHO, 2004.

25. Rolfe, U., and Partlow, D. (2022). Mental health care in paramedic practice. Class Publishing.

26. Increasing access to treatment for women with common maternal mental health problems – A sound investment: Maternal Mental Health Alliance. (2022). LSE Care policy and evaluation centre.

Non-Traumatic Chest Pain/Discomfort

1. Introduction

- Chest pain is one of the most common symptoms of acute coronary syndrome (ACS).
- It is also a common feature in many other conditions such as aortic dissection, chest infection with pleuritic pain, pulmonary embolus, reflux oesophagitis, indigestion and simple musculoskeletal chest pain.
- There must be a high index of suspicion that any chest pain is cardiac in origin.
- There are a number of specific factors that may help in reaching a reasoned working diagnosis, and applying appropriate management measures to the patient. ACS cannot be excluded on clinical examination alone (refer to **Acute Coronary Syndrome**).
- Do not assess symptoms differently in women and men or patients from different ethnic groups.

2. Assessment and Management

Assessing the type of pain is particularly important in the management of non-traumatic chest pain. For the types of pain typical for each cause, refer to Table 3.96.

TABLE 3.96 – Descriptions of Non-traumatic Chest Pain

Features which suggest a diagnosis of myocardial ischaemia include:
- Central chest pain.
- Crushing or constricting in nature.
- Persists for >15 minutes.
- Pain may also present in:
    - the shoulders
    - upper abdomen
    - referred to the neck, jaws and arms.

Features which suggest a diagnosis of stable angina include:
- Pain is typically related to exertion and tends to last minutes but should it persist for >15 minutes, or despite usual treatment, ACS is more likely.

Features of pleuritic-type pain:
- Stabbing.
- Generally one-sided.
- Worse on breathing in.
- Usually have cough with sputum.
- Raised temperature (>37.5°C) indicative of infection.

Features of indigestion-type pain:
- Central.
- Related to food.
- May be associated with belching and burning.

NB Some patients with ACS may also suffer indigestion-type pain and belching.

Features of muscular-type pain:
- Sharp/stabbing.
- Worse on movement.
- Often associated with tenderness on palpation.

Features of aneurysm-type pain:
- Sudden, severe pain.
- Pulsing sensation in the abdomen (like a heartbeat).
- Sudden, intense and persistent abdominal or back pain, which can be described as a tearing sensation.
- Pain that radiates to the back or legs.

Non-Traumatic Chest Pain/Discomfort

For the assessment and management of non-traumatic chest pain/discomfort, refer to Table 3.97.

TABLE 3.97 – ASSESSMENT and MANAGEMENT of: Non-Traumatic Chest Pain/Discomfort

NB A defibrillator must always be taken at the earliest opportunity to patients with symptoms suggestive of a myocardial infarction. Remain with the patient until handover to hospital staff.

Assess <C>ABCDE

- If any of the following **TIME-CRITICAL** features are present:
  - Major <C>ABCDE problems (refer to **Medical Emergencies in Adults – Overview** and **Medical Emergencies in Children – Overview**).
  - Suspected ACS, especially ST-segment-elevation myocardial infarction (STEMI) (refer to **Acute Coronary Syndrome**).
  - Aortic dissection.
- Start correcting any **<C>ABCDE** problems.
- Undertake a **TIME-CRITICAL** transfer to the nearest appropriate receiving hospital.
- Continue management en route.
- Provide an ATMIST information call.

ECG

- If required, monitor and record 12-lead ECG. Assess for abnormality (refer to **Cardiac Arrhythmia and Sudden Cardiac Death**).

NB For non-traumatic chest pain, an ECG should be taken as soon as practically possible to diagnose a STEMI requiring immediate conveyance to a centre able to provide Primary Percutaneous Coronary Intervention.

NB DO NOT exclude an ACS when patients have a normal resting 12-lead ECG – a normal ECG cannot reliably exclude ACS.

Assess for Specific Accompanying Features

- Nausea/vomiting.
- Sweating.
- Pallor.
- Cough.
- Breathlessness – **NB** If breathlessness is a predominant symptom/sign with tightness in the chest, then causes of breathlessness must also be considered (refer to **Dyspnoea**).

Undertake a Clinical Assessment Specifically for:

- Heart failure.
- Cardiogenic shock.
- Ask the patient if they have a previous history of coronary heart disease.

Other Conditions

- If clinical examination and a 12-lead ECG make a diagnosis of ACS less likely, assess for other acute conditions such as:
  - pulmonary embolism (refer to **Pulmonary Embolism**).
  - aortic dissection
  - pneumonia (refer to **Medical Emergencies in Adults – Overview** and **Medical Emergencies in Children – Overview**).

Respiratory Rate

- Measure and record respiratory rate.

Oxygen Saturation

- Monitor the patient's SpO_2; administer oxygen to achieve saturations of >94% if the patient presents as hypoxemic on air (refer to **Oxygen**).

Non-Traumatic Chest Pain/Discomfort

TABLE 3.97 – ASSESSMENT and MANAGEMENT of: Non-Traumatic Chest Pain/Discomfort *(continued)*

Blood Pressure and Fluids
- Measure and record blood pressure; if required, administer fluids (refer to **Intravascular Fluid Therapy in Adults** and **Intravascular Fluid Therapy in Children**).

Blood Glucose
- If appropriate, measure and record blood glucose for hypo/hyperglycaemia (refer to **Glycaemic Emergencies in Adults and Children**).

Temperature
- Measure and record temperature.

NEWS2
- These observations will enable you to calculate a NEWS2 Score (refer to **Sepsis**).

Assess Patient's Pain
- For the features of specific types of pain, refer to Table 3.96.
- Where present, assess the **SOCRATES** of pain and record initial and subsequent pain scores.
- Consider analgesia if appropriate (refer to **Pain Management in Adults and Children**).

Documentation
- Complete documentation to include all clinical findings, advice from other clinicians, onward referral and worsening advice given.

KEY POINTS!

Non-traumatic Chest Pain/Discomfort
- Most chest pain is not ACS – but this possibility needs to be excluded rapidly.
- Is there another life-threatening cause (e.g. aortic dissection)?
- Have a low threshold for recording a 12-lead ECG.
- A normal ECG cannot reliably exclude ACS.

Bibliography

1. National Institute for Health and Clinical Excellence. *Chest Pain of Recent Onset: Assessment and diagnosis of recent onset chest pain or discomfort of suspected cardiac origin* (CG95). London: NICE, 2010. Available from: https://www.nice.org.uk/guidance/cg95.
2. Porter A, Snooks H, Youren A, Gaze S, Whitfield R, Rapport F et al. 'Covering our backs': ambulance crews' attitudes towards clinical documentation when emergency (999) patients are not conveyed to hospital. *Emergency Medicine Journal* 2008, 25(5): 292–295.
3. NHS. *Abdominal aortic aneurysm*. London: NHS, 2017. Available from: https://www.nhs.uk/conditions/abdominal-aortic-aneurysm.

Overdose and Poisoning in Adults and Children

1. Introduction

Overdose and poisoning is a common cause of calls to the ambulance service. When dealing with overdose and poisoning, advice is available from the National Poisons Information Service (NPIS) database TOXBASE®. Consult your local procedures on how to use TOXBASE. The TOXBASE® app can be downloaded to Android/iOS systems and contains the same information as the website – this app can be used offline/in poor areas of mobile coverage. A 24-hour, seven-day telephone advice line is also available from NPIS: 0344 892 0111. Toxbase can also help if you have a patient you believe has been poisoned but are uncertain of the cause.

1.1 Overdose and Poisoning

- Exposure may occur by ingestion, inhalation, topical absorption or injection and may result in mortality or morbidity.
- Exposure in children generally occurs as a result of ingestion but can arise from eye and skin contact; exposure can arise via multiple routes.
- Overdose can result from both accidental and deliberate overdose.

Drugs/Medications

- Prescribed medication, over-the-counter medication, traditional medicines and health supplements can all cause poisoning. In particular, beta blockers such as propranolol, tricyclic antidepressants such as amitriptyline and calcium channel blockers can be substantially toxic.
- Some medicines have a narrow therapeutic range e.g. Lithium.
- Recreational drugs include depressants, stimulants, and hallucinogens.

Chemicals

- Consumer products for example, washing powders, washing-up liquids, fabric cleaning liquid/tablets, bleaches, hand gels, screen-washes, anti-freeze, de-icers, silica gel, batteries, petroleum distillates, white spirit (e.g. paints and varnishes), descalers and glues.
- Domestic, agricultural and industrial chemicals and substances. For example, cyanide, sodium nitrite, Orthochlorobenzalmalononitrile (CS gas) and gases such as carbon monoxide. Consider CBRN!

Natural substances

- Naturally occurring toxins such as plants and venomous creatures.

Foreign bodies

- Button batteries and magnets.

NB These are presented as examples only and should not be accepted as an exhaustive list. Refer to TOXBASE®.

Exposure may be:

Accidental (unintentional):

- This typically occurs in young children aged under 5 years. For children, ingestion of tablets and household products are most common, although almost anything, however unpalatable, may be ingested. Fortunately, most ingestions and exposures in young children result in no or very mild symptoms. Many common ingestions involve low toxicity substances, but there is the potential for significant toxicity with some substances. Exploratory ingestion may raise the possibility of safeguarding concerns, because of either inadequate supervision or the nature of the ingested substance, even in the absence of a toxic effect on the child. If suspected, this must be reported (refer to **Safeguarding Children** and **Safeguarding Adults at Risk**).
- Older adults, patients with cognitive impairment, learning difficulties and mental health conditions may be at risk of unintentional therapeutic excess. Attention to the risk of accidental overdose or poisoning when assessing these patients should be considered. Dispensing dates on pharmacy labels can be a good indication of the number of tablets a patient may have taken.
- Accidental exposure may also be a consequence of an industrial accident or exposure to fire.

Intentional:

- Attempted poisoning to oneself is an act of deliberate self-harm. Intentional poisoning may also result from intentional risk-taking behaviour such as excess alcohol ingestion or use of recreational drugs or inhalants.

Non-accidental (or deliberate) by a third party:

- This type of poisoning is less likely to be detected by the ambulance service, but if it is suspected it must be reported to the police and a safeguarding referral should be made (refer to **Safeguarding Adults at Risk** and **Safeguarding Children**).

2. Incidence

- It is difficult to estimate the exact number of overdose and poisoning incidents that occur, as not all cases are reported. In 2022/2023, there were 38,709 telephone calls to the National Poisons Information Service, 721,092 accesses to the TOXBASE® website and 9,145 accesses to the TOXBASE® app. 25% of calls to NPIS were in relation to children under the age of nine. Most of these incidents were accidental and occurred in the home.

Overdose and Poisoning in Adults and Children

3. Severity and Outcome

- There are a number of factors that affect severity and outcome following exposure: in particular, age and weight of the patient, toxicity of the agent, quantity taken, route of exposure, co-ingestion of multiple substances, delay in seeking medical help and underlying co-morbidities or physical injury.

- Death from poisoning is often due to airway obstruction and respiratory arrest, secondary to a decreased level of consciousness or severe cardiovascular toxicity with significant hypotension or cardiac arrest.

- Overdoses including slow, or modified-release medicines are likely to have a delayed onset of clinical effects.

4. Pathophysiology

- The pattern of clinical features following exposure will depend primarily on the individual substance.

- For details of the effects of specific substances, refer to TOXBASE®, contact the National Poisons Information Service or follow locally agreed procedures.

5. Assessment and Management

For the assessment and management of overdose and poisoning, refer to Tables 3.98 and 3.99.

TABLE 3.98 – ASSESSMENT of: Overdose and Poisoning in Adults and Children

Safety First – DO NOT put yourself in danger – carry out a dynamic risk assessment and undertake measures to preserve your own safety.

Consider if PPE is required to access, treat or transport the patient. Request specialist support early.

Avoid mouth-to-mouth ventilation.

Assess <C>ABCDE

- Many poisoned patients can be effectively managed by addressing the following **TIME-CRITICAL** features:
  - major **<C>ABCDE** problems (refer to **Medical Emergencies in Adults – Overview** or **Medical Emergencies in Children – Overview**)
  - cardiac and respiratory arrest (refer to the Resuscitation guidelines)
  - decreased level of consciousness – **NB** Most poisons that impair consciousness also depress respiration (refer to **Altered Level of Consciousness**)
  - respiratory depression (refer to **Airway and Breathing Management**)
  - arrhythmias and brady/tachycardia (refer to **Cardiac Arrhythmia and Sudden Cardiac Death**)
  - hypotension (systolic BP less than <9 0 mmHg) (refer to **Intravascular Fluid Therapy in Adults** and **Intravascular Fluid Therapy in Children**)
  - convulsions (refer to **Seizures in Adults** and **Seizures in Children**)
  - hypothermia (refer to **Hypothermia**)
  - hyperthermia (refer to **Heat Related Illness**)

- Start correcting any **<C>ABCDE** problems.
- Consider the need for specialist/enhanced critical care teams.
- Agitation can be challenging and difficult to manage and there are a number of options, including safe holding techniques or the use of appropriate medications. Refer to **Acute Behavioural Disturbance**, **Agitated Patients** and **Delirium**.
- Undertake a **TIME-CRITICAL** transfer to nearest appropriate receiving hospital.
- Continue patient management en route.
- Provide an ATMIST information call.

Oxygen

- Apply pulse oximeter.
- If indicated, administer oxygen, particularly in patients with evidence of impaired respiratory effort/rate, hypoxia, carbon monoxide poisoning or following inhalation of irritant gases (refer to **Oxygen**).
- Patients with paraquat poisoning may be harmed by supplemental oxygen, so avoid oxygen unless the patient is hypoxaemic. Target saturation 85–88%.

(continued)

Overdose and Poisoning in Adults and Children

TABLE 3.98 – ASSESSMENT of: Overdose and Poisoning in Adults and Children *(continued)*

Safety First – DO NOT put yourself in danger – carry out a dynamic risk assessment and undertake measures to preserve your own safety.

Consider if PPE is required to access, treat or transport the patient. Request specialist support early.

Avoid mouth-to-mouth ventilation.

Respirations
- Document and monitor respiratory rate.
  - Consider assisted ventilation if necessary.

Blood Pressure
- Hypotension is common in severe cases of poisoning.
- Monitor blood pressure.
- In cases of drug-induced symptomatic hypotension or asymptomatic hypotension refer to **Intravascular Fluid Therapy in Adults** and **Intravascular Fluid Therapy in Children**.

ECG
- Undertake continuous cardiac monitoring in patients with exposure to any drug that may be associated with cardiotoxicity and in patients with altered level of consciousness. Refer to **Altered Level of Consciousness**.
- A 12-lead ECG may be of diagnostic value and/or a rhythm strip should also be reviewed and handed over to the ED staff. However, do not delay on scene if the condition of the patient is time critical.

Blood Glucose Concentration
- Measure blood glucose concentration – especially in cases of alcohol intoxication, which is a common cause of hypoglycaemia or in any patient with an altered level of consciousness.
- Correct hypoglycaemia (refer to **Glycaemic Emergencies in Adults and Children**, **Glucagon** and **Glucose 10%**).
- Glucagon is not suitable for the pre-hospital treatment of betablocker overdose.

Specific Considerations
- Ascertain what has been ingested/inhaled/absorbed/injected – ask relatives, friends, work colleagues etc.
- Estimate the quantity taken.
- Ascertain what, if any, treatment has been given.
- Document the time the incident occurred.
- If possible, take and hand over to staff at the hospital the ingested substance/container/packet (if safe and feasible to do so).
- Remember to take the patients normal medications (including inhalers) to hospital as well.

TABLE 3.99 – MANAGEMENT of: Overdose and Poisoning in Adults and Children

Activated Charcoal
- Consider activated charcoal (refer to **Activated Charcoal**) – TOXBASE® can advise on potentially toxic doses of a substance where activated charcoal may be appropriate.

Naloxone
- Opioids (such as morphine, heroin, methadone). can cause respiratory depression; in cases of respiratory depression consider naloxone (refer to **Naloxone Hydrochloride**) and/or ventilation monitor vital signs closely.
- **NB** Repeated doses of naloxone may be required. If repeat doses of naloxone are required consider ventilation and time-critical transfer to hospital.
- **NB End of Life Patients – Naloxone is only** indicated in circumstances where a clinician suspects opioid-induced toxicity, from intentional or unintentional overdose. The aim is to reverse life-threatening respiratory depression only i.e. if the respiratory rate is <8 breaths per minute and the patient is unconscious and or cyanosed. Refer to **End of Life Care**.

Overdose and Poisoning in Adults and Children

TABLE 3.99 – MANAGEMENT of: Overdose and Poisoning in Adults and Children *(continued)*

Chemical Exposure
- If a Chemical, Biological, Radiological or Nuclear (CBRN) incident is suspected, refer to **CBRN** for management.
- Consider requesting specialist support as per local procedures (e.g. HART, SORT, MERIT)

Thermoregulation
- Hypo- or hyperthermia can occur (refer to **Heat Related Illness** or **Hypothermia**).
- Consider the need for active cooling, particularly if the body temperature is >39° or if there are features of heat stroke.

Carbon Monoxide Exposure

Acute and chronic exposure to carbon monoxide can present with non-specific symptoms that make recognition of exposure outside of known exposure difficult. The types of symptoms that can be associated with carbon monoxide exposure include:

- Acute: headache, dizziness, nausea, vomiting, general lethargy, ataxia, chest pain, confusion, shortness of breath, drowsiness and coma
- Chronic: headache, dizziness, nausea, vomiting, general lethargy, flu-like symptoms, confusion, memory issues, visual issues, ataxia

The following questions may suggest exposure to chronic carbon monoxide:
- **C**ohabitants/companions: Does anyone else feel unwell? Are any pets behaving abnormally?
- **O**utdoors: Do you feel better if you go outside or when you are away from the property for a prolonged time?
- **M**aintenance: Are any heating appliances properly maintained?
- **A**larms: Do you have a working carbon monoxide alarm? Has it activated?

Action to be taken if carbon monoxide poisoning is suspected:
- Remove crew/patient/others from immediate exposure and into a safer environment for continued assessment and management.
- Apply high-flow oxygen, regardless of pulse oximeter reading.
- If safe to do so, ensure the area is ventilated.
- Call fire service and/or HART teams to measure levels of carbon monoxide at the location.
- Consider contacting/advising to contact gas services.

Mental Health Presentations
- In cases of self-harm, assess the patient's emotional and mental state – undertake a rapid mental health assessment. Where appropriate, conversations should occur alone initially, to maintain confidentiality and help build trust (refer to **Mental Health Presentations**).
- Do not delay treatment, but if possible, document the following information:
    - the patient's home environment
    - the patient's social and family support network
    - the patient's emotional state and level of distress
    - the events leading to the incident.

Transfer to Further Care
- In all cases where non-conveyance is being considered TOXBASE® should be consulted via the TOXBASE® website/app.
- If appropriate, consider signposting or referring the patient to substance misuse services as per local pathways.
- All cases of self-harm, even if the substance (or amount of substance) is not associated with significant toxicity and the patient does not require emergency treatment, should result in a psychological assessment (except where the patient does not consent and has capacity to decline this). Consider alternative pathways (e.g. specialist mental health service) as per local procedures. **NB This decision should take into account the patient's preferences, and the inclusion criteria of the service.**

(continued)

Overdose and Poisoning in Adults and Children

TABLE 3.99 – MANAGEMENT of: Overdose and Poisoning in Adults and Children *(continued)*

Following an unintentional or accidental exposure, **some patients may be considered safe to be non-conveyed if**:

- the reported ingestion has been reviewed on TOXBASE®/NPIS, the patient is well and there are no significant concerns; **AND**
- the history given by the patient is deemed to be credible **AND**
- the incident is/was accidental or unintentional; **AND**
- if applicable, there is a responsible adult present and there are no safeguarding concerns; **AND**
- the patient has been appropriately safety netted.
- in paediatric exposures, a safeguarding referral must be made. Refer to **Safeguarding Children**.

NB Seek senior/specialist advice should there be any doubt.

Refusal to treatment and transport including Duty of Care (Refer to Duty of Care)

- On occasions patients who have taken an overdose either accidentally or intentionally indicate that they do not wish to travel to hospital against the advice of attending staff.
- An assessment of capacity should be undertaken (Refer to **Mental Capacity Act 2005**).
- An assessment of their mental health state and suicide risk should also be made (refer to **Mental Health Presentations**).
- Where the patient has capacity to make this decision, the reason for refusal should be determined and information about the potential consequences of not receiving further care should be provided to the patient.
- Specific consideration should be given during an assessment of capacity as to whether the substance(s) involved may directly or indirectly impair the patient's functional ability to make a decision owing to their physiological or cognitive impacts, or whether any psychological distress or underlying mental health condition may be impairing the ability of the patient to weigh and use information in order to make decision.
- If after all the relevant information has been provided to the patient, enabling them to make an informed decision, and the patient is felt to have capacity but still refuses to attend hospital, senior clinical support must be sought as per local procedures.
- Attendance of the police and/or local mental health services may be required, especially if the safety of the patient or others are at risk.

KEY POINTS!

Overdose and Poisoning in Adults and Children

- **Establish the event: if there are drugs, chemicals or other substances involved, establish the quantity, route of exposure and if alcohol has been consumed.**
- **NEVER induce vomiting.**
- **Bring the substance or substances and any containers for inspection at hospital, if it is safe to do so.**
- **Anyone with deliberate overdose must be transferred to hospital. Seek senior clinical support if the patient refuses to attend hospital.**
- **After confirmed unintentional or accidental exposure to a low toxicity substance, if they are asymptomatic some patients may be considered for home management.**
- **Consider exposure to carbon monoxide.**
- **Agitation can be challenging and difficult to manage and there are a number of options, including safe holding techniques or the use of appropriate medications. Advanced/specialist paramedics may have received additional training in this area. Refer to local procedures.**

Overdose and Poisoning in Adults and Children

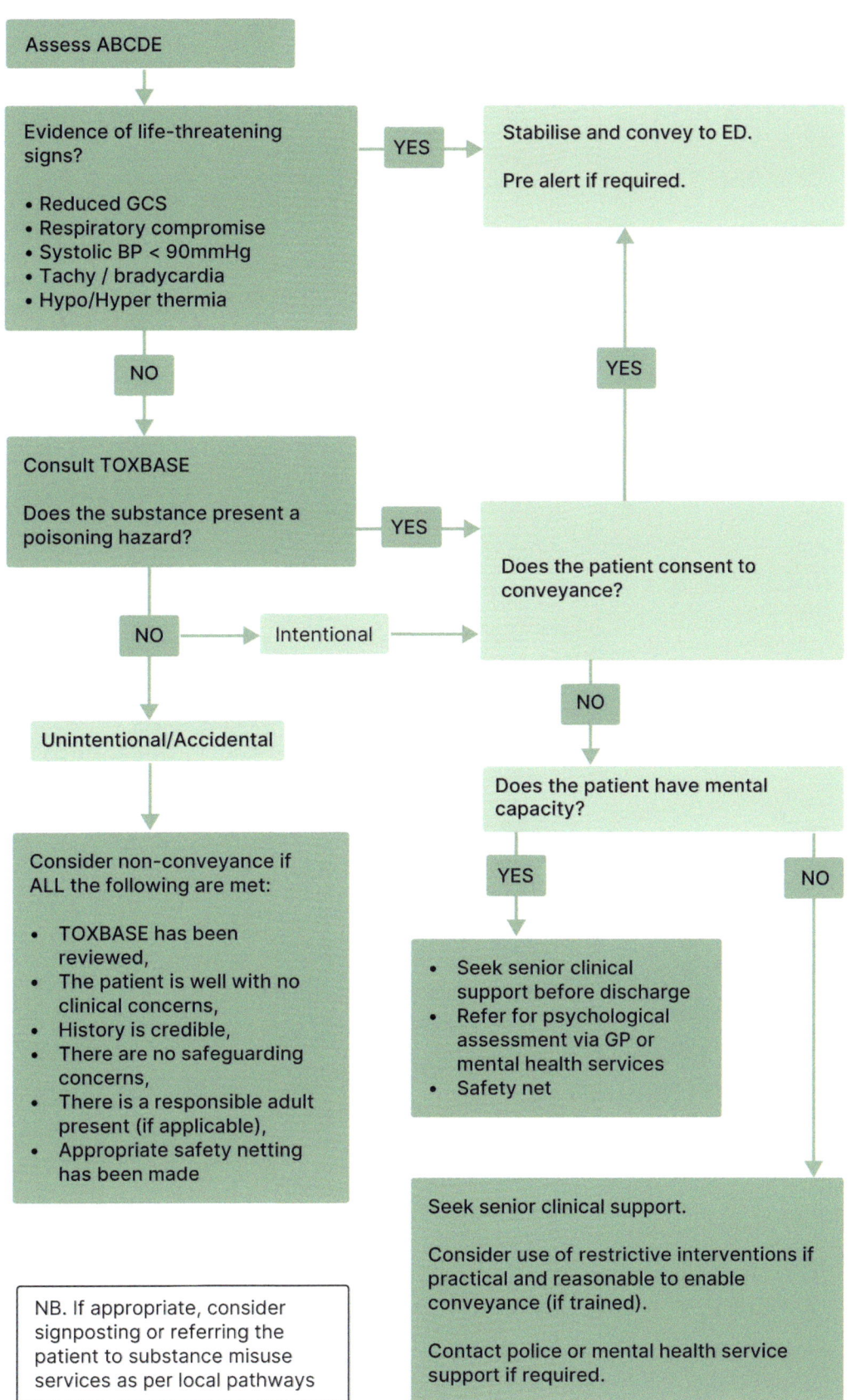

Figure 3.38 – Management of overdose and poisoning

Overdose and Poisoning in Adults and Children

Acknowledgements

We would like to gratefully acknowledge the Royal College of Emergency Medicine and National Poisons Information Service for their contributions, comments and input to this JRCALC guideline.

Bibliography

1. Soar J, Perkins GD, Abbas G, Alfonzo A, Barelli A, Bierens JJLM, et al. European Resuscitation Council Guidelines for Resuscitation 2010 Section 8: Cardiac arrest in special circumstances: electrolyte abnormalities, poisoning, drowning, accidental hypothermia, hyperthermia, asthma, anaphylaxis, cardiac surgery, trauma, pregnancy, electrocution. *Resuscitation* 2010, 81(10): 1400–1433.

2. National Institute for Health and Clinical Excellence. *Self-harm in over 8s: short-term management and prevention of recurrence* (NG225). London: NICE, 2022. Available from: https://www.nice.org.uk/guidance/ng225

3. Gunnell D, Bennewith O, Peters TJ, House A, Hawton K. The epidemiology and management of self-harm amongst adults in England. *Journal of Public Health* 2005, 27(1): 67–73. http://www.nice.org.uk/CG16

4. Gwini SM, Shaw D, Iqbal M, Spaight A, Siriwardena AN. Exploratory study of factors associated with adverse clinical features in patients presenting with non-fatal drug overdose/self-poisoning to the ambulance service. *Emergency Medicine Journal* 2011, 28(10): 892–894.

5. National Poisons Information Service. TOXBASE. Available from: L https://www.toxbase.org/login/?ReturnUrl=/

6. National Poisons Information Service. Available from: http://www.npis.org/index.html, 2020.

7. Coulson JM, Thompson JP. Investigation and management of the poisoned patient. *Clin Med* (Lond) 2008. 8(1): 89–91.

8. Afanag R, Jatana K. pH-neutralizing esophageal irrigations as a novel mitigation strategy for button battery injury. *The Larynscope* 2018. 129: 49–57. Available from: https://onlinelibrary.wiley.com/doi/abs/10.1002/lary.27312

9. UK Health Security Agency. National Poisons Information Service Annual Report 2022–2023. Crown, 2023.

Paediatric Gastroenteritis

1. Introduction

- Every year 10% of the UK's under-5s will have an episode of infective gastroenteritis.
- Characteristically they present with sudden onset of diarrhoea (with or without vomiting), which usually resolves without any specific treatment.
- When severe, dehydration can occur, which can be life-threatening. Younger children are most at risk of dehydration.
- Children should not simply be viewed as 'little adults'. They pose many pitfalls for the unwary and inexperienced, and present healthcare providers with significant challenges whatever the setting.
- Children display important differences in their anatomy, their physiology, their immunity and the illnesses they encounter, as well as the ways in which these conditions present, develop and progress.
- Difficulties verbalising and communicating their condition further add to these challenges.

1.1 'Major' and 'minor' illnesses

- Before considering 'minor' illnesses in children, it is crucial to both appreciate and understand that 'major' childhood illnesses – including life-threatening conditions such as meningococcal disease – rarely present in extremis, but more commonly present with relatively innocent features that can easily be mistaken for minor illnesses.
- Children with advanced major illness (or significant injury) typically have deranged vital signs that are usually readily detected. Earlier in their illness, these children may well have had normal physiology and appeared relatively well – if assessed early in their illness, these children might be misdiagnosed as only having a minor illness.

2. Severity and Outcome

In children with gastroenteritis:

- vomiting usually lasts 1–2 days, and stops within 3 days.
- diarrhoea usually lasts 5–7 days, and stops within 2 weeks.

3. Pathophysiology

- Many viruses, bacteria or other microbes can cause gastroenteritis. However, the most common cause in children is the Rotavirus. This virus can be spread easily through close contact as it is passed out in an infected person's diarrhoea.
- Once exposed to the virus, the incubation period is approximately 48 hours before symptoms start to show. It is thought that almost every child in the UK suffers a rotavirus infection at some point before they turn 5 years old. However, it is most common in children aged 6 months to 2 years old.
- In the UK, 18,000 children each year present at a hospital with a rotavirus infection. Ten percent will need admission due to dehydration.
- Other causes include bacterial infection such as *Escherichia Coli* (*E. coli*), Salmonella and Campylobacter bacteria that produce toxins that the food we eat. Once exposed to the virus, normally immunity is developed; hence it is uncommon in adults.

3.1 *Escherichia coli* O157:H7 infection

- *E. coli* O157:H7 is a bacterium found in the intestines of healthy cattle that can cause serious human infections, especially in the young and older people.
- It often leads to bloody diarrhoea and occasionally kidney failure (referred to as haemolytic uraemic syndrome or HUS). Outbreaks have occurred following school farm visits or following consumption of undercooked, contaminated beef. (Beef burgers are notorious, as the meat comes from many animals.)
- When *E. coli* O157:H7 infection is suspected (e.g. contact with a confirmed case), urgent specialist advice must be sought.

4. Assessment

- Gastroenteritis is diagnosed on clinical findings and should be suspected where there is a sudden change in stool consistency to loose or watery stools and/or a sudden onset of vomiting.
- History: consider the diagnosis when the child has had:
  - recent contact with someone with acute diarrhoea and/or vomiting
  - exposure to a known source of enteric infection (farm visits, contaminated water or food – see *Escherichia coli* 0157 infection above)
  - recent overseas travel.

4.1 Differential diagnosis

Apart from gastroenteritis, alternative diagnoses must be considered when the following features are found, and a more experienced paediatric assessment should be sought:

- Fever:
  - temp ≥38°C in child <3 months old
  - temp ≥39°C in child ≥3 months old.
- Shortness of breath or tachypnoea.
- Altered consciousness.
- Neck stiffness.
- Bulging fontanelle in infants.
- Non-blanching rash.
- Blood and/or mucus in stool.

Paediatric Gastroenteritis

- Bilious (green) vomit.
- Severe or localised abdominal pain.
- Abdominal distension or rebound tenderness.
- History/suspicion of poisoning.
- History of head injury.
- Appears systemically unwell.

Examination: clinical assessment for dehydration and shock

- Establish whether the child is red, amber or green on the traffic light system in Table 3.100.

TABLE 3.100 – Traffic Light System for Clinical Dehydration and Shock

	Green Low Risk	Amber Intermediate Risk	Red High Risk
Activity	• Responds normally to social cues • Content/smiling • Stays awake/awakens quickly • Strong normal cry/not crying	• Aged less than 1 year old • Altered response to social cues • Decreased activity • No smile	• Not responding normally to or no response to social cues • Appears ill to a healthcare professional • Unable to rouse or if roused does not stay awake • Weak, high-pitched or continuous cry
Skin	• Normal skin colour • Normal turgor	• Warm extremities	• Pale/mottled/ashen/blue • Cold extremities • Reduced skin turgor
Respiratory	• Normal breathing		• Tachypnoeic (refer to **Page for Age**)
Hydration	• CRT≤ 2 secs • Moist mucous membranes • Normal urine	• CRT 2–3 secs • Dry mucous membranes (except after a drink) • Reduced urine output • Clinically dehydrated (refer to Table 3.101)	• CRT >3 seconds • Clinically shocked (refer to Table 3.101)
Pulses/ Heart Rate	• Heart rate normal (refer to **Page for Age**) • Peripheral pulses normal		• Tachycardic (refer to **Page for Age**) • Peripheral pulses weak
Blood Pressure	• Normal, refer to **Page for Age**		• Hypotensive (refer to **Page for Age**)
Eyes	• Normal eyes	• Sunken eyes	
Other		• At risk of dehydration	

Children most at risk of dehydration include:

- Infants of low birth weight (i.e. <2.5 kg).
- Children <1 year, especially those aged <6 months.
- >5 diarrhoeal stools in the previous 24 hours.
- >2 vomits in the previous 24 hours.
- Those who have not been offered/not been able to tolerate oral fluids.
- Breastfed infants who have stopped feeding.
- Malnourished children.

Paediatric Gastroenteritis

TABLE 3.101 – Symptoms and Signs of Clinical Dehydration and Shock

Increasing severity of dehydration →

Symptoms No clinically detectable dehydration	Clinically dehydrated	Clinically shocked
Appears well	Appears to be unwell or deteriorating	–
Alert and responsive	Altered responsiveness (e.g. irritable, lethargic)	Decreased level of consciousness
Normal urine output	Decreased urine output. Output often decreased in those with normal hydration as a compensatory mechanism Unreliable in those in nappies with diarrhoea	–
Skin colour unchanged	Skin colour unchanged	Pallor, reduction in normal skin colour or mottling to skin. Mottling may not be easily detectable in all skin tones
Warm extremities	Warm extremities	Cold extremities
Signs **No clinically detectable dehydration**	**Clinically dehydrated**	**Clinically shocked**
Alert and responsive	Altered responsiveness (e.g. irritable, lethargic)	Decreased level of consciousness
Skin colour unchanged	Skin colour unchanged	Pallor, reduction in normal skin colour or mottling to skin. Mottling may not be easily detectable in all skin tones
Warm extremities	Warm extremities	Cold extremities
Eyes not sunken	Sunken eyes	–
Moist mucous membranes (except after a drink)	Dry mucous membranes (except for 'mouth breather')	–
Normal heart rate	Tachycardia	Tachycardia
Normal breathing pattern	Tachypnoea	Tachypnoea
Normal peripheral pulses	Normal peripheral pulses	Weak peripheral pulses
Normal capillary refill time	Normal capillary refill time	Prolonged capillary refill time
Normal skin turgor	Reduced skin turgor	–
Normal blood pressure	Normal blood pressure	Hypotension (decompensated shock)

(continued)

Paediatric Gastroenteritis

> **TABLE 3.101** – Symptoms and Signs of Clinical Dehydration and Shock *(continued)*
>
> **NB** Rectal examinations should never be performed in the pre-hospital assessment of the paediatric acute abdomen.
>
> Consider dehydration risk factors when interpreting symptoms and signs.
>
> Within the category of 'clinical dehydration', there is a spectrum of severity indicated by increasingly numerous and more pronounced symptoms and signs.
>
> Within the category of 'clinical shock', one or more of the symptoms and/or signs listed would be expected to be present.
>
> Dashes (–) indicate that these clinical features do not specifically indicate shock but may still be present. Symptoms and signs with red flags may help to identify children at increased risk of progression to shock.
>
> If uncertain, manage as if the child has those red flag symptoms and/or signs.

5. Management

Most children with gastroenteritis can be managed at home with oral fluids, although dehydrated children require NG or IV fluid replacement and those in shock may require urgent intravenous fluid resuscitation. Fluid losses can be replaced via the oral route, via a nasogastric tube or intravenously.

- Oral (and nasogastric) fluids:
  - oral rehydration salt (ORS) solutions are given orally or via a nasogastric (NG) tube.
  - they should be given as small, frequent volumes.
  - response to oral rehydration must be monitored by regular clinical assessment.
  - Over-the-counter (OTC) commercially available ORS solutions include Dioralyte, Dioralyte Relief, Electrolade and Rapolyte.
- Intravenous interventions (IV):
  - IV fluids are required when shock is suspected or confirmed and requires urgent hospital transfer.
  - when intravenous access cannot be established, intraosseous fluids may be required.
- Other treatments:
  - antibiotics, antidiarrhoeals and anti-emetics are not routinely used in the management of gastroenteritis.

Consider the outcome for the child identified by clinical assessment

- In those children who can be managed in the community:
  - fluid intake should be actively encouraged (e.g. milk, water, squash) – under-fives need approximately 10 ml of fluid every 10 minutes.
  - in infants, breastfeeding and other milk feeds should be continued.
  - in older children, fruit juices and fizzy drinks must be stopped.
  - ORS solutions should be offered to those at increased risk of dehydration as supplemental fluids, although toddlers and small children frequently refuse ORS because of the taste!
  - if oral intake is insufficient or if the child is persistently vomiting, they should be transferred to secondary care for NG or IV fluid replacement. (Inpatient management often includes a trial of ORS or NG fluids prior to IV fluid replacement.)
- Any child found to be **in shock** must be taken to hospital (refer to red flag system, 🚩 see Table 3.100). They will need additional fluids to not just **maintain** their normal body water but also to replace their fluid losses.
- **Clinically shocked** children require intravenous fluid resuscitation and urgent hospital transfer:
  - a rapid 10 ml/kg IV of infusion sodium chloride 0.9% may be given but should not delay hospital transfer.
  - clinical response to fluid boluses must be monitored.
  - if shock persists, this infusion should be repeated and other causes of shock considered (refer to **Sodium Chloride 0.9%**).
- Stool samples are not normally required but should be obtained in certain situations:
  - Diarrhoea ≥7 days
  - Recent overseas travel
  - Possible septicaemia
  - Blood/mucus in stool
  - Immunocompromise
  - Persisting diagnostic uncertainty
  - Contact the GP or out-of-hours service where this is thought to be necessary.

See Figure 3.39 for a decision support tool.

Paediatric Gastroenteritis

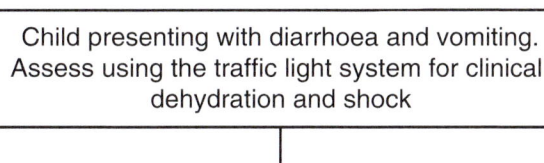

Figure 3.39 – Decision support tool for the assessment of children with gastroenteritis.

6. Referral Pathway

Children with gastroenteritis that are not dehydrated or shocked can initially be managed at home; if their condition progresses, seek an additional medical opinion (GP, OOH, emergency department, paediatrician) (see 'Safety netting' below).

- Hospital transfer is required if:
  - Oral intake is insufficient.
  - The child is persistently vomiting.
  - A child is found to be clinically dehydrated.
  - A child is found to be clinically shocked (Emergency Transfer).
  - A child requires intravenous therapy.
  - Suspicion of an alternative cause for the child's symptoms, e.g. UTI, meningococcal disease.
  - Additionally, some children's social circumstances will dictate additional/continued involvement of healthcare professionals.
- Give the following advice for non-dehydrated children managed at home.

6.1 Nutritional considerations

- During rehydration:
  - Continue breastfeeding.
  - Give full-strength milk straight away.
  - Continue the child's usual solid food.
  - Avoid fruit juices and fizzy drinks until the diarrhoea has stopped.
  - Consider giving an extra 5 ml/kg of ORS solution after each large watery stool in children at increased risk of dehydration.
  - If dehydration recurs after rehydration, restart oral rehydration therapy.

Safety Netting' should be provided for children who do not require referral, giving written information to parents and carers on how to:

- Recognise developing red flag symptoms (refer to Table 3.101), and get immediate help from an appropriate healthcare professional if red flag symptoms develop and, if necessary, make arrangements for follow-up at a specified time and place, that is face-to-face assessment.

Information and advice for parents and carers

Advise parents, carers and children that:

- good hand washing is essential to prevent the spread of gastroenteritis to themselves and other family members; use soap (liquid if possible) in warm, running water followed by careful drying.
- hands should be washed after going to the toilet (children) or changing nappies (parents/carers) and before preparing, serving or eating food.
- infected children should not share towels.
- children should not go to school or other childcare facility while they have diarrhoea or vomiting caused by gastroenteritis and must stay away for at least 48 hours after the last episode of diarrhoea or vomiting.
- children should not swim in swimming pools for 2 weeks after the last episode of diarrhoea.

Paediatric Gastroenteritis

> **KEY POINTS!**
>
> **Paediatric Gastroenteritis**
>
> - Gastroenteritis is common, frequently viral and usually self-limiting.
> - When severe, shock and life-threatening dehydration can occur.
> - Clinical assessment determines whether dehydration or shock is present (seek Red Flag (🚩) symptoms and signs).
> - Non-dehydrated children can frequently be managed at home with oral fluids or ORS.
> - Failed oral rehydration requires either NG or IV fluid replacement in secondary care.
> - Shocked children need urgent hospital treatment.
> - Early meningococcal disease is known to mimic gastroenteritis in small children. An urgent second opinion should be sought if meningococcal disease cannot be excluded.
> - Provide a 'safety net', with written information, for all children with gastroenteritis not transferred to hospital.
> - If uncertain, seek advice from the child's GP, an out-of-hours doctor or specialist advice line where available.

Bibliography

1. National Institute for Health and Clinical Excellence. *Diarrhoea and Vomiting in Children: Diarrhoea and vomiting caused by gastroenteritis: Diagnosis, assessment and management in children younger than 5 years* (CG84). Available from: https://www.nice.org.uk/guidance/cg84, 2009.
2. South Western Ambulance Service Trust. *Paediatric Gastroenteritis Clinical Guideline*. 2018.
3. Sandell JM, Charman SC. Can age-based estimates of weight be safely used when resuscitating children? *Emergency Medicine Journal* 2009, 26(1): 43–47.
4. Armon K, Stephenson T, MacFaul R, Eccleston P, Werneke U. An evidence and consensus based guideline for acute diarrhoea management. *Archives of Disease in Childhood* 2001, 85(2): 132–142.
5. Health Protection Agency. *Avoiding Infection on Farm Visits: Advice for the public*. 2011. Available from: http://www.hpa.org.uk/webc/HPAwebFile/HPAweb_C/1270122184581.

Pulmonary Embolism

1. Introduction

- Pulmonary embolism (PE) is an obstruction of the pulmonary vessels which usually presents as one of four types:

1. **Multiple small pulmonary emboli** – characterised by progressive breathlessness more commonly identified at outpatient appointments than through emergency presentation due to the long standing nature of the problem.
2. **Segmental emboli with pulmonary infarction** – may present with pleuritic pain and/or haemoptysis but with little or no cardiovascular compromise.
3. **Major pulmonary emboli obstruction of the larger branches of the pulmonary tree** – may present with sudden onset of shortness of breath with transient rise in pulse and/or fall in blood pressure. Often a precursor to a massive PE.
4. **Massive pulmonary emboli** – often presenting with loss of consciousness, tachypnoea and intense jugular vein distension, and may prove immediately or rapidly (within 1 hour) fatal or unresponsive to cardiopulmonary resuscitation.

- PE can present with a wide range of symptoms (refer to Table 3.102). The presence of predisposing factors (refer to Table 3.103) increases the index of suspicion of PE. However, in approximately 30% of cases, the presentation is idiopathic.
- Symptoms such as dyspnoea, tachypnoea or chest pain have been found in >90% of cases of patients with PE; pleuritic chest pain is one of the most frequent symptoms of presentation.
- There may be sudden collapse with no obvious physical signs, other than cardiorespiratory arrest.
- Lesser risk factors include air, coach or other travel leading to periods of immobility, especially whilst sitting, oral oestrogen (some contraceptive pills) and central venous catheterisation.
- Over 70% of patients who suffer PE have peripheral vein thrombosis and vigilance is therefore of great importance – it may not initially appear logical to check the legs of a patient with chest pain but can be of great diagnostic value in such cases.

TABLE 3.102 – Signs and Symptoms of PE

Symptoms
- Dyspnoea.
- Pleuritic chest pain.
- Substernal chest pain.
- Apprehension.
- Cough.
- Haemoptysis.
- Syncope.

Signs
- Respiratory rate >20 breaths per minute.
- Pulse rate >100 beats per minute.
- SpO_2 <92%.
- Signs of deep vein thrombosis (DVT).

TABLE 3.103 – Predisposing Factors

Factor

Surgery especially recent
- Abdominal.
- Pelvic.
- Hip or knee surgery.
- Post-operative intensive care.

Obstetrics
- Pregnancy. (Refer to **Maternal Resuscitation**)

Cardiac
- Recent acute myocardial infarction.

Limb problems
- Recent lower limb fractures.
- Varicose veins.
- Lower limb problems secondary to stroke or spinal cord injury.

Malignancy
- Abdominal and/or pelvic in particular advanced metastatic disease.
- Concurrent chemotherapy.

(continued)

Pulmonary Embolism

TABLE 3.103 – Predisposing Factors *(continued)*

Other
- Risk increases with age.
- ≥60 years of age.
- Previous proven PE/DVT.
- Immobility.
- Thrombotic disorder.
- Neurological disease with extremity paresis.
- Thrombophilia.
- Hormone replacement therapy and oral contraception.
- Prolonged bed rest >3 days.
- Other recent trauma.
- Long-duration travel (for example air travel).
- Obesity.

2. Incidence

- PE is a relatively common cardiovascular condition affecting approximately 21 per 10,000 per annum.

3. Severity and Outcome

- PE can be life-threatening leading to death in approximately 7–11% of cases; however, treatment is effective if given early.
- Patients with a previous episode(s) of PE are three times more likely to experience a recurrence.

4. Pathophysiology

- The development of a PE occurs when a blood clot (thrombus), comprising red cells, platelets and fibrin, forms in a vein, subsequently dislodges (embolism) and travels in the circulation. This is known as venous thromboembolism (VTE). If the embolism is small it may be filtered in the pulmonary capillary bed, but if the embolism is large it may occlude pulmonary blood vessels. The development of a VTE can also lead to DVT.
- The haemodynamic problems occur when >30–50% of the pulmonary arterial bed is occluded.
- The probability of a PE can be assessed using a clinical predication tool such as the Wells Criteria (refer to Table 3.104). Even if the Wells score indicates a PE is unlikely, any patient where a PE is suspected requires further investigation including a D-dimer test performed and the result acted upon within 4 hours.

TABLE 3.104 – Wells Criteria for PE

Item	Score
Clinical signs and symptoms of DVT (leg swelling and pain with palpation of the deep veins).	3
An alternative diagnosis is less likely than PE.	3
Pulse rate >100 beats per minute.	1.5
Immobilisation or surgery in the previous 4 weeks.	1.5
Previous DVT/PE.	1.5
Haemoptysis.	1
Malignancy (treatment ongoing or within previous 6 months or palliative).	1
Clinical Probability of PE	**Total**
Likely	>4 points
Unlikely	4 points or less

5. Assessment and Management

For the assessment and management of PE, refer to Table 3.105 and Figure 3.40.

TABLE 3.105 – ASSESSMENT and MANAGEMENT of: Pulmonary Embolism

Assess <C>ABCDE

- If any of the following **TIME-CRITICAL** features are present:
  - major **<C>ABCDE** problems
  - extreme breathing difficulty
  - cyanosis
  - severe hypoxia (SpO_2) <90% – unresponsive to oxygen.
- Start correcting any **<C>ABCDE** problems.
- Undertake a **TIME-CRITICAL** transfer to nearest appropriate receiving hospital.
- Continue patient management en route.
- Provide an ATMIST information call.

Pulmonary Embolism

TABLE 3.105 – ASSESSMENT and MANAGEMENT of: Pulmonary Embolism *(continued)*

Specifically Assess
- Respiratory rate and effort.
- Signs and symptoms combined with predisposing factors.
- Lower limbs for unilateral swelling; may also be warm with a change in skin colour – a darker area, purple or red.
- Calf tenderness/pain may be present – extensive leg clots may also lead to femoral tenderness.
- Differential diagnoses include pleurisy, pneumothorax or cardiac chest pain.

Position
- Position patient for comfort and ease of respiration – often sitting forwards – but be aware of potential hypotension.

Respiratory Rate
- Measure and record respiratory rate.

Oxygen Saturation
- Monitor the patient's SpO_2; administer oxygen to achieve saturations of >94% if the patient presents as hypoxaemic on air (refer to **Oxygen**).

Ventilation
- Consider assisted ventilation if indicated (refer to **Airway and Breathing Management**).

Pulse
- Measure and record pulse.

Blood Pressure and Fluids
- Measure and record blood pressure; if required, administer fluids (refer to **Intravascular Fluid Therapy in Adults** and **Intravascular Fluid Therapy in Children**).

Blood Glucose
- If appropriate, measure and record blood glucose for hypo/hyperglycaemia (refer to **Glycaemic Emergencies in Adults and Children**).

Temperature
- Measure and record temperature.

NEWS2
- These observations will enable you to calculate a NEWS2 score (refer to **Sepsis**).

ECG
- Monitor and record 12-lead ECG – be aware that the classic S1 Q3 T3 12-lead ECG presentation is often NOT present, even during massive PE. The most common finding is a sinus tachycardia (refer to **Cardiac Arrhythmia and Sudden Cardiac Death**).

Assess the Patient's Pain
- Where present, assess the **SOCRATES** of pain and record initial and subsequent pain scores.
- Consider analgesia if appropriate (refer to **Pain Management in Adults and Children**).

Documentation
- Complete documentation to include all clinical findings, advice from other clinicians, onward referral and worsening advice given.

Transfer to Further Care
- Transfer rapidly to nearest appropriate hospital.
- Clinically stable patients may be suitable for assessment at a SDEC (Same Day Emergency Care) facility according to local pathways, providing the four hours timeline can be met.
- Provide an alert/information call.
- Continue patient management en route.

(continued)

Pulmonary Embolism

TABLE 3.105 – ASSESSMENT and MANAGEMENT of: Pulmonary Embolism *(continued)*

ADDITIONAL INFORMATION

Whilst there is no specific pre-hospital treatment available, there may be a window of opportunity to manage massive PE before the patient progresses to cardiac arrest. Other in-hospital treatments may be effective, including: haemodynamic and respiratory support, thrombolysis, surgical pulmonary embolectomy, percutaneous catheter embolectomy and fragmentation and anticoagulation.

KEY POINTS!

Pulmonary Embolism

- **Common symptoms of PE are dyspnoea, tachypnoea, pleuritic pain, apprehension, tachycardia, cough, haemoptysis and leg pain/clinical DVT.**
- **Risk factors may be identifiable from the history.**
- **Ensure <C>ABCDE assessment and apply a pulse oximetry monitor early.**
- **Patients may present with unilateral swelling of the lower limbs; they may also be warm and red.**
- **Apply oxygen and if in respiratory distress, transfer to further care as a medical emergency.**

Bibliography

1. National Institute for Health and Clinical Excellence. *Venous thromboembolic diseases: diagnosis, management and thrombophilia testing* (NG158). London: NICE, 2020. Last updated: 02 August 2023. Available from: https://www.nice.org.uk/guidance/NG158.
2. BMJ Best Practice 2022. Pulmonary embolism. BMJ Publishing Group. Available from: https://bestpractice.bmj.com/info.
3. Di Nisio M, van Es N, Buller HR. Deep vein thrombosis and pulmonary embolism. *Lancet* 2016, 388: 3060–3073.
4. Resuscitation Council UK. *Special circumstances guidelines*. Published May 2021. Available from: https://www.resus.org.uk/library/2021-resuscitation-guidelines/special-circumstances-guidelines.
5. National Institute for Health and Clinical Excellence. *Venous thromboembolism in over 16s: reducing the risk of hospital-acquired deep vein thrombosis or pulmonary embolism* (NG 89). London: NICE, 2018. Available from: https://www.nice.org.uk/guidance/ng89.
6. Torbicki A, Perrier A, Konstantinides S, Agnelli G, Galie N, Pruszczyk P, et al. Guidelines on the diagnosis and management of acute pulmonary embolism. *European Heart Journal* 2008, 29(18): 2276–315.
7. Wells PS, Anderson DR, Rodger M, Ginsberg JS, Kearon C, Gent M. Derivation of a simple clinical model to categorize patients' probability of pulmonary embolism: increasing the models utility with the SimpliRED D-dimer. *Thrombosis and Haemostasis* 2000, 83: 416–420.
8. Cohen AT, Agnelli G, Anderson FA, Arcelus JI, Bergqvist D, Brecht JG, et al. Venous thromboembolism (VTE) in Europe: the number of VTE events and associated morbidity and mortality. *Thrombosis and Haemostasis* 2007, 98(4): 756–764.
9. Farmer RDT, Lawrenson RA, Todd JC, Williams TJ, MacRae KD, Tyrer F, et al. A comparison of the risks of venous thromboembolic disease in association with different combined oral contraceptives. *British Journal of Clinical Pharmacology* 2000, 49(6): 580–590.
10. Goldhaber SZ, Morrison RB. Pulmonary embolism and deep vein thrombosis. *Circulation* 2002, 106(12): 1436–1438.
11. Meyer G, Roy P-M, Gilberg S, Perrier A. Pulmonary embolism. *British Medical Journal* 2010, 340: c1421.
12. White RH. The epidemiology of venous thromboembolism. *Circulation* 2003, 107: I-4–8.
13. Wolf SJ, McCubbin T, Feldhaus KM, Faragher JP, Adcock DM. Prospective validation of Wells Criteria in the evaluation of patients with suspected pulmonary embolism. *Annals of Emergency Medicine* 2004, 44(5): 503–510.

Pulmonary Embolism

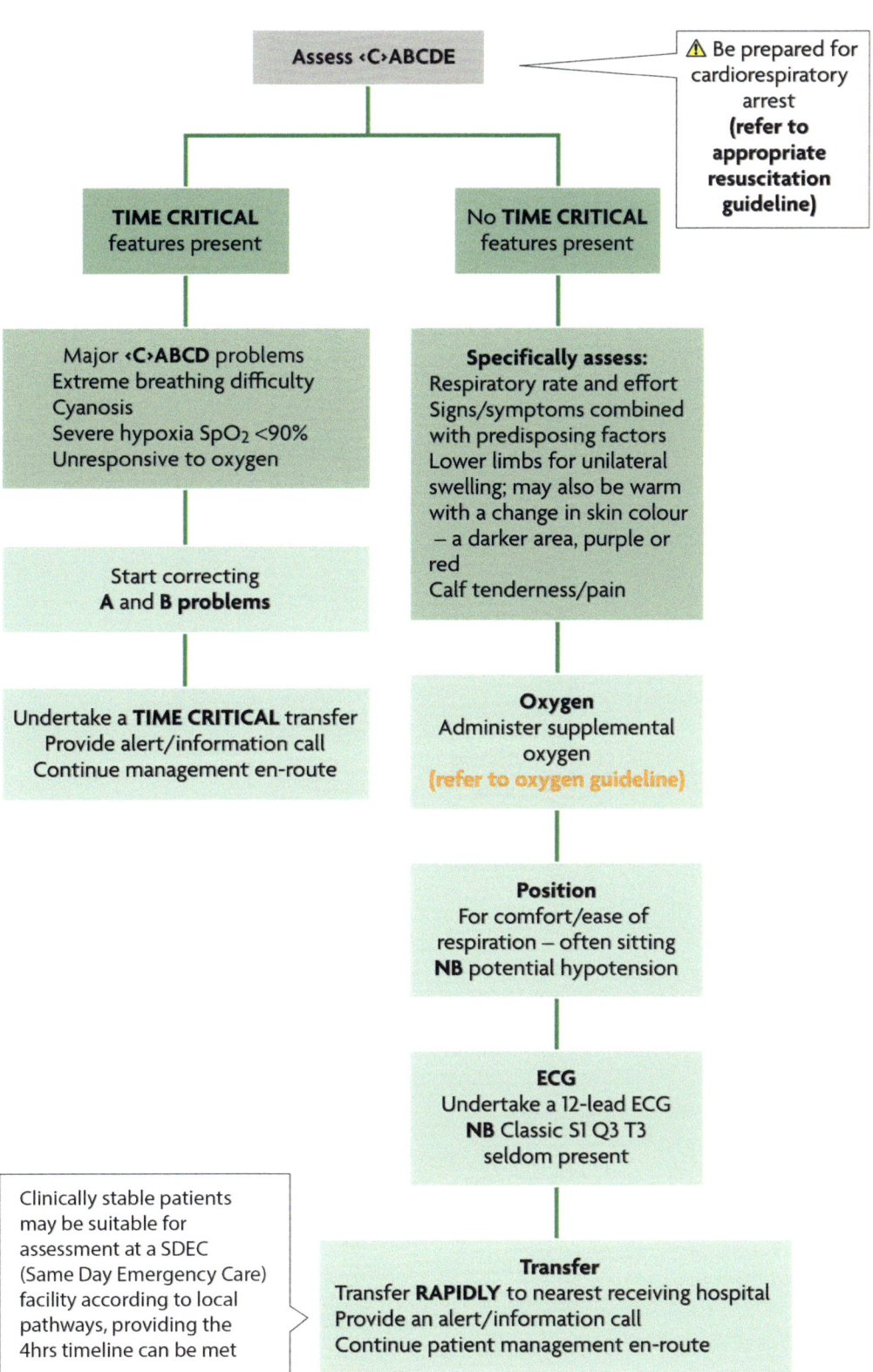

Figure 3.40 – Assessment and management algorithm of pulmonary embolism.

Respiratory Illness in Children

1. Introduction

- Children should not be viewed simply as 'little adults'. The assessment and management of paediatric patients may include potential pitfalls for the unwary and inexperienced and present healthcare providers with significant challenges wherever the setting.
- There are many important differences between children and adults in their anatomy, their physiology and their immunity. There may also be differences in the types of illnesses they encounter, as well as the ways in which these conditions present, develop and progress.
- Children may have difficulties verbalising and communicating their condition, presenting an additional challenge to clinicians.

1.1 'Major' and 'Minor' Illnesses

- Before considering 'minor' illnesses in children, it is crucial to both appreciate and understand that 'major' childhood illnesses (including life-threatening conditions such as meningococcal disease) rarely present in extremis, but more commonly present with relatively innocent features that can easily be mistaken for minor illnesses.
- Children with advanced major illness (or significant injury) typically have deranged vital signs that are usually readily detected. Earlier in their illness, these children may well have had normal physiology and appeared relatively well. If they were assessed early in their illness, there is a risk they might be misdiagnosed with only a minor illness.

This guideline on childhood respiratory illnesses includes:

1. Asthma.
2. Bronchiolitis.
3. Croup.
4. URTIs (tonsillitis, otitis media).
5. Pneumonia.

For the management of mild, moderate, severe and life-threatening asthma, refer to **Asthma in Adults and Children**.

Asthma is rare in very young children (under 1 year), and other causes of wheeze (such as bronchiolitis or viral-induced wheeze) should be considered.

2. Bronchiolitis

2.1 Introduction

Bronchiolitis is an acute, self-limiting respiratory infection that is usually caused by respiratory syncytial virus (RSV) and occurs predominantly in the autumn and winter months. It is characterised by inflammation of the bronchioles.

It is more prevalent during the winter months, peaking over a 6–8 week period, and is the most common lower respiratory tract infection during the first year of life.

Most children will recover without intervention. However, some may have difficulty breathing and need more input, especially very young babies.

2.2 Assessment

Bronchiolitis is commonly preceded by coryzal prodrome (upper respiratory infection, characterised by a non-specific cough, rhinorrhea and fever) for 1 to 3 days.

- Clinical presentation: a coryzal baby (peak age 2–5 months) with their first wheezy episode.
- Irregular breathing and apnoeas are frequently reported.
- During the first 72 hours, bronchiolitic infants may deteriorate clinically, before symptomatic improvements are seen.
- The baby's parents and siblings often have concurrent respiratory illnesses and may report sore throats or dry coughs.

TABLE 3.106 – Signs and Symptoms

↓Oxygen saturations
↑Respiratory rate
Recession
Fine, bilateral inspiratory crackles
High-pitched expiratory wheezes
Low-grade fever
Rhinorrhoea (runny nose)
Cough
Poor feeding
Vomiting
Pyrexia
Apnoea
Cyanosis

- Consider bronchiolitis as the provisional diagnosis if **all** of the following symptoms are present:
  - persistent cough
  - either tachypnoea or chest recession (or both)
  - either wheeze or crackles on chest auscultation (or both).
- When diagnosing bronchiolitis, take into account that the following symptoms are common in children with this disease:
  - fever (in around 30% of cases, usually of less than 39°C)
  - poor feeding (typically after 3 to 5 days of illness)

Respiratory Illness in Children

- young infants may present with apnoea without other clinical signs.
- **NB** Consider a diagnosis of pneumonia if the child has high fever (over 39°C) and/or persistently focal crackles.

2.3 Management

- Give oxygen supplementation to children with bronchiolitis if their oxygen saturation is persistently less than 94%.
- Treatments aim to provide respiratory support and support feeding/hydration.
- Antivirals, antibiotics, steroids, nebulisers, physiotherapy, steam treatments, nasal decongestants, homeopathy and complementary therapies have not been shown to be effective.
- Acute bronchiolitis lasts approximately 2 weeks from its onset, but can last up to 4 weeks.
- Ongoing cough and persisting wheeze are not uncommon after the initial illness has passed but should prompt further medical assessment.
- Generally, management of bronchiolitis will be conservative, with oxygen being the only drug administered in the pre-hospital environment. In most cases, medication is not needed to manage bronchiolitis because it is usually self-limiting (i.e. it settles without the need for treatment).
- Helping parents and carers to understand this can increase their confidence in caring for their child at home. It can also help them understand why medicines are not being administered en route to hospital.
- Clinicians should be aware of the increased need for hospital admission in infants fulfilling the following criteria:
  - pre-existing lung disease, congenital heart disease, neuromuscular weakness, immunodeficiency
  - aged under 3 months
  - prematurity
  - family anxiety
  - re-attendance or re-contact for the same presentation
  - duration of illness is less than 3 days.
- Preterm babies, those with chronic lung disease, children with congenital heart disease, cystic fibrosis, congenital or acquired immune deficiency (HIV) and those either aged <2 months or having apnoeas are at highest risk and must be transferred to further care.
- Previously well babies with diminished feeding, irregular breathing, hypoxia (O_2 saturations <94% on air), tachypnoea or tachycardia should also be transferred to further care where they will receive respiratory support and help with feeding/hydration.
- If the patient is managed on scene, robust safety-netting advice should be provided on how to recognise developing red flag symptoms such as:
  - worsening work of breathing such as grunting, nasal flaring, marked chest recession
  - fluid intake is 50–75% of normal or no wet nappy for 12 hours
  - apnoea or cyanosis
  - exhaustion (e.g. not responding normally to social cues; wakes only with prolonged stimulation).
- Safety-netting advice should also include:
  - advice that people should not smoke in the child's home because it increases the risk of more severe symptoms in bronchiolitis
  - instructions on how to get immediate help from an appropriate professional should any red flag symptoms develop.
- Salbutamol is not indicated in bronchiolitis. It will not benefit the condition, and the resultant tachycardia may confuse subsequent clinical assessment in hospital.

3. Croup

3.1 Introduction

- Croup is a common, acute, respiratory illness of gradual onset, characterised by stridor that typically is mild and self-limiting.
- Viral infections can spread to the larynx and trachea, causing inflammation and therefore compromise of the airway in severe cases.
- Croup is less common in older children, who are more likely to have epiglottitis, a more serious condition, and need to be admitted.

3.2 Incidence

- Croup mostly affects children between the ages of 6 months and 3 years, presenting most commonly in the second year of life.[11] However, children up to 15 years of age may be affected.
- It can occur all year round but peaks are seen in both spring and autumn.

3.3 Pathophysiology

- Croup results from viral infections, most commonly parainfluenza, but also RSV, influenza A and B, as well as *Mycoplasma pneumoniae*.
- Stridor, hoarseness and a barking 'seal-like' cough result from inflammation and narrowing around the subglottic region of the larynx. (This is the narrowest point of the paediatric airway).

NB Stridor is also seen in epiglottitis, bacterial tracheitis, retropharyngeal abscesses, foreign-body ingestion, anaphylaxis and angio-oedema, blunt trauma, glandular fever, hot gases inhalation and diphtheria – all children with any of these conditions should be transferred to further care.

Respiratory Illness in Children

3.4 Assessment

- Croup commonly has a gradual onset. Initial symptoms include a mild fever and a runny nose. This progresses to a sore throat and a barking cough, typical of the condition. Young children have smaller air passages and inflammation in the voice box leads to a narrowing of the gap between the vocal cords.
- Croup develops over a period of 1 or 2 days; the severity varies over that period but it is normally worse on the second night of the cough.
- Stridor associated with croup can also be caused by other conditions. Clinicians should consider differential diagnoses, such as:
  - epiglottitis
  - bacterial tracheitis
  - foreign bodies
  - anaphylaxis
  - angio-oedema
  - glandular fever
  - blunt trauma
  - retropharyngeal abscesses
  - inhalation of hot gases
  - diphtheria.
- All children with these conditions should be transferred to further care.
- The child with croup may have mild clinical features in keeping with a simple, upper respiratory tract infection, although they can present with more worrying features including respiratory distress, respiratory failure and respiratory arrest.
- The features of respiratory distress – increased respiration rate, increased work of breathing, recession, nasal flaring, grunting, use of accessory muscles and stridor – are described in **Medical Emergencies in Children – Overview**.

3.5 Management

- Keep the child in a position of comfort, sat upright and supported on a parent's lap – children often 'know' how to maintain their own airways in an optimal position (they often adopt a so-called 'tripod' posture).
- A calm approach is to be encouraged at all times. Any intervention likely to upset the child – examining their ears, nose or throat, blood sugar measurement, cannulation and even nebulisation (see below) – must be avoided, as distressing procedures can precipitate acute deterioration and complete airway obstruction. This is of particular importance in the pre-hospital environment where skills for expert airway intervention are not readily available.
- Steroids are the mainstay of treatment – usually oral dexamethasone (nebulised budesonide may be used as an alternative but may distress the child, adversely worsening their symptoms) – and work by relieving subglottic inflammation.
- Children with croup may benefit from early steroid treatment.
- Oral dexamethasone (refer to **Dexamethasone**) is preferred to nebulised budesonide, as nebulisation frequently distresses small children, producing further airway narrowing.

3.6 Referral Pathway

As above, irrespective of whether steroids are given, all children with stridor must still be transferred to further care for subsequent observation, even if clinical improvements are noted at home.

- All children under the age of two with croup must be conveyed to hospital
- All children with a respiratory rate above 40 breaths/min with croup must be conveyed to hospital.

If the patient is to be discharged on scene, it is important to give parents/guardians appropriate advice:

- Explain that croup is self-limiting and that symptoms usually resolve within 48 hours, although occasionally they may last for up to a week. Resolution of croup symptoms is usually followed by symptoms of upper respiratory tract infection.
- Advise the use of paracetamol or ibuprofen to control fever and pain/distress.
  - do not over- or under-dress a child with fever
  - tepid sponging is not recommended
  - do not routinely give antipyretic drugs to a child with fever with the sole aim of reducing body temperature.
- Explain that cough medicines, decongestants and short-acting beta-agonists are not effective. Croup is usually a viral illness and antibiotics are not needed.
- Ensure an adequate fluid intake.
- Do not advise humidified air (e.g. steam inhalation).
- Arrange for a clinician to review the child within a few hours, either by face-to-face consultation or by telephone. Advise parents to seek urgent medical advice if:
  - There is progression from mild to moderate airways obstruction, such as development of intermittent stridor at rest or increased effort of breathing (chest and suprasternal in-drawing), as the child may need to be observed in hospital.
  - If the child becomes toxic (pale, very high fever, tachycardic) as this may mean the child has an alternative diagnosis (e.g. bacterial tracheitis or epiglottitis).

Respiratory Illness in Children

- Advise the parents to call 999 or take the patient immediately to the emergency department (ED) if the child:
  – Becomes cyanosed.
  – Is unusually sleepy.
  – Is struggling to breathe and cannot be calmed down quickly.
  – Is restless, agitated or upset.
  – Or if stridor can be heard continually and recession is seen (the skin between the ribs is pulling in with every breath).
  – Has a significant reduction in normal skin colour, e.g. pallor or grey (includes blue lips) for more than a few seconds.
  – Is not responding.
  – Is having a lot of trouble breathing (e.g. the belly is sinking in while breathing, or the skin between the ribs or over the windpipe is pulling in with each breath; the nostrils may also be flaring in and out).
  – Wants to sit instead of lie down.
  – Cannot talk.
  – Is drooling.
  – Is having trouble swallowing.

Ensure that there is a communication to the patient's registered GP to inform them about the episode, the outcomes reached and any treatment given.

4. Upper Respiratory Tract Infections (URTIs), e.g. Tonsillitis (Sore Throat, Acute Pharyngitis, Acute Exudative Tonsillitis), Otitis Media, etc.

4.1 Introduction

Upper respiratory tract infections (URTIs) are one of the commonest reasons for paediatric presentation, especially during the winter months.

4.2 Incidence

25% of all under five year olds will see their GPs each year for tonsillitis.

4.3 Assessment

- Children with URTIs frequently complain of:
  – sore throat
  – cough
  – fever
  – headache
  – earache
  – systemic illness
  – anorexia and lethargy.
- Physical examination may reveal:
  – cervical lymphadenopathy
  – offensive breath
  – inflamed, purulent tonsils.

Breathing may also be compromised by either stridor or respiratory distress. In these circumstances, avoid attempts to examine the throat (see croup guidance above) and transfer urgently to further care.

The child's hydration status should be estimated, as fluid intake can be significantly decreased.

4.4 Management

URTIs are usually self-limiting. Parents should be offered simple advice about managing their child's symptoms (rest, extra fluids, analgesia, antipyretics etc.) and informed about the likely duration of their child's illness (refer to Table 3.107).

Antibiotics are not prescribed routinely. Most URTIs are viral and do not respond to antibiotics. Bacteria (e.g. streptococci) also cause URTIs but even in these cases antibiotics are rarely needed; they don't improve the child's symptoms and they can often cause diarrhoea, vomiting and rashes.

TABLE 3.107 – Typical Duration of Acute Respiratory Illnesses

Condition	Duration
Acute otitis media	4 days
Acute sore throat/pharyngitis/tonsillitis	1 week
Common cold	1½ weeks
Acute rhinosinusitis	2½ weeks
Acute cough/bronchitis	3 weeks

GPs tend to use one of three antibiotic strategies:

1. No antibiotics are needed where the URTI is thought likely to be self-limiting.
2. Delayed antibiotics are useful when symptoms fail to improve or worsen.
3. Immediate antibiotic prescriptions are reserved for the most severe cases, including:
   – Under twos with acute bilateral otitis media.
   – Children with acute otitis media and otorrhoea (ear discharge).
   – Children with acute streptococcal URTIs (no cough but fever, pustular tonsils and tender lymph nodes).

Antibiotics are also prescribed for children who are:
– Systemically very unwell.
– At high risk of serious complications because of pre-existing illnesses (heart, lung, renal, liver or neuromuscular disease, diabetes, cystic fibrosis, prematurity, immunosuppression or previous hospitalisations).

Over-the-counter cough and cold preparations often contain sedatives and antihistamines that are dangerous if taken accidentally by small children in overdose. As a result, these medicines are no longer available for children aged two years or

Respiratory Illness in Children

under. Children in this age group with colds and fever should now only be offered paracetamol or ibuprofen to manage their temperature, if needed.

Simple cough syrups containing glycerol, and honey and lemon may still be given, as well as vapour rubs and inhalant decongestants (see individual labelling).

4.5 Referral Pathway

Hospital admission may also be indicated when:

- There is diminished fluid intake (e.g. young child with severe tonsillitis or teenager with glandular fever).
- Where concerns regarding the diagnosis persist (**NB** early meningococcal disease is frequently misdiagnosed as an URTI in small children – where this diagnosis cannot be excluded, arrangements for an urgent medical opinion should be made). Refer to **Febrile Illness in Children**.
- Children with 'muffled' voices – they sound as if they have something hot in their mouths. These children must be transferred to further care to exclude quinsy (peritonsillar abscess).
- Tenderness behind the ear (over their mastoid process) in a child with otitis media, whose ear may or may not be starting to 'stick out', suggests mastoiditis (a dangerous infection of the bone around the ear) and must be transferred to further care.

4.6 Management in the Community

As when managing the febrile child, if a decision not to transfer a child to further care has been reached, a clinically justifiable reason should be present and properly documented. Refer to **Febrile Illness in Children**.

'Safety netting', with written advice, should again be encouraged and follow-up arrangements should be provided.

Where doubts persist, seek senior advice or review.

5. Pneumonia (Lower Respiratory Tract Infections, 'Chest Infections')

Children with pneumonia are likely to have the following signs and symptoms:

- Fever.
- Cough.
- Tachypnoea.
  - RR > 60 breaths/min, age 0–5 months
  - RR > 50 breaths/min, age 6–12 months
  - RR > 40 breaths/min, age > 12 months
- Nasal flaring.
- Chest indrawing.
- Oxygen saturations <95%.
- Crackles in the chest.
- Cyanosis.

Such children are likely to require antibiotics and additional oxygen and should be seen by either their GP or a paediatrician.

Table 3.108 indicates severity of disease by age of the patient. This should be used to determine whether urgent referral in the community is appropriate or transfer to the Emergency Department. Children with severe symptoms (oxygen saturations <92% or where auscultation demonstrates absent breath sounds or percussion presents as dull) should be transferred to the Emergency Department.

TABLE 3.108 – Severity Assessment

	Mild to moderate	Severe
Infants	Temperature <38.5°C	Temperature >38.5°C
	Respiratory rate <50 breaths/min	Respiratory rate >70 breaths/min
	Mild recession	Moderate to severe recession
	Taking full feeds	Nasal flaring
		Cyanosis (assess carefully for peripheral cyanosis using natural light, and examine the mucous membranes, lips and tongue)
		Intermittent apnoea
		Grunting respiration
		Not feeding
		Tachycardia*
		Capillary refill time ≥2s

Respiratory Illness in Children

TABLE 3.108 – Severity Assessment *(continued)*

Older children	Temperature <38.5°C Respiratory rate <50 breaths/min Mild breathlessness No vomiting	Temperature >38.5°C Respiratory rate >50 breaths/min Severe difficulty in breathing Nasal flaring Cyanosis (assess carefully for peripheral cyanosis using natural light, and examine the mucous membranes, lips and tongue) Grunting respiration Signs of dehydration Tachycardia* Capillary refill time ≥2s

* Values to define tachycardia vary with age and with temperature how to present the citation.

KEY POINTS!

Respiratory Illness In Children

- Childhood respiratory illnesses are common and usually self-limiting.
- Antibiotics are rarely indicated.
- Children with underlying conditions (e.g. prematurity, chronic lung disease, congenital heart disease, cystic fibrosis, congenital or acquired immune deficiency (HIV), cerebral palsy) are especially vulnerable and must be seen either by their GP or a paediatrician in hospital.
- Tachypnoea is a feature in all respiratory illnesses.
- Respiratory distress causes increased respiratory rate, increased work of breathing, recession, nasal flaring, grunting, use of accessory muscles and stridor.
- Exhaustion suggests respiratory failure and respiratory arrest may rapidly follow.
- Stridor can progress rapidly to complete upper airway obstruction and respiratory arrest.
- Approach a child with stridor calmly and gently. Sit them upright in a position of comfort and avoid painful/distressing procedures.
- Transfer all children with stridor for further medical assessment and observation.
- Steroids (dexamethasone) are frequently used to treat croup.
- Children with pneumonia require antibiotics and possibly oxygen therapy. They should be seen by either their GP or a paediatrician.
- Whilst URTIs are very common, early meningococcal disease can easily be misdiagnosed as an URTI. (When unable to exclude this diagnosis, make arrangements for an urgent second opinion.)
- Provide a 'safety net' (with written information) for all children with respiratory illness not transferred to hospital.
- If uncertain, seek advice from either the child's GP or the out-of-hours doctor.
- Asthma is rare in very young children (under 1 year), and other causes of wheeze (such as bronchiolitis or viral-induced wheeze) should be considered.

Bibliography

1. Godden CW, Campbell MJ, Hussey M, Cogswell JJ. Double blind placebo controlled trial of nebulised budesonide for croup. *Archives of Disease in Childhood* 1997, 76(2): 155–158.
2. Russell KF, Liang Y, O'Gorman K, Johnson DW, Klassen TP. Glucocorticoids for croup. *Cochrane Database of Systematic Reviews* 2011(1): CD001955.
3. Scottish Intercollegiate Guidelines Network. *Management of Sore Throat and Indications for Tonsillectomy* (Guideline 117). Edinburgh: SIGN, 2010. Available from: https://www.sign.ac.uk/sign-117-management-of-sore-throat-and-indications-for-tonsillectomy.html.
4. Sparrow A, Geelhoed G. Prednisolone versus dexamethasone in croup: a randomised equivalence

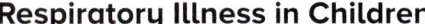

Respiratory Illness in Children

trial. *Archives of Disease in Childhood* 2006, 91(7): 580–583.

5. Baumer JH. Glucocorticoid treatment in croup. *Archives of Disease in Childhood Education and Practice Edition* 2006, 91(2): ep58–60.

6. Sandell JM, Charman SC. Can age-based estimates of weight be safely used when resuscitating children? *Emergency Medicine Journal* 2009, 26(1): 43–47.

7. Taussig LM, Castro O, Beaudry PH, Fox WW, Bureau M. Treatment of laryngotracheobronchitis (croup): use of intermittent positive-pressure breathing and racemic epinephrine. *American Journal of Diseases of Children* 1975, 129(7): 790–793.

8. Centre for Clinical Practice at the National Institute for Health and Clinical Excellence. *Acutely Ill Patients in Hospital: Recognition of and response to acute illness in adults in hospital* (CG50). London: NICE, 2007. Available from: https://www.nice.org.uk/guidance/cg50.

9. National Institute for Health and Clinical Excellence. *Respiratory Tract Infections – Antibiotic Prescribing: Prescribing of antibiotics for self-limiting respiratory tract infections in adults and children in primary care* (CG 69). London: NICE, 2008. Available from: https://www.nice.org.uk/guidance/cg69.

10. National Institute for Health and Care Excellence. *Bronchiolitis in Children: Diagnosis and management*.2015. Available from: https://www.nice.org.uk/guidance/ng9.

11. National Institute for Health and Clinical Excellence. *Croup. NICE Clinical Knowledge Summaries* London: NICE, 2012. Available from: https://cks.nice.org.uk.

Seizures in Adults

1. Introduction

- A seizure is a 'sudden attack of illness' (Oxford English Dictionary) but in contemporary neurology the term seizure means episodes involving sudden, temporary and subjectively involuntary neurological symptoms which may include movements, sensations, and imparemet of consciousness (refer to **Altered Level of Consciousness**).

- The differential diagnosis of seizure includes a single unprovoked seizure (which does not meet the definition of epilepsy), symptomatic seizures (provoked) due to acute brain pathology, functional or dissociative (nonepileptic) seizures, psychogenic non-epileptic seizures (also known as Nonepileptic Attack Disorder or Psychogenic Nonepileptic Seizures), vasovagal syncope and cardiogenic events. The full list of causes is long and beyond the scope of this guideline. Other JRCALC guidelines are potentially relevant to the assessment of the patients experiencing a seizure and are cited here where appropriate. There is often significant diagnostic uncertainty during and after a seizure and the term 'suspected sei-zure' is often appropriate to reflect the uncertainty.

- Eclampsia is a complication of pregnancy which may occur in women who are ≥20 weeks pregnant (including up to 14 days post-partum) and can give rise to seizures. Eclamptic seizures are beyond the scope of this guideline. Refer to **Pre-eclampsia and Eclampsia** and **Magnesium Sulfate** for the assessment and management of epileptic seizures in patients who are ≥20 weeks pregnantor within 14 days post-partum.

2. Epileptic Seizures

- Epileptic seizures are caused by abnormal electrical activity in the brain. There are many types of epileptic seizures. The manifestations of seizures depend on which part of the brain is affected. This guideline focuses on bilateral tonic-clonic seizures (BTCS), which are the most common type of seizure presenting in emergency services, and present as stiffening of the whole body (tonic phase), gradually merging into vigorous bilateral limb shaking (clonic phase). During BTCS, patients are unresponsive to commands or sensory stimuli and typically have their eyes open. Most BTCS terminate within 90 seconds of their onset. Afterwards patients are often confused and/or drowsy (postictal).

- BTCS that have not stopped after 5 minutes, or a series of such seizures without recovery in between and that have lasted for 5 minutes or more, are defined as convulsive status epilepticus (CSE). This is a medical emergency and requires rapid treatment. Long-term consequences may occur if CSE is not controlled within 30 minutes. However, many patients with prolonged seizures are having functional or dissociative seizures, which can resemble BTCS; see section 3. It may be difficult to distinguish between BTCS and functional/dissociative seizures, but some features are important in making this distinction (refer to Table 3.109).

- Seizures often start in only one part of the brain (a focal seizure) and then spread through the brain to cause BTCS. Consciousness may be retained in focal seizures (also called an aura). The manifestations of all types of epileptic seizures are very diverse and their description is beyond the scope of this guideline which focuses on BTCS.[1,2]

- If a patient suffers focal seizures that last over 10 minutes with some element of convulsion (e.g. muscle or mylonic twitch) AND impairment of consciousness, then these should be treated in the same way as BTCS. However, long-term consequences are only likely if the focal seizure continues for over 60 minutes.

- Epilepsy is a chronic disorder in which patients are at increased risk of unprovoked seizures. Epileptic seizures also occur as 'provoked' (acute symptomatic) seizures caused by irritation of the brain, for instance by head injury, stroke, alcohol, hypoglycaemia, drug overdose or infection. The provoking factor may itself require emergency treatment.

- Many patients with epilepsy have an emergency care plan. They may also have a supply of emergency medication (usually midazolam), which can be administered by carers or healthcare professionals according to the care plan. **Following an individual emergency care plan takes precedence over the generic advice provided here.**

TABLE 3.109 – Features Which Help to Distinguish Between BTCS and Functional/Dissociative Seizures.

Signs that favour Bilateral Tonic-Clonic (Epileptic) Seizures	Signs that favour Functional/Dissociative seizures
BTCS: during seizure	**Functional seizures: during seizure**
• Consistent, repeated, rhythmic myoclonic jerking	• Fluctuating intensity/location

(continued)

Seizures in Adults

TABLE 3.109 – Features Which Help to Distinguish Between BTCS and Functional/Dissociative Seizures. *(continued)*

Signs that favour Bilateral Tonic-Clonic (Epileptic) Seizures	Signs that favour Functional/Dissociative seizures
• 'Shock-like' movement	• Brief pauses, tremor or slow flexion/extension movements
• Arm & leg movements mostly synchronised/symmetrical	• Arm & leg movements often not synchronised/symmetrical
• Convulsive movements may spread from focal to generalised and tonic merging to clonic	• Convulsive movements may move from one body area to another
• Unresponsive (GCS 3–4 if grunting)	• May respond in some way (e.g. to speech, blink reflex or on NPA or IV insertion)
• Lateral tongue-biting common	• Tongue-biting rare/minor/involves tip
• Eyes often open	• Eyes mostly shut (opening may be resisted)
• Mouth often open	• Mouth often shut
• Pupils not reacting	• Pupils reacting
• No purposeful movements	• May carry out purposeful movements
• Low SpO_2 or cyanosis	• Normal SpO_2, no cyanosis, hyperventilation
• Typically short (<90 secs) or repeated without recovery between (constant prolonged rare)	• May be prolonged (>3 mins)
• Pelvic thrusting rare	• Pelvic-thrusting common
• Arching of the head, neck and spine rare	• Arching of the head, neck and spine common
• Clonic head movements to one side may occur	• Side-to-side movements of the head/body
• Initial scream, then grunting	• Crying during/after seizure
• Plantar response may be abnormal (big toe up)	• Plantar response normal (big toe flexed down)
BTCS: post-ictal	**Functional seizures: post-ictal**
• Gradual slowing down of seizure	• Rapid end to seizure
• Gradual post-ictal recovery	• Rapid post-ictal recovery
• Noisy/laboured post-ictal breathing	• Normal post-ictal breathing (or slow after hyperventilation)
BTCS: history	**Functional seizures: history**
• Onset under 10 years old	• Onset over 15 years old
• Alcohol misuse	• Recurrent 'status epilepticus' (a misdiagnosis)
• Provoked seizure (e.g. brain injury, infection)	• PTSD or other manifestations of functional neurological disorder

3. Functional/Dissociative Seizures

- Functional or dissociative seizures are a common cause of prolonged convulsive seizures. They are the most important differential diagnosis of epileptic seizures in the emergency setting. Functional seizures are an involuntary psychological response to distress and are commonly associated with a history of emotional trauma (e.g. abuse or neglect, potentially in childhood). Many patients with functional seizures have received an erroneous diagnosis of epilepsy. Such patients may be receiving antiseizure medications intended for epilepsy which are ineffective for functional seizures. Those who have received a diagnosis of functional seizures may know their condition by another name, e.g. non-epileptic attack disorder (NEAD), psychogenic seizures, conversion disorder or pseudo-seizures. The term pseudo-seizures should be avoided by health care professionals as it suggests the events are made up or put on, which can be upsetting for patients. (Involuntary) functional seizures are much more common than (voluntary) malingered seizures (deliberately acted out for some kind of personal gain).

- In contrast to seizures caused by epilepsy, convulsive activity in functional or dissociative

Seizures in Adults

seizures often continues for more than 5 minutes and functional seizures are commonly mistaken for status epilepticus. See Table 3.109 for a guide on distinguishing functional seizures from status epilepticus. Even prolonged functional seizures do not put the patient at risk of physiological derangement or brain damage. Emergency treatment with medication intended epilepsy is not effective and is potentially dangerous because it puts patients at risk of the side effects including respiratory depression, aspiration and death. Many patients with functional seizures have an emergency care plan which should be taken into account in decisions about treatment.

- Because of the similarity of functional seizures and CSE, it is important to note and record the characteristics of the seizures as accurately as possible. This aids assessment and treatment, and it also assists specialists in making the diagnosis in retrospect. For the same reason, families and carers may have been asked by specialists to video-record the events, and they should be encouraged to do so.

4. Syncope

- Vasovagal syncope (fainting) is the most common cause of transient loss of consciousness (refer to **Altered Levels of Consciousness**). People who faint usually feel dizzy and sweaty, get visual symptoms (blurred/white/black vision, seeing stars) and may experience distortion of hearing before they collapse. Brief but vigorous jerking may occur. This can mimic an epileptic seizure, although the jerking usually stops within less than 20 seconds, once normal cerebral circulation is restored and patients are rapidly reorientated after an event.

5. Alcohol

- Alcohol withdrawal is an important cause of seizures. Acute intoxication is a cause of reduced/loss of consciousness. Alcohol withdrawal and delirium tremens is a cause of seizures and requires urgent medical treatment and assessment in hospital. Treat ongoing seizures as below.

- Chronic alcohol overuse predisposes to seizures. Consider referring the patient to an alcohol misuse service as per locally agreed pathways. Refer to **Alcohol-Use Disorders**.

6. Driving

- The DVLA has specific and legal regulations regarding seizures and other causes of lost/altered consciousness. Epileptic seizures and the other conditions mentioned in this guideline are a common medical cause of collapse at the wheel. It is a legal requirement for drivers to inform the DVLA themselves if they have a medical condition that could affect driving.

- When it is appropriate, particularly when discharging a patient who is a driver and not conveying them to a healthcare facility, ambulance clinicians should:
    - advise the patient on the possible impact of their medical condition on their driving ability.
    - advise the patient on their legal requirement to notify the DVLA about seizures.
    - document any of the above if it is discussed with the patient.

Note that the patient could be fined up to £1,000 if they do not tell the DVLA about a medical condition that affects their driving, and they could be prosecuted if they are involved in an accident as a result.

If an ambulance clinician is concerned that the patient cannot or will not notify the DVLA themselves, it would be appropriate to liaise with the patient's GP and to document these actions.

7. Assessment and Management

Assessment and management of seizures varies according to:

- whether the seizure is ongoing/recurrent or has stopped (see Figure 3.41)
- what the manifestations of the seizure are; see Figure 3.41 to ascertain the presentation. If the convulsive seizure is ongoing or recurrent, refer to Table 3.110. If the seizure has stopped, refer to Table 3.111

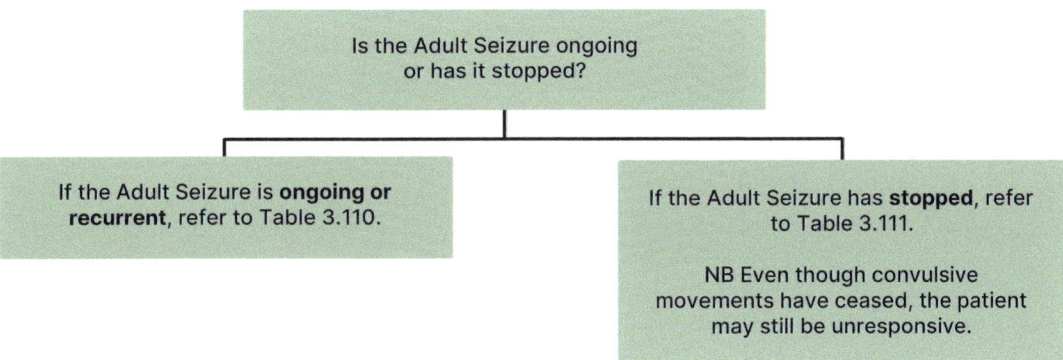

Figure 3.41 – Initial assessment and management of seizures in adults.

Seizures in Adults

TABLE 3.110 – ASSESSMENT and MANAGEMENT of: ONGOING/RECURRENT Adult Seizures

General

Assess <C>ABCDE

- Assess for, and simultaneously manage, immediately life-threatening conditions using the <C>ABCDE approach.

Correct Position

- Position the patient for safety and comfort. Protect from dangers, especially aspiration and head injuries, during the seizure.

History

- Take a focused history while simultaneously managing **<C>ABCDE**. Establish key information from carers/witnesses (if available). Consider all causes of seizures, especially potential provoking factors for epileptic seizures. Try to establish:
  - an estimate of the duration of the seizure.
  - if this is an isolated seizure or if there has been a cluster of seizures.
  - whether the patient already has a diagnosis of epilepsy or functional/dissociative seizures (and if there is a history of previous seizures regardless of formal diagnoses made by doctors).
  - whether there is a personalised seizure emergency management plan if the patient is already known to have a seizure disorder.
  - if the patient is compliant with antiseizure medication.
  - if the patient has a usual pattern (e.g. frequency and duration) to their seizures (is this different?).
  - whether any medication has already been administered to terminate the seizure.
  - if there were any symptoms preceding the seizure providing hints to its underlying cause and the need for additional emergency interventions (e.g. treatment of hypoglycaemia, thiamine deficiency, meningitis).
  - if the patient is pregnant and if the gestational age is ≥20 weeks, or within 14 days post-partum, suspect eclampsia and refer to **Pre-eclampsia and Eclampsia** and **Magnesium Sulfate**. In unknown or uncertain gestation, if the top of the uterus (fundus) is at or above the level of the umbilicus treat the patient as though they are over 20 weeks gestation.
  - relevant past medical history (including diabetes, hypertension, heart disease, cerebrovascular disease, dementia) and medication use.
  - any other potential provoking factors such as alcohol intake and illicit drug use.

Observe/Inspect

Description of the Seizure

Because of the similarity of functional seizures to convulsive status epilepticus (CSE) it is important to note and record the characteristics of the seizures as accurately as possible. This aids assessment and treatment during the seizure, but it also assists specialists in making the diagnosis in retrospect. For the same reason, families and carers may have been asked by specialists to video-record the events, and they should be encouraged to do so.

- Observe and record types of movements and record the parts of the body that are affected (see Table 3.109).
- Are they focal (affecting only part of the body) or bilateral (generalised) seizures. Do they involve rhythmic muscle spasms (myoclonic jerks) or only some focal effect like lip smacking or plucking at clothes?
- Assess the level of consciousness. What is the GCS? If it is a focal seizure, does the patient have impaired awareness?

Airway

Assess and Manage as Appropriate

- Consider an oropharyngeal airway but do not attempt to force an oropharyngeal airway into a convulsing patient if there is trismus or if it is not tolerated. Inability to tolerate an airway adjunct is suggestive of a GCS >3, which is not consistent with a bilateral tonic-clonic seizure (BTCS). A nasopharyngeal airway can be a useful adjunct. Use caution in patients who may have a basal skull fracture or facial injury.

Seizures in Adults

TABLE 3.110 – ASSESSMENT and MANAGEMENT of: ONGOING/RECURRENT Adult Seizures
(continued)

Breathing

Assess Breathing Rate and Quality

- BTCS causes cessation of effective respiration. Functional/dissociative seizures may involve breath-holding interspersed with periods of hyperventilation. Refer to **Hyperventilation Syndrome** guideline if relevant.
- For BTCS administer high-concentration oxygen using a reservoir mask at 15 l/min, until a reliable oximetry measurement can be obtained; clinicians should then aim for an oxygen saturation of 94–98% (or 88–92% if the patient is at risk of hypercapnic respiratory failure, e.g. COPD). Refer to **Oxygen**.
- If assessment indicates the patient has a functional/dissociative seizure, then oxygen should **not** normally be administered; measure oxygen saturation and only administer oxygen if it is actually required (SpO_2 of 93% or less).
- In convulsive state epilepticus (CSE), if pulse oximetry is low and/or end tidal CO_2 is high, and respirations are ineffective, then assist ventilation with a bag-valve-mask device (with suitable airway adjuncts, and supplemental oxygen); this may be difficult during the convulsive phase of seizure (but will be possible if there are pauses between seizures, or in the post-ictal period).
- Benzodiazepines can cause respiratory depression or apnoea, always anticipate this and be prepared to assist ventilations if required.

Circulation

Blood Pressure

- Measure BP as soon as possible. Suspect eclampsia as a cause of hypertension if the patient is pregnant (gestational age ≥20 weeks) or within 14 days post-partum. Refer to **Pre-eclampsia and Eclampsia** and **Magnesium Sulfate**.
- Benzodiazepines can cause hypotension (especially in the elderly or frail) and this should be anticipated.

Heart Rate and Rhythm

- Monitor heart rate and rhythm. Cardiac dysrhythmia can cause transient loss of consciousness and convulsive seizures (hypoxic seizures). However, sinus tachycardia is normal during epileptic or functional seizures. Refer to **Cardiac Arrhythmia and Sudden Cardiac Death** if relevant. Record a 12-lead ECG when possible, where the diagnosis is unclear. Document your interpretation of the ECG.
- Rarely, epileptic seizures or status epilepticus can trigger abnormal heart rhythms requiring ECG monitoring or even defibrillation.
- Rarely benzodiazepines can also cause arrhythmias.

IV Access

- Assess the need for IV access, taking into account individual circumstances. Consider the possible need for IV administration of emergency drugs, taking into account the choice of drug and alternative routes of administration.
- If a first dose of benzodiazepine (IM, buccal or PR) has been administered, and the seizure is ongoing, prepare to administer a further dose of benzodiazepine.

Disability

Consciousness

- Assess consciousness using AVPU and GCS. Take special care to record how the patient responds to voice and provide an opportunity for the patient to respond by grunting or moving part of a limb (e.g. squeezing the hand of the examiner). Ongoing convulsive seizures in patients who are responsive are likely to be functional seizures. Refer to Table 3.109.

Pupils

- Check pupillary light response. Observing eye movements during testing of the pupillary light response is more effective than painful stimuli in detecting responsivity in patients with functional seizures. Resisted eye opening or pupils that are responding may suggest functional/dissociative seizures, unequal pupils suggest a seizure provoked by intra-cranial pathology.

(continued)

Seizures in Adults

TABLE 3.110 – ASSESSMENT and MANAGEMENT of: ONGOING/RECURRENT Adult Seizures *(continued)*

Neurological deficit
- Assess for neurological deficit, motor and sensory, which may indicate a temporary postictal deficit (Todd's paralysis) or that the seizure may be secondary to a stroke.

Blood Glucose Level
- Measure capillary blood glucose and document the result. If glucose is <4 mmol/l, treat according to **Glycaemic Emergencies in Adults and Children**.

Exposure

Temperature
- Measure temperature. A raised temperature may indicate that the patient has an infection. Consider cerebral infections, especially meningococcal meningitis. Refer to **Meningococcal Meningitis and Septicaemia** if this is suspected. Epileptic seizures can cause a rise in body temperature in the absence of infection.

Injuries
- A head injury may be the cause of a seizure, i.e. a provoked seizure or may have occurred as a consequence of the seizure.
- This may have occurred in the context of a major trauma, RTC or could be due to a fall. Treat the head injury and the seizure in parallel.
- Seizures may cause injuries. Treat injuries as appropriate. Common minor injuries are facial contusions, dental injuries, joint dislocation and trauma to the tongue and lips. These should be noted even if they do not require immediate treatment because they are important factors for specialists to consider when trying to make a diagnosis in retrospect.

Incontinence
- Urinary incontinence regularly occurs in epileptic seizures but may also also occur in functional seizures or vasovagal episodes (rarely). It is not a good discriminator between epileptic seizures and functional seizures, but it is an important feature and it should be noted.

Rash
- Assess closely for a non-blanching rash using natural light if possible (or non-fluorescent light to avoid a blue tinge). Consider moistening the skin (if unbroken) to enhance the visibility of skin changes. A purpuric rash and fever is highly predictive of meningococcal infection/meningitis, which can cause seizures (refer to **Meningococcal Meningitis and Septicaemia**).

Pregnancy
- Examine the abdomen of female patients. Is there a palpable uterus? Is there possibility of eclampsia?
- If the top of the uterus (fundus) is at or above the level of the umbilicus treat the patient as though they are over 20 weeks gestation and refer to **Pre-eclampsia and Eclampsia** and **Magnesium Sulfate**.

Medications
- Benzodiazepines (midazolam or diazepam) are indicated for patients who are currently having bilateral tonic-clonic seizures (at the time of medication administration) AND who have:
  - Seizures lasting 5 minutes or more **OR**
  - 2 or more seizures without recovery between (lasting over 5 minutes) **OR**
  - 3 or more seizures in the last 24 hours (if this is abnormal for them)

OR

- Treat patients currently having focal seizures (lasting over 10 minutes) with some element of convulsion (e.g. muscle or myoclonic twitch) AND impairment of consciousness.
- Where a patient presents with focal motor seizures that evolve into BTCS the total seizure time including both focal and BTCS activity should be counted when determining the time at which anticonvulsants should be administered.

Seizures in Adults

TABLE 3.110 – ASSESSMENT and MANAGEMENT of: ONGOING/RECURRENT Adult Seizures *(continued)*

- Do not routinely treat adults suffering from focal aware seizures if they have a normal GCS. Adults suffering from focal aware seizures (with or without some element of seizure activity) should be conveyed for further assessment without treatment or (if the seizure is severe, causing distress or is prolonged) seek advice from a senior clinician.
- When attending a patient who has had previous administration of benzodiazepine:
  - If less than 4 hours since their first dose move to second dose. If the patient has already had two doses, seek senior support.
  - If over 4 hours since last dose of benzodiazepine, start treatment regimen again. Refer to patient's individual care plan if available.
- The maximum dose is two administrations of full recommended doses within 4 hours.
- In those who require emergency medical treatment for CSE; many will respond to pre-hospital treatment and the seizure will terminate. A priority is therefore timely and effective delivery of a dose(s) of a benzodiazepine drug via the optimal route of administration and then appropriate supportive care.
- If the seizure continues 10 minutes after the maximum dose of benzodiazepines, then consider the following:
  - alternative diagnosis, including functional seizures.
  - reasons for lack of effect, such as poor administration/absorption, patient size or inadequate dose.
  - any access to alternative route or second-line anti-convulsants (e.g. pre-hospital critical care).
- After prolonged seizures or drug treatment, anticipate and prepare for airway obstruction, respiratory depression/apnoea, hypotension and cardiac arrhythmia – resuscitation equipment **must** be immediately available at all times.
- In CSE when drug treatment is required, consider the following key points:
  - Time is crucial, benzodiazepines become less effective as time passes, **do not delay administration**.
  - The correct timing of administration is more important than the route.

Do not titrate them to effect, give the entire dose (once started) even if the seizure then stops. This will reduce the chance of the seizure recurring.

Conveyance and Referral

- All patients having their first seizure should be transported to hospital for investigation.
- All pregnant patients must be conveyed to the nearest hospital with consultant-led obstetric service. Refer to **Pre-eclampsia and Eclampsia**.
- A small proportion of patients will not respond to two doses of benzodiazepine treatment and will require time-critical transport to hospital. Preparing and transferring the patient for conveyance is therefore a competing priority; decisions about how long to treat at the scene, when to transport and to what extent the treatment and conveyance can happen simultaneously need to be made on a case-by-case basis. Second line agents may be required via a prehospital critical care team. Seek senior support if required.
- The following factors should be taken into account:
  - Time since onset of seizure(s).
  - Diagnosis (status epilepticus, functional seizure, uncertainty).
  - Pre-existing personalised seizure management plans.
  - Relative ease or difficulty of extricating the patient to the ambulance.
  - Distance from hospital and transport time.
  - Availability of an effective drug and route of administration.
  - Co-existing acute or chronic medical conditions.

Seizures in Adults

TABLE 3.111 – ASSESSMENT and MANAGEMENT of: STOPPED Adult Seizures

General

Assess <C>ABCDE

- Assess for, and simultaneously manage, immediately life-threatening conditions using the **<C>ABCDE** approach.
- Most patients will spontaneously make a full recovery after a seizure. The aim for these patients is to support them as they recover. However, all patients should undergo a careful assessment once their seizure has stopped to identify the small number with a serious underlying illness as well as those patients who have sustained serious injuries during the seizure.
- In Convulsive Status Epilepticus (CSE) it is common for seizures to pause, then restart, with no recovery in-between. If the patient is still unresponsive (but is no longer convulsing), be prepared for a further convulsive episode to recur.

Correct Position

- Position the patient for comfort and protect from dangers, especially aspiration if the patient remains obtunded. Consider placing in the recovery position.

History

- Take a focused history from patients and other informants, including previous episodes, while simultaneously managing **<C>ABCDE**. After an epileptic seizure, patients are often confused, drowsy and agitated. It can take minutes or hours for them to return to normal consciousness and they are unlikely to be able to give a reliable history immediately after a seizure. After functional seizure or syncope, the recovery is usually more rapid. Establish key information from carers/witnesses (if there are any available). Consider all causes of seizures, especially potential provoking factors for epileptic seizures. Try to establish:
  – an estimate of the duration of the seizure.
  – whether the patient already has a diagnosis of epilepsy or functional seizures (and if there is a history of previous seizures regardless of formal diagnosis).
  – whether there is a personalised seizure emergency management plan if the patient is already known to have a seizure disorder.
  – if the patient is compliant with antiseizure medication.
  – if this is an isolated seizure or if there has been a cluster of seizures.
  – if the patient has a usual pattern (e.g. frequency and duration) to their seizures (is this different?).
  – whether any medication has already been administered to terminate the seizure.
  – if there were any symptoms preceding the seizure providing hints to its underlying cause/need for additional emergency interventions (e.g. treatment of hypoglycaemia, thiamine deficiency, meningitis).
  – if the patient is ≥20 weeks pregnant or within 14 days post-partum suspect eclampsia and refer to **Pre-eclampsia and Eclampsia** and **Magnesium Sulfate**. In unknown or uncertain gestation, if the top of the uterus (fundus) is at or above the level of the umbilicus treat the patient as though they are over 20 weeks gestation.
  – relevant past medical history (including diabetes, hypertension, heart disease, cerebrovascular disease, dementia) and medication use.
  – any other potential provoking factors such as alcohol intake and illicit drug use.

Description of the Seizure

- An accurate assessment, including a detailed description of events, is very important during and after a seizure. Based on witness accounts and the events that you witnessed, write a detailed account of the events.

Airway

Assess and Manage as Appropriate

- Consider an oropharyngeal or nasopharyngeal airway.

Seizures in Adults

TABLE 3.111 – ASSESSMENT and MANAGEMENT of: STOPPED Adult Seizures *(continued)*

Breathing

Assess Breathing Rate and Quality

- Respiration usually rapidly returns to normal after cessation of a seizure.
- Measure oxygen saturations and only administer oxygen if it is actually required (SpO_2 of 93% or less). Refer to **Oxygen**.
- Benzodiazepines can cause respiratory depression or apnoea, even after the seizure has terminated, always anticipate this, monitor carefully and be prepared to assist ventilations if required.

Circulation

Blood Pressure

- Measure BP. Suspect eclampsia as a cause of hypertension if the patient is pregnant (gestational age ≥20 weeks) or within 14 days post-partum. Refer to **Pre-eclampsia and Eclampsia** and **Magnesium Sulfate**.
- Benzodiazepines can cause hypotension (especially in the elderly or frail) and this should be anticipated.

Heart Rate and Rhythm

- Monitor heart rate and rhythm. Perform a 12-lead ECG if the diagnosis is unclear. Document your interpretation of the ECG. Cardiac arrhythmias are an important cause of transient loss of consciousness and suspected seizures, so an ECG is an important part of the assessment of a patient after an undifferentiated seizure.
- Rarely benzodiazepines can also cause arrhythmias.

IV Access

- Assess the risk of another seizure and the potential need for IV access, taking into account individual circumstances. Consider the possible need for IV administration of emergency drugs, taking into account the choice of drug and the alternative routes of administration.

Disability

Consciousness

- Assess consciousness using AVPU and GCS. If improving, wait 10 minutes and repeat. Take special care to record how the patient responds to voice, and provide an opportunity for the patient to respond by grunting or moving part of a limb (e.g. squeezing the hand of the examiner). Refer to Table 3.109.
- Check pupillary response.
- After an epileptic seizure, patients are often left confused, tired and aching (this is the post-ictal state). The confusion usually resolves relatively rapidly, leaving the patient alert with a GCS of 15/15. Tiredness, aching and amnesia may persist longer than this, but it is not a cause for concern.

Neurological deficit

- Assess for neurological deficit, motor and sensory, which may indicate a temporary postictal deficit (Todd's paralysis) or that the seizure may be secondary to a stroke.

Blood Glucose Level

- Measure capillary blood glucose and document the result. If glucose is <4 mmol/l, treat according to **Glycaemic Emergencies in Adults and Children**.

Exposure

Temperature

- Measure temperature. A raised temperature may indicate that the patient has an infection. Consider cerebral infections, especially meningococcal meningitis. Refer to **Meningococcal Meningitis and Septicaemia** if this is suspected. Epileptic seizures can also lead to a temporary rise in body temperature in the absence of infection.

(continued)

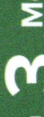

Seizures in Adults

TABLE 3.111 – ASSESSMENT and MANAGEMENT of: STOPPED Adult Seizures *(continued)*

Injuries
- Treat injuries as appropriate.
- A head injury may be the cause of a seizure, i.e. a provoked seizure or may have occurred as a consequence of the seizure.
- This may have occurred in the context of a major trauma, RTC or could be due to a fall. Treat the head injury and the seizure in parallel.
- Seizures may cause injuries. Common minor injuries are facial contusions, dental injuries, joint dislocation and trauma to the tongue from biting. These should be noted even if they do not require immediate treatment because they are important factors for specialists to consider when trying to make a diagnosis in retrospect.

Incontinence
- Urinary incontinence regularly occurs in epileptic seizures. It is also reported by patients with functional seizures and (more rarely) vasovagal episodes. It is not a good discriminator between epileptic and functional, but it is an important feature and it should be noted.

Rash
- Assess closely for a non-blanching rash using natural light if possible (or non-fluorescent light to avoid a blue tinge). Consider moistening the skin (if unbroken) to enhance the visibility of skin changes. A purpuric rash and fever is highly predictive of meningococcal infection/meningitis, which can cause seizures. Refer to **Meningococcal Meningitis and Septicaemia**.

Pregnancy
- Examine the abdomen of female patients. Is there a palpable uterus? Is there a possibility of eclampsia?
- If the top of the uterus (fundus) is at or above the level of the umbilicus treat the patient as though they are over 20 weeks gestation and refer to **Pre-eclampsia and Eclampsia** and **Magnesium Sulfate**.

Conveyance and Referral
- All patients with a first seizure must be conveyed to hospital.
- All pregnant patients must be conveyed to the nearest hospital with consultant-led obstetric service. Refer to **Pre-eclampsia and Eclampsia**.
- The decision whether to convey a patient to hospital after a convulsive seizure is difficult. The overall risk of adverse events is low, and most patients do not require the facilities of a hospital emergency department. But it is important to accurately identify those patients who do need transport to hospital. The following factors should be considered when making this decision:
  - First time seizure as this may be related to significant neurological event.
  - Single or serial seizures.
  - Known seizure disorder.
  - Extent of neurological recovery.
  - Whether the seizures have followed their normal pattern (e.g. frequency or duration).
  - Level of support/supervision. Availability of suitable care pathways.
  - Care plan.
  - Injuries.
  - Treatment with benzodiazepines (these patients should always be transported to hospital unless their care plan states otherwise).
  - Comorbidities including frailty.
  - Access to, and compliance with prescribed anti-seizure medications.
  - The patient's wishes, assuming that they have mental capacity. Refer to **Mental Capacity Act 2005**.

Seizures in Adults

> **TABLE 3.111** – ASSESSMENT and MANAGEMENT of: STOPPED Adult Seizures *(continued)*
>
> - For patients who are not conveyed:
>   – Document the rationale for the decision not to convey.
>   – Advise the patient to make an appointment with their epilepsy specialist or GP to discuss the events and provide them with a copy of the PRF if possible.
>   – Use an alternative care pathway if one is available, for example referral to an epilepsy specialist nurse team.
>   – Advise patients/carers to dial 999 if there are further seizures.
>   – Provide written advice if possible or leave a relevant patient information leaflet.
>   – Advise the patient about driving and DVLA regulations.

8. Emergency Medical Treatment

First-dose benzodiazepines

Consult an individual's emergency care plan if available. Refer to **Midazolam** and **Diazepam Injection** and **Diazepam Rectal**.

- Where a patient presents with focal motor seizures that evolve into BTCS the total seizure time including both focal and BTCS activity should be counted when determining the time at which anticonvulsants should be administered.

Other doses of benzodiazepines previously administered during this episode of care (within 4 hours) for example by carers, should be considered and subtracted from the maximum cumulative dose unless there was clear evidence it was not absorbed.

Midazolam

- If IM or buccal midazolam is immediately available, use this (do not use PR diazepam or delay administration by attempting IV access). IM midazolam is comparative to IV lorazepam used in hospital.
- Ambulance clinicians can administer the patient's own buccal midazolam provided they are competent to administer buccal medications and are familiar with midazolam's indications, actions and side effects, which are very similar to diazepam although midazolam is shorter acting.

Diazepam

- If midazolam is not available, administer IV/PR diazepam. Do not delay administration in an attempt to gain IV access.
- If IV access has been achieved, IV diazepam should be given in preference to the rectal preparation.

After the 1st dose

- Convulsive status epilepticus is an emergency, and can cause permanent brain damage or even death. If the patient continues to seize then move to second dose benzodiazepine.

Second-dose benzodiazepines

- If the seizure is continuing **5–10 minutes** after the first benzodiazepine has been given, a further dose of buccal/IM midazolam or IV/PR diazepam should be administered.
- When using midazolam most seizures will be terminated by the first dose, typically within 10 minutes of administration. Some patients will require a second dose at the 10-minute point (do not delay). However, it is acceptable to give a second dose of midazolam (IM or buccal) after 5 minutes at the clinician's discretion (subject to your PGD). Examples may be if the patient continues to have a severe bilateral tonic-clonic seizure without signs of resolution, has a history of requiring large/repeat doses of benzodiazepines, or who is significantly hypoxic because of the seizure. If the timing between doses is shortened this increases the risk of side effects e.g. respiratory depression/apnoea and/or hypotension.
- **The maximum dose is two administrations of full recommended doses within 4 hours.**
- If the convulsion continues 10 minutes after the maximum dose of benzodiazepines, then seek senior clinical advice to consider the following:
  – an alternative diagnoses, including functional seizure.
  – reason for lack of effect, such as poor administration/absorption, patient size or inadequate dose.
  – any access to alternative route or second-line anticonvulsants (e.g. from pre-hospital critical care).
- After prolonged seizures or drug treatment, anticipate and prepare for airway obstruction, respiratory depression/apnoea, hypotension and cardiac arrhythmia – resuscitation equipment must be immediately available at all times. This risk is significantly increased if they have also received opiates, additional benzodiazepines or alternative central nervous system depressants.

Seizures in Adults

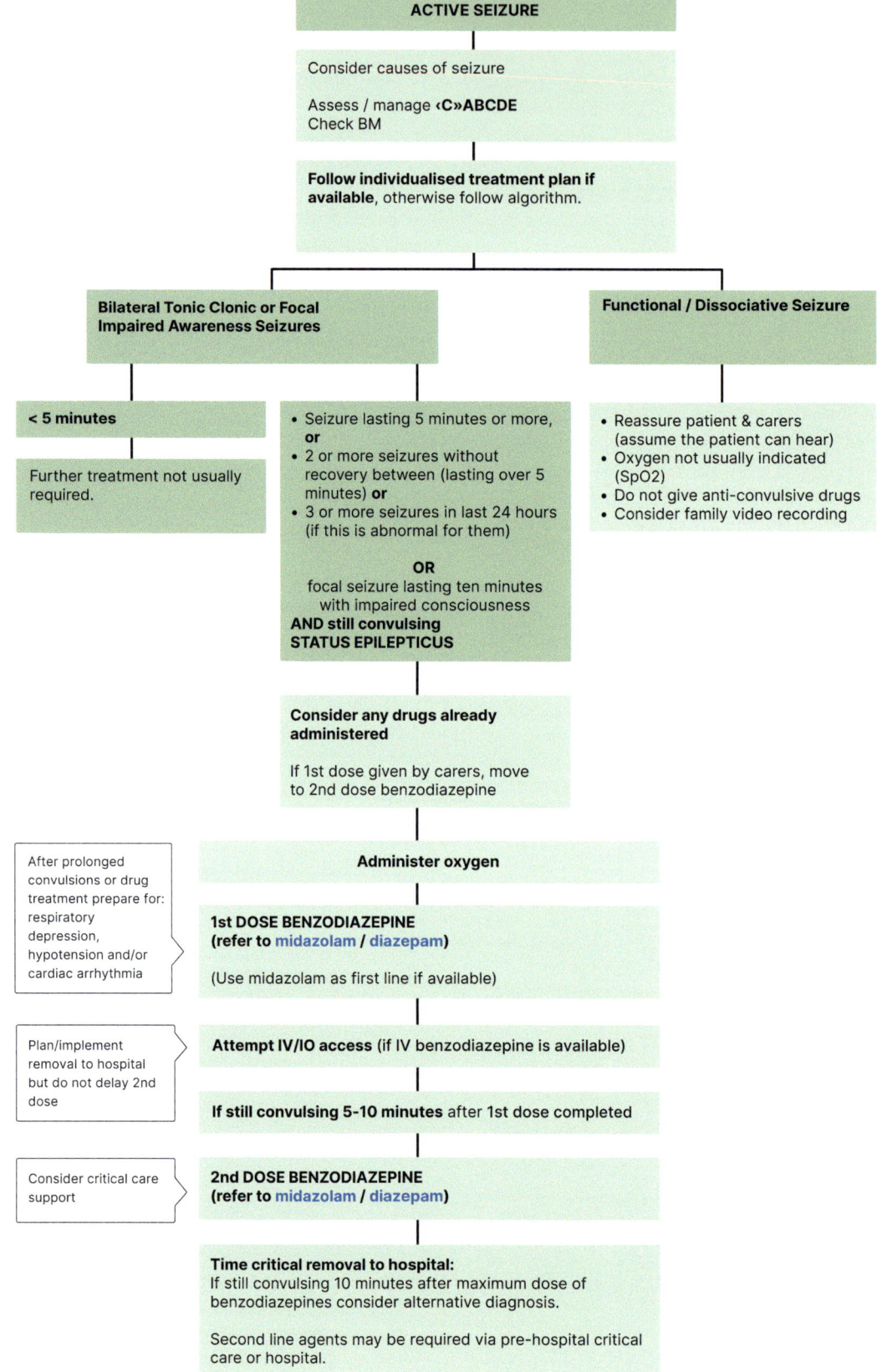

Figure 3.42 – Emergency medical treatment algorithm for adult seizures: ongoing or recurrent.

Seizures in Adults

> **KEY POINTS!**
>
> **Seizures in Adults**
> - Functional/dissociative seizures superficially resemble convulsive epileptic seizures and are the most important differential diagnosis of bilateral tonic-clonic seizures (BTCS) and convulsive status epilepticus (CSE).
> - Most BTCS are self-limiting and do not require drug treatment.
> - All patients with a first seizure should be conveyed to hospital.
> - Individual emergency care plans take precedence over these guidelines.
> - Treat uncorrected hypoglycaemia or hypoxia (where possible) before administering benzodiazepines.
> - Consider referral to an epilepsy specialist nurse team or an alternative care pathway for patients who are not conveyed.
> - If the patient is ≥20 weeks pregnant or within 14 days post-partum suspect eclampsia and refer to Pre-eclampsia and Eclampsia and Magnesium Sulfate.

Bibliography

1. Aldharman SS, Alayed FT, Almutairi FA, Aljohani BS, Alhumaidi KA, Alayyaf AS, Alismail RM, Binshalhoub FH, Alsahil SJ, Alnaaim SA. Intramuscular Versus Intravenous Treatment of Status Epilepticus: A Systematic Review. *Cureus*. 2023 Apr 27, 15(4): e38212.

2. Falco-Walter JJ, Bleck T. Treatment of established status epilepticus. *Journal of Clinical Medicine* 2016, 5(5): 49.

3. Meierkord H, Boon P, Engelsen B, Göcke K, Shorvon S, Tinuper P, Holtkamp M, European Federation of Neurological Societies. EFNS guideline on the management of status epilepticus in adults. *European Journal of Neurology* 2010, 17(3): 348–355.

4. APLS (2021) Bacon et al., Review of the new APLS guidelines (2021): management of the convulsing child. review-of-the-new-apls-guideline.pdf (scot.nhs.uk)

5. APLS Australia and New Zealand (2024) 'Advanced Paediatric Life Support: The Practical Approach 7th Edition', Algorithms | Status epilepticus (apls.org.au)

6. Brigo F, Nardone R, Tezzon F and Trinka E. 'Nonintravenous midazolam versus intravenous or rectal diazepam for the treatment of early status epilepticus: A systematic review with meta-analysis'. *Epilepsy & behavior* 2015, 49: 325–336. Available at: https://doi.org/10.1016/j.yebeh.2015.02.030.

7. Glauser T, Shinnar S, Gloss D, Alldredge B, Arya R, Bainbridge J, Bare M, Bleck T, Dodson WE, Garrity L, Jagoda A, Lowenstein D, Pellock J, Riviello J, Sloan E, Treiman DM. Evidence-Based Guideline: Treatment of Convulsive Status Epilepticus in Children and Adults: Report of the Guideline Committee of the Ameri-can Epilepsy Society. *Epilepsy Curr*. 2016 Jan-Feb, 16(1): 48–61. doi: 10.5698/1535-7597-16.1.48. PMID: 26900382; PMCID: PMC4749120.

8. Jain P, Sharma S, Dua T, Barbui C, Das RR and Aneja S. Efficacy and safety of anti-epileptic drugs in patients with active convulsive seizures when no IV access is available: Systematic review and meta-analysis. *Epilepsy Research* 2016, 122: 47–55.

9. McMullan J, Sasson C, Pancioli A and Silbergleit R. Midazolam versus diazepam for the treatment of status epilepticus in children and young adults: a meta-analysis. *Academic Emergency +-Medicine* 2010, 17(6): 575–82

10. McTague A, Martland T and Appleton R. (2018) 'Drug management for acute tonic-clonic convulsions including convulsive status epilepticus in children'. Cochrane Database of Systematic Reviews, 10;1:CD001905. doi: 10.1002/14651858.CD001905.pub3.

11. National Institute for Health and Clinical Excellence. *Epilepsies in children, young people and adults* (NG217). London: NICE, 2022. Available from: https://nice.org.uk/guidance/ng217.

12. Sathe AG, Tillman H, Coles LD, Elm JJ, Silbergleit R, Chamberlain J, et al. Underdosing of Benzodiazepines in Patients With Status Epilepticus Enrolled in Established Status Epilepticus Treatment Trial. *Acad Emerg Med* 2019, 26: 940–3.

13. Silbergleit R, Durkalski V, Lowenstein D, Conwit R, Pancioli A, Palesch Y and Barsan W. Intramuscular versus intravenous therapy for pre-hospital status epilepticus. *New England Journal Medicine* 2012, 366(7): 591–600 http://www.nejm.org/toc/nejm/366/7/

14. Zhao ZY et al. 'A Comparison of midazolam, lorazepam, and diazepam for the treatment of status epilepticus in children: a network meta-analysis', Journal Child Neurology 2016, 31(9): 1093-107. Available from: https://pubmed.ncbi.nlm.nih.gov/27021145/

Seizures in Children

1. Introduction

- Seizures arise from abnormal electrical activity in the brain. They are usually **bilateral/generalised** (affecting both sides of the body), but may also be **focal**, affecting just one part of the body.
- Seizures may be convulsive (tonic, clonic, or tonic-clonic) or non-convulsive. This guideline relates to convulsive seizures whether they are continuous or intermittent.[5]
- Fever is the commonest cause of seizures (febrile seizures) in children but they can also be caused by epilepsy, CNS infections (meningitis or encephalitis), metabolic conditions, brain tumours, hypoxia, electrolyte imbalances, head injuries or (rarely) hypertension.
- Most seizues stop on their own within 5 minutes (>90%). After 5 minutes, a seizure is unlikely to stop spontaneously. Prolonged seizures become harder to stop with antiseizure medication. As a consequence, if a seizure has not stopped within 5 minutes of its start, emergency (rescue) medication should be given.
- During febrile illnesses not caused by a CNS infection, small children (aged 6 months to 5 years) may develop febrile seizures. This is not epilepsy. They can occur in up to 1 in 20 children.
- A child having seizures that are not triggered by fever requires further investigation.
- Children can suffer functional/dissociative seizures, although this is more common after about 15 years of age. See **Seizures in Adults** for more information.
- Eclampsia is a complication of pregnancy which may occur in women who are ≥20 weeks pregnant (including up to 14 days post-partum) and can give rise to seizures. Refer to **Pre-eclampsia and Eclampsia** for more information.

2. Incidence

- 1 in 100 to 1 in 200 children have active epilepsy.
- It is twice as common in children as in adults.
- It can be related to another underlying condition such as cerebral palsy or a genetic disorder.

3. Severity and Outcome

Febrile Seizures

- Febrile seizures affect between 2–5% of children under 5 years of age.
- Approximately two thirds of children will only ever have one febrile seizure; the remaining third may have further episodes during subsequent febrile illnesses.
- Only a small proportion (reported 5%) of children with febrile seizures will go on to have epilepsy.

Convulsive Status Epilepticus (CSE)

- Convulsive status epilepticus (CSE) is the most common life-threatening neurological emergency in children.
- CSE may occur due to acute illness in children who do not have epilepsy.
- CSE is defined as tonic, clonic, or tonic-clonic seizure (continuous convulsive status epilepticus), or two or more such seizures between which consciousness was not regained (intermittent convulsive status epilepticus) lasting at least 5 minutes.[5]
- CSE lasting at least 30 minutes is associated with an increased risk of irreversible neuronal injury (permanent brain damage) and even death. The short term mortality after CSE in children is approximately 4%. Adverse outcomes are more common in those who have not received adequate prehospital treatment, those who have pre-existing neurological problems and children less than 5 years of age.
- In convulsive status epilepticus 30–40% start as focal. There is a wide spectrum of presentations for focal seizures. In a focal seizure only one side of the body is affected. Focal motor (shaking) signs are more concerning, whether intermittent or continuous, as it may represent a focal brain abnormality which may be developmental (e.g. cortical malformation) or acquired (e.g. brain tumour) and requires treatment.

4. Assessment

(Refer to Table 3.112)

- Correct hypoxia, ensure the child is not hypoglycaemic and seek an underlying cause for the seizure.
- Children with epilepsy in the UK may carry individualised 'Epilepsy Passports', containing essential information about their epilepsy, their emergency care plan and key professional contacts. These should be located, where possible, without delaying treatment.
- Document if the child was unwell or feverish, any serious past medical history and any important events immediately preceding the seizure (e.g. head injury).
- It is not sufficient to simply manage the seizure – the underlying cause for the seizure should also be sought (although this should not delay immediate treatment priorities).
- Seizures can be a feature of meningococcal meningitis/infection. Assess (i) closely for a non-blanching rash using natural light if possible (or non-fluorescent light to avoid a blue tinge) and (ii) examine for neck stiffness (provided there are no concerns of neck injury), since

Seizures in Children

neck stiffness can be a sign of meningitis, and treat if present. Sometimes, moistening the skin (if unbroken) can enhance the visibility of skin changes.

- Establishing that a seizure has fully stopped can be difficult. Following a tonic-clonic seizure, the repeated, regular, rhythmic jerks of the limbs (the clonic phase of the seizure) become less frequent and eventually stop. In the following minutes, the child may show some or all of the following features:
  - brief and irregular jerks of one or more limbs
  - eye deviation
  - nystagmus (jerky eye movements to one side and then back to the midline)
  - noisy breathing.
- Since these features do not **necessarily** mean the child is still seizing, if you are uncertain if there are continued epileptic seizures, do not give further benzodiazepines as further doses may increase risk of respiratory depression and respiratory arrest. Instead transfer the child rapidly to hospital, for further assessment and ongoing treatment.
- Although rare, if you are confident that the seizure is actually a functional/dissociative seizure, consult **Seizures in Adults** for advice on seizure management. If clinically uncertain, then treat for CSE.
- If the patient is pregnant and if the gestational age is ≥20 weeks or within 14 days post-partum, suspect eclampsia and refer to **Pre-eclampsia and Eclampsia** and **Magnesium Sulfate**. In unknown or uncertain gestation, if the top of the uterus (fundus) is at or above the level of the umbilicus treat the patient as though they are over 20 weeks gestation.

5. Management
(Refer to Table 3.112 and Figures 3.43)

- This section describes management of convulsive seizures. If you are treating for functional/dissociative seizures, refer to **Seizures in Adults** (section 3).
- Management follows <C>ABCDE priorities, treating the seizure once ABC issues have been addressed.
- Manage airway, breathing and circulation as usual (also remember to measure the blood glucose, as hypoglycaemia can cause seizures). Essential airway adjuncts may be required to maintain the airway. Administer oxygen and treat shock in the usual way. Oxygen saturation monitoring and capnography (if available) should be applied.
- If the child has an epilepsy passport or emergency care plan, then following it should take precedence over the following guidance.

- Most seizures stop spontaneously (within 5 minutes).
- Benzodiazepines (e.g. Midazolam or Diazepam) are indicated for children who are **currently having bilateral tonic-clonic seizures** (at the time of medication administration) **AND** who have:
  - seizures lasting 5 minutes or more **OR**
  - 2 or more seizures without recovery between (lasting over 5 minutes) **OR**
  - 3 or more seizures in the last 24 hours (if this is abnormal for them)

OR
  - Patients currently having focal seizures (lasting over **5** minutes) **with** some element of convulsion (e.g. muscle or myoclonic twitch) **regardless of whether they have an altered GCS or not (i.e. treat focal aware and focal impaired awareness seizures).**

- Where a patient presents with focal motor seizures that evolve into BTCS the total seizure time including both focal and BTCS activity should be counted when determining the time at which anticonvulsants should be administered.
- Children suffering focal aware seizures that do not have a convulsive element e.g. lip smacking, plucking at clothes or absences should not be treated with benzodiazepines unless their individual treatment plan states otherwise.
- Pre-hospital treatments include Midazolam (IM or buccal) and **Diazepam** (PR). Midazolam (by either route) is more effective than rectal Diazepam (which is the least effective at terminating seizures) so rectal Diazepam should only be used if Midazolam is not available.
- All benzodiazepines may cause respiratory depression/apnoea and rarely hypotension or arrhythmia. Anticipate these side effects, monitor carefully and continuously and be prepared to intervene.
- Do not delay the first dose of antiseizure medication.
- Before administering medication, ensure that the appropriate dose for the child's weight (or age if their weight is not known) is chosen, giving the **full** dose at the appropriate times. Do **not** either i) gradually 'titrate the dose upwards' or ii) only give a partial dose if the seizure stops (even if the seizure has stopped, a full dose must be given since this approach reduces the risk of seizure recurrence).
- If the seizure is continuing 5–10 minutes after the first dose of medication has been given, a second dose of benzodiazepine should be given intravenously or intra-osseously e.g. **diazepam** IV/IO (refer to **Diazepam**) but if this

Seizures in Children

is not possible a second dose can be given IM, buccally or rectally (the least effective route). This also applies if a carer has given the first dose of medication before the clinician arrives on scene.

- Children who continue to seize should have two (and normally only two) appropriate doses of benzodiazepine, regardless of medication or route.
- The maximum dose is two administrations of full recommended doses within 4 hours.
- If the seizure continues 10 minutes after the maximum dose of benzodiazepines have been given, then consider the following:
  - pharmacological reasons for the lack of effect, such as poor administration/absorption, patient size or inadequate dose.
  - availability of alternative second-line antiseizure medication (e.g. pre-hospital critical care Levetiracetam).
  - alternative diagnosis (including functional/dissociative seizures; refer to **Seizures in Adults** and **Pre-eclampsia and Eclampsia**).
- After prolonged seizures or drug treatment, anticipate and prepare for airway obstruction, respiratory depression/apnoea, hypotension and cardiac arrhythmia – resuscitation equipment must be immediately available at all times.

5.1 Hospital transfer/Transfer to further care

- In CSE, after initial assessment, the next priority is to administer benzodiazepines. A plan to extricate the child and transfer to hospital can be made simultaneously. The second dose of benzodiazepines (if required) should be administered after 5–10 minutes and this should not be delayed.
- Pre-alert the hospital if the child continues to seize during the journey or has other features of clinical concern requiring emergency treatment.
- All children having their first seizure should be transported to hospital for investigation.
- If the child has fully recovered and is known to have epilepsy and has only had one dose of benzodiazepine, it may not be necessary to take them to hospital.

TABLE 3.112 – ASSESSMENT and MANAGEMENT of: Seizures in Children

Assess <C>ABCDE

Treat problems as they are found.

- The airway must be cleared – oropharyngeal or nasopharyngeal airways may be helpful.
- Administer high levels of supplemental oxygen (refer to **Oxygen**).
- Assist ventilations with a BVM if necessary.
- Check blood glucose level, and manage if low (refer to **Glycaemic Emergencies in Adults and Children**).
- Monitor vital signs.
- Manage the seizure with medications when indicated (see below).

Medication

- If the child has an Epilepsy Passport or Emergency Care Plan, follow their pre-determined treatment plan (rather than the management described in this guideline, e.g. some children might respond better to a prescribed non-benzodiazepine alternative medication, such as paraldehyde).
- Benzodiazepines (Midazolam or Diazepam) are indicated for patients who are currently having a convulsive status epileptic seizure (at the time of medication administration) **AND** who have:
  - seizures lasting 5 minutes or more **OR**
  - 2 or more seizures without recovery between (lasting over 5 minutes) **OR**
  - 3 or more seizures in the last 24 hours (if this is abnormal for them)

OR
  - Patients currently having focal seizures (lasting over 5 minutes) with some element of convulsion (e.g. muscle or myoclonic twitch) regardless of whether they have an altered GCS or not (i.e. treat focal aware and focal impaired awareness seizures).
- Where a patient presents with focal motor seizures that evolve into BTCS the total seizure time including both focal and BTCS activity should be counted when determining the time at which anticonvulsants should be administered.

Seizures in Children

TABLE 3.112 – ASSESSMENT and MANAGEMENT of: Seizures in Children *(continued)*

First dose of benzodiazepine

Option 1:

- If the child **has** their own supply of medication (detailed on an Epilepsy Passport or an Emergency Care Plan) ask those present if they have already received a dose; if not, administer the patient's own medication.

Option 2:

- If the child does **not** have their own buccal midazolam medication give **IM** or **buccal Midazolam** (if carried) or (if Midazolam is not available) **IV** or **rectal Diazepam** (refer to **Midazolam/Diazepam**).*

* Be ready to support ventilation, as respiratory depression may occur.

Second dose benzodiazepine

If the child **has already received an anticonvulsant** (e.g. patient's own **buccal Midazolam** or **rectal Diazepam** or administration of benzodiazepine by HCP) and the seizure is continuing **5–10 minutes** after administration, the child **should** be given another full dose of IM or buccal Midazolam for their second dose of medication (or IV/rectal Diazepam if Midazolam is not available).

- When using midazolam most seizures will be terminated by the first dose, typically within 10 minutes of administration. Some patients will require a second dose at the 10-minute point (do not delay). However, it is acceptable to give a second dose of midazolam (IM or buccal) after 5 minutes at the clinician's discretion (subject to your PGD). Examples may be if the patient continues to have a severe bilateral tonic-clonic seizure without signs of resolution, has a history of requiring large/repeat doses of benzodiazepines, or who is significantly hypoxic because of the seizure. If the timing between doses is shortened this increases the risk of side effects e.g. respiratory depression/apnoea and/or hypotension.
- When attending a patient who has had previous administration of benzodiazepine:
  - If less than 4 hours since their first dose move to second dose. If the patient has already had two doses, seek senior support.
  - If over 4 hours since last dose of benzodiazepine, start treatment regimen again. Refer to patient's individual care plan if available.
- **The maximum dose is two administrations of full recommended doses within 4 hours.**
- If the seizure continues 10 minutes after the maximum dose of benzodiazepines, then consider the following:
  - pharmacological reasons for the lack of effect, such as poor administration/absorption, patient size or inadequate dose.
  - availability of alternative route or second-line antiseizure medication (e.g. pre-hospital critical care Levetiracetam).
- Alternative diagnosis (including functional/dissociative seizures; refer to **Seizures in Adults** and **Pre-eclampsia and Eclampsia**).
- After prolonged seizures or drug treatment, anticipate and prepare for airway obstruction, respiratory depression/apnoea, hypotension and cardiac arrhythmia.

Other Care

- Record the child's temperature.
- If transporting to hospital, ongoing assessments of ABCDEs and continuous ECG and oxygen saturation monitoring (and $EtCO_2$ if available) should be undertaken, continuing **oxygen** therapy as needed.
- If meningococcal meningitis is suspected, treat with **Benzylpenicillin** en route to hospital (refer to **Benzylpenicillin Sodium**).
- A child who has suffered a seizure and has a fever is likely to be distressed, therefore Paracetamol should be considered (refer to **Paracetamol**).
- A febrile child should wear light clothing only. If the child begins to shiver (e.g. after stripping off all layers down to a nappy), this will potentially raise core temperature and will be counterproductive.

(continued)

Seizures in Children

TABLE 3.112 – ASSESSMENT and MANAGEMENT of: Seizures in Children *(continued)*

Transfer to Further Care

The following should all be transported to hospital:

- Any child who is still seizing (convulsive status epilepticus) must be transferred to further care as soon as possible, preferably after the first dose of benzodiazepine – undertake a **TIME-CRITICAL** transfer, provide an alert/information call. Do not delay the second dose of benzodiazepine.
- Any child with suspected meningococcal septicaemia or meningitis – undertake a **TIME-CRITICAL** transfer, provide an alert/information call.
- All first febrile seizures, even if the child has recovered.
- Any seizure described as atypical for the patient.
- All children with seizures who have required more than one dose of antiseizure medication.
- Any child one year old or less who has had a seizure (even if fully recovered).
- Any child who has not fully recovered from their seizure.
- Where there is any difficulty accessing or compliance to prescribed medication.
- Any child where safeguarding concerns are suspected during medical assessment. The concerns should be documented and reported according to local procedures. (Refer to **Safeguarding Children**).

The following children (over one year old) may not require transport to hospital:

- Children following a febrile seizure:
    - that is **not their first** and
    - **who have completely recovered** and
    - **where the carer is happy for the child not to be transported**
- Children known to have epilepsy, who have recovered from a seizure, have followed their normal pattern and have not required more than one dose of medication do not need to be transported if they are otherwise well and this is consistent with their care plan. A responsible adult must be with the child.

Age 1 years to 5 years - If considered for non-conveyance all clinicians must make a direct referral to another registered HCP as per local trust procedures. If this cannot be arranged by the attending crew, the child must be transported to hospital.

Age 6 to 17 years - The patient's GP should be informed of the child's need for an emergency ambulance attendance.

KEY POINTS!

Seizures in Children

- **Convulsive status epilepticus (CSE) is a medical emergency and is associated with an increased risk of death and serious neurological impairment.**
- **Febrile seizures are a very common cause for a childhood seizure and occur between the ages of 6 months and 5 years.**
- **Most seizures stop spontaneously within 5 minutes.**
- **A seizure lasting 5 minutes (or more) should be treated with benzodiazepines.**
- **Buccal or IM Midazolam or rectal Diazepam are the most widely available emergency medications for childhood seizures in the UK.**
- **First-choice antiseizure medications are usually given buccally/IM or rectally, with buccal/IM Midazolam being the preferred treatment option.**
- **A second benzodiazepine dose should not be delayed.**
- **The full dose for the child's weight (or age if their weight is not known) must be given when treating a seizure.**
- **A child should not usually receive more than two doses of pre-hospital benzodiazepine medication.**
- **Always consider (and actively seek) the underlying cause for the seizure.**
- **All first seizures must be transported to hospital.**

Seizures in Children

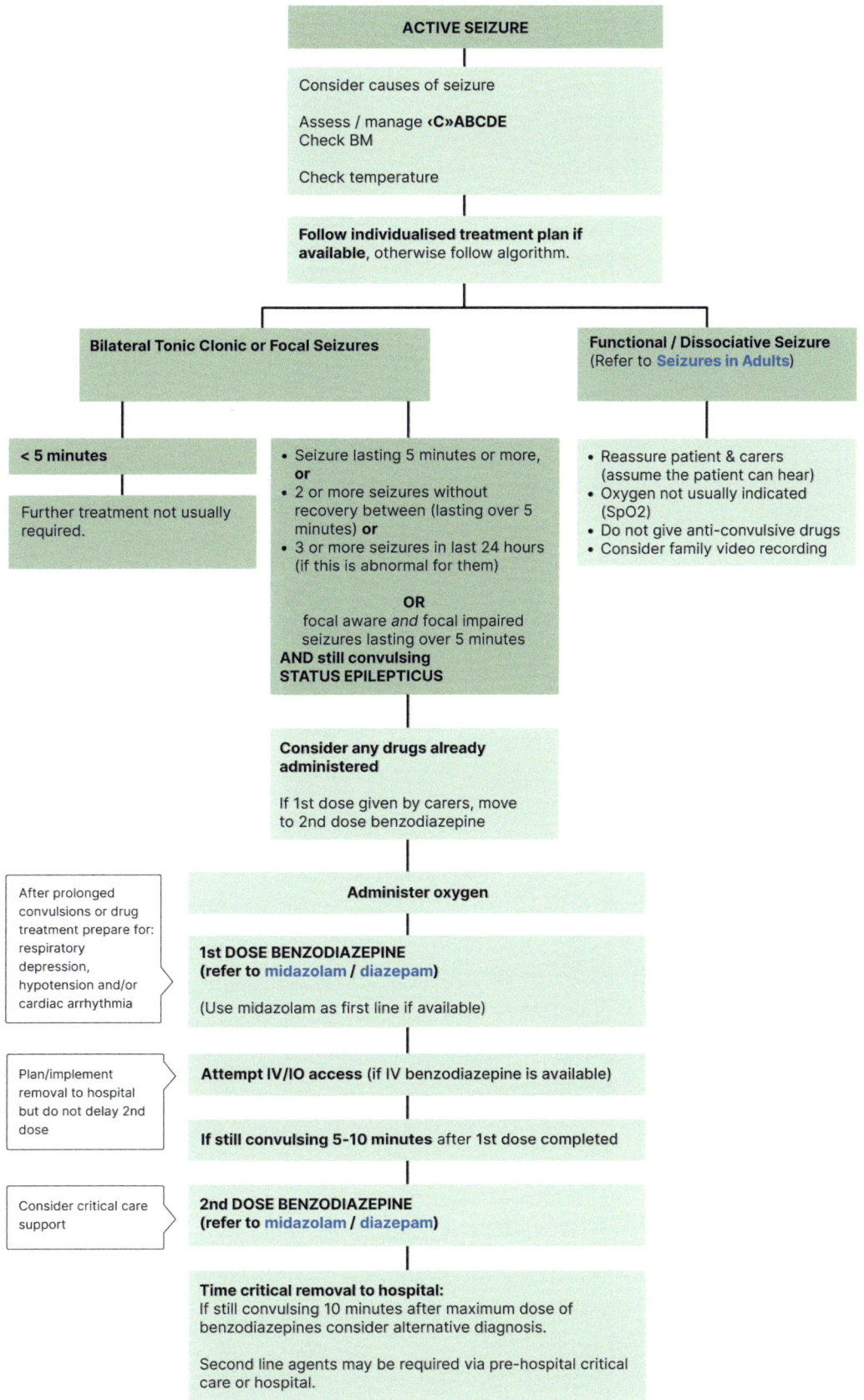

Figure 3.43 – Emergency medical treatment algorithm for child seizures.

Seizures in Children

Bibliography

1. APLS (2021) Bacon et al., Review of the new APLS guidelines (2021): management of the convulsing child. review-of-the-new-apls-guideline.pdf (scot.nhs.uk)

2. APLS Australia and New Zealand (2024) 'Advanced Paediatric Life Support: The Practical Approach 7th Edition', Algorithms | Status epilepticus (apls.org.au)

3. Baysun S, Aydin ÖF, Atmaca E, Gürer YKY. A comparison of buccal Midazolam and rectal Diazepam for the acute treatment of seizures. Clinical Pediatrics 2005, 44(9): 771–776.

4. Brigo F, Nardone R, Tezzon F and Trinka E. 'Nonintravenous Midazolam versus intravenous or rectal Diazepam for the treatment of early status epilepticus: A systematic review with meta-analysis'. Epilepsy & behavior 2015, 49: 325–336. Available at: https://doi.org/10.1016/j.yebeh.2015.02.030.

5. Chin RFM, Neville BGR, Peckham C, Bedford H, Wade A, Scott RC. Incidence, cause, and short-term outcome of convulsive status epilepticus in childhood: prospective population-based study. The Lancet 2006, 368(9531): 222–29. Available from: https://www.sciencedirect.com/science/article/pii/S0140673606690430?via%3Dihub

6. Dreier JW, Li J, Sun Y, Christensen J. Evaluation of Long-term Risk of Epilepsy, Psychiatric Disorders, and Mortality Among Children With Recurrent Febrile Seizures: A National Cohort Study in Denmark. JAMA Pediatr. 2019, 173(12): 1164–1170. doi:10.1001/jamapediatrics.2019.3343

7. Glauser T, Shinnar S, Gloss D, Alldredge B, Arya R, Bainbridge J, Bare M, Bleck T, Dodson WE, Garrity L, Jagoda A, Lowenstein D, Pellock J, Riviello J, Sloan E, Treiman DM. Evidence-Based Guideline: Treatment of Convulsive Status Epilepticus in Children and Adults: Report of the Guideline Committee of the American Epilepsy Society. Epilepsy Curr. 2016 Jan-Feb, 16(1): 48–61. doi: 10.5698/1535-7597-16.1.48. PMID: 26900382; PMCID: PMC4749120.

8. Jain P, Sharma S, Dua T, Barbui C, Das RR and Aneja S. Efficacy and safety of anti-epileptic drugs in patients with active convulsive seizures when no IV access is available: Systematic review and meta-analysis. Epilepsy Research 2016, 122: 47–55.

9. McMullan J, Sasson C, Pancioli A and Silbergleit R. Midazolam versus Diazepam for the treatment of status epilepticus in children and young adults: a meta-analysis. Academic Emergency Medicine 2010, 17(6): 575–82.

10. McTague A, Martland T and Appleton R. (2018) 'Drug management for acute tonic-clonic convulsions including convulsive status epilepticus in children'. Cochrane Database of Systematic Reviews, 10;1:CD001905. doi: 10.1002/14651858.CD001905.pub3.

11. National Institute for Health and Clinical Excellence. Epilepsies in children, young people and adults (NG217). London: NICE, 2022. Available from: https://nice.org.uk/guidance/ng217.

12. Sadleir LG, Scheffer IE. Febrile seizures. British Medical Journal 2007, 334(7588): 307–311.

13. Sathe AG, Tillman H, Coles LD, Elm JJ, Silbergleit R, Chamberlain J, et al. Underdosing of Benzodiazepines in Patients With Status Epilepticus Enrolled in Established Status Epilepticus Treatment Trial. Acad Emerg Med 2019, 26: 940–3.

14. Silbergleit R, Durkalski V, Lowenstein D, Conwit R, Pancioli A, Palesch Y and Barsan W. Intramuscular versus intravenous therapy for pre-hospital status epilepticus. New England Journal Medicine 2012, 366(7): 591–600 http://www.nejm.org/toc/nejm/366/7/

15. The Status Epilepticus Working Party, Appleton R, Choonara I, Martland T, Phillips B, Scott R, et al. The treatment of convulsive status epilepticus in children. Archives of Disease in Childhood 2000, 83(5): 415–419.

16. Woollard M, Pitt K. Antipyretic pre-hospital therapy for febrile convulsion: does the treatment fit? A literature review. Health Education 2003, 62(1): 23–28.

17. Yoong M, Chin RFM, Scott RC. Management of convulsive status epilepticus in children. Archives of Disease in Childhood Education and Practice Edition 2009, 94(1): 1–9.

18. Zhao ZY et al. 'A Comparison of Midazolam, lorazepam, and Diazepam for the treatment of status epilepticus in children: a network meta-analysis', Journal Child Neurology 2016, 31(9): 1093-107. Available from: https://pubmed.ncbi.nlm.nih.gov/27021145/

Sepsis

1. Introduction

1.1 Terminology

- Sepsis is a presentation that may be caused by a number of infective conditions encompassing a pathophysiology of which understanding is still developing. It is identified by multiple clinical signs or symptoms in a sick patient with an infection.

- The diagnosis of sepsis is only confirmed following the analysis of blood cultures and/or hospital admission. However, due to the high risk nature of sepsis, treatment is often instigated prior to a confirmed diagnosis.

- National Early Warning Scores (NEWS) are the best physiological scoring system for assessing sepsis and all causes of clinical deterioration.

- A NEWS2 score greater than or equal to 5 highlights a sick patient who needs urgent clinical review; it does not represent a diagnosis, only a patient at significant risk.

- Not all infections are sepsis. Infection is a continuum from mild to moderate to severe (sepsis) therefore clinical observations should be regularly checked for any deterioration.

1.2 Clinical Judgement

- Clinical decision making is critical in determining suspected sepsis.

- Clinicians can rule out suspected sepsis in mimic conditions (e.g. asthma, diabetic ketoacidosis), and rule in suspected sepsis when they are concerned.

- Over 70% of sepsis cases start in the community, and ambulance clinicians are often the first point of contact.

- If left untreated, sepsis can lead to shock, multi-organ failure and death.

- Ambulance clinicians can help improve clinical outcomes by recognising sepsis early, providing a pre-alert and undertaking a time-critical transfer to an emergency department (ED). Management may include (if indicated) high-flow oxygen, fluid resuscitation and benzylpenicillin if meningitis or meningococcal septicaemia is suspected. (Refer to **Meningococcal Meningitis and Septicaemia**.)

- **Suspect sepsis in adult patients if they:**
  - Look or feel unwell with a history of infection (actively seek a history of a source of infection, e.g. respiratory, urinary, skin)
  - NEWS2 greater than or equal to 5

NB Do not use NEWS2 score for children or for pregnant women up to 4 weeks post-partum. Refer to the **Prehospital Maternity Decision Tool**.

NB A raised NEWS2 score may be due to other conditions, consider a wide differential diagnosis (refer to **Medical Emergencies in Adults**). The higher the NEWS score, the more likely the patient is to be critically unwell.

2. Sepsis Definitions

2.1 Surviving Sepsis Campaign (2016)

- Sepsis is defined as life-threatening organ dysfunction caused by a dysregulated host response to infection.[1] Infections can affect patients in different ways and factors such as a patient's gender, age, race or other genetic determinants. Comorbidities and the patient's environment have a significant effect on the development and progression of an infection. These variations can result in patients with similar infections, having different presentations and different outcomes.[1]

2.2 NICE (2016)

- Sepsis is a clinical syndrome caused by the body's immune and coagulation systems being switched on by an infection. Sepsis with shock is a life-threatening condition that is characterised by low blood pressure despite adequate fluid replacement, and organ dysfunction or failure.

3. Incidence

- There are an estimated 150,000 cases of sepsis each year in the UK, with approximately 44,000 deaths attributed to sepsis. Half of ED sepsis patients arrive by ambulance.[2,3]

4. Severity and Outcome

- Patients transported to hospital by ambulance services are likely to be sicker than those arriving by other means, and 80% of patients in ITU due to sepsis admitted from ED arrive by ambulance services.[47]

- Determining the true incidence of sepsis in the UK is difficult due to inconsistencies in definitions, data sources, and other confounding factors.[37,38,39]

- The UK Sepsis Trust estimated that 200,000 people were admitted to hospitals in England with sepsis during 2017/18,[40] and the mortality rate is approximately 25–30%, with hospital mortality for septic shock approaching 40–60%.[38] In the UK and other middle/high-income countries, sepsis-related deaths primarily occur in the elderly, frail, those with comorbid diseases, and the immunocompromised, many of whom are at or near the end of life.[37] In England and Wales in 2022, sepsis was the underlying cause of 3,770 deaths and was either the underlying cause or a contributory factor in 25,542 deaths.[41]

- Sepsis can affect any age, but it is most common in the elderly and the very young,[42] with 77% of sepsis-related deaths in England occurring in people aged 75 years or older, while approximately 150 sepsis-related deaths occur annually in children aged 0–18 years.[39]

Sepsis

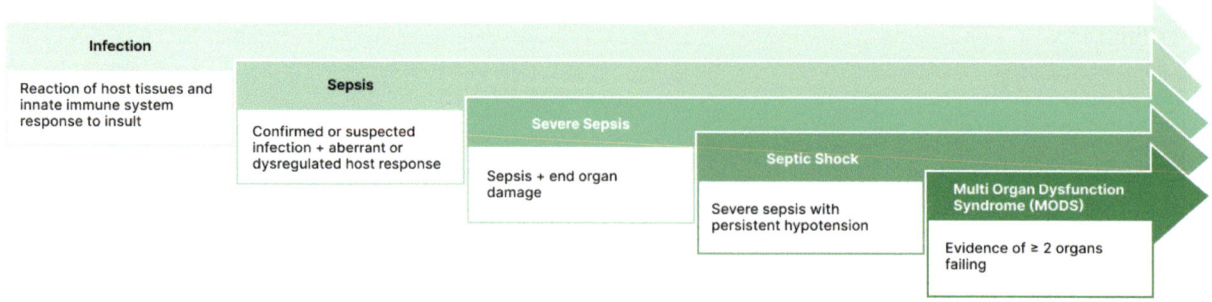

5. Pathophysiology

Sepsis is a multifaceted host response to the invasion of normally sterile tissue by pathogenic, or potentially pathogenic, micro-organisms.[1,12,13] The clinical manifestations of sepsis are highly variable between individuals due to age, underlying comorbidities, the causative pathogen and medications.[1,14]
Small amounts of cytokines are released into the circulation, leading to recruitment of inflammatory cells and an acute-phase response normally limited by anti-inflammatory mediators. In sepsis, there is a failure to control the inflammatory cascade, leading to a loss of capillary integrity, abnormal distribution of microvascular blood flow and stimulation of nitric oxide production, all leading towards organ injury and dysfunction.[12,13] Hypotension usually occurs in the latter stages of the disease process and ambulance clinicians will infrequently encounter patients at this stage of illness.

6. Risk Factors for Sepsis

The following groups of patients are at higher risk of developing sepsis:

- The very young (under 1 year), older people (over 65 years) or people who are very frail.
- People who have impaired immune systems because of illness or medicines, including those:
  - being treated for cancer with chemotherapy/immunotherapy/radiotherapy (refer to Section 7 below on Neutropenic Sepsis)
  - who have impaired immune function (for example, people with diabetes, people who have had a splenectomy or people with sickle cell disease)
  - taking long-term steroids
  - taking immunosuppressant drugs to treat non-malignant disorders.
- People who have had surgery, or other invasive procedures, in the past 6 weeks.
- People with any breach of skin integrity (for example, cuts, burns, blisters or skin infections).
- People who are intravenous substance users.
- People with indwelling lines or catheters.
- Pregnant women and up to 4 weeks post-partum (refer to Section 8 below on Women and Pregnancy).

Consider the following risk factors for sepsis in a new born baby:
  - History of maternal fever during labour or in the 24 hours before and after birth or maternal treatment with intravenous antibiotics for suspected infection.
  - History of having a previous baby with sepsis during the new born period.
  - History of ruptured membranes before labour.
  - Preterm birth following spontaneous labour (before 37 weeks' gestation).
  - Suspected or confirmed sepsis in another baby in the case of a multiple pregnancy.
  - Mother with suspected/confirmed sepsis in the puerperium (up to 4 weeks after birth).

7. Neutropenic Sepsis

- Neutropenic sepsis is a potentially fatal complication of cancer treatments, such as chemotherapy/immunotherapy/radiotherapy. Mortality rates of as high as 52% have been reported in adults.[1545] Patients can have neutropenia as a side effect of the cancer therapy, which increases their risk of developing severe infections. Cancer patients can become neutropenic and not develop normal signs or symptoms of severe infections or sepsis. If a patient is neutropenic and not showing signs of infection but is unwell, this should be taken seriously. Many patients develop this serious complication; therefore, always suspect neutropenic sepsis in patients having cancer treatment who become unwell.
- A neutropenic patient at risk of sepsis can look deceptively well and can deteriorate rapidly. A high index of suspicion is necessary, particularly if a patient who has recently undergone chemotherapy has an increased temperature. Patients who have received treatment within 6–8 weeks are at risk and at higher risk within the first 10 days after treatment.

Sepsis

- Patients may have been given an advice line telephone number to ring by their oncology service. Consider ringing advice lines such as this in line with your local procedures, as it may inform the appropriate destination or care pathway for the patient.
- Any of the following features could indicate that a neutropenic patient has an infection and is at risk of sepsis:
  – tachypnoea
  – tachycardia
  – hypotension
  – temperature greater than 37.5°C
  – pleuritic chest pain
  – shivering episodes/rigors
  – flu-like symptoms
  – catheter site infections
  – cellulitis.
- Note that neutropenic patients are unable to produce the pus normally associated with skin infections.
- Neutropenic sepsis is a medical emergency and all patients should be transported to the nearest emergency department or locally agreed pathway (oncology) with a hospital pre-alert.

8. Women and Pregnancy

- Have a very high index of suspicion for pregnant women who are unwell and have signs of infection (refer to the **Prehospital Maternity Decision Tool**).
- Take into account that women who are pregnant, have given birth or had a termination of pregnancy or miscarriage in the past 4 weeks are in a high-risk group for sepsis.[10] In particular, women who:
  – have impaired immune systems because of illness or drugs
  – have gestational diabetes, Type 1 or Type 2 diabetes or other comorbidities
  – needed invasive procedures (for example, caesarean section, forceps delivery, removal of retained products of conception)
  – had prolonged rupture of membranes
  – have or have been in close contact with people with group A streptococcal infection, for example scarlet fever
  – have continued vaginal bleeding or an offensive vaginal discharge.
- Note that the baseline heart rate in pregnancy is 10–15 beats per minute more than normal and there may be a decrease in systolic and diastolic blood pressure by an average of 10–15 mmHg. Therefore, this should be taken into account when considering sepsis, and rapid transport to definitive care is the priority and not extended on-scene times.
- These physiological changes in pregnancy can mask signs of significant sepsis and shock, and so can also 'render the existing NEWS2 inappropriate because the physiological response to acute illness can be modified in children and by pregnancy'.[16] Therefore, a strong index of suspicion must be maintained and transfer to hospital considered when underlying sepsis is suspected during or after pregnancy.
- Refer to **Maternity Care** for other changes in pregnancy.

9. Assessment

- Assess **ABCD** (refer to **Medical Emergencies in Adults – Overview** and **Medical Emergencies in Children – Overview**).
- Take extra care if the patient cannot provide a history, consider other ways to communicate e.g. language line. Refer to **Patients with Communication Difficulties**.
- Consider sepsis in all patients with non-specific, non-localised presentations, for example feeling very unwell, with a high temperature. Patients may present with an abnormally low temperature, but this is unlikely to be in isolation and will likely be accompanied by signs of peripheral shutdown and organ dysfunction.
- Think about potential infection causing general deterioration, particularly in older patients presenting with new confusion (delirium), falls or new immobility.
- Pay particular attention if concerns are expressed by the patient, or their family/carers, regarding changes in behaviour.
- Examine people with suspected sepsis for a change in their in normal skin colour. Look for cyanosis of the skin, lips or tongue, a non-blanching rash of the skin, any breach of skin integrity (for example, cuts, burns, ulcers or skin infections) or other rash indicating potential infection. Skin mottling may be difficult to detect in dark skin tones.
- If possible, try to identify a source of infection, but do not delay treatment and transfer to do so.
- Use a structured screening tool and NEWS2 score to stratify risk if sepsis is suspected.

10. Signs of Infection

Look for signs of infection by conducting a systems assessment, with particular regard for the areas covered in Table 3.113.

Sepsis

TABLE 3.113 – Signs of Infection

The review of systems should cover the following areas:

• General	• Lethargy
	• Fever
	• Rigors.
• Neurological system	• Severe headache
	• New or increased confusion
	• Signs of meningitis or encephalitis (neck stiffness/photophobia).
• Cardiovascular	• Shortness of breath, shortness of breath on exertion.
• Respiratory	• Shortness of breath, shortness of breath on exertion, increased respiratory rate or effort
	• Cough, productive or non-productive
	• Haemoptysis
	• Pleuritic pain.
• Gastrointestinal	• Abdominal pain or distension
	• Diarrhoea or vomiting.
• Genito-urinary	• A history of UTI symptoms (offensive urine, frequency, dysuria)
	• Reduced urine output
	• Abdominal, flank and back pain.
• Musculoskeletal	• Hot painful joint
	• Non-weight bearing.
• Skin	• Cellulitis
	• Infected ulcer
	• Diabetic foot ulcers, burns, purpuric or other ulcers
	• Burns
	• Non-blanching rash
	• Reduction in normal skin colour.
• Other	• Recent travel abroad
	• Dental infection
	• Exposure to an unwell contact.

NB This is not an exhaustive list and clinical judgement should be used when considering whether a sign or symptom of a serious infection is present.

11. Respiratory Rate

- An increased respiratory rate is an early indicator of illness, and can be one of the first clinical observations to become abnormal. Therefore, accurately measuring respiratory rate (e.g. at least over 30 seconds) is essential. The respiratory rate will increase due to a compensatory mechanism to reduce metabolic acidosis, a consequence of sepsis. Development of sepsis screening tools has demonstrated that respiration rates will be higher in patients with sepsis compared to non-septic patients.[17,18]

- Be aware of underlying illnesses that affect resting respiratory rate, e.g. patients with chronic illnesses, such as COPD, heart failure or pulmonary fibrosis may normally have higher respiratory rates and may not tolerate any new increased respiratory rate well.

- Respiratory rate is particularly important to assess in children, and is a very early sign of illness. It is recommended that children presenting with signs and symptoms of an infection have an accurate respiratory rate measured as it can be an important marker for serious illness.[19]

- Always refer to the relevant '**Page for Age**' for vital signs of normal parameters.

12. Oxygen Saturation in Suspected Sepsis

- Take into account that if peripheral oxygen saturation is difficult to measure in a person

Sepsis

with suspected sepsis, this may indicate poor peripheral circulation because of shock.

- In some groups of patients, taking a pulse oximetry reading may be difficult, for example in children, or those with existing chronic respiratory disease, due to lack of appropriate or suitable equipment, chronic low saturations or patient compliance.
- Patients with chronic airway disease may be at risk of hypercapnic respiratory failure (where normal oxygen saturations are 88–92%) and may have a lower oxygen saturation target that must be taken into account.[44] When assessing oxygen saturation, NEWS2 oxygen saturations scale 2 should be used for patients at risk of hypercapnic respiratory failure. Refer to **Chronic Obstructive Pulmonary Disease**.
- Pulse oximetry can over-estimate oxygen levels, and this inaccuracy is more likely to occur in patients with a dark skin tone than a light skin tone. The SpO_2 reading may misleadingly suggest the patient is within a normal oxygenation range despite oxygen saturations being low. Use caution and a wide clinical assessment to assess for possible hypoxia, particularly reviewing the respiratory rate.

13. Heart Rate in Suspected Sepsis

Interpret the heart rate of a person with suspected sepsis in context, taking into account that:

- Baseline heart rate may be lower in young people and adults who are fit.
- Older people with an infection may not develop an increased heart rate.
- Older people may develop a new arrhythmia in response to infection rather than an increased heart rate.
- Heart rate response may be affected by medicines, such as beta-blockers which may keep heart rate artificially low.

Always refer to the children's '**Page for Age**' for vital signs of normal parameters.

14. Blood Pressure in Suspected Sepsis

- Interpret blood pressure in the context of a person's usual blood pressure, if known.
- Patients may present with a normal BP but still have sepsis, particularly children and young people.

15. Confusion, Mental State and Cognitive State in Suspected Sepsis

- Interpret a person's mental state in the context of their normal function and treat any new changes as potentially significant.
- Be aware that changes in cognitive function may be subtle and assessment should include history from the patient and family or carers.
- Changes in cognitive function may present as changes in behaviour or irritability in both children and in adults with dementia.
- Changes in cognitive function in older people may present as acute changes in functional abilities.

16. Temperature in Suspected Sepsis

- Fever is an important clue in diagnosing illness, but should be evaluated alongside other symptoms and clinical findings. A high fever might reflect a strong immune response rather than illness severity, and absence of a fever does not rule out a serious condition.
- Do not use a person's temperature as the sole predictor of sepsis.
- Do not rely on fever or hypothermia to rule sepsis either in or out.
- Ask the person with suspected sepsis and their family or carers about any recent fever or rigors.
- Take into account that some groups of people with sepsis may not develop a raised temperature. These include:
  - people who are older or very frail
  - people on current or recent treatment for cancer
  - people deteriorating with sepsis
  - infants or young children.

Do not ignore a high temperature or symptoms of fever/rigors as they are useful in highlighting patients with infection.

17. Prehospital Sepsis Screening Tools

- Several pre-hospital sepsis screening tools have been proposed/developed; however, none have been validated in pre-hospital clinical practice.
- JRCALC recommends using tools that have been agreed locally in your own organisation, or across a network or region, and use of a NEWS2 score.

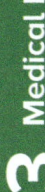

Sepsis

Physiological parameter	3	2	1	Score 0	1	2	3
Respiration rate (per minute)	≤8		9–11	12–20		21–24	≥25
SpO_2 Scale 1 (%)	≤91	92–93	94–95	≥96			
SpO_2 Scale 2 (%)	≤83	84–85	86–87	88–92 ≥93 on air	93–94 on oxygen	95–96 on oxygen	≥97 on oxygen
Air or oxygen?		Oxygen		Air			
Systolic blood pressure (mmHg)	≤90	91–100	101–110	111–219			≥220
Pulse (per minute)	≤40		41–50	51–90	91–110	111–130	≥131
Consciousness				Alert			CVPU
Temperature (°C)	≤35.0		35.1–36.0	36.1–38.0	38.1–39.0	≥39.1	

Figure 3.44 – NEWS2 chart. Reproduced from: Royal College of Physicians. *National Early Warning Score (NEWS) 2: Standardising the assessment of acute-illness severity in the NHS*. Updated report of a working party. London: RCP, 2017. Available from: https://www.rcplondon.ac.uk/projects/outputs/national-early-warning-score-news-2.

18. National Early Warning Score (NEWS2)

- NEWS2 should be undertaken for all patients who are ill, including suspected sepsis. However, NEWS2 should **NOT** be used for pregnant women up to 4 weeks post-natal or children under 16 years[16] (refer to the **Prehospital Maternity Decision Tool**).
- NEWS2 is designed as a system to help to identify a seriously ill or deteriorating patient in a standardised way across the NHS. It is not designed to identify the cause of the clinical deterioration. Its strength is its simplicity and pragmatism – using routine physiological measurements.
- NEWS2 allows healthcare workers to communicate in a common language.
- With regard to sepsis, a NEWS2 score of 5 or more predicts at least a twofold increase in the risk of adverse outcomes, **BUT** NEWS2 does not diagnose sepsis – it simply identifies sick patients who need urgent senior medical review and intervention. The nature of the intervention requires confirmation of the diagnosis.
- NEWS2 is the first step in a two-step process: (1) identification of the sick and/or deteriorating patient, and (2) a timely and appropriate clinical response.
- NEWS2 scores may record lower than the real severity of illness in patients who are taking beta-blockers and/or steroids.
- NEWS2 SpO_2 scale 2 score is only to be used where there is evidence hypercapnic respiratory failure has been confirmed.

National Early Warning Score (NEWS2)

Suspect sepsis in patients:

- Looks/feels unwell with a history of infection (actively seek a history of a source of infection, e.g. respiratory, urinary, skin)
- NEWS2 greater than or equal to 5

NB Do not use NEWS for children or pregnant women or up to 4 weeks post-partum. Refer to the **Prehospital Maternity Decision Tool**.

Where it is suspected a patient has sepsis:

- a score of 7 or more suggests high risk of severe illness or death from sepsis. These patients are critically unwell and need urgent conveyance to ED and pre-alert
- a score of 5 or 6 suggests a moderate risk of severe illness or death from sepsis
- a score of 1 to 4 suggests a lower risk of severe illness or death from sepsis*
- a score of 0 suggests a very low risk of severe illness or death from sepsis*

Sepsis

* unless on beta-blockers, steroids, or recent cancer therapy

NB Patients with a NEWS score of 4 or less with a suspected infection are lower risk, but not at zero risk.

Additional considerations for high risk:

- If a single parameter contributes 3 points to their NEWS2 score.
- New onset of confusion or responds only to voice or pain or is unresponsive.
- Non-blanching rash (petechial or purpuric).
- Cyanosis of skin, lips or tongue.
- Reduction in normal skin colour (mottled or ashen appearance; mottling may be difficult to detect in dark skin tones).
- Not passed urine in last 18 hours.
- Recent chemotherapy (in past 6 weeks).
- Acute kidney injury.
- Bone marrow transplant within last year.
- Recent trauma/surgery/intervention (6 weeks).

Additional considerations for moderate risk:

- History from friend/family of new altered mental behaviour/state.
- Impaired immune system.
- Significant trauma or surgery in the past 6 weeks.
- Not passed urine in the last 12–18 hours.

TABLE 3.114 – Adult Sepsis Risk Levels

High Risk Sepsis – Time-Critical Emergency	Moderate Risk Sepsis
• New onset of confusion or responds only to voice or pain or is unresponsive. • Systolic BP ≤90 mmHg (or drop ≥40 from normal) or mean arterial pressure less than 65 mmHg. • Heart rate ≥130 per minute. • Respiratory rate ≥25 per minute. • Needs oxygen to keep SpO2 ≥92% (or more than 88% in known chronic obstructive pulmonary disease). • Reduction in normal skin colour (mottled or ashen appearance; mottling may be difficult to detect in dark skin tones). • Non-blanching rash (petechial or purpuric). For signs and symptoms of meningococcal disease, refer to **Meningococcal Meningitis and Septicaemia**. • Cyanosis of skin, lips or tongue. • Not passed urine in last 18 hours. • Recent chemotherapy (in past 6 weeks).	The following are markers to indicate sepsis is likely: • History from friend/family of new altered mental behaviour/state. • Impaired immune system (illness or drugs including oral steroids). • History of acute deterioration of functional ability. • Trauma/surgery or invasive procedures in past 6 weeks. • Respiration rate 21–24 per minute or increased work of breathing. • Heart rate 91–130 per minute or new-onset arrhythmia (100 to 130 beats per minute in pregnancy). • Systolic BP 91–100 mmHg. • Not passed urine in the last 12–18 hours. • Tympanic temperature <36°C/axillary temperature <35°C. • Signs of potential infection, including redness, swelling or discharge at surgical site or breakdown of wound.

19. Children and Sepsis

Suspect sepsis in:

- children <16 years that present with fever/feeling unwell

OR

- children with abnormal observations

OR

- children with very worried parents/carers.

In children under 16, grade risk of severe illness or death from sepsis using the child's:

- history
- physical examination results, and
- criteria based on age

If children under 16 with suspected sepsis do not meet any high or moderate to high risk criteria, see them as being at lower risk of severe illness or death from sepsis. However lower risk is not zero risk and patients should be referred to an appropriate care pathway.

NB If children under 16 have two or more moderate to high risk criteria, consider treating as high risk.

Sepsis

TABLE 3.115 – CHILDREN UNDER 5

Criteria for stratification of risk of severe illness or death from sepsis

Category	Age	High risk criteria	Moderate to high-risk criteria
Behaviour	Any	<ul><li>No response to social cues</li><li>Appears ill to a healthcare professional</li><li>Does not wake, or if roused does not stay awake</li><li>Weak high-pitched or continuous cry</li></ul>	<ul><li>Not responding normally to social cues</li><li>No smile</li><li>Wakes only with prolonged stimulation</li><li>Decreased activity</li><li>Parent or carer concern that child is behaving differently from usual</li></ul>
Respiratory	Any	<ul><li>Grunting</li><li>Apnoea</li><li>Oxygen saturation of less than 90% in air or increased oxygen requirement over baseline*</li></ul>	<ul><li>Oxygen saturation of less than 92% in air or increased oxygen requirement over baseline*</li><li>Nasal flaring</li></ul>
Respiratory	Under 1 year	<ul><li>Raised respiratory rate: 60 breaths per minute or more</li></ul>	<ul><li>Raised respiratory rate: 50 to 59 breaths per minute</li></ul>
Respiratory	1 to 2 years	<ul><li>Raised respiratory rate: 50 breaths per minute or more</li></ul>	<ul><li>Raised respiratory rate: 40 to 49 breaths per minute</li></ul>
Respiratory	3 to 4 years	<ul><li>Raised respiratory rate: 40 breaths per minute or more</li></ul>	<ul><li>Raised respiratory rate: 35 to 39 breaths per minute</li></ul>
Circulation and hydration	Any	<ul><li>Bradycardia: heart rate less than 60 beats per minute</li></ul>	<ul><li>Capillary refill time of 3 seconds or more</li><li>Reduced urine output</li><li>For catheterised patients, passed less than 1 ml/kg of urine per hour</li></ul>
Circulation and hydration	Under 1 year	<ul><li>Rapid heart rate: 160 beats per minute or more</li></ul>	<ul><li>Rapid heart rate: 150 to 159 beats per minute</li></ul>
Circulation and hydration	1 to 2 years	<ul><li>Rapid heart rate: 150 beats per minute or more</li></ul>	<ul><li>Rapid heart rate: 140 to 149 beats per minute</li></ul>
Circulation and hydration	3 to 4 years	<ul><li>Rapid heart rate: 140 beats per minute or more</li></ul>	<ul><li>Rapid heart rate: 130 to 139 beats per minute</li></ul>
Skin	Any	<ul><li>Reduction in normal skin colour (mottled or ashen appearance; mottling may be difficult to detect in dark skin tones).</li><li>Cyanosis of skin, lips or tongue</li><li>Non-blanching rash (petechial or purpuric). For signs and symptoms of meningococcal disease, refer to **Meningococcal Meningitis and Septicaemia**.</li></ul>	<ul><li>Pallor of skin, lips or tongue</li></ul>
Temperature	Any	<ul><li>Less than 36°C</li></ul>	-
Temperature	Under 3 months	<ul><li>38°C or more</li></ul>	-
Temperature	3 to 6 months	-	<ul><li>39°C or more</li></ul>
Other	Any	-	<ul><li>Leg pain</li><li>Cold hands or feet</li></ul>

Sepsis

TABLE 3.116 – CHILDREN AGED 5 to 11

Criteria for stratification of risk of severe illness or death from sepsis

Category	Age	High risk criteria	Moderate to high-risk criteria
Behaviour	Any	• Objective evidence of altered behaviour or mental state • Appears ill to a healthcare professional • Does not wake or if roused does not stay awake	• Not behaving normally • Decreased activity • Parent or carer concern that the child is behaving differently from usual
Respiratory	Any	• Oxygen saturation of less than 90% in air or increased oxygen requirement over baseline*	• Oxygen saturation of less than 92% in air or increased oxygen requirement over baseline*
	Aged 5 years	• Raised respiratory rate: 29 breaths per minute or more	• Raised respiratory rate: 24 to 28 breaths per minute
	Aged 6 to 7 years	• Raised respiratory rate: 27 breaths per minute or more	• Raised respiratory rate: 24 to 26 breaths per minute
	Aged 8 to 11 years	• Raised respiratory rate: 25 breaths per minute or more	• Raised respiratory rate: 22 to 24 breaths per minute
Circulation and hydration	Any	• Heart rate less than 60 beats per minute	• Capillary refill time of 3 seconds or more • Reduced urine output • For catheterised patients: passed less than 1 ml/kg of urine per hour
	Aged 5 years	• Raised heart rate: 130 beats per minute or more	• Raised heart rate: 120 to 129 beats per minute
	Aged 6 to 7 years	• Raised heart rate: 120 beats per minute or more	• Raised heart rate: 110 to 119 beats per minute
	Aged 8 to 11 years	• Raised heart rate: 115 beats per minute or more	• Raised heart rate: 105 to 114 beats per minute
Temperature	Any	-	• Tympanic temperature less than 36°C
Skin	Any	• Reduction in normal skin colour (mottled or ashen appearance; mottling may be difficult to detect in dark skin tones). • Cyanosis of skin, lips or tongue. • Non-blanching rash (petechial or purpuric). For signs and symptoms of meningococcal disease, refer to **Meningococcal Meningitis and Septicaemia**.	-
Other	Any	-	• Leg pain • Cold hands or feet

Sepsis

TABLE 3.117 – CHILDREN aged 12 to 15

Criteria for stratification of risk of severe illness or death from sepsis

Category	High risk criteria	Moderate to high-risk criteria
History	• Objective evidence of new altered mental state	• History from patient, friend or relative of new onset of altered behaviour or mental state • History of acute deterioration of functional ability • Impaired immune system (illness or drugs including oral steroids) • Trauma, surgery or invasive procedures in the last 6 weeks
Respiratory	• Raised respiratory rate: 25 breaths per minute or more • New need for oxygen to maintain saturation more than 92%	• Raised respiratory rate: 21 to 24 breaths per minute*
Blood pressure	• Systolic blood pressure 90 mmHg or less or systolic blood pressure more than 40mmHg below normal	• Systolic blood pressure 91 to 100 mmHg
Circulation and hydration	• Raised heart rate: more than 130 beats per minute • Not passed urine in previous 18 hours. • For catheterised patients, passed less than 0.5 ml/kg of urine per hour	• Raised heart rate: 91 to 130 beats per minute (100 to 130 beats per minute in pregnancy) or new-onset arrhythmia • Not passed urine in the past 12 to 18 hours • For catheterised patients, passed 0.5 ml/kg to 1 ml/kg of urine per hour
Temperature	-	• Tympanic temperature less than 36°C
Skin	• Reduction in normal skin colour (mottled or ashen appearance; mottling may be difficult to detect in dark skin tones). • Cyanosis of skin, lips or tongue • Non-blanching rash (petechial or purpuric). For signs and symptoms of meningococcal disease, refer to **Meningococcal Meningitis and Septicaemia**.	• Signs of potential infection, including redness, swelling or discharge at surgical site or breakdown of wound

*Take into account that if peripheral oxygen saturation is difficult to measure in a person with suspected sepsis, this may indicate poor peripheral circulation because of shock, still needing urgent clinical management.

Patients who meet the high-risk criteria should be immediately transferred to an appropriate hospital with paediatric capability. These patients should be treated as time-critical and a pre-alert message passed to the receiving unit.

Clinical observations in children <12 years with suspected sepsis:

- Assess temperature, heart rate, respiratory rate, level of consciousness, oxygen saturation and capillary refill time.
- Measure blood pressure if equipment is available, i.e. a correctly-sized cuff, are available and taking a measurement does not cause a delay in assessment or treatment.

Sepsis

TABLE 3.118 – Sepsis Risk In Children In Relation to Respiratory and Heart Rates

AGE	TACHYPNOEA		TACHYCARDIA	
	Severe	Moderate	Severe	Moderate
1 year	≥60	50–59	≥160	150–159
1–2 years	≥50	40–49	≥150	140–149
3–4 years	≥40	35–39	≥140	130–139
5 years	≥29	24–28	≥130	120–129
6–7 years	≥27	24–26	≥120	110–119
8–11 years	≥25	22–24	≥115	105–114

20. Management

TABLE 3.119 – Management of Sepsis

• Oxygen therapy	• Sepsis is categorised as critical illness and requires supplemental oxygen regardless of initial oxygen saturation reading (SpO$_2$). Administer the initial oxygen dose until the vital signs are normal, then reduce oxygen dose and aim for target saturation within the range of 94–98%. • Oxygen should be given to children with suspected sepsis who have signs of shock or oxygen saturation (SpO$_2$) of less than 95% when breathing air. Treatment with oxygen should be given to ensure oxygen saturation is greater than 94%.
• Fluid therapy	• The choice of fluid is crystalloid, which should ideally be started prior to transportation but should not delay on scene time, then continued en route to hospital. • For adults and children aged ≥12 years with suspected sepsis and systolic blood pressure less than 90 mmHg or mean arterial pressure (MAP) less than 65 mmHg, give an intravenous fluid bolus of 250ml ideally over 10–15 minutes and monitor response but without delaying on scene. A 250 ml fluid bolus can be repeated up a total of 1000ml [49,50] • If the patient remains haemodynamically unstable after 1000ml, the patient should be referred to or discussed with a senior clinical decision maker. • IV fluids should be given to children if haemodynamically shocked or via IO route if unresponsive. Ensure on scene times are not increased or delayed by multiple attempts to gain IV access in children. • For children, give a bolus of 10 ml/kg over less than 10 minutes up to a maximum of 20 ml/kg. Assess response to fluids. Take into account pre-existing conditions (for example, cardiac disease or kidney disease), because smaller fluid volumes may be needed – seek clinical advice. Do not delay on scene gaining intravenous access in seriously ill children.
• Vasopressors	• If a patient remains haemodynamically unstable post administration of 1000ml of fluids, consideration can be given to escalation to critical care. Seek senior clinical advice as per local procedures but do not delay on scene.
• Rapid transport to hospital with pre-alert	• Keep on-scene times to a minimum. • Make a **TIME-CRITICAL** transfer. • Provide a pre-alert and NEWS2 score to the receiving hospital – 'patient has suspected sepsis' – in line with local arrangements. • Handover to hospital using local handover tools, such as SBAR, and give a NEWS2 score:

Sepsis

20.1 Further Management Considerations

Antibiotic Therapy

- If meningococcal disease is specifically suspected (fever and purpuric rash), give appropriate doses of parenteral benzylpenicillin and refer to **Meningococcal Meningitis and Septicaemia**.
- Early studies suggested significant survival benefit from early antibiotic administration in sepsis.[11] However, more recent studies fail to demonstrate such significant benefit. The recent PHANTASi trial, a multicentre randomised control trial, failed to demonstrate a reduction in mortality at 28 or 90 days.[48]
- Recent systematic reviews of prehospital antibiotics in sepsis did not demonstrate a decrease in mortality at 28, 30 or 90 days and did not reduce ICU or general hospital stay.[46, 47]

Paracetamol

- Paracetamol should not be given solely for reducing a high temperature but may be considered if the patient is in pain or to relieve distressing symptoms such as rigors.
- Paracetamol should only be given intravenously if the patient is unable to take anything orally or is in severe pain, otherwise oral paracetamol remains the first-line choice.
- Antipyretics such as paracetamol are often used in ICUs to manage fever in critically unwell patients by reducing the physiological stress fever causes; however, there is limited evidence to show any improvement in mortality.[28,29,30] Paracetamol is not part of any agreed sepsis pathway,[31] may not be beneficial and does not improve outcomes in septic patients.[29,32]
- Paracetamol may mask the abnormal physiology (such as a raised temperature) and therefore treatment opportunities for sepsis may be missed in hospital due to dampening of signs.
- If paracetamol is given this should be highlighted in the SBAR handover at hospital and documented.

Measurement of Lactate and Point of Care Testing (POCT)

- Currently there is insufficient evidence to make a robust recommendation in favour of changing current practice to include pre-hospital lactate measurement.
- NICE have not recommended measuring pre-hospital lactate for suspected sepsis.
- Lactate itself is not a predictor of sepsis. Lactate may be elevated in a number of clinical conditions, and may be normal in cases of septic shock.

Vasopressors

- The use of vasopressors in the pre-hospital setting for sepsis is a topic of ongoing national debate, with limited but emerging evidence. Vasopressors are used to maintain blood pressure in septic shock, a life-threatening condition. Studies suggest that early administration of vasopressors may improve outcomes by reducing time to haemodynamic stability, which is crucial for preventing organ damage.
- However, most research to date is focused on hospital settings, and pre-hospital use remains less established. Some trials have indicated potential benefits, such as improved survival and quicker resuscitation, but there are concerns over safety, including the risk of arrhythmias and complications related to peripheral administration.
- Current guidelines support adequate fluid resuscitation as the first step before the use of vasopressors (which should ideally be started in a controlled critical care environment). More research is needed to determine the safety and efficacy of pre-hospital vasopressor use.
- Critical/enhanced care teams may be able to offer this support and could be considered if a patient has an extended journey time to hospital and has evidence of haemodynamic instability, as per local procedures.

KEY POINTS!

Sepsis

- **Suspect sepsis in patients:**
  - Looks/feels unwell with a history of infection (actively seek a history of a source of infections, e.g. respiratory, urinary, skin)
  - NEWS2 greater than or equal to 5
  - Anyone with a NEWS greater than or equal to 7 should be deemed time-critical
- NEWS2 does not diagnose sepsis – it simply identifies sick patients who need urgent senior clinical review and interventions.
- Keep on-scene times to a minimum.

Sepsis

- **Provide a pre-alert and NEWS2 score to the receiving hospital – 'patient has suspected sepsis' – in line with local arrangements.**
- **Fever is an important clue in diagnosing illness, but its degree should be evaluated alongside other symptoms and clinical findings. A high fever may reflect a strong immune response rather than illness severity, and the absence of a fever does not rule out sepsis.**

Further Reading

Further important information and evidence in support of this guideline can be found in the Bibliography.[33,34,35,36] Other useful resources include:

http://sepsistrust.org/
https://www.nice.org.uk/guidance/ng51

Bibliography

1. Singer M, Deutschman CS, Seymour CW, Shankar-Hari M, Annane D, Bauer M, Bellomo R et al. The Third International Consensus definitions for sepsis and septic shock (Sepsis-3). *JAMA* 2016, 315: 801–810.
2. Wang HE, Weaver MD, Shapiro NI, Yealy DM. Opportunities for emergency medical services care of sepsis. *Resuscitation* 2010, 81: 193–197.
3. Guerra WF, Mayfield TR, Meyers MS, Clouatre AE, Riccio JC. Early detection and treatment of patients with severe sepsis by prehospital personnel. *Journal of Emergency Medicine* 2013, 44: 1116–1125.
4. Van der Wekken LC, Alam N, Holleman F, Van Exter P, Kramer MH, Nanayakkara PW. Epidemiology of sepsis and its recognition by emergency medical services personnel in the Netherlands. *Prehosp Emerg Care* 2016, 20(1): 90–96.
5. Groenewoudt M, Roest AA, Leijten FMM, Stassen PM. Septic patients arriving with emergency medical services: A seriously ill population. *European Journal of Emergency Medicine* 2014, 21: 330–335.
6. Roest AA, Stoffers J, Pijpers E, Jansen J, Stassen PM. Ambulance patients with nondocumented sepsis have a high mortality risk: a retrospective study. *Eur J Emerg Med* 2017, 24(1): 36–43.
7. Gray A, Ward K, Lees F, Dewar C, Dickie S, McGuffie C, Committee SS. The epidemiology of adults with severe sepsis and septic shock in Scottish emergency departments. *Emergency Medicine Journal* 2013, 30: 397–401.
8. Ibrahim I, Jacobs IG. Can the characteristics of emergency department attendances predict poor hospital outcomes in patients with sepsis? *Singapore Med J* 2013, 54: 634–638.
9. Martin GS, Mannino DM, Eaton S, Moss M. The epidemiology of sepsis in the United States from 1979 through 2000. *N Engl J Med* 2003, 348(16): 1546–1554.
10. National Institute for Health and Clinical Excellence. *Sepsis: Recognition, Diagnosis and Early Management* (NG51). London: NICE, 2017.
11. Liu VX, Fielding-Singh V, Greene JD, Baker JM, Iwashyna TJ, Bhattacharya J, Escobar GJ. The timing of early antibiotics and hospital mortality in sepsis. *American Journal of Respiratory and Critical Care Medicine*, 2017. Available from: http://atsjournals.org/doi/abs/10.1164/rccm.201609-1848OC.
12. Bone RC, Balk RA, Cerra FB, Dellinger RP, Fein AM, Knaus WA, Schein RM, Sibbald WJ. Definitions for sepsis and organ failure and guidelines for the use of innovative therapies in sepsis. The ACCP/SCCM Consensus Conference Committee. American College of Chest Physicians/Society of Critical Care Medicine. *Chest* 1992, 101: 1644–1655.
13. Bone RC, Sibbald WJ, Sprung CL. The ACCP-SCCM consensus conference on sepsis and organ failure. *Chest* 1992, 101: 1481–1483.
14. Angus DC, Van der Poll T. Severe sepsis and septic shock. *N Engl J Med* 2013, 369: 2063.
15. Herbst C, Naumann F, Kruse EB, Monsef I, Bohlius J, Schulz H, Engert A. Prophylactic antibiotics or G-CSF for the prevention of infections and improvement of survival in cancer patients undergoing chemotherapy, *Cochrane Database Syst Rev* 2009, 21(1): CD007107.
16. NICE. *National Early Warning Score Systems That Alert to Deteriorating Adult Patients in Hospital [MIB205]*. 2020. Available from: https://www.nice.org.uk/advice/mib205.
17. Polito CC, Isakov A, Yancey AH, Wilson DK, Anderson BA, Bloom I, Martin GS, Sevransky JE. Prehospital recognition of severe sepsis: development and validation of a novel emergency medical services screening tool. *Am J Emerg Med* 2015, 33(9): 1119–1125.
18. Goerlich CE, Wade CE, McCarthy JJ, Holcomb JB, Moore LJ. Validation of sepsis screening tool using StO$_2$ in emergency department patients. *J Surg Res* 2014, 190: 270–275.
19. Davis T. NICE guideline: feverish illness in children--assessment and initial management in children younger than 5 years. *Arch Dis Child Educ Pract Ed* 2013, 98: 232–235.
20. Bayer O, Schwarzkopf D, Stumme C, Stacke A, Hartog CS, Hohenstein C, Kabisch B, Reichel J, Reinhart K, Winning J. An early warning scoring system to identify septic patients in the prehospital setting: The PRESEP Score. *Acad Emerg Med* 2015, 22: 868–871.
21. Wallgren UM, Castren M, Svensson AE, Kurland L. Identification of adult septic patients in the prehospital setting: a comparison of two screening tools and clinical judgment. *Eur J Emerg Med* 2014, 21: 260–265.
22. Seymour CW, Kahn JM, Cooke CR, Watkins TR, Heckbert SR, Rea TD. Prediction of critical illness during out-of-hospital emergency care. *JAMA* 2010, 304: 747–754.
23. Sterling SA, Miller WR, Pryor J, Puskarich MA, Jones AE. The impact of timing of antibiotics on outcomes in severe sepsis and septic shock: A systematic review and meta-analysis. *Crit Care Med* 2015, 43: 1907–1915.

Sepsis

24. Band RA, Gaieski DF, Hylton JH, Shofer FS, Goyal M, Meisel ZF. Arriving by emergency medical services improves time to treatment endpoints for patients with severe sepsis or septic shock. *Academic Emergency Medicine* 2011, 18: 934–940.

25. Seymour CW, Gesten F, Prescott HC, Friedrich ME, Iwashyna TJ, Phillips GS et al. Time to treatment and mortality during mandated emergency care for sepsis. *New England Journal of Medicine* 2017. Available from: http://www.nejm.org/doi/full/10.1056/NEJMoa1703058?query=featured_home#t=articleTop.

26. Shaw J, Fothergill RT, Clark S, Moore F. Can the prehospital National Early Warning Score identify patients most at risk from subsequent deterioration? *EMJ Online First*, 13 May 2017.

27. Jarvis S, Kovacs C, Briggs J, Meredith P, Schmidt PE, Featherstone PI et al. Aggregate National Early Warning Score (NEWS) values are more important than high scores for a single vital signs parameter for discriminating the risk of adverse outcomes. *Resuscitation* 2015, 87: 75–80.

28. Anderson HA, Young J, Marrelli D, Black R, Lambreghts K, Twa MD. Training students with patient actors improves communication: a pilot study. *Optom Vis Sci* 2014, 91: 121–128.

29. Lee BH, Inui D, Suh GY, Kim JY, Kwon JY, Park J, Tada K et al. Association of body temperature and antipyretic treatments with mortality of critically ill patients with and without sepsis: multi-centered prospective observational study. *Crit Care* 2012, 16: R33.

30. Janz DR, Bastarache JA, Rice TW, Bernard GR, Warren MA, Wickersham N, Sills G et al. Randomized, placebo-controlled trial of acetaminophen for the reduction of oxidative injury in severe sepsis: the Acetaminophen for the Reduction of Oxidative Injury in Severe Sepsis trial. *Crit Care Med* 2015, 43: 534–541.

31. Daniels R, Nutbeam T, McNamara G, Galvin C. The sepsis six and the severe sepsis resuscitation bundle: a prospective observational cohort study. *Emerg Med J* 2011, 28: 507–512.

32. Young P. Acetaminophen to treat fever in intensive care unit patients with likely infection: a response from the author of the HEAT trial. *J Thorac Dis* 2016, 8: E631–632.

33. Boland LL, Hokanson JS, Fernstrom KM, Kinzy TG, Lick CJ, Satterlee PA, Lacroix BK. Prehospital lactate measurement by emergency medical services in patients meeting sepsis criteria. *West J Emerg Med* 2016, 17: 648–655.

34. Brown AFT, Cadogan MD. *Emergency Medicine: Diagnosis and Management.* London: Hodder Arnold, 2001.

35. Chamberlain D. Prehospital administered intravenous antimicrobial protocol for septic shock: A prospective randomized clinical trial. *Critical Care* 2009, 13: S130–S131.

36. Tobias AZ, Guyette FX, Seymour CW, Suffoletto BP, Martin-Gill C, Quintero J, Kristan J, Callaway CW, Yealy DM. Pre-resuscitation lactate and hospital mortality in prehospital patients. *Prehosp Emerg Care* 2014, 18: 321–327.

37. AoMRC. 2022. Statement on the initial antimicrobial treatment of sepsis. Academy of Medical Royal Colleges. https://www.aomrc.org.uk.

38. Cecconi M, Evans L, Levy M, et al. Sepsis and septic shock. *Lancet* 2018, 392(10141): 75–87

39. Singer M, Inada-Kim M. and Shankar-Hari M. Sepsis hysteria: excess hype and unrealistic expectations. *Lancet* 2019, 394(10208): 1513–1514.

40. Daniels R and Nutbeam T 2024. The sepsis manual 7th edition. UK Sepsis Trust. https://sepsistrust.org

41. ONS. 2023. Deaths from sepsis in the UK 2001 to 2022. Office for National Statistics. https://www.ons.gov.uk

42. NHS England. 2015. Improving outcomes for patients with sepsis: a cross-system action plan. www.england.nhs.uk/. www.england.nhs.uk/wp-content/uploads/2015/08/Sepsis-Action-Plan-23.12.15-v1.pdf.

43. Lambden, S., Creagh-Brown, B. C., Hunt, J., Summers, C., & Forni, L. G. (2018). Definitions and pathophysiology of vasoplegic shock. *Critical Care*, 22(1). https://doi.org/10.1186/s13054-018-2102-1

44. Royal College of Physicians. (2017, December 19). National Early Warning Score (NEWS) 2. Royal College of Physicians London; Royal College of Physicians. https://www.rcplondon.ac.uk/projects/outputs/national-early-warning-score-news-2

45. Hill JA, Park SY, Gajurel K, Taplitz R. 2023. A Systematic Literature Review to Identify Diagnostic Gaps in Managing Immunocompro-mised Patients with Cancer and Suspected Infection. Open Forum Infectious Diseases. https://doi.org/10.1093/ofid/ofad616

46. Poynter ME, Farrugia A, Kelly E, Simpson P. Prehospital administration of antibiotics in addition to usual care versus usual care alone for patients with suspected sepsis – a systematic review. *Paramedicine* 2023, 21(2). https://doi.org/10.1177/27536386231207055

47. Smyth M, Brace-McDonnell S, Perkins G. Impact of Prehospital Care on Outcomes in Sepsis: A Systematic Review. *Western Journal of Emergency Medicine* 2016, 17(4): 427–437. https://doi.org/10.5811/westjem.2016.5.30172

48. Alam N, Oskam E, Stassen PM, et al. Prehospital antibiotics in the ambulance for sepsis: a multicentre, open label, randomised trial. *The Lancet Respiratory Medicine* 2018, 6(1): 40–50. https://doi.org/10.1016/s2213-2600(17)30469-1

49. Sivapalan P, Ellekjær KL, Jessen MK, Meyhoff TS, Cronhjort M, Hjortrup PB, Wetterslev J, Granholm A, Møller MH, Perner A. Lower vs Higher Fluid Volumes in Adult Patients With Sepsis. *Chest* 2023, 164(4): 892–912. https://doi.org/10.1016/j.chest.2023.04.036

50. Beran A, Altorok N, Srour O, Malhas S-E, Khokher W, Mhanna M, Ayesh H, Aladamat N, Abuhelwa Z, Srour K, Mahmood A, Altorok N, Taleb M, Assaly R. Balanced Crystalloids versus Normal Saline in Adults with Sepsis: A Comprehensive Systematic Review and Meta-Analysis. *Journal of Clinical Medicine* 2022, 11(7): 1971. https://doi.org/10.3390/jcm11071971

51. Ware LB, Files DC, Fowler A, Aboodi MS, Aggarwal NR, Brower RG, Chang SY, Douglas IS, Fields S, Foulkes AS, Ginde, AA, Harris ES, Hendey GW, Hite RD, Huang W, Lai P, Liu KD, Thompson BT, Matthay MA, & National Heart L, and Blood Institute Prevention and Early Treatment of Acute Lung Injury Clinical Trials Network. 2024. Acetaminophen for Prevention and Treatment of Organ Dysfunction in Critically Ill Patients With Sepsis: The ASTER Randomized Clinical Trial. JAMA. https://doi.org/10.1001/jama.2024.8772

52. Ley Greaves R, Bolot R, Holgate A, Gibbs C. Safety of pre-hospital peripheral vasopressors: The SPOTLESS study (Safety of PrehOspiTaL pEripheral vaSopreSsors). *Emerg Med Australas*. 2024 Aug, 36(4):547–553. doi: 10.1111/1742-6723.14396. Epub 2024 Feb 29. PMID: 38423993

Sepsis

53. Jouffroy R, Hajjar A, Gilbert B, Tourtier JP, Bloch-Laine E, Ecollan P, Boularan J, Bounes V, Vivien B, Gueye PN. Prehospital norepineph-rine administration reduces 30-day mortality among septic shock patients. *BMC Infect Dis*. 2022 Apr 6, 22(1):345. doi: 10.1186/s12879-022-07337-y. PMID: 35387608; PMCID: PMC8988327.

54. Dinarello CA. Infection, fever, and exogenous and endogenous pyrogens: some concepts have changed. *The Journal of Infectious Diseases* 2004, 179(Supplement 2): S341–S346.

55. Mackowiak PA, Wasserman SS, and Levine MM. A critical appraisal of 98.6°F, the upper limit of the normal body temperature, and other legacies of Carl Reinhold August Wunderlich. *JAMA* 1997, 268(12): 1578–1580.

56. Saper CB and Breder CD. The neurologic basis of fever. *New England Journal of Medicine* 1994, 330(26): 1880–1886.

57. Young P, Saxena M, and Bellomo R. Fever management in intensive care patients with infections. *Critical Care* 2019, 23(1): 1–9.

58. Klein Klouwenberg PM, Ong DS, Bos LD, de Beer FM, van Hooijdonk RT, Huson MA, and van der Poll T. Interpreting critically ill patients' body temperature. *Intensive Care Medicine* 2015, 41(7): 1213–1225.

Sickle Cell Disease

1. Introduction

- Sickle cell disease is a hereditary condition affecting the haemoglobin contained within red blood cells. As a result, the patient's red blood cells form an abnormal sickle shape which results in increased risk of blockage of the small blood vessels (vaso-occulsion) and red cell breakdown resulting in anaemia.

- A previous history of sickle cell disease and complications will be present in most cases, with the patient almost always being aware of their condition and how best to manage their health and care. Sickle cell disease is a lifelong condition and patients often suffer chronic complications of their disease. They are often the best source of advice on how to manage their condition.

- The signs and symptoms include, but are not limited to, any of the following:
  - Severe pain, most commonly in the long bones and/or joints of the arms and legs, but also in the back, chest and abdomen
  - Fever/high temperature
  - Difficulty in breathing
  - Reduced oxygen (O_2) saturation
  - Cough
  - Chest pain
  - Pallor or jaundice
  - Tiredness/weakness
  - Inability to move a limb
  - Change in level of consciousness
  - Dehydration
  - Headache
  - Priapism – a prolonged erection of the penis.

2. Incidence

- There are different types of sickle cell disease (HbSS, HbSC, HbS Thalassaemia, HbSD, HbSO) which can vary in severity. Sickle cell disease is found most commonly in people of African or Caribbean origin, but can also affect people of Mediterranean, Middle Eastern and Asian origin. In the United Kingdom it is estimated that 15,000 adults and children suffer from sickle cell disease, with 1 in every 2,000 babies born with the condition.

3. Medical Emergencies

- Painful episodes are the commonest symptom, due to vaso-occlusion from sickled red cells in the small capillaries in the long bones. In the long term, vaso-occlusion also results in damage to the lungs, heart, kidneys, bones and other organs and tissues. Most patients will know what pain relief works best for them and if an ambulance has been called it is because the pain is severe.

- Painful crises are the commonest symptom due to vaso-occlusion of small blood vessels. Patients with sickle cell disease normally manage these episodes at home, however they can be severe and require emergency management and hospitalisation. Patients often understand which pain relief works best for them during these episodes.

- Acute chest syndrome is the leading cause of death amongst sickle cell patients. This is a common and potentially life-threatening complication of painful crises and is often precipitated by a chest infection. Patients present with shortness of breath, hypoxia and tachypnoea and tachycardia. Chest pain is often present, and the hypoxia responds poorly to inhaled oxygen. Crackles are often present in the lung bases and will ascend rapidly to involve the whole lung fields in severe cases. Patients with acute chest syndrome should be managed on intensive care and require exchange transfusion.

- Patients with sickle cell disease are at a high risk of thrombosis. Pulmonary embolus is an important differential diagnosis when patients complain of shortness of breath or chest pain.

- A stroke should be suspected in patients with any change in consciousness, a seizure, severe headache, loss of movement in a limb or loss of speech, and treated accordingly (refer to **Stroke/Transient Ischaemic Attack**). Stroke in children is usually due to a thrombotic event and may not present as a medical emergency.

- Overwhelming infection – sickle cell disease causes splenic atrophy and children, in particular, may die very suddenly due to pneumococcal infection or other bacteria.

- Sepsis and infection – sickle cell disease causes splenic atrophy which reduces the patient's immune response to encapsulated bacteria. In particular, children may quickly develop severe sepsis due to pneumococcal infection or other bacteria. Similarly, osteomyelitis is a common infective complication of sickle cell disease and is associated with fever and bone pain.

4. Pathophysiology

- The red cells of patients with sickle cell disease are prone to assuming an abnormal sickled shape when exposed to a variety of factors including hypoxia, extreme temperatures (cold and hot), dehydration and a variety of other factors that cause physiological and psychological stress. Sickle cells are prone to mechanical damage, hence haemolytic anaemia is common in this group of patients. Sickled cells pass less easily through blood vessels and this can lead to occlusion of the microvasculature resulting in tissue hypoxia, pain and end organ damage. Sickle cell symptoms can therefore occur in all organs of the body.

Sickle Cell Disease

- A crisis may follow as a result of an infection, during pregnancy, following surgery or a variety of other causes including physiological and psychological stress.

5. Assessment and Management

For the assessment and management of patients with sickle cell crisis, refer to Table 3.120 or Figure 3.45.

TABLE 3.120 – ASSESSMENT and MANAGEMENT of: Sickle Cell Disease

Assess <C>ABCDE

- If any of the following **TIME-CRITICAL** features present:
  - Major **<C>ABCDE** problems (refer to **Medical Emergencies in Adults – Overview** and **Medical Emergencies in Children – Overview**).
  - Acute chest syndrome, then:
    - Start correcting **<C>ABCDE** problems.
    - Undertake a **TIME-CRITICAL** transfer to nearest receiving hospital.
    - Continue patient management en route.
    - Provide an ATMIST information call.

Ask the Patient If They Have an Individualised Treatment Plan

- Be aware that the patient may have a treatment plan and follow this if it is available. Some patients have Coordinate My Care records which are easily accessible to clinicians. Check if the patient has a care record as part of the assessment.
- Patients with long-term conditions will often be able to guide their care.
- Follow **Medical Emergencies in Adults – Overview** and **Medical Emergencies in Children – Overview** in addition to the specific management detailed below.

Pulse

- Measure and record pulse rate.

Respiratory Rate

- Measure and record respiratory rate.

Oxygen

- Measure oxygen saturations.
- Administer supplemental oxygen to **ALL** patients as per **Oxygen** guidelines, including those with chronic sickle lung disease; oxygen helps to counter tissue hypoxia and reduce cell clumping.
- Administer high levels of supplemental oxygen via an appropriate mask/nasal cannula until a reliable SpO_2 measurement is available; then adjust the oxygen flow to aim for target saturation within the range of 94–98%. Refer to **Oxygen**.

NB It is safer to over-oxygenate until a reliable SpO_2 measurement is available.

Blood Glucose

- If appropriate, measure and record blood glucose for hypo/hyperglycaemia (refer to **Glycaemic Emergencies in Adults and Children**).

Temperature

- Measure and record temperature.

NEWS2

- These observations will enable you to calculate a NEWS2 Score (refer to **Sepsis**).

ECG

- If required, monitor and record 12-lead ECG. Assess for abnormality (refer to **Cardiac Arrhythmia and Sudden Cardiac Death**).

Blood Pressure and Fluids

- Patients with a sickle cell crisis will not have acute fluid loss but may present with dehydration if they have been ill for an extended period of time.
- Measure and record blood pressure; if required, administer fluids (refer to **Intravascular Fluid Therapy in Adults** and **Intravascular Fluid Therapy in Children**).

(continued)

Sickle Cell Disease

TABLE 3.120 – ASSESSMENT and MANAGEMENT of: Sickle Cell Disease *(continued)*

Pain Management

- Where present, assess the **SOCRATES** of pain and record initial and subsequent pain scores. Offer ALL patients pain relief. Consider any pain relief the patient may have taken prior to calling the ambulance service. Note that the patient will often understand which pain relief works best for them during a crisis.
- **Entonox** – administer initially but do not administer for extended periods (refer to **Nitrous Oxide (Entonox® or Nitronox™)**).
- **Opiate analgesia** – administer via the oral, subcutaneous or intramuscular route (refer to **Morphine Sulfate**), but not intravenously. The dose should be guided by the patient's individualised treatment plan if available; otherwise refer to **Pain Management in Adults and Children**.
- Always assess the effectiveness of any pain relief administered.

Conveyance to Hospital

- Consider conveying direct to specialist unit where the patient is usually treated, as per local pathways.
- Patients should not walk to the ambulance as this will exacerbate the effects of hypoxia in the tissues.
- Consider conveyance to hospital for patients with:
    - A temperature >38°C, as there is a risk of rapid deterioration.
    - Chest symptoms, as acute chest syndrome may develop quickly.
    - Unmanageable pain.
    - Severe vomiting/diarrhoea.
- Consider management in the community or referral to other services for:
    - Adult patients who are well and have only mild or moderate pain and a temperature of <38°C.
    - Paediatric patients who are well, have only mild or moderate pain and do not have an increased temperature. Consider referral in line with local pathways.
    - Admission is not necessarily required if the source of infection is obvious (such as a viral illness) and can be managed in the community.

Appropriate Advice

- Make sure that patients are aware of chest symptoms and/or their parents/carers understand the importance of seeking urgent medical advice if their clinical condition deteriorates, especially if breathing becomes faster or more laboured.
- Advice to be given includes:
    - Increase fluid intake, as dehydration will prolong a painful episode.
    - Avoid other factors that may trigger acute painful crisis, such as cold weather and excessive physical activity.
    - For pain management, use distraction techniques, such as games, computers and television.
- If the patient has no individualised treatment plan for pain, advise over-the-counter analgesia techniques, such as Paracetamol and Ibuprofen. **NB** Avoid Ibuprofen if the patient has renal impairment.
- Advise the patient and/or their parents/carer to seek urgent medical advice or go straight to hospital if they:
    - Become unwell or develop a fever with a temperature greater than 38°C (or any increased temperature in a child).
    - Develop chest symptoms, such as breathlessness or pain.
    - Have severe vomiting or diarrhoea, due to the risk of dehydration.
    - Are unable to control their pain at home.

Documentation

- Complete documentation to include all clinical findings, advice from other clinicians, onward referral and worsening advice given.

Sickle Cell Disease

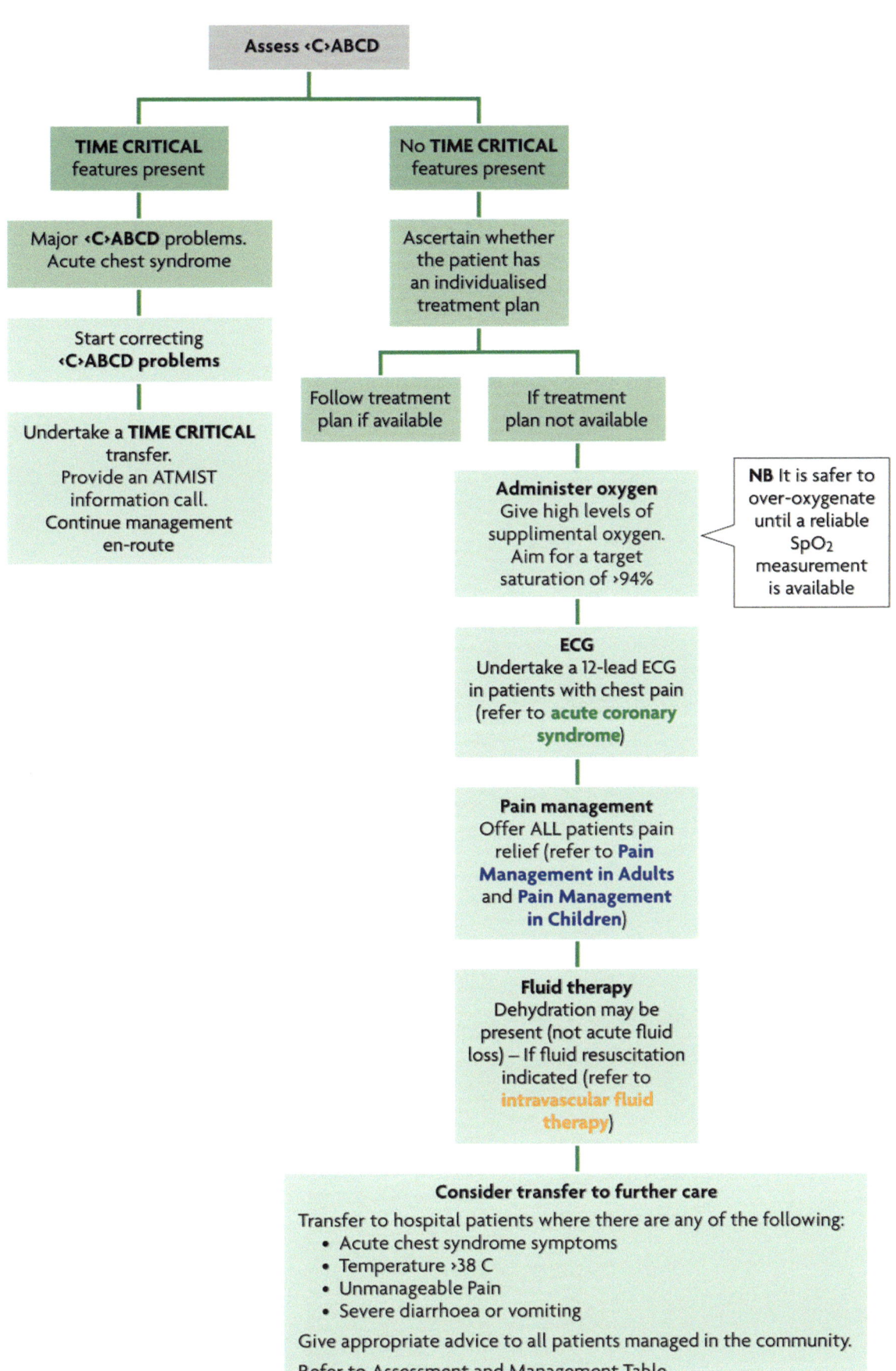

Figure 3.45 — Assessment and management algorithm for sickle cell disease.

Sickle Cell Disease

> **KEY POINTS!**
>
> **Sickle Cell Disease**
> - Sickle cell disease is a hereditary condition affecting the haemoglobin contained within red blood cells; the cells are irregular in shape and occlude the microvasculature, leading to tissue ischaemia.
> - The management of pain should be undertaken as early as possible.
> - Sickle cell crises can result in damage to the lungs, heart, kidneys, liver, bones and other organs and tissues.
> - Sickle cell crises can be very painful and patients should be offered pain relief as soon as possible.
> - In sickle cell crisis and acute chest syndrome, aim for an oxygen saturation of 94–98% or the saturation level that is usual for the individual patient.
> - Patients with sickle cell disease can be dangerously unwell but in no pain (e.g. aplastic crisis, stroke, hepatic sequestration, PE, etc.).
> - Acute chest syndrome is a leading cause of death amongst sickle cell patients and is characterised by hypoxia and tachypnoea.

Acknowledgements

We would like to gratefully acknowledge the Sickle Cell Society for their contributions, comments and input to this JRCALC guideline.

Bibliography

1. Johnson AG. *Report of a Working Party of the Standing Medical Advisory Committee on Sickle Cell, Thalassaemia and other Haemoglobinopathies: Policy in confidence.* London: HMSO, 1993.
2. Maxwell K, Streetly A, Bevan D. Experiences of hospital care and treatment-seeking behavior for pain from sickle cell disease: qualitative study. *Western Journal of Medicine* 1999, 171(5–6): 306–313.
3. Vichinsky EP, Neumayr LD, Earles AN, Williams R, Lennette ET, Dean D, et al. Causes and outcomes of the acute chest syndrome in sickle cell disease. National Acute Chest Syndrome Study Group. *The New England Journal of Medicine* 2000, 342(25): 1855–1865.
4. Yale SH, Nagib N, Guthrie T. Acute chest syndrome in sickle cell disease: crucial considerations in adolescents and adults. *Postgraduate Medicine* 2000, 107(1): 215–222.
5. National Institute for Health and Care Excellence. *Sickle Cell Disease.* Clinical Knowledge Summaries. 2016. Available from: https://cks.nice.org.uk/sickle-cell-disease#!references/1381889.

Stroke and Transient Ischaemic Attack

1. Introduction

- Stroke is a major health problem in the UK. Improving care for patients with stroke and transient ischaemic attack (TIA) is a key national priority. The most recent national clinical guideline for stroke was developed by the Intercollegiate Stroke Guideline Working Party and published by the Royal College of Physicians in 2016, under a process accredited by the National Institute for Health and Care Excellence (NICE). The JRCALC guidelines draw heavily on these. NICE published an updated guideline (NG128) in May 2019.

- The Intercollegiate Stroke Guideline Working Party (2016) and JRCALC acknowledge the paucity of evidence for pre-hospital assessment and management of patients with suspected stroke. Many recommendations are therefore based on expert consensus and accepted practice. Ambulance services are increasingly engaging with stroke specialists and academic partners on high-quality research to help develop the evidence to inform future guidelines and practice.

2. Pathophysiology

2.1 Acute Stroke

- Stroke is defined as a clinical syndrome, of presumed vascular origin, typified by rapidly developing signs of focal or global disturbance of cerebral functions lasting more than 24 hours or leading to death. Cerebrovascular disease is the third leading cause of disability in the UK. Approximately 85% of strokes are caused by cerebral infarction resulting from ischaemic stroke, 10% by primary intracerebral haemorrhage (ICH) and 5% by subarachnoid haemorrhage. The risk of recurrent stroke is 26% within 5 years of a first stroke and 39% by 10 years.

- Acute stroke is a **TIME-CRITICAL** medical emergency. For eligible patients with ischaemic stroke, treatment with thrombolytic therapy with alteplase is highly time dependent. Data from the Sentinel Stroke National Audit Programme (SSNAP) shows that in 2019–20 only 11.7% of all UK stroke patients received thrombolysis and 1.8% underwent thrombectomy. In order to determine suitability for treatment, patients must undergo a CT brain scan; therefore, patients need to be transferred to an appropriate hospital as rapidly as possible once the diagnosis is suspected. As an additional treatment for a specific cohort of selected patients, interventional arterial therapy is available. Mechanical Intra-Arterial Thrombectomy (IAT) is becoming increasingly available in specialist centres (now known as comprehensive stroke centres).

- According to the Intercollegiate Stroke Working Party (2016): 'There is strong evidence that specialised stroke unit care initiated as soon as possible after the onset of stroke provides effective treatments that reduce long-term brain damage, disability and healthcare costs'.

- The vast majority (95%) of people with stroke present in the community setting. Public information campaigns, notably the Stroke Association's FAST campaign, have raised awareness of stroke symptoms and encourage early call for help using the 999 system. Research has helped to inform procedures in ambulance Emergency Operations Centres to recognise stroke symptoms as early and accurately as possible to facilitate an appropriate emergency response. Reducing time from symptom onset by calling for help, and by speeding up pre-hospital assessment and reducing on-scene time, can expedite admission to an appropriate hospital. This reduces overall time to treatment and helps improve patient outcomes. The recently published Utstein recommendation for Emergency Stroke Care describes a 'Chain of Survival' for stroke care.

- The most sensitive features associated with diagnosing stroke in the pre-hospital setting are unilateral facial weakness, arm or leg weakness and speech disturbance.

- It is important to remember that thrombolysis and/or thrombectomy are not the only management proven to benefit stroke patients. Admission to a stroke unit for early specialist care is known to be life saving and to reduce disability.

- Not all stroke symptoms can be identified by using the FAST test in isolation.

- Have a high index of suspicion of acute stroke in patients presenting with new, sudden onset of the signs and symptoms listed in Table 3.121.

TABLE 3.121 – Signs and Symptoms

- Sudden onset numbness or weakness of the face, arm, or leg, especially on one side of the body.
- Sudden onset new confusion, trouble speaking, difficulty understanding speech, or difficulty swallowing.
- Sudden onset visual disturbance including in one or both eyes, blurred or double vision or loss of visual field.

(continued)

Stroke and Transient Ischaemic Attack

> **TABLE 3.121** – Signs and Symptoms *(continued)*
>
> - Sudden onset trouble walking, changes in gait, loss of balance, or lack of coordination.
> - Sudden onset severe headache resulting in a blinding pain//photophobia unlike anything experienced before (unlike their usual pattern of headaches).
> - Sudden onset of dizziness, nausea or vomiting.
> - Reduced level of consciousness, or altered mental status including transient loss of consciousness or behavioural changes.
> - Acute onset focal neurological deficit, or witnessed acute focal neurological deficit which has since resolved, or new onset focal seizures.
> - Acute onset neck pain or neck stiffness with no known cause.
> - Locked-in syndrome (full body paralysis below the neck)

- Be aware that the following non-specific symptoms may occur in a child presenting with stroke:
  - nausea or vomiting
  - fever
  - neck pain.
- Acute focal neurological signs may be absent, and attention should be given to parental or young person concerns about the presentation of unusual symptoms.
- However, there may be other non-neurological causes for these symptoms, referred to as 'stroke mimics', which are commoner than acute stroke:
  - seizures
  - syncope
  - sepsis
  - hypoglycaemia
  - migraine
  - decompensation of previous stroke
  - functional disorders.
- About 40% of suspected strokes are eventually diagnosed as a stroke 'mimic'. However, it is extremely difficult to distinguish a stroke mimic from a true stroke in the pre-hospital environment.

2.2 Suspected TIA

- TIA is defined as an acute loss of focal cerebral or ocular function with symptoms lasting less than 24 hours. It is thought to be caused by inadequate cerebral or ocular blood supply as a result of low blood flow, thrombosis or embolism associated with diseases of the blood vessels, heart or blood. TIA is associated with a very high risk of stroke in the first month and up to one year after the event. A suspected cerebrovascular event needs to be urgently followed up with investigation and treatment at a timely TIA specialised clinic.
- During the first few hours of a patient's symptoms it is not possible to differentiate between a TIA or stroke. Therefore, patients presenting with any ongoing facial weakness, arm weakness, speech impairment, loss of focal cerebral or ocular function should immediately be taken to hospital and investigated as suspected stroke.
- Patients with a suspected TIA must have completely returned to their normal level of functioning. Any remaining signs or symptoms, however slight, must be treated as ongoing stroke symptoms and be conveyed to definitive care.
- The 2019 update of NICE guidelines states:
  - Immediately refer patients who have had a suspected TIA for specialist assessment and investigation, to be seen within 24 hours of onset of symptoms. Follow local pathways; these may include ensuring that aspirin is administered to patients who are not conveyed to hospital.
- Do not use scoring systems, such as ABCD2, to assess risk of subsequent stroke or to inform urgency of referral for people who have had a suspected or confirmed TIA.

2.3 Intracerebral and Subarachnoid Haemorrhage

- Haemorrhagic strokes are generally more severe and are associated with a considerably higher risk of dying within the first three months and beyond when compared to ischaemic strokes. Around 1 in 10 patients who have a haemorrhagic stroke die before reaching hospital.
- Intracerebral haemorrhage (ICH) is a type of stroke often due to a spontaneous rupture of a vessel, causing bleeding within the brain itself. Uncontrolled hypertension (HTN) is the most common risk factor for spontaneous ICH. Ten to twenty percent of acute ICH occurs in patients taking oral anticoagulants and this brings an association with a high risk of early haematoma expansion. Rapid transportation to normalise coagulation can reduce this risk.
- Subarachnoid haemorrhage (SAH) is a haemorrhage from a cerebral blood vessel, aneurysm or vascular malformation into the subarachnoid space, which is the space

Stroke and Transient Ischaemic Attack

surrounding the brain where blood vessels lie between the arachnoid and pia mater. The presentation of SAH is usually different from other types of stroke as it typically presents with the sudden onset of severe headache and vomiting, and with non-focal neurological signs that may include loss of consciousness and neck stiffness.

- Sudden onset (thunderclap) occipital headache is a common presentation, the significance of which can be all too easily overlooked. Refer to guideline.

3. Incidence

3.1 Stroke

- According to the *State of the Nation* report published by the Stroke Association in 2018, there are more than 100,000 strokes in the UK each year. That is calculated at approximately one stroke every 5 minutes. The *Burden of Stroke in Europe* report published by King's College, London using 2015 data highlighted 39.3 strokes per 100,000 inhabitants annually within the UK. There are over 1.2 million stroke survivors residing within the UK. Stroke is the fourth biggest killer in England and Wales, and the third biggest killer in Scotland and Northern Ireland.

3.2 Childhood Stroke

- There are over 400 childhood strokes a year in the UK, which is more than one child every day. Anyone of any age can have a stroke, including babies and children. The causes of stroke in children are very different from those in adults, including cardiovascular malformations and genetic causes (such as clotting disorders). Although the risk of stroke in healthy children is extremely low, the risk of a thrombotic stroke is six times higher following a recent illness, such as cold/flu or chickenpox. For children having had none or only some of their routine vaccinations, the risk of a thrombotic stroke is eight times higher compared to those who have had all of their routine vaccinations. The risk of stroke in children is 19 times higher in children with congenital heart disease. Newborns are the most likely to have a stroke.

3.3 TIA

- The estimated incidence of first-ever TIA in the UK is 50 people per 100,000 population each year. This is likely to be an underestimate. One in twelve people (8%) will have a full stroke within a week of having a TIA.

3.4 Haemorrhage

- SAH incidence is 6–12 people per 100,000 population each year in the UK. Approximately 85% of patients bleed from an intracranial aneurysm, 10% from a non-aneurysmal peri-mesencephalic haemorrhage and 5% from other vascular abnormalities including arteriovenous malformation.

4. Severity and Outcome

- The case fatality of ischaemic stroke in adults aged 45 or older is estimated at 10.4 per 100 discharges, suggesting 53,004 deaths, or 41.5 per 100,000 inhabitants, due to stroke each year.

5. Assessment and Management

- The FAST (Face, Arms, Speech, Time) assessment tool should be used and carried out on **ALL** patients with suspected stroke/TIA. A deficit in any one of the face, arms or speech domains is sufficient for the patient to be identified as 'FAST positive'.

- A suspected acute stroke patient should be considered a **TIME-CRITICAL** patient. Perform a brief secondary survey but do not allow this, or any other non-essential pre-hospital interventions, to delay transport to hospital.

- Clinicians may consider using the PASTA (Paramedic Acute Stroke Treatments Assessments) structured assessment and handover as per local arrangements (see Price et al).

TABLE 3.122 – FAST Test

Facial weakness	Ask the patient to smile or show teeth. Look for **NEW** lack of symmetry.
Arm weakness	Ask the patient to lift their arms together and hold for 5 seconds. Does one arm drift or fall down? The arm with motor weakness will drift downwards compared to the unaffected limb.
Speech	Ask the patient to repeat a phrase. Assess for slurring or difficulty with the words or sentence, hesitation or even an inability to speak at all.
Time	Note the time of onset, if known, and pass this to the hospital as this has been shown to expedite time to CT scan.

- The FAST test is well established in UK practice for both clinicians and the general public. FAST has recognised limitations in that it will not identify all patients with stroke, such as those with sudden-onset visual disturbance/lateralising cerebellar dysfunction. The Intercollegiate Working Party (2016) recommends clinicians continue to treat a person as having a suspected

Stroke and Transient Ischaemic Attack

stroke if they are suspicious of the diagnosis despite a negative FAST test.

- The majority of strokes are ischaemic. Distinguishing between ischaemic and haemorrhagic strokes is not currently feasible clinically in the pre-hospital setting.
- Prehospital brain imaging is being evaluated in other countries (and in one UK centre) but the evidence is not sufficient to recommend wider implementation at this time.
- Video-conferencing is currently being evaluated in some parts of the UK to determine whether it assists in the triage and treatment of patients suffering some symptoms of stroke. (See: https://aace.org.uk/wp-content/uploads/2025/02/Stroke-Video-Conferencing.pdf)

TABLE 3.123 – ASSESSMENT and MANAGEMENT of: Stroke/TIA

Assess <C>ABCDE

- If any of the following **TIME-CRITICAL** features are present:
  - Major **<C>ABCDE** problems (refer to **Medical Emergencies in Adults – Overview** and **Medical Emergencies in Children – Overview**).
  - Fast positive or suspected stroke.
  - May have airway and breathing problems (refer to **Airway and Breathing Management**).
  - Level of consciousness may vary (refer to **Altered Level of Consciousness**).
  - Assess blood glucose level, as hypoglycaemia may mimic a stroke.
- Start correcting any **<C>ABCDE** problems.
- Undertake a **TIME-CRITICAL** transfer to a Hyper Acute Stroke Unit (HASU) or a thrombectomy-capable hospital, as per local pathway.
- Continue patient management en route.
- Provide an ATMIST pre-alert call including time of onset of symptoms, if known.

NB A UK study (Sheppard et al.) reported that providing a hospital pre-alert message is the most influential pre-hospital factor in facilitating timely assessment for acute stroke patients upon arrival in hospital and confirms in a UK setting the findings of previous work elsewhere. However, patients were only pre-alerted where stroke was recognised and symptom onset time recorded.

GCS

- Assess Glasgow Coma Scale (GCS) on unaffected side. Eye and motor assessments may be more readily assessed if speech is badly affected.

Respiratory Rate

- Measure and record respiratory rate.

Pulse

- Measure and record pulse.

Oxygen Saturation

- Monitor the patient's SpO_2, administer oxygen to achieve saturations of >94% if the patient presents as hypoxaemic on air (refer to **Oxygen**).

NB Among non-hypoxaemic patients with acute stroke, the prophylactic use of low-dose oxygen supplementation does not reduce death or disability at 3 months. Oxygen therapy is not recommended unless the patient is hypoxaemic.

Blood Pressure and Fluids

- Measure and record blood pressure; if required, administer fluids (refer to **Intravascular Fluid Therapy in Adults** and **Intravascular Fluid Therapy in Children**).

NB The BP will be used as a baseline in hospital.

- Intravenous access is not essential unless the patient requires specific interventions as it may delay transport to hospital.

Blood Glucose

- Measure and record blood glucose for hypo/hyperglycaemia (refer to **Glycaemic Emergencies in Adults and Children**).

NB Hypoglycaemia may mimic a stroke.

Stroke and Transient Ischaemic Attack

TABLE 3.123 – ASSESSMENT and MANAGEMENT of: Stroke/TIA (continued)

Temperature
- Measure and record temperature en route to hospital.

NEWS2
- These observations will enable you to calculate a NEWS2 Score (refer to **Sepsis**).

ECG
- **Do NOT delay transfer to hospital to record a 12-lead ECG. A 12-lead ECG is not necessary for stroke patients unless there are specific reasons (such as concurrent chest pain).**
- The recording of a pre-hospital 12-lead ECG has been associated with delay and worse outcomes in stroke patients.
- **Patients should have continuous (e.g. 3-lead) cardiac monitoring en route to capture arrhythmias** and specifically AF which increases the risk of stroke fivefold. This valuable information will help during any subsequent specialist assessment.

Assess the Patient's Pain
- Where present, assess the **SOCRATES** of pain and record initial and subsequent pain scores.
- Consider analgesia if appropriate (refer to **Pain Management in Adults and Children**).

Transfer
- A suspected acute stroke is a **TIME-CRITICAL** condition. Every effort **MUST** be made to minimise on-scene time.
- The destination hospital will depend on local pathways. For example, bypassing local hospitals and taking the patient direct to a HASU or a thrombectomy-capable hospital may be appropriate, as per local pathways.
- Pre-alert the receiving hospital for all suspected acute stroke patients within locally agreed treatment windows of care.
- Conscious patients should be conveyed in the most comfortable position for them. A large international randomised trial of hospitalised stroke patients reported that outcomes after acute stroke did not differ significantly between patients assigned to a lying-flat position and those assigned to a sitting-up position with the head elevated.
- Patients with suspected acute stroke should remain nil by mouth until they have a swallowing assessment in hospital. Have suction available for patients who are aphagic to protect their airway from secretions if necessary.
- Where possible, a witness should be asked to accompany the patient to hospital, to assist with further assessment.

Documentation
- Complete documentation to include all clinical findings, advice from other clinicians, onward referral and worsening advice given.

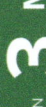

6. Audit Information

- Ambulance services are required to monitor aspects of stroke care through the National Ambulance Quality Indicators, and all are linking pre-hospital data to SSNAP to capture the entire acute patient journey. Careful documentation of your assessment and management, including accurate timings, is essential to improving care for this group of patients.
- SSNAP are currently working with NHS England on an ambulance-linkage project to complement and extend the current dataset, incorporating pre-hospital data.

Stroke and Transient Ischaemic Attack

> **KEY POINTS!**
>
> **Stroke and Transient Ischaemic Attack**
> - Time is of the essence in suspected acute stroke. Time is brain. Every effort MUST be made to minimise on-scene time, including avoidance of interventions that do not add value to the stroke patient, e.g. 12-Lead ECG and IV access, unless clearly indicated.
> - Record time of onset if known or last-seen-well time and pre-alert the appropriate hospital.
> - Stroke is common and may be due to either cerebral infarction or haemorrhage — it is not possible to distinguish haemorrhagic or ischaemic stroke clinically.
> - Mechanical Intra-Arterial Thrombectomy (IAT) is becoming increasingly available.
> - The most sensitive features associated with diagnosing stroke in the pre-hospital setting are facial weakness, arm and leg weakness and speech disturbance — the FAST test.
> - The FAST test should be carried out on ALL patients with suspected stroke or TIA.
> - Patients with TIA may be at high risk of stroke and require urgent specialist assessment, and local pathways should be followed.

Bibliography

1. Royal College of Physicians. *Stroke Guidelines*. London: RCP, 2016. Available from: https://www.rcplondon.ac.uk/guidelines-policy/stroke-guidelines.
2. National Institute for Health and Clinical Excellence. *Stroke and Transient Ischaemic Attack in over 16s: Diagnosis and initial management*. NICE guideline [NG128]. 2019. Available from: https://www.nice.org.uk/guidance/ng128.
3. Stroke Audit. Pre-hospital Care Concise Stroke Guide for Stroke 2016. Available from: https://www.strokeaudit.org/SupportFiles/Documents/Guidelines/Profession-Specific-Guides/5-Pre-Hospital.aspx.
4. Kobayashi A, Czlonkowska A, Ford GA, Fonseca AC, Luijckx GJ, Korv J, de la Ossa NP, Price C, Russell D, Tsiskaridze A, Messmer-Wullen M, De Keyser J. European Academy of Neurology and European Stroke Organization consensus statement and practical guidance for pre-hospital management of stroke. Eur J Neurol 2018, 25(3): 425–433. Available from: https://onlinelibrary.wiley.com/doi/epdf/10.1111/ene.13539
5. Stroke Association. *State of the Nation: Stroke statistics 2018*. Available from: https://www.stroke.org.uk/resources/state-nation-stroke-statistics.
6. SAFE. *Burden of Stroke in Europe*. Available from: http://strokeeurope.eu/data-comparison/results/?country1=United+Kingdom&country2=Belgium&criteria=StrokeEpidemilogy.
7. Stroke Audit. *Sentinel Stroke National Audit Programme*. Available from: https://www.strokeaudit.org/.
8. Watkins CL, Jones SP, Leathley MJ, Ford GA, Quinn T, McAdam JJ, Gibson JME, Mackway-Jones KC, Durham S, Britt D, Morris S, O'Donnell M, Emsley HCA, Punekar S, Sharma A, Sutton CJ. *Emergency Stroke Calls: Obtaining Rapid Telephone Triage (ESCORTT) — A programme of research to facilitate recognition of stroke by emergency medical dispatchers*. Southampton: NIHR Journals Library, 2014. Available from: https://www.ncbi.nlm.nih.gov/books/NBK262723/.
9. Nor AM, McAllister C, Louw SJ, Dyker AG, Davis M, Jenkinson D, et al. Agreement between ambulance paramedic- and physician-recorded neurological signs with Face Arm Speech Test (FAST) in acute stroke patients. Stroke: A Journal of Cerebral Circulation 2004, 35(6): 1355–1359.
10. Harbison J, Hossain O, Jenkinson D, Davis J, Louw SJ, Ford GA. Diagnostic accuracy of stroke referrals from primary care, emergency room physicians, and ambulance staff using the face arm speech test. Stroke: A Journal of Cerebral Circulation 2003, 34(1): 71–76.
11. Wilson C, Harley C, Steels S. Systematic review and meta-analysis of pre-hospital diagnostic accuracy studies. Emerg Med J 2018, 35: 757–764. Available from: https://emj.bmj.com/content/35/12/757.long
12. McClelland G, Rodgers H, Flynn D, Price C. The frequency, characteristics and aetiology of stroke mimic presentations: a narrative review. Eur J Emerg Med 2019, 26(1): 2–8. Available from: https://insights.ovid.com/pubmed?pmid=29727304
13. Neves Briard J, Zewude RT, Kate MP, Rowe BH, Buck B, Butcher K, Gioia LC. Stroke mimics transported by emergency medical services to a comprehensive stroke center: the magnitude of the problem. J Stroke Cerebrovasc Dis. 2018, 27(10): 2738–2745. Available from: https://www.strokejournal.org/article/S1052-3057(18)30293-3/fulltext
14. Fothergill RT, Williams J, Edwards MJ, Russell IT, Gompertz P. Does use of the recognition of stroke in the emergency room stroke assessment tool enhance stroke recognition by ambulance clinicians? Stroke 2013, 44(11): 3007–3012.
15. Morris S, Hunter RM, Ramsay AI, Boaden R, McKevitt C, Perry C, Pursani N, Rudd AG, Schwamm LH, Turner SJ, Tyrrell PJ, Wolfe CD, Fulop NJ. Impact of centralising acute stroke services in English metropolitan areas on mortality and length of hospital stay: difference-in-differences analysis. BMJ 2014, 349: g4757.
16. Ramsay AI, Morris S, Hoffman A, Hunter RM, Boaden R, McKevitt C, Perry C, Pursani N, Rudd AG, Turner SJ, Tyrrell PJ, Wolfe CD, Fulop NJ. Effects of centralizing acute stroke services on stroke care provision in two large metropolitan areas in England. Stroke 2015, 46(8): 2244–2251.
17. Rodrigues FB, Neves JB, Caldeira D, Ferro JM, Ferreira JJ, Costa J. Endovascular treatment versus medical care alone for ischaemic stroke: systematic review and meta-analysis. BMJ 2016, 353: i1754.
18. Zerna C, Thomalla G, Campbell BCV, Rha JH, Hill MD. Current practice and future directions in the diagnosis and acute treatment of ischaemic stroke. Lancet

Stroke and Transient Ischaemic Attack

2018, 392(10154): 1247–1256. Available from: https://www.thelancet.com/journals/lancet/article/PIIS0140-6736(18)31874-9/fulltext

19. Evans BA, Ali K, Bulger J, Ford GA, Jones M, Moore C, Porter A, Pryce AD, Quinn T, Seagrove AC, Snooks H, Whitman S, Rees N; TIER Trial Research Management Group. Referral pathways for patients with TIA avoiding hospital admission: a scoping review. Available from: https://bmjopen.bmj.com/content/7/2/e013443.long.

20. Bulger JK, Ali K, Edwards A, Ford G, Hampton C, Jones C, Moore C, Porter A, Quinn T, Seagrove A, Snooks H, Rees N. Care pathways for low-risk transient ischaemic attack. *Journal of Paramedic Practice* 2018,10(6).

21. Roffe C Nevatte T, Sim J, Bishop J, Ives N, Ferdinand P, Gray R; Stroke Oxygen Study Investigators and the Stroke OxygenStudy Collaborative Group. Effect of Routine Low-Dose Oxygen Supplementation on Death and Disability in Adults With Acute Stroke: The Stroke Oxygen Study Randomized Clinical Trial. *JAMA* 2017, 318(12): 1125–1135. Available from: https://jamanetwork.com/journals/jama/fullarticle/2654819

22. Munro SF, Cooke D, Kiln-Barfoot V, Quinn T. The use and impact of 12-lead electrocardiograms in acute stroke patients: a systematic review. *Eur Heart J Acute Cardiovasc Care* 2018, 7(3): 257–263. Available from: https://journals.sagepub.com/doi/full/10.1177/2048872615620893?url_ver=Z39.88-2003&rfr_id=ori%3Arid%3Acrossref.org&rfr_dat=cr_pub%3Dpubmed

23. Bobinger T, Kallmünzer B, Kopp M, Kurka N, Arnold M, Heider S, Schwab S, Köhrmann M. Diagnostic value of prehospital ECG in acute stroke patients. *Neurology* 2017, 88(20): 1894–1898. Available from: http://n.neurology.org/content/88/20/1894.long

24. Anderson CS, Arima H, Lavados P, Billot L, Hackett ML, Olavarría VV, Muñoz Venturelli P, Brunser A, Peng B, Cui L, Song L, Rogers K, Middleton S, Lim JY, Forshaw D, Lightbody CE, Woodward M, Pontes-Neto O, De Silva HA, Lin RT, Lee TH, Pandian JD, Mead GE, Robinson T, Watkins C; HeadPoST Investigators and Coordinators. Cluster-Randomized, Crossover Trial of Head Positioning in Acute Stroke. *N Engl J Med* 2017, 376(25): 2437–2447. Available from: https://www.nejm.org/doi/10.1056/NEJMoa1615715?url_ver=Z39.88-2003&rfr_id=ori:rid:crossref.org&rfr_dat=cr_pub%3d www.ncbi.nlm.nih.gov

25. Royal College of Paediatrics and Child Health. *Stroke in Childhood – Clinical guideline for diagnosis, management and rehabilitation*. London: Royal College of Paediatrics and Child Health, 2017. Available from: https://www.rcpch.ac.uk/resources/stroke-childhood-clinical-guideline-diagnosis-management-rehabilitation.

26. Royal College of Paediatrics and Child Health. *Management of children and young people with an acute decrease in conscious level – Clinical guideline*. London: Royal College of Paediatrics and Child Health, 2016. Available from: https://www.rcpch.ac.uk/resources/management-children-young-people-acute-decrease-conscious-level-clinical-guideline.

27. AACE. *Stroke Video Conferencing*. 2020. Available from: https://aace.org.uk/initiatives/stroke-video-conferencing/.

28. Lumley HA, Flynn D, Shaw L, McClelland G, Ford GA, White PM, Price CI. A scoping review of pre-hospital technology to assist ambulance personnel with patient diagnosis or stratification during the emergency assessment of suspected stroke. *BMC Emergency Medicine* 2020, 20(30). Available from: https://bmcemergmed.biomedcentral.com/articles/10.1186/s12873-020-00323-0

29. Stroke Audit. *The Seventh SSNAP Annual Report: Stroke care received for patients admitted to hospital between April 2019 to March 2020*. Available from: https://www.strokeaudit.org/Documents/National/Clinical/Apr2019Mar2020/Apr2019Mar2020-AnnualReport.aspx.

30. Feldborg Lyckhage L, Hansen ML, Procida K, Wienecke T. Prehospital continuous ECG is valuable for very early detection of atrial fibrillation in patients with acute stroke. *Journal of Stroke and Cerebrovascular Diseases* 2020, 29(9).

31. Fassbender K, Walter S, Grunwald I, Merzou F, Mathur S, Lesmeister M, Liu Y, Bertch T, Grotta J. Prehospital stroke management in the thrombectomy era. *Lancet Neurology* 2020, 19.

32. Li T, Cushman JT, Shah MN, Kelly AG, Rich DQ, Jones CMC. Prehospital time intervals and management of ischemic stroke patients. *American Journal of Emergency Medicine* 2020, 7.

33. Hifumi T, Yamakawa K, Shiba D, Okazaki T, Kobata H, Gotoh J, Unemoto K, Kondo Y, Yokobori S, for the Japan Resuscitation Council (JRC) Neuroresuscitation Task Force and the Guidelines Editorial Committee. Head positioning in suspected patients with acute stroke from prehospital to emergency department settings: a systematic review and meta-analysis. *Acute Medicine & Surgery* 2021, 8(1). DOI: 10.1002/ams2.631.

34. Rudd AG, Bladin C, Carli P, De Silva DA, Field TS, Jauch EC, Kudenchuk P, Kurz MW, Lærdal T, Ong M, Panagos P, Ranta A, Rutan C, Sayre MR, Schonau L, Shin SD, Waters D, Lippert F. Utstein recommendation for emergency stroke care. *International Journal of Stroke* 2020, 15(5).

35. Ashton C, Sammut-Powell C, Birleson E, Mayoh D, Sperrin M, Parry-Jones AR. Implementation of a prealert to improve in-hospital treatment of anticoagulant-associated strokes: analysis of a prehospital pathway change in a large UK centralised acute stroke system. *BMJ Open Quality* 2020,9: e000883. DOI: 10.1136/bmjoq-2019-000883.

36. Price CI, Shaw L, Islam S, Javanbakht M, Watkins A, McMeekin P, Snooks H, Flynn D, Francis R, Lakey R, Sutcliffe L, McClelland G, Lally J, Exley C, Rodgers H, Russell I, Vale L, Ford GA. Effect of an enhanced paramedic acute stroke treatment assessment on thrombolysis delivery during emergency stroke care: A cluster randomized clinical trial. *JAMA Neurology* 2020. DOI: 10.1001/jamaneurol.2020.0611.

37. Lally J, Vaittinen A, McClelland G, Price CI, Shaw L, Ford GA, Flynn D, Exley C. Paramedic experiences of using an enhanced stroke assessment during a cluster randomised trial: a qualitative thematic analysis. *Emergency Medicine Journal* 2020, 37: 480–485. DOI: 10.1136/emermed-2019-209392.

Vascular Emergencies

Table of Abbreviations

Abbreviation	Meaning
AAA	Abdominal Aortic Aneurysm
rAAA	Ruptured abdominal aortic aneurysm
ADD-RS	Aortic Dissection Detection Risk Score
AC	Arterial Centre
CLTI	Chronic Limb-threatening Ischaemia
CVD	Cardiovascular disease
PAD	Peripheral Arterial Disease
SpO2	Saturation oxygen measured by pulse oximetry
ALI	Acute Limb Ischaemia
AVF or AV fistula	Arteriovenous fistula
AVG or AV graft	Arteriovenous graft

1. Introduction

- Vascular services deal with disorders of the arteries, veins and lymphatics.
- In the emergency setting, this includes aortic aneurysm and aortic dissection, except those of the ascending aorta or aortic arch, which are managed by cardiac surgeons.
- Cardiovascular disease (CVD) affects not only the heart but also the aorta and the arteries to the brain (ischaemic stroke), to the gastrointestinal tract (mesenteric ischaemia) and to the legs (peripheral arterial disease, PAD). Acute ischaemia could involve the upper limbs, gut, brain or lower limbs.
- Acute limb ischaemia is a common cause of emergency vascular admission when due to acute arterial occlusion by an embolus or thrombus.

1.1 Conveyance Destinations

- Many regions have vascular services networks. Vascular emergencies are treated at an arterial centre (AC). Some but **NOT** all of these manage thoracic aortic pathology. Some patients require referral for cardiac/aortic surgery in a regional cardiac surgical centre. Refer to local pathways on destination decisions.

2. Incidence

- The prevalence of CVD is set to rise nationally due to an increasingly ageing population with rising levels of obesity and diabetes.
  - Over 40% of admitted patients under a vascular team have diabetes.
  - Over 80% of all vascular patients are current or ex-smokers.
- In England, one in five people over the age of 65 years have peripheral arterial disease; 20% of these will deteriorate to develop chronic limb-threatening ischaemia (CLTI).
- The incidence of aortic aneurysm rupture was decreasing even before the introduction of the NHS abdominal aortic aneurysm (AAA) screening programme for men aged 65 years or older.
- The number of emergency admissions for aortic dissection, acute limb ischaemia and new diabetic foot problems has risen.
- Aortic disease is less likely to be routinely diagnosed in women and therefore the diagnosis of ruptured AAA or acute aortic dissection is more likely to be missed in an emergency presentation.

3. Severity and Outcome

- There are around 3,000 deaths each year from ruptured AAAs in men aged 65 and over in England and Wales, which accounts for 1.7% of all deaths in this age group.
- The national screening programme for AAAs aims to reduce the death rate by 50%.

4. Aortic Aneurysm

- Aneurysms occur within four main areas of the aorta (refer to Table 3.124 and Figure 3.46). However, they are most common in the abdominal aorta, where they are referred to as abdominal aortic aneurysm (AAA).

4.1 Pathophysiology

- An aneurysm occurs when the artery wall weakens and stretches as a result of atherosclerotic degeneration. As the aneurysm expands, the aorta dilates, increasing the risk of rupture. Overall mortality, including out-of-hospital mortality, is 85%.
- As AAAs expand in size, they may become painful in the chest, lower back, loin or groin.

Vascular Emergencies

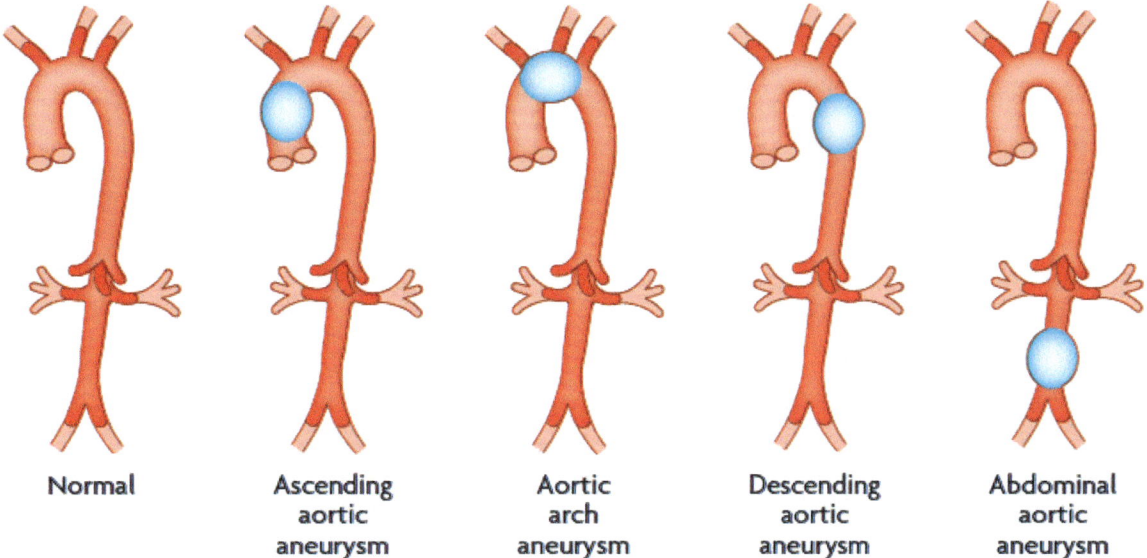

Figure 3.46 – Various aortic aneurysms.

They may also lead to new pulsating sensations in the abdomen. The risk of rupture is high in a symptomatic aneurysm, which is therefore considered an indication for urgent surgery (for assessment and management of ruptured AAA (rAAA), refer to Table 3.125 and Figure 3.47).

TABLE 3.124 – Complications of Aortic Aneurysm by Site

AORTIC AREA	COMPLICATIONS/PROGNOSIS
Ascending aorta	• Haemopericardium, which leads to syncope or sudden death. • Right haemothorax, which invariably leads to sudden death.
Arch of aorta	• Mediastinal haematoma. • Compression of pulmonary trunk or artery.
Descending thoracic aorta	• Compression of pulmonary trunk or artery. • Left haemothorax, which leads to sudden death. • Rarely, erosion into the oesophagus, which leads to profuse haematemesis.
Abdominal aorta	• Retroperitoneal haemorrhage, which leads to back pain with shock. • Intraperitoneal haemorrhage, which leads to acute abdominal pain and shock. Rarely, erosion into the intestine (small 'herald' or profuse GI bleed).

TABLE 3.125 – ASSESSMENT and MANAGEMENT of: Ruptured Aortic Aneurysms

Assess <C>ABCDE

- If any of the following **TIME-CRITICAL** features are present:
  – major **<C>ABCDE** problems (refer to Medical Emergencies in Adults – Overview).
- Start correcting any **<C>ABCDE** problems; see blood pressure targets below.
- Undertake a **TIME-CRITICAL** transfer to the nearest appropriate receiving arterial centre.
- Continue patient management en route.
- Provide an **ATMIST** information call.

(continued)

Vascular Emergencies

TABLE 3.125 – ASSESSMENT and MANAGEMENT of: Ruptured Aortic Aneurysms *(continued)*

History
- Patients presenting with a suspected rAAA will commonly present with one of the following:
  - syncope
  - back pain
  - abdominal pain
  - groin pain.

Risk Factors
- Known AAA.
- Cardiovascular disease.
- Peripheral arterial disease.
- Smoker or ex-smoker.
- History of hypertension.
- Marfan syndrome, Loeys-Deitz syndrome, Vascular Ehlers-Danlos syndrome, and other connective tissue disorders.
- Family history of aortic dissections, AAA or connective tissue disorders.

Respiratory Rate
- Measure and record respiratory rate.

Pulse
- Measure and record bi-lateral radial and femoral pulses.

Oxygen Saturation
- Monitor the patient's SpO_2, and administer oxygen to achieve saturations of 94–98% if the patient presents as hypoxemic on air (refer to **Oxygen**).

Blood Pressure
- Measure and record blood pressure in both upper limbs.

Blood Glucose
- If appropriate, measure and record blood glucose for hypoglycaemia or hyperglycaemia (refer to **Glycaemic Emergencies in Adults and Children**).

Temperature
- Measure and record temperature.

NEWS2
- These observations will enable you to calculate a NEWS2 score (refer to **Sepsis**).

ECG
- If appropriate, monitor and record a 12-lead ECG. Assess for abnormality (refer to **Cardiac Arrhythmia and Sudden Cardiac Death**).

Assess the Patient's Pain
- Where present, assess the **SOCRATES** of pain and record initial and subsequent pain scores.
- Consider analgesia if appropriate (refer to **Pain Management in Adults and Children**).

Physical Examination
- May be a reduction in normal skin colour/pallor or appear unwell.
- Tachycardia, possibly weak femoral pulses.
- Palpable abdominal pulsating mass may not be present in approximately 50% of cases. If present, this will be in the epigastric area. It is normal to be able to palpate the abdominal aorta in slim patients and this is not necessarily diagnostic of a AAA in absence of other symptoms or signs.
- Abdominal tenderness.
- Hypotension.

Vascular Emergencies

TABLE 3.125 – ASSESSMENT and MANAGEMENT of: Ruptured Aortic Aneurysms *(continued)*

Management

- Patients presenting with the following symptoms should be conveyed directly to an arterial centre as per local pathways:
  - Sudden onset of abdominal, lower back, loin or groin pain with or without collapse or hypotension in a patient with a previously diagnosed AAA which has not been repaired. A collapse may not occur if the rupture is initially into the retroperitoneal area and contained rather than into the abdominal cavity.
  - Sudden onset of abdominal, lower back, loin or groin pain and collapse or hypotension in a patient aged 50 years or older with a palpable AAA.
- Patients outside of this presentation, even with a known AAA, should be transported to the nearest ED for further assessment.
- The following are considered exclusions to ED bypass in the case of a suspected rAAA. In these cases, the patient should be conveyed to the nearest ED or managed at home as per patient-specific pathway:
  - Patient has had a cardiac arrest, or a cardiac arrest is imminent.
  - Airway unable to be safely managed.
  - Patient was recognised prior to this event as approaching the end of their life and is on an end-of-life care pathway. Consider if appropriate to manage the patient at home, with appropriate support.
  - Patient has an advanced directive specifically declining surgery even if their life is at risk.
  - Patients where it has been previously agreed that they are not for surgical intervention as are not likely to survive elective or emergency aortic surgery.
  - Avoid intravenous fluid therapy where possible, as raising the blood pressure will increase the bleeding. If there are signs of impaired cerebral perfusion such as confusion, cautious administration of **Sodium Chloride 0.9%** can be given.

Differentials

- A common differential is ureteric (renal) colic. Patients who are presenting with ureteric colic pain will not be hypotensive.

Documentation

- Complete documentation to include all clinical findings and advice from other clinicians.

5. Aortic Dissection

- Aortic dissection is classified into dissection of the ascending aorta, Type A, and dissection of the descending thoracic and/or abdominal aorta, Type B (refer to Table 3.126). Occasionally, a Type B dissection extends into the aortic arch and is then classified 'Non-A Non-B'.
- Type A dissection is more common, occurring in 70% of patients, and has a higher rate of early mortality. The mortality increases by 1–2% every hour patients are untreated.
- Refer to Table 3.127 for calculating the possibility of an occurrence of an aortic dissection in the patient.

5.1 Pathophysiology

- Aortic dissection originates as a **tear** within the intimal layer of the aorta, with blood flow occurring within the outer layer of the tunica media. Blood then flows both through the new channel, the 'false' lumen, and along its original channel, the 'true' lumen. The aorta may dissect down from the aortic root to the bifurcation of the common iliac arteries in a matter of seconds.
- The majority of these tears occur within the ascending aorta because of higher stresses on the aortic wall due to being closer to the aortic valve.
- Acute dissection causes sudden onset of severe pain, which is often described as '**tearing**' or '**ripping**' in nature.
- The aortic wall can rupture, leading to blood loss within the mediastinum or thoracic cavity and hypotension – patients may require **immediate surgery**.
- Refer to Table 3.128 for the assessment and management of an aortic dissection.
- Pain is typically maximal at onset and then improves.

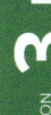

Vascular Emergencies

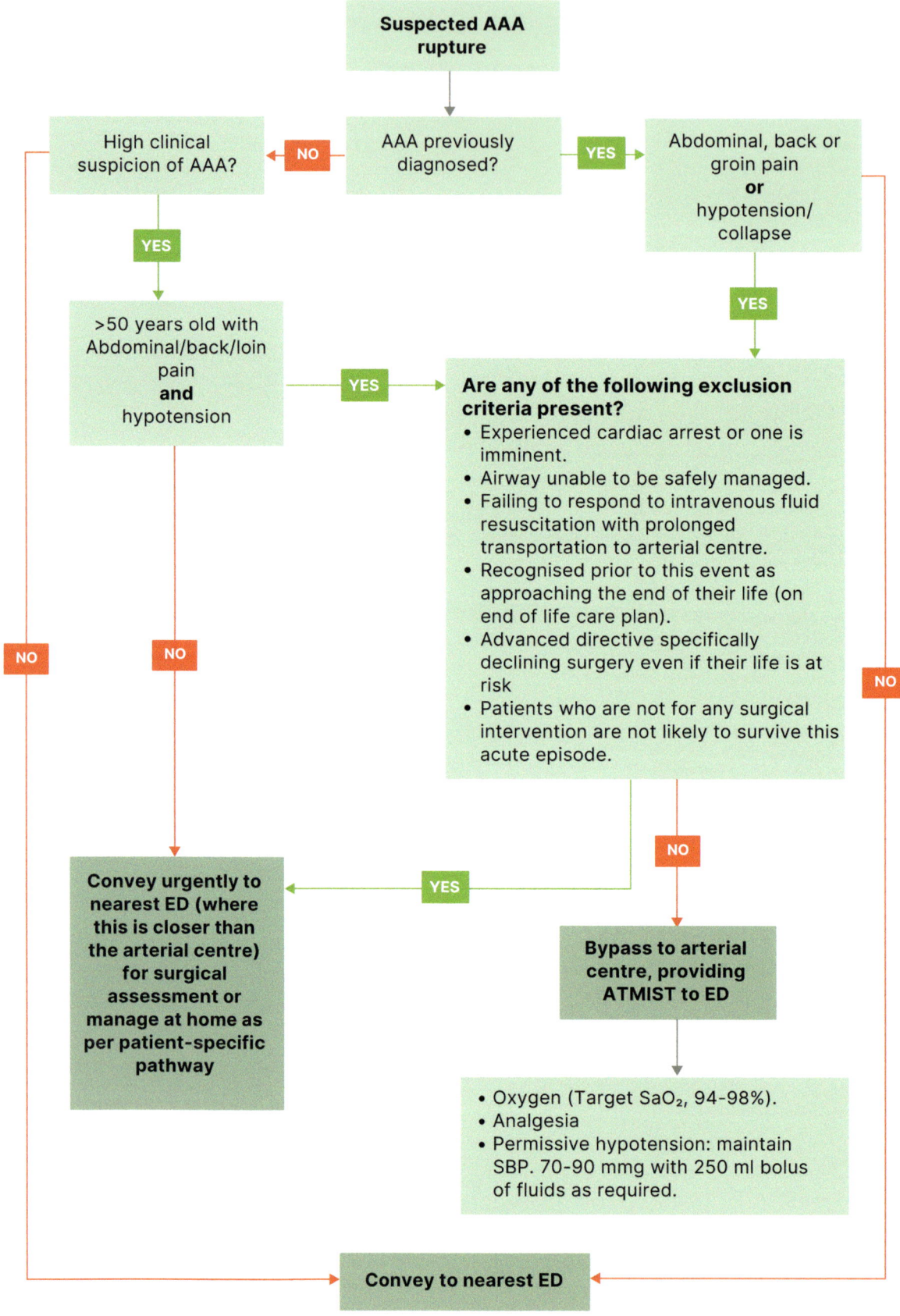

Figure 3.47 — Assessment and management of rAAA.

Vascular Emergencies

TABLE 3.126 – Complications of Dissection

Type A aortic dissection	• Cardiac tamponade, which leads to hypotension and/or sudden death. • Haemothorax, which leads to hypotension and/or sudden death. • Myocardial ischaemia or infarction. • Severe acute aortic regurgitation. • Renal, intestinal or lower limb underperfusion.
Type B aortic dissection	• Mediastinal haematoma. • Renal, intestinal or lower limb underperfusion. • Spinal cord infarction (leg numbness or weakness).

TABLE 3.127 – Aortic Dissection Detection Risk Score (ADD-RS)

PREDISPOSING CONDITIONS	PAIN FEATURES	EXAMINATION FINDINGS
• Marfan syndrome • Family history of aortic disease • Known aortic valve disease • Recent aortic surgery • Known aortic aneurysm	• Abrupt or rapid onset • Severe • Ripping or tearing	• Pulse deficit or BP differential between upper limbs • Focal neurological deficit and pain • New aortic regurgitant murmur and pain • Hypotension or shock

If any positive in any column, convey to hospital.

THINK AORTA

TABLE 3.128 – ASSESSMENT and MANAGEMENT of: Aortic Dissection

Assess ABCDE
- If any of the following **TIME-CRITICAL** features are present:
  – Major **ABCDE** problems (refer to **Medical Emergencies in Adults – Overview**).
- Start correcting any **ABCDE** problems.
- Undertake a **TIME-CRITICAL** transfer to nearest arterial or cardiac centre, as per local pathways.
- Continue patient management en route.
- Provide an **ATMIST** information call.

History
- Mediastinal haematoma.
- Renal, intestinal or lower limb underperfusion.
- Spinal cord infarction (leg numbness or weakness).

Risk Factors
- Marfan syndrome, Loeys-Deitz syndrome and Vascular Ehlers Danlos syndrome, and another connective tissue disease.
- Family history of aortic disease.
- Known aortic valve disease (i.e. bicuspid aortic valve).
- Recent aortic surgery.
- Known thoracic aortic aneurysm.
- Hypertension, which is often poorly controlled.
- Age 60 years or older.
- Smoker or ex-smoker.
- Recent cocaine use.

(continued)

Vascular Emergencies

TABLE 3.128 – ASSESSMENT and MANAGEMENT of: Aortic Dissection *(continued)*

- Can be precipitated by exercise, such as lifting weights or cycling.
- Can complicate blunt thoracic trauma.
- Aortic dissection can be a cause of maternal death during pregnancy.

Respiratory Rate
- Measure and record respiratory rate.

Pulse
- Measure and record bi-lateral radial and femoral pulses.

Oxygen Saturation
- Monitor the patient's SpO$_2$, and administer oxygen to achieve saturations of 94–98% (refer to **Oxygen**).

Blood Pressure
- Measure and record blood pressure in both upper limbs, which may be high as a consequence of the dissection.
- Hypotension is a prognostic sign for a poor patient outcome.
- Differential blood pressures may be present in around 30% of ascending or descending thoracic aortic dissections. A difference of 20 mmHg or greater between the right arm and a site beyond the dissection (left arm or leg) is considered diagnostic.

Blood Glucose
- If appropriate, measure and record blood glucose for hypoglycaemia or hyperglycaemia (refer to **Glycaemic Emergencies in Adults and Children**).

Temperature
- Measure and record temperature.

NEWS2
- Calculate a NEWS2 score (refer to NEWS2).

ECG
- If appropriate, monitor and record 12-lead ECG. Assess for abnormality (refer to **Cardiac Arrhythmia and Sudden Cardiac Death**).
- A 12-lead ECG is not a diagnostic tool to distinguish between aortic dissection and acute coronary syndrome. A patient with dissection may present with a normal ECG, ST depression or ST elevation.

Assess the Patient's Pain
- Where present, assess the **SOCRATES** of pain and record initial and subsequent pain scores.
- Consider analgesia if appropriate (refer to **Pain Management in Adults and Children**).
- Sudden onset of severe chest pain or back pain or both occurs in 80% of patients. This pain is often described as sharp, ripping, tearing or knife-like pain.
- This maximum onset sharp, knife-like pain assists in differentiating between aortic dissection and the classic cardiac chest pain that builds up in intensity over a few minutes.

Physical Examination
- Faint or absent heart sounds.
- Distended neck veins.
- Restlessness, anxiety, feeling of impending doom.
- Signs of clinical shock, including hypotension.
- Chest auscultation for signs of pleural effusion representing a haemothorax.

Vascular Emergencies

TABLE 3.128 – ASSESSMENT and MANAGEMENT of: Aortic Dissection (continued)

Management

- Minimise time spent on scene, with rapid transportation to hospital, ideally an arterial/cardiac centre. Refer to local pathways.
- Ensure effective analgesia to minimise pain and reduce the sympathetic nervous response which can worsen the dissection. For inter-hospital transfer **after the diagnosis of acute aortic dissection has been made on CT aortogram**, IV beta-blockade is prescribed and titrated to achieve pulse rate and blood pressure control.

Documentation

- Complete documentation to include all clinical findings, and advice from other clinicians.

6. Ischaemic Limbs

- **Acute limb ischaemia** (ALI) is a vascular emergency that can result in the loss of life or limb if not treated promptly. Ischaemia is considered 'acute' when symptoms have developed over 2 weeks or less.
- ALI is the result of **embolic**, **thrombotic** or **traumatic** arterial occlusion.
- In the most severely ischaemic limbs, hospital treatment within **6 hours** is required to prevent permanent damage or amputation.
- ALI is most common in patients aged 60 years or older but can occur in younger patients due to rare pre-existing conditions such as haematological or connective tissue disorders.
- Refer to Table 3.129 for the assessment and management of ALI.

TABLE 3.129 – ASSESSMENT and MANAGEMENT of: Acute Limb Ischaemia

Assess <C>ABCDE

- If any of the following **TIME-CRITICAL** features are present:
  - major **<C>ABCDE** problems (refer to **Medical Emergencies in Adults – Overview**).
- Start correcting any **<C>ABCDE** problems; see blood pressure targets below.
- Undertake a **TIME-CRITICAL** transfer to the nearest appropriate receiving arterial centre.
- Continue patient management en route.
- Provide an **ATMIST** pre-alert.

History

- Assess the patient for history associated with vascular concerns. Specific history related to ALI includes:
  - sudden onset of limb pain
  - limb has a reduction in normal skin colour
  - limb feels cold to touch
  - reduced sensation
  - inability to move limb
  - mottling of skin which may be difficult to detect in dark skin tones (severe or late ischaemia) compared to other limb. The patient may have weak or absent unilateral pulses.
  - sudden onset or deterioration of pain in the limb of patient who has recently undergone vascular surgery
  - sudden onset of painful, cold, insensate limb, which patient may be unable to move, with absent pulses.

(continued)

Vascular Emergencies

TABLE 3.129 – ASSESSMENT and MANAGEMENT of: Acute Limb Ischaemia *(continued)*

Risk Factors
- The following risk factors are associated with an increased risk of an ALI:
  - peripheral artery disease
  - aortic or popliteal aneurysm
  - recent vascular surgery, previous vascular graft or angioplasty
  - cardiac arrhythmias (e.g. AF)
  - valve replacement
  - recent MI
  - malignancy
  - smoker or ex-smoker
  - diabetes

Respiratory Rate
- Measure and record respiratory rate.

Pulse
- Measure and record pulse.

Oxygen Saturation
- Monitor the patient's SpO_2, and administer oxygen to achieve saturations of 94–98% if the patient presents as hypoxemic on air (refer to **Oxygen**).

Blood Pressure
- Measure and record blood pressure.

Blood Glucose
- If appropriate, measure and record blood glucose for hypoglycaemia or hyperglycaemia (refer to **Glycaemic Emergencies in Adults and Children**).

Temperature
- Measure and record temperature.

NEWS2
- These observations will enable you to calculate a NEWS2 score (refer to **Sepsis**).

ECG
- If required, monitor and record a 12-lead ECG. Assess for abnormality (refer to **Cardiac Arrhythmia and Sudden Cardiac Death**).

Assess the Patient's Pain
- Where present, assess the **SOCRATES** of pain and record initial and subsequent pain scores.
- Consider analgesia if appropriate (refer to **Pain Management in Adults and Children**).

Physical Examination
- The 6 'P's on physical examination are associated with identifying ALI, **but note not all 6 'Ps' may be present in a patient with clinically significant ALI**:
  - **P**ain, the majority of patients will have persistent pain
  - **P**aresthesia, reduced sensation or numbness
  - **P**allor, cyanosis or a reduction in normal skin colour
  - **P**ulselessness
  - **P**aralysis
  - **P**erishing with cold or cooler than other limb.

Vascular Emergencies

TABLE 3.129 – ASSESSMENT and MANAGEMENT of: Acute Limb Ischaemia *(continued)*

Management
- For patients presenting with any of the following presentations, consider direct conveyance to an arterial centre as per local pathway:
  - sudden onset or deterioration of pain in the limb of patient who has recently undergone vascular surgery or angioplasty
  - sudden onset of painful, cold, numb limb, which patient may be unable to move, with absent pulses
  - mottling (which may be difficult to detect in dark skin tones) of a limb with absent pulses
  - recent onset of rest pain in a patient with known peripheral vascular disease.
- Intravenous access should be gained in a limb that is not suspected to be affected by neurovascular compromise.
- The following are considered exclusions to primary bypass in the case of a suspected ALI:
  - patient recognised prior to the acute event as approaching the end of their life, on an end-of-life care pathway.
  - patient with an advanced directive in place specifically declining any vascular intervention even if their life is at risk.

Documentation
- Complete documentation to include all clinical findings, advice from other clinicians and onward referral.

7. Diabetic Foot Problem

- Diabetes is increasingly common in the UK, and a major cause of foot problems leading to lower limb amputation.
- When people with diabetes present with sepsis, both the person's life and limb are at risk if it is not recognised as a matter of urgency that the foot is the source.

7.1 Pathophysiology
- Diabetes is associated with more rapid progression of CVD. Type II diabetes specifically is associated with a high rate of peripheral arterial disease.
- People with diabetes often have reduced sensation in their feet (neuropathy), meaning that ulcers may develop, minor injuries may be missed and sepsis can develop.
- People with diabetes are more prone to infections and less able to fight them.
- Refer to Table 3.130 for a summary of this.

TABLE 3.130 – ASSESSMENT and MANAGEMENT of: Acute Diabetic Foot Problems

Assess <C>ABCDE
- If any of the following **TIME-CRITICAL** features are present:
  - major **<C>ABCDE** problems (refer to **Medical Emergencies in Adults – Overview**).
- Start correcting any **<C>ABCDE** problems; see blood pressure targets below.
- Undertake a **TIME-CRITICAL** transfer to the nearest appropriate receiving arterial centre.
- Continue patient management en route.
- Provide an **ATMIST** pre-alert.

History
- New or recurrent foot ulcer.
- Pain or swelling in the foot.

Risk Factors
- Diabetes, especially if blood sugar control has been poor.
- History of foot ulceration.
- Peripheral arterial disease.
- Peripheral neuropathy.

(continued)

Vascular Emergencies

TABLE 3.130 – ASSESSMENT and MANAGEMENT of: Acute Diabetic Foot Problems *(continued)*

Respiratory Rate
- Measure and record respiratory rate.

Pulse
- Measure and record pulse.

Oxygen Saturation
- Monitor the patient's SpO$_2$, and administer oxygen to achieve saturations of 94–98% (refer to **Oxygen**).

Blood Pressure
- Measure and record blood pressure.

Blood Glucose
- Measure and record blood glucose for hypoglycaemia or hyperglycaemia (refer to **Glycaemic Emergencies in Adults and Children**).

Temperature
- Measure and record temperature.

NEWS2
- These observations will enable you to calculate a NEWS2 score (refer to **Sepsis**).

ECG
- If appropriate, monitor and record a 12-lead ECG. Assess for abnormality (refer to **Cardiac Arrhythmia and Sudden Cardiac Death**).

Assess the Patient's Pain
- Where present, assess the **SOCRATES** of pain and record initial and subsequent pain scores.
- Patients may have little to no pain, after sensation has been lost in the foot.
- Consider analgesia if appropriate (refer to **Pain Management in Adults and Children**).

Physical Examination
- **Examination of the feet of patients with diabetes is essential when a foot problem could be a cause of pain or sepsis:**
  - foot ulceration
  - foot abscess
  - necrosis or dry gangrene
  - local infection or cellulitis or both
  - blistering
  - nail abnormalities with infection or ischaemia
  - painful, hot, swollen foot with break in the skin
  - spreading cellulitis
  - clinical shock.
- Severity of diabetic foot infections is classified as:
  - Mild – local, superficial infection less than 2 cm from ulcer edge
  - Moderate – local infection with more than 2 cm erythema or involving deeper structures (such as abscess, osteomyelitis, septic arthritis or fasciitis)
  - Severe – local infection with signs of a systemic inflammatory response. Refer to **Sepsis**.

Management
- Transfer to hospital immediately if there are limb- or life-threatening problems such as:
  - Foot ulceration with fever or sepsis
  - Foot ulceration with limb ischaemia
  - Suspected deep-seated soft tissue or bone infection, or 'If patient has already been taking antibiotics and symptoms have worsened rapidly or significantly, the person has become systemically very unwell, or if they have severe pain out of proportion to the infection'.
- Ensure effective analgesia to minimise pain.
- For all other active diabetic foot problems, refer to local pathways.

Vascular Emergencies

TABLE 3.130 – ASSESSMENT and MANAGEMENT of: Acute Diabetic Foot Problems *(continued)*

Differentials
- Other sources of sepsis, limb ischaemia, osteomyelitis or necrotising fasciitis.

Documentation
- Complete documentation to include all clinical findings and advice from other clinicians.

8. AV Fistula Bleeds

8.1 What Is an AV Fistula/Graft?

- An arteriovenous fistula or arteriovenous graft is a surgically constructed connection of an artery and a vein to allow haemodialysis. When a vein is joined directly to the artery, this is an arteriovenous fistula (also known as an AV fistula, or fistula, or AVF for short).
- Both AVFs and AVGs are commonly sited in the forearm (wrist area); they may also be sited in the upper arm (above the elbow) or even in the upper leg.
- Both AVFs and AVGs are deliberately sited just a few millimetres below the skin surface and can carry between 500 ml and 4000 ml of blood every minute.
- Patients should have been given first-aid instructions about what to do if bleeding occurs and what the warning signs of bleeding are. They may also have been given a patient information sheet or advice leaflet.

8.2 Why May an AV Fistula Haemorrhage?

- Over time, repeated needling of the AVF or AVG can result in weakening or thinning of the skin over them and/or the wall of the AVF or AVG itself. The AVF or AVG can also become infected, this can lead to scabs, ulcers and/or false aneurysms forming. If the AV fistula/graft ruptures, is punctured or cut, it is likely to bleed very heavily.

8.3 Complications and Increased Risks of Bleeding Associated with AV Fistulas and AV Grafts

- Infection of the AV fistula/graft site – indicated by a change in skin colour (red, maroon, purple or darker than the surrounding area), redness or painful swelling, discharge or pus. This increases the risk of the fistula/graft rupturing and the patient bleeding catastrophically. An infected fistula/graft needs urgent treatment in hospital.
- Damage or injury to the AV fistula/graft due to trauma or infection – anything which damages the fistula/graft (direct blow to the AV fistula/graft), increased pressure in the arm (e.g. lying on the arm when asleep or wearing a tight shirt above the fistula) or infection can cause serious damage.
- Alteration in the fistula/graft, skin or arm, e.g. damaged skin, any abnormal lumps, a swollen or painful area or altered sensation in the arm, may indicate a serious problem with the AV fistula/graft.
- Any non-healing scab/wound over the AV fistula/graft.
- Bleeding between dialysis sessions.
- Aneurysms that are increasing in size – either at cannulation sites or elsewhere.
- Shiny, thin skin over the fistula/graft – particularly over aneurysms.

8.4 Management of AV Fistulas and AV Grafts Haemorrhage

- Management should be the same as for any external bleeding by applying continuing direct pressure.
- The quickest and simplest first aid measure to control bleeding from an AVG or AVF is to use an inverted plastic bottle top (the concave/inside part of the bottle top applied to the skin) to seal it – sterility is not an issue in an emergency. Direct pressure can also be applied with the limb elevated directly over the artery feeding the fistula. The objective is to stop the bleeding, not to save the fistula/graft.
- Do NOT use multiple ambulance absorbent dressings as these do not apply adequate pressure and therefore do not arrest the haemorrhage. Tourniquets are not generally recommended, as incorrect placement can exacerbate the bleeding significantly, they should only be used if other options have been unsuccessful. If used, a tourniquet should be positioned 'above' the bleeding site and as near to the axilla as possible, i.e. between the heart and the bleeding site. The intention is to occlude the arterial blood flow, which may be challenging due to the calcification of vessels. If applying a tourniquet, failure to occlude arterial flow can result in a venous tourniquet exacerbating haemorrhage.
- If available, an Olaes® dressing is a suitable option, utilising the plastic cup component of the dressing (refer to Figure 3.49). The cup should be applied directly to the skin over the bleeding point and secured in place using the elasticated dressing to seal and tamponade the bleeding. It may be easiest to do this having removed the

Vascular Emergencies

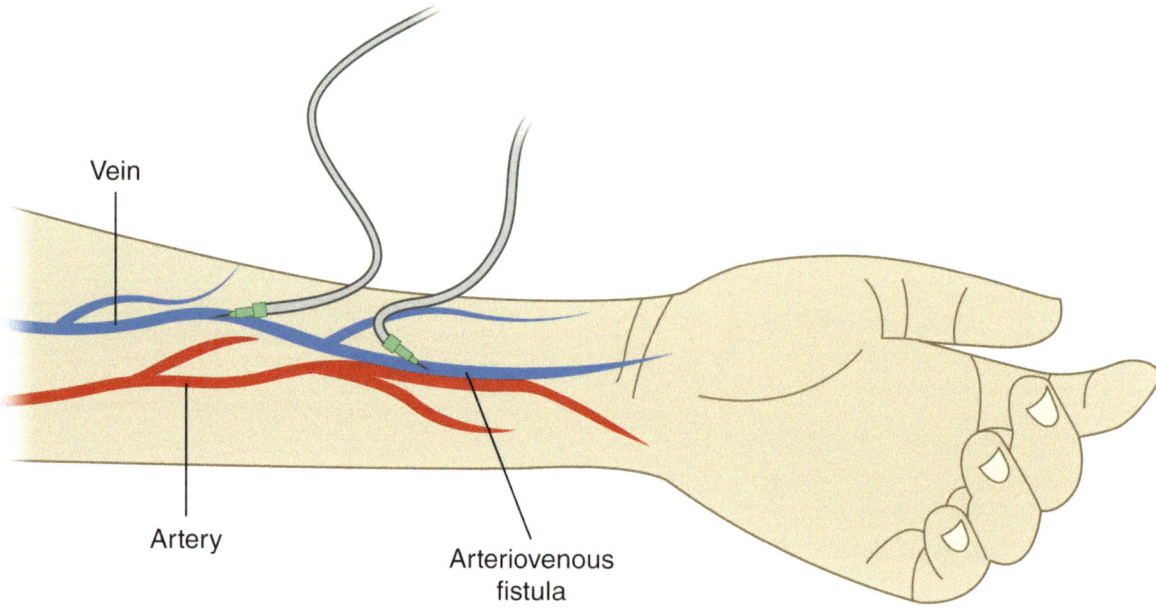

Figure 3.48 – AV fistula site.

gauze from the dressing pocket of the dressing to debulk it.
- All patients experiencing a spontaneous bleed from their AV fistula/graft (however minor) and/or felt to be at immediate risk of a bleed or further bleed MUST be conveyed to hospital for review.
- Consider direct admission to the regional renal transplant centre as per locally agreed care pathways.

8.5 Other Considerations
- If you need to cannulate a patient with an AV fistula/graft, never cannulate the fistula or the arm or in the limb the AVF is sited in.
- Do not record a blood pressure on the arm with the fistula/graft.
- Patients with a fistula/graft may be prescribed anticoagulant medications during their dialysis treatment.

9. Other Vascular Bleed Considerations

Complications from surgical wounds:
- Patients that have had specific vascular surgery or procedures involving insertion of cannulas into vessels can be at higher risk of bleeding.
- If any surgical wound is at or near the site of a blood vessel (particularly large blood vessels) there is a risk of erosion into the blood vessel and the potential for catastrophic bleeding. Infection or wound breakdown in-creases this risk.
- One example is an infected wound after a carotid endarterectomy (a surgical procedure to remove a build-up of plaques which cause narrowing of a carotid artery).
- Local wound complications may include; delayed or non-healing of the wound, infection, abscess formation, osteomyelitis or further wound breakdown. Systemic complications include bacteraemia and sepsis.
- Patients that have had (any) surgery and have complications related to the surgical wound may have been given advice about what to watch out for, what to do and who to contact. Follow this advice if appropriate.
- The need for conveyance or management in the community should be considered depending on the wound complication. Referral or liaison with community/UCR teams or liaison with a clinician/surgeon/unit that per-formed the surgery may be appropriate, as per local pathways.
- Drug users who inject can be at risk of internal and external bleeding. Some drug users may develop pseudo-aneurysms at an injection site (e.g. this may present as a pulsatile swelling in the groin. Catastrophic bleeding can occur if these rupture).

Vascular Emergencies

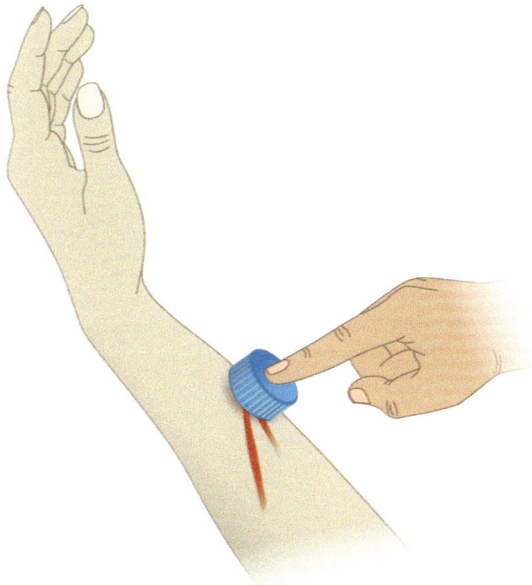

Figure 3.49 – AV fistula bleed.

KEY POINTS!

Vascular Emergencies

- Vascular emergencies require TIME-CRITICAL transfers. Refer to local pathways for destination decisions for the nearest ED, arterial centre or cardiac unit.
- Ruptured abdominal aortic aneurysm should be considered in people aged over 50 years with abdominal, back, loin, groin pain or hypotension.
- Acute aortic dissection causes sudden onset maximum initial pain, which is often described as 'tearing' in nature.
- Acute limb ischaemia is a vascular emergency that may result in a loss of life or limb if not treated promptly. People with diabetes often have reduced sensation in their feet and neuropathy, meaning that ulcers develop, minor injuries are missed and sepsis develops.
- To control bleeding from an AV fistula, direct local pressure should be used rather than dressings or a tourniquet. There is a risk of catastrophic blood loss if not controlled.
- All patients with a spontaneous bleeding from their AV fistula/graft must be conveyed to hospital.
- Patients with a small spontaneous bleed following vascular surgery or vascular procedural cannulation may be at risk of a more pronounced or even catastrophic bleed later. Does the patient have a specific advice leaflet from their surgery? Consider if need to convey to hospital for assessment.
- In patients with unexplained severe abdominal or back pain: **Think aorta!**

Bibliography

1. Lo RC, Lu B, Fokkema MTM, Conrad M et al. Relative importance of aneurysm diameter and body size for predicting abdominal aortic aneurysm rupture in men and women. *Journal of Vascular Surgery* 2014 59(5): 1209–1216. DOI: 10.1016/j.jvs.2013.10.104.
2. DoH. Cardiovascular Disease Outcomes Strategy: Improving Outcomes for People with or at risk of Cardiovascular Disease. 2013. Available from: https://www.gov.uk/government/publications/cardiovascular-disease-outcomes-strategy-improving-outcomes-for-people-with-or-at-risk-of-cardiovascular-disease.
3. Royal College of Emergency Medicine. *Best Practice Guidelines for the Management and Transfer of Patients with a diagnosis of Ruptured Abdominal Aortic Aneurysm to a specialist Vascular Centre*. 2012. Available from: www.rcem.ac.uk/docs/.
4. The Vascular Society of Great Britain and Ireland at the Royal College of Surgeons. *The Provision of Services for Patients with Vascular Disease*. 2015. London.
5. Brearley S. Acute leg ischaemia. *BMJ* 2013, 346.
6. Cumberbatch G. *Aortic Dissection*. 2017. Available from: https://www.rcemlearning.co.uk/references/aortic-dissection/.

Vascular Emergencies

7. Dr Joseph, TM. *Thoracic Aortic Aneurysm*. 2017. Available from: http://drjosephtm.blogspot.com/2017/04/thoracic-aortic-aneurysms.html#!/2017/04/thoracic-aortic-aneurysms.html.

8. Erbel R, Aboyans V, Boileau C, Bossone E, Di Bartolomeo R, Eggebrecht H et al. ESC Guidelines on the diagnosis and treatment of aortic diseases. *European Heart Journal* 2014, 35: 2873–2926.

9. French C. *CBP: Aortic Aneurysm*. 2016. Available from: http://slideplayer.com/slide/6845630/.

10. Wheatley G. *Acute Aortic Dissections: 'It's complicated'.* 2015. Available from: https://badaorta.com/acute-aortic-dissections-its-complicated/.

11. British Renal Society. Vascular Access Special Interest Group — A multi professional initiative. *Kidney Care* 2016, 1(3): 150–152.

12. Ellingson KD, Palekar RS, Lucero CA et al. Vascular hemorrhages contribute to deaths among hemodialysis patients. *Kidney Int.* 2012, 82(6): 686–692.

13. Inston N, Mistry H, Gilbert J, et al. Aneurysms in vascular access: State of the art and future developments. *J Vasc Access* 2017, 18(6): 464–472.

14. Bossone E, Carbone A, Eagle KA. Gender Differences in Acute Aortic Dissection. *J Pers Med.* 2022, Jul 15;12(7): 1148. doi: 10.3390/jpm12071148. PMID: 35887644; PMCID: PMC9324420.

15. BMJ 2024. BMJ Best Practice, Abdominal aortic aneurysm. Available from: https://bestpractice.bmj.com/topics/en-gb/3000088.

16. BMJ 2024. BMJ Best Practice, Aortic dissection. Available from: https://bestpractice.bmj.com/topics/en-gb/3000226.

17. NICE 2020. National Institute for Health and Care Excellence. Abdominal aortic aneurysm: diagnosis and management [NG156]. Available from: https://www.nice.org.uk/guidance/ng156

4

Trauma

Trauma Emergencies in Adults – Overview

1. Introduction

For references, refer to individual trauma guidelines.

- Trauma is a leading cause of death in the UK. The wide range of traumatic injuries encountered in pre-hospital care can present a complex challenge. Research suggests that assessing and managing patients in a systematic way can lead to improved outcomes.
- This overview will outline the process of assessment and management of trauma patients. This guideline supports the following related guidelines:
  - abdominal trauma
  - head trauma
  - limb trauma
  - spinal injury and spinal cord injury
  - pelvic trauma
  - thoracic trauma
  - trauma in pregnancy
  - traumatic cardiac arrest
  - airway management
  - burns and scalds
  - electrical injuries
  - fluid therapy
  - oxygen therapy
  - pain management.

This guideline uses mechanism of injury (MOI) and primary survey as the basis of care for all trauma patients.

2. Incidence

- In England it is estimated that there are approximately 20,000 cases of major trauma annually. Road traffic collisions (RTC) are the most common cause.

3. Severity and Outcome

- In England major trauma accounts for approximately 5,400 deaths each year, with many more cases leading to significant short- and long-term morbidity. In Scotland (1992–2002) there were 5,847 deaths resulting from trauma. Major trauma is the leading cause of death in patients under 45 years of age.

4. Incident Management

- Overall control of the incident allows paramedics to concentrate on patient assessment and management and it is recommended that a model, such as SCENE, is used to assess the initial trauma scene so that it can be managed effectively (refer to Table 4.1).

TABLE 4.1 – SCENE	
S	**Safety** Perform a dynamic risk assessment: are there any dangers now or will there be any that become apparent during the incident? This needs to be continually re-assessed throughout the incident. Appropriate personal protective equipment should be utilised according to local guidelines.
C	**Cause including MOI** Establish the events leading up to the incident. Is this consistent with your findings?
E	**Environment** Are there any environmental factors that need to be taken into consideration? These can include problems with access or egress, weather conditions or time of day.
N	**Number of patients** Establish exactly how many patients there are during the initial assessment of the scene.
E	**Extra resources needed** Additional resources should be mobilised now. These can include additional ambulances, helicopter or senior medical support. Liaise with the major trauma advisor according to local protocols.

5. Patient Assessment

A primary survey should be undertaken for **ALL** patients as this will rapidly identify patients with actual or potential **TIME-CRITICAL** injuries (refer to Table 4.3).

A secondary survey is a more thorough 'head-to-toe' assessment of the patient. It should be undertaken following completion of the primary survey, where time permits. The secondary survey will usually be undertaken during transfer to further care; however, in some patients with time-critical trauma, it may not be possible to undertake the secondary survey before arrival at further care (refer to Table 4.4).

Trauma Emergencies in Adults – Overview

5.1 Primary Survey

- The primary survey should take no more than 60–90 seconds and follow the **<C>ABCDE** approach. Document the vital signs and the time they were taken.
- Consider MOI and the possible injury patterns that may result, but be aware that mechanism alone cannot predict or exclude injury and physiological signs should be utilised as well.
- Assessment and management should proceed in a '**stepwise**' manner and life-threatening injuries should be managed as they are encountered, i.e. do not move onto breathing and circulation until the airway is secured. Every time an intervention has been carried out, re-assess the patient.
- As soon as a life-threatening injury is identified and managed, it is recommended that transport should be immediately instigated to the appropriate trauma facility according to local procedures.
- If immediate transfer is not possible, consider mobilising senior clinical support if not already done during the SCENE assessment.

MANAGEMENT OVERVIEW

If the patient has a life-threatening condition, start immediate transfer to an appropriate trauma facility according to local procedures, with treatment undertaken en route to hospital.

- Provide an alert/information call.
- Continue patient re-assessment and management.
- If a patient requires IV fluids (refer to **Intravascular Fluid Therapy in Adults**) and triggering local network major trauma criteria then they should receive a bolus of tranexamic acid if available (refer to **Tranexamic Acid**).
- **Pain management** – if analgesia is indicated, refer to **Pain Management in Adults and Children**.
- Hand over – it is recommended that the patient is handed over to receiving clinicians using the ATMIST format (refer to Table 4.2).

If the patient is **NON-TIME-CRITICAL**, undertake a secondary survey (refer to Table 4.4).

5.2 Secondary Survey

- A secondary survey should only commence after the primary survey has been completed and in critical patients only during transport.

TABLE 4.2 – ATMIST

A	**A**ge
T	**T**ime of incident
M	**M**echanism
I	**I**njuries
S	**S**igns and symptoms
T	**T**reatment given/immediate needs

TABLE 4.3 – ASSESSMENT and MANAGEMENT of: Trauma Emergencies

- All stages should be considered but some may be omitted if not considered appropriate.
- To reduce clot disruption, avoid unnecessary movements.
- When available, consider administration of tranexamic acid to all patients who require **TIME-CRITICAL** transfer.

At each stage, consider the need for:

- **TIME-CRITICAL** – transfer to nearest appropriate hospital as per local trauma care pathway.
- **Early senior clinical support.**

<C> – Catastrophic Haemorrhage

- Assess for the presence of **LIFE-THREATENING EXTERNAL BLEEDING**
- Follow the management in Figures 4.2 and 4.3.

A – Airway

- Assess the airway and **AT ALL TIMES** consider C-spine injury and the need to immobilise (refer to **Spinal Injury and Spinal Cord Injury**).
- **Look for** obvious obstructions (e.g. teeth/dentures, foreign bodies, vomit, blood, trauma, soot/burns/oedema in burn patients).
- **Listen for** noisy airflow (e.g. snoring, gurgling or no airflow).
- **Feel for** air movement.

(continued)

Trauma Emergencies in Adults – Overview

TABLE 4.3 – ASSESSMENT and MANAGEMENT of: Trauma Emergencies *(continued)*

- Correct any airway problems immediately by:
  - jaw thrust, chin lift (no neck extension).
  - suction (if appropriate).
  - nasopharyngeal airway.
  - oropharyngeal airway.
  - supraglottic airway (if appropriate).
  - endotracheal intubation (only if trained/authorised and waveform capnography available).
  - needle cricothyroidotomy.

B – Breathing

- Assess rate, depth and quality of respiration.
- Grade breathing 1–5:
1. patient not breathing
2. slow <12 per min
3. normal 12–20 but check depth
4. fast 20–30 observe very closely
5. very fast >30.
- Feel for depth and equality of chest movement, any instability of chest wall.
- Look for obvious chest injuries, wounds, bruising or flail segment.
- Auscultate lung fields assessing air entry on each side.
- Percuss the chest wall checking the pitch of the percussion note.
- In addition, assess the chest and neck for the following using the mnemonic **TWELVE**:
  - **T**racheal deviation
  - **W**ounds, bruising or swelling
  - **E**mphysema (surgical)
  - **L**aryngeal crepitus
  - **V**enous engorgement
  - **E**xcluding open/tension pneumothorax, flail segment, massive haemothorax.
- Administer 100% O_2 in all patients with critical trauma to target O_2 sats of 94–98%, even if there are risk factors such as COPD.
  - Breathing graded at 1,2 should receive O_2 via BVM, as should grade 5 if clinically appropriate.
  - Breathing graded at 3,4 should receive supplemental 100% O_2 but be monitored very closely.
  - Apply non-occlusive dressing to sucking chest wounds (refer to **Thoracic Trauma**).
  - Decompress a tension pneumothorax (refer to **Thoracic Trauma**).
  - Flail segments should not be splinted (refer to **Thoracic Trauma**).

NB Restraint (POSITIONAL) asphyxia – If the patient is required to be physically restrained (e.g. by police officers) in order to prevent them injuring themselves or others, or for the purpose of being detained under the Mental Health Act, then it is paramount that the method of restraint allows both for a patent airway and adequate respiratory volume. **Under these circumstances it is essential to ensure that the patient's airway and breathing are adequate at all times.**

C – Circulation

- If massive external haemorrhage was controlled at start of assessment, re-assess this now.
- Assess for radial and carotid pulses, noting rate, rhythm and volume, assess central and peripheral capillary refill time, note skin colour, texture and temperature.
- Remain alert to the possibility of internal bleeding and assess for signs of blood loss in five places (blood on the floor and four more):
1. External
2. Chest (already done during breathing assessment)
3. Abdomen by palpation and observation of bruising or external marks

Trauma Emergencies in Adults – Overview

TABLE 4.3 – ASSESSMENT and MANAGEMENT of: Trauma Emergencies *(continued)*

4 Pelvis – do not manipulate the pelvis – MOI may suggest a fracture

5 Long bones – assess for but do not be distracted by limb trauma.

- Consider hypovolaemic shock but be aware that blood loss of 1000–1500 ml is required before classical signs start to appear. Signs of hypovolaemic shock include pallor, cool peripheries, anxiety and abnormal behaviour, increased respiratory rate and tachycardia. Signs of shock also appear much later in certain patient groups (e.g. pregnant women, patients on beta-blockers and the physically fit). There may well be little evidence of shock.
- Follow the management for haemorrhage control in Figures 4.2 and 4.3.
- Consider splinting:
  - In the critical patient, **long bone fractures** should be splinted en route to the trauma facility.
  - **Pelvic fractures** should be stabilised at the earliest possible opportunity, preferably before the patient is moved (refer to **Pelvic Trauma**).

Fluid therapy

- If fluid replacement is indicated, refer to **Intravascular Fluid Therapy in Adults**.

TRANEXAMIC ACID

- If a patient requires IV fluids and triggering local network major trauma criteria then they should receive a bolus of tranexamic acid (refer to **Tranexamic Acid**).
- A study around use of TXA in major trauma concluded that administration of TXA to patients with bleeding trauma reduces mortality to a similar extent in women and men, but women are substantially less likely to be treated with TXA and if they are treated it is at a later stage than for men.
- In cases of internal or uncontrolled haemorrhage, undertake a **TIME-CRITICAL** transfer to appropriate hospital according to local procedures.
- To minimise clot disruption, avoid unnecessary movement in victims of blunt trauma:
  - Log roll should be avoided wherever possible.
  - Patients should be lifted from the ground using a scoop (bivalve) stretcher.
  - Once on a scoop (bivalve) stretcher, patients should be transported on it.
  - A long spinal board is an extrication device and should not be used unless required (refer to **Spinal Injury and Spinal Cord Injury**).
  - A patient with penetrating trauma who has no neurology and no possibility of direct trauma to the spinal column should NOT be immobilised.

D – Disability

- Obtain a full GCS (refer to Table 4.5) for the patient.
- Assess and note pupil size, equality and response to light.
- Altered mental status:
  - Check blood glucose level to rule out hypo/hyperglycaemia as the cause (refer to **Glycaemic Emergencies in Adults and Children**).

E – Exposure and Environment

- At this stage, further monitoring may be applied.
- Exposure:
  - Ensure patient does not suffer from exposure to cold/wet conditions.
- Trapped patient:
  - Consider mobilising early senior clinical support.

- The secondary survey is a more thorough 'head-to-toe' survey of the patient; however, it is important to monitor the patient's vital signs during the survey.
- In some patients with critical trauma it may not be possible to undertake a secondary survey before arriving at a trauma facility. However, in patients with altered mental status it is recommended that a blood glucose reading should be taken during transport.
- Consider scoring a patient's level of frailty. Refer to Figure 4.1.[7]
  - The Rockwood Clinical Frailty Scale (CFS) is a judgement-based frailty assessment tool. It is not validated for people under the age of 65 years or those with long-term disabilities.

Trauma Emergencies in Adults – Overview

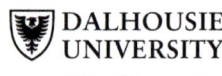

Figure 4.1 – Clinical Frailty Scale. Used with permission from Dr. Rockwood and the Geriatric Medicine Research Unit.

Frailty must be sensed, described and measured: not guessed. If the patient you are assessing is acutely unwell and over 65 years, consider using the CFS, as per local pathways.
- The score is based on the patient's baseline, so use the tool to score how the patient was 2 weeks ago (prior to deterioration) or their usual level of functioning when well, rather than how they present today. If possible, cross-reference what the patient describes to you with a description from relatives/carers.
- Do NOT compare the patient to the pictures (e.g. person using walking aids) alone to make a judgement on the level of frailty.

TABLE 4.4 – Secondary Survey

ASSESSMENT

Head
- Re-assess airway.
- Check skin colour and temperature.
- Palpate for bruising/fractures.
- Check pupil size and reactivity.
- Examine for loss of cerebrospinal fluid.
- Establish Glasgow Coma Scale (refer to Table 4.5).
- Assess for other signs of basal skull fracture.

NB For further information, refer to **Head Injury**.

Trauma Emergencies in Adults – Overview

TABLE 4.4 – Secondary Survey *(continued)*

Neck
- The collar will need to be loosened for proper examination of the neck.
- Re-assess for signs of life-threatening injury using the mnemonic **TWELVE**:
  - **T**racheal deviation
  - **W**ounds, bruising or swelling
  - **E**mphysema (surgical)
  - **L**aryngeal crepitus
  - **V**enous engorgement (jugular)
  - **E**xcluding open/tension pneumothorax, flail segment, massive haemothorax.
- Assess and palpate for spinal tenderness; particularly note any bony tenderness.

NB For further information, refer to **Spinal Injury and Spinal Cord Injury**.

Chest
- Assess rate, depth and quality of respiration and grade breathing 1–5:

1. patient not breathing
2. slow <12 per min
3. normal 12–20 but check depth
4. fast 20–30 observe very closely
5. very fast >30

- Breathing graded at 1,2 should receive O_2 via BVM, as should grade 5 if clinically appropriate.
- Breathing graded at 3,4 should receive supplemental 100% O_2 but should be monitored very closely.
- Feel for rib fractures, instability and surgical emphysema.
- Look for contusions, seat-belt marks and flail segments.
- Auscultate lung fields for signs of:
  - Pneumothorax
  - Tension pneumothorax
  - Haemothorax
  - Cardiac tamponade
  - Assess for signs of pulmonary contusion.
- Examine the front and as much of the back as is possible.

NB for further information, refer to **Thoracic Trauma**.

Abdomen
- Examine for open wounds, contusions and seat-belt marks.
- Palpate the entire abdomen for tenderness and guarding.
- Examine the front and as much of the back as is possible.

NB For further information, refer to **Abdominal Trauma**.

Pelvis
- Blood loss may be visible either from the urethra or per vaginum (PV).
- The patient may have the urge to urinate.

NB For further information, refer to **Pelvic Trauma**.

Lower/upper limbs
- Examine lower limbs then upper limbs.
- Look for wounds and evidence of fractures.
- Check for MSC in **ALL** four limbs:
  - **MOTOR** – Test for movement.
  - **SENSATION** – Apply light touch to evaluate sensation.
  - **CIRCULATION** – Assess pulse and skin temperature.

NB For further information, refer to **Limb Trauma**.

Trauma Emergencies in Adults – Overview

TABLE 4.5 – Glasgow Coma Scale

Item	Element	Score
Eyes Opening:		
	Spontaneously	4
	To speech	3
	To pain	2
	None	1
Verbal Response:		
	Orientated	5
	Confused	4
	Inappropriate words	3
	Incomprehensible sounds	2
	No verbal response	1
Motor Response:		
	Obeys commands	6
	Localised pain	5
	Withdraws from pain	4
	Abnormal flexion	3
	Extensor response	2
	No response to pain	1

6. The Trapped Patient

Entrapment can be:

- **Relative:** trapped by difficulty in access/egress from the wreckage, including the physical injury stopping normal exit.
- **Absolute:** firmly trapped by a vehicle and its deformity, necessitating specialised cutting techniques to free the patient.

All patients with evidence of injury should be considered time-dependent and their entrapment time should be minimised.

6.1 Management

- Conduct a thorough assessment of the incident using SCENE or similar model.
- Consider mobilising senior clinical support at the earliest opportunity.
- Mobilise and liaise with other emergency services.
- Perform primary survey and manage as per Table 4.3. Clinical care during entrapment should be limited to necessary critical interventions to expedite safe extrication.
- Develop a bespoke patient centred extrication plan with the primary focus of minimising entrapment time.
- Provide analgesia (refer to **Pain Management in Adults and Children**).

6.2 Extrication

- The Emergency services on scene should work together to develop a bespoke patient centred extrication plan with the primary focus of minimising entrapment time.
- Independent of actual or suspected injuries patients should be handled gently. A focus on absolute movement minimisation is not justified.
- Self-extrication or minimally assisted extrication should be the standard 'first line' extrication unless one of the following contraindications are present:
  – An inability to understand or follow instructions
  – Injuries or baseline function that prevents the patient standing on one leg.

(Some injuries that may prevent self-extrication are: unstable pelvic fracture, impalement, or bilateral leg fractures)

Immobilisation:

- Longboards are extrication devices and should not be used beyond the extrication phase
- Pelvic slings/binders to be applied when this can safely be done with minimal handling. This will often be after extrication
- Cervical collars should only be used following clinical assessment. After extrication, consider loosening or removing the cervical collar
- Standard practice is to immobilise the spine. There are two common approaches to this within UK paramedic practice:
  – head blocks and scoop with collar
  – head blocks and scoop without collar

Care during entrapment:

Patient-focused extrication:

- Communicate with patients, explain actions, and use their name
- Where appropriate, reassure patients as to the safety of others involved in the incident (including animals)
- Provide an 'extrication buddy': this is a member of the emergency services team dedicated to communication, reassurance and explanation to the entrapped patient.
- Allow communication with family members or other close contacts
- Rescuers should be aware that clinical observations may prolong entrapment time and a pragmatic decision regarding their frequency should be made on a case-by-case basis

Trauma Emergencies in Adults – Overview

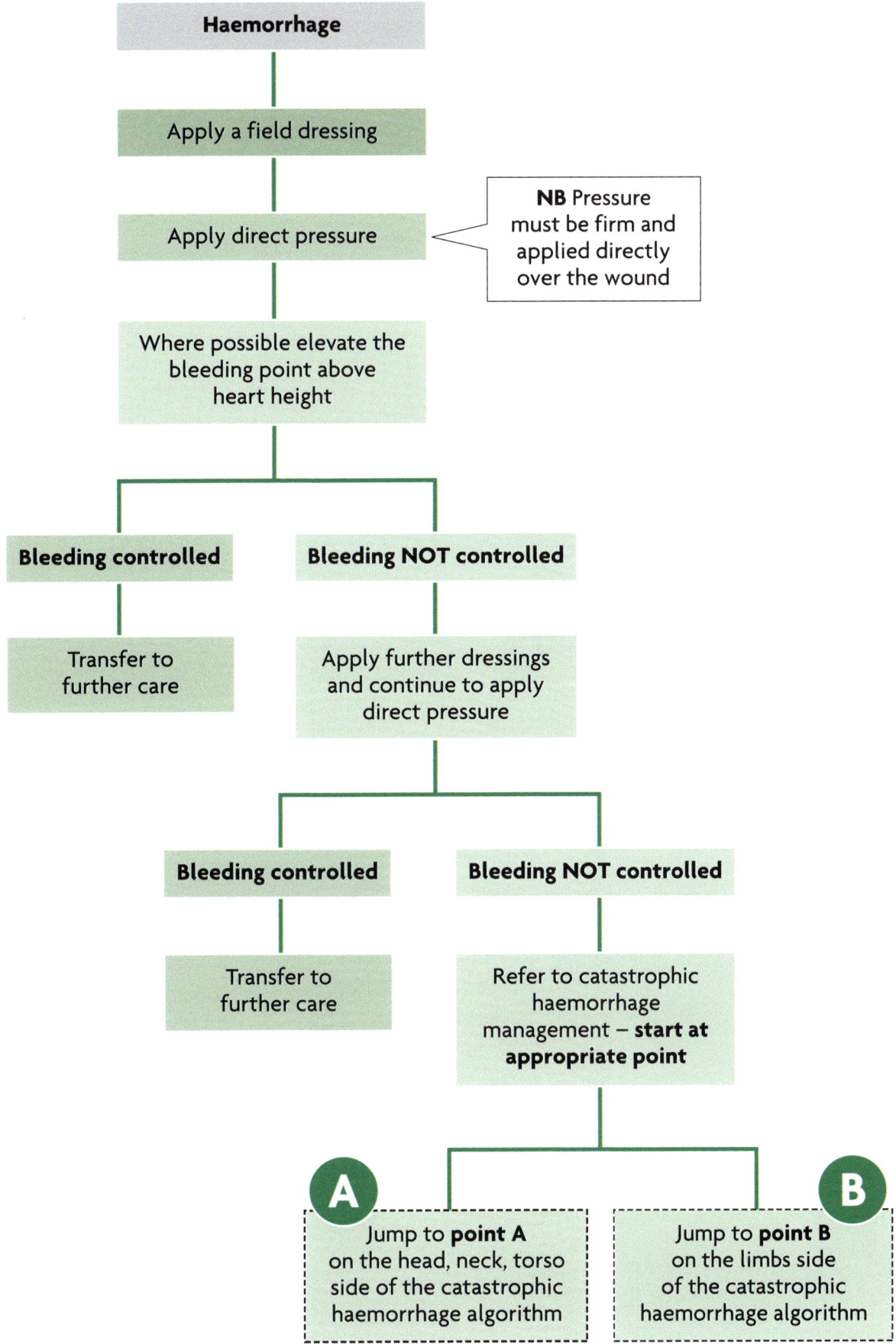

Figure 4.2 – The management of haemorrhage algorithm.

Trauma Emergencies in Adults – Overview

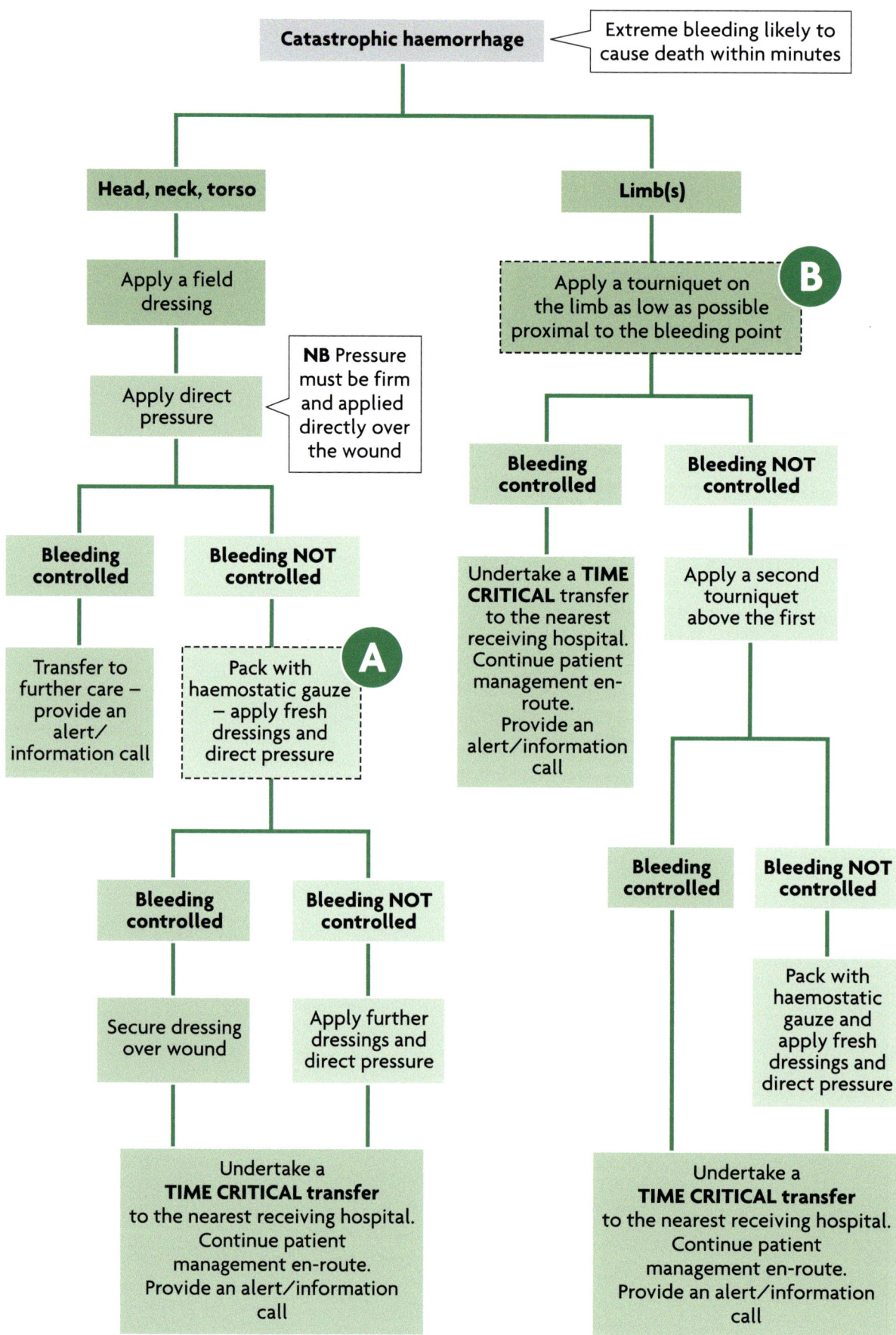

Figure 4.3 – The management of catastrophic haemorrhage algorithm.

Trauma Emergencies in Adults – Overview

7. Hanging

7.1 Introduction
- Hanging is the most common method of suicide, accounting for 61% of all suicides in those aged 10 years and above (Apr–Jul 2020). Males outnumber females by roughly 3:1 and ages 45–64 have the highest rate.[1] Hanging may be accidental or deliberate.

7.2 Mechanisms and Definitions
- Hanging may be defined as a short drop or long drop, fully suspended or partially supported (where the entire weight of the body is not supported by the ligature). A long drop can lead to sudden death as a result of a fracture-dislocation of the upper cervical vertebrae. A short drop may lead to death by asphyxia. There is no agreed definition of the height required for a long or short drop; the approximate height of the drop should be handed over to other clinicians and documented.
- In a short-drop or partially supported hanging, the patient may asphyxiate and may not have a cervical spine fracture. The mechanism of death in short drop is compression of the airway and blood vessels of the neck. This can also cause vagal discharge through pressure on the baroreceptors in the carotid sinus and the carotid body.[2]

7.3 Assessment & Management
- Undertake a risk assessment with regards to whether you are able to safely get access to the patient.
- Identify if there are any conditions unequivocally associated with death (refer to **Termination of Resuscitation and Verification of Death in Adults**).
- Identify if there are signs of life or the need for resuscitation.
- Remove (and if necessary, cut) ligatures.
- Consider dispatching or calling for additional specialist teams or critical care resources at an early stage, as per local procedures.
- Consider the need for requesting additional support, particularly for the management of the post-ROSC agitated patient and for advanced airway management.
- Safely move the patient into an appropriate position for further assessment and management, protecting the cervical spine if a cervical spine or serious laryngeal injury is suspected.
- Refer to **Trauma Emergencies in Adults – Overview** and **Trauma Emergencies in Children – Overview** for assessment and management of injuries.
- Airway management should be prioritised over cervical spine management (refer to **Advanced Life Support**).
- Ventilation and/or intubation may be difficult due to the potential for airway injury and laryngeal swelling.

7.4 Hanging and Cardiac Arrest
- Manage as per **Advanced Life Support** and refer to **Termination of Resuscitation and Verification of Death in Adults**.
- If CPR is not commenced, where possible clinicians should not disturb the scene to assist police investigations.

7.5 Post-ROSC Care
- Be aware that patients are likely to be hypoxic and agitated, and may benefit from interventions by specialist or critical care teams.
- Consider the possibility of spinal or spinal cord injury (refer to **Spinal Injury and Spinal Cord Injury**).

7.6 Staff Wellbeing
- All staff may be affected by this type of incident. This could affect them immediately after the incident or in the longer term. Always offer support to all staff that have attended and follow local procedures for this. Undertake post-incident debriefs as per local procedures. Refer to **Staff Health and Wellbeing**.
- Consider the need to signpost bystanders/witnesses/family to support as well.
- A study around use of TXA in major trauma concluded that administration of TXA to patients with bleeding trauma reduces mortality to a similar extent in women and men, but women are substantially less likely to be treated with TXA and if they are treated it is at a later stage than for men.

Acknowledgements

We would like to gratefully acknowledge the contribution of Tim Nutbeam, John JM Black, Paul Gibbs, Graham McClelland, Lee Thompson, and Gary Shaw to this JRCALC guideline.

Trauma Emergencies in Adults – Overview

> **KEY POINTS!**
>
> **Trauma Emergencies in Adults – Overview**
> - Overall assessment of safety is of prime importance: self, scene, casualties.
> - The primary survey forms the basis of patient assessment, with due consideration for C-spine immobilisation.
> - Arrest of external haemorrhage can be life-saving.
> - Consider seeking senior clinical advice/support at the earliest opportunity.
> - Standard paramedic practice still includes collars and head blocks as an option.
> - A study around use of TXA in major trauma concluded that administration of TXA to patients with bleeding trauma reduces mortality to a similar extent in women and men, but women are substantially less likely to be treated with TXA and if they are treated it is at a later stage than for men.

Further Reading

British Renal Society. Vascular Access Special Interest Group – a multi professional initiative. *Kidney Care* 2016, 1(3): 150–152.

Ellingson KD, Palekar RS, Lucero CA et al. Vascular hemorrhages contribute to deaths among hemodialysis patients. *Kidney International* 2012, 82(6): 686–692.

Inston N, Mistry H, Gilbert J, et al. Aneurysms in vascular access: state of the art and future developments. *Journal of Vascular Access* 2017, 18(6): 464–472.

Bibliography

1. Office for National Statistics (ONS). *Deaths from Suicide That Occurred in England and Wales: April to July 2020*. 2021. Available from: https://www.ons.gov.uk/peoplepopulationandcommunity/birthsdeathsandmarriages/deaths/articles/deathsfromsuicidethatoccurredinenglandandwales/aprilandjuly2020.
2. Gubbins K. The hanging/hanged patient and relevance to pre-hospital care. *Journal of Paramedic Practice* 2016, 8(6). DOI: 10.12968/jpar.2016.8.6.290.
3. Alqahtani S, Nehme Z, Williams B, Bernard S, and Smith K. Temporal Trends in the incidence, characteristics, and outcomes of hanging-related out-of-hospital cardiac arrest. *Prehospital Emergency Care* 2020, 24(3): 369–377. DOI: 10.1080/10903127.2019.1666944.
4. Paul SP, Paul R, Heaton PA. Accidental hanging injuries in children: recognition and management. *British Journal of Hospital Medicine* 2017, 78(10): 572–577. DOI: 10.12968/hmed.2017.78.10.572.
5. Shaw G, Thompson L, McClelland G. Hangings attended by emergency medical services: a scoping review. *British Paramedic Journal* 2021, 5(4): 40–48. DOI: 10.29045/14784726.2021.3.5.4.40.
6. Turner J, et al. Out-of-hospital cardiac arrest due to hanging: a retrospective analysis. *Emergency Medicine Journal* 2021. DOI: 10.1136/emermed-2020-210839.
7. Rockwood, K et al. (2005) A global clinical measure of fitness and frailty in elderly people. *Canadian Medical Association Journal* 173(5): 489–495.
8. Nutbeam, T., Fenwick, R., Smith, J.E. et al. A Delphi study of rescue and clinical subject matter experts on the extrication of patients following a motor vehicle collision. *Scand J Trauma Resusc Emerg Med* 30, 41 (2022). https://doi.org/10.1186/s13049-022-01029-x

Trauma Emergencies in Children – Overview

1. Introduction
- Paediatric trauma is managed following the standard <C>ABCDE approach to trauma, taking into account differences in the child's anatomy, relative size and physiological response to injury. These differences are addressed below.

2. Incidence
- 700 children die as a result of accidents in England and Wales each year.
- 50% of child trauma deaths occur in motor vehicle incidents. Children travelling by car should legally be restrained but this law is not always followed and many deaths and serious injuries occur following vehicular ejection. Additionally, child deaths from cycle and pedestrian incidents are also very common.
- 30% of child trauma deaths occur at home, with burns and falls being the leading causes.
- Child death reviews often identify circumstances that could potentially have been avoided had injury prevention methods been rigorously applied.
- Hanging is the most common method of suicide, accounting for 61% of all suicides in those aged 10 years and above (Apr–Jul 2020). Hanging may be accidental or deliberate. Please refer to Section 7 in **Trauma Emergencies in Adults – Overview**.

3. Assessment: The Basic Trauma Approach

3.1 SCENE
Overall control of the incident allows paramedics to concentrate on patient assessment and management and it is recommended that a model, such as SCENE, is used to assess the initial trauma scene so that it can be managed effectively (see below).

S	Safety
	Risk assessment. Perform a dynamic risk assessment. Are there any dangers now or will there be any that become apparent during the incident? This needs to be continually re-assessed throughout the incident. Appropriate personal protective equipment should be utilised according to local protocols.
C	Cause including MOI
	Establish the events leading up to the incident. Is this consistent with your findings? Read the scene/wreckage looking for evidence that children were involved (e.g. toys or child seats). These may provide a clue that a child has been ejected from the vehicle or wandered off from the scene but may still require medical attention or other care. Ask if children were involved.
E	Environment
	Are there any environmental factors that need to be taken into consideration? These can include problems with access or egress, weather conditions or time of day.
N	Number of patients
	Establish exactly how many patients there are during the initial assessment of the scene
E	Extra resources needed
	Additional resources should be mobilised now. These can include additional ambulances, helicopter or senior medical support. Liaise with the major trauma advisor according to local protocols.

3.2 Primary Survey
- Catastrophic haemorrhage (refer to Figure 4.5).
- Airway with cervical spine control (refer to **Spinal Injury and Spinal Cord Injury**).
- Breathing.
- Circulation.
- Disability.
- Exposure.

The management of a child suffering a traumatic injury requires a careful approach, with an emphasis on explanation, reassurance and honesty. Trust of the carer by the child makes management much easier.

If possible, it is helpful to keep the child's parents/carers close by for reassurance, although their distress can exacerbate that of the child.

3.3 Stepwise Primary Survey Assessment
As for all trauma care, a systematic approach, managing problems as they are encountered before moving on, is required.

4. Catastrophic Haemorrhage
Catastrophic blood loss must be arrested immediately (refer to Figure 4.5).

5. Airway
- In small children, the relatively large occiput tends to flex the head forward. In order to return the head to the neutral position it may be necessary to insert a small amount of padding under the shoulders.
- Vomit, blood or foreign material may obstruct the airway. Apply gentle suctioning under direct vision. Blind finger sweeps are contra-indicated.
- Head tilt should be avoided in trauma and a chin lift alone or a jaw thrust used to open the airway.
- If an airway adjunct is needed, then an oropharyngeal airway should be inserted

Trauma Emergencies in Children – Overview

under direct vision. If it is necessary to insert a nasopharyngeal airway (e.g. because of trismus), care must be taken in all head-injured children in case there is an underlying skull fracture, causing a risk of misplacement through the cribriform plate into the brain. It is also important to avoid damage to the adenoidal tissue. This can cause considerable bleeding, making the airway even more difficult to manage.

- High concentration oxygen (O_2) (refer to **Oxygen**) should be administered routinely, whatever the oxygen saturation, in children sustaining major trauma or long bone fractures.
- Administer high concentration O_2 via a non-rebreathing mask, to maintain an oxygen saturation of at least 94%. If a high-flow mask is not tolerated, the mask (or just the oxygen tubing) may be held near the child's nose or mouth.
- Airway burns are considered as a 'special case' (refer to **Burns and Scalds**). Examine for soot in the nostrils and mouth, erythema and blistering of the lips and hoarseness of the voice. These suggest potential airway injury. These children require early endotracheal intubation and may deteriorate faster than adults due to the smaller diameter of their airway. Unless there is somebody at the scene who is trained in pre-hospital paediatric anaesthesia and difficult paediatric airway management who can electively intubate the child, it is best to transport the child rapidly (time-critical transfer) and to pre-alert the hospital so they can have suitable experts standing by. If the airway swelling becomes life-threatening, and the airway cannot be controlled any other way, needle cricothyroidotomy may be required. Surgical airways should be avoided for those under the age of 12 years.

6. Cervical Spine

- Cervical spinal immobilisation is essential when an injury to the neck has possibly occurred. Manual immobilisation is initially used, although the subsequent use of a correctly sized cervical collar, head blocks and forehead/chin tapes and a scoop stretcher or a long board where the child has to be extricated is recommended. If the child is combative, this may not be possible and manual immobilisation may be the only possible method (refer to **Spinal Injury and Spinal Cord Injury**).

7. Breathing

- A child's chest wall is readily deformable and may withstand significant force. As a result, significant intra-thoracic injuries can occur without any apparent external chest wall signs.
- **Auscultate** the chest if practical.

- **Look at** the chest for bruising and record the rate and adequacy of breathing. Chest wall movement and the presence of any wounds should be sought. Poor excursion may suggest an underlying pneumothorax.
- **Feel** for rib fractures, or surgical emphysema.
- This should reveal good, bilateral air entry and the absence of any added sounds. Listen specifically to the following three areas:
1. above the nipples in the mid-clavicular line
2. in the mid-axilla under the armpits
3. at the rear of the chest, below the shoulder blades when it is possible to access this area.

TABLE 4.6 – Normal Respiratory Rates

Age	Respiratory rate
<1 year	40–60 breaths per minute
1–2 years	25–35 breaths per minute
2–5 years	25–30 breaths per minute
5–11 years	20–25 breaths per minute
>12 years	15–20 breaths per minute

- Percuss the chest if possible assessing for hyporesonance or hyperresonance.
- Assess for:
  - Tension pneumothorax.
  - Massive haemothorax.
  - Sucking chest wounds (open pneumothorax).
  - Flail chest.

NB Refer to **Thoracic Trauma** for the management of these conditions.

NB Distended neck veins are very difficult to see in children and in shock may be absent.

7.1 Management

- If ventilation is inadequate (see below) the child's respiratory effort may require support from bag-valve-mask ventilation and high-flow oxygen. Assist ventilation at a rate equivalent to the normal respiratory rate for the age of the child (refer to Table 4.6) if:
  - The child is hypoxic (SpO_2 <90%) and remains so after 30–60 seconds on high concentration O_2.
  - Respiratory rate is <50% normal or >3 times normal.
- Treat life-threatening chest injuries as per appropriate guideline (see above).

8. Circulation

- Refer to Medical Emergencies – Recognition of Circulatory Failure.

Trauma Emergencies in Children – Overview

- Look firstly for evidence of significant external haemorrhage and treat as per haemorrhage guideline (refer to Figures 4.4 and 4.5).
- Assess the:
  - Brachial or carotid pulses; record rate and volume (refer to Table 4.7):
    - tachycardia (with a poor pulse volume) suggests shock
    - bradycardia also occurs in the shocked child but is a **PRE-TERMINAL SIGN**.
- Respiratory rate: elevated due to compensatory mechanisms in shock.
- Capillary refill time: measure on the forehead or sternum.
- Colour.
- Conscious level.
- Examine the abdomen for signs of intra-abdominal bleeding (if present, assume a pelvic fracture).
- Remember cardiac tamponade in a rapidly deteriorating child where chest injury has occurred and where the cause of the deterioration is not clear (refer to **Thoracic Trauma**).

TABLE 4.7 – Normal Heart Rates

Age	Heart rate
<1 year	110–160 beats per minute
1–2 years	100–150 beats per minute
2–5 years	95–140 beats per minute
5–11 years	80–120 beats per minute
>12 years	60–100 beats per minute

- Significant blood losses are seen in long bone fractures, with even greater losses (double the volume) seen when the fracture is open, when compared to a corresponding closed fracture; for example, in a closed femoral fracture 20% of the circulating blood volume may bleed into the surrounding tissues compared to losses of 40% from an open femoral shaft fracture.

8.1 Management

- Splintage, traction and full immobilisation can reduce blood loss and pain.
- Where possible, vascular access can be gained en route to hospital, reducing the time spent on scene. Use the widest possible cannula for the veins available.
- In paediatric trauma, **5 ml/kg fluid boluses** are used and repeated as needed to improve clinical signs (e.g. RR, HR, capillary refill, conscious level) **towards normal**. Seek advice to exceed maximum dose in trauma.

NB Hypotensive resuscitation practices (as used in adult trauma) should not be used in children.

- Due to their physiological reserves, children maintain their systolic blood pressures in the face of major blood loss, with hypotension only occurring at a very late stage. Significant cardiovascular compromise and even cardiac arrest may occur if volume resuscitation were to be delayed until a child had reached such an advanced state of hypovolaemia.
- Following IV fluid resuscitation, in paediatric major trauma with catastrophic haemorrhage, a bolus of tranexamic acid should be given, if available (refer to **Tranexamic Acid**).

9. Disability – Assessment

Record the initial level of consciousness using the AVPU Scale (below):

A	Alert
V	Responds to voice
P	Responds to painful stimulus
U	Unresponsive

as well as:
- The time of the AVPU assessment.
- Pupil size, shape, symmetry and response to light.
- Whether the child was moving some or all limbs. If there is no movement, then ask the child to 'wiggle' their fingers and toes, paying particular note to movements peripheral to any injury site.
- Any abnormalities of posture.
- If the child is not **alert** they should be considered time-critical. A formal GCS (see Appendix) en route may be valuable to the receiving hospital but should only be recorded if it can be accurately done and does not delay transfer.

9.1 Stepwise Disability Management

- Confusion or agitation in an injured child may result directly from a significant head injury, but equally may be secondary to hypoxia from an impaired airway or compromised breathing or else hypoperfusion due to blood loss and shock.
- The management of any child with impaired consciousness is based on ensuring an adequate airway, oxygenation, ventilation and circulation.
- Always measure the blood glucose level in any child with altered consciousness. If hypoglycaemia is detected, refer to **Glycaemic Emergencies in Adults and Children** for treatment.

Trauma Emergencies in Children – Overview

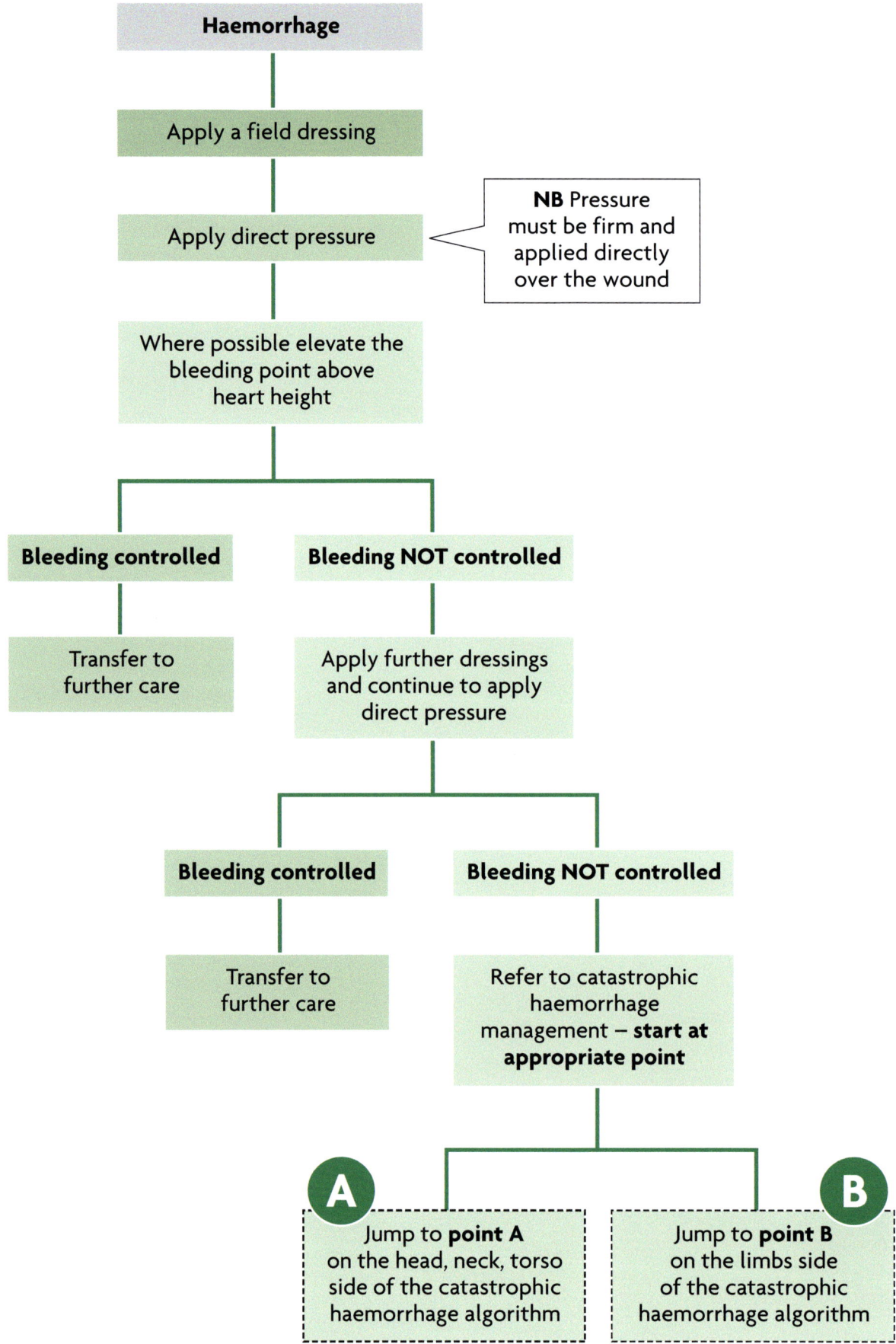

Figure 4.4 – The management of haemorrhage algorithm.

Trauma Emergencies in Children – Overview

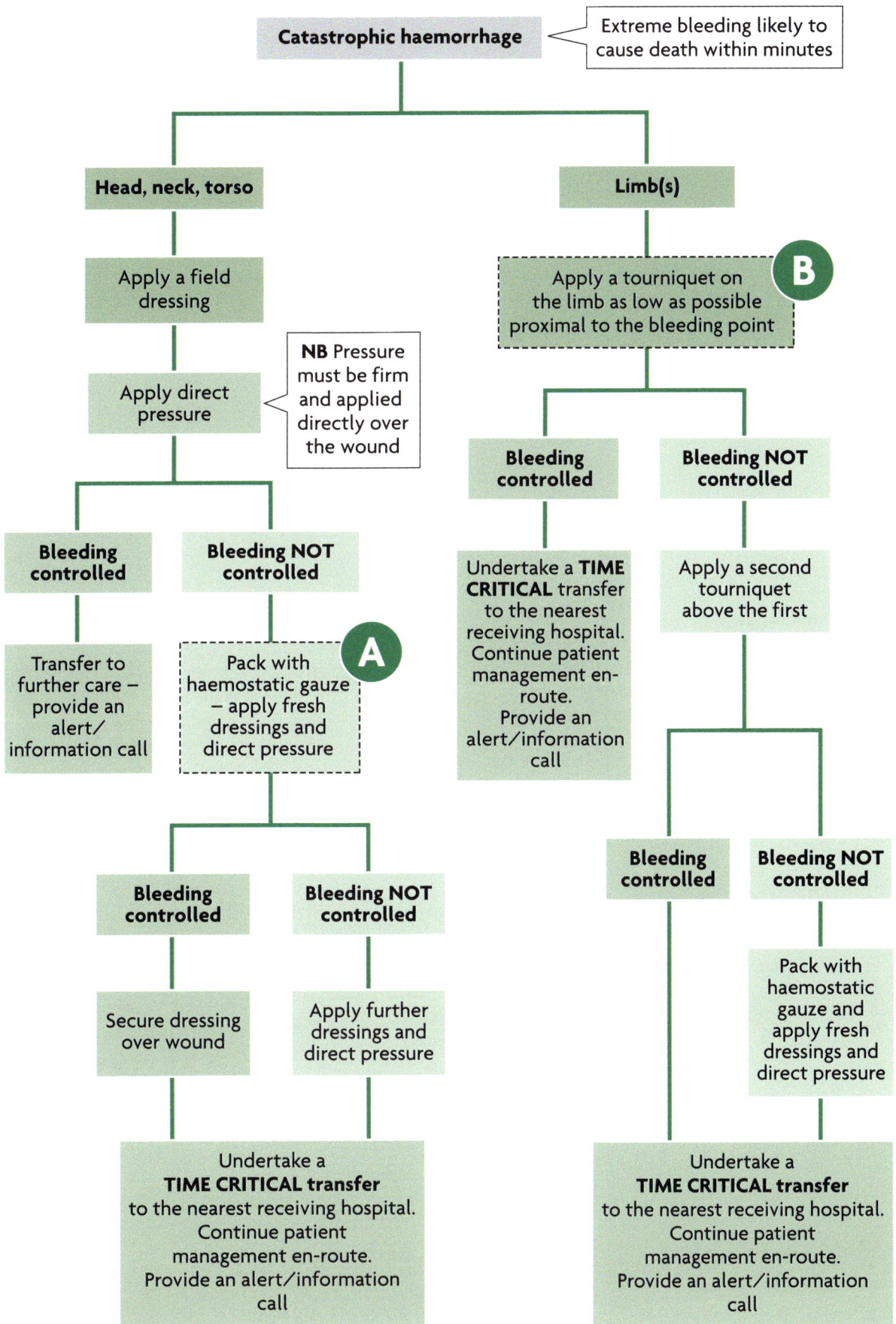

Figure 4.5 – The management of catastrophic haemorrhage algorithm.

Trauma Emergencies in Children – Overview

10. Exposure

- Children will lose heat rapidly when exposed for examination and immobilised during trauma care. Do protect the child from a cold environment during your assessment.
- Expose children 'piecemeal' if possible, replacing a piece of clothing before removing the next, as stripping a child may cause insecurity or embarrassment as well as exposing them to cold.
- If the child is **TIME-CRITICAL** they must be packaged appropriately (with full spinal immobilisation – or improvisation as tolerated – and pelvic splint if pelvic injury suspected) and transported rapidly to hospital.
- An **alert/information call should be given for all TIME-CRITICAL children** en route.
- If there is no apparent problem with the primary survey, a secondary survey may be commenced en route. This should not delay the transfer to definitive care.

10.1 Secondary Survey

- This is a systematic and careful review of each part of the injured child looking for non-critical and/or occult injuries. It is rarely possible to complete this before hospital in a seriously injured child.
- Any deterioration in the child's condition mandates an immediate return to the primary survey and the problem sought and treated.
- Dress and immobilise any injuries found as required. Perform a simple **MSC** check of **ALL** four limbs (see below):

M	MOTOR	Test for movement
S	SENSATION	Apply light touch to evaluate sensation
C	CIRCULATION	Assess pulse and skin temperature

11. Analgesia in Trauma

- As would happen for an adult, a child's pain must be addressed once their life-threatening problems have been attended to (refer to **Pain Management in Adults and Children**).
- **Note:** Paediatric drug doses are expressed as mg/kg (refer to **specific drug protocols/Page-for-Age** for dosages and information). Drug doses **MUST** be checked prior to **ANY** drug administration, no matter how confident the practitioner may be.

12. Summary

- Read the scene for mechanism of injury and the presence of children.
- Trauma emergencies in childhood are managed using similar priorities and techniques to those used in adult practice. Remember the important anatomical and physiological differences encountered in children whilst performing primary (and/or secondary) surveys.
- Children may **conceal** serious underlying injuries using compensatory mechanisms, so a high index of clinical suspicion is required. Agitation and/or confusion may indicate primary brain injury, but may also be due to inadequate ventilation and/or cerebral perfusion.

APPENDIX – Glasgow Coma Scale and Modified Glasgow Coma Scale

TABLE 4.8 – Glasgow Coma Scale

Item	Element	Score
Eyes Opening:		
	Spontaneously	4
	To speech	3
	To pain	2
	None	1
Verbal Response:		
	Orientated	5
	Confused	4
	Inappropriate words	3
	Incomprehensible sounds	2
	No verbal response	1

Trauma Emergencies in Children – Overview

TABLE 4.8 – Glasgow Coma Scale *(continued)*

Motor Response:		
	Obeys commands	6
	Localised pain	5
	Withdraws from pain	4
	Abnormal flexion	3
	Extensor response	2
	No response to pain	1

TABLE 4.9 – Modification of Glasgow Coma Scale for Children Aged Under Four Years Old

Item		Score
Eyes Opening:		As per adult scale
Best Verbal Response:	Appropriate words or social smiles, fixes on and follows objects	5
	Cries, but is consolable	4
	Persistently irritable	3
	Restless, agitated	2
	Silent	1
Motor Response:		As per adult scale

KEY POINTS!

Trauma Emergencies in Children – Overview

- Important anatomical and physiological differences exist between children and adults – a different approach will often be needed.
- Read the wreckage – toys or child seats may indicate that children have been involved in the incident.
- Assess and continuously re-assess <C>ABCDE.
- Detect time-critical problems as part of the primary survey and transport urgently with a hospital pre-alert.

Bibliography

1. Office for National Statistics (ONS). Deaths from Suicide That Occurred in England and Wales: April to July 2020. 2021. Available from: https://www.ons.gov.uk/peoplepopulationandcommunity/birthsdeathsandmarriages/deaths/articles/deathsfromsuicidethatoccurredinenglandandwales/aprilandjuly2020.

Abdominal Trauma

1. Introduction

- Trauma to the abdomen can be extremely difficult to assess even in a hospital setting. In the field, identifying which abdominal structure(s) has been injured is less important than identifying that abdominal trauma itself has occurred.
- It is therefore of major importance to note abnormal signs associated with blood loss and to establish that abdominal injury is the probable cause, rather than being concerned with, for example, whether the source of that abdominal bleeding originates from the spleen or liver.
- There may be significant intra-abdominal injury with very few, if any, initial indications of this at the time the abdomen is examined by the paramedic at the scene.

2. Severity and Outcome

Abdominal trauma (blunt/penetrating) is a leading cause of morbidity and mortality.

3. Pathophysiology

- The abdomen may be described as three anatomical areas:
  - **Abdominal cavity** – extends from the diaphragm to the pelvis. It contains the stomach, small intestine, large intestine, liver, gall bladder and spleen.

    The upper abdominal organs are partly in the lower thorax and lie under the lower ribs; therefore, fractures of lower ribs may damage abdominal structures such as the liver and spleen.
  - **Pelvis** – contains the bladder, the lower part of the large intestine and, in the female, the uterus and ovaries. The iliac artery and vein overlie the posterior part of the pelvic ring and may be torn in pelvic fractures, adding to already major bleeding.
  - **Retro-peritoneal area** – lies against the posterior abdominal wall, and contains the kidneys and ureters, pancreas, abdominal aorta, vena cava and part of the duodenum. These structures are attached to the posterior abdominal wall, and are often injured by shearing due to rapid deceleration forces.

4. Abdominal Injuries

Blunt trauma – the most common pattern of injury seen; results from direct blows to the abdomen or rapid deceleration. Blunt trauma may also result from all phases of a blast.

- The spleen, liver (hepatic tear) and 'tethered' structures such as the duodenum are the most commonly injured. The small bowel, mesentery and aorta may also sustain injury.

Penetrating trauma – stab wounds, gunshot wounds, blast injuries and other penetrating injuries.

- **Stab wounds** – stab injures should be assumed to have caused serious damage until proved otherwise. Damage to liver, spleen or major blood vessels may cause massive haemorrhage. **NB** Upper abdominal stab wounds may have caused major intra-thoracic damage if the weapon was directed upwards (refer to). Similarly, chest-stabbing injuries may also cause intra-abdominal injury.
- **Gunshot wounds** – tend to cause both direct and indirect injury, due to the forces involved and the chaotic paths that bullets may take. The same rules apply to associated intra-thoracic injuries.
- **Blast injuries** – can lead to both blunt and penetrating injuries. Where an explosion occurs in a confined space, the blast wave can cause injuries to the bowel (perforation and haemorrhage) and penetrating ballistics can lead to organ damage.

5. Assessment and Management

For the assessment and management of abdominal trauma, refer to Table 4.10.

- When managing critically ill or injured patients, early consideration should be given to the requirement for additional critical care resources, they should be requested promptly. Consideration should be given to the following factors in reaching these decisions:
  1. Clinical scope of practice such as the ability to deliver emergency anaesthesia or blood products
  2. Transport platform (road versus air and the ability to undertake aeromedical transfer)
  3. Balance time for interventions on scene against delay reaching definitive care
  4. Ability to rendezvous with the transporting ambulance en route to hospital
- These decisions should be made in conjunction with remote clinical support where possible, for example via an ambulance control room critical care, trauma, HEMS desk or senior clinician. Delaying on scene time in critically ill or injured patients may not be justifiable if care can be escalated more quickly and safely by rapidly transferring the patient to hospital.
- If patient is known or suspected to be pregnant, refer to **Trauma in Pregnancy**.

Abdominal Trauma

TABLE 4.10 – ASSESSMENT and MANAGEMENT of: Abdominal Trauma

Assess <C>ABCDE
- Control any external catastrophic haemorrhage – refer to **Trauma Emergencies in Adults – Overview** and **Trauma Emergencies in Children – Overview**.
- If any of the following **TIME-CRITICAL** features are present:
  - major <C>ABCDE problems
  - haemodynamic compromise
  - decreased level of consciousness
  - neck and back injuries – refer to **Spinal Injury and Spinal Cord Injury**, then:
- Start correcting **A** and **B** problems.
- Undertake a **TIME-CRITICAL** transfer to nearest appropriate receiving hospital. This may be a major trauma centre; refer to local pathways.
- Provide an alert/information call.
- Continue patient management en route.
- Minimise ongoing heat loss in patients with major trauma.

Assess
Ascertain the mechanism of injury:
- **Road traffic collision:** look for impact speed and severity of deceleration; seat-belt and lap-belt use are particularly associated with torn or perforated abdominal structures.
- **Stabbing and gunshot wound(s):** consider the length of the weapon used or the type of gun and the range.
- **Blast injuries:** blast wave injuries and penetrating ballistics.

Assess the chest and abdomen. **NB** Some abdominal organs (e.g. liver and spleen) are covered by lower ribs/chest margins.

ABDOMEN:
- Examine for signs of tenderness.
- Examine for external signs of injury (e.g. contusions, seat/lap-belt abrasions).
- Examine for evisceration (protruding abdominal organs).

GENTLY palpate the four quadrants of the abdomen for signs of tenderness, guarding and rigidity. Shoulder-tip pain should increase suspicion of injury or internal bleeding.

NB Significant **INTRA-ABDOMINAL TRAUMA** may show little or no evidence in the early stages, therefore DO NOT rule out injury if initial examination is normal.

CHEST:
- Fractures of the lower ribs – if confirmed or suspected, refer to **Thoracic Trauma**.

Evisceration
- **DO NOT** push protruding abdominal organs back into the abdominal cavity.
- Cover protruding abdominal organs with warm moist dressings.

Impaling Objects
- Leave impaling objects (e.g. a knife) **IN SITU**.
- Handle and move the patient very carefully, address bleeding with appropriate treatment. Avoid rigid fixation or handling of the impaling object where possible. **NB** Be vigilant – the patient may try to remove the object and this could be used as a weapon.

Haemorrhage
- In the case of external haemorrhage, apply a large non-adherent wound pad, and bandage to secure in place and direct pressure (refer to **Trauma Emergencies in Adults – Overview** and **Trauma Emergencies in Children – Overview**).

Consider Tranexamic Acid
- Tranexamic acid should be given where appropriate as early as possible (refer to **Tranexamic acid**).

(continued)

Abdominal Trauma

TABLE 4.10 – ASSESSMENT and MANAGEMENT of: Abdominal Trauma *(continued)*
Oxygen
• Administer high levels of supplemental oxygen (aim for SpO$_2$ 94–98%) (refer to **Oxygen**).
Ventilation
Consider assisted ventilation at a rate of 12–20 respirations per minute if:
• Oxygen saturation (SpO$_2$) is <90% on high levels of supplemental oxygen.
• Respiratory rate is <10 or >30 breaths per minute.
• Inadequate chest expansion.
Refer to **Airway and Breathing Management**.
Vital Signs
• Monitor vital signs.
• Monitor ECG.
Pelvic Injuries
• Consider pelvic injuries – if suspected, refer to **Pelvic Trauma**.
Thoracic Injuries
• If the injury affects the chest, refer to **Thoracic Trauma**.
Pain Management
• If pain relief is indicated, refer to **Pain Management in Adults and Children**.
Fluid
• If fluid resuscitation is indicated, refer to **Intravascular Fluid Therapy in Adults** and **Intravascular Fluid Therapy in Children**.
• **DO NOT** delay on scene for fluid replacement.
Transfer to Further Care
• Continue patient management en route.
• Provide an alert/information call.

KEY POINTS!

Abdominal Trauma

- **Abdominal trauma can be difficult to assess.**
- **Identifying that abdominal trauma has occurred is more important than identifying which structure(s) has been injured, therefore note signs associated with blood loss.**
- **Observe mechanism of injury.**
- **Ensure <C>ABCDEs are assessed and managed; consider C-spine immobilisation.**
- **Transport to the nearest appropriate facility, providing an alert/information call en route. This may be a major trauma centre; refer to local pathways.**
- **Tranexamic acid should be given where appropriate as early as possible (refer to Tranexamic acid).**

Bibliography

1. National Institute for Health and Clinical Excellence. *Major Trauma: Assessment and Initial Management* (NG39). London: NICE, 2016. Available from: https://www.nice.org.uk/guidance/ng39.

2. Jorgensen H, Jensen CH, Dirks J. Does pre-hospital ultrasound improve treatment of the trauma patient? A systematic review. *European Journal of Emergency Medicine* 2010, 17(5): 249–253.

3. Best Evidence Topics. Does the 'Seatbelt Sign' predict intra-abdominal injury after motor vehicle trauma in children? *Emergency Medicine Journal* 2012, 29(2): 163–164.

4. Demetriades D, Murray J, Brown C, Velmahos G, Salim A, Alo K, et al. High-level falls: type and severity of injuries and survival outcome according to *age*. *Journal of Trauma and Acute Care Surgery* 2005, 58(2): 342–345.

Abdominal Trauma

5. England RJ, Dalton R, Walker J. Penetrating handlebar injury causing bowel evisceration. *Injury Extra* 2004, 35(4): 40–41.

6. Hardcastle TC, Coetzee GJN, Wasserman L. Evisceration from blunt trauma in adults: an unusual injury pattern: 3 cases and a literature review. *Scandinavian Journal of Trauma, Resuscitation & Emergency Medicine* 2005, 13: 234–235.

7. Holmes IF, Sokolove PE, Brant WE, Palchak MJ, Vance CW, Owings JT, et al. Identification of children with intra-abdominal injuries after blunt trauma. *Annals of Emergency Medicine* 2002, 39(5): 500–509.

8. Mulholland SA, Cameron PA, Gabbe BJ, Williamson OD, Young K, Smith KL, et al. Pre-hospital prediction of the severity of blunt anatomic injury. *Journal of Trauma and Acute Care Surgery* 2008, 64(3): 754–760. DOI: 10.1097/01.ta.0000244384.85267.c5.

9. Newgard CD, Lewis RJ, Kraus IF. Steering wheel deformity and serious thoracic or abdominal injury among drivers and passengers involved in motor vehicle crashes. *Annals of Emergency Medicine* 2005, 45(1): 43–50.

10. Nishijima DK, Simel DL, Wisner DH, Holmes JF. Does this adult patient have a blunt intra-abdominal injury? *Journal of the American Medical Association* 2012, 307(14): 1517–1527.

11. Owers C, Morgan JL, Garner JP. Abdominal trauma in primary blast injury. *British Journal of Surgery* 2011, 98(2): 168–179.

12. Plurad DS. Blast injury. *Military Medicine* 2011, 176(3): 276–282.

13. Sugrue M, Balogh Z, Lynch J, Bardsley J, Sisson G, Weigelt J. Guidelines for the management of haemodynamically stable patients with stab wounds to the anterior abdomen. *ANZ Journal of Surgery* 2007, 77(8): 614–620.

14. Royal College of Emergency Medicine. *Abdominal Trauma*. 2010. Available from: https://www.rcemlearning.co.uk/references/abdominal-trauma/.

Burns and Scalds

1. Introduction

- Burns arise in a number of accident situations, and may have a variety of presentations (refer to Table 4.11), accompanying injuries or pre-existing medical problems associated with the burn injury. Scalds, flame or thermal burns and chemical and electrical burns will all produce a different burn pattern, and inhalation of smoke or toxic chemicals from the fire may cause serious accompanying complications.

- A number of burn patients will also be seriously injured following falls from a height in fires, or injuries sustained as a result of road traffic collision where a vehicle ignites after a collision or crash.

- Explosions will often induce flash burns and other serious injuries due to the effect of the blast wave or flying debris.

- Inhalation of superheated smoke, steam or gases in a fire will induce major airway swelling and respiratory obstruction – refer to Table 4.12 for signs of airway burns. The likelihood of an airway injury increases with the presence of multiple risk factors or signs.

- Non-accidental injury should always be considered when burns have occurred in children and vulnerable adults including older people, in particular where the mechanism of injury described does not match the injury sustained, or there is inconsistency in the history (refer to **Safeguarding Children** and **Safeguarding Adults at Risk**).

TABLE 4.11 – Burns/Scalds

Electrical

Search for entry and exit sites. Assess ECG rhythm. The extent of burn damage in electrical burns is often impossible to assess fully at the time of injury (refer to **Electrical Injuries**).

Thermal

The skin contact time and temperature of the source determine the depth of the burn. Scalds with boiling water are frequently of short duration as the water flows off the skin rapidly. Record the type of clothing (e.g. wool retains the hot water). Those resulting from hot fat and other liquids that remain on the skin may cause significantly deeper and more serious burns. Also the time to cold water and removal of clothing is of significant impact.

TABLE 4.11 – Burns/Scalds *(continued)*

Chemical

It is vital to note the nature of the chemical. Alkalis in particular may cause deep, penetrating burns, sometimes with little initial discomfort. Certain chemicals such as phenol or hydrofluoric acid can cause poisoning by absorption through the skin and therefore must be irrigated with COPIOUS amounts of water for a minimum of 20 minutes (this should be continued until definitive care is available if patient condition and water supply allows) (refer to **CBRN**).

TABLE 4.12 – Signs/Increased Risk of Airway Burns

Signs

- Facial or neck burns.
- Soot in the nasal and oral cavities.
- Coughing up blackened sputum.
- Cough and hoarseness.
- Difficulty with breathing and swallowing.
- Blistering around the mouth and tongue.
- Scorched hair, eyebrows or facial hair.
- Stridor or altered breath sounds such as wheezing.
- Loss of consciousness.
- Fires/blasts in enclosed spaces.

- Preceding long-term illness, especially chronic bronchitis and emphysema, will seriously worsen the outcome from airway burns.
- Remember that a burn injury may be preceded by a medical condition causing a collapse (e.g. elderly patient with a stroke collapsing against a radiator).
- Burns can be very painful (refer to **Pain Management in Adults and Children**).

2. Burn Severity

- Refer to Wallace's Rule of Nines or the Lund and Browder chart to assess total body surface area (TBSA).
- For small or large burns (<15% or > 85%), it is acceptable to use the patient's palmar surface including the fingers as a size estimate. This equates to approximately 1% TBSA.
- Be aware of the risk of underestimating the size of burns with patients with large breasts or who are obese. These factors can significantly affect the proportion of TBSA using standardised charts.

Burns and Scalds

- Use all of the burn area, but do not consider areas of erythema as this is often transient in the initial phases of a burn. Do not try to differentiate between levels of burn (superficial, partial thickness, full thickness etc.) as it is impractical to estimate the depth of burns in the initial hours following injury.

- Only a rough estimate is required; an accurate measure is not possible in the early stages. However, the size of a burn may well influence referral and management pathways.

3. Assessment and Management

- For the assessment and management of burns and scalds in adults, refer to Table 4.13.

TABLE 4.13 – ASSESSMENT and MANAGEMENT of: Burns and Scalds

Ensure Scene Safety for Rescuer and Patient
If safe to do so, stop the burning process:
- Remove from the burn source.
- Brush off dry chemical.

Assess <C>ABCDE
- If any of the following **TIME-CRITICAL** features present:
    - major **<C>ABCDE** problems
    - airway burns (soot or oedema around the mouth and nose)
    - history of hot air or gas inhalation; these patients may initially appear well but can deteriorate very rapidly and need complex airway intervention
    - respiratory distress
    - evidence of circumferential (completely encircling) burns of the chest, neck, limb
    - significant facial burns
    - burns >15% in adults and >10% in children TBSA
    - presence of other major injuries, then:
- Start correcting A and B and undertake a **TIME-CRITICAL** transfer to nearest appropriate hospital according to local care pathways.
- Continue patient management en route.
- Provide an alert/information call.

Specifically Assess
- Airway patency as early intervention may be required with inhalational burns; if intubation is impossible, needle cricothyroidotomy is the management of choice.
- Waveform capnography should be used whenever intubation is performed.
- Breathing for rate, depth and any breathing difficulty (refer to **Airway and Breathing Management**).
- Evidence of trauma – for neck and back trauma, refer to **Spinal Injury and Spinal Cord Injury**.
- Co-existing or precipitating medical conditions.

Oxygen
- Administer supplemental **oxygen** via a non-rebreathing mask – SpO_2 readings may be false due to carboxyhaemoglobin.

Cool/Irrigate the Burn
- Irrigate with copious amounts of water as soon as is practicable; this can still be effective up to 3 hours after the injury. Irrigate the burn for a maximum of 20 minutes, except for chemical burns (acid, alkalis and other corrosive substances) where the irrigation can be continued up to 1 hour.
- Cut off burning or smouldering clothing, providing it is not adhering to the skin.
- Remove any constricting jewellery, including rings.
- **DO NOT** use ice or ice water, as this can worsen the burn injury and exaggerate hypothermia.
- Use saline if no other irrigant available.
- Gel-based dressings may be used but water treatment is preferred.
- Alkali burns require prolonged irrigation – continue until definitive care.

(continued)

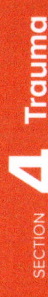

Burns and Scalds

TABLE 4.13 – ASSESSMENT and MANAGEMENT of: Burns and Scalds *(continued)*

Assess Burn Size
- Rule of Nines or Lund and Browder Chart.
- Patient's palmar surface, including adducted fingers.
- Consider obesity and large breasts when estimating burn size.

Dress the Burn
- Use small sheets of clingfilm – do not wrap around limbs but layer the film.
- In the absence of clingfilm, use a clean cotton sheet.

Elevate the affected area if possible, to reduce the risk of oedema.

NB Do not apply creams, ointments, wet gauze or non-adherent dressings; they interfere with the assessment process.

Fluid Resuscitation
- Large burns (>10% in children and >15% in adults) require intravenous fluids (refer to **Intravascular Fluid Therapy in Adults** and **Intravascular Fluid Therapy in Children**).
- If IV access is required, obtain on a non-affected limb where possible.

Wheezing
If the patient is wheezing as a result of smoke inhalation:
- Administer nebulised salbutamol (refer to **Salbutamol**) 6–8 litres of O_2 per minute.

Assess the Need for Analgesia
If indicated (refer to **Pain Management in Adults and Children**).

NB Cooling and application of dressings frequently eases pain.

Documentation
- How the patient was burned.
- Time the burn occurred and how long patient was exposed to source of burning.
- Temperature of the source of burning (e.g. boiling water, hot fat etc.).
- Whether first aid was undertaken.
- Time and volume of infusions.

Transfer to Further Care
- The following patients should be conveyed to the nearest Emergency Department (ED), from where transfer to a regional burns unit may be arranged, if necessary, or transfer in accordance with local referral pathways:
    - Any full-thickness burns.
    - Deep dermal burns affecting more than 5% of TBSA in adults, and all deep dermal burns in children.
    - All chemical and electrical burns (including lightning injuries).
    - Any high-pressure steam injury.
    - Any burn associated with suspected non-accidental injury, regardless of the complexity.
    - Burns affecting the face, hands, feet, genitalia perineum or any flexural surface such as the neck, axilla, elbow or knee.
    - Circumferential deep dermal burns.
    - Burns associated with suspected inhalation injury.
    - Burns associated with co-morbidities that may affect wound healing or increase the risk of complications.
    - Burns associated with significant other injuries.
    - Burns associated with sepsis.
    - People who may require admission due to social circumstances or inadequate pain control.
- Complete documentation.

Burns and Scalds

TABLE 4.13 – ASSESSMENT and MANAGEMENT of: Burns and Scalds (continued)

Alkali Burns to the Skin and Eye(s)
- When irrigating the eyes, ensure that the fluid runs away from the contralateral eye to avoid contamination.
- Irrigate with water and continue en route to hospital – it may take hours of irrigation to neutralise the alkali. This also applies to eyes, which require copious and continual irrigation, ideally with water or saline in the absence of a water source.

Acid/Chemical Burns to the Skin and Eye(s)
- When irrigating the eyes, ensure that the fluid runs away from the contralateral eye to avoid contamination.
- Irrigate copiously, ideally with water or otherwise with saline if no water source available.

NB Specific treatment agents may be available in industrial settings with on-site medical/first aid.

Chemical Burns
- **DO NOT** wrap in clingfilm.

NB Do not attempt to neutralise chemicals, as additional heat will be generated, which may increase tissue damage.

Circumferential Burns
- Encircling completely a limb or digit. Full thickness burns may be 'limb threatening', and require early in-hospital incision/release of the burn area along the length of the burnt area of the limb (surgical escharotomy).

Corrosive Substances
- Following a significant increase in the frequency of serious criminal assaults using acids and corrosive substances, the National Ambulance Resilience Unit (NARU) has advised:

Personal Safety
- Make a dynamic risk assessment and ensure your own safety.
- Exercise extreme caution if there appear to be multiple patients or an ongoing attack.
- Ensure accurate updates are provided to ensure awareness of the severity of the incident, so this can be escalated if necessary.
- Activate specialist resources early where there appear to be multiple patients or extensive contamination.
- Wear eye protection and double-glove nitrile gloves.
- Protect any exposed skin by wearing a jacket to provide a barrier.
- Do not carry out sniff tests on contaminants or containers.
- If attacked, use hands to protect face; skin may blister and scar, but corrosives in the eyes may cause irreversible loss of vision.
- Corrosive vapours should be considered in terms of ventilation from around any contaminants.

Patient Management
- Irrigate freely with clean water for 20 minutes; this includes utilisation of the fire brigade if required.
- If a shower is available, use this with a mild soap which can be used safely on skin.
- Try to ensure any run-off does not come into contact with other uncontaminated parts of the body.
- Early and thorough irrigation of the face and eyes is important to reduce the risk of long-term damage.
- Eye irrigation can be achieved by using a bag of saline, giving set (maximum half open) and washing with a gentle stream.
- Contaminated clothing should be cut off whenever possible and left on scene. Do not pull contaminated clothing over the head or remove clothing that is adhering to the skin.
- Contaminated jewellery should be removed, rinsed and placed in a bag or wrapped to avoid skin contact and then handed back to the patient.
- If possible, get the patient to do as much as possible with directions; this may not always be possible but will greatly reduce the exposure to the first responders.
- Do not apply any form of dressing or gel until the burn has been adequately irrigated.
- Minimise on-scene duration for patients with large burns or burns on the face, eyes or hands.

Burns and Scalds

> **KEY POINTS!**
>
> **Burns and Scalds**
> - Airway status can deteriorate rapidly and may need complex interventions available at the emergency departments.
> - Stopping the burning process is essential.
> - The time from burning is an essential piece of information.
> - Pain relief is important.
> - Consider non-accidental injury in children and vulnerable adults, including older people.
> - When irrigating the eyes, ensure that the fluid runs away from the contralateral eye to avoid contamination.

Bibliography

1. The Royal Children's Hospital Melbourne. *Burns/Management of Burn Wounds*. 2018. Available from: https://www.rch.org.au/clinicalguide/guideline_index/Burns/.

2. National Institute for Health and Care Excellence. *Burns and Scalds*. Clinical Knowledge Summaries. 2017. Available from: https://cks.nice.org.uk/burns-and-scalds#!scenario.

3. Porter A, Snooks H, Youren A, Gaze S, Whitfield R, Rapport F et al. 'Covering our backs': ambulance crews' attitudes towards clinical documentation when emergency (999) patients are not conveyed to hospital. *Emergency Medicine Journal* 2008, 25(5): 292–295.

4. Ayers DE, Kay AR. Management of burns in the wilderness. *Travel Medicine and Infectious Disease* 2005, 3(4): 239–248.

5. Boots RJ, Dulhunty JM, Paratz J, Lipman J. Respiratory complications in burns: an evolving spectrum of injury. *Clinical Pulmonary Medicine* 2009, 16(3): 132–138.

6. Cancio LC. Airway management and smoke inhalation injury in the burn patient. *Clinics in Plastic Surgery* 2009, 36(4): 555–567.

7. Enoch S, Roshan A, Shah M. Emergency and early management of burns and scalds. *British Medical Journal* 2009, 338(7700): 937–941.

8. Hassan Z, Wong JK, Bush J, Bayat A, Dunn KW. Assessing the severity of inhalation injuries in adults. *Burns: Journal of the International Society for Burn Injuries* 2010, 36(2): 212–216.

9. Hermans MHE. A general overview of burn care. *International Wound Journal* 2005, 2(3): 206–220, 222–223.

10. Karpelowsky JS, Rode H. Basic principles in the management of thermal injuries. *South African Family Practice* 2008, 50(3): 24–31.

11. Karpelowsky JS, Wallis L, Madaree A, Rode H. South African Burn Society burn stabilisation protocol. *South African Medical Journal* 2007, 97(8): 574–547.

12. Marek K, Piotr W, Stanislaw S, Stefan G, Justyna G, Mariusz N, et al. Fibreoptic bronchoscopy in routine clinical practice in confirming the diagnosis and treatment of inhalation burns. *Burns: Journal of the International Society for Burn Injuries* 2007, 33(5): 554–560.

13. Mlcak RP, Suman OE, Herndon DN. Respiratory management of inhalation injury. *Burns: Journal of the International Society for Burn Injuries* 2007, 33(1): 2–13.

14. Muehlberger T, Ottomann C, Toman N, Daigeler A, Lehnhardt M. Emergency pre-hospital care of burn patients. *The Surgeon: Journal of the Royal Colleges of Surgeons of Edinburgh & Ireland* 2010, 8(2): 101–104.

15. New Zealand Guidelines Group. *Management of Burns and Scalds in Primary Care*. Wellington: Accident Compensation Corporation, 2007. Available from: http://www.moh.govt.nz/notebook/nbbooks.nsf/0/BD-251444C120DC0FCC2573210070271D/$file/burns_full.pdf.

16. Palmieri TL. Inhalation injury: research progress and needs. *Journal of Burn Care and Research* 2007, 28(4): 549–554.

17. Pham TN, Gibran NS. Thermal and electrical injuries. *Surgical Clinics of North America* 2007, 87(1): 185–206.

18. Singh S, Handy J. The respiratory insult in burns injury. *Current Anaesthesia and Critical Care* 2008, 19(5–6): 264–268.

19. Spanholtz TA, Theodorou P, Amini P, Spilker G. Severe burn injuries: acute and long-term treatment. *Deutsches Arzteblatt* 2009, 106(38): 607–613.

20. Suzuki M, Aikawa N, Kobayashi K, Higuchi R. Prognostic implications of inhalation injury in burn patients in Tokyo. *Burns: Journal of the International Society for Burn Injuries* 2005, 31(3): 331–336.

21. Walton JJ, Manara AR. Burns and smoke inhalation. *Anaesthesia & Intensive Care Medicine* 2005, 6(9): 317–321.

22. Wasiak J, Cleland H, Campbell F. Dressings for superficial and partial thickness burns. *Cochrane Database of Systematic Reviews* 2007, 3: CD002106.

23. Durrant CAT, Simpson AR, Williams G. Thermal injury: the first 24 h. *Current Anaesthesia and Critical Care* 2008, 19(5–6): 256–263.

24. Freiburg C, Igneri P, Sartorelli K, Rogers F. Effects of differences in percent total body surface area estimation on fluid resuscitation of transferred burn patients. *Journal of Burn Care and Research* 2007, 28(1): 42–48.

25. Hackenschmidt A. Burn trauma priorities for a patient with 80% total body surface area burns. *Journal of Emergency Nursing* 2007, 33(4): 405–408.

26. Hussain S, Ferguson C. Assessing the size of burns: which method works best? *Emergency Medicine Journal* 2009, 26(9): 664–666.

27. Singer AJ, Dagum AB. Current management of acute cutaneous wounds. *New England Journal of Medicine* 2008, 359(10): 1037–1046.

Burns and Scalds

28. Williams C. Successful assessment and management of burn injuries. *Nursing Standard* 2009, 23(32): 53–54.
29. Allison K, Porter K. Consensus on the pre-hospital approach to burns patient management. *Emergency Medicine Journal* 2004, 21(1): 112–114.
30. Williams G, Dziewulski P. Intravascular fluid therapy in burns injury. In Group. TJRCALGD, editor, 2011.
31. Blackhurst H. Estimation of burn surface area using the hand. *BestBets* 2007. Available from: http://www.bestbets.org/bets/bet.php?id=01516.
32. Jose RM, Roy DK, Vidyadharan R, Erdmann M. Burns area estimation: an error perpetuated. *Burns: Journal of the International Society for Burn Injuries* 2004, 30(5): 481–482.
33. Jose RM, Roy DK, Wright PK, Erdmann M. Hand surface area: do racial differences exist? *Burns: Journal of the International Society for Burn Injuries* 2006, 32(2): 216–217.
34. Lee J-Y, Choi J-W, Kim H. Determination of hand surface area by sex and body shape using alginate. *Journal of Physiological Anthropology* 2007, 26(4): 475–483.
35. Liao C-Y, Chen S-L, Chou T-D, Lee T-P, Dai N-T, Chen T-M. Use of two-dimensional projection for estimating hand surface area of Chinese adults. *Burns: Journal of the International Society for Burn Injuries* 2008, 34(4): 556–559.
36. Yu C-Y, Hsu Y-W, Chen C-Y. Determination of hand surface area as a percentage of body surface area by 3D anthropometry. *Burns: Journal of the International Society for Burn Injuries* 2008, 34(8): 1183–1189.
37. Hidvegi N, Nduka C, Myers S, Dziewulski P. Estimation of breast burn size. *Plastic and Reconstructive Surgery* 2004, 113(6): 1591–1597.
38. Ichiki Y, Kato Y, Kitajima Y. Assessment of burn area: most objective method. *Burns: Journal of the International Society for Burn Injuries* 2008, 34(3): 425–426.
39. Singer AJ, Brebbia J, Soroff HH. Management of local burn wounds in the ED. *American Journal of Emergency Medicine* 2007, 25(6): 666–671.
40. Cuttle L, Kravchuk O, Wallis B, Kimble RM. An audit of first-aid treatment of pediatric burns patients and their clinical outcome. *Journal of Burn Care & Research: Official publication of the American Burn Association* 2009, 30(6): 1028–1034.
41. Health Protection Agency. *HPA Compendium of Chemical Hazards*. London: HPA, 2007. Available from: http://www.hpa.org.uk/Topics/ChemicalsAndPoisons/CompendiumOfChemicalHazards.

Drowning

1. Introduction

- Drowning is a common cause of accidental death, particularly at the extremes of age.
- **Drowning** is a type of suffocation induced by the submersion of the mouth and nose in a liquid. As a result, the person is prevented from inhaling air due to liquid occluding the entrance of the airway (mouth and nose). NB. Drowning does not infer that the patient has died. Outdated terms such as near drowning, secondary drowning, dry drowning are no longer in use.
- Associated terminology includes:
  - **Submersion** which is the airway being occluded by liquid; the remainder of the body does not necessarily have to be below the surface of the liquid.
  - **Immersion** which means being covered in a liquid medium and does not necessarily imply the entire body has to be submerged; in this situation, the main problem will be hypothermia. Following prolonged immersion of most of the body, there may be cardiovascular collapse, most commonly if the patient is rescued vertically from the liquid medium in which they find themselves; the cause of cardiovascular collapse being the result of removal from the hydrostatic pressure of the surrounding liquid as they are rescued – "circum-rescue collapse".
- The main problems associated with drowning are asphyxia and subsequent hypoxia.
- **Exacerbating factors:** Intoxication from alcohol or drugs often accompanies incidents. Occasionally, an immersion incident may be precipitated by a medical cause, such as a convulsion, or traumatic injuries.
- Drowning incidents frequently involve a multi-agency response.

2. Incidence

- Worldwide there are approximately 236,000 deaths per year[2] with 659 water related fatalities in the UK in 2023.[3] Many more experience a "non-fatal drowning" event.[4]

3. Severity and Outcome

- The outcome of a non-fatal drowning event varies from full recovery to severe neurological deficit and disability. The duration and severity of hypoxia sustained as a result of drowning is the most important determinant of outcome.[5, 6, 7]
- Following prolonged immersion/submersion hypothermia may be a contributing factor to outcome, even in relatively warm weather.
- Concomitant trauma may occur. Consider the mechanism of the incident in determining the likelihood of injury. E.g. consideration for spinal injury if patient is described as having dived into shallow water immediately before the drowning event.

4. Pathophysiology

- Following submersion, a conscious patient will initially attempt to hold their breath. They will then preferentially swallow water rather than aspirate it, until the urge to breathe takes over. They will then aspirate water into the lungs. In some patients, water may also cause spasm of the vocal cords (laryngospasm) which acts to mechanically occlude the airway. Aspiration of water and laryngospasm may both contribute to the final common pathway of hypoxia, with associated hypercapnia.
- Any water aspirated will wash away surfactant in the alveoli, resulting in alveolar collapse. This atelectasis decreases lung compliance, increasing the work of breathing, and requiring higher pressures to ventilate the lungs if supported ventilation is required.
- The patient will become bradycardic as hypoxia progresses, which eventually results in cardiac arrest. Timely rescue and correction of hypoxaemia are critical interventions for survival.
- Those immersed in water who remain conscious may have aspirated water due to wave splash or following short periods of submersion during their drowning event. Look for clinical signs of aspiration which may indicate the need for hospital admission. E.g. "Foam" at the mouth, persistent cough, crepitations or crackles heard on auscultation, or any evidence of respiratory distress.[5, 8]
- In some circumstances a medical or traumatic event proceeding the immersion or submersion will have resulted in cardiac arrest without aspiration of water. More than one pathology may be present and require management.
- Whilst there are subtle differences in the physiology associated with salt water versus fresh water drowning, there are no differences in the initial clinical management of the patient, and it has no bearing on survival to hospital discharge.
- Following prolonged immersion, the patient is at risk of circum-rescue collapse. Conscious casualties should be encouraged to keep fighting for their survival. Semi-conscious or unconscious casualties, where possible, should be removed from the water in a horizontal position but this should not delay the rescue attempt.[9]
- In water temperatures below 15°C, the cold shock response peaks. Upon immersion/submersion there is an involuntary gasp (2–3 Litres) and uncontrollable hyperventilation lasting up to 90 seconds. Loss of respiratory control means the lethal dose of water for drowning can be quickly aspirated. The sympathetic nervous system surge

Drowning

associated with the cold shock response can also result in cardiac arrest with agonal gasping mimicking drowning.[5, 8, 10, 11]

5. Rescue and Resuscitation

⚠ Safety first – **DO NOT** put yourself in danger.

- Additional specialist rescue resources may be required
- A dynamic risk assessment should be undertaken to preserve your own safety, members of public present, and that of other rescuers:[12]
    - Ensure safe distance from the water's edge is maintained.
    - Establish number of patients involved.
    - Gather available history or mechanism of the incident.
    - Specific details to include:
        - Age, older than 12?
        - Size of the patient(s)? (small/thin)
        - Time of immersion/submersion? (Duration of submersion strong indicator of probability of survival)
        - Any potential air pockets? E.g. Trapped inside a car which is submerged.
        - Approximate temperature of the water.
- Consider calling for senior clinical advice early in incidents that may require termination of rescue attempts based on futility of resuscitation, particularly if the patient is a child.

5.1 Aquatic Rescue

- Maintain personal safety at all times.
- Shout to the casualty and encourage them to float on their back. When their breathing is under control encourage them to move towards the edge.
- Throw buoyancy aids (i.e. any suitable object that floats) and/or throw lines towards the patient from a safe position.
- In general, only those trained in rescue should attempt entry into the water following a dynamic risk assessment.
- If spinal injury precautions are indicated based on mechanism of the incident these should be applied after extrication from the water. Refer to **Spinal Injury and Spinal Cord Injury**.

5.2 Spontaneously Breathing Drowning Patient

- Alleviate hypoxaemia as soon as possible.
- Administer supplemental oxygen:
    - Conscious patients – Oxygen mask with reservoir bag (10–15 l/min^{-1}).
    - Reduced conscious level – Perform assisted ventilation via bag-valve-mask with supplemental oxygen.
- If the conscious patient does not respond to initial oxygen therapy, assisted ventilation via bag-valve-mask with supplemental oxygen should be used. Non-invasive ventilation can also be considered where this is available and the patient is conscious and compliant with therapy.[5, 13–18]
- Ventilation may be difficult due to reduced lung compliance. Mechanical drainage of water from the lungs should not be carried out.
- Consider requesting specialist clinical services to assist with airway and resuscitation management.
- Adequate oxygenation and ventilation may restore cardiac activity.
- Foam in the airway can be ignored, but suction is required if fluid or vomit is obstructing the airway.
- Approximately 80% of patients will aspirate water into their stomach. There is a high risk of regurgitation of the stomach contents, especially if the patient has ingested alcohol/drugs – have suction at hand. Be prepared to take action for vomit.
- Measure respiratory rate and assess the work of breathing. Apply a pulse oximeter, but be aware that a poor signal is commonly seen with cold, wet peripheries.[19]
- Tympanic temperature measurement in wet patients is unreliable. Use clinical assessment of temperature e.g. conscious level and absence or presence of shivering. Wet patients will begin to cool rapidly. Carefully remove wet clothes and commence re-warming strategies. Refer to **Hypothermia**.

5.3 Cardiac Arrest Following Drowning Event

- Conditions unequivocally associated with death also apply to drowning incidents.
- Incidents involving prolonged submersion, resuscitation attempts may be withheld as per the submerged person tool Figure 4.6.
- Refer to **Advanced Life Support**.
- Modifications to standard Advanced Life Support:
    - As soon as the patient is rescued – clear airway, provide 5 initial ventilations (critical importance of alleviating hypoxia) and then commence CPR.
    - Foam in the airway can be ignored, but suction is required if fluid or vomit is obstructing the airway.
    - Supraglottic airways (SGA) can be used successfully in this patient group. Capnography should be used to confirm and optimise position of a SGA. Ventilation may be difficult due to reduced lung compliance.
    - Consider requesting specialist clinical services to assist with airway and resuscitation management.

Drowning

- Defer defibrillator/AED use until after CPR is underway.
- Adequate oxygenation and ventilation may restore cardiac activity.
- There is a high risk of regurgitation of the stomach contents. Be prepared to take action for vomit if there is return of spontaneous circulation.
- Prolonged immersions/submersions are associated with hypothermia. Temperature management targets as per standard post-ROSC care.
• Discontinuing resuscitation following drowning event:
  - Adults: If following 30 minutes of ALS interventions, the patient has been **persistently and continuously** asystolic and all reversible causes (including hypothermia) have been identified and corrected, resuscitation can be terminated. Termination of resuscitation at 30 minutes if other rhythms are present should be discussed with senior clinical advice.
  - Children: Resuscitation of children should be continued to hospital unless there are conditions unequivocally associated with death.

5.4 Management of Hypothermia Associated with Drowning

• Refer to **Hypothermia** and **Advanced Life Support** (Hypothermia).
• UK sea water is generally 6–10°C throughout winter and early spring, being warmest in late summer. Commercial swimming pools are generally maintained at about 27°C. Immersion in most circumstances therefore risks a varying degree of hypothermia, depending on water temperature and duration.

5.5 Intravascular Fluid Therapy

• Consider elevation of the legs in patients who are initially hypotensive following an immersion/submersion incident.
• Persistent hypotension may benefit from intravenous fluid boluses to support the circulation. If fluid resuscitation is indicated, refer to **Intravascular Fluid Therapy in Adults** and **Intravascular Fluid Therapy in Children**.

5.6 Submersion and Survival

• The strongest predictor of survival following a drowning event is the duration and severity of hypoxia.
• In adults and children, there are no cases in the literature of survival where the duration of continual submersion (airway below the surface of the liquid and therefore hypoxic) has been greater than 30 minutes when the water temperature is greater than 6°C.
• In water colder than 6°C, "Icy Cold", the period of submersion during which successful resuscitation may be possible extends from 30 minutes up to 90 minutes.[5, 13, 20, 21] This is due to the potential neuroprotection associated with rapid, selective cooling of the brain prior to the effects of hypoxia taking effect. Rapid brain cooling is due to:
  - Aspiration of large volumes of very cold water during the initial period of cold shock following submersion.
  - Cooling from the surface of the body. Lightly clothed and smaller individuals (children and small adults), with low levels of insulation and higher surface area to mass ratios, are more likely to survive protracted periods of submersion.
• If moving to (body) recovery phase (<90 minutes), clinical input (paramedic level or equivalent) is required for verification of death or withholding resuscitation.
• Consider remote and/or senior clinical support to aid decision making in complex cases.
• In general, resuscitation should be commenced on all children and continued to hospital. In cases where a child is likely to be recovered after 30 minutes of continual submersion <u>and</u> starting resuscitation is considered futile, senior clinical advice should be sought to support decision making. Any decisions to withhold, or commence resuscitation outside the submerged person tool should be agreed by all responders present.
• Search and Rescue of submerged persons is technically very difficult with significant associated risk. Any decision to extend rescue operations must balance the probability of survival against the risk to rescuers.
• Actions in submersion incidents:
  - Follow JESIP principles and co-locate with other emergency services and agree on plan based on Joint Decision Model (JDM).
  - Share information gathered.
  - Use Submerged Person Decision Tool (Figure 4.6) to support continuous risk assessments.
  - If there are any discrepancies amongst services present on timing of transition from rescue attempts to body recovery, seek remote and/or senior clinical advice to aid decision making.

Drowning

5.7 Submerged Person Tool

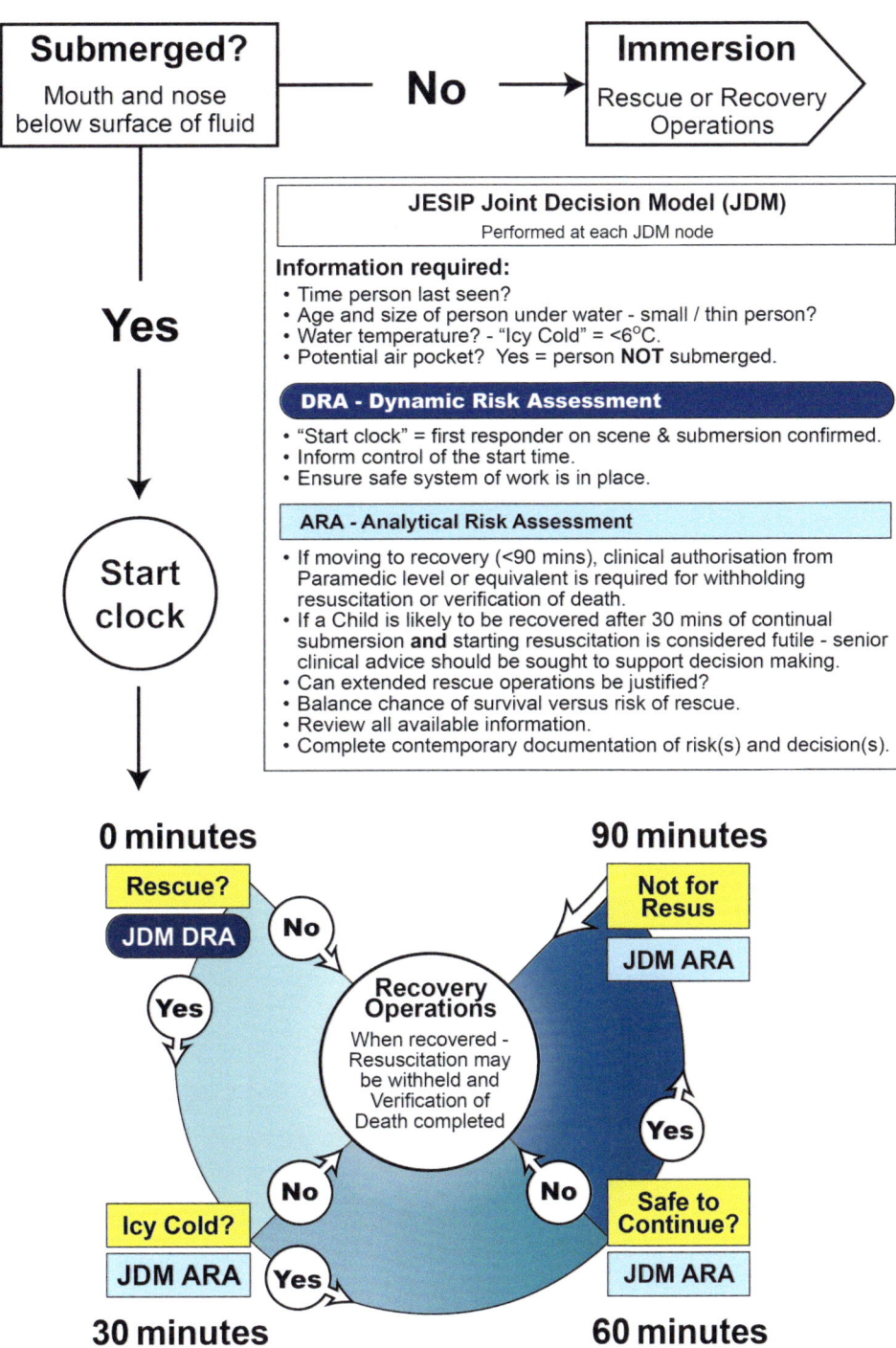

Figure 4.6 – Submerged person tool

Drowning

6. Safeguarding

- There is an association with suicide attempts and drowning. In 2023 there were 208 fatalities due to suicide, and a similar number associated with criminal intent.[3]
- Consider child maltreatment and submit a safeguarding referral if:
  - A child has a non-fatal or fatal drowning incident, and the explanation is absent or unsuitable, or if the child's presentation is inconsistent with the account.
  - If the incident suggests a lack of supervision.
- Refer to **Safeguarding Children**.[22, 23]

7. Discharge on Scene

- Patients can be discharged on scene with safety net advice and signposting if certain criteria are met:[13, 24–26]
  - No clinical concerns.
  - No safeguarding concerns.
  - No evidence of "foam" at the mouth.
  - No persistent cough.
  - No increased work of breathing or adverse clinical signs found on examination of the respiratory system.
  - No requirement for supplementary oxygen.
  - All clinical observations are within normal range. (NEWS2 score of 0, or equivalent normal range in children). Refer to **National Early Warning Score (NEWS2)**.
  - The patient will be accompanied by a responsible adult who can refer to medical services on their behalf if they deteriorate.
- Safety net advice as a minimum should include reference to:
  - During a non-fatal drowning event small amounts of water may have been inhaled (aspirated), which are not clinically detectable in the few hours following the event. On rare occasions the patient's lungs may produce an inflammatory response within the following 72 hours which presents as increasing shortness of breath.
  - If the patient feels at all unwell or short of breath up to 72 hours post incident, they should attend the emergency department as soon as possible and explain they have been involved in a drowning incident.

KEY POINTS!

Drowning

- **Ensure own personal safety.**
- **Duration and severity of hypoxia associated with drowning is strongest predictor of outcome.**
- **Successful resuscitations have occurred after prolonged submersions in icy cold water.**
- **Hypothermia is a condition often associated with drowning incidents.**
- **Severe complications may develop several hours after a submersion/immersion incident.**

Bibliography

1. van Beeck EF, Branche CM, Szpilman D, Modell JH, Bierens JJLM. A new definition of drowning: towards documentation and prevention of a global public health problem. *Bull World Health Organ*. 2005 Nov, 83(11): 853–6.
2. WHO fact sheet on drowning [Internet]. [cited 2024 Feb 20]. Drowning. Available from: https://www.who.int/news-room/fact-sheets/detail/drowning
3. Annual reports and data – National Water Safety Forum [Internet]. [cited 2021 Mar 29]. Available from: https://www.nationalwatersafety.org.uk/waid/annual-reports-and-data/
4. Meddings D. Clarification and categorization of non-fatal drowning [Internet]. [cited 2024 Jul 2]. Available from: https://www.who.int/publications/m/item/clarification-and-categorization-of-non-fatal-drowning.
5. Szpilman D, Morgan PJ. Management for the Drowning Patient. *CHEST*. 2021 Apr 1, 159(4): 1473–83.
6. Bierens J, Abelairas-Gomez C, Barcala Furelos R, Beerman S, Claesson A, Dunne C, et al. Resuscitation and emergency care in drowning: A scoping review. *Resuscitation*. 2021 May 1, 162: 205–17.
7. European Resuscitation Council Guidelines 2021: Cardiac arrest in special circumstances – Resuscitation [Internet]. [cited 2021 Apr 26]. Available from: https://www.resuscitationjournal.com/article/S0300-9572(21)00064-2/fulltext
8. Bierens JJLM, Lunetta P, Tipton M, Warner DS. Physiology Of Drowning: A Review. Physiol Bethesda Md. 2016 Mar;31(2): 147–66.
9. Golden F, Tipton MJ. Essentials of Sea Survival. Human Kinetics; 2002. 324.
10. Tipton MJ. The initial responses to cold-water immersion in man. *Clin Sci Lond Engl 1979*. 1989 Dec, 77(6): 581–8.
11. Shattock MJ, Tipton MJ. 'Autonomic conflict': a different way to die during cold water immersion? *J Physiol*. 2012 Jul 15, 590(14): 3219–30.
12. Nutbeam T, Boylan M, Leech C, Bosanko C, editors. 2023. ABC of prehospital emergency medicine. 2nd edition. Hoboken, NJ: John Wiley & Sons.

Drowning

13. Davis CA, Schmidt AC, Sempsrott JR, Hawkins SC, Arastu AS, Giesbrecht GG, et al. Wilderness Medical Society Clinical Practice Guidelines for the Treatment and Prevention of Drowning: 2024 Update. *Wilderness Environ Med*. 2024 Mar 1, 35(1_suppl): 94S–111S.

14. Thompson J, Petrie DA, Ackroyd-Stolarz S, Bardua DJ. Out-of-Hospital Continuous Positive Airway Pressure Ventilation Versus Usual Care in Acute Respiratory Failure: A Randomized Controlled Trial. *Ann Emerg Med*. 2008 Sep 1, 52(3): 232–241.e1.

15. Dottorini M, Eslami A, Baglioni S, Fiorenzano G, Todisco T. Nasal-Continuous Positive Airway Pressure in the Treatment of Near-Drowning in Freshwater. CHEST. 1996 Oct 1;110(4): 1122–4.

16. Nava S, Schreiber A, Domenighetti G. Noninvasive Ventilation for Patients With Acute Lung Injury or Acute Respiratory Distress Syndrome. *Respir Care*. 2011 Oct 1, 56(10): 1583–8.

17. Michelet P, Bouzana F, Charmensat O, Tiger F, Durand-Gasselin J, Hraiech S, et al. Acute respiratory failure after drowning: a retrospective multicenter survey. *Eur J Emerg Med*. 2017 Aug, 24(4): 295.

18. Ruggeri P, Calcaterra S, Bottari A, Girbino G, Fodale V. Successful management of acute respiratory failure with noninvasive mechanical ventilation after drowning, in an epileptic-patient. *Respir Med Case Rep*. 2016 Jan 1, 17: 90–2.

19. Montenij LJ, de Vries W, Schwarte L, Bierens JJLM. Feasibility of pulse oximetry in the initial prehospital management of victims of drowning: A preliminary study. *Resuscitation*. 2011 Sep 1, 82(9): 1235–8.

20. Truhlář A, Deakin CD, Soar J, Khalifa GEA, Alfonzo A, Bierens JJLM, et al. European Resuscitation Council Guidelines for Resuscitation 2015: Section 4. Cardiac arrest in special circumstances. *Resuscitation*. 2015 Oct 1, 95: 148–201.

21. Tipton MJ, Golden FSC. A proposed decision-making guide for the search, rescue and resuscitation of submersion (head under) victims based on expert opinion. *Resuscitation*. 2011 Jul, 82(7): 819–24.

22. Overview | Child maltreatment: when to suspect maltreatment in under 18s | Guidance | NICE [Internet]. NICE; [cited 2021 Apr 30]. Available from: https://www.nice.org.uk/guidance/cg89

23. Child maltreatment: when to suspect maltreatment in under 18s. *Child Maltreat*. 2017, 32.

24. Szpilman D. Near-drowning and drowning classification: a proposal to stratify mortality based on the analysis of 1,831 cases. *Chest*. 1997 Sep, 112(3): 660–5.

25. Causey AL, Tilelli JA, Swanson ME. Predicting discharge in uncomplicated near-drowning. *Am J Emerg Med*. 2000 Jan 1, 18(1): 9–11.

26. Auerbach PS, Cushing TA, Harris NS $q (Norman S, editors. Auerbach's wilderness medicine. Seventh edition. Philadelphia, PA: Elsevier/Mosby; 2017. 2.

Electrical Injuries

1. Introduction
- Electrical injury is potentially life-threatening.
- Incidents can occur in domestic or industrial settings.
- Electrical injury may also result from a lightning strike, which may deliver up to 300,000,000 volts.
- The severity of injury and injury pattern can vary, depending on the current, voltage and alternating (AC) or direct (DC) current direction. Electrical injuries can be caused by a wide range of voltages, but the risk of injury is generally greater with higher voltages.[1]

2. Incidence
- In the UK, approximately 14 fatalities are caused by electrical injuries each year. Those most likely to be fatally electrocuted are males between the ages of 20–24.[2]

3. Severity and Outcome
- Electrical injury can cause serious multi-system damage, leading to morbidity and mortality. This results from a combination of tissue damage from the thermal effects along the current pathway, arrhythmias and on occasion secondary traumatic injuries.
- The nature and extent of injury depends on:
  - The voltage and whether it is alternating (AC) or direct (DC).
  - The magnitude of the current.
  - Resistance to current flow, related to age or body mass.
  - Duration of exposure to the current.
  - Pre-existing medical conditions.
  - The pathway of the current – current traversing the myocardium is more likely to be fatal and hand-to-hand travel is more dangerous than hand-to-foot or foot-to-foot.

4. Pathophysiology
- **Cardiovascular:** This may include myocardial ischaemia i.e. angina, myocardial infarction; cardiac arrhythmias both initial (most commonly ventricular fibrillation) and delayed,[3] and cardiorespiratory arrest.
- **Respiratory:** Lung tissue damage can occur in both low and high-voltage electrical injury resulting in dyspnoea and haemoptysis.
- **Muscular paralysis:** May occur from contact with high-voltage electricity affecting the central respiratory control system or respiratory muscles, causing respiratory and then cardiorespiratory arrest.
- **Burns:** May be apparent on the skin at the point of contact (entry and exit). However burns may also affect deeper tissues including viscera, muscles, blood vessels and nerves as thermal energy and associated thermal impacts traverse the body via neurovascular bundles. Unusual burn patterns may be left on the body following a lightning strike.
- **Neurological:** May range from altered mental status, paralysis, seizures, amnesia, headache, temporary blindness or deafness which can be transient and tend to resolve within a few hours.[4]
- **Trauma:** May include joint dislocation, fracture or compartment syndrome. This may occur from sustained tetanic muscle contraction or secondary trauma from falling or being thrown. Injuries may be similar to those seen in primary blast injury (barotrauma/rupture of air filled cavities).[4]
- **Pregnancy:** Due to the complexities of fetal/maternal injury it is strongly recommended that pregnant patients are conveyed to hospital for further assessment.[5,6]

Other considerations:
- Internal implanted cardioverter-defibrillators (ICD) and cardiac pacemakers, can be sensitive to low voltages. (Refer to **Implantable Cardioverter Defibrillator**).
- Successful deployment of a Taser is considered both an electrical injury and a penetrating injury if the skin is broken. (Refer to **Police Incapacitants**).

5. Assessment and Management
For the assessment and management of electrical injuries, refer to Table 4.14 and Figure 4.7.

Electrical burns may have very small entry and exit wounds that mask very extensive internal tissue and organ damage. Do not therefore assume that minimal surface injury is indicative of overall minor tissue damage.

Electrical Injuries

TABLE 4.14 – ASSESSMENT and MANAGEMENT of: Electrical Injuries

⚠ **Ensure Scene Safety for Rescuer and Patient**

- ⚠ !!! DO NOT approach the patient until the electricity supply is cut off (isolated) and you have confirmation from appropriate safety officers, as per local protocol.

NOTE: Attach defibrillator pad at the earliest opportunity to ALL patients and keep defibrillator with the patient until handover to hospital staff.

Assess <C>ABCDE

- If any of the following major **TIME-CRITICAL** features are present:
  - cardiorespiratory arrest (refer to **Advanced Life Support**)
  - facial/airway burns (refer to Airway and Breathing Management)
  - cardiac arrhythmia (refer to **Cardiac Arrhythmia and Sudden Cardiac Death**)
  - significant trauma (refer to appropriate **Trauma** guideline)
  - extensive burns (refer to **Burns and Scalds**), then:
- Start correcting <C>ABCDE and undertake a **TIME-CRITICAL** transfer to nearest receiving hospital or specialist burns unit or major trauma unit if appropriate.
- Continue patient management en route.
- Consider a pre-hospital alert call.

Specifically Consider

- Mechanism – likely magnitude of the current and voltage.
- Airway patency, as early intervention may be required.
- Breathing – rate, depth and any breathing difficulty (refer to Airway and Breathing Management).
- Circulation – undertake an initial 12-lead ECG and consider continuous monitoring as arrhythmias may also develop. Cardiorespiratory resuscitation may require repeated defibrillation, especially in children.[7]
- Exposure – to understand the extent of burns or trauma (refer to appropriate **Trauma** guideline).

Oxygen

- Monitor the patient's SpO_2, and if the patient presents as hypoxemic on air then administer oxygen with a target saturation of 94–98% (refer to **Oxygen**).

Fluid

- Consider fluid resuscitation (refer to **Intravascular Fluid Therapy in Adults** and **Intravascular Fluid Therapy in Children**).

Assess the Need for Pain Relief

- Assess and manage as appropriate (refer to **Pain Management in Adults and Children**).

Definitive Care

- **ALL** patients believed to have been exposed to a large current/high voltage electrical injury should be conveyed. Patients who have been exposed to a small current/low voltage injury, who are asymptomatic, with no injuries and have normal initial 12-lead ECG may not require hospital assessment.

Consider

- If there may be a safeguarding need or whether onward signposting to local health promotion services may be beneficial.[8]

Electrical Injuries

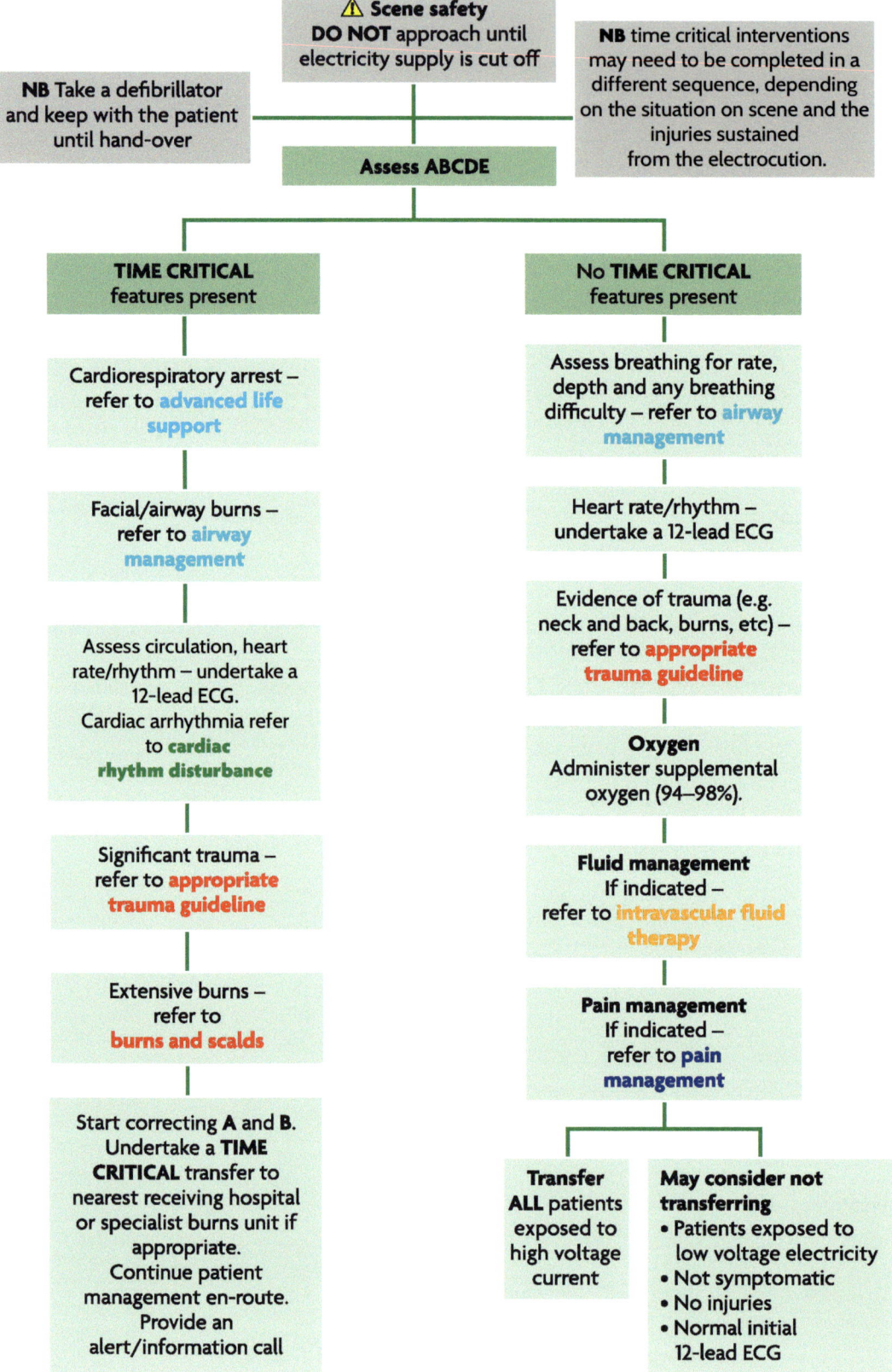

Figure 4.7 – Assessment and management of electrical injuries algorithm.

Electrical Injuries

> **KEY POINTS!**
>
> **Electrical Injuries**
> - Scene safety.
> - Undertake an initial 12-lead ECG and consider continuous monitoring.
> - Consider trauma.
> - Severe tissue damage may be present despite apparently minor injury.
> - Exposure to low voltage may not require hospitalisation.

Bibliography

1. Health and Safety Executive. *Electrical Injuries*. 2010. Available from: http://www.hse.gov.uk/electricity/injuries.htm.

2. Office for National Statistics. 2022. *Deaths where ICD-10 codes W86 or W87 were recorded as the underlying cause, England: 2019 to 2020 registrations*. Available from: https://www.ons.gov.uk/file?uri=/peoplepopulationandcommunity/birthsdeathsandmarriages/deaths/adhocs/14400deathswhereicd10codesw86orw87wererecordedastheunderlyingcauseengland2019to2020registrations/deathsw86w87201920englandfinal.xlsx

3. Ghazal Asswad, A, et al. Delayed, unprovoked, hemodynamic collapse with following asystole in a pediatric patient following a high-voltage injury: a case report and literature review. *Pediatric cardiology* 2022, 43(5): 1163–1168.

4. Hawkins E, Gostigian G, & Diurba S (2024). Lightning Strike Injuries. Emergency medicine clinics of North America. https://doi.org/https://doi.org/10.1016/j.emc.2024.02.021

5. Caballero-Carvajal, JA, et al. Secondary maternal-fetal consequences to electrical injury: A literature review. *Taiwanese journal of obstetrics & gynecology* 2020, 59(1): 1–7.

6. Sparić R, et al. Electric shock in pregnancy: a review. *The journal of maternal-fetal & neonatal medicine : the official journal of the European Association of Perinatal Medicine, the Federation of Asia and Oceania Perinatal Societies, the International Society of Perinatal Obstetricians* 2016, 29(2): 317–323.

7. Rodríguez-Núñez, A., et al. Shockable rhythms and defibrillation during in-hospital pediatric cardiac arrest. *Resuscitation* 2014, 85(3): 387–391.

8. Roberts S and Meltzer JA. An evidence-based approach to electrical injuries in children. *Pediatric emergency medicine practice* 2013, 10(9): 1–16.

9. Royal College of Emergency Medicine. *Electrical Injuries – Lightning*. Clinical Knowledge Summaries. 2017. Available from: https://www.rcemlearning.co.uk/references/electrical-injuries-lightning/.

10. Soar J, Perkins GD, Abbas G, Alfonzo A, Barelli A, Bierens JJLM, et al. European Resuscitation Council Guidelines for Resuscitation 2010 Section 8: cardiac arrest in special circumstances: electrolyte abnormalities, poisoning, drowning, accidental hypothermia, hyperthermia, asthma, anaphylaxis, cardiac surgery, trauma, pregnancy, electrocution. *Resuscitation* 2010, 81(10): 1400–1433.

11. Gauglitz GG, Herndon DN, Jeschke MG. Emergency treatment of severely burned pediatric patients: current therapeutic strategies. *Pediatric Health* 2008, 2(6): 761–775.

12. Yarrow J, Moiemen N, Gulhane S. Early management of burns in children. *Paediatrics and Child Health* 2009, 19(11): 509–516.

13. Ritenour AE, Morton MJ, McManus JG, Barillo DJ, Cancio LC. Lightning injury: a review. *Burns: Journal of the International Society for Burn Injuries* 2008, 34(5): 585–594.

14. Dollery W. Cardiac monitoring not needed in household electrical injury if the patient is asymptomatic and has a normal ECG. *BestBets*, 2003. Available from: http://www.bestbets.org/bets/bet.php?id=9.

15. Bailey B, Gaudreault P, Thivierge RL. Cardiac monitoring of high-risk patients after an electrical injury: a prospective multicentre study. *Emergency Medicine Journal* 2007, 24(5): 348–352.

16. Adukauskiene D, Vizgirdaite V, Mazeikiene S. Electrical injuries. [In Lithuanian]. *Medicina (Kaunas)* 2007, 43(3): 259–266. Abstract in English available from: http://www.ncbi.nlm.nih.gov/pubmed/17413256.

17. Spies C, Trohman RG. Narrative review: electrocution and life-threatening electrical injuries. *Annals of Internal Medicine* 2006, 145(7): 531–537.

18. Vierhapper MF, Lumenta DB, Beck H, Keck M, Kamolz LP, Frey M. Electrical injury: a long-term analysis with review of regional differences. *Annals of Plastic Surgery* 2011, 66(1): 43–46. DOI: 10.1097/SAP.0b013e3181f3e60f.

Falls in Older Adults

1. Introduction

- Falls are defined as an unintentional or unexpected loss of balance resulting in coming to rest on the floor, the ground or an object below knee level. The impact of a fall on the individual and their family is not to be underestimated, with falls often leading to a fear of falling and potentially having psychological as well as physical effects. A fall is distinguished from a collapse, which occurs as a result of an acute medical problem such as an acute arclirhythmia, a transient ischaemic attack or vertigo.[2] A fall can be precipitated by an acute medical condition, and the actual cause of the fall can be very difficult to establish on initial presentation. This guideline covers falls from a standing height. Falls from above standing height or 2 metres above the ground are not covered in this guideline (refer to **Section 4 – Trauma**).

- The term 'mechanical fall' is **not** an appropriate term to use when describing a fall; it implies that a benign aetiology for an older person's fall exists and it is inaccurate, is inconsistently used, is not associated with a discrete fall evaluation and does not predict outcomes.[3]

- Older people in contact with healthcare professionals for any reason should be asked routinely whether they have fallen in the past year, asked about the frequency, context and characteristics of the falls and referred to appropriate falls prevention pathways as per local arrangements. Recently, the SAFER 2 study (a large multi-centre cluster randomised controlled trial) has shown that a paramedic protocol for assessment of older patients (aged ≥65) who have fallen, with an option to refer direct to a community-based falls service (in place of conveyance to the ED), is safe, inexpensive and reduced subsequent 999 calls in those patients. There was no overall difference in outcomes (whether taken to hospital or managed at home) between the trial arms.

2. Incidence

- Falls are the leading cause of emergency calls in the over 65s and account for 10–25% of emergency ambulance responses each year for adults aged over 65 years.[4] In the London Ambulance Service alone, there were 70,380 incidents of people aged 65 and over who were coded as presenting with a fall in the period for 2015–16.

- Falls represent the second leading cause of accidental injury death worldwide and the leading cause of injury-related mortality in the UK.[5] Every year 1 in 3 people aged over 65 and up to 1 in 2 aged over 80 will fall at least once.[6] By 2025, it is estimated that this will account for over 3.2 million falls in people over the age of 65 in England alone.[7] Up to 14,000 people will die each year as a result of a fall and a subsequent fractured neck or femur.[8]

- A fall of <2 metres is the commonest mechanism of injury in older patients.[9]

3. Severity and Outcome

- As part of the normal ageing process, there are a loss of bone density, loss of muscle tone, skin changes and often increased poly-pharmacy. A simple fall in an older person may result in a much more significant injury than would be seen in a younger person. Clinicians should have a higher index of suspicion of injury in older people. However, falls are not a part of normal ageing and are typically due to pathological changes described earlier.

- The *Silver Book*[10] recommends ways in which emergency admissions for older people can be reduced and emphasises that health and social care services must adapt to meet older people's urgent care needs, including ambulance services.

- Falls can be a marker of frailty, which is associated with common syndromes of ageing including immobility, incontinence, susceptibility to the side effects of medication, delirium and dementia, all of which increase the complexity of the presentation and may indicate a change in normal health status. Frail older people typically suffer falls indoors. For a person with frailty, a relatively small event (e.g. a minor infection, a new medication or constipation) may trigger a sudden and dramatic functional decline. Frailty is a clinically recognised state of increased vulnerability. It results from ageing associated with a decline in the body's physical and psychological reserves. This can cause the person to fall and also to struggle to recover following a fall. It is important to recognise the presence of frailty in weighing the benefits and risks of any intervention or treatment plan. Even if no injury has been sustained, further assessment and support post-fall will enable the provision of the right care and support for the person.

4. Risk Factors for Falls

Refer to Table 4.15.

- Risk factors for falls can be broadly classified into three categories:
  - intrinsic factors – relating to the person
  - extrinsic factors – relating to the person's environment
  - exposure to risk.

- However, it is recognised that falls often result from the dynamic interactions of risks in all categories.

- Intrinsic risk factors include changes in the body caused by the normal ageing process, certain medical conditions, excessive alcohol, being physically inactive or a combination of these.

Falls in Older Adults

- It is important to consider dementia and cognitive impairment in the assessment of a patient who has fallen. As many as 11–26% of patients presenting with a fall will have cognitive impairment, some of which will be undiagnosed.[11, 12] Patients with dementia are more likely to fall, to have more falls and to sustain an injury (such as a hip fracture or head injury) from the fall. If sustaining an injury, the outcomes are worse for the patient, their family, the health service and society at large. It is therefore vital to recognise this as a high-risk group.
- It is important that the cause of the fall is considered so that the correct pathways are chosen or excluded; red flags should always be excluded and modifiable factors considered.

TABLE 4.15 – Intrinsic and Extrinsic Falls Risk Factors[13]

Common intrinsic risks of falls[14]	Common extrinsic risk factors of falls
- lower extremity weakness - previous falls - gait and balance disorders - visual impairment - depression - functional and cognitive impairment - dizziness - low body mass index - urinary incontinence - postural hypotension - female sex - being over age 80. **Other intrinsic causes of falls** - sensory deficit (poor vision, peripheral neuropathy) - musculoskeletal disease (osteoarthritis, proximal muscle weakness, previous joint replacement) - other neurodegenerative conditions - central nervous system disease (cognitive dysfunction, vestibular hypofunction, cerebrovascular disease, cerebral hypoperfusion) - Parkinson's disease and Parkinsonism.	- polypharmacy (use of multiple medications) - psychotropic medications - poor lighting (especially on stairs), glare and shadows - low ambient temperature - wet, slippery or uneven floor surfaces - thresholds at room entrances - obstacles and tripping hazards, including clutter - chairs, toilets or beds being too high, low or unstable - inappropriate or unsafe walking aids - inadequately maintained wheelchairs, for example brakes not locking - improper use of wheelchairs, for example failing to clear foot plates - unsafe or absent equipment, such as handrails - pets, such as cats and dogs - loose-fitting footwear and clothing, such as trailing dressing gowns - access to the property, wheelie bins, the garden, uneven ground.

Many medicines cause postural hypotension and may contribute to over 20% of extrinsic falls. Common causes are:

- cardiac drugs:
  - antiarrhythmics (e.g. digoxin)
  - alpha-blockers (e.g. doxazosin)
  - beta-blockers (e.g. bisoprolol, atenolol)
  - ACE inhibitors (e.g. ramipril, lisinopril)
  - angiotensin 2 blockers (e.g. losartan, candesartan)
  - diuretics (e.g. furosemide, bumetanide, spironolactone, bendroflumethiazide)
  - calcium channel blockers (e.g. amlodipine, diltiazem)
- urological drugs (e.g. oxybutynin)
- neuropsychiatric drugs:
  - Parkinson's drugs (e.g. madopar, sinemet, ropinirole)
  - tricyclic antidepressants (e.g. amitriptyline)
  - antipsychotics (e.g. haloperidol, risperidone)
  - painkillers (e.g. opioids)
- In these patients, a formal medicines optimisation review may be indicated by the GP practice or another clinical lead (following local guidance).

Certain activities can be 'high risk' because of the specific interaction of risk factors involved, for example poor balance combined with standing on a stool to change a light bulb or reach a high shelf. To understand falls risk in the environment fully, it is important to observe a person moving around in their environment; referral for a falls assessment in line with local pathways/guidelines will facilitate this.

Falls in Older Adults

4.1 Risks Related to a 'Long Lie'
- A 'long lie' is usually defined as someone who has been on the floor for over 1 hour and has been unable to get up. However, the estimated time on the floor, and mobility while there, may vary greatly and will influence clinical decision making, i.e. a patient who has been completely immobile on the floor for several hours will be at higher risk than someone who can move across the floor but cannot pull themselves up onto a chair or bed or into a standing position.
- Anyone who has experienced a long lie is at a higher risk of complications, such as pneumonia, pressure areas, rhabdomyolysis, dehydration and hypothermia.
- Increasing age and other co-morbidities will increase the risk of complications from a long lie; each patient will need to be assessed on an individual basis, to plan ongoing management.

5. Psychology of Falling
- Depression, fear of falling and other psychological problems are common effects of falls. Loss of confidence as well as social withdrawal and loneliness can occur, even when there is no injury. A person who is fearful about falls will often avoid physical activity, become weaker and may fall more as a result. Social isolation can also result if the person stops going out.
- Some older people are fearful that a fall may lead to a loss of independence, being admitted to hospital, loss of control over their life or being rehoused. These well-documented fears can lead to patients not reporting falls, masking symptoms or being reluctant to attend an emergency department or be referred to their GP. Clinicians should be aware of these issues and help to promote independence. Positive conversations should emphasise the simple things that can be done to reduce falls risk, regain confidence and maintain independence through referral to other services for further assessment and support.

6. Assessment and Management

6.1 Specific History and Examination Considerations
- A thorough and careful physical examination is required, along with a high index of suspicion, to exclude common but easily missed injuries, such as rib fractures, spinal fractures and delayed presentation of a previous head injury.
- A perceived minor injury, such as a fractured rib, may have more serious long-term consequences for an older person, e.g. pulmonary contusions. Minor injuries can also lead to a temporary loss of independence, which, for a person with frailty, can become permanent without aggressive management and rehabilitation. Every rib fracture increases the risk of dying by 15% in frail older people.
- The history taken on scene needs to be thorough and well documented in the patient record; where possible it should be corroborated with relatives, carers or associated healthcare professionals.
- Initial assessment should exclude the possibility of syncope. Transient loss of consciousness should be assumed to have occurred unless proven otherwise (refer to **Altered Level of Consciousness**).
- Clinical history should include:
  – details of any previous altered level of consciousness, including number and frequency
  – the person's medical history and family history of cardiac disease (for example, personal history of heart disease and family history of sudden cardiac death)
  – current medication that may have contributed to altered level of consciousness (for example, diuretics)
  – vital signs and NEWS2 score (for example, pulse rate, respiratory rate and temperature) – repeat if clinically indicated
  – lying and standing blood pressure if clinically appropriate
  – other cardiovascular and neurological signs.
- Consider scoring a patient's level of frailty. Refer to Figure 4.8.[1]
  – The Rockwood Clinical Frailty Scale (CFS) is a judgement-based frailty assessment tool. It is not validated for people under the age of 65 years or those with long-term disabilities. Frailty must be sensed, described and measured: not guessed. If the patient you are assessing is acutely unwell and over 65 years, consider using the CFS, as per local pathways.
  – The score is based on the patient's baseline, so use the tool to score how the patient was 2 weeks ago (prior to deterioration) or their usual level of functioning when well, rather than how they present today. If possible, cross-reference what the patient describes to you with a description from relatives/carers.
  – Do NOT compare the patient to the pictures (e.g. person using walking aids) alone to make a judgement on the level of frailty.
- It is important to consider that medications prescribed for co-morbidities may complicate the clinical picture and presentation.

6.2 12-Lead ECG
- Older people who fall should have a 12-lead ECG (with auto-interpretation) recorded. This must be interpreted by the assessing clinician unless they are confident the patient has complete

Falls in Older Adults

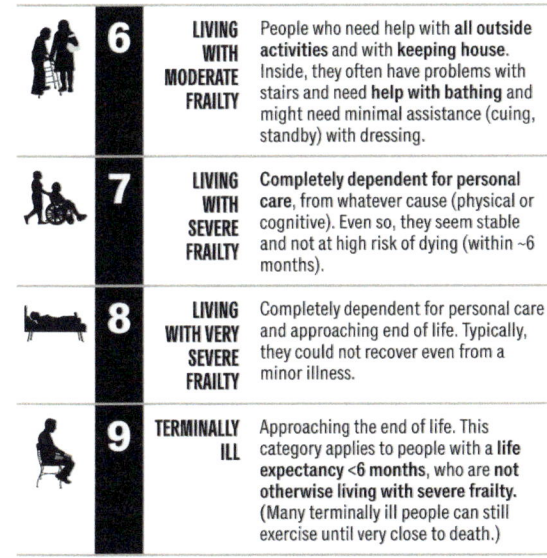

Figure 4.8 – Clinical Frailty Scale. Used with permission from Dr. Rockwood and the Geriatric Medicine Research Unit.

recall of the event and clearly describes an extrinsic factor that caused the fall. Transient loss of consciousness (TLoC) should be assumed unless proven otherwise; refer to TLOC and NICE guidance.

> **'Red flags' for syncope seen in a 12-lead ECG include:**
> 🚩 conduction abnormality (for example, complete right or left bundle branch block, atrial fibrillation or any degree of heart block)
> 🚩 evidence of a long or short QT interval
> 🚩 any ST segment or T wave abnormalities.

6.3 Atrial Fibrillation (AF) and Falls

- Ensure that a 12-lead ECG is performed on any patient with an irregular pulse felt on palpation to identify the underlying rhythm.
- It may be difficult to determine if AF is new or not. The patient may know themselves or have been told that they have an irregular heartbeat/AF, or you may be able to contact the patient's health professional/GP or review care plans/medical notes.
- If the patient is asymptomatic and has a heart rate below 120/minute, and an extrinsic cause of the fall has been identified, consider contacting a GP to have a clinical discussion and agree a care plan.
- Consider conveyance to hospital as a priority if the patient is found to be in atrial fibrillation (AF) after a fall and has symptoms such as:
  – altered mental status
  – dizziness
  – chest pain
  – heart rate above 120/minute
  – dyspnoea
  – palpitations
  – hypotension.
- If the patient has AF and has had a potential syncope, refer to local syncope pathways or follow local guidance.

6.4 Postural Hypotension

- Postural hypotension should be checked for if there is no clear extrinsic cause of the fall, if there are no features to suggest an alternative cause, if symptoms are typical such as light-headedness, dizziness or feeling weak and faint

Falls in Older Adults

on standing and if the patient is being considered for management at home.
- Procedure for checking postural hypotension:
  1. Identify if you are going to need assistance to stand the patient and simultaneously record a BP. Use a manual sphygmomanometer if possible and definitely if the automatic machine fails to record.
  2. Explain procedure to the patient.
  3. The first BP should be taken after lying for at least 5 minutes.
  4. The second BP should be taken after standing in the first minute.
  5. A third BP should be taken after standing for 3 minutes.
  6. This recording can be repeated if the BP is still falling.
  7. Symptoms of dizziness, light-headedness, vagueness, pallor, visual disturbance, feelings of weakness and palpitations should be documented.
  8. A positive result is: a. A drop in systolic BP of 20 mmHg or more (with or without symptoms) b. A drop to below 90 mmHg on standing even if the drop is less than 20 mmHg (with or without symptoms) c. A drop in diastolic BP of 10 mmHg with symptoms (although clinically much less significant than a drop in systolic BP).
- If the patient is unable to stand, a sitting reading may be taken; however, the sensitivity of the test is reduced in this case.
- Symptomatic postural hypotension is a significant finding that requires further investigation and medication review but rarely requires admission (refer to local guidance for further assessment). Asymptomatic postural hypotension may be managed through primary care.

6.5 Confusion/Delirium
- Confusion is routinely encountered with older adults who have fallen. Often associated with dementia, confusion can also be an indication of an acute pathology presenting as delirium. The patient may be either more (hyperactive delirium) or less (hypoactive delirium) active than normal, although the mixed type is the commonest. However, dementia is characterised by a gradual onset and is not reversible, whereas delirium typically is described as having a rapid onset and is attributed to a reversible cause.
- Be mindful that the confusion may pre-exist and even contribute to the fall, or may occur as a consequence of the fall. This makes gaining a comprehensive and corroborated history very important.
- Where a patient presents with confusion, apply the principles of assessing capacity to consent and be prepared to modify your communication to the needs of the patient. Look for documents such as 'This is me'.[15] Listening to the family, carers or friends who know the patient best may provide clear indications regarding the onset and severity of the confusion, and any changes to it as this is the most reliable single indicator of delirium, especially in patients who cannot communicate. Where concerns are expressed, you should have a high index of suspicion that the confusion is new and requires further investigation or referral.
- New onset confusion can be due to physiological changes resulting from head injury, hypoxia, infection, stroke or transient ischaemic attack (TIA), hypoglycaemia, ketoacidosis, side effects of medications or drugs and the effects of withdrawal from drugs or alcohol. In addition, other causes could include carbon monoxide poisoning, encephalitis or meningitis, electrolyte imbalance, post-seizure and, more rarely, an underactive thyroid gland, tumour, thiamine deficiency, hypo/hyperparathyroidism and Cushing's disease.

6.6 Skin Assessment for Adults
- Consider performing an assessment of the patient's skin after a fall to ensure that the skin is intact. Gain the patient's consent or act in their best interests. Consider patient dignity and body temperature as you examine them. Pay attention to areas of bony prominence that are subject to pressure when lying on a hard surface, such as the back of head and ears, shoulders, elbows, lower back and buttocks, hips, inner knees and heels.
- A skin assessment in adults should take into account:
  - any pain or discomfort reported by the patient
  - skin integrity in areas of pressure
  - colour changes or discoloration
  - variations in heat, firmness and moisture (due to incontinence, oedema or dry or inflamed skin).
- If any concerns are identified, consider referral to community nursing teams in line with local pathways/guidance.
- Refer to Figure 4.9 for an aid to assessing skin breakdown.

6.7 Continence
- Confirm the patient's usual toileting/continence regime. Consider new symptoms, including dysuria, increased frequency of urination, suprapubic tenderness, urgency and polyuria, but do not carry out a urine dipstick in the absence of symptoms of UTI.[16]

Falls in Older Adults

- If continent/partially continent, consider if they are likely to be able to locate and physically get to the toilet/commode, rearrange clothes and clean the genital area and hands.
- If incontinent/partially continent, consider if the patient/carer is able to manage pads/catheter care, rearrange clothes, clean the genital area and hands and dispose of waste safely. Community nursing services may be available to provide rapid continence assessment including recatheterisation.

6.8 How to Decide If the Patient Could Be Managed in the Community

- Decisions on whether to manage a patient at home/in the community can be challenging and should be made following a comprehensive history, clinical assessment and examination. Decisions on the best management of an older person who has fallen are made on a risk/benefit basis and may benefit from discussion with locally agreed clinical contacts. These could include ambulance service clinical advice lines or other healthcare professionals clinical advice lines using a shared decision making approach, and should always consider the views of the patient and relatives/carers. The final referral decision will also depend on the availability and responsiveness of local community health and social care services. Well-structured advice on how to assess and make decisions related to choosing an appropriate clinical pathway improves patient safety and outcomes.[17]
- There are also risks in taking an older person to hospital, including institutionalisation and/or deconditioning (the consequence of prolonged bed rest, leading to loss of functional status through reduced muscle mass and strength). The decline in muscle mass and strength has been linked to falls, functional decline, increased frailty, immobility and healthcare-associated infection.[18]
- Some older people who fall may prefer to be managed in the community or at home, and where possible this should be supported, particularly where family/carers can also provide support. Following a comprehensive patient assessment and wider review of the circumstances of the fall (having excluded injuries/acute illness), ambulance clinicians should provide the referral for this to occur in line with local pathways and guidance.

6.9 Ongoing Referral

- All older people who have fallen resulting in an ambulance call/attendance, but who are then managed at home, should be offered referral pathways as per local guidelines. The purpose of referral/re-referral is to prevent further falls and injury.
- Referrals should take into account current care plans and other health and social care organisations already involved in the patient's care.
- Decision making should be a shared process, including the patient and their family/carers/other health and social care professionals/any person holding their lasting power of attorney for health and welfare.
- Referral to services via locally agreed pathways may result in:
  – multifactorial falls risk assessment
  – frailty assessment
  – assessment of care needs, including telecare.

6.10 Falls Prevention[5]

- Ambulance clinicians have a role to play in having conversations with people who are at risk of falling, or who have fallen, to try and prevent further falls. The evidence-based Making Every Contact Count (MECC) approach[19] can be applied or other locally agreed methods of ensuring health prevention messages can be given. A MECC interaction takes a matter of minutes and is not intended to add to busy workloads, but should be part of the conversations after a fall or with patients who have been identified as at risk of falling. Evidence suggests that the broad adoption of the MECC approach could potentially have a significant impact on the health of the population.
- Support can be given to older people at risk of falling by routinely asking them about falls and encouraging them to stay active and connected, eat well and reduce alcohol intake, to reduce the risk of falling and to improve outcomes if a fall happens. Consider discussing the measures a person can take to reduce their risk factors for falling, the exercises recommended by falls teams or other healthcare professionals, the preventable nature of some falls and where they can seek further advice and assistance.
- Consider leaving the patient with an information leaflet about falls prevention and suggesting telecare options, such as a pendant-type alarm so help can be summoned for any further falls, or simple solutions to providing a safer physical environment. Conversations can take place with carers/family members if the person has cognitive impairment.
- Older people in contact with healthcare professionals for any reason should be asked **routinely** whether they have fallen in the past year and asked about the frequency, context and characteristics of the falls. Referrals should be made in line with local guidance.

Falls in Older Adults

Early warning sign - blanching erythema
Areas of discoloured tissue that blanch when fingertip pressure is applied and the colour recovers when pressure is released, indicating damage is starting to occur but can be reversed.

On darkly pigmented skin, blanching does not occur and changes to colour, temperature and texture of skin are the main indicators.

Grade 1	Grade 2	Grade 3	Grade 4
Non-blanchable erythema	**Partial thickness skin loss**	**Full thickness skin loss**	**Full thickness tissue loss**
Intact skin with non-blanchable redness, usually over a bony prominence. Darker skin tones may not have visible blanching but the colour may differ from the surrounding area. The affected area may be painful, firmer, softer, warmer or cooler than the surrounding tissue.	Loss of the epidermis/dermis presenting as a shallow open ulcer with a red/pink wound bed without slough or bruising.[1] May also present as an intact or open/ruptured blister.	Subcutaneous fat may be visible but bone, tendon or muscle is not visible or palpable. Slough may be present but does not obscure the depth of tissue loss. May include undermining or tunnelling.[2]	Extensive destruction with exposed or palpable bone, tendon or muscle. Slough may be present but does not obscure the depth of tissue loss. Often includes undermining or tunnelling.[2]

Moisture lesions
Moisture lesions are skin damage due to exposure to urine, faeces or other body fluids.

a) Location: Located in peri-anal, gluteal, cleft, groin or buttock area. Not usually over a bony prominence.

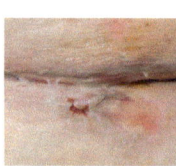

b) Shape: Diffuse often multiple lesions. May be 'copy', 'mirror' or 'kissing' lesion on adjacent buttock or anal cleft. Linear.

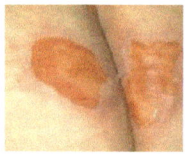

c) Edges: Diffuse irregular edges.

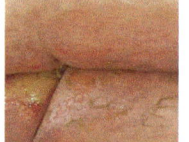

d) Necrosis: No necrosis or slough. May develop slough if infection present.

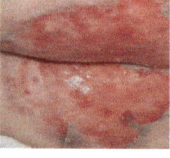

e) Depth: Superficial partial thickness skin loss. Can enlarge or deepen if infection present.

f) Colour: Change in skin colour may not be uniform. Patients with a light skin tone may have pink or white skin areas (maceration) whereas patients with a dark skin tone may show maroon, lighter or darker skin areas. Peri-anal redness/maroon/darker skin may be present.

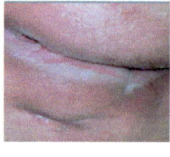

Where pressure ulcers commonly occur

The shaded points indicate vulnerable areas of the body with regards to pressure ulcers

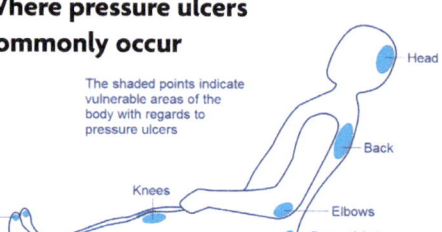

[1] Bruising can indicate deep tissue injury

[2] The depth of a Grade 3 or 4 pressure ulcer varies by anatomical location. Areas such as the bridge of the nose, ears, occiput and malleolus do not have fatty tissue so the depth of these ulcers may be shallow. In contrast areas which have excess fatty tissue can develop deep Grade 3 pressure ulcers where bone, tendon, muscle is not directly visible or palpable.

Figure 4.9 – Grading tool for assessing skin breakdown. Reproduced with kind permission of Healthcare Improvement Scotland.

Falls in Older Adults

TABLE 4.16 – ASSESSMENT and MANAGEMENT of: Falls in Older People

Primary Survey

- Assess **<C>ABCDE**
- Are any of the following **TIME-CRITICAL** features present?
  - major **<C>ABCDE** problems
  - altered level of consciousness
  - neck and back injuries.
- Refer to:
  - **Airway and Breathing Management**
  - **Trauma Emergencies in Adults – Overview**

SECONDARY ASSESSMENT – TRAUMA

Assess for Trauma/Injuries

- Make a careful physical assessment, as relatively minor injury can have significant consequences in older people; all should include a pain assessment.

Caution

- Older adults can present with major trauma with seemingly minor mechanism of injury and kinetic energy transfer.
- Assess specifically for evidence or risk of occult bleeding (intracranial, intrathoracic and intra-abdominal).
- Be mindful of apparently minor head injuries in the context of concurrent anticoagulant, clopidogrel or combination anti-platelet therapy and other coagulopathies. Refer to local policies around minor head injuries.

Consider Spinal Injuries[20, 21, 22, 23, 24, 25]

- Falls are a more frequent cause of spinal 'cord' injury in the older patient.
- Central Cord Syndrome (CCS) may occur in susceptible older individuals with degenerative spinal disease who sustain hyperextension of the cervical spine during trauma.
- CCS can result from ground height/level surface falls and is also associated with flexion and compression trauma mechanisms.

Specifically Assess

- Motor weakness in the upper and lower extremities; any impairment will usually be greater in the upper extremities than in the lower extremities, especially in the muscle of the hands.
- Sensory impairment may be variable and limited to mild sensory impairment in the hands or feet.

Note

- In trauma, CCS may present with/without bony spinal injury.
- Assess carefully for fragility fractures.

Refer to:
  - **Head Injury**
  - **Spinal Injury and Spinal Cord Injury**
  - **Thoracic Trauma**
  - **Abdominal Trauma**
  - **Limb Trauma**.

Also consider:
  - skin integrity/turgor (long lies)
  - chest injuries, including thorough palpation of the chest to exclude rib fractures
  - osteoporosis.

(continued)

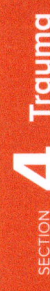

Falls in Older Adults

TABLE 4.16 – ASSESSMENT and MANAGEMENT of: Falls in Older People *(continued)*

SECONDARY ASSESSMENT – MEDICAL

Intrinsic Factors

- Take a detailed history of how the fall is described.
- Can the history be corroborated by a reliable third party?
- Document a NEWS2 score[26, 27]

Refer to:
- **Altered Level of Consciousness** (in particular transient loss of consciousness (TLoC))
- **Glycaemic Emergencies in Adults and Children**
- **Cardiac Arrhythmia and Sudden Cardiac Death**
- **Seizures in Adults**
- **Sepsis** (check for pyrexia or hypothermia as markers of possible infection)
- **Stroke/Transient Ischaemic Attack**
- **Overdose and Poisoning in Adults and Children** (intentional or unintentional).

Also consider:
- possible bleeding – intracranial, intrathoracic, intra-abdominal
- acute kidney injury
- delirium
- frailty, in line with local guidance
- polypharmacy – use of multiple medicines.

REVIEW OF SYSTEMS

- Cardiovascular (include postural hypotension assessment and consider 12-lead ECG).
- Respiratory system.
- Gastrointestinal (bowels, bladder, eating/drinking).
- Genitourinary (if a urinary infection is suspected clinically with signs such as increased frequency/dysuria and suprapubic tenderness, follow local guidelines).
- Neurological (stroke/TIA).
- Musculoskeletal.
- Hair, skin (look for pressure areas) and nails.
- Mental health (anxiety, depression, fear of falling).

HISTORY OF THE FALL

- Consider using a mnemonic such as SPLAT:[28]
  - **Symptoms** prior to and at the time of the fall.
  - **Previous** falls, near falls and/or fear of falling.
  - **Location** to identify contributing environmental factors (for example, was there poor lighting, was footing poor, did they trip or were they in a crowd?).
  - **Activity** the person was participating in when they fell (for example, were they turning, changing position or transferring?).
  - **Time** of day the fall occurred (falls in the morning could be due to postural hypotension and later in the day could be due to fatigue).
- Ascertain how the fall happened, considering the following:
  - Intrinsic factors (including pathological factors, e.g. collapse).
  - Extrinsic factors (including environment, trips and hazards).
  - Can the patient recall the fall in detail? Words such as 'I must have tripped' suggest no recollection (refer to **Altered Level of Consciousness**, especially transient loss of consciousness (TLoC)).
  - Can the history of the fall be corroborated by a reliable third party?
  - Is there a history of previous falls? When did these occur, with what frequency; were any injurious?
  - Is this fall consistent with previous falls or different?
  - Is there a new onset of confusion?
  - Are alcohol/drugs/medication involved?

Falls in Older Adults

TABLE 4.16 – ASSESSMENT and MANAGEMENT of: Falls in Older People *(continued)*

FUNCTIONAL ASSESSMENT – MOBILITY

- Mobility must be considered to:
  - help exclude injury
  - determine if mobility is a factor contributing to falls risk
  - ascertain a person's ability to function safely at home following the fall.
- Observe the person getting up from their chair, balancing on standing, walking round their home (including turning) and sitting down again – using their usual walking aid if applicable.
- A formal test may be used as per local guidance, such as the 'get up and go' test or the 'turn 180 degrees' test.[29, 30, 31]
- A mobility assessment should also take into account the use and state of repair of walking aids.
- While the person is moving around, check they can weight-bear and consider how steady, safe and confident they are.
- Where possible, find out the person's normal mobility status; it may be that a person has limited mobility normally but is managing well with regular visits from family or carers and/or with equipment such as a commode.
- Consider whether the person is able to:
  - get to the toilet/commode and transfer on and off it safely
  - access a drink or simple snack
  - manage on the stairs if this is essential to get to the toilet/bed or other rooms
  - take essential medications as prescribed
  - summon help.
- If the person receives care, consider the timing of the next visit. Contact the agency if possible. Information may be found in a care plan.
- Consider local services that may be available to respond to support the person in remaining at home and avoiding hospital admission.

OTHER CONSIDERATIONS

General

- Look/ask for other information about the patient, such as anticipatory care plans that may detail preferences for place of care, clinical management, home care input, nursing/therapy input, including access to electronic care records.
- Ask about lasting power of attorney/end of life and DNACPR/ReSPECT decisions.
- In cases of worsening chronic confusion, consider referral back to GP/local pathway.
- Consider frailty in line with local guidance.
- Consider the need for senior clinical advice/support.

Extrinsic Factors

- Walking aids (consider correct use, state of repair, suitability for the patient).
- Footwear (good fit, not worn out, adequate grip and support).
- Floor surfaces (clear of obstructions, carpets and rugs not frayed or lifted, not slippery or wet/greasy).
- Lighting.
- Temperature.
- Spectacles and hearing aids, telecare alarm (worn, clean and working, regular check-ups).
- Home safety, smoke alarms, clutter and other trip hazards, exit routes, crime risks, ability to self-evacuate, home adaptations.
- Shared decision making with patients and families/carers/other health and social care professionals.
- Respect the autonomy of the individual.

(continued)

Falls in Older Adults

TABLE 4.16 – ASSESSMENT and MANAGEMENT of: Falls in Older People *(continued)*
Safeguarding
• Ask the patient if they feel safe.
• Consider the need for additional support, protection or referral for safeguarding.
• Refer to **Safeguarding Adults at Risk**.
Social Context
• Housing type.
• Living alone or with spouse/family/partner.
– What is the level of support offered by the above?
– Does the patient have caring responsibilities? What are they and are they affected by the fall?
– What are the existing support/care packages in place? When is the next planned visit of carers?
– Are the patient/relatives and carers coping or in denial?
• Is support/care assessment required?
• Does the family and carer burden/need require assessment?
• Does the patient suffer social isolation/loneliness?
Referral and Safety-Netting
• Follow local policies or guidelines.
• Patients who have fallen should be offered referral to a community-based falls service to enable secondary prevention as per local policies.[17]
Prevention
• Self-care and links to the voluntary sector.
• Signposting.
• Local leaflets, contacts and information.
• Written advice for non-injury falls.
• Advice for the patient, their relatives and carers.
• Make Every Contact Count (MECC) opportunities.

KEY POINTS!

Falls in Older Adults

- The term 'mechanical fall' is not an appropriate term to use when describing a fall.
- Initial assessment should exclude the possibility of syncope.
- A thorough and careful physical examination is required along with a high index of suspicion, to exclude common but easily missed injuries.
- Some older people who fall may prefer to be managed in the community or at home, and where possible this should be supported, particularly where family/carers can also provide support.
- All older people who have fallen resulting in an ambulance call/attendance, but are then managed at home, should be offered referral pathways as per local guidelines.
- Ambulance clinicians have a role to play in talking with people who are at risk of falling, or who have fallen, to try and prevent further falls.

Further Reading

Further important information and evidence in support of this guideline can be found in the Bibliography.[32]

Other useful resources include:

http://www.sciencedirect.com/science/article/pii/S096663621400705X

Falls in Older Adults

Bibliography

1. Rockwood K et al. A global clinical measure of fitness and frailty in elderly people. *Canadian Medical Association Journal* 2005, 173(5): 489–495.: https://pubmed.ncbi.nlm.nih.gov/16129869/.

2. National Institute for Health and Clinical Excellence. *Falls in Older People* (QS86). London: NICE, 2017. Available from: https://www.nice.org.uk/guidance/qs86/chapter/Quality-statement-6-Medical-examination-after-an-inpatient-fall.

3. Tirrell GP, Lipsitz LA, Liru SW. Is there such a thing as a mechanical fall? *American Journal of Emergency Medicine* 2016, 34(3): 582–585. DOI: 10.1016/j.ajem.2015.12.009.

4. Ambulance Service Network Community Health Services Forum. Falls prevention: new approaches to integrated falls prevention services. *Briefing* 2012: 234. NHS Confederation. Available from: http://www.nhsconfed.org/~/media/Confederation/Files/Publications/Documents/Falls_prevention_briefing_final_for_website_30_April.pdf.

5. National Institute for Health and Clinical Excellence. *Falls in Older People: Assessing Risk and Prevention* (CG161). London: NICE, 2013.

6. Department of Health. *National Service Framework for Older People*. London: The Stationery Office, 2001.

7. Projecting Older People Population Information Systems. Available from: http://www.poppi.org.uk/index.php?pageNo=315&PHPSESSID=eujokv2jii3d1vj7q70s8eh5c4&sc=1&loc=8640&np=1.

8. Age UK. *Stop Falling: Start Saving Lives and Money*. London: Age UK, 2012.

9. Trauma Audit and Research Network. *Major Trauma in Older People*. Manchester: University of Manchester, 2017.

10. British Geriatrics Society. *Quality Care for Older People with Urgent and Emergency Care Needs: The 'Silver Book'*. London: British Geriatric Society, 2012.

11. Davies AJ, Kenny RA. Falls presenting to the accident and emergency department: types of presentation and risk factor profile. *Age and Ageing*. 1996, 25(5): 362–366.

12. Bloch F, Jegou D, Dhainaut J-F et al. Do ED staffs have a role to play in the prevention of repeat falls in elderly patients? *American Journal of Emergency Medicine* 2009, 27(3): 303–307.

13. College of Occupational Therapists. *Occupational Therapy in the Prevention and Management of Falls in Adults* (Practice Guideline). London: COT, 2015.

14. American Geriatrics Society. *AGS/BGS Clinical Practice Guideline: Prevention of Falls in Older Persons*. 2010. Available from: http://www.medcats.com/FALLS/frameset.htm.

15. Alzheimer's Society. *This Is Me*. Available from: https://www.alzheimers.org.uk/download/downloads/id/3423/this_is_me.pdf.

16. Scottish Intercollegiate Guidelines Network. *Management of Suspected Bacterial Urinary Tract Infection in Adults* (SIGN Guideline 88). Edinburgh: Healthcare Improvement Scotland, 2012.

17. Snooks HA et al. Support and assessment for fall emergency referrals (SAFER) 2. *Health Technol Assess* 2017, 21(13): 1–218. Available from: https://www.ncbi.nlm.nih.gov/pubmed/28397649.

18. Gillis A, McDonald B. Deconditioning in the hospitalised elderly. *Canadian Nurse* 2005, 101(6): 16–20. Available from: https://www.ncbi.nlm.nih.gov/pubmed/16121472.

19. Health Education England. *Making Every Contact Count*. Available from: http://www.makingeverycontactcount.co.uk/.

20. Shadler P, Shue J, Giradi F. Central Cord Syndrome, A review of epidemiology, treatment and prognostic factors. *JSM Neurosurg Spine* 2016, 4(3): 1075.

21. National Association of Emergency Medical Technicians. *Prehospital Trauma Life Support*. Spinal Trauma, Chapter 17 Geriatric Trauma, St Louis, MO: Mosby JEMs Elsevier, 2016. Especially Ch. 11, Spinal trauma and Ch. 17 Geriatric trauma.

22. McKinley M, Santos K, Meade M et al. Incidence and outcomes of spinal cord injury clinical syndromes. *J Spinal Cord Med* 2007, 30: 215–224.

23. Ryan M, Henderson J. The epidemiology of fractures and fracture-dislocations of the cervical spine. *Injury* 1992, 23: 38–40.

24. Mandavia D, Newton K. Geriatric trauma. *Emerg Med Clin North Am* 1998, 16: 257–274.

25. Wagner R, Jagoda A. Spinal cord syndromes. *Emerg Med Clin North Am* 1997, 15: 699–711.

26. Cei M et al. In-hospital mortality and morbidity of elderly medical patients can be predicted at admission by the modified early warning score: a prospective study. *Int J Clin Pract* 2009, 63(4): 591–595.

27. Romero-Ortunoa R, Wallisa S, Birama R, Keevila V, Clinical frailty adds to acute illness severity in predicting mortality in hospitalized older adults: an observational study. *European Journal of Internal Medicine* 2016, 35: 24–34.

28. Bauman CA, Milligan JD, Patel T et al. Community-based falls prevention: lessons from an Inter-professional Mobility Clinic. *J Can Chiropr* 2014, 58(3): 300–311.

29. Mathias S, Nayak USL, Isaacs B. Balance in elderly patients: the 'get-up and go' test. *Arch Phys Med Rehabil*. 1986, 67: 387–389.

30. Nevitt MC, Cummings SR, Kidd S, Black D. Risk factors for recurrent nonsyncopal falls. A prospective study. *Journal of the American Medical Association* 1989, 261(18): 2663–2668.

31. Simpson JM, Worsfold C, Reilly E, Nye N. A standard procedure for using TURN180: testing dynamic postural stability among elderly people. *Physiotherapy* 2002, 88(6): 342–353.

32. Murdoch I, Turpin S, Johnson B, MacLullich A, Losman E. *Geriatric Emergencies*. London: Wiley-Blackwell, 2015.

Head Injury

1. Introduction

- Head injury is a common presentation to the ambulance service. This can range from a trivial head injury through to severe life-threatening injuries.
- Head injury is defined as any trauma to the head other than superficial injuries to the face. Each year, 1.4 million people attend emergency departments (EDs) in England and Wales with a recent head injury. Between 33% and 50% of these are children aged under 15 years. Annually, about 200,000 people are admitted to hospital with head injury. Of these, 20% have features suggesting skull fracture or have evidence of brain injury. Most patients recover without specific or specialist intervention, but others experience long-term disability or even die from the effects of complications that could potentially be minimised or avoided with early detection and appropriate treatment. While there are a range of patients who require further assessment in hospital, a number of patients may be safely discharged at the scene, providing the patient, family members and carers are given appropriate verbal and written head injury advice.
- The incidence of death from head injury is low, with as few as 0.2% of all patients attending Emergency Departments with a head injury dying as a result of this injury. Ninety-five percent of people who have sustained a head injury present with a normal or minimally impaired conscious level (Glasgow Coma Scale (GCS) greater than 12) but the majority of fatal outcomes are in the moderate (GCS 9–12) or severe (GCS 8 or less) head injury groups, which account for only 5% of attenders at ED.
- It is estimated that 25–30% of children aged under 2 years who are hospitalised with head injury have an abusive head injury (refer to **Safeguarding Children**).
- Ambulance clinicians need to consider early detection and treatment of life-threatening brain injury, where present, but also be able to safely discharge patients with negligible risk of brain injury.

2. Pathophysiology

- Primary brain injury occurs at the time of injury. Prevention strategies include the wearing of motorcycle and cycle helmets, the use of vehicle restraint systems (e.g. seat belts and airbags) and public education.
- Secondary brain injury occurs following the primary event as a result of hypoxia, hypercarbia or hypoperfusion.
- A reduced level of consciousness may lead to airway obstruction or inadequate ventilation, resulting in poor oxygenation, carbon dioxide retention and acidosis.

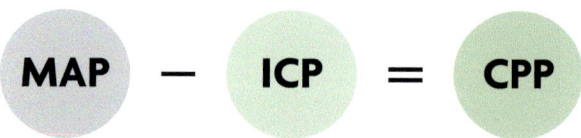

Figure 4.10 – Cerebral perfusion pressure.

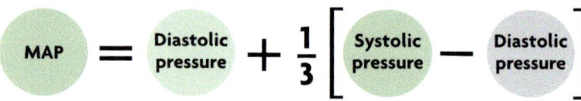

Figure 4.11 – Mean arterial pressure.

- Impact brain apnoea is an immediate transient cessation of breathing following a head injury, often without significant anatomical insult. The sudden mechanical force exerted on the head can cause autonomical dysfunction, resulting in neurogenic shock characterised by a period of apnea. Hypoxia is the leading cause of mortality in these patients, and priority should be given to airway and breathing.
- Blood loss from other injuries in a patient with multisystem trauma may lead to hypovolaemia, hence a fall in mean arterial pressure (MAP) and consequently cerebral perfusion pressure (CPP).
- CPP needs to be maintained to ensure normal brain physiology and prevent oedema. It is determined by the relationship between the MAP and the intracranial pressure (ICP). This is the mean pressure during the cardiac pumping cycle pushing blood into the brain against the resistance of the ICP (refer to Figures 4.10 and 4.11).

3. Assessment of Patients with Head Injury

- All patients should have an initial A–E assessment, including assessment of:
  - GCS
  - pupils (size and reactivity)
  - focal peripheral neurology (see below).
- Consider full cervical spine immobilisation for patients who have sustained a head injury, where appropriate (refer to **Spinal Injury and Spinal Cord Injury**).
- For patients aged 65 or older, and for older patients that have fallen from a height of greater than 1 metre or 5 stairs, be particularly aware of the potential for more severe brain injury and/or spinal cord injury as well as the increased risk of multiple traumatic injuries in this group (refer to **Falls in Older Adults**).

3.1 Glasgow Coma Scale

- In all communications, documentation and handovers, the individual components of the GCS should be given as well as the total GCS score.

Head Injury

- In some patients (for example, patients with dementia, underlying chronic neurological disorders or learning disabilities), the pre-injury baseline GCS may be less than 15. Establish this where possible and take it into account during assessment.
- Blood glucose level must be checked as part of initial assessment, as alteration in behaviour or conscious level may be attributed to this.
- History-taking must include assessment of medications (i.e. anticoagulants, antiplatelets) and other factors that either place the patient at higher risk of serious underlying injury or may suggest that the patient cannot be safely discharged at the scene.

3.2 Focal Neurological Deficit

- Focal neurological deficit covers problems restricted to a particular part of the body or a particular activity, for example difficulties with understanding, speaking, reading or writing; decreased sensation; loss of balance; general weakness; visual changes; abnormal reflexes; and problems walking.

3.3 Basal Skull fracture or Open fractures

- Signs of basal skull fracture include CSF clear fluid running from the ears or nose (late sign), bilateral peri-orbital haematoma (panda eyes), or mastoid bruising behind the ear (late sign). Signs of open head injury include a visible fracture of the skull through a scalp laceration or a penetrating foreign body to the scalp.

4. Management of Traumatic Brain Injury in the Pre-Hospital Setting

4.1 Airway with Cervical Spine Control

- It is well recognised that airway obstruction and aspiration are significant and often preventable causes of death in patients with severe traumatic brain injury (TBI). Basic airway manoeuvres are essential to prevent primary airway obstruction and associated brain hypoxia. These should be instigated with consideration for protecting the cervical spine, as it is estimated that up to 6.5% of TBIs are complicated by a cervical spine injury. However, there is also strong evidence to suggest that, probably due to compression of the jugular veins of the neck, tightly or poorly fitted rigid cervical spinal immobilisation collars create a detrimental rise in ICP. Such ICP rises should be avoided where possible in TBI. Patients should be immobilised using the methods found elsewhere in these practice guidelines.
- Once standard immobilisation has been achieved, with the head and body secured, consideration should be given to loosening or removing the collar. This is to mitigate the effects of the collar on ICP and may help to reduce agitation. The decision to loosen or remove the collar is in no way a decision to clear the C-spine and the reasons for collar removal should be clearly documented and handed over to the receiving hospital team.
- In addition to maintaining C-spine immobilisation, evidence suggests that placing the patient in a 30° head-up position reduces the effects of a raised ICP in patients with TBI, and this is traditionally employed once the cervical collar is removed in the intensive care unit . The logistical challenges of elevating a patient to 30° while immobilised in the pre-hospital setting probably render this process all but redundant. However, clinicians should remain aware of the effect of positioning, and ensure that the patient's head remains above, or at least level with, the feet throughout extrication and transfer.
- Patients with a severe head injury (GCS 8 or less) or those patients who are unable to maintain their own airway will benefit from advanced airway management and ventilation strategies to reduce secondary brain injury. Consideration should be given to whether an appropriately skilled and trained clinician is available to provide pre-hospital emergency anaesthesia at scene, or with a rendezvous en route to hospital, or whether immediate transfer should take place to hospital. The distance and journey time from an appropriate receiving unit should be considered in line with local procedures and pathways. Advice may be sought via senior advice systems within your employing service. The level of pre-hospital enhanced care available in any one area and at any time of the day is variable. Diverting to a trauma unit should only be for immediate airway compromise that cannot be managed in the pre-hospital setting.

4.2 Breathing and Ventilation

- Adequate ventilation is essential to the management of TBI through the avoidance of hypoxia and maintenance of 'normocapnia'. Numerous studies have demonstrated the correlation between arterial hypoxaemia and poor prognosis following TBI, with some even demonstrating increased mortality of up to 50% following only brief episodes of desaturation. Current evidence suggests that oxygen should initially be administered at 10–15 l/min via a non-rebreathing mask, with a target saturation of 94–98%.
- Evidence also demonstrates that those patients who remain normocapnic (4.6 and 6.0 kPa) following a TBI have significantly better outcomes. Hyperventilation reduces arterial carbon dioxide concentrations, and leads to a consequent vasoconstriction within the cerebral

Head Injury

vasculature, worsening cerebral hypoxia. Hypercapnia, associated with hypoventilation, increases the vasodilatation of the cerebral blood vessels, which increases intracranial volumes and therefore ICP.

4.3 Circulation

- It has been estimated that between 8 and 13% of patients with severe traumatic head injuries are hypotensive either at the scene of the injury or in the ED. In addition, a wealth of evidence demonstrates a strong correlation between hypotension and poor outcome in TBI, with some highlighting that a single episode of hypotension (SBP < 90 mmHg) is independently linked to a double increase in mortality rate.

- MAP is considered to be a better guide to CCP than systolic blood pressure alone, but ICP measurement is required to established the optimum MAP. This leads to the obvious conclusion that effective management of hypotension in the pre-hospital setting improves the outcomes of patients with TBI.

- Haemorrhage control (especially from the highly vascular scalp) should be established early to avoid the unnecessary consumption of coagulation products, and where hypotension is identified intravenous fluid resuscitation should be commenced. Unfortunately, there still remains a lack of clear research evidence to demonstrate the most appropriate fluid for resuscitation in TBI when blood products are unavailable, and in most cases it will be dictated by local service interpretations and current formulary restrictions.

- Patients with significant head injury, hypotension and evidence of other blunt injury should have intravenous fluids titrated to maintain a palpable radial pulse **OR** systolic BP of >90 mmHg. Patients with significant head injury, hypotension and evidence of penetrating injury to the torso should have intravenous fluids titrated to maintain a good volume central pulse **OR** systolic BP >60 mmHg. In patients with evidence of severe TBI but with no other objective signs of injury (i.e. apparent isolated head injury), the therapeutic goal should be to maintain a systolic BP of 110 mmHg. Refer to **Intravascular Fluid Therapy in Adults**.

- Patients with isolated head injury can present with cardiovascular instability due to neurogenic shock. Clinicians should be mindful of this and should have intravenous fluids titrated to maintain a palpable radial pulse OR systolic BP of >110 mmHg.

- NICE Head Injury guidance recommends Tranexamic acid (TXA) is administered as soon as possible to patients of all ages with a GCS of 12 or less. TXA is received on average 62 minutes earlier if given in the pre-hospital setting, highlighting the importance of pre-hospital administration. Refer to **Tranexamic acid**.

4.4 Disability

- The patient's GCS should be calculated, as this can be an important prognostic indicator and is useful for monitoring injury progression over time.

- Pupils should be examined for size, reaction and whether they are equal.

- Acute cerebral herniation, often referred to as 'coning', represents a serious neurosurgical emergency. Clinicians should be vigilant for the following clinical signs in a patient with reduced GCS:
  - Hypertension
  - Bradycardia
  - Unilateral or bilateral pupil dilatation, non-reactive to light.

- Patients demonstrating signs of cerebral herniation require **TIME-CRITICAL** transfer to a neurosurgical centre. Management of cerebral herniation in the pre-hospital setting is challenging. Clinicians should ensure that they are taking all reasonable steps to manage oxygenation, ventilation and circulation/perfusion. Osmotic diuretic fluid therapy (using hypertonic saline) should be considered as a temporising measure in accordance with locally agreed clinical guidelines, and clinicians should consider seeking senior clinical advice and support.

4.5 Exposure/Environment/Extricate

- There is a high incidence of associated injuries found in patients with TBI, and an attempt to identify these during the secondary survey should be made, while remaining aware of the severe impacts of prolonged scene delays.

- Over recent years, there has been a growing interest in the potential benefits of therapeutic hypothermia in TBI, although to date, research has failed to demonstrate any statistical benefit in long-term outcome. The key message therefore is that the patient should be maintained within a 'normothermic' range.

- Time on scene should be kept to a minimum.

4.6 Pain and Agitation

- Agitation in TBI has a number of potential causes. One commonly overlooked cause of agitation in patients with a TBI is pain, either from the head injury itself or from associated injuries sustained at the time of the TBI. Managing pain in TBI poses a challenge for the pre-hospital clinician; a patient in pain will be agitated and more difficult to manage, and may place themselves at risk of further cerebral hypoxia.

- The administration of opiates in severe TBI can be considered but there is a need to be aware of the potential for exaggerated respiratory

Head Injury

depression, hypoventilation, hypercapnia and increased ICP. The decision whether to use opiates in those with a TBI is therefore a clinical one, underpinned by careful assessment and close monitoring for adverse effects.

- Clinicians might consider requesting more senior assistance for patients whose TBI is complicated by agitation associated with acute pain. Midazolam can be considered as an adjunct to help settle an agitated patient (refer to Section 5 below).

4.7 Evacuation Considerations

- The underlying principles of effective pre-hospital management of TBI are rapid assessment; swift and appropriate management; and timely transportation to a receiving centre with sufficient expertise to manage the patient. This will be dependent upon local resources and operational plans for those sustaining significant trauma, but clinicians should consider the most appropriate mode of evacuation early in the incident, to reduce on-scene time as much as possible.

- Helicopter emergency medical services (HEMS) may be able to facilitate more rapid transfer and evacuation but the decision to wait for HEMS arrival should be a balanced decision based on journey time to receiving unit and the need for additional transfer to HEMS at both incident and hospital end.

- A pre-alert call and a detailed clinical handover using ATMIST to the receiving unit is imperative for all patients with a significant TBI.

5. Special Considerations – Head Injuries in the Older Person

- Although significant head injury is a condition seen in the younger generation, a second peak in incidence occurs in those >65 years. Cerebral atrophy due to age means that older people have an increased susceptibility to intracranial haemorrhage following what may be an apparently minor head injury. In addition, older people are at increased risk of intracranial bleeding due to the use of anticoagulants. Older patients may present to healthcare services in an atypical way following a head injury as significant extra or subdural bleeding may occur before the GCS drops and GCS assessment may be complicated in the context of pre-existing cognitive decline. Clinicians should consider and assess for TBI in all older patients who have sustained a traumatic injury.

- Ambulance clinicians should be able to undertake a comprehensive clinical and social assessment of older adults. Symptoms of a head injury can mimic other conditions (e.g. stroke, spinal cord injury, delirium, side effects of anticholinergic medication) and therefore, ambulance clinicians should be vigilant in differentiating between the symptoms caused by a head injury and those stemming from other underlying conditions or medication side effects.

- When assessing older adults with known cognitive impairments (e.g., dementia, Alzheimer's disease) for head injuries, it is crucial to utilise a comprehensive, multi-faceted assessment approach due to their limited ability to recall events. If there is low clinical suspicion of a head injury, based on observable signs and symptoms, and after consultation with caregivers for baseline behaviour comparisons, patients may be discharged on-scene with clear safety netting advice or referred to appropriate community services for follow-up. Ensure that the decision-making process for discharge or referral is documented, including the rationale and any advice given to caregivers or patients.

- Patients on anticoagulants and/or antiplatelets (other than aspirin monotherapy) attending the ED will be considered for a CT scan even if they have no other risk factors.

- Patients who are prescribed dual antiplatelet therapy (e.g. aspirin and clopidogrel) should be transported to an ED.

- The risk of intracranial bleeding in patients prescribed anticoagulants and antiplatelets (other than aspirin monotherapy) who do not have any other head injury symptoms is low but important. Ambulance clinicians should avoid basing the decision for ED referral solely on the anticipation of a head CT scan. The decision as to whether current anticoagultants will need to be paused must also be considered. In situations of uncertainty, immediately seek senior clinical advice to evaluate the necessity of ED attendance. This decision should involve the patient, clearly communicate potential risks, and align with the patient's health priorities and best interests.

- Clinical frailty is a multidimensional syndrome that describes a patient's physiological reserve to cope with everyday life and stressors and better reflects their status rather than their chronological age. When assessing an older adult with a head injury, their **Clinical Frailty** should be assessed, and consider transport of patients with a CFS >4 who have a head injury to the ED as these patients are at an increased risk of a worse outcome. Where patients are assessed as being very frail or end of life, ambulance clinicians should individually consider patients with advanced care and ReSPECT plans.

6. Midazolam in Traumatic Brain Injury

- Patients with TBI can pose a challenge for management in the pre-hospital setting, and any associated hypoxia, hypercapnia and intracranial

Head Injury

hypertension can contribute significantly to a poorer prognosis. Although not robust, the evidence suggests that the therapeutic benefits of midazolam for these patients can include amnesia, anxiolysis and, most critically, an ability to effectively provide oxygenation and ventilation, which may help reduce the detrimental secondary brain injury they incur. However, sedating agents will reduce systemic blood pressure, leading to a decrease in CPP, in addition to further jeopardising the patient's airway. Therefore, the decision to use midazolam to facilitate safe patient management needs to be carefully considered. Such interventions should only be undertaken after additional training and confirmation of ability to deal with the complications of midazolam use. Remember – Midazolam is a sedating agent with an unpredictable dose response relationship in a head-injured patient and may cause a patient to rapidly become deeply sedated requiring immediate enhanced care intervention. Any practitioner considering the use of midazolam in head injuries should be specifically trained in and capable of undertaking the additional interventions required or consideration should be given to calling enhanced critical care.

7. Assessment and Management of Mild to Moderate Head Injury

- Ambulance clinicians need to consider early detection and treatment of life-threatening brain injury, where present, but also be able to safely discharge patients with negligible risk of brain injury. Ninety-five percent of people who have sustained a head injury present with a normal or minimally impaired conscious level (GCS greater than 12).

- Additional care should be taken when assessing children, older people and other patient groups such as those with dementia, underlying chronic neurological disorders or learning disabilities. These can be more difficult to accurately assess and have a higher rate of additional and non-accidental injuries. In some patients, the pre-injury baseline GCS may be less than 15. Establish this where possible, and take it into account during assessment. History-taking must include assessment of medications (e.g. anticoagulants and antiplatelets) and other factors that either place the patient at higher risk of serious underlying injury or may suggest that the patient cannot be safely discharged at the scene.

- The following guidance is written to highlight key features of head injuries that require hospital attendance and those patients who can be safely cared for in the community. The list is not exhaustive – a holistic assessment of the patient, mechanism of injury, symptoms, observations and the scene in general must be made and combined with patient's priorities and wishes. Where any doubt exists regarding the suitability of a patient for discharge, they should be referred to the emergency department.

- Patients discharged from hospital will need to have suitable supervision arrangements at home to identify any changes which require further investigation. Ensure that any pertinent information regarding the home environment is passed on to the receiving hospital.

TABLE 4.17 – Conveyance Decision Tool

Red criteria

Refer to the local major trauma triage tool and consider the need for immediate transfer to a major trauma centre and/or for a pre-alert call.

Immediately transport to hospital if any one of the following is found:

- GCS score of less than 15 on initial assessment.
- Any loss of consciousness as a result of the injury.
- Any focal neurological deficit since the injury.
- Any suspicion of a skull fracture or penetrating head injury since the injury.
- Amnesia for events before or after the injury.
- Persistent headache since the injury.
- Any vomiting episodes since the injury (clinical judgement should be used regarding the cause of vomiting in those aged 12 years or younger and the need for referral).
- Any seizure since the injury.
- Any previous brain surgery.
- A high-energy head injury.
- Any history of bleeding or clotting disorders.

Head Injury

> **TABLE 4.17** – Conveyance Decision Tool *(continued)*
>
> - Current anticoagulant or antiplatelet therapy (except aspirin monotherapy).
> - Current drug or alcohol intoxication.
> - Any safeguarding concerns (for example, possible non-accidental injury or a vulnerable person is affected).
> - Continuing concern by the ambulance clinician about the diagnosis.
> - Irritability or altered behaviour, particularly in infants and children aged under five years.
> - No visible trauma to the head but still of concern to the clinician.
> - No one is able to observe the injured person at home.
> - Continuing concern by the injured person or their family or carer about the diagnosis.
>
> **Green criteria**
>
> Consider discharge where all of the following can be met:
>
> - No Red criteria are identified.
> - Able to appropriately safety-net the patient in the community with suitable supervision arrangements. If the patient has no carer at home or lives alone, only discharge them if suitable supervision arrangements have been organised (e.g. arranging for a relative, friend or neighbour to visit regularly) or when the risk of late complications is deemed negligible.
> - Verbal and written advice can be given to the patient and those supervising.
> - Patient, carers and clinician have no ongoing concerns.

Additional considerations

Patients currently undergoing anticoagulant therapy should be assessed in hospital. Common anticoagulants include:

- Warfarin
- Rivaroxaban
- Apixaban
- Dabigatran
- Edoxaban
- Heparin
- Dalteparin
- Enoxaparin
- Tinzaparin

Patients undergoing anti-platelet therapy require assessment in hospital unless they are on Aspirin monotherapy and no other criteria for hospital assessment are present and they fulfil the green criteria above. Common anti-platelets include:

- Clopidogrel
- Ticagrelor
- Prasugrel
- Dipyridamole

7.1 Discharge at the Scene

- Not all patients who have sustained a head injury will require further assessment in a hospital. Where no red features are present and where all green conditions can be met, patients may be discharged from the scene.
- Complications from head injuries can develop over a number of hours or days, and as such any decision to discharge a patient from the scene needs to be supported by appropriate safety-netting. At a minimum this should include a period of time, for example up to 24 hours, in which the patient can be supervised by a suitable adult who is able to call for help should there be any deterioration. Verbal and written advice that is age appropriate should be given in line with NICE Guideline NG232 (2023) (see Head injury and concussion – NHS). Guidance should refer, at a minimum, to any potential for a developing head injury that would require further assessment, common symptoms that do not require further treatment and guidance around what the patient can or cannot do while recovering from the injury.

Head Injury

Assessment

C - Catastrophic haemorrhage
manage catastrophic haemorrhage (see management of catastrophic haemorrhage algorithm)

A - Airway and C-Spine
Establish current or impending airway loss. Consider C-Spine status

B - Breathing
Assess rate, pattern and effectiveness of respiration. Obtain oxygen saturations and CRT

C - Circulation
Assess pulse rate, rhythm and volume. Assess BP. Confirm control of significant haemorrhage

D - Disability
Assess GCS.
Measure temperature and blood glucose.
Identify associated injuries taking account of mechanism and injury patterns.
Check pupil reaction

Evacuation considerations

Management

- See guidelines for management of catastrophic haemorrhage

- Establish and maintain a patent airway
- Protect cervical spine to prevent secondary spinal cord injury

- Maintain O_2 saturations with supplemental O_2 as required **(See target values)**
- Instigate capnographic monitoring if available
- Avoid hyper / hypoventilation of mechanically ventilated patients **(See target values)**

- Instigate and maintain haemorrhage control
- Avoid any episodes of unmanaged hypotension **(See target values)**
- Obtain IV access
- Adult: use 250ml boluses of selected fluid to ensure BP remains in target range **(See target values)**
- Children: avoid hypotension (see age specific systolic BP targets)
- Avoid excessive dilution of clotting factors through excessive fluid

- Administer Tranexamic acid if GCS is 12 or less - see Tranexamic acid
- Cover patients to prevent heat loss during extrication and evacuation
- Avoid using cool or cold infusions
- Correct abnormalities of blood glucose
- Manage pain in accordance with local or national guidelines
- Monitor level of consciousness and be prepared for impending management challenges in those with a diminishing GCS
- Treat seizures according to established JRCALC guidelines

- If meets local trauma bypass criteria transfer to Major Trauma Centre
- Monitor for deterioration Consider 30° head up tilt
- Early pre-alert call to receiving unit

Treatment goals (adults):
SpO_2: >94%
Blunt trauma: systolic BP >90 mmHg
Penetrating torso trauma: systolic BP >60 mmHg
Severe TBI: systolic BP >110 mmHg
$ETCO_2$: 35-40 mmHg, kPa 4.6-6.0

Treatment goals (children):
SpO_2: 95%
$ETCO_2$: 35-40 mmHg, kPa 4.6-6.0
Blood Pressure: see age-specific systolic BP targets

Age-specific systolic Blood Pressure targets (children)	
< 1 year	>80 mmHg
1-5 years	>90 mmHg
5-14 years	>100 mmHg
>14 years	>110 mmHg

Figure 4.12 – Assessment and management of head injury.

Head Injury

Bibliography

1. National Institute for Health and Clinical Excellence. *Head Injury: Assessment and early management.* London: NICE, 2023. Available from: https://www.nice.org.uk/guidance/ng232.

2. Bayless P, Ray VG. Incidence of cervical spine injuries in association with blunt head trauma. *Am J Emerg Med* 1989, 7: 139–142.

3. Boer C, Franschman G, Loer S. Prehospital management of severe traumatic brain injury: conecpts and ongoing controversies. *Curr Opin Anesthesio* l 2012, 25: 556–562.

4. Chestnut R, Marshall L, Klauber M et al. Early and late systemic hypotension as a frequent and fundamental source of cerebral ischaemia following severe brain injry in the Traumatic Coma Data Bank. *Acta Neurochir Suppl* 1993, 59: 121–1253.

5. Clifton G, Valadka A, Zygun D et al. Very early hypothermia induction in patients with severe brain injury (The National Acute Brain Injury Study: hypothermia II): a randomized trial. *Lancet Neurol* 2011, 10: 131–139.

6. Dubick MA, Shek P, Wade CE. ROC trials update on prehospital hypertonic saline resuscitation in the aftermath of the US-Canadian trials. *Clinics* 2013, 68(6): 883–886.

7. Dumont T, Visioni A, Rughani A et al. Inappropriate pre-hospital ventilation in severe traumatic injuries increases in-hospital mortality. *J Neurotrauma* 27: 1223–1241

8. Ferguson J, Mardel SN, Beattie TF, Wytch R. Cervical collars: a potential risk to the head-injured patient. *Injury* 1993, 24(7): 454–456.

9. Flanagan S, Hibbard M, Riordan B. Traumatic Brain Injury in the Elderly: Diagnostic and Treatment Challenges. Clin Geriatr Med 2006, 22: 449–468.

10. Gu J, Yang T, Kuang Y et al. Comparison of the safety and efficacy of propofol with midazolam for sedation of patients with severe traumatic brain injury: A meta-analysis. *Journal of Critical Care* 2014, 29: 287–290.

11. Ho AM, Fung KY, Joynt GM, Karmakar MK, Peng Z. Rigid cervical collar and intracranial pressure of patients with severe head injury. *J Trauma* 2002, 53: 1185–1188.

12. Holly LT, Kelly DF, Counelis GJ, Blinman T, McArthur DL, Cryer HG. Cervical spine trauma associated with moderate and severe head injury: Incidence, risk factors, and injury characteristics. *J Neurosurg* 2002, 96 (Suppl 3): 285–291.

13. Hunt K, Hallworth S, Smith M. The effects of rigid collar placement on intracranial and cerebral perfusion pressures. *Anaesthesia* 2001, 56: 511–513.

14. Langlois JA, Kegler SR, Butler JA, et al. Traumatic brain injury-related hospital discharges: results from a 14-state surveillance system, 1997. MMWR CDC Surveill Summ 2003, 52: 1–20.

15. Ng I, Lim J, Wong H. Effects of head posture on cerebral hemodynamics: its influences on intracranial pressure, cerebral perfusion pressure, and cerebral oxygenation. Neurosurgery 2004, 54(3): 593–597.

16. O'Driscoll B, Howard L, Davison A (On behalf of the British Thoracic Society Emergency Oxygen Guideline Development Group). Guidelines for Emergency Oxygen Use in Adult Patients. *Thorax* 2008, 63 (Suppl VI). DOI: 10.1136/thx.2008.102947.

17. Peterson K, Carson S, Carney N. Hypothermia treatment for traumatic brain injury: a systematic review and meta-analysis. *J Neurotrauma* 2008, 25: 62–71.

18. Piatt JH Jr Detected and overlooked cervical spine injury among comatose trauma patients: from the Pennsylvania trauma outcomes study. *Neurosurg Focus* 2005, 19: E6.

19. Piek J, Chesnut R, Marshall L et al. Extracranial complications of severe head injury. *J Neurosurg* 1992, 77: 901–907.

20. Stiver S, Manley G. Prehospital management of traumatic brain injury. *Neurosurg Focus* 2008, 25(4): E5.

21. Stocchetti N, Furlan A, Volta F. Hypoxemia and arterial hypotension at the accident scene in head injury. *J Trauma* 1996, 40: 764–767.

22. Tian HL, Guo Y, Hu J, Rong BY, Wang G, Gao WW, et al. Clinical characterization of comatose patients with cervical spine injury and traumatic brain injury. *J Trauma* 2009, 67: 1305–1310.

23. Trunkey D. Towards optimal trauma care. *Arch Emerg Med* 1985, 2: 181–195.

24. Urwin SC, Menon DK. Comparative tolerability of sedative agents in head-injured adults. *Drug Saf* 2004, 27: 107–133.

25. Carney N, Totten AM, O'reilly C, Ullman JS et. al. Brain Trauma Guidelines: Guidelines for the Management of Severe Traumatic Brain Injury, Fourth Edition. *Neurosurgery* 2016, 80(1).

26. Wilson MH, Hinds J, Grier G, Burns B, Carley S, and Davies G. Impact brain apnoea—A forgotten cause of cardiovascular collapse in trauma. *Resuscitation* 2016, 105: 52–58.

27. Pandrich, M. J., & Demetriades, A. K. (2020). Prevalence of concomitant traumatic cranio-spinal injury: a systematic review and meta-analysis. *Neurosurgical review*, 43(1), 69–77.

28. Pandrich, M. J., & Demetriades, A. K. (2020). Prevalence of concomitant traumatic cranio-spinal injury: a systematic review and meta-analysis. *Neurosurgical review*, 43(1), 69–77.

29. Coats TJ, Fragoso-Iñiguez M, Roberts I. Implementation of tranexamic acid for bleeding trauma patients: a longitudinal and cross-sectional study. *Emergency Medicine Journal* 2019; 36: 78–81. doi:10.1136/emermed-2018-207693

30. Santing, J. A., Lee, Y. X., van der Naalt, J., van den Brand, C. L., & Jellema, K. (2022). Mild traumatic brain injury in elderly patients receiving direct oral anticoagulants: a systematic review and meta-analysis. *Journal of Neurotrauma*, 39(7–8), 458–472.

31. Fuller, G., Sabir, L., Evans, R., Bradbury, D., Kuczawski, M., & Mason, S. M. (2020). Risk of significant traumatic brain injury in adults with minor head injury taking direct oral anticoagulants: a cohort study and updated meta-analysis. *Emergency medicine journal*, 37(11), 666–673.

32. Moffatt, S., Venturini, S., & Vulliamy, P. (2023). Does pre-injury clopidogrel use increase the risk of intracranial haemorrhage post head injury in adult patients? A systematic review and meta-analysis. *Emergency Medicine Journal*, 40(3), 175–181.

33. Mathieu, F., Malhotra, A. K., Ku, J. C., Zeiler, F. A., Wilson, J. R., Pirouzmand, F., & Scales, D. C. (2022). Pre-injury antiplatelet therapy and risk of adverse outcomes

Head Injury

after traumatic brain injury: a systematic review and meta-analysis. *Neurotrauma Reports*, 3(1), 308–320.

34. van den Brand, C. L., Tolido, T., Rambach, A. H., Hunink, M. G., Patka, P., & Jellema, K. (2017). Systematic review and meta-analysis: is pre-injury antiplatelet therapy associated with traumatic intracranial hemorrhage?. *Journal of neurotrauma*, 34(1), 1–7.

35. Galimberti, S., Graziano, F., Maas, A. I., Isernia, G., Lecky, F., Jain, S., ... & Otesile, O. (2022). Effect of frailty on 6-month outcome after traumatic brain injury: a multicentre cohort study with external validation. *The Lancet Neurology*, 21(2), 153–162.

36. Pandrich, M. J., & Demetriades, A. K. (2020). Prevalence of concomitant traumatic cranio-spinal injury: a systematic review and meta-analysis. *Neurosurgical review*, 43(1), 69–77.

37. Spaite, D. W., Hu, C., Bobrow, B. J., Chikani, V., Barnhart, B., Gaither, J. B., Denninghoff, K. R., Adelson, P. D., Keim, S. M., Viscusi, C., Mul-lins, T., & Sherrill, D. (2017). The Effect of Combined Out-of-Hospital Hypotension and Hypoxia on Mortality in Major Traumatic Brain Injury. *Annals of emergency medicine*, 69(1), 62–72. https://doi.org/10.1016/j.annemergmed.2016.08.007

38. Blanchard, I. E., Ahmad, A., Tang, K. L., Ronksley, P. E., Lorenzetti, D., Lazarenko, G., ... & Stelfox, H. T. (2017). The effectiveness of pre-hospital hypertonic saline for hypotensive trauma patients: a systematic review and meta-analysis. *BMC emergency medicine*, 17(1), 1–13.

39. Nunez-Patino, R. A., Rubiano, A. M., & Godoy, D. A. (2020). Impact of cervical collars on intracranial pressure values in traumatic brain injury: a systematic review and meta-analysis of prospective studies. *Neurocritical care*, 32, 469–477.

40. O'Driscoll BR, Howard LS, Earis J on behalf of the British Thoracic Society Emergency Oxygen Guideline Group, et al BTS guideline for oxygen use in adults in healthcare and emergency settings. Thorax 2017; 72: ii1–ii90.

41. Wu, X., Tao, Y., Marsons, L., Dee, P., Yu, D., Guan, Y., & Zhou, X. (2021). The effectiveness of early prophylactic hypothermia in adult patients with traumatic brain injury: A systematic review and meta-analysis. *Australian Critical Care*, 34(1), 83–91.

42. Shekhar, C., Gupta, L., Premsagar, I., Sinha, M., Kishore, J., Kamal, V., ... & Tung, P. (2019). Extracranial complications of traumatic brain injury: Pathophysiology—A review. *Journal of Neuroanaesthesiology and Critical Care*, 6(03), 200–212.

43. Lulla, A., Lumba-Brown, A., Totten, A. M., Maher, P. J., Badjatia, N., Bell, R., ... & Bobrow, B. J. (2023). Prehospital Guidelines for the Management of Traumatic Brain Injury–3rd Edition. *Prehospital Emergency Care*, 1–32.

Limb Trauma

1. Introduction

- There is one fundamental rule to apply to limb trauma cases and that is NOT to allow limb injuries, however dramatic in appearance, distract the clinician from less visible but potentially life-threatening problems, such as airway obstruction, compromised breathing, poor perfusion or spinal injury.
- Patients with limb trauma are likely to be in considerable pain and distress; consider pain management as soon as clinically possible (refer to **Pain Management in Adults and Children**).

2. Pathophysiology

- A fracture is an injury which involves the bony skeleton. The pathophysiology and potential for complications differs depending on the mechanism and type of injury (refer to Table 4.18).
- Blood loss from femoral shaft fractures can be considerable, involving loss of 500–2000 millilitres in volume. If the fracture is open, blood loss is increased.
- Nerves and blood vessels are at risk from sharp bony fragments, especially in very displaced fractures and dislocations, hence the need to return fractured and/or dislocated limbs to normal alignment as soon as possible. Fractures around the elbow and knee are especially likely to injure arteries, veins and nerves.
- The patella, a sesamoid bone that forms part of the anterior mechanism of the knee, sits in a vertical groove in front of the femoral and tibial bones called the trochlear groove. It protects the underlying femoral-tibial joint.
- The six 'P's of ischaemia are shown in Table 4.19.

TABLE 4.18 – Types of Limb Injury

There are several types of fracture (open & closed). Emphasis should be placed on identifying displaced (out of alignment) fractures which may require manipulation and non-displaced fractures (see Table 4.21).

Closed fracture

A fracture that is contained, the skin over the site of injury is unbroken.

Open fracture

Any fracture with an associated open wound.

The bone may protrude through an open wound, or fragments of bone may have broken through the skin but subsequently have been covered over by skin/soft tissues due to recoil.

Open fractures present a risk of significant haemorrhage, and risk of infection

Dislocation

Where the articular surfaces of the joint are not in continuity. Dislocation can affect the digits, wrist, elbow, shoulder, patella, knee, ankle, foot and occasionally the hip.

Patella Dislocation

Dislocation is usually lateral but can be superior, inferior or medial

In rare cases the patella can rotate around so it appears 'flipped over' and instead of looking flat under the skin as it does in a simple lateral dislocation, the patella appears like a 'dorsal fin' protruding sharply.

Compartment syndrome

A complication of limb fractures arising from increased pressure in closed osseofascial (muscle) compartments due to contained haemorrhage or oedema. This can lead to distal limb ischaemia with potentially catastrophic consequences for the limb.

Degloving

Traumatic injury (with or without underlying fractures) where layers of skin and underlying soft tissue are torn away from underlying structures by shearing forces. Degloving can be to the superficial fascia, partial depth into deeper soft tissues or full depth down to the bone.

Amputations/partial amputations

Amputations most frequently involve digits but can involve part or whole limbs. Partial amputations may still result in a viable limb, providing there is minimal crushing damage and survival of some vascular and nerve structures.

(continued)

Limb Trauma

TABLE 4.18 – Types of Limb Injury *(continued)*

Neck of femur/hip fractures

Fracture through the femoral neck, between the femoral shaft and femoral head.

Hip fractures occur more commonly in older people and are one of the most common limb injuries encountered in pre-hospital care. Patients often present with shortening and external rotation of the leg on the injured side, with pain in the hip and, sometimes, referred pain in the knee. Although shortening and rotation are a common sign, these are not always present. The circumstances of the injury must be considered – often the older person has been on the floor for some time, which increases the possibility of hypothermia, dehydration, pressure ulcers and chest infection, so careful monitoring of vital signs is essential (refer to **Falls in Older Adults**).

Patients (particularly older patients) with hip pain and the inability to weight bear to the extent they could prior to a fall should be considered as having a hip (or pubic ramus) fracture.

TABLE 4.19 – Six 'P's of Ischaemia

These signs and symptoms may indicate an ischaemic limb through injury or the development of compartment syndrome.

SIGN		SYMPTOM
Common	Pallor	Due to compromised blood flow to limb. Limb can appear pale, dusky or mottled (especially in children).
	Paraesthesia	Changes in sensation where there is pressure on the nerve.
	Pain	Out of proportion to the apparent injury; often in the muscle and with the slightest movement, which may not ease with splinting/analgesia.
Uncommon/ Late Signs	Paralysis	Loss of active movement.
	Pulselessness	The loss of peripheral pulses is a grave late sign caused by swelling, blood vessel rupture or occlusion, which can lead to the complete occlusion of circulation.
	Perishing cold	The limb is distally cold to the touch.

3. Incidence

- Limb trauma is a common injury in high energy impacts. Causes can be relatively simple and include but are not limited to; falls, sports incidents, road traffic collisions, occupational or intentional causes (assault, self-harm), and can occur at any age.
- In certain patient groups (e.g. frail, older or bariatric patients) injuries can occur from relatively minor trauma (e.g. falls from a standing height can lead to femoral fractures).
- Patellar dislocations are often caused by low energy mechanisms and more frequently affect children and adolescents. Lateral patella dislocation is usually caused by sports injuries with a lateral force applied to the patella or external tibial torsion which often occurs when the affected limb is planted.

4. Severity and Outcome

- Severity and outcome differ depending on the nature of the injury. However, limb trauma can have serious consequences; for example, infection following an open fracture can affect the future viability and long-term function of the limb.

4.1 Limb threatening injurues

- Limb trauma can be life and limb threatening, i.e., if not managed promptly and appropriately, there is increased risk of long term complications (e.g. loss of function or amputation), permanent limb damage and systemic effects on the patient.

Limb Trauma

- Features of limb threatening injury include:
  - Severe pain (even with analgesia)
  - Loss of pulses distal to injury and/or significantly delayed capillary refill (can be a late sign)
  - Impaired neurology
  - Critical skin: tension skin over the site of injury. Pale, white, discoloured, or blanching skin
  - Risk of a closed fracture becoming an open fracture
  - Significant haemorrhage in the presence of open fractures, amputation and/or degloving injury

4.2 Knee dislocation

- Knee dislocation often involves a large force (e.g. RTC) which moves the tibia relative to the femur and out of its normal position. This is always accompanied by rupture of the ligaments holding the joint in place.
- The knee may remain displaced or may return to its original position. Both are termed a knee dislocation, and both cause limb instability and many cause neurovascular damage. Long term consequences and/or osteoarthritis are likely.
- Knee dislocation can include fractures, and commonly have vascular injury.

4.3 Splinting

Splinting of the affected limb will contribute to 'circulation' care by reducing further blood loss and pain during extrication and transfer to hospital. A variety of different methods are available, depending on the injury site – see Table 4.20.

- Traction splint – a device for applying longitudinal traction to the femur, using the pelvis and the ankle as static points. Correct splintage technique using a traction splint reduces:
  - pain
  - further or neurovascular damage
  - bone fragment movement and the risk of a closed fracture becoming an open fracture
  - the risk of fat embolus
  - muscle spasm by pulling the thigh to a natural cylindrical shape
  - blood loss by compression of bleeding sites.
- Manufacturers' and Trust specific guidelines should be followed when applying traction splints
- If using vacuum splints, ensure that adequate immobilisation is achieved and maintained throughout transfer

TABLE 4.20 – Splinting

INJURY	SPLINTAGE TYPE
Fractured neck of femur	Padding between legs. Figure-of-eight bandage around ankles. Broad bandage: two above, two below the knee.
Fractured shaft of femur (open and closed)	Traction splint. **NB** Fractures of the ankle, tibia, fibula, knee or pelvis on the same side as the femoral fracture may limit use of a traction splint; Trust guidelines should be followed.
Fracture or fracture dislocation around the knee	Without reduction – vacuum splint the limb in the presenting position without causing further pain, avoiding putting pressure on protruding areas and blood vessels. Following reduction – vacuum splint the limb as straight as possible. Traction splint for straight limbs but without the application of traction.
Patella dislocation	Without reduction – vacuum splint the limb in the most comfortable position. Consider support on pillow (under the knee and thigh). If the patella has relocated – vacuum splint the limb in a straight position. Do not allow the patient to bend their knee or weight bear.
Tibia/fibula shaft fracture / Ankle fracture / Foot fracture	Moulded splint (e.g. vacuum splint or similar mouldable device). Box splint (in the absence of mouldable splint)
Clavicle / Humerus / Radius / Ulna	Self-splintage may be adequate and less painful than a sling. Broad-arm sling. Vacuum splints may be well suited to immobilising forearm fractures.

Limb Trauma

5. Crush Injury and Crush Syndrome

- Crush injury is a term used to describe the injury directly resulting from crushing of a limb and crush syndrome. It relates to the systemic manifestation of muscle cell damage resulting from pressure or crushing. Crush syndrome is relatively rare in the UK and the severity of the condition is related to the degree of force, duration of crush and bulk of tissue/muscle affected. Clinicians should be aware of the risks of crush syndrome in less obvious patient groups such as older or bariatric patients who fall and have a prolonged lie in the same position.

- Crush injuries without the risk of crush syndrome should be managed in accordance with the guidance for the injury as it presents: haemorrhage controlled, wounds dressed and fractures splinted. Intravenous fluid should only be administered if the patient is hypotensive (refer to **Intravascular Fluid Therapy in Adults** and **Intravascular Fluid Therapy in Children**).

- Crush syndrome occurs as a result of traumatic rhabdomyolysis (muscle breakdown) and leads to kidney injury. Metabolic acidosis combined with the release of nephrotoxic substances (myoglobin, urate and phosphate) can lead to the development of shock, cardiac arrhythmias and kidney injury. Early treatment reduces the risk of complications.

6. Assessment and Management

For the assessment and management of limb trauma, refer to Table 4.21.

TABLE 4.21 – ASSESSMENT and MANAGEMENT of: Limb Trauma

Assess <C>ABCDE

- Control any external catastrophic haemorrhage (refer to **Trauma Emergencies in Adults – Overview**).
- If any of the following **TIME-CRITICAL** features are present:
  - major **<C>ABC** complications
  - haemodynamic compromise/shocked (refer to **Intravascular Fluid Therapy in Adults**)
  - altered level of consciousness (refer to **Altered Level of Consciousness**)
  - neck and back injuries (refer to **Spinal Injury and Spinal Cord Injury**)
  - limb threatening injury – loss of neurovascular function (e.g. resulting from a dislocation that requires prompt realignment), then:
- Correct **<C>ABC** complications.
- Mid-shaft femoral fracture (open and closed) – give appropriate analgesia and then apply traction. Initial traction can be manual where sufficient personnel are available, but this should be changed to a traction splint at the earliest opportunity and always prior to transport.
- Threatened limb – where it is possible to do so, give appropriate analgesia then re-align the fracture/dislocation and splint the limb in its anatomical position with the aim of improving neurovascular function. The decision to do this must be based on the capability of the clinician and the degree of limb compromise. Delays on scene due to repeated unsuccessful attempts to reduce a fracture must be avoided.
- Refer to major trauma tool and where appropriate undertake a **TIME-CRITICAL** transfer to a major trauma centre. Provide a pre-alert using ATMIST.
- If the patient needs an immediate lifesaving intervention, transfer to nearest trauma unit.

Continue patient management en route.

Specifically Assess

- Determine the mechanism of injury and any factors indicating the forces involved (the pattern of fractures may indicate mechanism of injury):
  - fractures of the heel (calcaneum) in a fall from a height may be accompanied by pelvic and spinal crush fractures (refer to **Pelvic Trauma** and **Spinal Injury and Spinal Cord Injury**)
  - 'dashboard' injury to the knee may be accompanied by a fracture or dislocation of the hip
  - humeral fractures from a side impact are associated with chest injuries (refer to **Thoracic Trauma**)
  - tibial fractures are rarely isolated injuries and are often associated with high energy trauma and other life-threatening injuries.
- Assess all four limbs for injury to long bones and joints – in suspected fracture, expose limbs to fully assess swelling and deformity.

Limb Trauma

TABLE 4.21 – ASSESSMENT and MANAGEMENT of: Limb Trauma (continued)

- Assess neurovascular function of affected limb – motor, sensation and circulation, distal to the fracture site. Compare to unaffected site, if possible.
  - Assess pulses distal to injury (e.g. in leg injury, palpate dorsalis pedis pulse, in arm injury palpate radial pulse as capillary refill time can be misleading)
- Monitor vital signs.
- Assess general skin colour.
- Consider age of patient – consider greenstick fractures in children.
- Consider accompanying illnesses:
  - some cancers can spread to bones and result in pathological fractures (e.g. breast, lung, kidney, thyroid and prostate) from relatively minor or no apparent injuries
  - osteoporosis in older adults increases the risk of fractures.

Oxygen

- Administer high levels of supplemental oxygen (aim for SpO_2 94–98%) (refer to **Oxygen**).

Splintage

In pre-hospital care it is difficult to differentiate between ligament sprain and a fracture; ASSUME a fracture and immobilise.

- Where possible, remove jewellery from the affected limbs before swelling occurs, and document this.
- Check and document the presence/absence of pulses, motor, sensation and circulation distal to injury.
- Apply appropriate splintage (refer to Table 4.20).
- After any intervention, re-check and document the presence/absence of pulses, motor, sensation and circulation distal to the injury.

Fracture reduction

- If there is neurovascular compromise distal to the injury, or significant displacement of the injured limb, the limb may need to be reduced to improve circulation.
- Consider availability of enhanced care for additional analgesia, but do not delay on scene in time-critical patients.
- Refer to **Pain Management in Adults and Children**.
- Limb injuries and fractures involving joints (e.g. ankle, hip, shoulder) should not routinely be reduced in the pre-hospital environment without enhanced or specialist care.
- Only reduce displaced ankle fractures where there is clear neurovascular compromise or compromise of the overlying skin.
- The aim of fracture reduction is to return the limb to normal alignment and reduce tension/pressure on the overlying skin.
- Where deformity is minor and both distal sensation and circulation are intact, then realignment is not necessary before hospital.
- Document and record the fracture and position of the limb prior to re-alignment.

Fracture reduction procedure (long bones)

- Apply gentle but firm traction distal to the injury, whilst applying counter traction proximal to the injury.
- Re-assess and document the neurovascular status
  - Neurovascular status worse: return limb to original position and splint
  - Neurovascular status improved: apply appropriate splint

Fracture reduction of the ankle

- Deformed fracture/dislocation of the ankle is usually associated with fracture/ dislocation of the distal tibia/fibula and can be a complex injury.
- Reduction of these injuries will require significant analgesia and/or sedation.
- Indications to attempt ankle manipulation are:
  - Signs of vascular impairment (absent or very weak distal pulse, significantly prolonged capillary refill)
  - Impaired neurology
  - Critical skin over the fracture site (blanching or discolouration)
- The primary objective is to sufficiently reduce skin tension or restore bloody supply.

(continued)

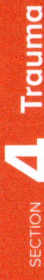

Limb Trauma

TABLE 4.21 – ASSESSMENT and MANAGEMENT of: Limb Trauma *(continued)*

Dislocation reduction
- In all cases, assess the mechanism of injury and any factors involved. It must be an acute injury to consider relocation.

Knee dislocation
- If grossly deformed with clear neurovascular compromise, then the limb should be reduced to as normal anatomical alignment as possible. Apply longitudinal traction and move the tibia relative to the femur.
- If there is a dimpling or 'pinching in' of the skin do not attempt reduction, due to likely involvement of soft tissues.

Patella dislocation and reduction
- The patient often describes a popping sensation followed by the knee giving way and the knee is often presented in some flexion with the patella clearly displaced laterally.
- Consider history, including:
  - age and general health
  - connective tissue disorders and hypermobile limbs
  - family history of dislocation
  - skeletal immaturity
  - previous dislocations and management
  - previous limb surgery including scars
  - previous limb instability
  - limb conditions such as patella alta (high-riding patella).
- Assess distal neurovascular function.
- Medial pain indicates damage to medial patello-femoral ligament (MPFL) which is one of the main stabilisers of the patella. Medial pain will likely prevent other examination of the knee from being performed.
- If there are likely to be any associated fractures or injuries: do not attempt a reduction.
- A simple, lateral dislocation is indicated by patella clearly visible laterally (outside the trochlear groove and an indentation where the patella should be).

Pain relief – (refer to Pain Management in Adults and Children guidelines)
- Treat pain early as it increases the chance of a successful relocation.
- Administer Entonox (or Penthrox where available) as a preference when relocation is to be attempted over morphine, as successful relocation itself is likely to significantly reduce the pain.
- Opioids can increase hospital stay, however if the patient is unable to get sufficient analgesia with Nitrous oxide or Penthrox, even when coached, then consider morphine and/or sedation. Consider enhanced/critical care involvement.
- Opioids and/or sedation are more likely to be needed if some time has passed since injury.
- Consider access to enhanced care for sedation/analgesia.
- If relocation is not going to be attempted or is unsuccessful then consider opioids early in the process.
- Keep the patient warm as cold is likely to induce shivers which can contract the muscles and increase the pain, reducing the likelihood of successful reduction.

Relocation
- Laterally displaced patellae should be relocated if possible to prevent hypoperfusion and further soft tissue damage. Time from injury to relocation has an impact on likelihood of relocation.
- One attempt to relocate a simple, lateral non-rotated patella dislocation with a clear mechanism of injury without suspicion of an underlying fracture may be attempted if the clinician is confident.

Limb Trauma

TABLE 4.21 – ASSESSMENT and MANAGEMENT of: Limb Trauma *(continued)*

- With the patient lying as flat as possible in a supine position (or seated if supine is not possible), the leg should be fully straightened out by gently lifting the foot and ankle up, without applying excessive force.
- If it does not spontaneously relocate on straightening the limb, with gentle anteromedial pressure applied from the lateral side to manoeuvre the patella back over to the anterior of the knee.
- If successful, it will appear to 'pop' back into position. On occasion the patella is stuck and will not move. Do not force it.
- Check distal neurovascular status after relocation.
- Splintage – see Table 4.20.
- All patients with patella dislocation should be conveyed to hospital for review and follow up.

Open Fracture
- Gross contamination can be removed from wounds but do not irrigate open fractures of the long bones, hindfoot or midfoot in pre-hospital settings.
- Consider taking photographs prior to applying dressings according to local policies.
- Where possible, apply a saline-soaked dressing and cover with an occlusive layer (e.g. transparent occlusive film, sterile field from blast dressing).
- Any gross displacement from normal alignment must, where possible, be corrected, and splints applied (refer to Table 4.20).

NB Document the nature of the contamination, as contamination may be drawn inside following realignment.

Amputations, partial amputations and degloving
- Do not irrigate grossly contaminated wounds.
- Immobilise a partially amputated limb in a position of normal anatomical alignment.
- Where possible dress the injured limb to prevent further contamination.
- Apply a saline-soaked dressing covered with an occlusive layer.

NB Reimplantation following amputation or reconstruction following partial amputation may be possible. In order that the amputated parts are maintained and transported in the best condition possible:

- remove any gross contamination
- cover the part(s) with a moist dressing
- secure in a sealed plastic bag
- place the bag in a container or another bag with ice – do not place body parts in direct contact with ice as this can cause tissue damage; the aim is to keep the temperature low but not freezing.

Neck of femur fractures
Giving/administering effective analgesia is one of the most important interventions in managing neck of femur fractures. Refer to **Pain Management in Adults and Children**.

- Assess for signs of potential neck of femur fracture:
  - History of fall, including a fall from standing height or low velocity falls, particularly in older or frail patients
  - Shortening and external rotation of the leg on the injured side (may not always be seen)
  - Pain in the hip and/or groin
  - Referred pain in the knee
- Assess the period the patient has been on the floor or immobile for signs of hypothermia, dehydration, pressure ulcers or infection.
- Consider a potential neck of femur fracture in patients who are unable to mobilise, have pain on moving, or have altered mobility following a fall.

(continued)

Limb Trauma

TABLE 4.21 – ASSESSMENT and MANAGEMENT of: Limb Trauma *(continued)*

- Caution should be applied with older patients, and those with cognitive impairment who may not be able to describe the history and/or focus on the assessment.
- Do not attempt to reduce or manipulate neck of femur fractures. The emphasis should be restoring normal anatomical position.
- Immobilise by strapping the injured leg to the normal one with padding between the legs – extra padding with blankets and strapping around the hips and pelvis can be used to provide additional support while moving the patient (refer to Table 4.20).
- Rhabdomyolysis is more common in older patients, particularly those who have prolonged immobility following a fall. Either can prolong hospital stay and may be fatal.
- There is evidence to suggest that fast-tracking patients in the emergency department improves outcomes in fractured neck of femur. Consider pre-alert (ATMIST) and follow local pathways/guidance

Trapped limbs

- The patient should be extricated as soon as possible.
- Tourniquets should only be used to control catastrophic external haemorrhage and not applied to trapped limbs otherwise.
- Refer to **Intravascular Fluid Therapy** guideline for management of crush injuries and crush syndrome.

Compartment syndrome

Assess for signs of compartment syndrome, which may include the six 'P's:

- Disproportionate pain relative to the injury
- Palpable tension across the skin
- Swelling of an anatomical compartment
- Skin pallor, weakness or paraesthesia, as well as difficulty in moving the affected body part.

Apparently normal signs of distal perfusion may still be present. Loss of distal pulse is a very late sign.

Consider the need for rapid transfer to nearest appropriate hospital. Follow local limb trauma pathway as appropriate. The patient may require urgent surgery. Consider appropriate analgesia and elevate the limb en route.

Pain management

- Pain management is an important intervention.
- Consider analgesia even where patients report a low pain score, reassess on minimal movement of the limb, and always prior to any significant movement, splinting or packaging.

Refer to **Pain Management in Adults and Children**.

Fluid

- If fluid resuscitation is indicated, refer to **Intravascular Fluid Therapy in Adults** and **Intravascular Fluid Therapy in Children**.
- **DO NOT** delay on scene for fluid replacement if peripheral pulses are present.

Antibiotic

- Administer prophylactic antibiotic (in line with local guidance) as soon as possible and preferably within 1 hour of injury to patients with open fractures (other than hands and distal foot injuries), without delaying transport to hospital.

Refer to local policy/PGD for administration of antibiotics.

Non-accidental Injury

- When assessing an injury in a patient, consider the possibility of non-accidental injury (refer to **Safeguarding Children** and **Safeguarding Adults at Risk**).

Limb Trauma

TABLE 4.21 – ASSESSMENT and MANAGEMENT of: Limb Trauma *(continued)*

Transfer to Further Care

- Transfer suspected open fractures of the long bone, hindfoot or midfoot directly to a major trauma centre or specialist centre for orthoplastic care, as per local policy.
- In some areas, intermediate care in a trauma unit may be required, according to local trauma network guidelines. Follow local policy.
- Transfer suspected open fractures of the hand, wrist or toes to nearest trauma unit, unless there are pre-hospital triage indications for direct transport to a major trauma centre. Follow local policy as appropriate.
- Seek advice on the transfer of patients with complex/open fractures according to local guidelines.
- Patients with shoulder, knee and patella dislocations should be transferred to further care with imaging facilities, even if the shoulder/knee or patella has been relocated.
- If the patella has not been relocated (with or without distal circulatory compromise), the patient should be transported to the nearest receiving ED.
- Handover of any reduction is important. Full documentation should include swelling and bruising and should be noted pre and post reduction.
- Continue patient management en route.
- Provide a pre-alert using ATMIST.
- At the hospital, inform staff of:
    - any skin wound relating to a fracture
    - any reduced fracture(s) that were initially open.
- Complete documentation.

KEY POINTS!

Limb Trauma

- Ensure <C>ABCDEs are assessed and managed first; follow appropriate C-spine immobilisation guideline (Spinal Injury and Spinal Cord Injury).
- DO NOT become distracted by the appearance of limb trauma from assessing less visible but life-threatening problems, such as airway obstruction, compromised breathing, poor perfusion and spinal injury.
- Do not irrigate open fractures.
- Limb trauma can cause life-threatening haemorrhage.
- Assess for neurovascular status distal to the fracture site. This should be re-assessed regularly and following any reduction.
- Any dislocation that threatens the neurovascular status of a limb must be treated with urgency.
- Splint to prevent further blood loss and to reduce pain.
- Limb trauma can cause considerable pain and distress – consider pain management as soon as clinically possible after arriving on scene.
- In cases of life-threatening trauma, commence a TIME-CRITICAL transfer and do not delay time on scene.

Bibliography

1. National Institute for Health and Clinical Excellence. *Fractures (Complex): Assessment and Management (NG37)*. London: NICE, 2016. Available from: https://www.nice.org.uk/guidance/ng37.
2. National Institute for Health and Clinical Excellence. *Fractures (Non-complex): Assessment and Management (NG38)*. London: NICE, 2016. Available from: https://www.nice.org.uk/guidance/ng38.
3. National Institute for Health and Clinical Excellence. *Major Trauma: Assessment and Initial Management (NG39)*. London: NICE, 2016. Available from: https://www.nice.org.uk/guidance/ng39.
4. National Institute for Health and Clinical Excellence. *Major Trauma: Service Delivery (NG40)*. London: NICE, 2016. Available from: https://www.nice.org.uk/guidance/ng40.

Limb Trauma

5. National Institute for Health and Clinical Excellence. *Spinal Injury: Assessment and Initial Management* (NG41). London: NICE, 2016. Available from: https://www.nice.org.uk/guidance/ng41.

6. National Institute for Health and Clinical Excellence. *When to Suspect Child Maltreatment* (CG89). London: NICE, 2009. Available from: https://www.nice.org.uk/guidance/cg89.

7. Porter A, Snooks H, Youren A, Gaze S, Whitfield R, Rapport F et al. 'Covering our backs': ambulance crews' attitudes towards clinical documentation when emergency (999) patients are not conveyed to hospital. *Emergency Medicine Journal* 2008, 25(5): 292–295.

8. Aflatooni J, & McKay SD. Efficient Recognition and Closed Reduction of Locked Lateral Patella Dislocation. *Cureus* 2023, 15(1): 1–7. DOI: https://doi.org/10.7759/cureus.33415

9. BMJ Best Practice. Joint Dislocation. *Definitions* 2020. DOI: https://doi.org/10.32388/92iq46

10. Danielsen O, Poulsen TA, Eysturoy NH, Mortensen ES, Hölmich P, & Barfod KW. Familial association and epidemilogical factors as risk factors for developing first time and recurrent patella dislocation: a systematic review and best knowledge synthesis of present literature. In *Knee Surgery, Sports Traumatology, Arthroscopy* (Issue 0123456789) 2023, Springer Berlin Heidelberg. DOI: https://doi.org/10.1007/s00167-022-07265-z

11. Folt J, & Vohra T. Case Report Low-velocity knee dislocation in the morbidly obese. *American Journal of Emergency Medicine* 2012, 30(9): 2090.e5-2090.e6. DOI: https://doi.org/10.1016/j.ajem.2011.12.031

12. Cooper C, Dennison FM, Leufkens HGM, Bishop N, van Staa TP. Epidemiology of childhood fractures in Britain: a study using the General Practice Research Database. *Journal of Bone and Mineral Research* 2004, 19(12): 976–981.

13. Daniels JM, Zook EG, Lynch JM. Hand and wrist injuries. Part II: Emergent evaluation. *American Family Physician* 2004, 69(8): 1949–1956.

14. Griffiths R, Alper J, Beckingsale A, Goldhill D, Heyburn G, Holloway J et al. Management of proximal femoral fractures 2011. *Anaesthesia* 2012, 67(1): 85–98.

15. Hodgetts TJ, Mahoney PF, Russell MQ, Byers M. ABC to <C>ABC: redefining the military trauma paradigm. *Emergency Medical Journal* 2006, 23(10): 745–746.

16. Jagdeep N, Durai N, Umraz K, Christopher M, Stephen B, Frances S et al. *Standards for the Management of Open Fractures of the Lower Limb*. London: British Association of Plastic Reconstructive and Aesthetic Surgeons, British Orthopaedic Association, 2009. Available from: http://www.bapras.org.uk/professionals/clinical-guidance/open-fractures-of-the-lower-limb.

17. Kaye JA, Jick H. Epidemiology of lower limb fractures in general practice in the United Kingdom. *Injury Prevention* 2004, 10(6): 368–374.

18. Klos K, Muckley T, Gras F, Hofmann GO, Schmidt R. Early posttraumatic rotationplasty after severe degloving and soft tissue avulsion injury: a case report. *Journal of Orthopaedic Trauma* 2010, 24(2): e1–5.

19. Kragh JF Jr, Walters TJ, Baer DG, Fox CJ, Wade CE, Salinas J et al. Practical use of emergency tourniquets to stop bleeding in major limb trauma. *Journal of Trauma* 2008, 64 (suppl. 2): S38–49; discussion S49–50.

20. Lee C, Porter KM. Pre-hospital management of lower limb fractures. *Emergency Medicine Journal* 2005, 22(9): 660–663.

21. Lee C, Porter KM, Hodgetts TJ. Tourniquet use in the civilian pre-hospital setting. *Emergency Medicine Journal* 2007, 24(8): 584–587.

22. Lisle DA, Shepherd GJ, Cowderoy GA, O'Connell PT. MR imaging of traumatic and overuse injuries of the wrist and hand in athletes. *Magnetic Resonance Imaging Clinics of North America* 2009, 17(4): 639–654.

23. National Library of Medicine. *Fractures*. 2011. Available from: http://www.nlm.nih.gov/medlineplus/fractures.html.

24. Pearse MF, Harry L, Nanchahal J. Acute compartment syndrome of the leg. *British Medical Journal* 2002, 325(7364): 557–558.

25. Taxter AJ, Konstantakos EK, Ames DW. Lateral compartment syndrome of the lower extremity in a recreational athlete: a case report. *American Journal of Emergency Medicine* 2008, 26(8): 973.e1–2.

26. van Staa TP, Dennison EM, Leufkens HGM, Cooper C. Epidemiology of fractures in England and Wales. *Bone* 2001, 29(6): 517–522.

27. Weinmann M. Compartment syndrome. *Emergency Medical Services* 2003, 32(9): 36.

28. Wood SP, Vrahas M, Wedel SK. Femur fracture immobilization with traction splints in multisystem trauma patients. *Pre-hospital Emergency Care* 2003, 7(2): 241–243.

29. British Orthopaedic Association, British Association of Plastic Reconstructive and Aesthetic Surgeons. *The Management of Severe Open Lower Limb Fractures*. 2009. Available from: http://www.boa.ac.uk.

30. Melamed E, Blumenfeld A, Kalmovich B, Kosashvili Y, Lin G, Israel Defense Forces Medical Corps Consensus Group on Pre-hospital Care of Orthopedic Injuries. Pre-hospital care of orthopedic injuries. *Pre-hospital Disaster Medicine* 2007, 22(1): 22–25.

31. Bragg S. Avulsion amputation of the hand. *Journal of Emergency Nursing* 2005, 31(3): 282.

32. Bragg S. The boxers' fracture. *Journal of Emergency Nursing* 2005, 31(5): 473.

33. Bragg S. Vertical deceleration: falls from height. *Journal of Emergency Nursing* 2007, 33(4): 377–378.

34. Greaves I, Porter K, Smith JE. Consensus statement on the early management of crush injury and prevention of crush syndrome. *J R Army Meds Corps* 2003, 149: 255–259. DOI: 10.1136/jramc-149-04-02.

Pelvic Trauma

1. Introduction

- Major pelvic injuries are predominantly observed where there is a high-energy transfer to the patient such as might occur following road traffic collision, pedestrian accident, fall from height or crush injury.
- Less-serious pelvic injuries may also occur following low-energy transfer events, particularly in the elderly (such as a simple fall), amongst patients with degenerative bone disease or receiving radiotherapy and rarely as a direct consequence of seizure activity.
- The majority of pelvic injuries do not result in major disruption of the pelvic ring, but rather involve fractures of the pubic ramus or acetabulum. Presentation of these injuries is very similar to neck of femur fractures.
- Mechanism of injury:
  - High-energy transfer
  - Fall from height
  - Crush injury.
- Risk factors:
  - Advancing age
  - Degenerative bone disease
  - Radiotherapy.

2. Incidence

- Pelvic fractures are present in 7% of UK trauma patients.[6]
- From 2013 to 2019, 23,823 patients with pelvic fractures (PAF) were admitted to major trauma centres in England. 12,480 (52%) underwent operative intervention.[7]

3. Severity and Outcome

- Major pelvic injuries can be devastating and are often associated with a number of complications that may require extensive rehabilitation.
- Pelvic trauma deaths frequently occur as a result of associated injuries and complications rather than the pelvic injury itself.
- Haemorrhage may be the cause of death in pelvic trauma patients. Bleeding is usually retroperitoneal; the volume of blood loss correlates with the degree and type of pelvic disruption.

4. Pathophysiology

4.1 Skeletal Anatomy

- Increasing pelvic volume allows for increased haemorrhage; conversely, reducing pelvic volume reduces potential for bleeding by realignment of broken bone ends.

4.2 Classification of Injury

- As with other fractures, pelvic fractures may be classified as open or closed, and benefit from being further described as either haemodynamically stable or unstable. Patients who are haemodynamically unstable are at greater risk of death and would benefit greatly from a suitable pre-hospital alert message.
- Pelvic ring disruptions (as identified by in-hospital imaging) can be subdivided into four classes by mechanism of injury: antero-posterior compression (APC), lateral compression (LC), vertical shear (VS) and combined mechanical injury (CMI), a combination of the aforementioned classes.

4.3 Vascular Injury

- The arteries most frequently injured are the iliolumbar arteries, the superior gluteal and the internal pudendal because of their proximity to the bone, the sacro-iliac joint and the inferior ligaments of the pelvis. Bleeding from the venous network after a pelvic fracture is more frequent than arterial bleeding because the walls of the veins are more fragile than arteries. Blood may pool in the retroperitoneal space and haemostasis may occur spontaneously in closed fractures, especially if there is no concomitant arterial haemorrhage.

4.4 Other Injuries

- Urogenital injury (urethral and vaginal injuries) are common in pelvic fractures. Vaginal lacerations result from either penetration of a bony fragment or from indirect forces from diastasis of the symphysis pubis. Injuries to the cervix, uterus and ovaries are rare.
- Bladder rupture and rectal injury can also occur in pelvic fractures.
- Pelvic injury is commonly associated with intra-thoracic and/or intra-abdominal injury.

5. Assessment and Management

For the assessment and management of pelvic trauma, refer to Table 4.22.

- When managing critically ill or injured patients, early consideration should be given to the requirement for additional critical care resources, they should be requested promptly. Consideration should be given to the following factors in reaching these decisions:

1. Clinical scope of practice such as the ability to deliver emergency anaesthesia or blood products
2. Transport platform (road versus air and the ability to undertake aeromedical transfer)
3. Balance time for interventions on scene against delay reaching definitive care

Pelvic Trauma

4. Ability to rendezvous with the transporting ambulance en route to hospital
- These decisions should be made in conjunction with remote clinical support where possible, for example via an ambulance control room critical care, trauma, HEMS desk or senior clinician.

Delaying on scene time in critically ill or injured patients may not be justifiable if care can be escalated more quickly and safely by rapidly transferring the patient to hospital.
- If patient is known or suspected to be pregnant, refer to **Trauma in Pregnancy**.

TABLE 4.22 – ASSESSMENT and MANAGEMENT of: Pelvic Trauma

Assess <C>ABCDE
- Control any external catastrophic haemorrhage (refer to **Trauma Emergencies in Adults – Overview** and **Trauma Emergencies in Children – Overview**).
- Evaluate whether patient is **TIME-CRITICAL** or **NON-TIME-CRITICAL** following criteria as per trauma emergencies guideline.
- If patient is **TIME-CRITICAL**:
  – correct **A** and **B** problems.
  – stabilise the pelvis on scene and rapidly transport to nearest suitable receiving hospital.
  – Provide an alert/information call.
  – Continue patient management en route.
- Minimise ongoing heat loss in patients with possible major trauma.
- In **NON-TIME-CRITICAL** patients, perform a more thorough patient assessment with a brief secondary survey.

Specifically Consider
- Pelvic fracture should be considered based upon the mechanism of injury.
- Clinical assessment of the pelvis includes observation for physical injury such as bruising, bleeding, deformity or swelling to the pelvis or genitalia. Shortening or splaying of a lower limb(s) may be present (see also **Limb Trauma**).
- Assessment by compression or distraction (e.g. springing) of the pelvis is unreliable and may both dislodge clots and exacerbate any injury and must not be performed. Any patient with a relevant mechanism of injury and concomitant hypotension **MUST** be managed as having a **time-critical pelvic injury** until proven otherwise.

Oxygen
- Major pelvic injury falls into the category of critical illness and requires high levels of supplemental oxygen regardless of initial oxygen saturation reading (SpO_2). Maintain high-flow oxygen (15 litres per minute) until vital signs are normal; thereafter, reduce flow rate, titrating to maintain oxygen saturations (SpO_2) in the 94–98% range (refer to **Oxygen**). Normalisation of vital signs in the context of an unstable pelvic injury is unlikely to occur in the prehospital phase.

Pelvic Trauma

TABLE 4.22 – ASSESSMENT and MANAGEMENT of: Pelvic Trauma *(continued)*
Pelvic Stabilisation
• There is currently no evidence to suggest that any particular pelvic immobilisation device or approach is superior in terms of outcome in pelvic trauma, and a number of methods have been reported. A pelvic immobilisation device should be applied, at the earliest practical opportunity, where there is a mechanism of injury suggestive of a pelvic ring fracture, along with suspicion of active bleeding (tachycardia and/or hypotension and/or decreased level of consciousness).
• This may be achieved by: – Use of an appropriate purpose-made pelvic binder/splint. – Apply the pelvic splint directly to skin, if this can be done easily with minimal handling. – Expert consensus suggests the use of an appropriate pelvic splint is preferable to improvised immobilisation techniques. In all methods, circumferential pressure is applied over the greater trochanters and not the iliac crests. Care must be exercised so as to ensure that the pelvis is not reduced beyond its normal anatomical position. Consider an improvised pelvic binder, but only if a purpose-made binder does not fit. – Pressure sores and soft tissue injuries may occur when immobilisation devices are incorrectly fitted. – Reduction and stabilisation of the pelvic ring should occur as soon as is practicable whilst still on scene, as stabilisation helps to reduce blood loss by realigning fracture surfaces, thereby limiting active bleeding and additionally helping to stabilise clots. Reduction of the pelvis may have a tamponade effect, particularly for venous bleeding; however, there is little evidence to support this belief. – Log rolling of the patient with possible pelvic fracture should be avoided as this may exacerbate any pelvic injury; where possible, utilise an orthopaedic scoop stretcher to lift patients off the ground and limit movement to a 15° tilt.
Consider Tranexamic acid
• Tranexamic acid should be given where appropriate as early as possible (refer to **Tranexamic acid**).
Fluid Therapy
• There is little evidence to support the routine use of IV fluids in adult trauma patients (refer to **Intravascular Fluid Therapy in Adults** and **Intravascular Fluid Therapy in Children**).
Pain Management
• Patients' pain should be managed appropriately (refer to **Pain Management in Adults and Children**).

6. Referral Pathway

The following cases should ALWAYS be transferred to further care:

- Any patient with hypotension and potential pelvic injury **MUST** be treated as a **TIME-CRITICAL** pelvic injury until proven otherwise. Transfer to a Major Trauma Centre should be considered as per local guidelines.
- Any patient with sufficient mechanism of injury to cause a pelvic injury.

The following cases MAY be considered suitable/safe to be left at home:

- None.

7. Special Considerations for Children

- There is a lower incidence compared with adults. In children, pelvic injuries have a lower mortality with fewer deaths occurring as a direct result of pelvic haemorrhage; blood loss is more likely to be from solid visceral injury than the pelvis.
- Different injury patterns in children; greater incidence of diaphragmatic injury.
- Principles of management are the same (refer to **Pain Management in Adults and Children** and **Tranexamic acid**), with the exception of fluid and oxygen therapy (refer to **Intravascular Fluid Therapy in Children** and **Oxygen**).
- Clinical findings in small children can be unreliable.

Pelvic Trauma

> **KEY POINTS!**
>
> **Pelvic Trauma**
> - Pelvic fracture should be considered based upon mechanism of injury.
> - The majority of pelvic fractures are stable pubic ramus or acetabular fractures.
> - Any patient with hypotension and relevant mechanism of injury MUST be considered to have a TIME-CRITICAL pelvic injury.
> - 'Springing' or distraction of the pelvis must not be undertaken.
> - Pelvic stabilisation should be implemented as soon as is practicable whilst still on scene.
> - Consider appropriate pain management.
> - Tranexamic acid should be given where appropriate as early as possible (refer to Tranexamic acid).
> - The use of a scoop stretcher is recommended to avoid log rolling the patient unless extrication is required.

Bibliography

1. National Institute for Health and Clinical Excellence. *Fractures (Complex): Assessment and Management* (NG37). London: NICE, 2016. Available from: https://www.nice.org.uk/guidance/ng37.

2. National Institute for Health and Clinical Excellence. *Fractures (Non-complex): Assessment and Management* (NG38). London: NICE, 2016. Available from: https://www.nice.org.uk/guidance/ng38.

3. National Institute for Health and Clinical Excellence. *Major Trauma: Assessment and Initial Management* (NG39). London: NICE, 2016. Available from: https://www.nice.org.uk/guidance/ng39

4. National Institute for Health and Clinical Excellence. *Major Trauma: Service Delivery* (NG40). London: NICE, 2016. Available from: https://www.nice.org.uk/guidance/ng40.

5. National Institute for Health and Clinical Excellence. *Spinal Injury: Assessment and Initial Management* (NG41). London: NICE, 2016. Available from: https://www.nice.org.uk/guidance/ng41.

6. Mostafa A, Kyriacou H, Chimutengwende-Gordon M, and Khan WS. An overview of the key principles and guidelines in the management of pelvic fractures. *Journal of Perioperative Practice* 2020, 31(9). https://doi.org/10.1177/1750458920947358

7. Martin A, McMaster J, Bretherton C, and Noyes D. Pelvic and acetabular fracture care in England: current workload and future directions. *The Annals of The Royal College of Surgeons of England* 2021, 103(6). https://doi.org/10.1308/rcsann.2021.0015.

8. Brown JK, Jing Y, Wang S, Ehrlich PF. Patterns of severe injury in pediatric car crash victims: Crash Injury Research Engineering Network database. *Journal of Pediatric Surgery* 2006, 41(2): 362–367.

9. O'Brien DP, Luchette FA, Pereira SJ, Lim E, Seeskin CS, James L, et al. Pelvic fracture in the elderly is associated with increased mortality. *Surgery* 2002, 132(4): 710–714.

10. Stein DM, O'Connor JV, Kufera JA, Ho SM, Dischinger PC, Copeland CE et al. Risk factors associated with pelvic fractures sustained in motor vehicle collisions involving newer vehicles. *Journal of Trauma* 2006, 61(1): 21–30.

11. Demetriades D, Karaiskakis M, Toutouzas K, Alo K, Velmahos G, Chan L. Pelvic fractures: epidemiology and predictors of associated abdominal injuries and outcomes. *Journal of the American College of Surgeons* 2002, 195(1): 1–10.

12. Demetriades D, Murray J, Brown C, Velmahos G, Salim A, Alo K et al. High-level falls: type and severity of injuries and survival outcome according to age. *Journal of Trauma* 2005, 58(2): 342–345.

13. Gustavo Parreira J, Coimbra R, Rasslan S, Oliveira A, Fregoneze M, Mercadante M. The role of associated injuries on outcome of blunt trauma patients sustaining pelvic fractures. *Injury* 2000, 31(9): 677–682.

14. Inaba K, Sharkey PW, Stephen DJG, Redelmeier DA, Brenneman FD. The increasing incidence of severe pelvic injury in motor vehicle collisions. *Injury* 2004, 35(8): 759–765.

15. Kimbrell BJ, Velmahos GC, Chan LS, Demetriades D. Angiographic embolization for pelvic fractures in older patients. *Archives of Surgery* 2004, 139(7): 728–732.

16. Tarman GJ, Kaplan GW, Lerman SL, McAleer IM, Losasso BE. Lower genitourinary injury and pelvic fractures in pediatric patients. *Urology* 2002, 59(1): 123–126.

17. Demetriades D, Murray J, Martin M, Velmahos G, Salim A, Alo K et al. Pedestrians injured by automobiles: relationship of age to injury type and severity. *Journal of the American College of Surgeons* 2004, 199(3): 382–387.

18. Hill RMF, Robinson CM, Keating JF. Fractures of the pubic rami. *Journal of Bone & Joint Surgery, British Volume* 2001, 83-B(8): 1141–1144.

19. Baxter NN, Habermann EB, Tepper JE, Durham SB, Virnig BA. Risk of pelvic fractures in older women following pelvic irradiation. Journal *of the American Medical Association* 2005, 294(20): 2587–2593.

20. Boufous S, Finch C, Lord S, Close J. The increasing burden of pelvic fractures in older people, New South Wales, Australia. *Injury* 2005, 36(11): 1323–1329.

21. Hauschild O, Strohm PC, Culemann U, Pohlemann T, Suedkamp NP, Koestler W et al. Mortality in patients with pelvic fractures: results from the German pelvic injury register. *Journal of Trauma* 2008, 64(2): 449–455.

22. Croce MA, Magnotti LJ, Savage SA, Wood IGW, Fabian TC. Emergent pelvic fixation in patients with exsanguinating pelvic fractures. *Journal of the American College of Surgeons 2007* , 204(5): 935–939.

23. Duane TM, Tan BB, Golay D, Cole FJ Jr, Weireter LJ Jr, Britt LD. Blunt trauma and the role of routine pelvic

Pelvic Trauma

23. radiographs: a prospective analysis. *Journal of Trauma* 2002, 53(3): 463–468.

24. Gonzalez RP, Fried PQ, Bukhalo M. The utility of clinical examination in screening for pelvic fractures in blunt trauma. *Journal of the American College of Surgeons* 2002, 194(2): 121–125.

25. Tien IY, Dufel SE. Does ethanol affect the reliability of pelvic bone examination in blunt trauma? *Annals of Emergency Medicine* 2000, 36(5): 451–455.

26. Heetveld MJ, Harris I, Schlaphoff G, Balogh Z, D'Amours SK, Sugrue M. Hemodynamically unstable pelvic fractures: recent care and new guidelines. *Journal of Surgery* 2004, 28(9): 904–909.

28. Grotz MRW, Gummerson NW, Gansslen A, Petrowsky H, Keel M, Allami MK et al. Staged management and outcome of combined pelvic and liver trauma: an international experience of the deadly duo. *Injury* 2006, 37(7): 642–651.

29. Sriussadaporn S. Abdominopelvic vascular injuries. *Journal of the Medical Association of Thailand* 2000, 83(1): 13–20.

30. Rowe SA, Sochor MS, Staples KS, Wahl WL, Wang SC. Pelvic ring fractures: implications of vehicle design, crash type, and occupant characteristics. *Surgery* 2004, 136(4): 842–847.

31. Dyer GSM, Vrahas MS. Review of the pathophysiology and acute management of haemorrhage in pelvic fracture. *Injury* 2006, 37(7): 602–613.

32. Bottlang M, Simpson T, Sigg J, Krieg JC, Madey SM, Long WB. Noninvasive reduction of open-book pelvic fractures by circumferential compression. *Journal of Orthopaedic Trauma* 2002, 16(6): 367–373.

33. Reiff DA, McGwin G Jr, Metzger J, Windham ST, Doss M, Rue LW III. Identifying injuries and motor vehicle collision characteristics that together are suggestive of diaphragmatic rupture. *Journal of Trauma* 2002, 53(6): 1139–1145.

34. Waydhas C, Nast-Kolb D, Ruchholtz S. Pelvic ring fractures: utility of clinical examination in patients with impaired consciousness or tracheal intubation. *European Journal of Trauma and Emergency Surgery* 2007, 33(2): 170–175.

35. Sauerland S, Bouillon B, Rixen D, Raum MR, Koy T, Neugebauer EAM. The reliability of clinical examination in detecting pelvic fractures in blunt trauma patients: a meta-analysis. *Archives of Orthopaedic and Trauma Surgery* 2004, 124(2): 123–128.

36. Lee C, Porter K. The pre-hospital management of pelvic fractures. *Emergency Medicine Journal* 2007, 24(2): 130–133.

37. Bottlang M, Krieg JC, Mohr M, Simpson TS, Madey SM. Emergent management of pelvic ring fractures with use of circumferential compression. *Journal of Orthopaedic Trauma* 2002, 16(6): 367–373.

38. Friese G, LaMay G. Emergency stabilization of unstable pelvic fractures. *Emergency Medical Services* 2005, 34(5): 65.

39. Jowett AJL, Bowyer GW. Pressure characteristics of pelvic binders. *Injury* 2007, 38(1): 118–121.

40. Katsoulis E, Drakoulakis E, Giannoudis PV. (iii) Management of open pelvic fractures. *Current Orthopaedics* 2005, 19(5): 345–353.

41. Krieg JC, Mohr M, Ellis TJ, Simpson TS, Madey SM, Bottlang M. Emergent stabilization of pelvic ring injuries by controlled circumferential compression: a clinical trial. *Journal of Trauma, Injury, Infection, & Critical Care* 2005, 59(3): 659–664.

42. Salomone JP, Ustin JS, McSwain NE Jr, Feliciano DV. Opinions of trauma practitioners regarding pre-hospital interventions for critically injured patients. *Journal of Trauma* 2005, 58(3): 509–515; discussion 515–517.

43. Simpson T, Krieg JC, Heuer F, Bottlang M. Stabilization of pelvic ring disruptions with a circumferential sheet. *Journal of Trauma, Injury, Infection, & Critical Care* 2002, 52(1): 158–161.

44. Nunn T, Cosker TDA, Bose D, Pallister I. Immediate application of improvised pelvic binder as first step in extended resuscitation from life-threatening hypovolaemic shock in conscious patients with unstable pelvic injuries. *Injury* 2007, 38(1): 125–128.

45. Krieg JC, Mohr M, Mirza AJ, Bottlang M. Pelvic circumferential compression in the presence of soft-tissue injuries: a case report. *Journal of Trauma, Injury, Infection, & Critical Care* 2005, 59(2): 470–472.

46. Junkins EPJ, Nelson DS, Carroll KL, Hansen K, Furnival RA. A prospective evaluation of the clinical presentation of pediatric pelvic fractures. *Journal of Trauma* 2001, 51(1): 64–68.

47. Silber JS, Flynn JM, Koffler KM, Dormans JP, Drummond DS. Analysis of the cause, classification, and associated injuries of 166 consecutive pediatric pelvic fractures. *Journal of Pediatric Orthopaedics* 2001, 21(4): 446–450.

48. Junkins EP, Furnival RA, Bake RG. The clinical presentation of pediatric pelvic fractures. *Pediatric Emergency Care* 2001, 17(1): 15–18.

Spinal Injury and Spinal Cord Injury

1. Introduction

- In the trauma patient, spinal injuries are uncommon compared to other time-critical injuries. The majority are stable; some are unstable, risking spinal cord damage, and a small number are associated with spinal cord injury (SCI) at the outset. Differentiation between stable and unstable injuries requires specific imaging in the ED.
- Effective management from the time of injury is important to ensure optimal outcomes. This guideline provides guidance for the assessment and initial management of cervical spine and spinal trauma, including indicators to guidance for related conditions.

2. Pathophysiology

- The spinal cord runs in the spinal canal down to the level of the second lumbar vertebra in adults.
- The amount of space in the spinal canal in the upper neck is relatively large, and risk of secondary injury in this area can be reduced by actions that reduce secondary spinal cord injury. In the thoracic area the cord is wide and the spinal canal relatively narrow; injury at this level is more likely to completely disrupt and damage the spinal cord.
- Spinal shock is a state of complete loss of motor function and often sensory function found sometimes after SCI. This immediate reaction may go on for some considerable time, but some recovery may well be possible. Complete and incomplete cord injury cannot be distinguished in the presence of spinal shock.
- Neurogenic shock is the state of poor tissue perfusion caused by sympathetic tone loss after spinal cord injury. This may cause bradycardia, vasodilatation and hypotension.

3. Incidence

- Falls are a frequent cause of SCI in the older person. Maintain a high index of suspicion in cases of older people who have had low-energy falls (e.g. falling from standing).
- SCI affects young and fit people and will continue to affect them to a varying degree for the rest of their lives.
- Road traffic collisions (RTCs), falls and sporting injuries are the most common causes of SCI – as a group, motorcyclists occupy more spinal injury unit beds than any other group involved in road traffic collisions. Rollover road traffic collisions where occupants are not wearing seat belts, and the head comes into contact with the vehicle body, and pedestrians struck by vehicles are likely to suffer SCI. Ejection from a vehicle increases the risk of injury significantly.
- UK Trauma Audit Research Network (TARN) data has shown that, in the presence of a cervical bony injury, 13.4% of patients have associated injuries elsewhere in the thoracic and lumbar spine.
- Unstable spinal injuries and cord injuries are rare and are commonly associated with other serious injuries. These injuries may impair measures to minimise secondary spinal cord injury e.g. the avoidance of hypoxia and/or hypoperfusion. Absolute movement minimisation takes additional time and needs to be balanced against other priorities for actual and suspected injuries.

3.1. Risk Factors

- RTCs:
  - rollover RTCs
  - non-wearing of seat belts
  - ejection from vehicle
  - struck by a vehicle.
- Sporting injuries:
  - diving into shallow water
  - horse riding
  - rugby
  - gymnastics and trampolining.
- Falls:
  - older people.
  - rheumatoid arthritis.
- Violent attacks and domestic incidents.
- Certain sporting accidents, especially diving into shallow water, horse riding, rugby, gymnastics and trampolining, have a higher than average risk of SCI. Rapid deceleration injury such as gliding and light aircraft accidents also increases the risk of SCI.
- Older people and those with rheumatoid arthritis are prone to odontoid peg fractures that may be difficult to detect clinically. Such injuries can occur from relatively minor trauma (e.g. falls from a standing height).

3.2. Cauda Equina Syndrome (CES)

- Cauda equina syndrome (CES) is caused by compression of the nerves in the spinal canal below the end of the spinal cord (at L2 vertebra level). It can occur in patients with trauma, a herniated disc, chronic or acute low back pain, tumours or infection.
- Clinical diagnosis of CES is not easy. Most cases are of sudden onset and progress rapidly within hours or days. However, CES can evolve slowly and patients do not always complain of pain. Roughly 50–70% of patients have urinary retention on presentation.
- CES is an acute surgical emergency; early diagnosis is essential and the patient requires

Spinal Injury and Spinal Cord Injury

immediate conveyance to hospital for investigation if CES is suspected. Early surgical decompression is crucial to prevent permanent neurological damage.

Refer to **Low Back Pain (Non-traumatic)**.

> **Red flag signs and symptoms of CES**
>
> 🚩 Loss of bladder and/or bowel dysfunction control, causing incontinence.
> 🚩 Reduced sensation in the saddle (perineal) area.
> 🚩 New onset sexual dysfunction.
> 🚩 Neurological deficit in the lower limb (motor/sensory loss, reflex changes, bilateral sciatica).

4. Severity and Outcome

- Injury most frequently occurs at the junctions of mobile and fixed sections of the spine. Hence fractures are more commonly seen in the lower cervical vertebrae, where the cervical and thoracic spine meets (C5, 6, 7/T1 area), and the thoracolumbar junction. Of patients with one identified spinal fracture, 10–15% will be found to have another.
- In the extreme, SCI may prove immediately fatal where the upper cervical cord is damaged, paralysing the diaphragm and respiratory muscles.
- Partial cord damage, however, may solely affect individual sensory or motor nerve tracts, producing varying long-term disability. It is important to note that there is an increasing percentage of cases where the cord damage is only partial and quality recovery is possible, providing the condition is recognised and managed appropriately.

5. Immobilisation

- All patients with the possibility of spinal injury and a reduced GCS should have manual immobilisation commenced at the earliest time, while initial assessment is undertaken.
- If immobilisation is indicated then the whole spine must be immobilised. There are two common approaches to this within UK paramedic practice:
  - head blocks and scoop with collar
  - head blocks and scoop without collar.

The following techniques may be used:

- Patient lying supine:
  - Use a scoop stretcher and cervical spine immobilisation. To minimise movement of the spine, utilise a maximum 10-degree tilt to the left and right if required.
  - Patients should be transported on the scoop stretcher unless there is a prolonged journey time, when a vacuum mattress should be utilised.
  - To utilise the vacuum mattress, lift the patient using the scoop stretcher, then insert the mattress underneath and remove the scoop stretcher.
- Patient lying prone:
  - Log roll the patient with manual immobilisation of the cervical spine to enable a scoop stretcher to be used.
  - Perform a two-stage log roll onto a vacuum mattress.
- Patient requiring extrication:
  - Extrication devices should be used if there is any risk of rotational movement.
  - Rearward extrication on an extrication board.
  - Side extrication invariably involves some rotational component and therefore has higher risks in many circumstances.
  - During extrication the cervical spine can be immobilised manually or with a semi-rigid collar. After extrication the whole spine should be fully immobilised with head blocks replacing the semi-rigid collar.

NB The longboard should only be used as an extrication device. Do not transport patients to hospital on a longboard.

5.1. Extrication

See Extrication section in **Trauma Emergencies in Adults – Overview**

5.2. Cautions/Precautions

Vomiting

- Vomiting and consequent aspiration are serious consequences of immobilisation. Ambulance clinicians must always have a plan of action in case vomiting should occur. Consider the use of anti-emetics where the patient complains of nausea or other symptoms where vomiting may occur.
- Head blocks may need to be removed and manual in-line immobilisation instituted. This may include:
  - suction
  - head-down tilt of the immobilisation device
  - rolling the patient onto one side on the immobilisation device.

Restless/Combative Patients

- There are many reasons for the patient to be restless and it is important to rule out reversible causes (e.g. hypoxia, pain, fear).
- If, despite appropriate measures, the patient remains restless, the use of spinal immobilisation devices may be difficult and could be counterproductive. A struggling patient is more likely to increase any injury, so think about letting

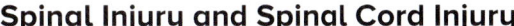

Spinal Injury and Spinal Cord Injury

them find a position where they are comfortable with manual in-line spinal immobilisation.
- The use of restraint can increase forces on the injured spine and therefore a 'best possible' approach should be adopted.

Head Injury
- Patients with a head injury may have raised intracranial pressure, which restraint and application of a cervical collar can increase; therefore a 'best possible' approach should be adopted.

Special Cases
- Some older patients, and those with known spinal deformities (e.g. severe kyphosis), may not be able to tolerate immobilisation or breathe adequately when positioned absolutely flat. Therefore a 'best possible' approach should be adopted, which may include manual in-line immobilisation or maintenance of the pre-existing spinal deformity where putting the patient in the in-line neutral position is unsafe.

Immobilisation of Spinal Injuries
- Soft collars do not limit movement and should not be used.
- Head blocks and tape should be used to immobilise the cervical spine.
- The application of devices is more important than the variation of devices.
- To achieve neutral position in an adult, the occuput should be raised by 2 cm.
- Extrication devices (e.g. KED) are better than extrication boards at reducing rotational movement.
- Vacuum mattresses are more comfortable, and give better immobilisation.
- Vacuum mattresses cannot be used for extrication and are vulnerable to damage.
- Long extrication/spinal boards should only be used as an extrication device. Patients should be immobilised using a scoop stretcher. Once on a scoop stretcher they should remain on it unless they are placed on a vacuum mattress when there is a prolonged journey time.

5.3. When Not to Apply Immobilisation

- Not all patients require immobilisation (refer to Figure 4.13). When assessing for spinal injury, it is important to consider whether the patient:
  - is under the influence of drugs or alcohol
  - is uncooperative or confused
  - has any bony spinal pain anywhere along the spine
  - has any significant distracting injuries
  - has a reduced level of consciousness
  - has a priapism (unconscious or exposed male)
  - has any foot or hand weakness (motor assessment)
  - has any absent or altered sensation in the limbs (sensory assessment)
  - has a history of past spinal problems, including previous spinal surgery or conditions that predispose to instability of the spine.
- If the assessment cannot be completed or **any of the above factors are present**, carry out full in-line immobilisation.
- Penetrating injury to the head has not been shown to be an indication for spinal immobilisation in the absence of altered neurology, and even penetrating injuries of the neck only rarely need selective immobilisation.
- The few patients missed with SCI are often at the extremes of age. Such criteria can be reproducibly used in the pre-hospital environment. Mechanism of injury was not shown to be an independent predictor of injury.
- Use of such guidelines can significantly reduce the use of unnecessary immobilisation.
- Some patients may sustain thoracic or lumbar injuries in addition to, or in isolation from, cervical spine injuries. If you suspect thoracic or lumbar injuries, whether the cervical spine has been cleared, then full spinal immobilisation should be undertaken whenever possible.

5.4. Hazards of Immobilisation

- The value of routine pre-hospital spinal immobilisation remains uncertain and any benefits may be outweighed by the risks of rigid collar immobilisation, including:
  - compromised airway
  - increased intracranial pressure
  - increased risk of aspiration
  - restricted ventilation
  - dysphagia
  - skin ulceration
  - inducement of pain, even in those with no injury
  - known spinal deformities.

5.5. Sequence for Immobilisation

- All patients should be initially immobilised if the mechanism of injury suggests the possibility of SCI.

Blunt Trauma
- Following assessment, it is possible to remove the immobilisation if ALL the criteria are met (refer to Figure 4.13).
- Spinal pain does not include tenderness isolated to the muscles of the side of the neck.

Penetrating Trauma
- Those with isolated penetrating injuries to limbs or the head do not require immobilisation.

Spinal Injury and Spinal Cord Injury

- Those with truncal or neck trauma should be immobilised if there is new neurology and/or the trajectory of the penetrating wound could pass near or through the spinal column.

5.6. Immobilisation of Children

- When carrying out in-line spinal immobilisation in children, manually stabilise the head with the spine in-line and consider the following:
  - If appropriate, involve family members and carers.
  - If possible, keep infants in their car seats.
  - Use a scoop stretcher with blanket rolls, vacuum mattress, vacuum limb splints or Kendrick extrication device.

6. Assessment and Management

For assessment and management of the cervical spine and spine, refer to Table 4.23 and Figure 4.13.

TABLE 4.23 – ASSESSMENT and MANAGEMENT of: Cervical Spine and Spinal Trauma

Assess <C>ABCDE while controlling the spine

- Control any external catastrophic haemorrhage (refer to **Trauma Emergencies in Adults – Overview** and **Trauma Emergencies in Children – Overview**).
- At all stages of the assessment, protect the patient's cervical spine with manual in-line immobilisation and avoid moving the remainder of the spine.

TIME-CRITICAL Patient

- Follow criteria in **Trauma Emergencies in Adult – Overview**.
- If the patient is **TIME-CRITICAL**:
  - Manage the airway.
  - Immobilise the spine.
  - Transfer to a major trauma centre; unless the patient needs an immediate lifesaving intervention, transfer to nearest trauma unit.
  - Provide a pre-alert using ATMIST.
  - Continue patient management en route (see below).

Assess Oxygen Saturation

(Refer to **Oxygen**)

- Adults – administer high levels of supplemental oxygen and aim for target saturation within the range of 94–98% – except for patients with COPD.
- Children – administer high levels of supplemental oxygen.

Determine mechanism of injury

- Forces causing injury include:
  - hyperflexion
  - hyperextension
  - rotation
  - compression
  - one or more of these.

Specific Symptoms of SCI

- The patient may complain of:
  - cervical and/or spinal pain
  - loss of sensory function in the limbs
  - loss of motor function in the limbs
  - sensation of burning in the trunk or limbs
  - sensation of electric shock in the trunk or limbs.

(continued)

Spinal Injury and Spinal Cord Injury

TABLE 4.23 – ASSESSMENT and MANAGEMENT of: Cervical Spine and Spinal Trauma *(continued)*

Rapidly Assess to Determine the Presence and Estimate the Level of Spinal Cord Injury

- The following signs may indicate injury:
  - diaphragmatic or abdominal breathing
  - hypotension (BP often <80–90 mmHg) with bradycardia
  - warm peripheries or vasodilatation in the presence of low blood pressure
  - flaccid (floppy) muscles with absent reflexes
  - priapism – partial or full erection of the penis.
- In a conscious patient – assess sensory and motor function:
  - use light touch and response to pain
  - examine upper limbs and hands
  - examine lower limbs and feet
  - examine both sides
  - undertake the examination in the MID-AXILLARY line, NOT the MID-CLAVICULAR line, as T2, T3 and T4 all supply sensation to the nipple line; use the forehead as the reference point to guide what is normal sensation.

NB Always presume a SCI in the unconscious trauma patient.

Non-TIME-CRITICAL Patient

- Perform a more thorough assessment with a brief secondary survey

Assess for Neurogenic Shock

- Diagnosis is difficult in pre-hospital care – the aim is to:
  - maintain blood pressure of approximately 90 mmHg systolic
  - obtain IV access
  - determine the need for fluid replacement but DO NOT delay on scene (refer to **Intravascular Fluid Therapy in Adults** and **Intravascular Fluid Therapy in Children**).
- In neurogenic shock, a few degrees of head-down tilt may improve the circulation, but remember that in cases of abdominal breathing, this manoeuvre may further worsen respiration and ventilation. This position is also unsuitable for a patient who has, or may have, a head injury.
- If bradycardia is present, consider atropine (refer to **Atropine Sulfate**) – but it is important to rule out other causes (e.g. hypoxia, raised ICP, severe hypovolaemia).

Assess the Need for Assisted Ventilation

- Refer to **Airway and Breathing Management**.

Steroids

- Steroids have no part to play in the pre-hospital management of acute spinal cord injuries.

At Hospital

- The patient should be on a scoop stretcher.
- Complete documentation and, if possible, record information whether the assessments show that the patient's condition is improving or deteriorating.

Additional Information

- Transportation of spinal patients:
  - Driving should balance the advantages of smooth driving and time to arrival at hospital. No immobilisation technique eliminates movement from vehicle swaying and jarring.
  - There is no evidence to show advantage of direct transport to a spinal injury centre.
  - Patients should be transported on the scoop stretcher unless there is a prolonged journey time, when a vacuum mattress should be utilised.
  - As half of all cases of spinal injuries have other serious injuries, any unnecessary delay at the scene or in transit should be avoided.

Spinal Injury and Spinal Cord Injury

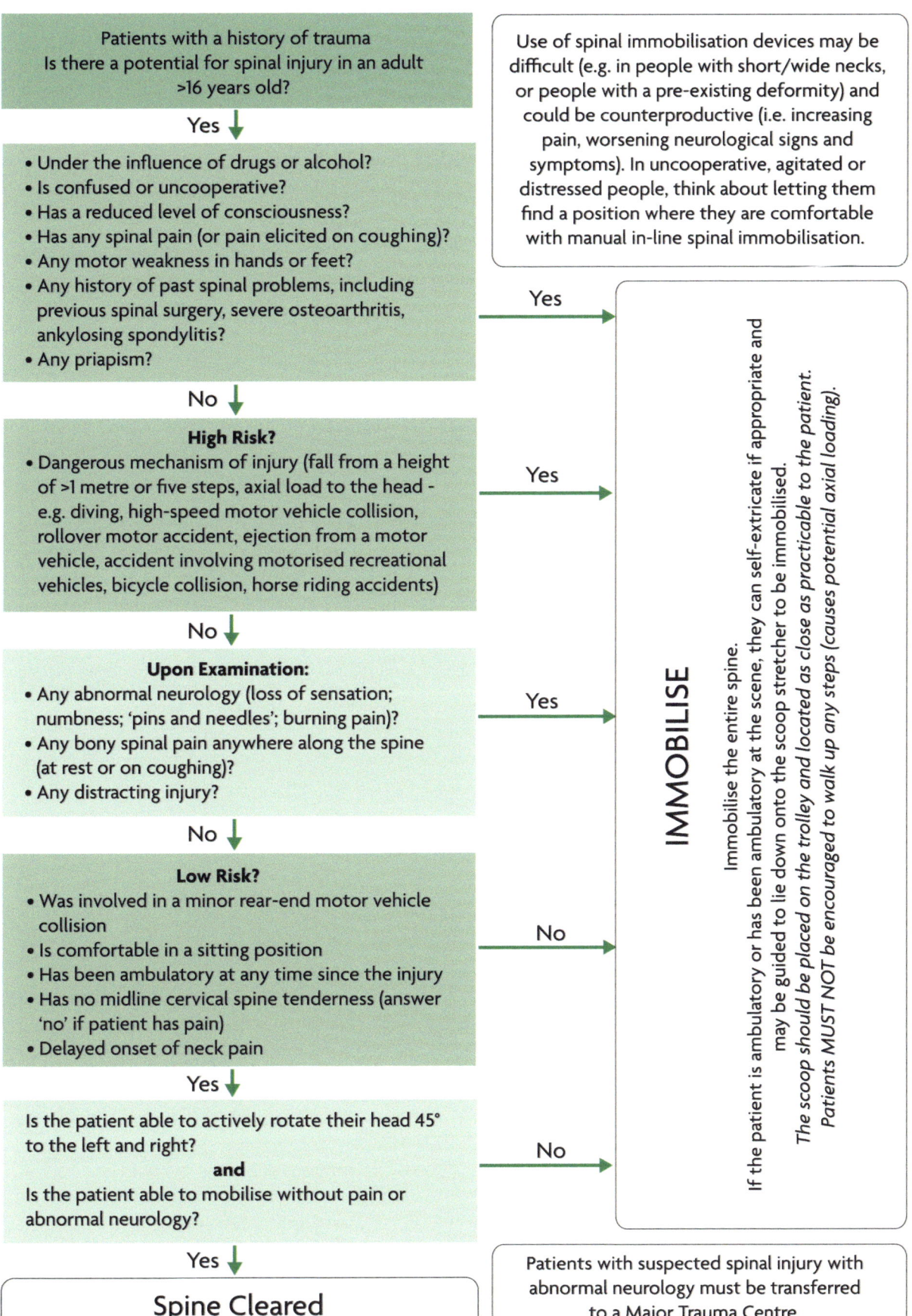

Figure 4.13 – Immobilisation algorithm.

Spinal Injury and Spinal Cord Injury

> **KEY POINTS!**
>
> **Spinal Injury**
> - Immobilise the whole spine until it is positively cleared.
> - Immobilise the whole spine in all unconscious blunt trauma patients.
> - If the cervical spine is immobilised, the thoracic and lumbar spine also need immobilisation.
> - Asking a patient to self-extricate is acceptable, but does not clear the cervical spine.
> - Standard immobilisation is by means of head blocks, tape and scoop.
> - The longboard is solely used as an extrication device, and not for transporting patients to hospital.
> - Aspiration of vomit, pressure sores and raised intracranial pressure are major complications of immobilisation.

Bibliography

1. National Institute for Health and Clinical Excellence. Fractures (Complex): Assessment and Management (NG37). London: NICE, 2016. Available from: https://www.nice.org.uk/guidance/ng37.
2. National Institute for Health and Clinical Excellence. Fractures (Non-complex): Assessment and Management (NG38). London: NICE, 2016. Available from: https://www.nice.org.uk/guidance/ng38.
3. National Institute for Health and Clinical Excellence. Major Trauma: Assessment and Initial Management (NG39). London: NICE, 2016. Available from: https://www.nice.org.uk/guidance/ng39.
4. National Institute for Health and Clinical Excellence. Major Trauma: Service Delivery (NG40). London: NICE, 2016. Available from: https://www.nice.org.uk/guidance/ng40.
5. National Institute for Health and Clinical Excellence. Spinal Injury: Assessment and Initial Management (NG41). London: NICE, 2016. Available from: https://www.nice.org.uk/guidance/ng41.
6. Hoffman JR, Wolfson AB, Todd K, Mower WR. Selective cervical spine radiography in blunt trauma: methodology of the National Emergency X-Radiography Utilization Study (NEXUS). *Ann Emerg Med*. 1998, 32(4): 461–469.
7. Canadian CT Head and C-Spine (CCC) Study Group. Canadian C-Spine Rule study for alert and stable trauma patients: I. Background and rationale. *CJEM*. 2004, 4(2): 84–90.
8. Trauma Audit and Research Network. *Major Trauma in Older People*. Manchester: University of Manchester, 2017.
9. Nutbeam, T., Fenwick, R., Smith, J.E. et al. A Delphi study of rescue and clinical subject matter experts on the extrication of patients following a motor vehicle collision. Scand J Trauma Resusc Emerg Med 30, 41 (2022). https://doi.org/10.1186/s13049-022-01029-x

Thoracic Trauma

1. Introduction

- In pre-hospital care, the most common problem associated with severe thoracic injuries is hypoxia, either from impaired ventilation (lung contusion, pneumothorax, pain) or secondary to hypovolaemia from massive bleeding into the chest (haemothorax) or major vessel disruption (e.g. ruptured thoracic aorta).

2. Incidence

- Severe thoracic injuries are one of the most common causes of death from trauma, accounting for approximately 25% of trauma-related deaths.

3. Severity and Outcome

- Despite the very high percentage of serious thoracic injuries, the vast majority of them can be managed in the pre-hospital setting and in hospital with chest drainage and resuscitation.

4. Pathophysiology

- The mechanism of injury is an important guide to the likelihood of significant thoracic injuries. Injuries to the chest wall usually arise from direct contact, for example intrusion of wreckage in a road traffic collision or blunt trauma arising from a direct blow. Seat-belt injuries fall into this category and may cause fractures of the sternum, ribs and clavicle.
- Rapid deceleration injuries may result in shearing forces sufficient to rupture great vessels such as the aorta and other vascular structures in the thorax.
- If the force/deceleration is sufficient, the deformity and the damage to the chest wall structures may induce tearing and contusion to the underlying lung and other structures. This may produce a combination of severe pain on breathing (pleuritic pain, pain from rib fractures) and a damaged lung, both of which will significantly reduce the ability to ventilate adequately. This combination is a common cause of hypoxia.
- Blunt trauma to the sternum may cause myocardial contusion, which may result in cardiac arrhythmia and sudden cardiac death and/or cardiac failure.
- Penetrating trauma may directly damage the heart, lungs and great vessels, either both in isolation and in combination. It must be remembered that penetrating wounds to the upper abdomen, neck or back may well cause injuries within the chest remote from the entry wound. Conversely, penetrating wounds to the chest may involve the liver, kidneys and spleen.
- The lung may be damaged, with bleeding causing a haemothorax or an air leak causing a pneumothorax. Penetrating or occasionally a blunt injury, may result in cardiac injuries. Blood can leak into the non-elastic surrounding pericardial sac and build up pressure to an extent that the heart is incapable of refilling to pump blood into circulation. This is known as cardiac tamponade and can be fatal if not rapidly treated at hospital (see additional information in Table 4.28).
- The five immediately life-threatening thoracic injuries encountered in the pre-hospital setting are:

1. tension pneumothorax
2. massive haemothorax (following uncontrolled haemorrhage into the chest cavity)
3. open chest wounds
4. flail chest
5. cardiac tamponade.

5. Assessment and Management

For the assessment and management of thoracic trauma, refer to Tables 4.24 to 4.30.

- When managing critically ill or injured patients, early consideration should be given to the requirement for additional critical care resources, they should be requested promptly. Consideration should be given to the following factors in reaching these decisions:

  1. Clinical scope of practice such as the ability to deliver emergency anaesthesia or blood products
  2. Transport platform (road versus air and the ability to undertake aeromedical transfer)
  3. Balance time for interventions on scene against delay reaching definitive care
  4. Ability to rendezvous with the transporting ambulance en route to hospital

- These decisions should be made in conjunction with remote clinical support where possible, for example via an ambulance control room critical care, trauma, HEMS desk or senior clinician. Delaying on scene time in critically ill or injured patients may not be justifiable if care can be escalated more quickly and safely by rapidly transferring the patient to hospital.
- If patient is known or suspected to be pregnant, refer to **Trauma in Pregnancy**.

Thoracic Trauma

TABLE 4.24 – ASSESSMENT and MANAGEMENT of: Thoracic Trauma

Assess <C>ABCDE

- Control any external catastrophic haemorrhage (refer to **Trauma Emergencies in Adults – Overview** and **Trauma Emergencies in Children – Overview**).
- If any of the following **TIME-CRITICAL** features are present:
  - major **<C>ABCD** complications
  - penetrating chest injury
  - flail chest
  - tension pneumothorax
  - cardiac tamponade
  - surgical emphysema
  - blast injury to the lungs.
- Correct **<C>ABC** problems.
- Undertake a **TIME-CRITICAL** transfer to a major trauma centre.[1]
- Major unmanageable **A** and **B** problems should be transferred to the nearest trauma unit.
- Provide a pre-alert using ATMIST.
- Continue patient management en route.
- Minimise ongoing heat loss in patients with major trauma.
- A load-and-go approach is particularly important with penetrating injuries, unless enhanced care support is likely to arrive before the patient can reach an appropriate hospital. Consider a rendezvous en route if appropriate. Reducing time to hospital with a safe transfer should be the priority.

Specifically Consider
  - rib fractures
  - tension pneumothorax
  - open chest wounds
  - flail chest
  - surgical emphysema
  - cardiac tamponade
  - impaling objects.
  - blast injury

- Refer to Tables 4.25 to 4.30 for the assessment and management of these conditions/situations.

Non-time-critical Patient

- Undertake a secondary survey.

Monitor SpO$_2$ and Assess for Signs of Hypoxia

- Administer high levels of supplemental oxygen until the vital signs are normal, then aim for a target saturation within the range of 94–98% (refer to **Oxygen**).

Assess Breathing Adequacy, Respiratory Rate, Effort and Volume and Equality of Air Entry

- Consider assisted ventilation at a rate of 12–20 respirations per minute if any of the following are present:
  - SpO$_2$ <90% on high levels of supplemental oxygen.
  - Respiratory rate is <10 per minute.
  - Inadequate chest expansion.

NB Exercise caution, as any positive pressure ventilation may increase the size of a pneumothorax and create tension.

Monitor Nasal EtCO$_2$

- EtCO$_2$ presents an immediate picture of the patient's condition.

Monitor Heart Rate and Rhythm

- Attach ECG monitor.

Thoracic Trauma

TABLE 4.24 – ASSESSMENT and MANAGEMENT of: Thoracic Trauma (continued)

Consider IV Fluids
- Obtain IV access.
- Refer to **Intravascular Fluid Therapy in Adults** and **Intravascular Fluid Therapy in Children** – **DO NOT** delay on scene.

Consider Tranexamic Acid
- Tranexamic acid should be given where appropriate as early as possible (refer to **Tranexamic acid**).

Assess Patient's Level of Pain
- Refer to **Pain Management in Adults and Children**.

NB Avoid Entonox in a patient with a suspected pneumothorax as there is a significant risk of enlarging a pneumothorax.

NB Adequate analgesia may improve ventilation by allowing better chest wall movement, but high doses of opiates may induce respiratory depression. Careful titration of doses is therefore required. Refer to **Pain Management in Adults and Children**.

Specific Considerations for Children

Assess and manage as above but consider:
- Children can have severe internal chest injuries with minimal or no external evidence of chest injuries.
- Children show signs of shock late due to good compensatory mechanisms.
- Always consider multiple injuries in children with rib fractures, as this suggests a significant mechanism of injury and isolated chest injuries are rare in children.
- Consider non-accidental injury.

Additional Information
- Chest trauma is treated with difficulty in the field, and prolonged treatment before transportation is **NOT** indicated if significant chest injury is suspected.
- Open chest wounds – seal the wound with a proprietary dressing with a valve, but if none are available use a three-sided dressing.
- Specifically consider the need for thoracic surgery intervention.
- Impaling objects – handle and move the patient very carefully, address bleeding with appropriate treatment. Avoid rigid fixation or handling of the impaling object where possible. **NB** Be vigilant – the patient may try to remove the object and this could be used as a weapon.
- Remember any stab or bullet wound to the chest, abdomen or back may penetrate the heart.
- Patients with significant chest trauma may often insist on sitting upright and this is especially common in patients with diaphragmatic injury who may get extremely breathless when lying down. In this instance, the patient is best managed sitting in a position in which they are most comfortable. Consider assessment of the c-spine and document rationale for management.
- In the rare incident of gunshot/stab injury to personnel wearing protection vests (e.g. ballistic and stab), these may protect from penetrating injury. However, serious underlying blunt trauma (e.g. pulmonary contusion) may be caused to the thorax and penetrating injury can still occur; a thorough examination of the front, back and sides of the chest should still be undertaken. Be aware that blast injury may still occur where a protective vest has been worn.
- **NEVER UNDERESTIMATE THESE INJURIES.** There is a strong link between serious blunt chest wall injury and thoracic spine injury. Maintain a high index of suspicion.

TABLE 4.25 – ASSESSMENT and MANAGEMENT of: Flail Chest

- Flail chest is usually the result of a significant blunt chest injury, causing two or more rib fractures in two or more places resulting in a segment of the rib cage becoming detached from the rest of the chest wall. A sternal flail can also occur where the ribs or costal cartilages are fractured on both sides of the chest. This results in a flail segment that moves independently of the rest of the chest during respiration, leading to inadequate ventilation. The ensuing pulmonary insufficiency is caused by three pathophysiological processes:

(continued)

Thoracic Trauma

TABLE 4.25 – ASSESSMENT and MANAGEMENT of: Flail Chest *(continued)*

1 The negative pressure required for effective ventilation is disrupted due to the paradoxical motion of the flail segment.
 2 The underlying pulmonary contusion, which causes haemorrhage and oedema of the lung. This can cause worsening hypoxia which may not be detectable for several hours.
 3 The pain associated with the multiple rib fractures will result in a degree of hypoventilation.
  – Small flail segments may not be detectable.
  – Large flail segments may impair ventilation considerably as a result of pain alone.

Assess for Signs of a Flail Chest   • Flail segments should not be immobilised and efforts to maintain ventilation are the priority.   • Allow the patient to sit in a position in which they are most comfortable, rather than trying to make them lie flat on a scoop stretcher.   **NB** Traditionally, the patient has been turned onto the affected side for transportation, but this CANNOT be achieved on a scoop stretcher.
Assess the Patient's Level of Pain   • Consider the need for analgesia (if indicated, refer to **Pain Management in Adults and Children**).
Transfer   • Undertake a **TIME-CRITICAL** transfer to a major trauma centre, unless the patient needs an immediate lifesaving intervention, in which case initially transfer to nearest trauma unit.   • Provide a pre-alert using ATMIST.   • Continue patient management en route.

TABLE 4.26 – ASSESSMENT and MANAGEMENT of: Rib Fractures
• Rib fractures are very common in patients with trauma, particularly in older adults who may sustain these in a fall from a standing height. Although a single rib fracture is painful and may cause significant immobility, multiple rib fractures are associated with underlying lung injuries, most commonly pulmonary contusions; the signs and symptoms of which may not appear for several hours e.g. hypoxia.   • Multiple rib fractures, displaced rib fractures, or those with underlying concomitant injuries may require inpatient monitoring for respiratory failure or surgical correction. Older patients with rib fractures tend to have a higher mortality rate than younger patients and may require closer monitoring. Even relatively minor chest injuries can lead to internal injury to the lung, collapse (pneumothorax), effusions (blood or fluid) and rarely hernias.
Assess   • Rib fractures may also be associated with other injuries such as spinal trauma (e.g. vertebral fractures) or abdominal injuries (e.g. splenic injury) which should also be examined for.   • As part of the primary survey the chest wall should be carefully palpated to detect rib fractures which may be splinted by intercostal muscle spasm.   Symptoms of rib fracture include: • Pain in chest area, particularly when patient breathes in or coughs.   • Shortness of breath is usually caused by the chest wall pain not allowing deep breaths to be taken, occasionally it can be associated with the lung collapsing after the injury; a build-up of fluid in the chest cavity (effusion) or a developing chest infection (pneumonia).   • Swelling or tenderness around the affected ribs.   • Sometimes bruising on the skin.   • Patient feeling or hearing a crack.
Transfer   • Older adults and patients with suspected multiple rib fractures should be assessed in hospital to allow for a period of respiratory monitoring and consideration of supplementary oxygen, possibly CT imaging and potentially rib fixation. Many of these patients also require support from specialist therapists as part of a prolonged recovery.   • Ribs cannot be easily splinted or supported like other bones, so they're usually left to heal naturally.

Thoracic Trauma

TABLE 4.26 – ASSESSMENT and MANAGEMENT of: Rib Fractures *(continued)*

Patients may be considered for home management if:
- Patient has access to analgesia
- No significant co-morbidities/frailty/other injuries
- Younger age
- Suspected simple/single (not multiple) rib fracture

Patients not conveyed must be given safety netting advice to include:
- Regularly take slow, deep breaths to help clear mucus from lungs
- Use painkillers, such as paracetamol, consider the need for stronger analgesia if required
- Hold an ice pack (or a bag of frozen peas) wrapped in a tea towel to the affected ribs regularly in the first few days to bring down swelling
- Breathe normally and cough when they need to – to help clear mucus from lungs to prevent chest infections
- Hold a pillow against chest if they need to cough
- Walk around and sometimes move shoulders to help them breathe and clear mucus from their lungs
- Try to sleep more upright for the first few nights

Patient advised to seek help if:
- worsening breathlessness
- abdominal or shoulder pain
- coughing up blood
- pain had not improved within a few weeks/chest pain getting worse
- coughing up yellow or green mucus
- a very high temperature or feeling hot and shivery

TABLE 4.27 – ASSESSMENT and MANAGEMENT of: Tension Pneumothorax

- This progressively builds up air under tension on the affected side, collapsing that lung and putting increasing pressure on the heart and great vessels and the opposite lung. Decreased venous return is significantly affected by compression of the vessels, especially the inferior vena cava, as the mediastinum is pushed towards the contralateral side. Coughing and shouting can make a situation worse. If this air is not released externally, the heart will be unable to fill and the other lung will no longer be able to ventilate, inducing cardiac arrest.
- Tension pneumothorax is most often related to penetrating trauma, but can arise spontaneously from blunt or crushing injuries to the chest and as the result of a blast wave. This will present rapidly with an increase in breathlessness and extreme respiratory distress (respiratory rate often >30 breaths per minute). Subsequently the patient may deteriorate and the breathing rate may rapidly slow to <10 breaths per minute before the patient arrests.
- Signs and symptoms:
    - The chest on the affected side may appear to be moving poorly or not at all.
    - At the same time, the affected chest wall may appear to be over-expanded (hyperexpansion).
    - Air entry will be greatly reduced or absent on the affected side.
    - In the absence of shock, the neck veins may become distended.
    - Later, the trachea and apex beat of the heart may become displaced away from the side of the pneumothorax, and cyanosis and breathlessness may appear.
    - Hyperresonance may be present.
    - Surgical emphysema may be present and evolve rapidly.
    - Occasionally, the patient will only present with rapidly deteriorating respiratory distress.
    - The patient may present appear shocked as a result of decreased cardiac output.
    - Patients are usually tachycardic and hypotensive.
- Ventilation of a patient with a chest injury is a common cause of tension pneumothorax in the pre-hospital setting. Forcing oxygenated air into the lung under positive pressure will progressively expand a small, undetected simple pneumothorax into a tension pneumothorax. This will take some minutes and may well be several minutes after ventilation has commenced. It is usually noticed by increasing back pressure during ventilation; either by the bag becoming harder to squeeze or the ventilator alarms sounding.

(continued)

Thoracic Trauma

TABLE 4.27 – ASSESSMENT and MANAGEMENT of: Tension Pneumothorax *(continued)*

Assess Breathing Adequacy, Respiratory Rate, Volume and Equality of Air Entry
- LOOK, FEEL, PERCUSS, and AUSCULTATE.
- View both sides of the chest and check they are moving; auscultate to ensure air entry is present and percuss on both sides.
- **Only perform needle thoracocentesis in a patient if there is haemodynamic instability, hypotension, or increasing respiratory compromise.**
- If a tension pneumothorax is likely, decompress rapidly by needle thoracocentesis.
- If the patient requires positive pressure ventilation, an open thoracostomy should be performed if an appropriately skilled practitioner is available

Observe the Patient for Signs of Recurrence of the Tension Pneumothorax
- If the procedure was unsuccessful, repeat the needle thoracocentesis.
- Consider the use of a longer needle in patients with a thicker chest wall, following your organisation's guidelines.

Transfer
- Undertake a **TIME-CRITICAL** transfer to a major trauma centre, unless the patient needs an immediate lifesaving intervention, in which case transfer to nearest trauma unit.
- Provide a pre-alert using ATMIST.

NB Needle thoracocentesis may not always decompress tension pneumothoraces in large patients. In such cases, a thoracostomy with or without a chest drain may need to be performed. This needs to be done either in hospital or by appropriately trained practitioners.

TABLE 4.28 – ASSESSMENT and MANAGEMENT of: Cardiac Tamponade

The heart is enclosed in a tough, non-elastic membrane called the pericardium. A potential space exists between the pericardium and the heart itself. If a penetrating wound injures the heart, the blood may flow under pressure into the pericardial space. As the pericardium cannot expand, a leak of as little as 20–30 ml of blood can cause compression of the heart. This decreases cardiac output and causes tachycardia and hypotension. Further compression reduces cardiac output and cardiac arrest may occur.

Assess for Signs of Cardiac Tamponade
- Signs of hypovolaemic shock, tachycardia and hypotension, accompanied by blunt or penetrating chest trauma, may be an indication of cardiac tamponade.
- Note the presence of distended neck veins and muffled heart sounds when listening with a stethoscope.
- Cardiac tamponade is a **TIME-CRITICAL**, **LIFE-THREATENING** condition that requires rapid surgical intervention, resulting in an open chest operation to evacuate the compressing blood.
- DO NOT delay on scene inserting cannulae or commencing fluid therapy.

Transfer
- Undertake a **TIME-CRITICAL** transfer to a major trauma centre, unless the patient needs an immediate lifesaving intervention, in which case transfer to nearest trauma unit.
- Provide a pre-alert using ATMIST.
- Re-assess **ABC** en route to hospital.

NB Needle pericardiocentesis is not recommended in the pre-hospital setting, as it is rarely successful, has significant complications and may delays definitive care

Thoracic Trauma

TABLE 4.29 – ASSESSMENT and MANAGEMENT of: Surgical Emphysema
• Surgical emphysema is the build-up of air withing the subcutaneous tissues that produces swelling of the chest wall, neck and face, with a cracking feeling under the fingers when the skin is pressed. This indicates an air leak from within the chest as a result of a pneumothorax, a ruptured large airway or a fractured larynx. • Normally it requires no specific treatment, but it does indicate potentially SERIOUS underlying chest trauma. Sometimes the surgical emphysema might be extensive and cause the patient to swell up. Where the emphysema is progressively increasing, look for a possible underlying tension pneumothorax. • In some cases, surgical emphysema may become so severe as to tighten the overlying skin and restrict chest movement. A tension pneumothorax must be excluded as above. If there is no improvement, the patient must be transferred to hospital as soon as possible.
Assess for Signs of Surgical Emphysema
• Assess for swelling of the chest wall, neck and face, with a cracking feeling under the fingers when the skin is pressed.
Consider Possible Underlying Tension Pneumothorax
• Refer to tension pneumothorax guidance above.

TABLE 4.30 – ASSESSMENT and MANAGEMENT of: Blast Injury
• Blast injury is caused by three mechanisms: 1 Rupture of air-filled organs. 2 Missiled debris. 3 Contact injury. • Although rare in survivors, strongly suspect a blast lung injury if the patient is suffering from tympanic injury. However, the absence of a tympanic injury DOES NOT exclude lung injury. **NB** Being shielded from blast debris DOES NOT exclude lung injury.
Assess for Blast Injury
• Pre-hospital management is supportive with oxygen, pain relief and careful monitoring whilst transferring to an MTC.

KEY POINTS!

Thoracic Trauma

- **Thoracic injury is commonly associated with hypoxia, either from impaired ventilation or secondary to hypovolaemia from massive bleeding into the chest (haemathorax) or major vessel disruption.**
- **Older adults may sustain multiple rib fractures from a fall from standing height and may need close monitoring in hospital due to increased risk of death.**
- **Count the respiratory rate and look for asymmetrical chest movement.**
- **Pulse oximetry and end-tidal CO_2 monitoring must be used as this will assist in recognising hypoxia/inadequate ventilation.**
- **The mechanism of injury is an important guide to the likelihood of significant thoracic injury.**
- **Blunt trauma to the sternum may induce myocardial contusion, which may result in ECG rhythm disturbances and cardiac failure.**
- **ECG monitoring should be used.**
- **Impaled objects – handle and move the patient very carefully, address bleeding with appropriate treatment. Avoid rigid fixation or handling of the impaling object where possible.**
- **Do not probe or explore penetrating injuries.**
- **Tranexamic acid should be given where appropriate as early as possible (refer to Tranexamic acid).**

Thoracic Trauma

Bibliography

1. National Institute for Health and Clinical Excellence. *Fractures (Complex): Assessment and Management* (NG37). London: NICE, 2016. Available from: https://www.nice.org.uk/guidance/ng37.

2. National Institute for Health and Clinical Excellence. *Fractures (Non-complex): Assessment and Management* (NG38). London: NICE, 2016. Available from: https://www.nice.org.uk/guidance/ng38.

3. National Institute for Health and Clinical Excellence. *Major Trauma: Assessment and Initial Management* (NG39). London: NICE, 2016. Available from: https://www.nice.org.uk/guidance/ng39.

4. National Institute for Health and Clinical Excellence. *Major Trauma: Service Delivery* (NG40). London: NICE, 2016. Available from: https://www.nice.org.uk/guidance/ng40.

5. National Institute for Health and Clinical Excellence. *Spinal Injury: Assessment and Initial Management* (NG41). London: NICE, 2016. Available from: https://www.nice.org.uk/guidance/ng41.

6. National Institute for Health and Clinical Excellence. *When to Suspect Child Maltreatment* (CG89). London: NICE, 2009. Available from: https://www.nice.org.uk/guidance/cg89.

7. Revell M, Porter K, Greaves I. Fluid resuscitation in pre-hospital trauma care: a consensus view. *Emergency Medicine Journal* 2002, 19(6): 494–498.

8. Lee C, Revell M, Porter K, Steyn R. The pre-hospital management of chest injuries: a consensus statement. Faculty of Pre-hospital Care, Royal College of Surgeons of Edinburgh. *Emergency Medicine Journal* 2007, 24(3): 220–224.

9. Warner KJ, Copass MK, Bulger EM. Paramedic use of needle thoracostomy in the pre-hospital environment. *Prehospital Emergency Care* 2008, 12(2): 162–168.

10. Waydhas C, Sauerland S. Pre-hospital pleural decompression and chest tube placement after blunt trauma: a systematic review. *Resuscitation* 2007, 72(1): 11–25.

11. Dretzke J, Sandercock J, Bayliss S, Burls A. Clinical effectiveness and cost effectiveness of pre-hospital intravenous fluids in trauma patients. *Health Technology Assessment* 2004, 8(23).

12. Turner J, Nicholl J, Webber L, Cox H, Dixon S, Yates D. A randomised controlled trial of prehospital intravenous fluid replacement therapy in serious trauma. *Health Technology Assessment* 2000, 4(31).

13. Stern SA. Low-volume fluid resuscitation for presumed hemorrhagic shock: helpful or harmful? *Current Opinion in Critical Care* 2001, 7(6): 422–430.

14. Pepe PE, Mosesso VNJ, Falk JL. Pre-hospital fluid resuscitation of the patient with major trauma. *Prehospital Emergency Care* 2002, 6(1): 81–91.

15. Borman JB, Aharonson-Daniel L, Savitsky B, Peleg K. Unilateral flail chest is seldom a lethal injury. *Emergency Medicine Journal* 2006, 23(12): 903–905.

16. BMJ Evidence Centre. Best Practice: Cardiac tamponade. 2012. Available from: http://bestpractice.bmj.com/best-practice/monograph/459.html.

17. Fitzgerald M, Spencer J, Johnson F, Marasco S, Atkin C, Kossmann T. Definitive management of acute cardiac tamponade secondary to blunt trauma. *Emergency Medicine Australasia* 2005, 17(5–6): 494–499.

18. Friend KD. Prehospital recognition of tension pneumothorax. *Prehospital Emergency Care* 2000, 4(1): 75–77.

19. Massarutti D, Trillo G, Berlot G, Tomasini A, Bacer B, D'Orlando L et al. Simple thoracostomy in pre-hospital trauma management is safe and effective: a 2-year experience by helicopter emergency medical crews. *European Journal of Emergency Medicine* 2006, 13(5): 276–280.

20. Wanek S, Mayberry JC. Blunt thoracic trauma: flail chest, pulmonary contusion, and blast injury. *Critical Care Clinics* 2004, 20(1): 71–81.

21. Blaivas M. Inadequate needle thoracostomy rate in the pre-hospital setting for presumed pneumothorax. *Journal of Ultrasound in Medicine* 2010, 29(9): 1285–1289.

22. Clinical Guidelines for Major Incidents and Mass casualty events (NHSE 2020) which may be of interest to clinicians wanting more in-formation – there are excellent graphics on blast, ballistic, crush and blunt injuries. https://www.england.nhs.uk/wp-content/uploads/2018/12/B0128-clinical-guidelines-for-use-in-a-major-incident-v2-2020.pdf

5

Maternity Care

Maternity Care (including Obstetric Emergencies Overview)

1. Introduction

- Any woman of childbearing age may be pregnant and, unless there is a history of hysterectomy, there must be a high index of suspicion that any abdominal pain or vaginal bleeding may be pregnancy related.
- There are three fundamental rules which must be followed at all times when dealing with a pregnant woman:
  a Resuscitation of the mother must always be the priority.
  b Manual uterine displacement must be employed to support resuscitation measures beyond 20 weeks gestation (refer to Figure 5.1).
  c Hypotension is a late sign of shock. Any signs of hypovolaemia during pregnancy are likely to indicate a 35% (class III) blood loss and must be treated aggressively.
- In cases of maternal cardiac arrest requiring ongoing cardiopulmonary resuscitation, pre-alert the nearest emergency department with an obstetric unit when transferring a pregnant woman in order to ensure preparedness for an emergency perimortem caesarean section (resuscitative hysterotomy), as delivering the fetus may be required to help facilitate maternal resuscitation. **NB Effective resuscitation of the mother will provide effective resuscitation of the fetus.**
- When ambulance clinicians attend an obstetric emergency, they should work as a team, with the paramedics responsible and accountable for the care of the woman or newborn baby and delegating tasks accordingly.
- When a midwife is present, paramedics and midwife must work together to act in the best interests of the woman and the newborn baby. If both mother and newborn baby are clinically well, the midwife is the responsible and accountable clinician. The midwife can either discharge the ambulance clinicians, and arrange for ongoing community midwifery care, or arrange conveyance of the mother and baby together to the most appropriate facility.
- In the event of a newborn requiring conveyance to hospital ahead of the mother, it may be preferable that the midwife remains on scene with the mother to manage the third stage of labour, assess for perineal trauma and manage any ongoing postpartum bleeding. Ambulance clinicians can manage ongoing care of the newborn, utilise the established communication channels and pre-alert the nearest emergency department (ED) where the baby can be assessed. The mother should be repatriated with the baby as soon as reasonably possible at the same location.
- The MBRRACE-UK annual report, *Saving Lives, Improving Mothers' Care,* reviews maternal deaths in the UK and produces recommendations relating to care provision. The report continues to show an overall decrease in the maternal death rate, which is currently 8.5 women per 100,000 maternities.
  - Maternal deaths from direct causes – complication from the pregnancy itself such as bleeding, blood clots, pre-eclampsia or infection – continue to decrease.
  - Maternal deaths from indirect causes – pre-existing conditions that are not direct pregnancy complications such as heart disease, epilepsy, mental health problems or cancer – remain high.
  - Deaths from mental health problems contribute to around a quarter of maternal deaths occurring between 6 weeks and 1 year after the end of pregnancy.
  - The focus of care must be upon establishing appropriate resuscitative measures, placing a pre-alert to the nearest emergency department with an obstetric unit attached, conveying the woman, with manual uterine displacement in place, and preparation for further assessment and treatment, including a perimortem caesarean section if necessary.
  - Effective communication is therefore essential to ensure clinical information being passed on is complete and relevant, utilising a structured communication tool.
- There is a three- to fourfold increased risk of myocardial infarction in pregnancy and the postpartum period.
- Pulmonary embolism is more common throughout pregnancy and the postpartum period.

2. Communication, Information-sharing and Consent

All women who are booked for maternity care should have access to their handheld maternity records. These will provide key information regarding medical history, previous and current pregnancies, obstetric problems as well as emergency contact details for care providers, including next of kin. Information within these notes may aid assessment during the primary and/or secondary survey. Maternity units may also have their own unique set of handheld records or, in some cases, these may be electronic.

2.1 Human Factors and 'SBAR'

- Clinical performance and safe practice can be enhanced through an understanding of the effects of teamwork, tasks, equipment, workspace, culture and organisation on human behaviour and abilities, and application of that knowledge within a clinical setting.
- Increasing situational awareness and the utilisation of communication tools (such

Maternity Care (including Obstetric Emergencies Overview)

as Situation, Background, Assessment, Recommendation, or SBAR) help to promote a safer environment and enhance clinical outcome. Awareness of what is happening around us can be reduced during emergency situations, and this can lead to near misses and/or adverse outcomes. It is therefore essential that enhanced communication skills, and an environment in which open and honest lines of communication are encouraged, are maintained.

- The use of the SBAR communication tool is recommended in order to optimise transfer of information between members of the multi-disciplinary team. The purpose of SBAR is to promote the accurate and unambiguous handover of clinically relevant information regarding care of the mother from one healthcare professional to another. The use of SBAR has the potential to improve the speed at which care is delivered and the quality of care that is ultimately provided.

2.2 Consent

- Consent to treatment is the principle that a person must give permission before they receive any type of medical treatment, investigation or examination. Consent from a woman is needed regardless of the procedure. For consent to be valid it must be voluntary and informed, and the person consenting must have the capacity to make the decision. If an adult has the capacity to make a voluntary and informed decision to consent to or refuse a particular treatment, their decision must be respected. This is still the case even if refusing treatment would result in their death, or the death of their unborn child.
- The provision of adequate information should include the benefits and risks of the proposed treatments, and alternative treatments. If the woman is not offered as much information as they reasonably need to make their decision, and in a format that they can understand, their consent will not be valid.
- Consent can be given verbally or in writing and should be given to the healthcare professional directly responsible for the person's current treatment.
- Consent may not be necessary if a person requires emergency treatment that is believed to be in their best interests or to save their life and they are unable to give consent due to a lack of capacity caused by either mental or physical complications.
- During obstetrics emergencies, it may be necessary to perform intimate examination in order to perform lifesaving treatment. Practitioners must, where possible, obtain informed consent and offer the woman a chaperone. All examinations must be carried out sensitively, with respect for the woman's dignity, cultural beliefs and confidentiality.

3. Physiological Changes in Pregnancy

Pregnancy is timed from the FIRST day of the last period and may last up to or in excess of 42 weeks. The pregnancy is divided into three trimesters (1–12 weeks +6 days, 13–25 weeks +6 days and 26 weeks+). These terms are used with the maternity handheld records; they will also detail the lead clinician, i.e. the midwife or the obstetrician who is responsible for the provision of maternity care with the woman.

There are a multitude of physiological and anatomical changes during pregnancy that may influence the management of the pregnant woman. These changes include:

- Cardiovascular system:
  - An increase in cardiac output by 20–30% in the first 10 weeks of pregnancy.
  - An increase in average maternal heart rate by 10–15 beats per minute.
  - A decrease in systolic and diastolic blood pressure by an average of 10–15 mmHg due to a reduction in peripheral resistance caused by an increase in the release of the progesterone hormone.
  - The weight of the gravid uterus, from 20 weeks gestation onwards, may cause compression of the inferior vena cava (IVC), reducing venous return and lowering cardiac output by up to 40% for women in the supine position; this in turn can reduce blood pressure. The combined effects of the gravid uterus on the IVC and a reduction in peripheral vascular resistance can result in the woman feeling faint or having an episode of syncope, resolved by repositioning her onto her side or into the lateral position.
  - An increase in blood volume through haemodilution (increasing by 45%) occurs together with a small increase in the numbers of red blood cells. The disproportionate increase of plasma volume relative to the increase in red cell mass can lead to a 'physiological' anaemia in the mother from around 27 weeks gestation. Due to the increase in blood volume, a pregnant woman is able to tolerate greater blood loss before showing signs of hypovolaemia. This compensation is at the expense of shunting blood away from the uterus and placenta, and therefore the fetus.
- Respiratory system:
  - An increase in breathing rate and effort and a decrease in vital capacity, as the gravid uterus enlarges and the diaphragm becomes splinted. Some shortness of breath is common during pregnancy but early consideration should be given to the need for increased oxygen requirements.

Maternity Care (including Obstetric Emergencies Overview)

- Oedema of the larynx may compromise airway management, and a collapsed pregnant woman requires the airway to be secured as soon as possible.
- Placement of an advanced airway (supraglottic airway or endotracheal intubation) should be secured in all maternal cardiac arrests (refer to **Maternal Resuscitation**).

• Gastrointestinal system:
- An increase in the acidity of the stomach contents, due to a delay in gastric emptying, caused by progesterone-like effects of the placental hormones.
- Relaxation of the cardiac sphincter makes regurgitation of the stomach contents more likely (refer to **Maternal Resuscitation**).
- Nausea and vomiting can occur around 4–8 weeks' gestation and continue until around 14–16 weeks. Some severe cases may continue for a longer period of time and can result in rapid dehydration (hyperemesis gravidarum) requiring hospital assessment/admission.

4. Appropriate Destination for Conveyance

• The choice of destination to convey mother and baby should be carefully considered and in line with local procedures. Ideally, mother and baby should be conveyed to the same destination. There are units, commonly called birth/birthing centres (or 'standalone' maternity units), that are solely midwifery-led. Be aware that there are no resident obstetricians, anaesthetists or neonatologists with the capability of performing advanced obstetric or neonatal interventions at these sites. There are no specialist neonatal facilities.

• The mother may choose to book for delivery at a particular unit and request to be conveyed there; however, in an emergency situation this may have to be overridden:
- The nearest emergency department (ED) will be the appropriate destination when there is cardiac arrest, major airway problems, ongoing eclamptic convulsions and severe uncontrollable bleeding.
- In other obstetric emergencies (e.g. shoulder dystocia, mild to moderate bleeding etc.), transfer to the nearest full obstetric unit (i.e. not a birthing centre or 'standalone' midwifery unit) will be appropriate. Remember that in many cases a full obstetric unit will be co-located with an ED but this may not always be the case.

• Careful consideration should always be given to the most appropriate destination in each case. Also consider carefully the accessibility of a unit (e.g. out-of-hours, locked doors, corridors and lifts). In line with local procedures, pre-alert arrangements and telephone numbers should be agreed and readily available to clinicians.

5. Assessment

• Critical assessment of the mother is vital in all situations, while fetal assessment may be indirect based on reported movements etc. Refer to Table 5.1.
• Neonatal assessment is also important, with particular reference to respiratory effort and maintaining body temperature. Refer to Table 5.3.

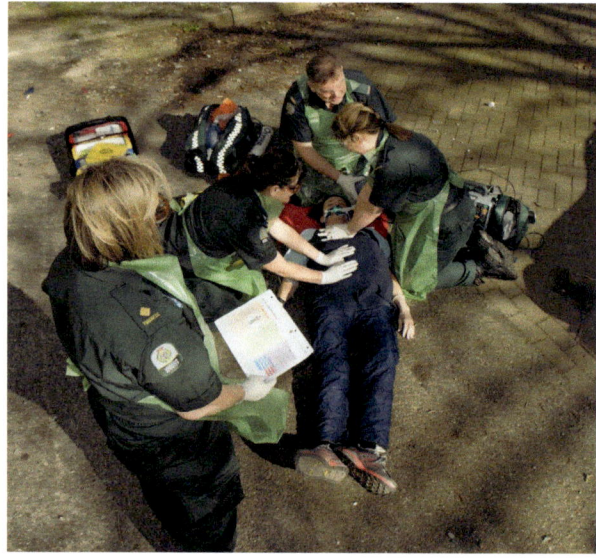

Figure 5.1 – Manual uterine displacement.

Maternity Care (including Obstetric Emergencies Overview)

TABLE 5.1 – Assessment
Quickly assess the woman and scene as you approach
Primary survey
• It is important to remember that a woman and, if born, a newborn baby will require assessment.
• The aim of the primary survey is to identify any life-threatening problems, to enable management to be commenced as rapidly as possible and to reach an early determination of the priority for transportation. The primary survey should be modified in the presence of actual or suspected trauma (refer to **Trauma in Pregnancy**).
Massive external haemorrhage

• Is there a significant volume of blood visible without the need to disturb the woman's clothing?
  – Is the woman's clothing soaked?
  – Is there blood on the floor?
  – Are there a number of blood-soaked sanitary pads visible?

Airway
• Is the woman able to talk? (Yes = airway open.) If the woman is unresponsive, refer to **Maternal Resuscitation**. • Is the woman making unusual sounds? (Gurgling = fluid in the airway.) • Is suction required? (Snoring = tongue/swelling/foreign body obstruction.) • If the woman is unresponsive, open the airway and look in – suction for fluids, manually remove solid obstructions.
Breathing
• Document respiratory rate and effort. (Are accessory muscles being used?) • Obtain oxygen saturations as soon as possible. • Auscultate for added sounds. (Wheeze = bronchospasm; coarse sounds = pulmonary oedema.) • Assess for the presence of cyanosis. • Give oxygen based on clinical findings (not routinely).
Circulation
• Document radial pulse rate and volume. (Capillary refill time (CRT) may be used if neither the radial nor carotid pulses can be palpated.) • Assess skin colour and temperature (to touch). (Pallor, or cold or damp skin = an adrenergic reaction to shock.) • Record blood pressure – the systolic is most valuable if you suspect shock. • Visually inspect the abdominal area and gently palpate for evidence of internal bleeding (indicated by tenderness, guarding, firm woody uterus).
Disability
• Perform an CVPU assessment of consciousness level (is the woman Conscious, responding only to Voice, responding only to Pain or Unresponsive?). • Document the woman's posture (normal, convulsing (state whether focal or generalised), abnormal flexion, abnormal extension). • Document pupil size and reaction (PEaRL – pupils equal and reacting to light).

(continued)

Maternity Care (including Obstetric Emergencies Overview)

TABLE 5.1 – Assessment *(continued)*

Expose/environment/evaluate

- Ensuring consent is obtained, expose and visually inspect the vaginal opening:
  - Is there any evidence of bleeding?
  - Can you see a presenting part of the baby?
  - Is there a prolapsed loop of cord?
  - Have the waters broken (and if so, is the amniotic fluid clear, blood stained or meconium stained)?
  - Does the perineum bulge with each contraction?
  - If the baby has been born, is there a significant perineal tear? Can you see any part of the uterus?
- Assess the environment:
  - Is the woman or baby at risk of hypothermia?
  - Are the surroundings as clean as you can make them if the birth is imminent?
  - Are there other children present (this may indicate a previous pregnancy with live birth)?
- Evaluate how time-critical the woman's condition is.
  - If it is time-critical, decide immediately whether you need to transport the woman urgently to the nearest hospital with an obstetric unit, placing a pre-alert as early as reasonably possible. (The nearest hospital with an obstetric unit may not be the booked unit; however, it is critical the woman has rapid obstetric or appropriate assessment at the nearest facility.)
  - If the birth is imminent, remember to call for additional clinical resource. This may include midwifery assistance, which may be deployed from the nearest maternity unit to the location of the woman (follow local guidelines).

Fundus

- Make a quick assessment of fundal height: a fundus at the level of the umbilicus equates to a gestation of approximately 22 weeks. By definition, if fundal height is below the umbilicus, this suggests that if the fetus is delivered, it is unlikely to survive.

Fetal activity

- Ask the mother when she last felt her baby move.

Secondary survey

- If any critical problems are identified during the primary survey, the secondary survey should only be undertaken when any <C>**ABCDE** problems have been addressed and transportation to definitive care has commenced (if this is possible). In many cases where critical problems are identified, it will not be possible or appropriate to undertake a secondary survey in the pre-hospital phase of care.

6. Prehospital Maternity Decision Tool

- This tool should always be used when attending patients who are **pregnant** (or suspected pregnant) **regardless of gestation** or up to **4 weeks post birth/pregnancy loss/termination**.
- Use to aid immediate clinical decision making on scene.
- NEWS2 should not be used in this group of patients.
- This tool should be used alongside clinical judgement and other relevant JRCALC guidelines and local guidance/pathways.
- If there is a high concern (red flag), do not ask for remote advice from the maternity service, act on the concern(s) using the table below.
- Clinical parameters are relevant during labour and should not be dismissed due to pain. If birth is imminent, use the Imminent Birth guideline. Patient observations should be recorded during and after birth, any concerns highlighted by the tool should be acted on as soon as possible following birth.

	High concern (red flag)	Medium concern (amber flag)	Low concern (green flag)	Medium concern (amber flag)	High concern (red flag)
Respiratory Rate (/min)	Below 7	7-8	9-21	22-24	Above 24
SpO₂ (%)	Below 93% / Any oxygen requirement	93-94%	95-100%	N/A	N/A
Pulse Rate (bpm) during pregnancy and up to 48 hours after birth	Below 63	63-70	71-112	113-121	Above 121
Pulse Rate from 48 hours AFTER birth (bpm)	Below 51	51-57	58-98	99-107	Above 107
Systolic Blood Pressure (mmHg)	Below 94	94-100	101-135	136-144	Above 144
Diastolic Blood Pressure (mmHg)	Below 57	57-61	62-88	89-96	Above 96
Temperature (°C)	Less than 35.7	35.7 - 36.1	36.2-37.2	37.3 - 37.4	Above 37.4

	Low concern (green flag)	Medium concern (amber flag)	High concern (red flag)
Consciousness	Alert	N/A	CVPU (Confusion, Voice, Pain, Unresponsive)
Cardiac symptoms	Nil	N/A	Chest Pain / Shortness of Breath / Palpitations
Abdominal pain	Nil	N/A	Any pain or contractions 20-37* weeks / Constant abdominal pain (any gestation) / Uterine scar pain (any gestation)
Symptoms prior to 20 weeks pregnant	Nil	Abdominal pain	Shoulder tip pain / One sided abdominal pain / Suspected/confirmed ectopic pregnancy
PV blood loss LESS THAN 20 weeks pregnant	Nil	Maternity sanitary pad not fully soaked within 30 minutes	Maternity sanitary pad fully soaked (50mls) within 30 minutes
PV loss MORE THAN 20 weeks pregnant	Sticky, pink, mucous plug (show) more than 37 weeks pregnant / Clear fluid over 36+6 weeks	Sticky, pink, mucous plug (show) less than 37 weeks pregnant	Any fresh red bleeding / Blood stained amniotic fluid / Meconium stained waters (green) / Offensive smelling waters / Waters broken under 37 weeks
Postnatal PV blood loss (lochia)	Maternity sanitary pad not fully soaked within 30 minutes	N/A	Maternity sanitary pad fully soaked (50mls) within 30 minutes / Offensive smelling lochia
Pre-eclampsia/Eclampsia symptoms (MORE THAN 20 weeks gestation)	Nil	Nausea & vomiting / Malaise	Severe pain just below ribs / Severe headache / Problems with vision / Sudden oedema to feet/hands/face
Neurological	Asymptomatic	N/A	Active seizure / History of recent seizure
Appearance	Looks well	N/A	Looks unwell

*Labour pain 37 weeks and above - refer to Imminent Birth guideline

Additional concerns:
Patient/family/clinician concerns should always be considered as part of the clinical assessment
Language barriers – use interpreting services and convey to hospital for further assessment
If recommended transfer is declined – escalate according to local protocols
Mental capacity concerns – follow local protocols
Safeguarding concerns – follow local protocols

	All green flags	1 amber flag	Any red flag or 2 amber flags
Action required	Follow local guidance.	Transport to hospital via ambulance.	Requires time critical assessment in hospital. Minimise time on scene.
Emergency pre-alert	No	Consider	Follow local guidance.
Destination	Follow local guidance.	Follow local guidance.	Follow local guidance.
Ongoing observations	If conveying continue regular observation	Observations every 15 minutes	Observations every 5 minutes

Figure 5.2 – Prehospital Maternity Decision Tool

Maternity Care (including Obstetric Emergencies Overview)

7. At-risk Ethnic Groups

7.1 At-risk Ethnic Groups and Maternal Deaths[6]

- The Mother and Babies: Reducing Risk through Audits and Confidential Enquiries across the UK (MBRRACE-UK) *Saving Lives, Improving Mothers' Care* report was released in 2020. The data was produced from looking at maternal deaths from 2016 to 2018. This confidential enquiry found that Black women are four times more likely to die during pregnancy than White women. Mixed ethnicity women are three times more likely and Asian women are twice as likely as White women to die during childbirth.

- Due to ongoing globalisation and migration patterns, clinicians are increasingly attending patients from diverse cultural and/or ethnic minority backgrounds. According to the Office for National Statistics, approximately a quarter of women giving birth in the UK are from ethnic minority groups.

- Despite the publication of a number of national policy documents and local initiatives to improve childbirth experiences, previous work streams have highlighted disparities within ethnic minority groups which indicate this group of women have worse pregnancy and birth outcomes than White women.[8]

- Whilst it is not known what causes the increased risk of mortality, it is important that we are aware as out-of-hospital clinicians of the increased risk to patients from ethnic minority groups.

- Communication is an important part of clinical assessment and history-taking. It is important that as clinicians we remember to remove barriers to communication; this may mean using simplified language. Translation services should also be utilised if English is not the patient's first language; family members translating can inadvertently lead to misinformation being given to the clinician. For example, women may struggle to describe in full their symptoms, extent of bleeding or mental health issues, due to cultural beliefs associated with those conditions, especially if partners or family members are acting as translators.

- As clinicians, it is important to recognise that in some cultures there may not be specific psychological terms directly associated with stress/anxiety/depression, or the patient may not be familiar with these terms, and so the patient will often describe having physical symptoms such as palpitations or shortness of breath.

- Once you have provided clinical advice, it is important to check the patient and family have fully understood the information provided. It is important to document specific condition worsening advice and potential consequences to the patient if they choose not to adhere to the advice provided.

- Women unfamiliar with the NHS, even if English-speaking, may not be familiar with the systems and processes in place to support their pregnancy, especially as other countries will often have very different healthcare models. For instance,

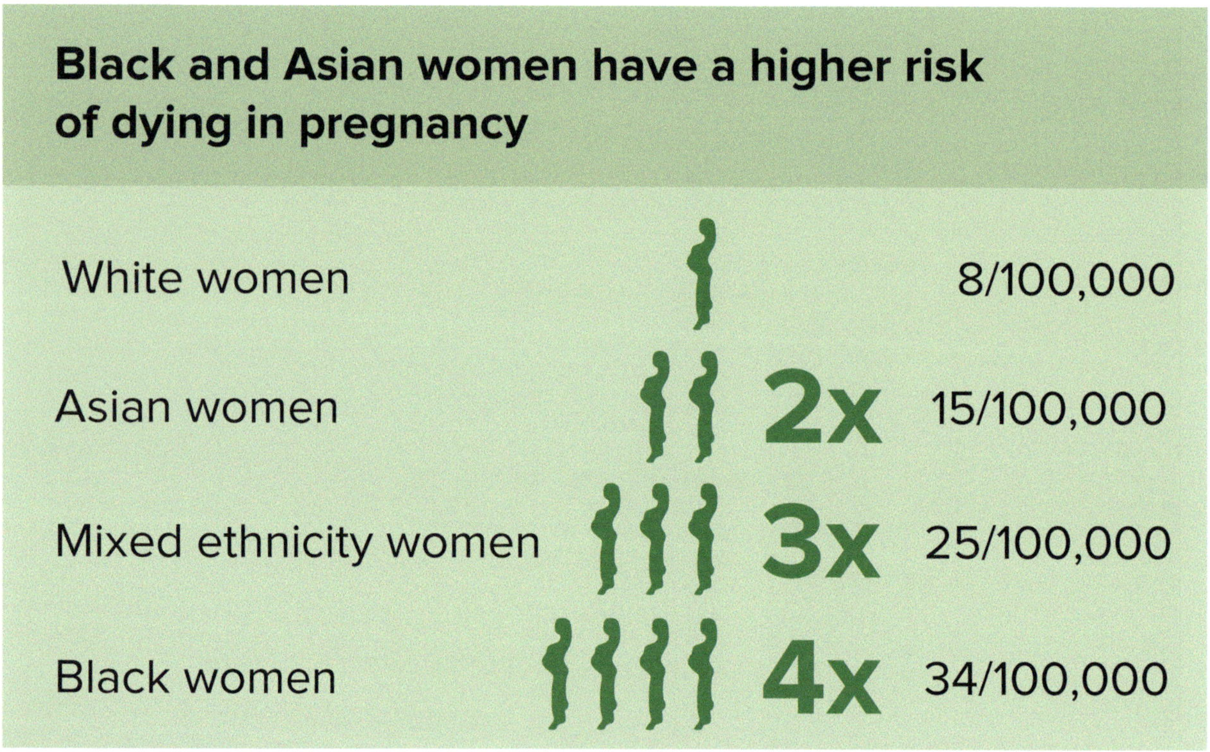

Black and Asian women have a higher risk of dying in pregnancy

White women		8/100,000
Asian women	2x	15/100,000
Mixed ethnicity women	3x	25/100,000
Black women	4x	34/100,000

Figure 5.3 – Maternal deaths.

Maternity Care (including Obstetric Emergencies Overview)

there may be a cultural expectation from the woman or partner that an all-female ambulance crew attend their emergency. It is important that clinicians respect the patient's wishes and explore the reason for this request. It is important to emphasise that delaying accessing definitive care or further assessment could directly impact the heath of baby and mother. However, in some situations it may be considered appropriate to request a second resource for a woman to attend.

7.2 Pain Management

- Pain management is a particularly important consideration in ethnic minority women, as 'the interpretation of pain behaviours is heavily dependent on the social and cultural learnings and understandings of both the person in pain and the observer'.[9]

- Women may present pain symptoms differently; some women may choose to be quiet, and others more vocal and expressive. As clinicians it is important that we recognise that people do respond differently to pain and it is equally important to remember our own responses to pain are not the only way pain can be expressed.

- Therefore, it is important to assess pain and manage it in accordance with what the patient is telling you. Refer to **Pain Management in Adults and Children**.

8. Special Cases

8.1 Concealment, Denial and Unknown Pregnancy

Occasionally, pregnancy may be concealed or denied until labour commences. In both situations there may have been no antenatal care. There may be mental health, drug and alcohol abuse issues and safeguarding concerns (refer to **Safeguarding Adults at Risk** and **Safeguarding Children**). Some concealed pregnancies may result in the birth occurring in secret. Ambulance clinicians must be aware that the consequences of concealment and denial can have a fatal outcome for both mother and baby.

- Always consider the possibility of pregnancy in any woman of reproductive age. Ask the woman if she could be pregnant. Be aware that a young teenage girl may not want to answer such a question in the presence of a parent or carer.

- It may be necessary to visually inspect and palpate the abdomen for evidence of a pregnant uterus.

- If labour is confirmed and birth is not imminent, determine if there is any relevant medical history. Transfer the woman to the nearest obstetric unit.

- Determine how many weeks pregnant the woman is if known, or by visual inspection of the abdomen; where the uterine fundus is at the level of the umbilicus the pregnancy may be more than 22 weeks.

- If birth is in progress or occurs en route, request a midwife from the nearest maternity unit, if this service is available, and additional resources and prepare for birth (see Table 5.1).

- Once the baby has been born and assessed, transfer mother and baby to the nearest obstetric unit.

- If the woman is unaware of pregnancy, consider birth/miscarriage in any significant per vaginum (PV) bleed that cannot be explained.

- Pre-alert the nearest obstetric unit or nearest ED with an obstetric unit, dependent upon considered gestation.

- Discuss at handover any safeguarding concerns identified when attending the home environment (refer to **Safeguarding Adults at Risk** and **Safeguarding Children**).

8.2 Female Genital Mutilation (FGM)

Overview

- Female Genital Mutilation (FGM), also known as 'female genital cutting', 'female genital mutilation/cutting' or 'cutting', refers to all procedures involving partial or total removal of the external female genitalia or other injury to the female genital organs for non-medical reasons.

- FGM is predominately practised in Africa, Yemen, Iraqi Kurdistan and parts of Malaysia and Indonesia.

- The World Health Organization classifies FGM into four categories (see Table 5.2).

TABLE 5.2 – Four Categories of Female Genital Mutilation (FGM) and Management

Type 1	Partial or total removal of the clitoris and/or the prepuce (clitoridectomy).
Type 2	Partial or total removal of the clitoris and labia minora, with or without excision of the labia majora (excision).
Type 3	Narrowing of the vaginal orifice with creation of a covering seal by cutting and appositioning the labia minora and/or the labia majora, with or without excision of the clitoris (infibulation).
Type 4	All other harmful procedures to the female genitalia for non-medical purposes, for example: pricking, piercing, incising, scraping and cauterisation.

Maternity Care (including Obstetric Emergencies Overview)

- FGM is practised for a variety of complex reasons. FGM has no health benefits but does increase health risks. FGM is a human rights violation and a form of child abuse. Refer to **Safeguarding Adults at Risk** and **Safeguarding Children** for guidance regarding when, as healthcare professionals, we are legally required to report and raise safeguarding under the Female Genital Mutilation Act 2003.[10]

FGM and Pregnancy

- Women with FGM are more prone to complications in pregnancy. Clinicians should be aware of the increased likelihood of urinary tract infections and other infections. During childbirth, women may also encounter additional complications; the more severe the type of FGM, the higher the risk. Infibulated (Type 3) cannot give birth unassisted; the scar tissue covering the introitus does not allow for the passage of the baby without de-fibulation.

- FGM can cause prolonged labour, increase the risk of a newborn requiring resuscitation and additional support and can cause significant vaginal and perineal tearing resulting in a postpartum haemorrhage.

- As clinicians, it is important to recognise a woman who has had FGM. Women may not know FGM has taken place, therefore clear communication and history-taking are important. Women who have been identified as having had FGM, if known

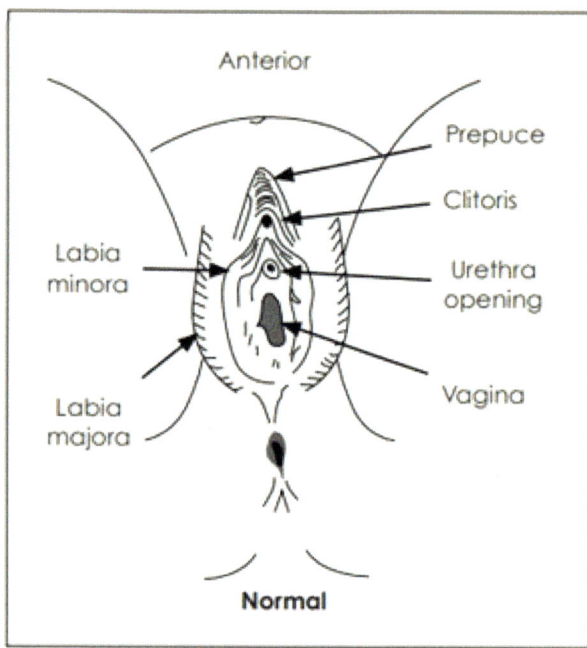
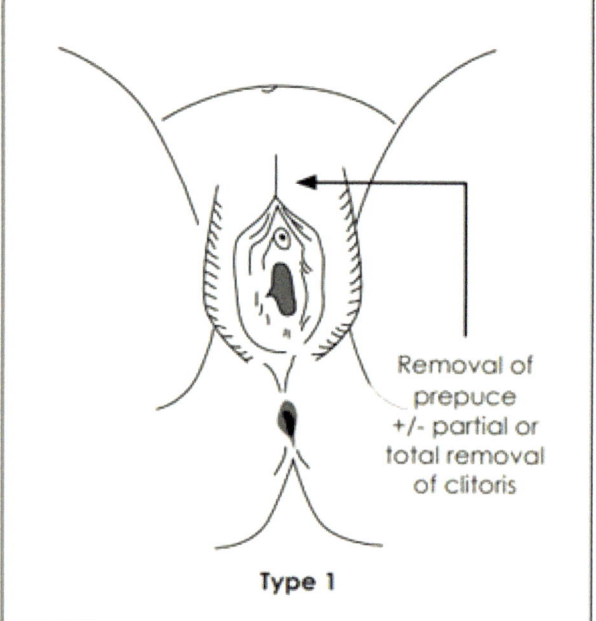
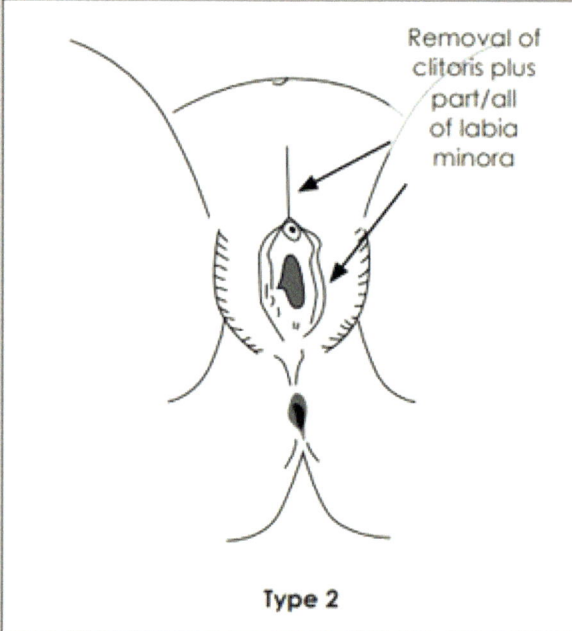
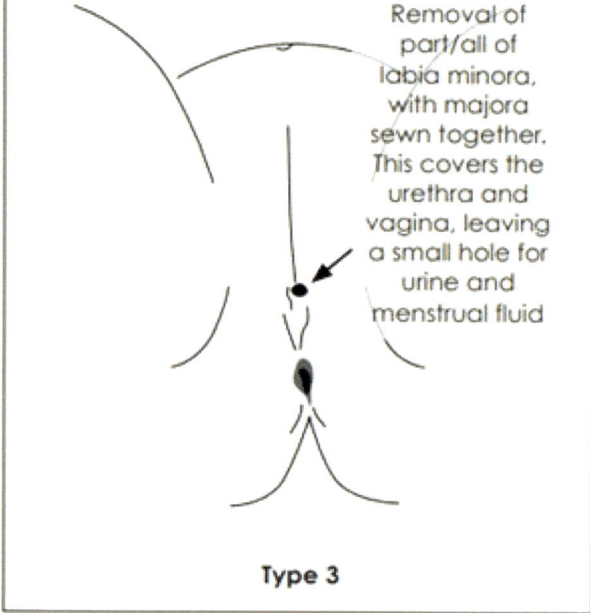

Figure 5.4 – The four FGM categories.

Maternity Care (including Obstetric Emergencies Overview)

to maternity services, will have their hospital care booked with a consultant obstetrician and a specialist midwife team. If de-fibulation is required, this may have been undertaken antenatally or be planned for once labour begins.

- If the woman has not received antenatal care and evidence of FGM is present, early recognition and early conveyance of these women is required. If birth is imminent, where possible rapid conveyance to the nearest obstetric unit must be undertaken. Further resources should be considered, but do not delay transportation. An information call should be placed to the identified obstetric unit informing them of the concerns and the estimated arrival time.

Obstetric Problems

- The narrowed vaginal opening in FGM types 3 and 4 is likely to cause obstetric problems.
- These include:
  – prolonged and obstructed labour
  – an increase in the number of episiotomies and perineal tears
  – a high caesarean section rate caused by the difficulty in fetal monitoring and lack of adequately trained obstetric staff
  – an increased incidence of postpartum haemorrhage
  – an increased incidence of postnatal wound infection
  – maternal death from obstructed labour and postpartum haemorrhage
  – increased stillbirth and early neonatal death rates
  – increased neonatal morbidity from hypoxia and brain damage.

9. Glossary of Terms

Table 5.3 provides a glossary of abbreviations specific to maternity and commonly used in handheld maternity records.

TABLE 5.3 – Glossary

ABBREVIATION	TERM
LMP	Last menstrual period.
EDD	Estimated date of delivery – the timing of the pregnancy is written in the notes in the format e.g. 12/40, i.e. 12 weeks have elapsed out of the 40-week pregnancy.
T or D	Term or expected date of delivery/pregnancy, therefore T+3 or D+3 in the notes is 3 days over the EDD.
CEPH	Cephalic (head).
BR	Breech.
G	Gravida, the number of times a woman has been pregnant (including the present pregnancy), e.g. G3.
P	Parity, the number of times a woman has given birth to a liveborn or stillborn baby, e.g. P3. A second figure implies previous miscarriages or terminations, e.g. P3+2.

KEY POINTS!

Maternity Care (including Obstetric Emergencies Overview)

- Any woman of childbearing age MAY be pregnant.
- Due to the increase in blood volume, the pregnant woman is able to tolerate greater blood or plasma loss before showing signs of hypovolaemia; establish large bore (16G) IV cannulation early.
- A pregnant woman in cardiac arrest must ideally be conveyed with left manual uterine displacement after 20 weeks' gestation (maintaining left lateral tilt is an alternative but may be more difficult to use effectively in the pre-hospital care environment).
- The use of SBAR to communicate between ambulance clinicians and maternity clinicians can optimise transfer of information.
- Black women are four times more likely to die during pregnancy than White women. Women with a mixed ethnic background are three times more likely than White women to die in childbirth, and Asian women are twice as likely.

Maternity Care (including Obstetric Emergencies Overview)

Bibliography

1. Knight M, Tuffnell D, Kenyon S, Shakespeare J, Gray R, Kurinczuk JJ (eds) on behalf of MBRRACE-UK. *Saving Lives, Improving Mothers' Care – Surveillance of maternal deaths in the UK 2011–13 and lessons learned to inform maternity care from the UK and Ireland Confidential Enquiries into Maternal Deaths and Morbidity 2009–13*. Oxford: National Perinatal Epidemiology Unit, University of Oxford, 2015.

2. Catchpole (2010), cited in Department of Health. *Human Factors Reference Group Interim Report, 1 March 2012*. National Quality Board, 2012. Available from: http://www.england.nhs.uk/ourwork/part-rel/nqb/ag-min/.

3. Woollard M, Hinshaw K, Simpson H, Wieteska S (eds) *Pre-hospital Obstetric Emergency Training*. Oxford: Wiley-Blackwell, 2009.

4. Centre for Maternal and Child Enquiries. Saving mothers' lives: reviewing maternal deaths to make motherhood safer: 2006–2008. *BJOG: An International Journal of Obstetrics & Gynaecology* 2011, 118 (suppl. 1).

5. Bourjeily G, Paidas M, Khalil H, Rosene-Montella K, Rodger M. Pulmonary embolism in pregnancy. *The Lancet* 2010, 375(9713): 500–512.

6. Race Disparity Unit, UK Government. *Writing About Ethnicity*. Available from: https://www.ethnicity-facts-figures.service.gov.uk/style-guide/writing-about-ethnicity.

7. Knight M, Bunch K, Tuffnell D, Shakespeare J et al. (eds). MBRRACE (2020) *Saving Lives, Improving Mothers' Care: Lessons learned to inform maternity care from the UK and Ireland Confidential Enquiries into Maternal Deaths and Morbidity 2016–18*. Available from: https://www.npeu.ox.ac.uk/assets/downloads/mbrrace-uk/reports/maternal-report-2020/MBRRACE- UK_Maternal_Report_Dec_2020_v10_ONLINE_VERSION_1404.pdf.

8. Henderson J, Gao H, Redshaw M (2013) Experiencing maternity care: the care received and perceptions of women from different ethnic groups. *BMC Pregnancy and Childbirth* 13. DOI: 10.1186/1471-2393-13-196.

9. Whitburn LY, Jones LE, Davey M, McDonald S (2019) The nature of labour pain: an updated review of the literature. *Women and Birth: Journal of The Australian College of Midwives* 32(1). DOI: 10.1016/j.wombi.2018.03.004.

10. Royal College of Obstetricians & Gynaecologists (2015) *Female Genital Mutilation and Its Management*. Available from: https://www.rcog.org.uk/globalassets/documents/guidelines/gtg-53-fgm.pdf.

Breech Birth

1. Incidence, Risk Factors and Diagnosis

Vaginal breech birth is where the feet or buttocks of the baby are born first, rather than the baby's head.

Breech presentation affects 3–4% of births at term (37 weeks onwards) and is more common in pre-term births.[10]

At onset of labour, breech presentation may be known and reported by the patient or recorded in the pregnancy notes.

In some circumstances, breech presentation is unknown and the first diagnosis is made when the buttocks/ or feet are visible and advancing through the vaginal entrance (introitus)

Breech birth can cause fetal hypoxia. It is therefore likely that the baby will require resuscitation (refer to **Newborn Life Support**).

Breech babies are more likely to pass meconium during the birth. Presence of meconium does not require different management, but should be documented and handed over to maternity/neonatal staff.

Cord prolapse is more common with a breech presentation (refer to **Imminent Birth**).

Consider seeking senior clinical support and advice as per local procedures. This should not cause further delay on scene if the appropriate decision is to transport rapidly.

Some manoeuvres specific to breech birth require the clinician to insert their fingers into the woman's vagina. It is essential for clinicians to gain appropriate consent prior to performing these manoeuvres.

2. When to Leave Scene Immediately

Rapid transport to the nearest hospital with an obstetric service with a pre-alert message (or alternative as agreed locally), is indicated in the following circumstances:

- Buttocks are not visible or not advancing through the vaginal entrance.
- A foot or feet are presenting, with the buttocks not immediately visible (i.e. 'footling' breech).
- A hand or arm is presenting, with the buttocks not immediately visible.

In these circumstances – do not progress with vaginal delivery on scene.

Footling breech

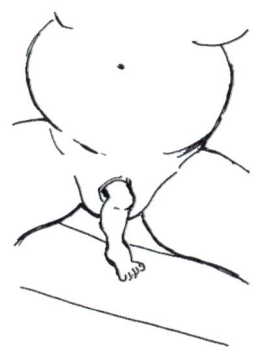
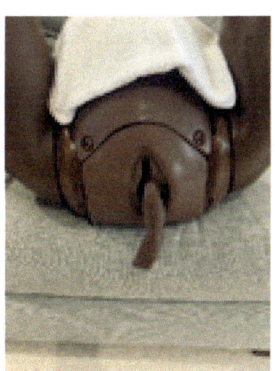

Breech Birth: Imminent/Not Imminent (See Figure 5.5)	
Birth imminent:	**Birth is not imminent:**
The buttocks are visible and advancing through the vaginal entrance (introitus). Clinicians should prepare for birth on scene.	Buttocks are not visible or not advancing through the vaginal entrance
	A foot or feet are presenting, with the buttocks not immediately visible (i.e. 'footling' breech)
	A hand or arm is presenting, with the buttocks not immediately visible

Breech Birth

3. Maternal Position During Imminent Breech Birth

Encourage the woman to adopt an upright position (e.g. edge of the bed/sofa, all-fours, squatting or kneeling) as gravity may assist with the birth. Ensure the woman's bottom is off the floor so there is room for the baby to hang down as it descends.

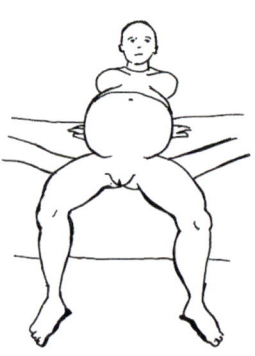 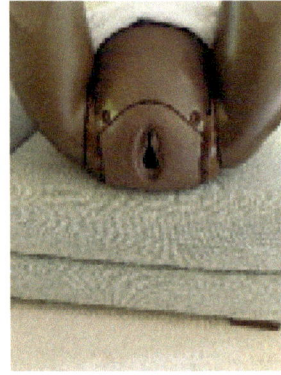

Mother in semi recumbent position

Note: In the Semi-recumbent position keep the mother's buttocks AT THE EDGE of the bed, to allow the baby to 'hang down' under its own weight during delivery.

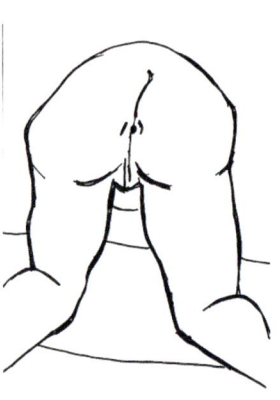 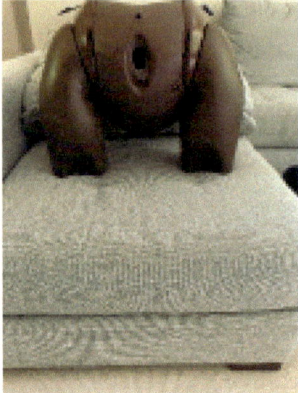

Mother in 'all fours' position

Note: In the all fours position the baby can be delivered on the floor or bed/sofa but ensure a safe landing area.

4. Timing

When both buttocks are born, the risk of hypoxia is increased as the baby descends further through the birth canal. The woman should be encouraged to push continuously from this point (do not wait for contractions as they may slow down/stop). It is crucial that clinicians recognise (and act upon) any delay in progress.

Allocate someone to start a timer. Where possible, this person should not be involved in the clinical management to aid situational awareness.

➜ When both buttocks are born, start the timer – **the baby must be fully born within 5 minutes**

Delay of more than 5 minutes from the birth of the buttocks is associated with poor outcomes. If manoeuvres do not result in the birth of the baby within this time rapid transport to hospital is indicated.

All timings and any manoeuvres performed should be clearly documented.

5. 'Hand Poised' Approach and When to Intervene

Many breech births occur spontaneously without intervention. Use a 'hands poised' approach, with a clinician ready to assist if required. If delay **does** occur at any stage, the baby is at high risk of hypoxia and manoeuvres must be used to assist the birth (see Figure 5.5).

Clinicians should observe the condition of the baby throughout the birth.

If any of the following signs are seen, it may indicate fetal hypoxia so manoeuvres should be performed:

- The parts of the baby that are born are not well perfused, and have no movement or tone
- White, empty umbilical cord
- No movement/absent tone

6. Handling the Baby

If the baby descends spontaneously with maternal pushing, there is no need to handle the baby. Do not touch the umbilical cord as this can cause vasospasm, interrupting the flow of oxygen to the baby.

The baby may need to be rotated to restore normal breech birth physiology and to be able to release the arms. If you do need to rotate the baby, hold the baby over the bony prominences of its' pelvis. **Do not apply pressure to the soft tissue of the abdomen** as this may cause internal injury. **Do not pull** on the baby as this may further complicate the birth and/or cause injury. **Rotate in the direction that keeps the baby's back facing towards the mother's abdomen** (i.e. 'bum to tum') – see images below:

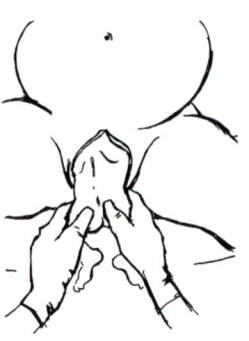 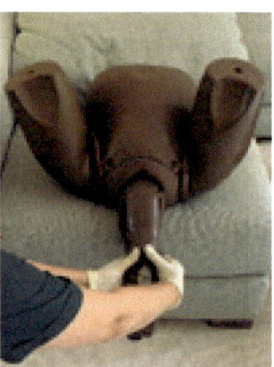

Mother in semi-recumbent – baby's back must face towards you.

Breech Birth

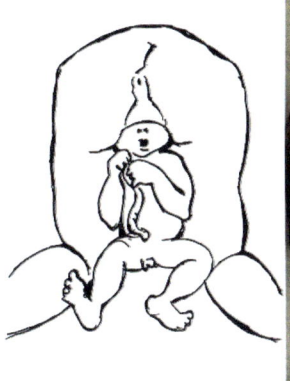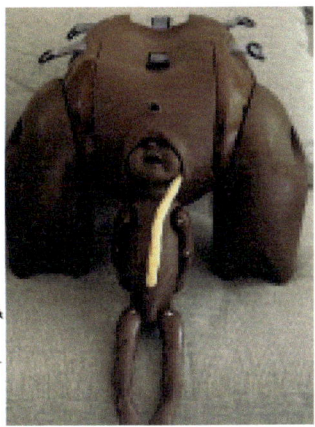

Mother in all fours – baby's abdomen must face towards you.

7. Transfer and Conveyance of the Woman

The woman should be advised to walk, with support, to the ambulance. Do not use a carry chair if the birth is in progress (i.e. when buttocks, legs or umbilical cord are externally visible).

If you have to move rapidly when a breech baby is partly delivered, consider using a towel or blanket as a sling to support parts of the baby that are exposed.

Once in the ambulance, position the woman on her side on the stretcher, with her upper leg supported with a folded pillow (or similar) to reduce pressure on the presenting parts.

Right or left lateral position is suitable for conveyance.[4,15] Positioning the woman on her right side offers reassurance, allowing her to face the clinician or relative:

- Continually observe for signs of imminent birth en route.
- Provide early pre-alert message to the nearest obstetric unit and request maternity staff to meet the ambulance at an agreed entrance to avoid any delays.
- Stop the vehicle to assist with the birth if required.

8. Management of Breech Birth (See Figure 5.5)

Recognition of Breech Birth imminent: remain on scene

If baby's buttocks are visible and advancing through the vaginal entrance (introitus), birth is imminent so remain on scene.

Prepare:

Request help and additional resources as per local procedures.

Prepare for newborn life support (**Newborn Life Support**).

Assist the woman into a position that aids gravity (position at the edge of the bed/trolley or all-fours).

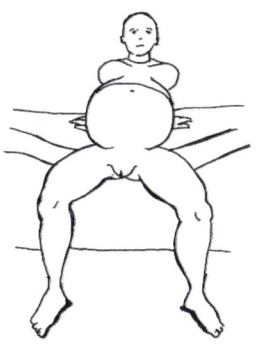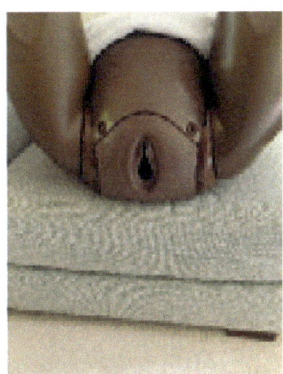

Mother semi-recumbent – vagina over edge of bed to allow birth.

Note: In the Semi-recumbent position keep the mother's buttocks AT THE EDGE of the bed, to allow the baby to 'hang down' under its own weight during delivery

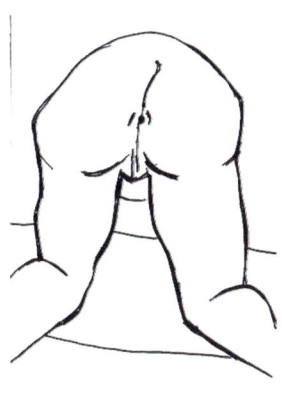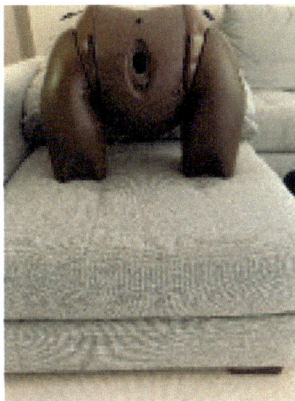

Mother in all fours – baby will birth onto bed

Note: In the all fours position the baby can be delivered on the floor or bed/sofa but ensure a safe landing area.

Clinical Management

Observe for descent of the baby, have your hands 'poised' ready to intervene or to receive the baby.

When the widest part of the buttocks are born, start a timer and encourage continuous pushing (do not wait for contractions or expect them to continue). The baby must be born within the next 5 minutes. Look for continuous progress – if descent stops use appropriate manoeuvres and be prepared to initiate rapid transfer if these are unsuccessful.

Once the legs are born, **ensure the baby's back faces the woman's abdomen** (i.e. 'tum to bum'). Do not pull on the baby or touch the cord. Look for continuous progress and descent.

Breech Birth

9. Legs Delayed

If the legs are delayed:

Apply gentle pressure behind the baby's knees to release the legs – see Figure 5.5. Look for continuous progress and descent.

10. Arms Delayed

If the arms are delayed:

When the scapula (shoulder blade) is seen – the elbows/arms should now be visible. When the baby's elbow is visible:

- Hook your finger into the antecubital fossa (inside the elbow) and draw the arm down and deliver alongside the baby's body. Do this for both sides to release the arms.
- If you cannot see the arms, you will need to rotate the baby to bring the arms into view.
- Place your hands around the baby's pelvis.
- Rotate the baby until the shoulder is uppermost.
- If the arm is not delivered, place your finger into the vagina (gain consent first) finding the axilla and feel down the humerus until you reach the elbow.
- Place your finger into the antecubital fossa (inside the elbow) and complete delivery as described above.
- If the second arm does not then deliver, rotate the baby in the other direction and repeat.
- Once both arms are released, rotate the baby to face in the correct direction – see images below:

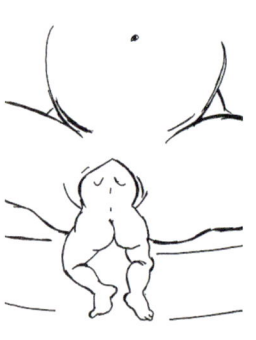 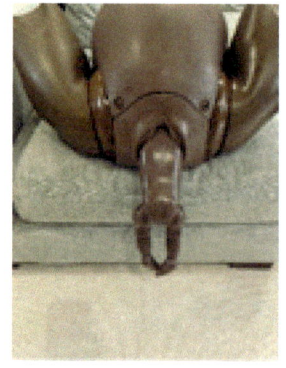

Mother semi-recumbent – baby's back must face towards you

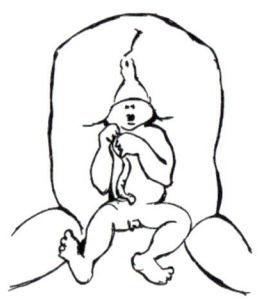 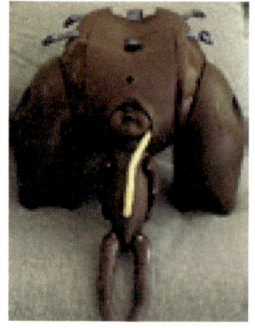

Mother in all fours – baby's abdomen must face towards you

11. Head Delayed

If head is delayed and the mother is in a semi recumbent position:

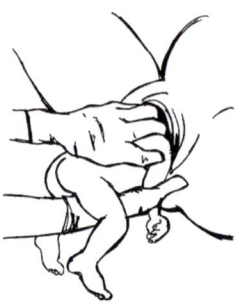 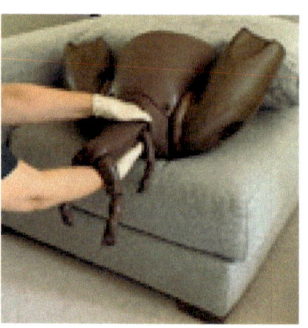

Baby's back should face towards you (see image above)

- Place one hand through the baby's legs to support baby's body along your arm, inserting the fingers into the woman's vagina.
- Place your two fingers on to the baby's cheekbones – avoid mouth and eyes.
- With the other hand, insert your fingers into the vagina (with mothers consent) along the nape of the baby's neck and apply firm pressure to the back of the baby's head to bring the chin toward the chest. Apply pressure with both hands at the same time to flex the baby's head.
- Raise the baby upward to lift through the curve of the pelvis to deliver the baby.

If the head is delayed and mother is in all fours position:

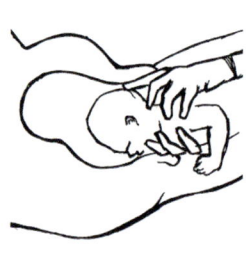 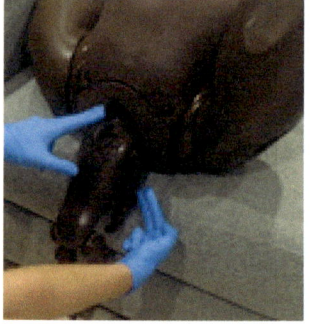

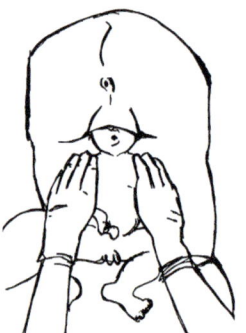 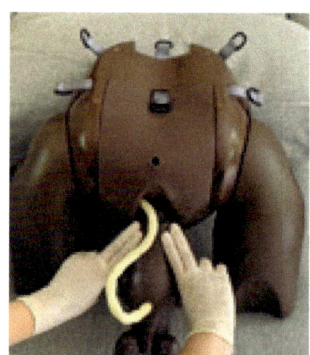

Baby's abdomen should face towards you.

- Place your hands against the front of the baby's shoulders and apply gentle pressure to flex the baby's head forward as it's born (i.e. apply a 'shoulder press' – see image below):

Breech Birth

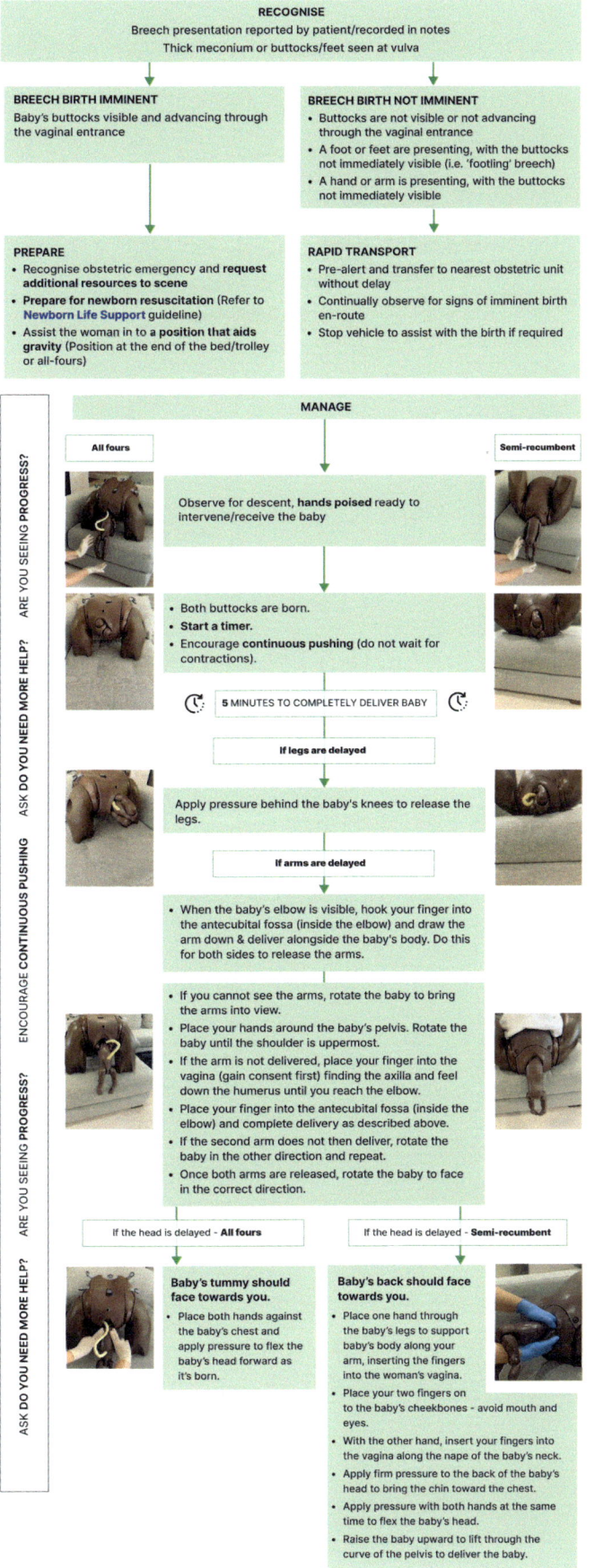

Figure 5.5 – Management of breech birth.

Breech Birth

References

1. Azria E et al. Factors associated with adverse perinatal outcomes for term breech fetuses with planned vaginal delivery. *American Journal of Obstetrics and Gynecology* 2012, 207(4). doi:10.1016/j.ajog.2012.08.027.

2. Azria E et al. Neonatal mortality and long-term outcome of infants born between 27 and 32 weeks of gestational age in breech presentation: The EPIPAGE Cohort Study. *PLOS ONE* 2016, 11(1). doi:10.1371/journal.pone.0145768.

3. Bogner G. et al. Breech delivery in the all fours position: A prospective observational comparative study with Classic Assistance. *Journal of Perinatal Medicine* 2014, 43(6): 707–713. doi:10.1515/jpm-2014-0048.

4. Carbonne B et al. Maternal position during labor: effects on fetal oxygen saturation measured by pulse oximetry. *Obstetrics & Gynecology* 1996, 88(5): 797–800. DOI: 10.1016/0029-7844(96)00298-0

5. Doyle NM et al. Outcomes of term vaginal breech delivery. *American Journal of Perinatology* 2005, 22(06): 325–328. doi:10.1055/s-2005-871530.

6. Hofmeyr GJ and Kulier R. (2012) Expedited versus Conservative approaches for vaginal delivery in breech presentation. Cochrane Database of Systematic Reviews [Preprint]. doi:10.1002/14651858.cd000082.pub2.

7. Louwen F et al. Does breech delivery in an upright position instead of on the back improve outcomes and avoid Cesareans? *International Journal of Gynecology & Obstetrics* 2017, 136(2): 151–161. doi:10.1002/ijgo.12033.

8. Pasupathy D et al. Time trend in the risk of delivery-related perinatal and neonatal death associated with breech presentation at term. *International Journal of Epidemiology* 2008, 38(2): 490–498. doi:10.1093/ije/dyn225.

9. Reitter A et al. Does pregnancy and/or shifting positions create more room in a woman's pelvis? *American Journal of Obstetrics and Gynecology* 2014, 211(6). doi:10.1016/j.ajog.2014.06.029.

10. Royal College of Obstetricians and Gynaecologists (RCOG) (2017) Management of breech presentation (green-top guideline no. 20B), RCOG. Available at: https://www.rcog.org.uk/guidance/browse-all-guidance/green-top-guidelines/management-of-breech-presentation-green-top-guideline-no-20b/(Accessed: 21 June 2023).

11. Spillane E, Walker S and McCourt C. (2021) Optimal time intervals for vaginal breech births: A case-control study [Preprint]. doi:10.22541/au.163251114.49455726/v1.

12. Su M et al. Factors associated with adverse perinatal outcome in the term breech trial. *American Journal of Obstetrics and Gynecology* 2003, 189(3): 740–745. doi:10.1067/s0002-9378(03)00822-6.

13. Walker S, Scamell M and Parker P. Principles of physiological breech birth practice: A Delphi Study. *Midwifery* 2016, 43: 1–6. doi:10.1016/j.midw.2016.09.003.

14. Walsh D. Physiological positions for breech birth. *International Journal of Childbirth* 2017, 7(2): 58–59. doi:10.1891/2156-5287.7.2.58.

15. Wu S et al. Effects of right lateral position on changes of fetal hemodynamics in late pregnancy. *J Ultrasound Med* 2023, 9999: 1–7. doi:10.1002/jum.16261

Care of the Newborn

1. Introduction

- The physiology of the fetus is fundamentally different from that of the newborn baby, with both structural and functional distinctions. The transition from intra- to extrauterine life is characterised by changes in circulatory pathways, initiation of ventilation and oxygenation via the lungs instead of the placenta and many changes in metabolism.

- The majority of term newborn babies complete this process in a rapid, smooth and organised fashion in the first few moments after birth. However, circulatory and pulmonary changes continue for up to 6 weeks after birth. Preterm babies or those with underlying disease may experience a delay in transition.

- Regular assessment is required to ensure that the baby who is experiencing problems with transition is recognised and appropriate interventions are initiated.

2. Thermal Care

- Thermoregulation is a crucial aspect of newborn care. Heat loss occurs by radiation, convection and conduction. A wet baby will also lose heat by evaporation. Babies have a large surface area relative to weight, so losses are proportionately greater. Preterm babies are at particular risk as their surface area to volume ratio is even larger. A cold baby has increased oxygen consumption and is at risk of hypoglycaemia and acidosis. For each degree below 36.5°C, the risk of mortality increases by 28%.

- Exclude any draughts, and heat the environment as much as possible. Babies should be thoroughly dried, a hat applied and be wrapped in towels or placed skin to skin. Use a pod or foil wrap if available. The ambulance should be kept well heated to prevent cooling during the transfer to hospital. Time with doors open or with the baby outside of a warm building/ambulance should be kept to a minimum (refer to **Newborn Life Support**).

- Normal newborn temperature is 36.5 to 37.5°C. Temperature recordings should be taken with an appropriately calibrated thermometer as soon as practical after birth, ideally at least once during transport and then on arrival at destination.

2.1 Skin to Skin

- Skin to skin (Figure 5.6) should be facilitated in line with the mother's wishes as long as mother and baby are well and the mother is able to hold the baby securely. If the mother is unwell, cold, shocked or does not want to do skin to skin, it can be done with a partner or other family member. Alternatively, the baby can be wrapped in towels.

- When skin to skin, the baby should be placed in a prone position with their head turned to one side so that the face is easily visible to the mother. The baby should have a hat on.

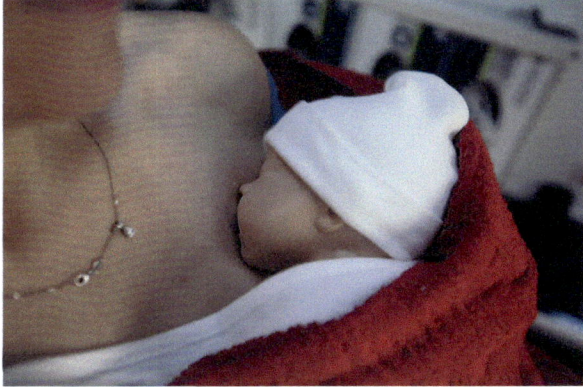

Figure 5.6 – Skin-to-skin care.
Note: The baby has a hat on and is covered with towel/blanket to keep warm. The position allows observation of airway and breathing efforts and may, if the situation permits, allow early breast feeding.

- Vigilant observation of the mother and baby should continue, with prompt removal of the baby if the health of mother or baby gives concern.

- Staff should have a conversation with the mother and family about recognising any changes in the baby's condition while the baby is skin to skin.

- The mother and baby will need regular observation by caregivers.

- Follow local guidance for any transport of the baby and mother to hospital.

3. Newborn Pathophysiology

3.1 Perinatal Hypoxia

- Perinatal hypoxia can occur for various reasons, including cord compression, cord prolapse, significant placental or umbilical bleeding. The presence of thick meconium may indicate an episode of perinatal hypoxia. Babies can cope with a degree of hypoxia at birth. However, severe perinatal hypoxia has a poor prognosis and is often associated with neurological deficit and cerebral palsy.

- Therapeutic hypothermia is used by neonatal teams in a hospital environment to reduce the risk of neurodevelopment impairment or death. It is not within the scope of pre-hospital clinicians to initiate therapeutic hypothermia. Unless carrying out an intra-facility transport and you have been specifically instructed to keep the ambulance cold, always heat the ambulance and follow the thermoregulation guidance above.

3.2 Hypoglycaemia

- Following birth, the baby undergoes a process of metabolic adaptation. Keeping the baby warm reduces metabolic stress and energy use to help maintain blood sugar. Breast milk is an ideal

Care of the Newborn

source of energy after birth, so if the baby is well and not requiring any support, women should be encouraged to breastfeed as soon as possible (within the first hour if possible/appropriate).

- The newborn baby has a relatively immature liver with limited glycogen stores. Therefore, hypoglycaemia must not be treated using intramuscular glucagon (glucagon works by stimulating the liver to convert glycogen into glucose). Buccal glucose 40% oral gel can be used (refer to **Glucose 40% Oral Gel**).

- Many hypoglycaemic babies are asymptomatic, so babies at risk of hypoglycaemia undergo blood sugar checks in the hospital setting.

- **Those at risk of hypoglycaemia include babies who are:**
  - preterm (<37 weeks)
  - small for gestational age
  - <2.5 kg at birth
  - in need of resuscitation at birth
  - born to diabetic mothers
  - born to mothers using beta-blockers (labetalol)
  - suffering from perinatal hypoxia
  - suffering from hypothermia
  - suffering from infection/sepsis.

- **Signs and symptoms of hypoglycaemia can be non-specific and include:**
  - jitteriness
  - irritability
  - lethargy
  - apnoeic episodes
  - convulsions
  - high-pitched cry
  - suspected or confirmed sepsis
  - hypotonia
  - cyanosis
  - altered level of consciousness
  - abnormal feeding behaviour (e.g. not waking for feeds after a period of feeding well).

- **Severe and prolonged hypoglycaemia can lead to convulsions and brain injury. Any baby at risk of hypoglycaemia or who has signs/symptoms of hypoglycaemia must be transported to hospital as soon as possible for further investigation and management. Seek advice/inform the receiving centre where the clinical situation is of concern.**

- While pre-hospital clinicians would not usually be expected to take blood glucose samples from a newborn baby, if the clinical situation or signs suggest possible hypoglycaemia or if advised to treat potential low blood sugar (despite feeding, or where feeds are not possible), then buccal glucose gel can be administered as per JRCALC guidance.

3.3 Neonatal Jaundice

- Jaundice refers to the yellow colouration of the skin, sclera and mucous membranes caused by a raised bilirubin level.

- Jaundice can be physiological or pathological. It is not possible to measure the level of bilirubin or to decipher between physiological or pathological causes in the pre-hospital environment.

- Babies at risk of pathological jaundice include:
  - those <38 weeks
  - those with a previous sibling with neonatal jaundice requiring phototherapy where there may be a familial predisposition, such as a blood group incompatibility
  - babies born by instrumental or caesarean birth where bruising has occurred
  - babies born to a diabetic mother.

- The following jaundiced babies justify transfer to hospital, as the cause may be pathological and the baby will require urgent investigation:
  - ≤24 hours of age
  - lethargic or sleepy
  - babies with chalky stools and/or dark urine
  - babies at risk of pathological jaundice
  - babies showing any other sign of being unwell
  - jaundice after 14 days.

- Jaundiced babies that do not meet the categories above still require a review by a midwife, GP, neonatal doctor or health visitor within the next 4 hours either in the community or in ED.

3.4 Preterm Birth

- Prematurity is defined as <37 weeks' gestation. Preterm infants are more likely to need increased assistance with thermoregulation, airway support and breathing, as well as feeding.

- Particularly at <32 weeks' gestation, spontaneous breathing will most likely be inadequate, as these babies have immature lungs which are deficient in surfactant.

- Pre-hospital clinicians should resuscitate/stabilise using the newborn life support algorithm and approach (refer to **Newborn Life Support**). Prioritise thermal care and airway breathing support. These babies require immediate transfer to the nearest emergency department (ED) with an obstetric unit.

- Premature babies can be born in good condition initially but may deteriorate quickly without support. Therefore, they require continuous monitoring, and clinicians need to be ready to intervene with airway/breathing support at any time.

Care of the Newborn

3.4.1 Extremely Preterm Birth: Survival-focused Care

- Ambulance clinicians may attend births at the extremes of prematurity and viability. These babies require intensive thermoregulation, ventilatory support and rapid transfer to hospital.
- **Newborn Life Support** outlines the survival-focused care that is justified in babies born above 22 weeks and those where the gestation is not known. Be aware that even an extremely premature neonate may initially have breathing efforts with a good heart rate but is at risk of rapid deterioration, so will require airway and breathing support with continuous monitoring until definitive care can be delivered in the hospital setting.
- Evident observed signs of life after birth include at least one of the following:
  - easily visible heartbeat seen through the chest wall,
  - visible pulsation of the cord,
  - breathing or sustained gasps and/or
  - definite movement of arms and legs.
- Short-lived fleeting reflex activity, including transient gasps, brief visible pulsation of the chest wall or brief twitches or involuntary muscle movement, can be observed in babies that have died shortly before birth, and so fleeting reflex activity observed only in the first minute after birth may not warrant classification as signs of life.[1]
- Where there are signs of life and the gestation is unknown, airway and breathing support with ventilation should be continued until a neonatal team can assess the gestation and weight of the baby. The team will then consider the ongoing management in the best interests of the baby and the family.
- Neither a midwife nor an ambulance clinician should discontinue resuscitative attempts; this decision should be made by the neonatal team.

3.4.2 Extremely Preterm Birth: Comfort Care

- Babies known to be born before 22 weeks are pre-viable and should receive comfort care. This includes:
  - Compassionately explaining to the parents that the baby has been born too early and will not be able to survive even with significant neonatal care. Express your condolences and sympathy. Give the parents time and be sensitive to the individualised needs of the parents.
  - Wrapping the baby sensitively and offering the baby to the parents to hold. Most parents will find this extremely challenging but very helpful within the grieving process.
  - Explaining to the parents that the baby may have the occasional movement or reflex but that the baby is not in pain or suffering and may continue to show signs of life for some time after birth.
  - The baby should be held firmly and can be cuddled but not receive too much stimulation.
  - Please see the following link for information for parents (SANDS Leaflet): https://www.sands.org.uk/sites/default/files/Sands_Bereavement_Book_June2021.pdf.

3.5 Congenital Abnormalities

- The outcome of babies born with congenital abnormalities varies but is improving with advancement in medical therapies and interventions. The abnormality may have been detected on antenatal scans or may have been undiagnosed until birth. All babies who are known to have a congenital abnormality should be transferred to hospital where the abnormality can be assessed and treated, even when the baby appears to be normal at birth.
- Where the abnormality involves a section of the internal organs being outside the body, use cling film to cover the defect to reduce fluid and heat losses and risk of infection. Do not wrap the cling film circumferentially around the newborn's body as this may inhibit breathing.

3.6 Early Onset Neonatal Sepsis

- Early onset neonatal sepsis can be life-threatening, and it is important that it is recognised and treated early.
- **If the mother has any of the following risk factors, the baby is more at risk of having early onset neonatal sepsis:**
  - Systemic antibiotic treatment given to the mother for confirmed or suspected invasive bacteria.
  - Group B Streptococcus (GBS) colonisation, bacteriuria or infection in CURRENT pregnancy.
  - A previous baby with invasive GBS infection.
  - Preterm, pre-labour rupture of membranes of any duration.
  - Suspected or confirmed intrapartum rupture of membranes >18 hours.
- If any of the following are recognised in the baby, early neonatal sepsis could be the cause:[13]
  - Hypoglycaemia.
  - Altered behaviour or responsiveness.
  - Altered muscle tone (e.g. floppiness).
  - Feeding difficulties (e.g. feed refusal).
  - Feed intolerance (including vomiting or abdominal distension).
  - Abnormal heart rate (bradycardia or tachycardia).
  - Signs of respiratory distress (including grunting, recession, tachypnoea).
  - Hypoxia (e.g. central cyanosis or reduced oxygen saturation level).
  - Jaundice within 24 hours of birth.

Care of the Newborn

- Temperature abnormality (lower than 36°C or higher than 38°C) unexplained by environmental factors.
- Unexplained excessive bleeding.

- If risk factors, signs or symptoms are identified, the baby should be transferred to the nearest ED with an obstetric unit.

4. Assessment and Management

Normal observations in a newborn baby

	Normal ranges	How to measure	Further information
Colour	Pink/ centrally perfused mucous membranes	Observation: It is normal for a baby to have a different skin colour for the first couple of minutes after birth, but the baby should be centrally perfused at all times following this.	For example, a baby with a light skin tone may appear blue initially but this colour change may be more difficult to detect in a baby with dark skin tone. Examine closely. Babies should rapidly perfuse after birth which will change their skin color. For example, changing from blue to pink in a baby with light skin tone. Or changing from pallor to a slight darkening/maroon tinge in dark skin tones.
Tone	Flexed	Observation: A baby born well-flexed and with good tone is normally well.	Babies who remain floppy require urgent medical attention.
Respiratory rate	40–60 breaths per minute	Observation: Count breaths over 1 minute. Irregular, abdominal breathing is normal in a neonate.	Observe for signs of increased work of breathing or inadequacy, such as grunting (noise on inspiration or expiration), intercostal recession, nasal flaring.
Heart rate	100–160 bpm	Auscultation: Listen to the heart rate for 1 minute with a stethoscope.	Palpating the cord is less accurate. Saturation and ECG monitoring (if suitable leads are available) can be effective but may not be available immediately after birth.
Temperature	36.5–37.5°C	Measure: Use an appropriately calibrated thermometer.	Maintain temperature throughout any assessment, resuscitation and transport.

TABLE 5.4 – ASSESSMENT and MANAGEMENT of: The Newborn

Place of Resuscitation
- Consider these factors in advance of birth if possible.
- Ensure room is warm and close doors and windows to minimise drafts.

Management of the Cord
- Unless there are concerns about mother or baby, the cord should remain intact until it has gone white (or for at least 60 seconds). It can then be clamped and cut approximately 5 cm from the umbilicus.
- If assessment indicates a need for immediate resuscitation of the newborn, clamp and cut the cord and move to the resuscitation area.
- If there is any evidence of a snapped cord, clamp the cord immediately and observe the baby for signs of hypovolaemia (for example, pale mucous membranes and respiratory issues).

Assess Need for Resuscitation at Birth (Refer to Newborn Life Support)
- Assess **colour**, **tone**, **breathing** and **heart rate** after birth and continue to observe until care is handed over to the maternity team.
- Undertake any necessary resuscitation/stabilisation according to **Newborn Life Support** guidance.

Care of the Newborn

TABLE 5.4 – ASSESSMENT and MANAGEMENT of: The Newborn (continued)

- Prioritise:
  - thermal care
  - airway and breathing
  - (circulation).
- Undertake a **TIME-CRITICAL** transfer to the nearest appropriate destination as agreed locally once available resources are secured. This may require transfer separately from the mother.
- Provide a pre-alert/information call detailing the neonatal emergency.

Thermoregulation

- Always optimise thermoregulation throughout.
- Ensure the newborn baby is dried thoroughly after birth, with particular attention to the head. Apply a hat, cover the baby with towels, foil wrap and increase the environmental temperature.
- Consider other adjuncts (plastic wrap/thermal mattress if required/available).
- If mother and baby are well, skin-to-skin contact can be used to optimise thermoregulation, but it is paramount to continuously monitor airway and breathing.

Preterm Babies

- Use **Newborn Life Support** guidelines to initiate resuscitation in babies ≥22 weeks or where the gestation is unknown and there are signs of life.
- Provide comfort care to babies known to be <22 weeks gestation.
- Be aware that preterm babies may often deteriorate quickly even if born in good condition, so be ready to ventilate at any point.

Meconium

- Babies born with thick meconium-stained amniotic fluid should receive the same care as all babies – stimulation, thermal care and resuscitation as required. If not responding to initial airway and breathing manoeuvres, inspection may be considered to exclude obstruction.
- It is important to inform hospital staff at handover so that accelerated monitoring of the baby can be initiated.

Suspected Hypoglycaemia

- Ensure early feeding and keep the baby warm to prevent hypoglycaemia.
- Transfer to hospital if the baby is at risk of hypoglycaemia or signs of hypoglycaemia are seen.
- IM glucagon will NOT work due to poor glycogen stores in the newborn. Buccal dextrose can be used.

Jaundice

- Jaundice babies require a timely assessment by an appropriate healthcare professional.

Safeguarding

- If there are safeguarding concerns on scene, these should instigate a referral as per local protocols. A woman who has had a BBA and declines transfer to hospital should not be left on scene with the baby without initiating discussions with safeguarding professionals (unless a midwife is present).

5. Interface with Maternity Care Providers

- History-taking and accessing maternity notes will support your on-scene decision making.
- Liaison with maternity services should occur within local recommended processes. If a mother and baby is well and there is a midwife en route, it may be appropriate to wait for the midwife. Your clinical assessment on scene will help you decide whether you need to escalate the care.
- Any baby born with a midwife unavailable will require hospital admission with their mother to receive ongoing care from the maternity team. The mother and baby should be promptly transported to the nearest obstetric maternity unit. Apply a wristband label to the mother and baby if available.
- If the mother declines conveyance to hospital, the priority is to explain that pre-hospital clinicians cannot discharge a mother and newborn baby on scene without a midwife or doctor present. Follow local guidelines on assessing maternal capacity. Once born, the baby has rights of its own, so should receive medical care that is in its best interests.

Care of the Newborn

> **KEY POINTS!**
>
> **Care of the Newborn**
> - Ensure the environment is optimised; consider cord management and the need for additional resources.
> - Dry baby thoroughly at birth and keep warm during assessment, resuscitation and transport using a hat, warm blankets and foil wrap/pod or other adjuncts (plastic wrap/thermal mattress) if available/necessary.
> - The need for resuscitation can be determined from an assessment of the baby's condition at birth, including colour, tone, breathing and heart rate.
> - Undertake any necessary resuscitation/stabilisation using the recommended Newborn Life Support approach.
> - Preterm babies need extra vigilance, get cold quicker and even if demonstrating breathing efforts and adequate HR at birth may deteriorate, so be prepared to provide additional thermal, airway and ventilatory support. They will require further management in hospital.
> - Consider and treat hypoglycaemia as soon as possible to prevent convulsions or long-term neurological damage.
> - All babies with congenital abnormalities should be transferred to hospital for assessment.
> - Identify jaundice and ensure that the neonate receives timely medical review.
> - Be aware of risk factors in mother or baby, which might suggest a high risk of early onset neonatal sepsis.

Bibliography

1. MBRRACE-UK. *Determination of Signs of Life Following Spontaneous Birth Before 24+0 Weeks of Gestation Where, Following Discussion with the Parents, Active Survival-focused Care Is Not Appropriate.* 2020. Available at: https://timms.le.ac.uk/signs-of-life/resources/signs-of-life-guidance-v1.2.pdf.
2. National Institute for Health and Care Excellence. *Neonatal Infection: Antibiotics for Prevention and Treatment* [NG195]. London: National Institute for Health and Clinical Excellence, 2021. Available from: https://www.nice.org.uk/guidance/ng195.
3. Beard L, Lax P, Tindall M. Physiological effects of transfer for critically ill patients. *Anaesthesia Tutorial of the Week* 2016, 330. Available from: http://anaesthesiology.gr/media/File/pdf/330-Physiological-effects-of-transfer-for-critically-ill-patients.pdf.
4. British Association of Perinatal Medicine. 2022. Available from: https://www.bapm.org/British Association of Perinatal Medicine. 2022. Available from: https://www.bapm.org/
5. Burakevych N, McKinlay CJD, Harris DL et al. Factors influencing glycaemic stability after neonatal hypoglycaemia and relationship to neurodevelopmental outcome. *Sci Rep* 2019, 9: 8132. Available from: https://doi.org/10.1038/s41598-019-44609-1.
6. Carter BS. Pediatric palliative care in infants and neonates. *Children* (Basel, Switzerland) 2018, 5(2): 21. Available from: doi:10.3390/children5020021.
7. Cornblath M, Hawdon JM, Williams AF, Aynsley-Green A, Ward-Platt MP, Schwartz R et al. Controversies regarding definition of neonatal hypoglycemia: suggested operational thresholds. *Pediatrics* 2000, 105(5): 1141–1145.
8. National Collaborating Centre for Women's and Children's Health. *Diabetes in Pregnancy (CG63).* London: National Institute for Health and Clinical Excellence, 2015.
9. Wyckoff MH, Wyllie J, Aziz K, de Almeida MF, Fabres J, Fawke J, Guinsburg R et al. and on behalf of the Neonatal Life Support Collaborators. Neonatal Life Support: 2020 International Consensus on Cardiopulmonary Resuscitation and Emergency Cardiovascular Care Science with Treatment Recommendations 2020, 142: S185–S221. Available from: https://doi.org/10.1161/CIR.0000000000000895Circulation.
10. National Institute for Health and Care Excellence. Jaundice in Newborn Babies under 28 Days [CG98]. London: National Institute for Health and Care Excellence, 2016. Available from: https://www.nice.org.uk/guidance/cg98
11. Polglase GR, Blank DA, Barton SK, Miller SL, Stojanovska V, Kluckow M, Gill AW, LaRosa D, Te Pas AB, Hooper SB. Physiologically based cord clamping stabilises cardiac output and reduces cerebrovascular injury in asphyxiated near-term lambs. *Arch Dis Child Fetal Neonatal Ed* 2018, 103: F530–F538. Available from: doi:10.1136/archdischild-2017-313657.
12. Madar J, Roehr CC, Ainsworth S, Ersdal H, Morley C et al. European Resuscitation Council Guidelines 2021: Newborn resuscitation and support of transition of infants at birth. *Resuscitation* 2021, 161: 291–326. Available from: doi:10.1016/j.resuscitation.2021.02.014.
13. Simonsen KA, Anderson-Berry AL, Delair SF, Davies HD. Early-onset neonatal sepsis. *Clin Microbiol Rev* 2014, 27(1): 21–47. Available from: doi:10.1128/CMR.00031-13
14. Van de Voorde P, Turner NM, Djakow J et al. European Resuscitation Council Guidelines 2021: Paediatric Life Support. Available from: https://cprguidelines.eu/assets/guidelines/European-Resuscitation-Council-Guidelines-2021-Pa.pdf

Cord Prolapse

1. Umbilical Cord Prolapse

- Umbilical cord prolapse occurs when the umbilical cord exits the cervical opening before the baby is born. The cord will be seen protruding from the vagina.
- The umbilical cord has the potential to get trapped in front of the baby, causing compression and reduced blood flow to the baby. It is therefore a **TIME-CRITICAL** obstetric emergency that carries a high rate of fetal morbidity and mortality. **It requires immediate recognition and rapid transfer with a pre-alert to the nearest consultant led obstetric unit.**

DO NOT DELAY TIME ON SCENE – ensure concurrent activity to expedite care.

- Assist woman to wear underwear and clean dry pad which will contain and cradle the cord against the woman's external genitalia.
- If attending as a solo responder, position the woman in the knee/chest position (below) while awaiting an ambulance.
- Once a conveying resource has arrived, leave immediately minimising time on scene.
- To enable rapid transfer to the ambulance, the woman **should** be walked.

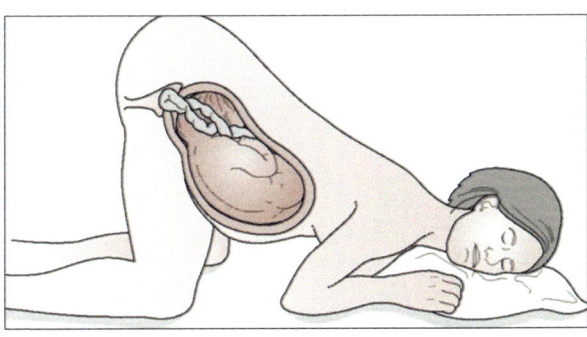

- Once in the ambulance, position the woman on either side with whatever is available (for example a blanket) under her hip to raise the pelvis and reduce pressure on the cord (sometimes known as the exaggerated Sims). Positioning the woman on her right side offers reassurance, allowing her to face the clinician or relative.
- Offer Entonox if the woman experiences pain. Refer to **Nitrous Oxide (Entonox® or Nitronox™)**.
- Continually observe for signs of imminent birth en route (if birth is imminent, stop the vehicle when safe to do so and assist the woman to birth). Refer to **Imminent Birth**.
- **It is not safe to convey the woman in the all-fours position in the ambulance.**

Transfer to the nearest obstetric unit. **DO NOT DELAY TIME ON SCENE.**

- Place an early pre-alert stating the obstetric emergency of cord prolapse.
- It may be necessary to request maternity staff to meet the ambulance clinicians at a suitable entrance to avoid any delays due to accessing lifts or entry to buildings.
- If a midwife is on scene, they may perform bladder filling as a midwifery intervention.

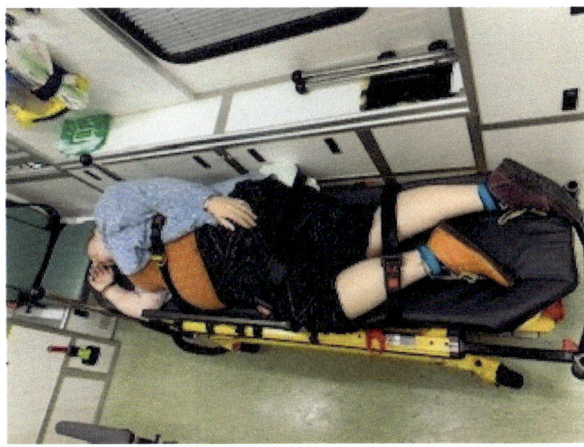

Cord Prolapse

2. Management of Cord Prolapse

Team preparation
En route review JRCALC obstetric guidelines if not driving, to achieve a shared mental model

↓

Assist woman to wear underwear and clean dry pad which will contain and cradle the cord against the woman's external genitalia.

↓

Position the woman in the knee chest position while awaiting ambulance.
Do not convey in this position.

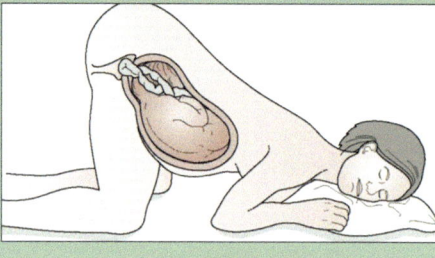

↓

Where possible, walk the woman to the ambulance

↓

Position the woman on either side elevating the pelvis using whatever is available, e.g. a blanket.
Ensure woman is secured using ambulance safety straps.

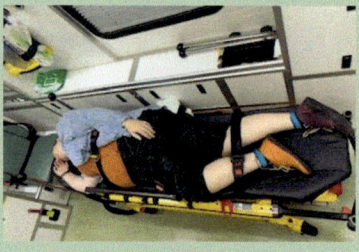

↓

Assess for imminent birth en-route
Administer Entonox if required

Transfer to nearest consultant led obstetric unit with pre-alert.

TIME CRITICAL - DO NOT DELAY TIME ON SCENE.

Figure 5.7 – Pre-hospital maternity emergency – management of cord prolapse.

Cord Prolapse

> **KEY POINTS!**
>
> **Cord Prolapse**
> - Cord prolapse is a TIME-CRITICAL emergency.
> - Minimise time on scene.
> - Avoid handling the cord.

References

1. Ahmed W and Hamdy M. Optimal management of umbilical cord prolapse. *International Journal of Women's Health* 2018, 10: 459–465.
2. Barrett. Funic reduction for the management of umbilical cord prolapse. *Am J Obstet Gynecol.* 1991, 165(3): 654–657.
3. Kwan A, Chaemsaithong P, Wong L, Tse W, Hui A and Leung T. Transperineal ultrasound assessment of fetal head elevation by manoeuvres used for managing umbilical cord prolapse. *Ultrasound in Obstetrics & Gynecology* 2020, 58(4): 603–608.
4. Murphy D and MacKenzie I. The mortality and morbidity associated with umbilical cord prolapse. *Br J Obstet Gynaecol.* 1995, 103(10): 826–830.
5. Royal College of Obstetricians and Gynaecologists. 2014. Umbilical Cord Prolapse – Green-top guideline No.50 URL: Layout Proof (rcog.org.uk)
6. Wong L, Kwan A, Lau S, Sin W and Leung T. Umbilical cord prolapse: revisiting its definition and management. *American Journal of Obstetrics and Gynaecology* 2021, 225(4): 357–366.
7. Wu S, Liao G, and Yang J. Effects of right lateral position on changes of fetal hemodynamics in late pregnancy. *J Ultrasound Med* 2023, 2(10): 2341–2347.

Imminent Birth

Introduction

This guidance is for cephalic presentations (when the head is presenting first).

If buttocks, a foot or feet are presenting refer to **Breech Birth**.

1. Assessing a Woman in Labour

Take a history (consider requirement for interpreter):
- Number of weeks gestation?
- Multiple or single pregnancy?
- Number of pregnancies (gravida)?
- Number of livebirths (parity) and modes of birth?
- Any medical conditions?
- Any complications in the current pregnancy?
- Any complications in previous pregnancies?
- Any bleeding?
- Any waters broken? When did they break? What colour are they?
- Any concerns voiced by patient or family?

2. Assessing Uterine Contractions

- Monitor the time that the contraction lasts and the time between the end of one contraction and the start of the next.
- If verbal communication is challenging then ask the patient to raise their hand at the start and end of the contraction.

Normal contractions – occurring after 36+6 weeks gestation; the pain comes and goes, the abdomen is soft in between contractions.

Abnormal contractions – occurring before 37 weeks OR constant pain and/or pain that is felt in an area of scarring from previous uterine surgery (e.g. caesarean section). This requires time critical conveyance to the nearest obstetric unit with a pre-alert.

2.1 High risk pregnancy identified

Time critical conveyance to the nearest obstetric unit is required where:
- Any current maternal risks are identified, even if the contractions are normal.
- The pregnancy is high risk even if the contractions are normal. Refer to Table 5.5.

TABLE 5.5 – Factors for High Risk Pregnancy

Maternal	Fetal
• Consultant led care in pregnancy	• Shoulder dystocia
• Diabetes (gestational or pre-existing)	• Cord prolapse
• Hypertensive disorders including pre-eclampsia and eclampsia	• Preterm (<37 weeks)
• Any bleeding in pregnancy after 20 weeks	• Twins or triplets
• Previous caesarean section	• Congenital abnormalities
• Limited antenatal care	• Born after 42 weeks of pregnancy
• Concealed pregnancy	• Small for gestational age
• Non-prescription drug use	• Meconium stained liquor
• Alcohol misuse	• Blood stained liquor
• Advanced maternal age (≥40 yrs)	• Offensive smelling liquor
• Smoking	• Abnormal ultrasound scan findings
• Infection	• Safeguarding concerns
• Use of beta-blockers	• If waters are broken prior to 37 weeks
• High BMI (≥30)	• If waters are broken more than 18 hours in a term pregnancy
• Cardiac conditions	
• Obstetric choleostasis	
• Polyhydramnios (excessive amniotic fluid)	
• Oligohydramnios (reduced amniotic fluid)	
• Placenta accreta spectrum	
• Placenta praevia	
• Auto-immune disease	

Imminent Birth

TABLE 5.5 – Factors for High Risk Pregnancy *(continued)*

Maternal	Fetal
• Transplant recipient	
• Kidney disease	
• Liver disease	
• Neurological conditions including epilepsy	
• Clotting disorders	
• Previous venous thromboembolic event	
• Previous obstetric emergency	
• Previous severe perineal trauma (3rd degree or 4th degree tear)	
• Immobility	
• Mental health conditions	
• Sickle cell disease	
• Current maternal infection	

NB If abnormal contractions or high risk pregnancy, imminent birth (see below) will take priority over any risk factors or red flags that are identified. Undertake time critical conveyance to appropriate destination according to local guidelines as soon as possible after the birth (once appropriate interventions have taken place); place pre-alert.

3. Signs of Imminent Birth

Clinicians should stay and prepare to facilitate birth on scene when the following are present:

- Regular contractions (1–2 minute intervals)

AND either of:

- Urge to push or bear down
- Head visible and advancing through the vaginal entrance (ask for consent, observe external vaginal area during a contraction)

Head visible (head may recede between contractions – this is normal):

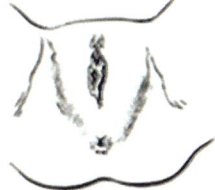

Crowning (head remains visible and doesn't slip back in between contractions):

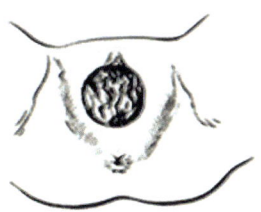

NB Internal vaginal examination for cervical assessment is not within the scope of any ambulance clinician.

3.1 What to do if birth is not imminent

- Any patient having contractions requires fetal monitoring and so should be recommended to be conveyed to hospital by ambulance. If a homebirth is planned, request a midwife to attend according to local guidelines.

3.2 Continuous dynamic assessment

- Continue to assess the signs of imminent birth during every contraction.
- If a decision is made to stay on scene but **there is no progress after 10 minutes**, including the same amount of presenting part visible, prepare to extricate and undertake a time critical transfer to the nearest obstetric unit with a pre-alert.
- Be ready for the situation to change during extrication and transport.

3.3 Birth becomes imminent en route to hospital

- Pull over and stop the ambulance to facilitate the birth then follow the Management of Imminent Birth guidance in Section 3.4.
- Call for additional resources according to local guidelines.
- Consider requirement for critical care if high risk pregnancy.
- Proceed to the nearest appropriate destination according to local guidelines. It is not necessary to await birth of the placenta before continuing with the conveyance to hospital. Provide pre-alert.

Imminent Birth

3.4 Management of Imminent Birth

Initial steps

- Call for help: ensure enough resources have been requested as per local procedure; at least one paramedic clinician should be present in one of the vehicles on scene. Consider escalating for critical care if this is a high risk pregnancy.
- Apply PPE and use universal precautions.
- Introduce team and establish rapport with patient and family.
- Identify a lead clinician for the patient and for each expected baby if possible.
- If it is a planned home birth then request a midwife from the patient's home birth team according to local guidelines.
- Be prepared to support the birth in the absence of the midwife.
- Allow the patient to adopt a position that is most comfortable for them. It is not advisable for them to lie completely flat on their back.
- Allow the patient to spontaneously push during contractions and gain consent to observe for progress externally.
- The patient should respond to signals from their body telling them how and when to push.
- Offer **Entonox** to assist with pain management.

3.5 Preparing environment and equipment

- Ensure lighting is adequate.
- Prepare equipment, including dry towels, maternity pack, thermal mattress (e.g. transwarmer) and additional warming equipment.
- Ensure the ambient temperature is as high as possible (aim for 25°C).
- Ensure windows/doors are closed and heating is set to maximum.
- Prepare an area for newborn life support; this should be a firm, flat area off the floor ideally in the same room as the patient giving birth. All newborn life support equipment should be available including airway adjuncts and newborn masks (refer to **Newborn Life Support**).

4. Supporting Birth of the Baby

- Once you see the head visible, one clinician must have their hands poised in preparation for the birth of the baby.
- At the point of crowning (head remains visible and doesn't slip back in between contractions) encourage the patient to **pant** to slow down the birth of the last bit of the head.
- After the head is born, the baby's head should turn to the side between or during the next contraction (restitution).
- Following the birth of the head; the remainder of the baby should be born during the next contraction – if this does not occur this is a shoulder dystocia – refer to **Shoulder Dystocia**.
- Following the birth of the head, allow the patient to spontaneously push guided by their body. Do not pull on the baby at any point.
- Support the baby as the shoulders and body are born, then lift the baby towards the patient's abdomen.
- The umbilical cord may be around the baby's neck and does not require removal during delivery, as the baby can be born with the cord left in place. If the cord remains around the neck or body following birth, unloop the cord.

5. Initial Newborn Assessment at Birth

- Place the baby directly onto the patient's abdomen and begin to dry and stimulate the baby with a dry towel (see section 12.2 for preterm management).
- Assess the newborn with the cord intact over the first 60 seconds following birth whilst providing adequate thermoregulation.
- Replace the wet towel with a dry towel and apply a hat to the baby.
- Assess colour, tone, breathing and heart rate. If any of these are abnormal, clamp and cut the cord and start **Newborn Life Support**.

	Normal ranges	Abnormal ranges Start **Newborn Life Support**
Colour	Centrally perfused mucous membranes (e.g. gums)	Centrally cyanosed (blue) mucous membranes more than 1 minute following birth
Tone	Flexed	Floppy
Breathing Rate	40–60 per minute	Below 40 per minute
Heart Rate (stethoscope)	100–160 per minute	Below 100

Imminent Birth

Do not use a defibrillator at any point for monitoring or for Newborn Life Support.

6. Thermoregulation

Promoting newborn thermoregulation is crucial during assessment, resuscitation and transport. Proactive measures should be taken at every birth for every baby.

- Ensure windows/doors are closed and heating is set to maximum (aim for 25°C).
- Ambulances should be kept well heated.
- If the baby is above 32 weeks gestation, at birth thoroughly dry the baby using dry towels; remove wet towels.
- If the baby is **32 weeks or below**, place undried in a clear plastic bag and onto a heat source: see Management of Extreme Preterm: altered approach (section 12.3).
- Apply a hat to a dry head.
- Whenever the baby is on the patient's abdomen ensure the patient's abdomen is dry.
- Apply a thermal mattress.
- Apply additional warming aids if available e.g. insulating wrap.

7. Optimal Cord Management – all gestations

At birth, a third of the baby's blood volume is in the placenta; morbidity and mortality is reduced if the baby's cord remains intact for at least 60 seconds following birth. Leaving the cord intact for the first 60 seconds is "optimal cord management".

Clamp the cord **immediately** if:

- The cord is snapped (if it is snapped at baby's abdomen, apply pressure, undertake time critical conveyance with pre-alert).
- The attached cord prevents the clinician from undertaking effective newborn life support.
- If there are further babies to be born (see Multiple Pregnancy).

Optimal cord clamping and cutting:

- If the baby is well at birth, keep the cord intact until it has gone **white**.
- If the cord is extremely short and prevents the baby being held clamp and cut at 60 seconds.
- Clamp the cord approximately 5 cm from the baby using a cord clamp in the maternity pack.
- Place another clamp approximately 5 cm further along the cord.
- Use the cord scissors from the maternity pack to cut the cord in the space **between** the clamps.
- Minimise amount of time the baby is exposed.
- If deemed suitable, offer a parent or birth partner to cut the cord. Assist them to do so safely.

CAUTION – ensure the newborn's fingers and genitals are clear of the scissors. Be aware of bodily fluid exposure as a result of blood spurting from the cord.

8. Third Stage of Labour (birth of the placenta)

Third stage of labour is the delivery of placenta and membranes and the control of maternal bleeding.

If midwives are present they may administer prophylactic uterotonics and undertake controlled cord traction ("active management of third stage"). This is not within the scope of ambulance clinicians.

The following actions following birth can promote placenta delivery:

- Supporting the patient to pass urine.
- Skin to skin and/or breastfeeding if desired.
- Upright positions to aid gravity.

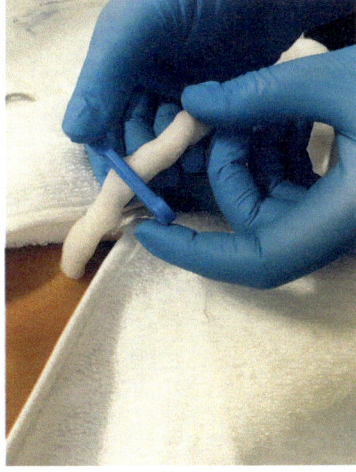
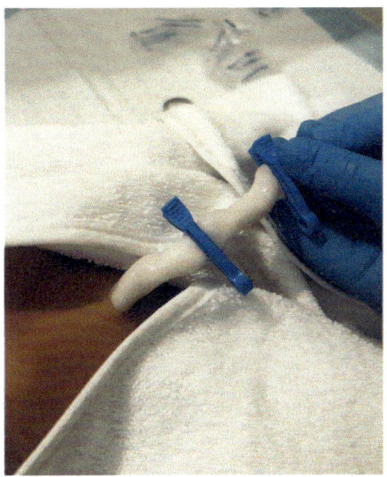
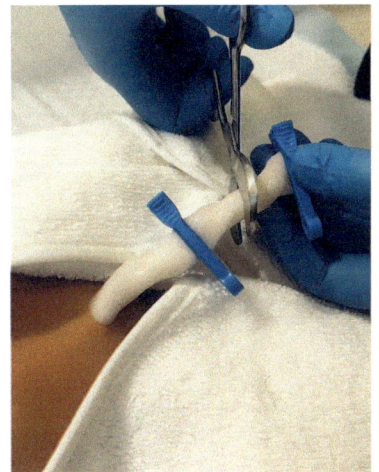

Imminent Birth

Management of third stage (without the presence of a midwife)

- Following delivery a clean incontinence sheet should be placed under the buttocks so that bleeding can be monitored.
- Regularly undertake patient's observations at scene and/or en route to hospital.
- Monitor the patient for excessive bleeding (500 mls or more or any blood loss that causes signs of hypovolaemic shock) and refer to **Management of Post-partum Haemorrhage (PPH)**.
- Do not pull on the cord at any point.
- If the placenta is still in situ **20 minutes** after birth, undertake time critical conveyance to the nearest obstetric unit with a pre-alert.
- Ensure the placenta and all items which contain blood are transported to the hospital, so that blood loss can be measured.
- Examining a placenta and membranes for completeness is not within the scope of ambulance clinicians.
- If the patient wishes to keep their placenta, transport the placenta to hospital and reassure the patient that the maternity staff will return the placenta to them after examination.

9. Skin-to-skin and Infant Feeding

- If desired by parents, the baby can have skin-to-skin with an adult who is warm. Place the baby prone and wrap the baby and the adult together keeping the face exposed.
- Ensure the airway is optimised by the head being turned to the side. Either a parent or a clinician needs to monitor the newborn continuously.
- Apply additional warming aids including a hat and thermal mattress.
- If the patient would like to breastfeed the baby they should do so unless there is a clinical need to convey.

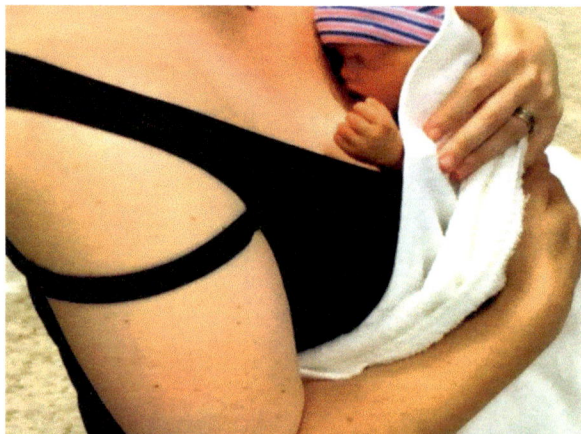

Figure 5.8 – Newborn being held skin-to-skin

- The need to transport should be prioritised over infant feeding.
- Providing breastfeeding guidance is not within the scope of ambulance clinicians.

10. Transport

- Request additional resources for transportation according to local guidelines.
- Safe transport to hospital is essential: follow local guidelines using appropriate available equipment.
- If there are any concerns with mum or baby, they should be conveyed in separate ambulances with clear, compassionate communication to the parents. This includes if there are risk factors for the mother or baby becoming unwell en route to hospital. A non-birthing parent or family member may travel with the baby.
- Ensure the mother/birthing person is conveyed to the same hospital as the baby.
- Preterm or newborns requiring additional support or monitoring should **not** be transported in a car seat.
- The baby should not travel skin-to-skin.
- Thermoregulation during transport is essential including using a thermal mattress and blizzard wrap if available.
- Babies should have ID bands applied with the mother/birthing person's name and postcode.
- If the mother/birthing person and baby are conveyed in separate ambulances ensure maternity staff are aware of the location of both mother/birthing person and baby so that they can reunite them as soon as possible/appropriate.

11. Observations of Mother and Baby Following Birth

After every birth the patient and baby(ies) require at least two sets of observations from either the ambulance service or midwives if they are present. Document the observations on **individual** patient records and act on any abnormalities.

Use the parameters on the **Prehospital Maternity Decision Tool** for ongoing assessment of the patient who has given birth.

Use the parameters on Page for Age and **Care of the Newborn** for ongoing assessment of the baby.

Temperature recordings should be taken with an appropriate, calibrated, thermometer as soon as practical after birth, *at least* once during transport and then on arrival at destination (see **Care of the Newborn**).

Oxygen saturation monitoring should be applied during transport of preterm babies, babies that have undergone newborn life support, babies with abnormal findings on assessment or babies that are requiring ongoing airway support.

Imminent Birth

12. Special Considerations

12.1 Waterbirth

Attending and managing planned births in water is outside the scope of practice for ambulance clinicians. On arrival you should **request the patient to leave the water and assist them to do so.**

If the patient declines to leave the water, explain the following risks (involve her birth partner in the conversation if present):

- Ambulance clinicians do not have training in waterbirth.
- Ambulance clinicians do not have training to resolve obstetric emergencies in the water. Therefore if there was an obstetric emergency in the water there is potential for a poor outcome.
- Ambulance services do not carry the equipment to monitor the water temperature (which is crucial for the baby's safety at birth).

Advise the patient to leave the water again.

If the patient makes an informed decision to stay in the water against your advice, perform the following actions:

- Contact senior clinical/medical advice and request a midwife to attend as per local procedures.
- Document the discussions with the patient and the senior clinical team.
- Request additional resources to scene anticipating the need to extricate the patient in an emergency.
- Warm the room and turn on the lights.
- Prepare several dry towels, the maternity pack and set up an area for newborn life support.
- Use sleeve protectors (if available) and gloves over the top, wear eye protection and an apron.
- Continuously assess for imminent birth and continue to recommend to the patient that they should exit the pool if the birth or head is not advancing or if there are new concerns such as meconium or fresh red bleeding.
- **If there is a shoulder dystocia** (body is not born during the next contraction after the head is born), ask the patient to promptly stand up and help them to exit the pool, stating that this is now an obstetric emergency. Refer to **Shoulder Dystocia**.
- Be aware that the action of standing up and stepping out of the pool may release the baby so keep hands poised at all times to catch the baby.

If the baby is born under the water, ask the patient to bring the baby's head above the water level.

If the patient cannot bring the baby to the surface of the water, you must put your hands in the water, lift the baby up and ensure the baby's head is above the water so that the baby can breathe spontaneously without inhaling the water.

- Clamp and cut the umbilical cord.
- Move the baby out of the water and assess the newborn and provide newborn thermoregulation and newborn life support if required.
- Assessment and care of the patient and the baby should be undertaken, preferably by two separate clinicians.
- Keep the baby in the same room as the patient, within eyesight if possible.
- Help the patient out of the pool.
- The third stage of labour should happen out of the water.
- Document all discussions and care management.

12.2 Preterm labour/birth

Babies born before 37 completed weeks are preterm.

Preterm babies born out of hospital are at high risk of morbidity and mortality. Time critical conveyance to the nearest obstetric maternity unit is required where the patient is having preterm contractions.

Be aware that preterm contractions may present atypically such as back pain, period pain, urinary tract symptoms or mild abdominal pain.

The assessment of whether to stay on scene and the actions during delivery are the same as for term babies (see section 4 – Supporting Birth of the Baby). If birth is imminent and advancing, then remain and prepare for birth and urgently request senior support as per local guidelines.

As soon as the baby is born, undertake thermoregulation and assessment, referring to **Newborn Life Support** if required. Once initial assessment is complete, thermoregulation is optimised and essential interventions have been undertaken, a time critical conveyance to definitive care is required as soon as possible, even if the baby is born in good condition. Preterm babies require constant monitoring as they are at risk of deterioration at any point. SpO_2 monitoring should be placed on the right hand/wrist for heart rate and oxygen saturation monitoring.

Preterm babies are at significant risk of death from hypothermia.[2] Every effort must be taken to keep them as warm as possible following birth and during extrication and transport.

12.3 Extremely preterm babies – Altered approach

Babies born between 22 and 32 completed weeks require an altered approach. Refer to **Newborn Life Support**. The following should be undertaken according to local guidelines:

- Following birth, place the wet baby in a clear plastic bag, provide 60 seconds of optimal cord management. During this time, wrap and place onto a heat source [thermal mattress] with a hat in situ.

Imminent Birth

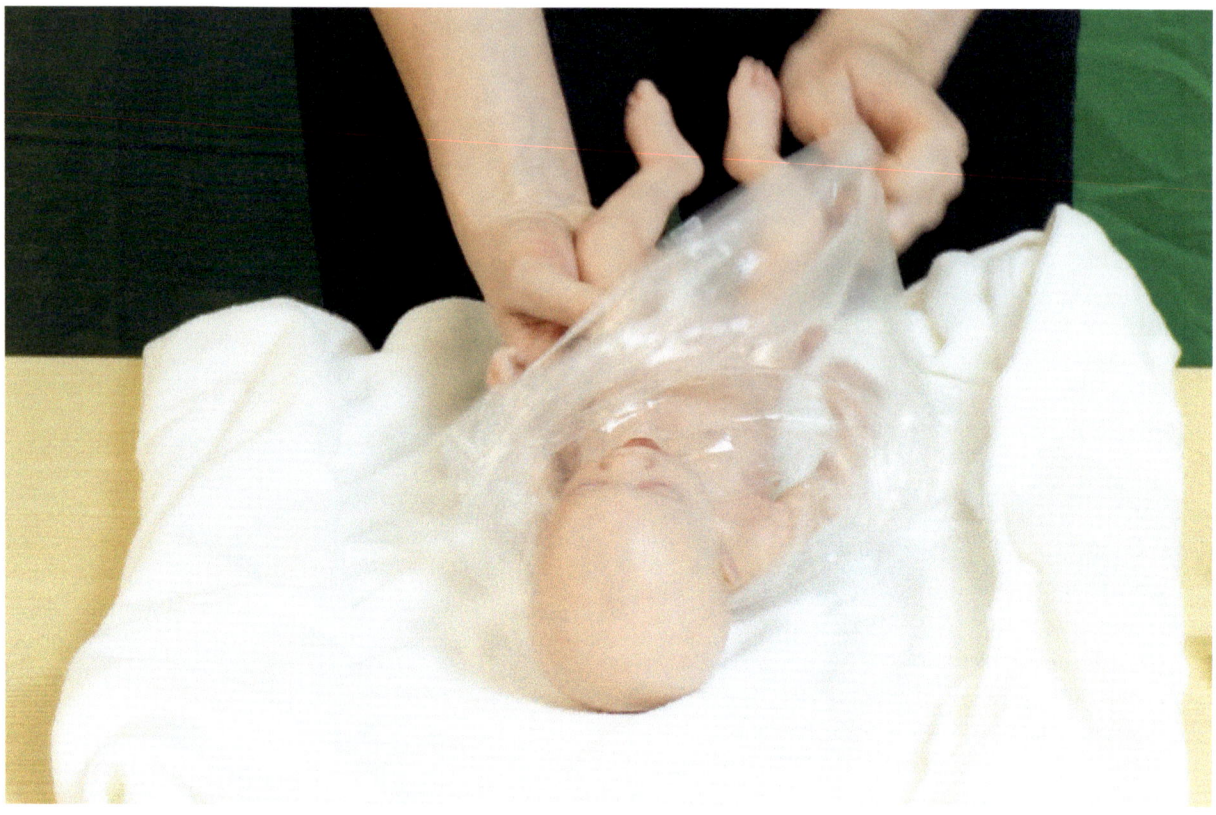

- Undertake newborn assessment (See Section 5) and newborn life support if required.
- The baby should only go into a plastic bag if there is a thermal mattress available.
- If a plastic bag and a heat source are not available use a dry towel to very gently dab-dry the baby. Wrap and keep warm.
- Handle preterm babies with extreme care at all times.
- Do not apply ECG stickers to preterm newborns due to skin fragility.
- An oxygen saturation monitor should be applied to the right hand/wrist to monitor heart rate and oxygen saturations.

The above applies to babies that appear smaller than expected for their gestation at birth (this may include multiples) or where the gestation is unknown and the baby is appearing as though they would fit in the plastic bag.

NB The plastic bag can be a transparent food-grade bag, plastic wrap or a designated neo-help bag.

If a foodgrade plastic bag is used, make a hole in the centre of the sealed end, gather up the bag and place over the baby's head like a poncho. Seal up the bag; SpO_2 monitoring can be placed with the wire out of the sealable end.

12.4 Planned homebirth (midwives not on scene)

Contact maternity services to attend the homebirth according to local guidelines. Ambulance clinicians should stay on scene until they arrive and provide a clinical handover.

If midwives are not able to attend within a locally agreed timescale, recommend conveyance to an appropriate destination according to local guidelines.

If the patient and/or baby has abnormal observations or red flags at any point, the patient and baby should be conveyed to hospital for further assessment with pre-alert. Do not wait for midwives to arrive if this is the case.

12.5 Freebirth

Freebirth is when a patient chooses to give birth without any trained healthcare professionals present. Freebirth is legal in the UK.

If the ambulance service is called to the property, the maternity service should be requested to attend even if the patient has previously declined their input. This is to facilitate informed choice and ongoing care planning.

- Provide clinical care and recommendations according to JRCALC guidelines.
- Escalate the situation to a senior clinician as per local guidelines.
- If the baby is born, care should be provided in the best interests of the child.
- If the baby is born, a midwife will be required for handover of care.
- Document all discussions and care provided.

Imminent Birth

The patient declines conveyance to hospital in labour or following birth:

- Explain and document the reasons why you are advising transportation.
- Request a midwife to attend according to local guidelines and inform them that the patient is declining conveyance to hospital against medical advice.
- **If the baby has been born, ambulance clinicians should not leave the scene before providing a face to face clinical handover to a midwife.**
- Document all discussions and escalate the situation as per local guidelines.

12.6 Multiple pregnancy and birth

- Follow imminent birth guidance (Section 3) to assess the need to stay and prepare for birth. If possible, extricate and undertake time critical conveyance to the nearest obstetric unit with a pre-alert.
- Ensure the pre-alert states multiple pregnancy.
- Constantly assess en route and take appropriate action to manage birth/s if the circumstances change.
- Offer **Entonox** to assist with pain management.

If twin birth is imminent or occurs en route:

- Request a second and third resource and consider advanced care teams (where available).
- Follow the Supporting birth of the baby (Section 4) for the birth of Twin 1.
- When Twin 1 has been born, clamp and cut the cord **immediately**.
- Undertake a newborn assessment (Section 5) and thermoregulation (Section 6). Refer to the **Newborn Life Support** if required.
- The placenta from Twin 1 may spontaneously deliver at any point.
- Communicate clearly with the patient.
- The contractions are likely to decrease following the birth of the first twin. Unless the birth of Twin 2 is imminent and advancing, attempt to extricate to an appropriate destination if possible for the birth of Twin 2 (Twin 2 is more at risk of hypoxia). Provide pre-alert.
- Continue to monitor the patient closely for signs of imminent birth of Twin 2 throughout extrication and transport.
- If the birth of Twin 2 is imminent and advancing immediately after Twin 1, support the birth of the baby (Section 4). If the baby is presenting breech, follow **Breech Birth**.
- If the birth of Twin 2 occurs en route to hospital, request additional resources as per local guidelines.
- At birth, Twin 2 can have cord clamping in line with the Newborn Life Support guidance (dry and assess for 60 seconds then clamp and cut if requiring resuscitation; if no resuscitation is required, wait for the cord to turn white).
- If the patient and both babies are well, convey all the patients to an appropriate destination according to local guidelines and provide a pre-alert stating the number of patients.
- Try to minimise time on scene.
- If either twin requires ongoing resuscitation, convey separately to an appropriate destination according to local guidelines with a pre-alert.
- Be mindful that the patient is at higher risk of PPH following a twin birth. Do not give any uterotonics with a second fetus in-situ.
- Apply a label to each twin stating the individual time they were born.

Triplets and more – in labour

- Time critical conveyance is a priority – caesarean section is the preferred mode of birth for triplets.
- Follow guidance above for Multiple Pregnancy and birth.
- Immediately clamp cord after each baby; the last baby can have optimal cord management (Section 7).

12.7 Amniotic membranes presenting

- Do not attempt to burst the amniotic membranes at any point prior to birth.
- If a presenting part cannot be visualised behind the amniotic sac, prepare for time critical conveyance.
- Monitor continuously for any progress.
- If the sac bursts at any point observe for the presenting part. If the presenting part is a foot, feet or hands, or cord, convey under time critical conditions to the nearest maternity unit as per **Breech Birth**.
- If the head is presenting and the birth is progressing, stay on scene/stop the ambulance and prepare for birth and refer to Section 4 – Supporting birth of the baby.

12.8 En caul (born with membranes and placenta intact)

- Apply appropriate PPE.
- Pull some membranes away from the baby's body using your index finger and thumb.
- Tear the membranes with your fingers.
- If the membranes are too tough to tear, use the tips of a pair of scissors from the maternity pack to carefully make a small incision in the membranes close to your pinched finger and thumb. Once ruptured, the amniotic fluid will rapidly drain away.
- Carefully peel the remaining membranes away from the baby's mouth and nose in order to ensure the airway is clear.

Imminent Birth

- Remove the membranes from the baby, clamp and cut the cord and undertake newborn assessment (Section 5) and thermoregulation (Section 6).

- Note in the clinical record the status of the amniotic fluid — clear, blood stained, meconium present or offensive smelling.

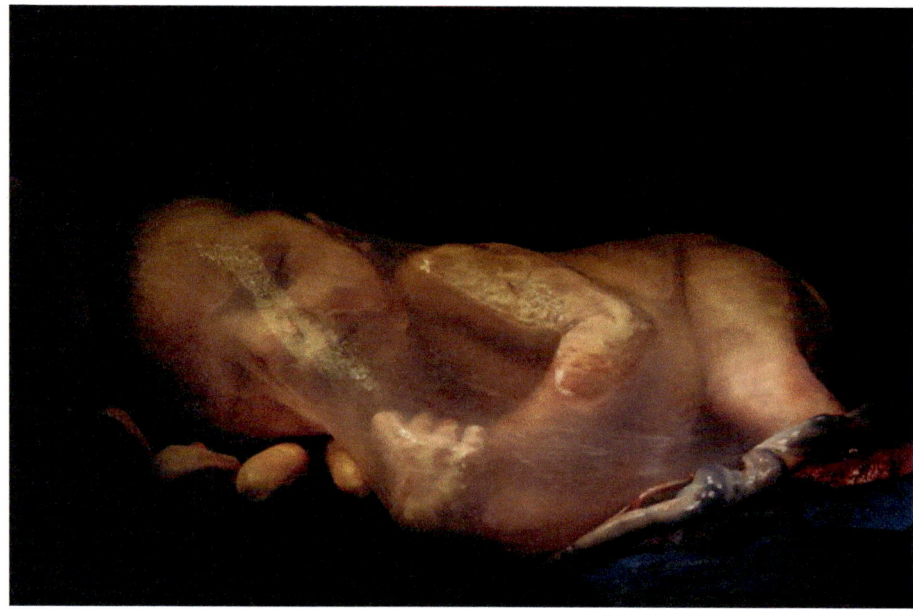

Image reproduced with kind permission from Daniela Justus.

13. Birth Complications

Refer to individual guidelines:

- Breech Birth
- Cord Prolapse
- Pre-eclampsia and Eclampsia
- Shoulder Dystocia

APPENDIX 1 – Estimating Volumes of Blood Loss

Different blood volumes to aid with estimation.

Reproduced with kind permission from PROMPT maternity foundation.

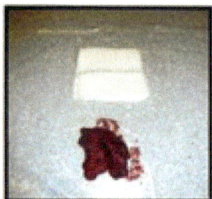
Small swab: 50mls

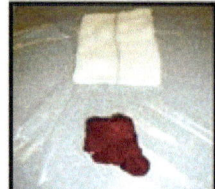
Medium swab: 100mls

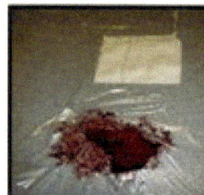
Large swab: 350mls

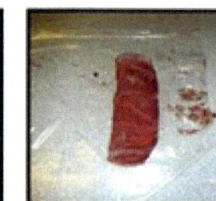
Sanitary towel: 100mls

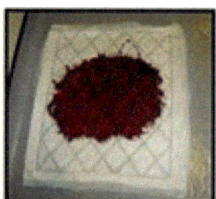
Inco sheet: 250mls

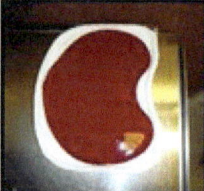
Kidney dish: 600mls

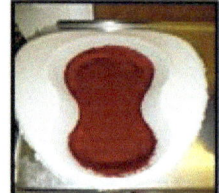
Bedpan: 500mls

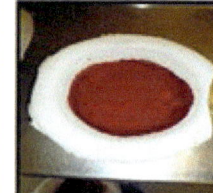
Vomit bowl: 300mls

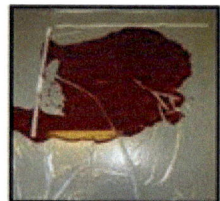
Floor spills:
50 x 50 (500mls)
75 x75 (1000mls)
100 x 100 (1500mls)

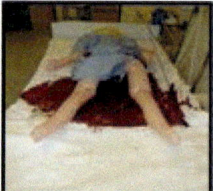
PPH:
On bed only (1000mls) Spilling to floor (2000mls)

Imminent Birth

Further Resources

- Watch this video with more information about the amniotic sac.
- Image sequence showing how to open a membrane.

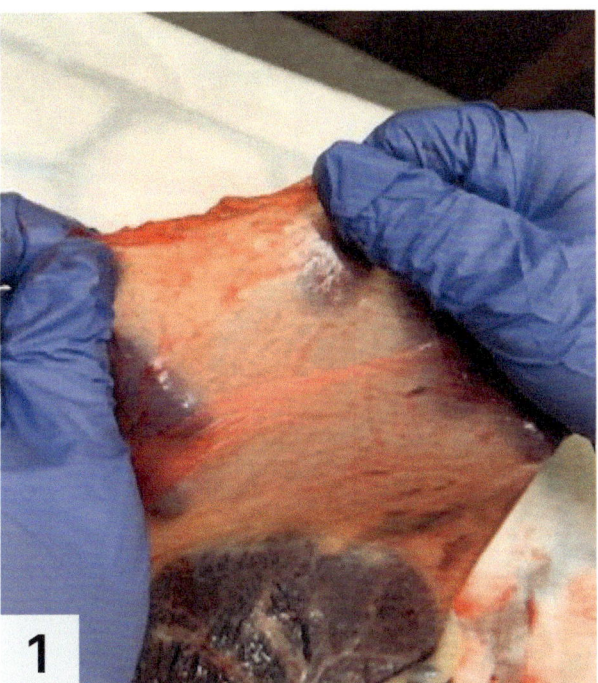
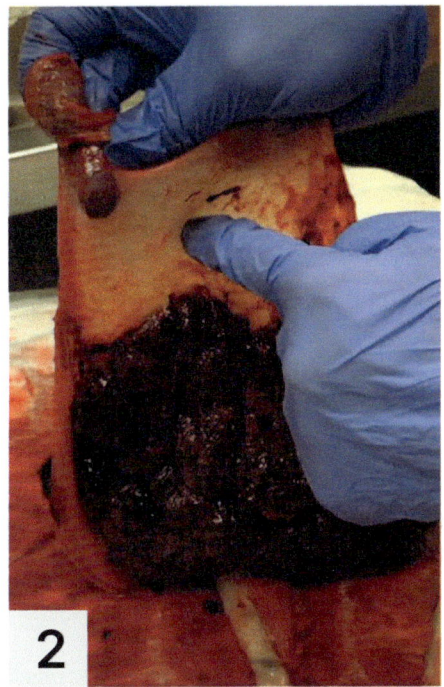
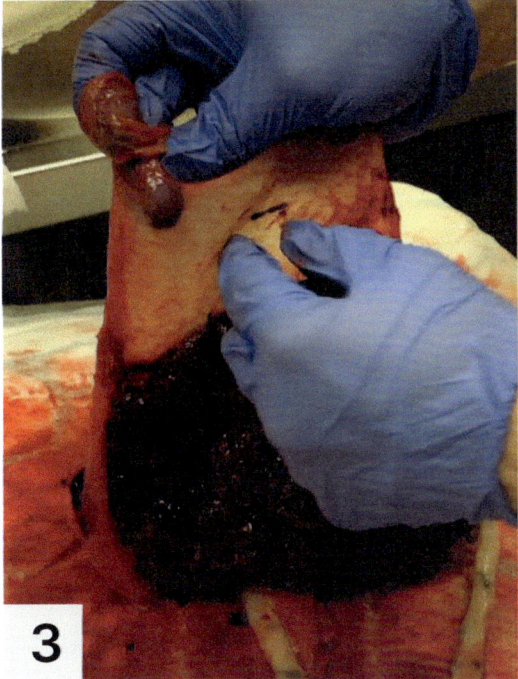
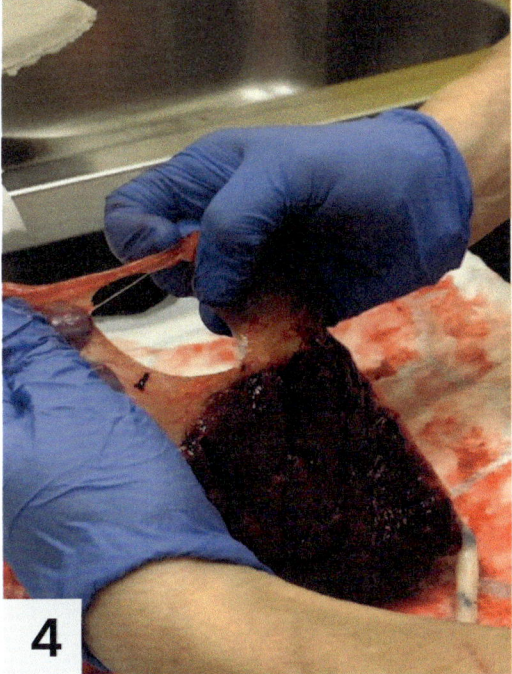

Imminent Birth

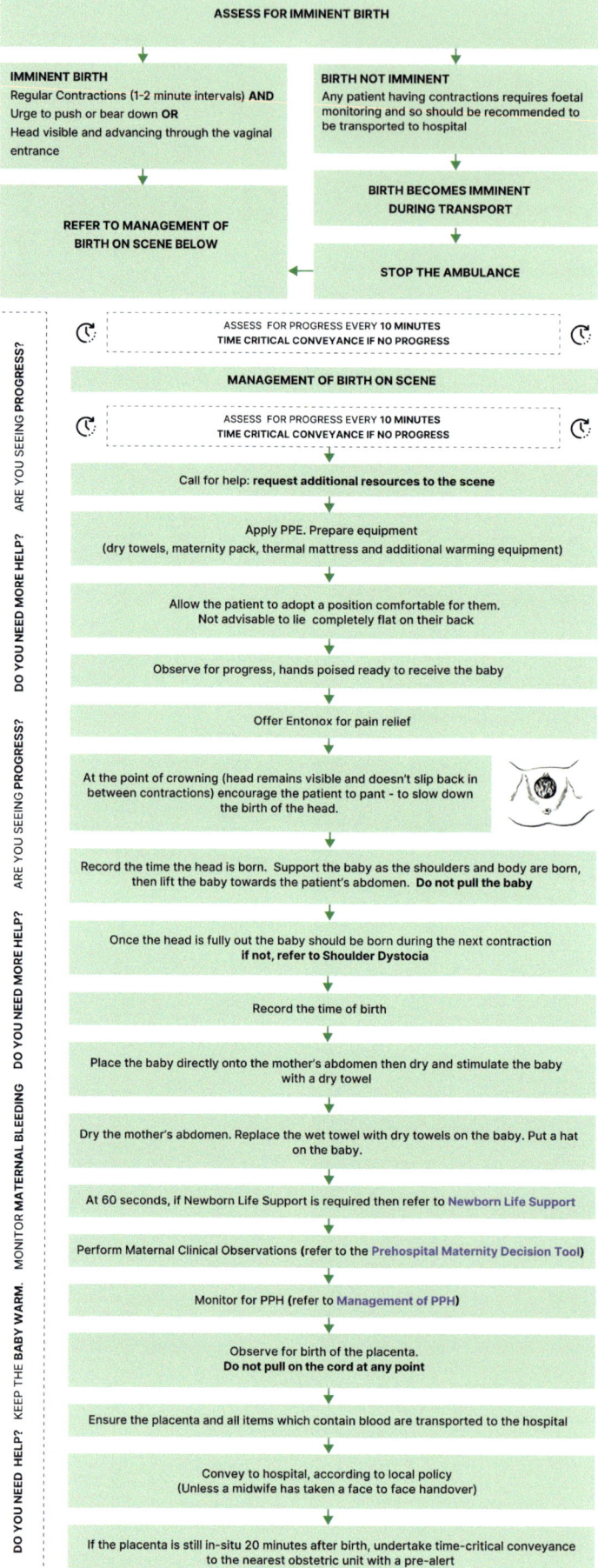

Figure 5.9 – Management of imminent birth

Imminent Birth

> **KEY POINTS!**
>
> **Imminent Birth**
> - Clinicians should perform a continuous dynamic assessment regarding staying on scene. If a decision is made to stay on scene but there is no progress after 10 minutes, including the same amount of presenting part visible, prepare to extricate and undertake a time critical transfer to the nearest obstetric unit with a pre-alert.
> - If the placenta is still in situ 20 minutes after birth, undertake time critical conveyance to an appropriate destination with a pre-alert.
> - In most situations, the cord should remain intact for at least 60 seconds following birth whilst performing thermoregulation and an assessment of the baby.
> - Maintaining normothermia in the newborn is critical while on scene and during conveyance. The optimum body temperature of the baby should be between 36.5 and 37.5 degrees.

Bibliography

1. Fawke J, Wyllie J, Madar J, Ainsworth S, Tinnion R, Chittick R, Wenlock N, Cusack J, Monnelly V, Lockey A, Hampshire S. 2021. Newborn resuscitation and support of transition of infants at birth Guidelines. Resuscitation Council [UK].

2. Goodwin L, Voss S, McClelland G, Beach E, Bedson A, Black S, Deave T, Miller N, Taylor H, Benger J. Temperature measurement of babies born in the pre-hospital setting: analysis of ambulance service data and qualitative interviews with paramedics. *Emergency Medical Journal* 2022, Nov; 39(11): 826–832.

3. National Institute of Child Health and Human Development. *What is a high-risk pregnancy?* Rockville NICHD, 2017.

4. Laptook AR, Salhab W, Bhaskar B; Neonatal Research Network. Admission temperature of low birth weight infants: predictors and associated morbidities. *Pediatrics* 2007 Mar, 119(3): e643-9. doi: 10.1542/peds.2006-0943. Epub 2007 Feb 12. PMID: 17296783.

5. Woollard M, Hinshaw K, Simpson H, Wieteska S. Normal delivery. In Pre-hospital Obstetric Emergency Training. Oxford: Wiley-Blackwell, 2009: 28–37.

6. Woollard M, Hinshaw K, Simpson H, Wieteska S. Structured approach to the obstetric patient. In Pre-hospital Obstetric Emergency Training. Oxford: Wiley-Blackwell, 2009: 38–52.

7. Woollard M, Hinshaw K, Simpson H, Wieteska S. Emergencies in late pregnancy. In Pre-Hospital Obstetric Emergency Training. Oxford: Wiley-Blackwell, 2009: 62–110.

8. Woollard M, Hinshaw K, Simpson H, Wieteska S. Emergencies after delivery. In Pre-hospital Obstetric Emergency Training. Oxford: Wiley-Blackwell, 2009: 111–124.

9. Woollard M, Hinshaw K, Simpson H, Wieteska S. Care of the baby at birth. In Pre-hospital Obstetric Emergency Training. Oxford: Wiley-Blackwell, 2009: 125–135.

10. Health and Care Professions Council. Standards of Conduct, Performance and Ethics: Your Duties as a Registrant. London: Health Professions Council, 2003.

Management of Post-partum Haemorrhage (PPH)

1. Introduction

- **Primary PPH:** Blood loss of 500 mls or more or any blood loss that results in clinical signs of hypovolemic shock. Occurs within 24 hours of birth.
- **Secondary PPH:** Excessive bleeding from the birth canal between 24 hours and 6 weeks post birth (if a maternity sanitary pad is soaked within 30 minutes).

If Primary or Secondary PPH is diagnosed, complete ALL parts of the following management package (regardless of the cause or whether the placenta has delivered).

(Refer to the algorithm)

If PPH is diagnosed, complete all parts of the following management package (regardless of cause or whether the placenta has been delivered).

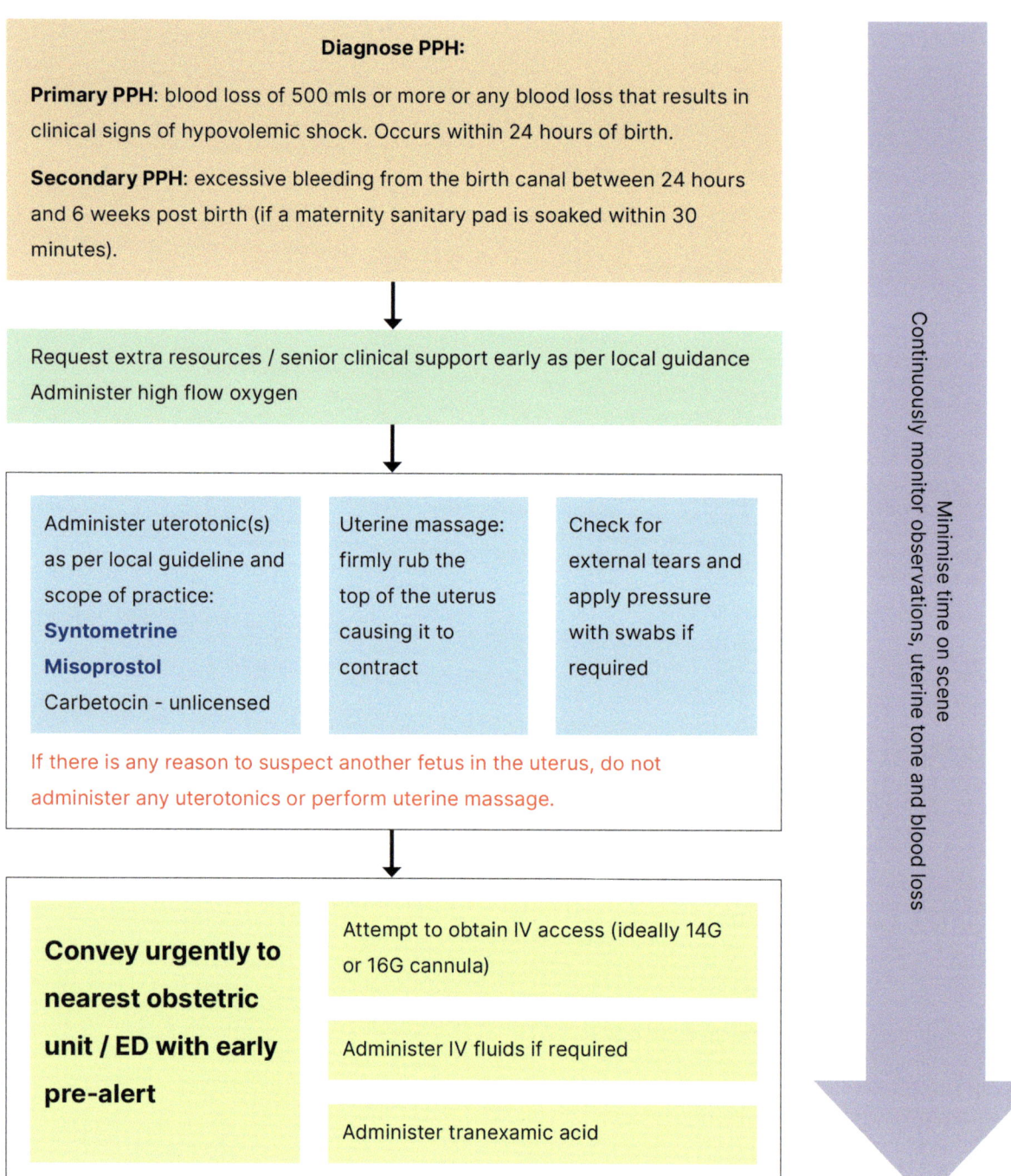

Figure 5.10 – Management of primary and secondary PPH.

Management of Post-partum Haemorrhage (PPH)

2. Pathophysiology

(For reference only; management is the same regardless of the cause)

TONE: The uterine muscle needs to contract post birth in order to close off placental arteries. If there is lack of uterine tone following birth the placental bed will continue to bleed. 70% of primary PPH are from uterine atony.

TRAUMA: Any tear to the genital tract. Inspect externally with consent.

TISSUE: Retained products of conception including placenta, membranes and/or blood clots. This is the cause of the majority of secondary PPH; retained products may also result in infection.

THROMBIN: A clotting disorder may reduce the woman's ability to form sufficient clots for haemostasis.

NB Patients that weigh less will be compromised quicker than patients that weigh more.

3. Management

Immediately:

- Request senior clinical support early as per local guidance
- Administer high flow oxygen

Perform Uterine massage:

- Palpate the abdomen and feel for the top of the uterus (fundus).
- Assess uterus for size/height – if it is below the level of the umbilicus tone is likely to be good.
- Assess tone of the uterus: it should feel hard like a cricket ball.

If unable to feel a hard central structure at or below the umbilicus assume poor tone and commence uterine massage. Massage with a cupped hand in a circular motion.

- The uterus should become firm as massage is applied. Provide pain relief as required (refer to **Pain Management in Adults and Children**).

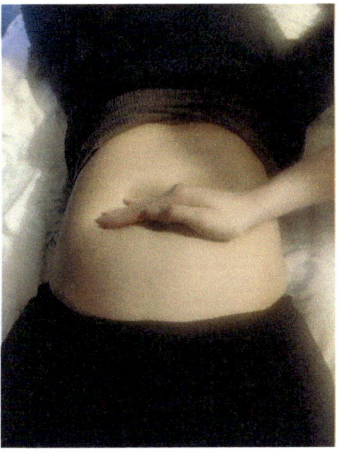

- When performing uterine massage, initially PV blood loss/clots may be observed as the uterus starts to contract. Continue to massage and observe PV loss, which should then reduce.
- Ideally one clinician should be allocated to perform uterine massage whenever there is poor tone or if the woman is bleeding. Keep hand in place whenever possible so you can feel immediately if uterine tone relaxes. Recommence uterine massage if there is poor tone or bleeding continues.

Administer Uterotonic Drugs:

- "Uterotonics" such as syntometrine and misoprostol are drugs to manage PPH. They sustain a uterine contraction for the control of bleeding after birth.
- If there is any specific reason to suspect another fetus is in the uterus, do not administer any uterotonics or perform uterine massage.
- **Administer uterotonics** available locally according to scope of practice:
  – Refer to **Syntometrine**.
  – Refer to **Misoprostol**.
  – Carbetocin: may be available in some ambulance trusts (as an alternative to syntometrine; unlicensed).
- Clinicians that have multiple uterotonics available to them should use one agent at a time and observe for any effect. They can be used in any order. If the haemorrhage is catastrophic they can be given in quick succession. Do not delay time on scene.

Administer Anti-fibrinolytic drug:

- Establish intravenous access (ideally with two large bore (14G or 16G) cannulae). If cannulation is unsuccessful prioritise extrication and conveyance.
- Following administration of uteronic(s), administer **Tranexamic Acid** (TXA).
- Tranexamic acid should be administered within 3 hours of onset of excessive bleeding.
- Administration of tranexamic acid should not delay transport; consider administering en route.
- Tranexamic acid is ideally given intravenously. However, it can be given intramuscularly if intravenous access is not possible; follow local guidelines.

Ongoing management:

- Continuously monitor all observations for signs of hypovolaemic shock and treat accordingly.
- If there is an obvious external tear use swabs to apply sustained pressure.
- Administer fluid replacement if required to maintain systolic blood pressure of 90 mmHg (refer to **Intravascular Fluid Therapy in Adults**).

Management of Post-partum Haemorrhage (PPH)

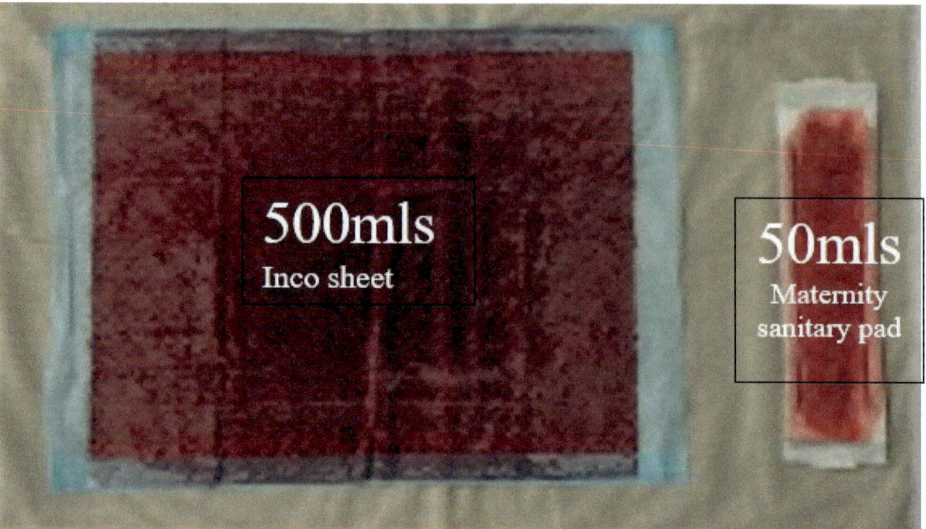

Figure 5.11 – Examples of blood volumes.

- Undertake a time critical conveyance to hospital according to local guidelines. Provide a pre-alert stating "postpartum haemorrhage".
- The patient should be conveyed in any supine position.
- Use the first available transporting resource to convey the patient.
- During conveyance provide ongoing assessment and uterine massage if required to maintain uterine tone.
- Provide emotional support to the patient and family throughout and listen to any concerns.

Continuously estimate blood loss:
- PPH diagnosis should be based on estimated blood loss but also on the clinical picture (observations).
- If in doubt, diagnose PPH and deliver the management package above.

Management of the cord and placenta during primary PPH:
- Complete all the management steps above regardless of whether the placenta has delivered or not.
- The cord should remain intact until the cord has gone white (if the baby is well) or for at least 60 seconds following birth. However, if the patient is having a PPH the cord can be clamped and cut earlier if required to logistically facilitate the delivery of PPH management.
- Do not pull on the cord/placenta before it has delivered. If the placenta delivers, transport it to hospital in an appropriate clinical waste bag.
- Do not wait on scene for the placenta to deliver if there is a PPH; undertake a time critical conveyance to hospital according to local guidelines with an early pre-alert.

4. Bimanual Compression

- Bimanual compression is an internal manoeuvre only performed during major ongoing haemorrhage when other measures have failed and regardless of whether placenta is delivered or not.
- It may be considered by paramedics that have received appropriate training to undertake this intervention (follow local policy).

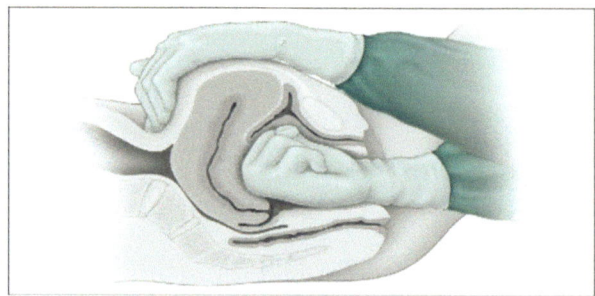

(Reprinted with permission from Beckmann CRB, Ling FW, Smith RP et al. Obstetrics & Gynecology. 6th ed. Philadelphia, PA: Lippincott Williams & Wilkins, 2009)

Management of Post-partum Haemorrhage (PPH)

> **KEY POINTS!**
>
> **Management of Post-partum Haemorrhage (PPH)**
> - Request senior clinical support early as per local guidance.
> - If there is any specific reason to suspect another fetus is in the uterus, do not administer any uterotonics or perform uterine massage.
> - Perform uterine massage.
> - Administer uterotonic drugs.
> - Following administration of uteronic(s), administer tranexamic acid (TXA).

References

1. Püchel J, Sitter M, Kranke P, Pecks U. Procedural techniques to control postpartum hemorrhage. *Best Practice & Research Clinical Anaesthesiology* 2022, 10.1016/j.bpa.2022.09.002.

2. Jones AJ, Federspiel JJ, Eke AC. Preventing postpartum hemorrhage with combined therapy rather than oxytocin alone pharmacologic therapy. *American Journal of Obstetrics & Gynecology MFM* 2022, 10.1016/j.ajogmf.2022.100731, (100731).

3. Fernanda M, Nassar A, Theron G, Barnea G. FIGO recommendations on the management of postpartum hemorrhage. *Int J Gynecol Obstet.* 2022, 157(Suppl. 1): 3–50.

4. Mavrides E, Allard S, Chandraharan E, Collins P, Green L, Hunt BJ, Riris S, Thomson AJ on behalf of the Royal College of Obstetricians and Gynaecologists. Prevention and management of postpartum haemorrhage. *BJOG* 2016, 124: e106–e149.

5. Chandraharan E, Krishna A (2017). Diagnosis and management of postpartum haemorrhage, BMJ British Medical Journal Publishing Group. Available at: http://www.bmj.com/content/358/bmj.j3875.abstract. Accessed 20/04/2023.

6. WHO Recommendations on prevention and treatment of postpartum haemorrhage and the WOMAN trial. https://www.who.int/reproductivehealth/topics/maternal_perinatal/pph-woman-trail/en/. Accessed 20/04/2023.

7. Mousa H, Blum J, El Senoun G, Shakur H, Alfirevic Z. Treatment for primary postpartum hemorrhage. Cochrane Database Syst Rev. 2014, 2(CD0003249). https://doi.org/10.1002/14651858.CD003249.pub3.

8. Leonardsen ACL, Helgesen AK, Ulvøy L. et al. Prehospital assessment and management of postpartum haemorrhage- healthcare personnel's experiences and perspectives. *BMC Emerg Med* 2021, 21(98). https://doi.org/10.1186/s12873-021-00490-8. 9

Maternal Resuscitation

1. Introduction

- As outlined by the Mother and Babies: Reducing Risk through Audits and Confidential Enquiries Across the UK (MBRRACE) report, 'for women in the United Kingdom, giving birth remains safer than ever – less than 9 in every 100,000 women die in pregnancy and around childbirth. Overall the maternal mortality rate in the UK continues to fall'.
- Between 2012 and 2014, deaths from 'indirect' causes were the largest group of deaths; these are deaths from conditions not directly due to pregnancy but due to existing conditions which are exacerbated by pregnancy, for example women with heart problems. Given the very gradual rate of decline and the complexity of medical conditions now experienced by women during pregnancy, achieving the Government's ambition to reduce maternal deaths by 20% by 2020 and 50% by 2030 presents a major challenge for the health service that will require co-ordination of care across multiple specialities.[1]
- A maternal death is defined internationally as the death of a woman during or up to 6 weeks (42 days) after the end of pregnancy (whether the pregnancy ended by termination, miscarriage or a birth, or was an ectopic pregnancy) through causes associated with, or exacerbated by, pregnancy.[2]
- A late maternal death is one that occurs between 6 weeks and 1 year after the end of pregnancy.
- Deaths are further subdivided on the basis of cause into:
    - direct deaths, from pregnancy-specific causes, such as pre-eclampsia
    - indirect deaths, from other medical conditions made worse by pregnancy, such as cardiac disease
    - coincidental deaths, where the cause is considered to be unrelated to pregnancy, such as road traffic accidents.

These definitions are summarised in Table 5.6.

TABLE 5.6 – Definitions of Maternal Deaths[2]

Maternal Death is the death of a woman while pregnant or within 42 days of the end of the pregnancy, including giving birth, ectopic pregnancy, miscarriage or termination of pregnancy, from any cause related to or aggravated by the pregnancy or its management, but not from accidental or incidental causes.

Direct Death	Resulting from obstetric complications of the pregnant state (pregnancy, labour and puerperium), from interventions, omissions, incorrect treatment or from a chain of events resulting from any of the above.
Indirect Death	Resulting from previous existing disease, or disease that developed during pregnancy and which was not the result of direct obstetric causes but which was aggravated by the physiological effects of pregnancy.
Late Death	Occurring between 42 days and 1 year after the end of pregnancy, including giving birth, ectopic pregnancy, miscarriage or termination of pregnancy, as the result of Direct or Indirect maternal causes.
Coincidental Death	From unrelated causes that happen to occur in pregnancy or the puerperium. Termed 'Fortuitous' in the International Classification of Diseases (ICD).

- It is important to recognise that there are two patients.
- Effective resuscitation of the mother may provide effective resuscitation of the fetus.
- Resuscitation of the mother is the primary concern.
- If there is no response to CPR after 5 minutes, undertake a **TIME-CRITICAL** transfer to the nearest emergency department (ED), ideally with an obstetric unit attached. Place a pre-alert as soon as possible to enable the ED team to organise a maternity team, as an immediate peri-mortem caesarean section (resuscitative hysterotomy) may be performed.

2. Cardiac Arrest

Undertake a TIME-CRITICAL transfer as soon as ventilation is achieved and CPR commenced.

2.1 Introduction

- The approach to resuscitating a pregnant woman is the same as that of any adult in cardiac arrest. However, from 20 weeks gestation onwards, the weight of the gravid uterus can cause 30% of cardiac output to be sequestered into the lower limbs with a woman lying supine.
- Immediately manually displace the uterus to the maternal left side (relieving pressure on the inferior vena cava (refer to Figure 5.12)).
- CPR should not be terminated in the pre-hospital setting on a pregnant woman.

Maternal Resuscitation

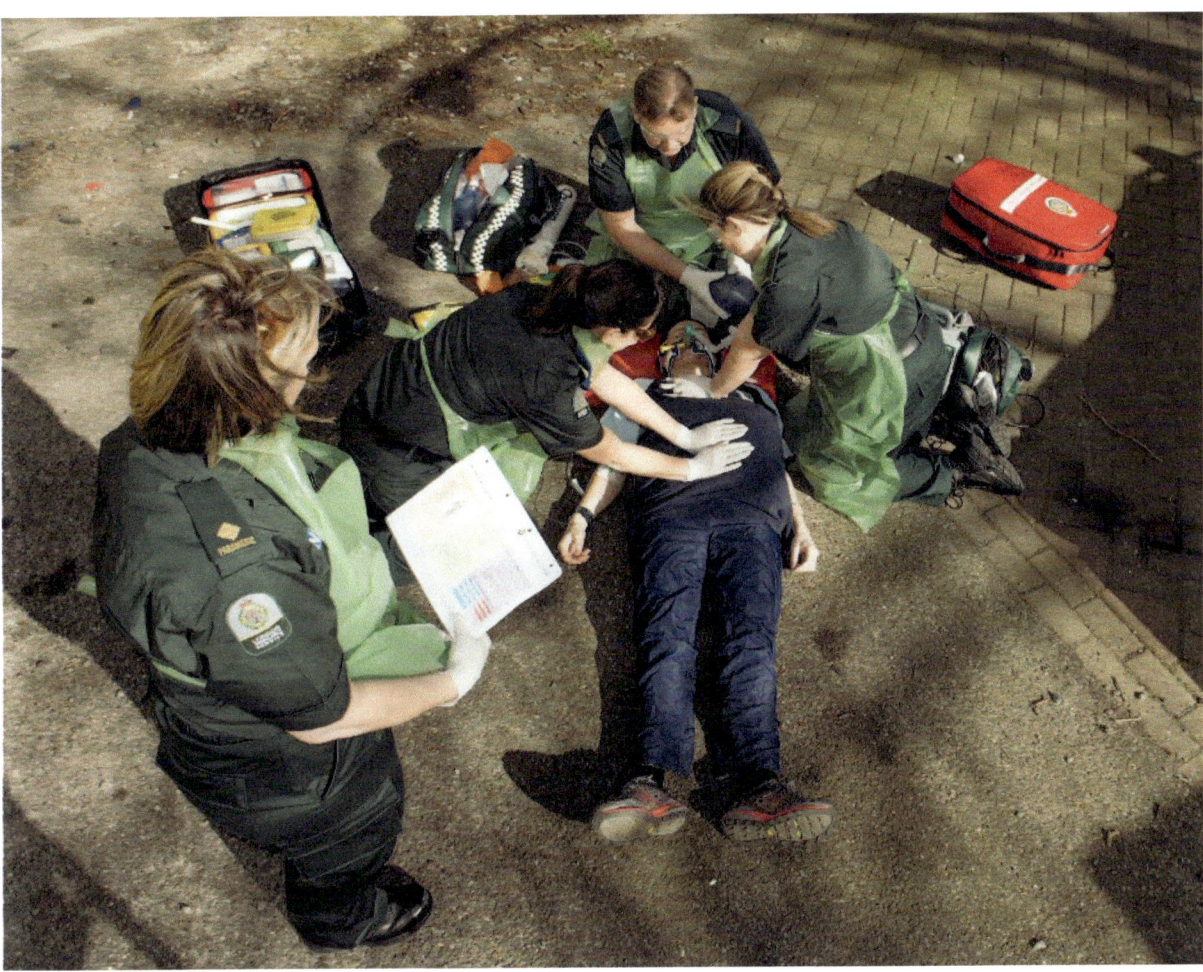

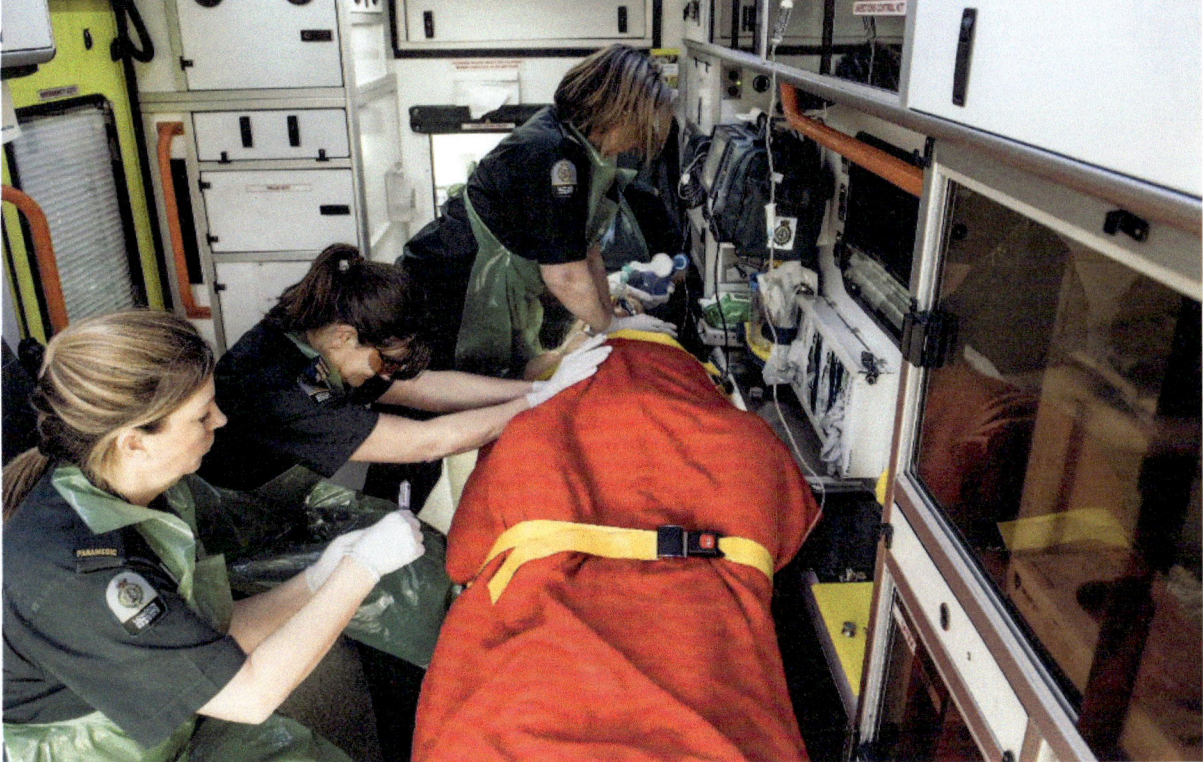

Figure 5.12 – Manual uterine displacement during resuscitation.

Maternal Resuscitation

2.2 Pathophysiology

Cardiac arrest in pregnancy is very rare. Common causes of sudden maternal death include haemorrhage, embolism (thromboembolic and amniotic fluid) and hypertensive disorders. Figure 5.13 and Table 5.7 detail the common reversible causes of maternal collapse in the pregnant woman.

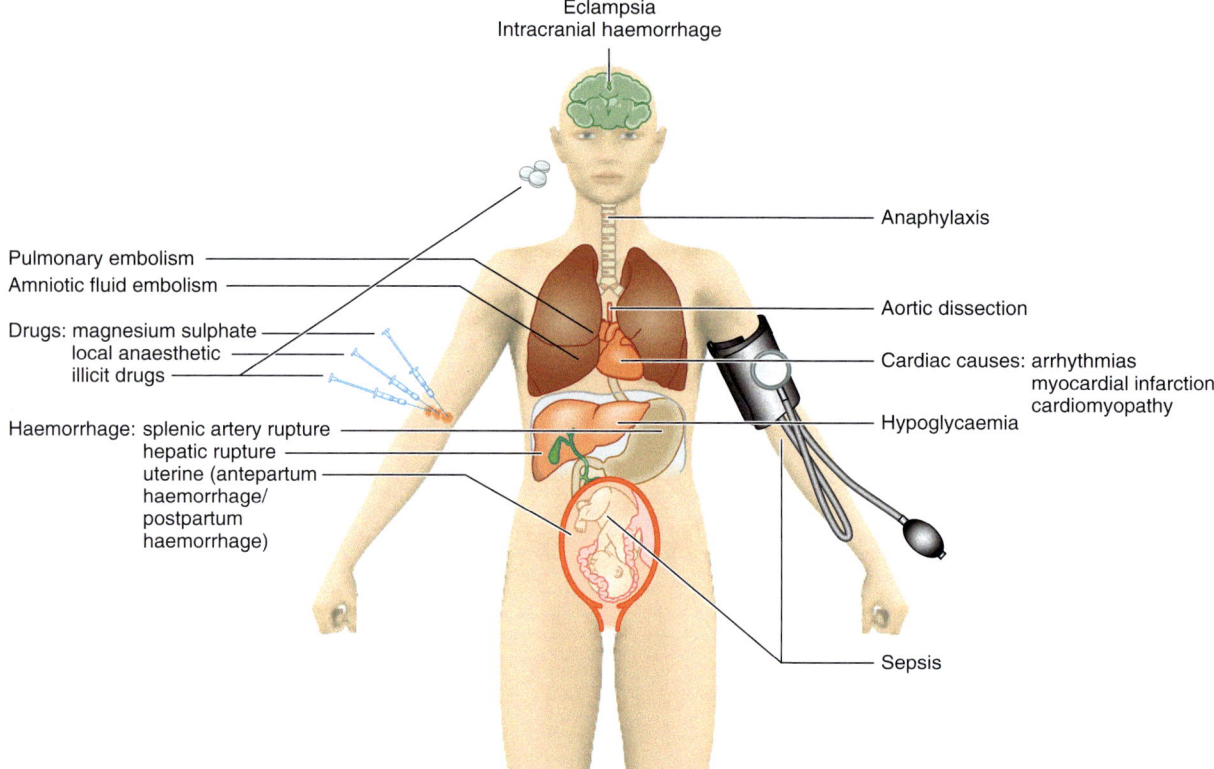

Figure 5.13 – Causes of maternal collapse.[3] Republished with kind permission of the Royal College of Obstetricians and Gynaecologists.

TABLE 5.7 – Reversible Causes of Maternal Collapse[3]

REVERSIBLE CAUSE		CAUSE IN PREGNANCY
4Hs	• Hypovolaemia • Hypoxia • Hypo/hyperkalaemia and other electrolyte disturbances • Hypothermia	• Bleeding (may be concealed) (obstetric/other) or relative hypovolaemia of dense spinal block; septic or neurogenic shock. • Pregnant women become hypoxic rapidly. • Cardiac events: peripartum cardiomyopathy, myocardial infarction, aortic dissection, large-vessel aneurysms. • No more likely.
4Ts	• Thromboembolism • Toxicity • Tension pneumothorax • Tamponade (cardiac)	• Amniotic fluid embolus, pulmonary embolus, air embolus, myocardial infarction. • Local anaesthetic, magnesium, other. • Following trauma/suicide attempt
	• Eclampsia and pre-eclampsia	• Includes intracranial haemorrhage.

Maternal Resuscitation

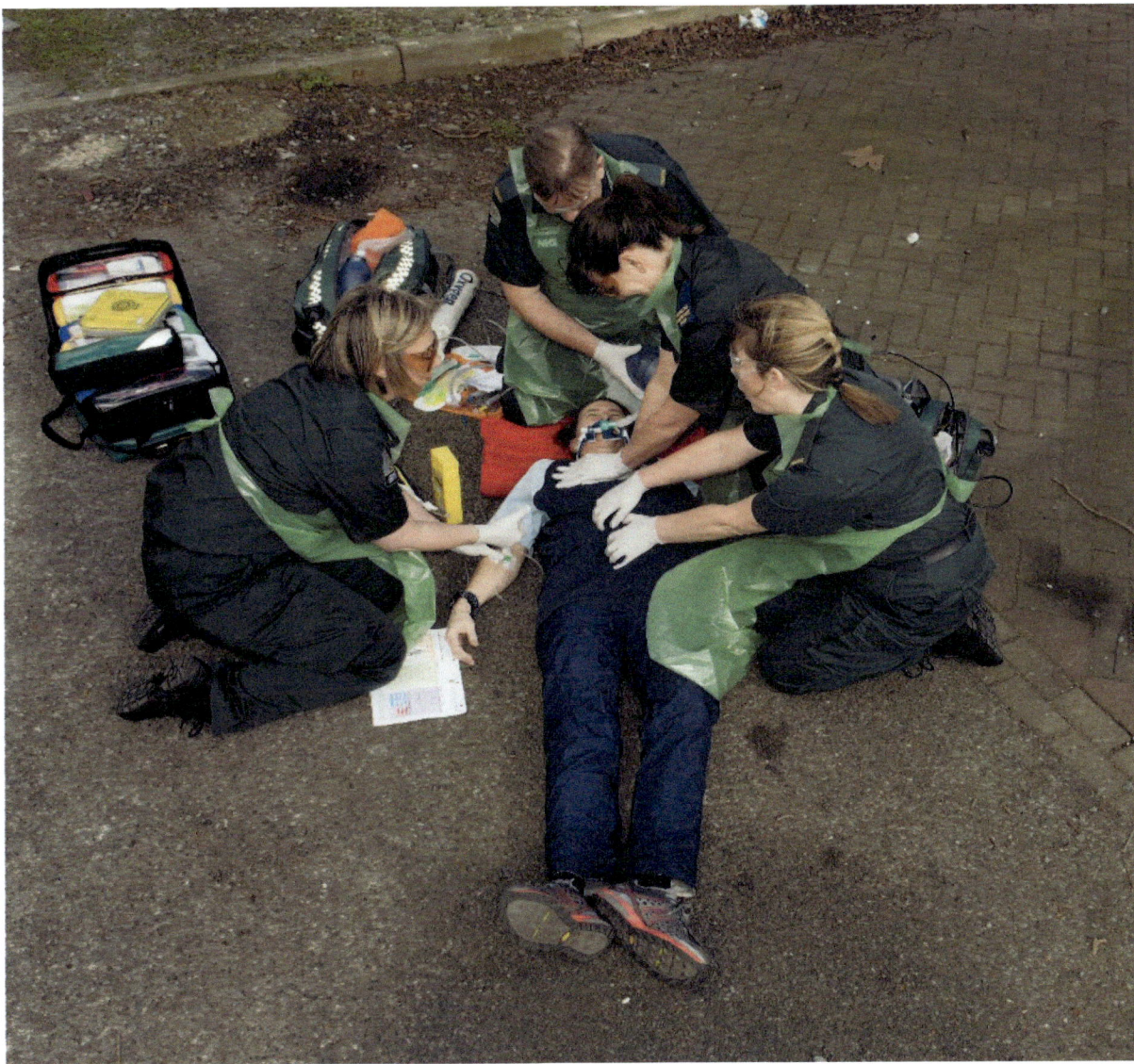

Figure 5.14 – Working as a team.

2.3 Modifications for Cardiac Arrest in Pregnancy

For the assessment and management of cardiac arrest during pregnancy, refer to Table 5.8.

Key points are listed below:

- Start resuscitation according to standard ALS guidelines, with manual displacement of the uterus to the maternal left to minimise inferior vena caval compression (spinal board will not achieve the required left lateral tilt).
- The hand position for chest compressions may need to be slightly higher (2–3 cm) on the sternum for patients with advanced pregnancy (e.g. >28 weeks).
- Consider using a tracheal tube 0.5–1.0 mm smaller than usual as the trachea can be narrowed by oedema and swelling. Supraglottic airway devices are a suitable alternative in the pre-hospital setting and may provide a more rapid means of oxygenation than potentially prolonged intubation attempts.[4]
- Defibrillation energy levels are as recommended for standard defibrillation. If large breasts make it difficult to place an apical defibrillator electrode, use an antero-posterior or bi-axillary electrode position.
- Establish IV or IO access as soon as possible, preferably at a level above the diaphragm.
- Identify and correct the cause of the arrest using 4Hs and 4Ts as appropriate.
- Administer 100% supplemental oxygen (refer to **Oxygen**).
- Undertake a **TIME-CRITICAL** transfer to the nearest ED, ideally with an obstetric unit attached. Place a pre-alert as soon as possible to enable the ED team to organise a maternity team, as an immediate peri-mortem caesarean section (resuscitative hysterotomy) may be performed.

Maternal Resuscitation

2.4 The Team Approach to Pre-hospital Resuscitation (Resuscitation Council 2015)

- Resuscitation requires a system to be in place to achieve the best possible chance of survival. The system requires technical and non-technical skills (teamwork, situational awareness, leadership, decision making) in the pregnant woman; this will also involve consideration for manual uterine displacement.

Allocation of Roles

- Appoint a team leader as early as possible; ideally they should be a paramedic or clinician experienced in pre-hospital resuscitation.
- The team leader should assign team members specific roles, which they clearly understand and are capable of undertaking. This will promote teamwork, reduce confusion and ensure organised and effective management of resuscitation.
- A minimum of four trained staff are required to deliver high-quality resuscitation. This will necessitate dispatch of more than one ambulance resource.
- Ensure there is 360° access to the patient ('Circle of Life'):
  - Position 1: Airway (at head of patient) – the person must be trained and equipped to provide the full range of airway skills.
  - Position 2: High-quality chest compressions and defibrillation if needed – at patient's left side. Be prepared to alternate with the operator at position 3 to avoid fatigue.
  - Position 3: High-quality chest compressions and access to the circulation (intravenous, intraosseous) – at patient's right side.
  - Position 4: Team leader – stand back and oversee the resuscitation attempt, only becoming involved if required. The team leader should have an awareness of the whole incident and ensure high-quality resuscitation is maintained and appropriate decisions made.

The team leader will need to allocate the role of manual uterine displacement and may need the involvement of additional resources where available.

TABLE 5.8 – ASSESSMENT and MANAGEMENT of: Cardiac Arrest During Pregnancy

Undertake a primary survey ABCDE

- At 20 weeks, the uterine fundus will be below the umbilicus.
- Manage as per standard advanced life support (refer to **Advanced Life Support**).
- Assess and exclude reversible causes (see Table 5.7).
- Caution – ventilation with a bag-valve-mask may lead to regurgitation and aspiration. A supraglottic airway device may reduce the risk of gastric aspiration and make ventilation of the lungs easier (refer to **Airway and Breathing Management**).
- If there is no response to CPR after 5 minutes, undertake a **TIME-CRITICAL** transfer to the nearest ED, ideally with an obstetric unit attached. Place a pre-alert as soon as possible to enable the ED team to organise a maternity team, as an immediate peri-mortem caesarean section (resuscitative hysterotomy) may be performed.
- For pregnant women at 20 weeks gestation or more, use manual uterine displacement (to the maternal left side) to avoid compression of the inferior vena cava.
- Manual displacement can be applied from either the maternal left or right side, with the assistant ensuring the uterus is displaced towards the maternal left (Resuscitation Council, 2015).
- Within the ambulance saloon, manual uterine displacement must be maintained.
- Establish IV or IO access as soon as possible, preferably at a level above the diaphragm.

KEY POINTS!

Maternal Resuscitation

- **DO NOT withhold or terminate maternal resuscitation.**
- **ALWAYS manage pregnant women in cardiac arrest at greater than 20 weeks' gestation with manual displacement of the uterus to the maternal left.**
- **If resuscitation attempts fail to achieve ROSC within 5 minutes of the cardiac arrest, undertake a TIME-CRITICAL transfer to the nearest ED, ideally with an obstetric unit attached.**
- **Provide an early pre-alert to enable the ED team to summon the maternity team, as an immediate peri-mortem caesarean section (resuscitative hysterotomy) may be performed.**

Maternal Resuscitation

Further Reading

Further important information and evidence in support of this guideline can be found in the Bibliography.[5,6,7,8]

Bibliography

1. Knight M, Tuffnell D, Kenyon S, Shakespeare J, Gray R, Kurinczuk JJ (eds) on behalf of MBRRACE-UK. *Saving Lives, Improving Mothers' Care – Surveillance of maternal deaths in the UK 2011–13 and lessons learned to inform maternity care from the UK and Ireland Confidential Enquiries into Maternal Deaths and Morbidity 2009–13*. Oxford: National Perinatal Epidemiology Unit, University of Oxford, 2015.

2. World Health Organization. *International Classification of Diseases (ICD) 10*. Available from: http://apps.who.int/classifications/icd10/browse/2016/en#/XV, 2010.

3. Royal College of Obstetricians and Gynaecologists. *Maternal Collapse in Pregnancy and the Puerperium* (Green-top Guideline 56). London: RCOG, 2010, updated 2014. Available from: https://www.rcog.org.uk/globalassets/documents/guidelines/gtg_56.pdf.

4. Resuscitation Council. *Prehospital Resuscitation*. Available from: https://www.resus.org.uk/resuscitation-guidelines/prehospital-resuscitation, 2015.

5. Deakin CD, Nolan JP, Soar J, Sunde K, Koster RW, Smith GB, et al. European Resuscitation Council Guidelines for Resuscitation 2010 Section 4: adult advanced life support. *Resuscitation* 2010, 81(10): 1305–1352.

6. Koster RW, Baubin MA, Bossaert LL, Caballero A, Cassan P, Castren M, et al. European Resuscitation Council Guidelines for Resuscitation 2010 Section 2: adult basic life support and use of automated external defibrillators. *Resuscitation* 2010, 81(10): 1277–1292.

7. Soar J, Perkins GD, Abbas G, Alfonzo A, Barelli A, Bierens JJLM, et al. European Resuscitation Council Guidelines for Resuscitation 2010 Section 8: cardiac arrest in special circumstances: electrolyte abnormalities, poisoning, drowning, accidental hypothermia, hyperthermia, asthma, anaphylaxis, cardiac surgery, trauma, pregnancy, electrocution. *Resuscitation* 2010, 81(10): 1400–1433.

8. Deakin CD, Nolan JP, Sunde K, Koster RW. European Resuscitation Council Guidelines for Resuscitation 2010 Section 3: electrical therapies: automated external defibrillators, defibrillation, cardioversion and pacing. *Resuscitation* 2010, 81(10): 1293–1304.

Newborn Life Support

This section of the newborn guidance focuses on the resuscitation/stabilisation of a baby immediately after birth. The guideline will discuss recognition and management of a baby born in poor condition and the immediate actions that should be taken.

1. Introduction

- Passage through the birth canal is a hypoxic event for the fetus, since placental respiratory exchange is prevented for the 50–75 seconds' duration of the average contraction. Mature babies have energy stores to help cope with this.
- Most, but not all, infants adapt well to extra-uterine life, but some require help with stabilisation, and some require resuscitation. Up to 85% breathe spontaneously without intervention; a further 10% respond after drying, stimulation and airway opening manoeuvres; approximately 5% receive positive pressure ventilation. Intubation rates vary between 0.4% and 2%. Fewer than 0.3% of infants receive chest compressions and only 0.05% receive adrenaline.[1]
- The approach to Newborn Life Support guideline outlines this help and comprises the following elements:
  - umbilical cord management
  - thermal care – drying and covering the baby to conserve heat
  - assessing the need for any intervention
  - opening the airway
  - lung aeration
  - ventilation breaths
  - chest compressions.

2. Assessment and Management

TABLE 5.9 – ASSESSMENT and MANAGEMENT of: Newborn Life Support

Environment

In all cases:

- Ensure the ambient temperature is as high as possible.
- Close windows and doors to reduce cold draughts.
- Prepare a firm, flat environment for potential resuscitation.
- Prepare equipment, including warm towels, and consider extra warming equipment if possible.
- Are additional resources required?

Cord Management

Delayed clamping of the cord improves haemodynamic stability and may have survival and longer-term benefits, especially in the preterm. Warm placental blood may improve thermal stability.

Planning is required:

- The cord can remain intact while the baby is assessed at birth. If the baby initiates breathing spontaneously and does not require immediate intervention, wait at least 60 seconds or ideally for the cord to become white as blood stops flowing from the placenta to the baby.
- If immediate resuscitation is required, then the cord should be clamped and cut, the baby moved to the resuscitation area and appropriate measures taken to stabilise the baby.
- Initial thermal measures and assessment can take place on the perineum with the cord intact. Do not leave the baby exposed in a cold environment.
- If there is any evidence of a snapped cord, clamp the cord immediately and observe the baby for signs of hypovolaemia (for example, pale mucous membranes and respiratory issues).

Thermal Care

Outcomes are poorer and mortality increased if babies get cold. Babies are born wet and can become cold very easily, particularly if they remain wet and exposed.

- Term and late preterm infants:
  - Dry the baby, ideally with pre-warmed towels, paying particular attention to the head; remove the wet towel, and cover with a dry towel.
  - Apply a hat – a lot of heat can be lost from the head.
  - A newborn that does not require resuscitation can be placed with the mother and skin-to-skin contact provided. Use a blanket covering the baby to protect from drafts.
- Preterm infants (<32 weeks):[2]
  - In the preterm infant, the same measures may be used. Where airway and breathing are stable, skin to skin can be an effective way of providing warmth.

With skin-to-skin care, continuous observations of the baby's airway position and breathing are needed, to ensure these are maintained. Where interventions are needed, this may not be practical.

Newborn Life Support

TABLE 5.9 – ASSESSMENT and MANAGEMENT of: Newborn Life Support *(continued)*

Skin to skin affords the opportunity for early feeding to reduce the risk of hypoglycaemia. If available, other measures may be considered, such as:

- Plastic bag/[3, 4] wrap:
  - There is evidence from hospital and low-resource settings that placing babies under 32 weeks' gestation undried into a plastic wrap or a bag with radiant heat can improve thermal stability.
  - A plastic wrap reduces evaporative heat loss and where a radiant heat source (exothermic mattress, skin to skin) is not available may still be used with conventional measures, such as wrapping in a towel. It is not necessary to dry the baby if a plastic wrap or bag is used in a timely manner.
  - **Babies must never be placed in plastic wrap and left exposed.**
- Thermal mattress:
  - Exothermic mattresses are an effective way of providing radiant heat to help keep babies warm and may be used in conjunction with plastic wrap and towels.
  - Activate in advance of the delivery according to manufacturer recommendations.
  - The heat is unregulated. Never place a baby directly onto a mattress, as this may cause burns; ensure the mattress and/or baby is wrapped with a towel.
- The use of such devices should be under specific agreed local guidance.
- Care needs to be taken in the unregulated environment of the pre-hospital setting and ambulance where monitoring of temperature may be more of a challenge.
- Record the temperature as soon as is practical. Check at regular intervals if able to do so without unwrapping the baby. Beware of overheating the baby.
- If in transit, ensure cabin temperature is high. (If uncomfortable for the attendants, then likely more appropriate for the baby.)

Assessment

The initial assessment should be carried out as soon as possible after the birth of the baby. It establishes whether interventions are required.

Assessment can be carried out with the cord intact and while measures are being undertaken to keep the baby warm.

- **Colour** – Examine the lips, tongue and mucous membranes. Babies will display cyanosis immediately after delivery in these areas, but central perfusion improves leading to the development of enhanced skin colour. A baby that continues to show cyanosis is of potential concern. A baby with pallor is of immediate concern as this suggests significant distress.
- **Tone** – A flexed baby with muscle tone has a functioning nervous system. Of concern are floppy unconscious babies who need immediate help and who may not be able to maintain their airway.
- **Breathing** – If a baby is breathing with visible chest movement, this suggests the brain is working. Ensure the baby has an open airway – breathing efforts may be adequate or inadequate/absent, in which case support is required.
- **Heart rate** – Listen to the heart rate with a stethoscope – a fast heart rate (>100) suggests adequate oxygenation; a slower heart rate (60–100) suggests that there is a degree of hypoxia. A very slow HR (<60) indicates significant fetal hypoxic stress and a need to intervene.

Try not to expose the baby when checking the heart rate. A stethoscope is the best immediate tool.

Breathing and heart rate determine whether actions are required.

Pulse oximeter: If a suitable probe is available, then attaching to the right wrist using an infant probe can give an accurate heart rate and provides an indication of oxygenation. It does not provide immediate information at the time of birth but takes approximately 90 seconds to establish a satisfactory signal where the circulation is adequate. It can help guide subsequent interventions.

ECG leads can be used to monitor heart rate (see below).

Defibrillator pads are not required for newborn life support (NLS) and should not be used to monitor heart rate.

Airway

Having an open airway is critical. In the unconscious or floppy baby, the prominent occiput may lead to flexion and compromise of the airway of an infant on their back. Position rather than particulate matter is the commonest problem.

- Place the baby on their back with the head in a neutral position, neither flexed nor extended.

(continued)

Newborn Life Support

> **TABLE 5.9 – ASSESSMENT and MANAGEMENT of: Newborn Life Support** *(continued)*
>
> - If the baby is very floppy, a chin support or jaw thrust may be required.
> - A small pad (2 cm thick) can be placed under the shoulders to assist in maintaining the neutral position. Be careful not to over-extend.

Breathing

Inflation (aeration) of the lungs by delivery of air is essential to displace lung fluid in order to establish effective ventilation – longer breaths are delivered to achieve this.

If a baby is crying vigorously, this suggests an adequate airway and breathing effort. Feeble or intermittent cries or silence indicate that help may be required.

If the breathing is inadequate after initial assessment, it is necessary to support (use two people if resources permit).

- Select an appropriate (best-fit) mask and 500 ml paediatric bag-valve system.
- Start on air.
- Give five inflation breaths, sustaining the inflation pressure for 2–3 seconds with each breath.
- Be careful when squeezing the bag. Aim for consistent but not forceful delivery.
- Where it is possible to measure the inflation pressure, aim for 30 cm of water peak pressure for a term baby (25 cm initially for a preterm baby <32 weeks) – otherwise aim for enough pressure to see the chest rise gently.

Note – The first two or three breaths replace the fluid in the lungs with air without changing the volume in the chest. Therefore, you may not observe the chest wall rise until the fourth or fifth breath.

Reassess

- After any intervention, reassess.
- Check the **heart rate** and whether there is **chest movement**.

If the heart rate is fast (>100), assume lung aeration has been successful.

- If the baby does not breath spontaneously, then breathe for the baby.
- Deliver ventilation breaths – 30/minute.
- Reassess heart rate and chest movement every 30 seconds.
- Continue until the baby is breathing on their own.

If the heart is slow (60–100), very slow (<60) or absent, either lung aeration has not been adequate **or** the baby requires more than lung aeration alone.

- It is most likely that you have not aerated the lungs effectively.
- It is vital to achieve effective lung inflation and chest movement before moving on to chest compressions.

If the chest is **not** moving:

- Reposition
  - Is the head in the neutral position?
  - Do you need to do a jaw thrust?
- Repeat inflation breaths.
- Reassess **heart rate** and **chest movement**.

If there is no heart rate response and no visible chest movement:

- Consider:
  - Do you need help with the airway from a second person (if not used already)?
  - Is there obstruction in the oropharynx? (Where an appropriately sized laryngoscope is available with suction and where the clinician has the expertise, inspect the airway and remove any obvious obstruction under direct vision.)
  - An oropharyngeal airway can be used in babies >32 weeks' gestation but must be sized correctly.
  - Do you need to consider a supraglottic airway device? For babies of around 2 kg or more, an appropriate size laryngeal mask (e.g. size 1 i-gel) may be used.
  - Do you need a longer inflation time or higher pressure?

Newborn Life Support

TABLE 5.9 – ASSESSMENT and MANAGEMENT of: Newborn Life Support (continued)

- Repeat five inflation breaths after each manoeuvre.
- Reassess heart rate and chest movement.

If the chest is moving but the heart rate remains slow/very slow, ensure that the lungs have been successfully aerated:

- Ventilate for 30 seconds.
- Check the **heart rate** and confirm **chest movement**.

Cardiac Compressions

Should only be commenced after the lungs have been successfully inflated and the HR remains very slow or absent.

- **If the heart rate remains very slow or absent despite the chest moving and after 30 seconds of ventilation, commence cardiac compressions.**
- Ensure the baby is on a flat, hard surface (not a mattress or sofa).
- Encircle the lower chest with both hands in such a way that the two thumbs can compress the lower third of the sternum, at a point just below an imaginary line joining the nipples, with the fingers over the spine at the back.
- Compress the chest quickly and firmly in such a way as to reduce the antero–posterior diameter of the chest by a third.
- The ratio of compressions to inflations in newborn resuscitation is synchronised at 3:1 – 15 cycles in 30 seconds.
- If available, supplement oxygen 100% (flow approx. 6–8 l/min into reservoir bag).
- If baby is in a plastic bag, leave in the bag. Try and maintain the baby's temperature.

Reassess

Reassess every 30 seconds.

- If the heart rate increases and is greater than 60 bpm:
  - Stop cardiac compressions.
  - Continue ventilation unless the baby is breathing effectively.
  - Monitor the heart rate.
  - Wean oxygen if saturations are satisfactory (>95%).
- ECG complexes do not indicate the presence of a cardiac output and should not be the sole means of monitoring the infant. However, improving heart rate on ECG is likely to indicate successful ventilation and some cardiac output.
- If the heart rate continues to be very slow or absent:
  - Continue cardiac compressions and ventilation.
  - Consider next steps.

Next Steps

- Undertake a TIME-CRITICAL transfer.
- Provide a pre-alert and convey to the nearest appropriate destination, as agreed locally.
- Consider securing the airway if not done previously by placing a supraglottic airway device if the infant is of sufficient maturity/size and this will not significantly delay transport.

Venous Access and Drugs

- Attempting to gain IV/IO access must not distract from maintaining high-quality chest compressions and effective lung inflation, and it should only be undertaken when crew numbers and resources are sufficient.
- Early enhanced care support should be requested as per local procedures.
- Where fluid and drugs are required, they may be administered to the neonate as per **Page for Age.**
- Very rarely, the heart rate cannot increase because the infant has lost significant blood volume. If this is the case, there is often a history of blood loss from the infant, but not always. In the presence of hypovolaemia, a fluid bolus of 0.9% sodium chloride may be given over 10–20 seconds.[2] Refer to **Sodium Chloride.**

(continued)

Newborn Life Support

TABLE 5.9 – ASSESSMENT and MANAGEMENT of: Newborn Life Support *(continued)*

Meconium

- Babies born with thick meconium-stained amniotic fluid should receive the same care as all babies – stimulation, thermal care and resuscitation as required. If not responding to initial airway and breathing manoeuvres, inspection may be considered to exclude obstruction.

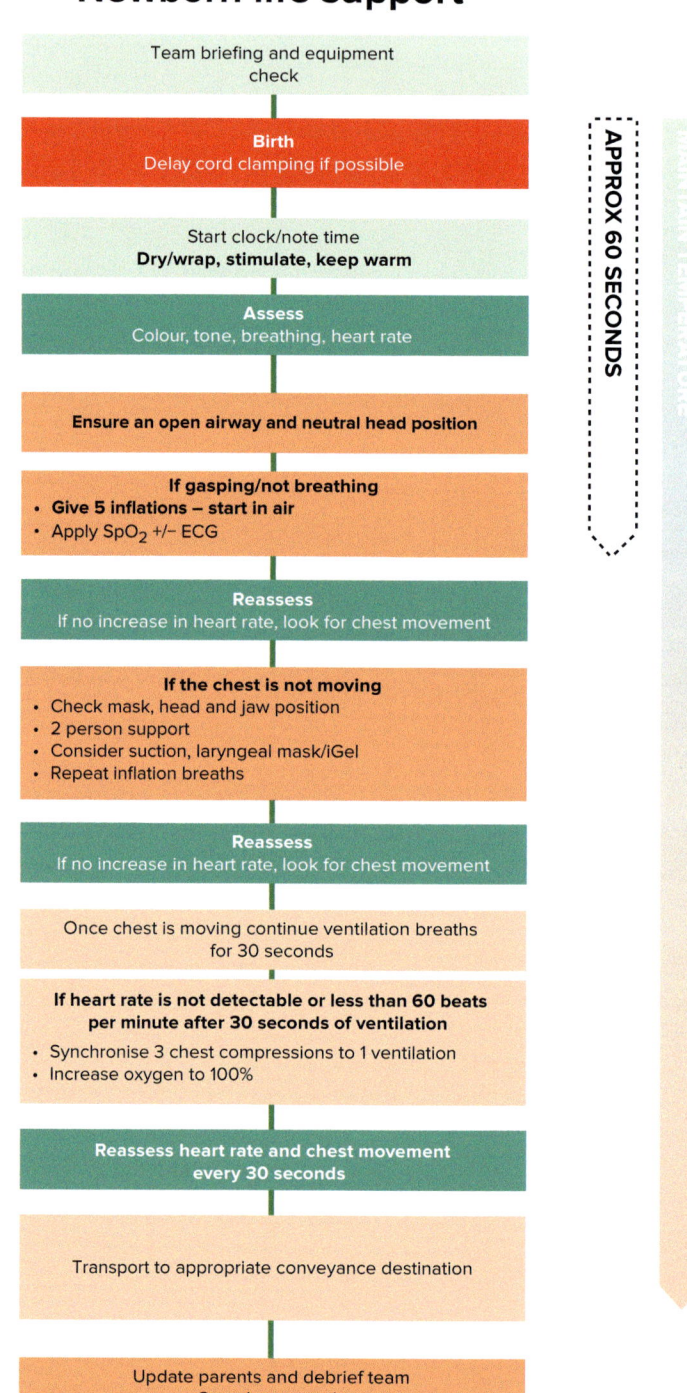

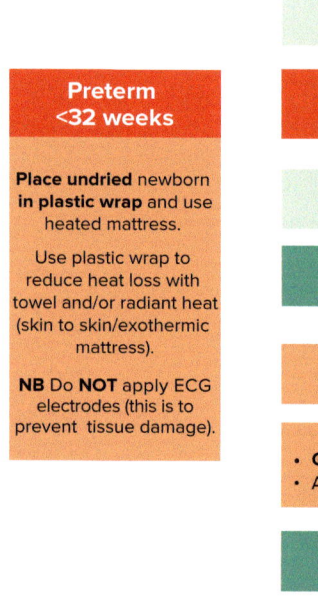

Figure 5.15 – Newborn life support algorithm – modified from the Resuscitation Council (UK) Guidelines 2021 algorithm (www.resus.org.uk).

Newborn Life Support

3. Resuscitation/Stabilisation of the Preterm Baby

This section of the newborn life support guidance focuses on the care of babies born at preterm and extreme preterm gestations. This includes the care of babies born at 22 weeks.

As stated within **Care of the Newborn**, a preterm infant is any baby born at <37 weeks' gestation. For the purpose of this guidance, an extreme preterm baby is any baby born at <32 weeks' gestation, in line with the UK Resuscitation Council guidelines. These babies are vulnerable and require an altered approach in resuscitation.

Why an altered approach?

- **Delayed cord clamping (DCC):** Many preterm babies do not need resuscitation but stabilisation to help them adapt to birth. DCC confers greater advantages in this vulnerable population and should be considered unless immediate intervention is required.
- **Size:** Babies born <32 weeks are smaller and can get cold very quickly. They also have fewer reserves and hypothermia will take effect sooner. It is vital that measures are taken to help them keep warm.
- **Fragile lungs:** Surfactant will not be present in the lungs and a preterm may not breathe effectively. Even if making breathing efforts or initially crying, preterm babies may still need help as the breathing efforts may be inadequate and they get tired. Care needs to be taken with smaller inflation volumes and gentle breaths.
- **Oxygen requirement:** These babies may require oxygen and ideally under pulse oximetry guidance. This can be difficult in the out-of-hospital setting without blenders.
- Clinicians should use the NLS algorithm (Figure 5.15) for resuscitation/stabilisation.
- It is not appropriate to resuscitate babies known to be at <22 weeks' gestation; however, in other situations the approach is towards 'survival-focused care' for the extreme preterm baby with measures as recommended above. Separate guidance exists for comfort care of the extreme preterm baby[2] (see Figure 5.16).
- Early communication with specialist teams is important to ensure destination and receiving teams are prepared for the arrival of the baby.

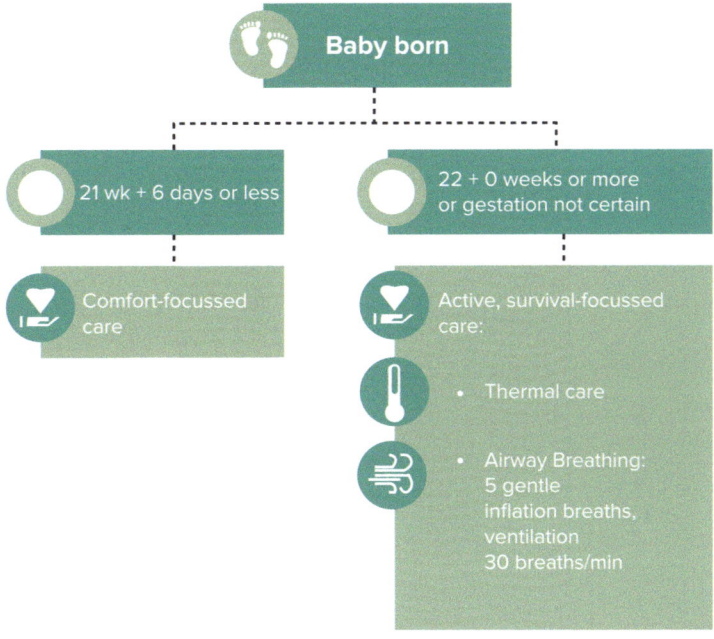

Figure 5.16 – Stabilisation versus non-intervention. Reproduced with permission from the British Association of Perinatal Medicine (BAPM) 2022 (www.bapm.org).

Newborn Life Support

> **KEY POINTS!**
>
> **Newborn Life Support**
> - Passage through the birth canal is a hypoxic event and some babies may require help to establish normal breathing after birth.
> - Keep the environment as warm as possible, prepare an area for potential resuscitation/stabilisation.
> - Consider delayed cord clamping unless immediate resuscitation is required.
> - Assess colour, tone, breathing and heart rate.
> - Babies become cold very easily; dry the baby, remove any wet towels and wrap with dry ones. Use a hat and other thermal measures if required. Skin to skin for well babies. Preterm babies need extra help.
> - If intervention is required, ensure the airway is open by placing the baby on their back with the head in a neutral position. If the baby is very floppy, apply jaw support/thrust.
> - If the baby is not breathing adequately, give five 2–3-second inflation breaths.
> - Check heart rate and chest movement.
> - If the chest does not move and the heart rate is not fast/increasing, repeat airway manoeuvres and inflation breaths.
> - Once lung aeration is achieved, if the baby is not spontaneously breathing, give 30 seconds of ventilation breaths — approx. 30 breaths/min — and confirm chest movement.
> - Check heart rate and chest movement.
> - If the chest is moving with ventilation breaths (no spontaneous breathing) and the heart rate is fast, continue ventilation.
> - If the chest is moving but the heart rate remains very slow (< 60 beats/min), chest compressions are necessary. Compress the chest quickly and firmly at a synchronised ratio of three compressions: one inflation ideally with two thumb encircling technique. Fifteen cycles per 30 seconds. 100% oxygen if available.
> - On transfer, once in the ambulance keep the compartment as warm as possible.
> - Liaise with the receiving unit to inform of situation of baby and mother.

Further Reading

Further important information and evidence in support of this guideline can be found in the Bibliography.[3, 4]

Bibliography

1. Fawke J, Wyllie J, Madar J et al. *Newborn Resuscitation and Support of Transition of Infants at Birth*. London: Resuscitation Council UK, 2021. Available from: https://www.resus.org.uk/library/2021-resuscitation-guidelines/newborn-resuscitation-and-support-transition-infants-birth.

2. British Association of Perinatal Medicine. *Pre-hospital Management of the Baby Born at Extreme Preterm Gestation: A BAPM Framework for Practice.* 2022. Available from: https://www.bapm.org/.

3. Belsches TC, Tilly AE, Miller TR, Kambeyanda RH, Leadford A, Manasyan A, Chomba E et al. Randomised trial of plastic bags to prevent term neonatal hypothermia in a resource-poor setting. *Pediatrics* 2013, 132(3). Available from: http://pediatrics.aappublications.org/content/132/3/e656.

4. Leadford AE, Warren JB, Manasyan A, Chomba E, Salas AA, Schelonka R, Carlo WA. Plastic bags for prevention of hypothermia in preterm and low birth weight infants. *Pediatrics* 2013, 132(1). Available from: http://pediatrics.aappublications.org/content/132/1/e128.

5. Wyllie J, Bruinenberg J, Roehr CC, Rüdiger M, Trevisanuto D, Urlesberger B. European Resuscitation Council Guidelines for resuscitation 2015: Section 7. resuscitation and support of transition of babies at birth. *Resuscitation* 2015, 95: 249–263.

6. Wyllie J, Perlman JM, Kattwinkel J, et al. Part 7: neonatal resuscitation: 2015 International Consensus on Cardiopulmonary Resuscitation and Emergency Cardiovascular Care Science with Treatment Recommendations. *Resuscitation* 2015, 95: e169–201.

Pre-eclampsia and Eclampsia

1. Definitions

- **Pre-eclampsia** is a multi-organ disorder of pregnancy that usually develops after 20 weeks' gestation, most commonly near term (37 weeks' gestation). The condition can also present or worsen in the postnatal period (up to 14 days following birth).
- It is usually characterised by an increase in blood pressure and/or proteinuria or symptoms listed in section 3 (refer to **Prehospital Maternity Decision Tool**).
- **Eclampsia** is a tonic-clonic seizure, a serious neurological complication of pre-eclampsia. Patients with eclampsia may present without any prior blood pressure concerns or diagnosis of pre-eclampsia.
- Patients with eclampsia can present after 20 weeks' gestation. They can also present for the first time in the postnatal period, usually within 48 hours following birth.

2. Assessment

- The **Prehospital Maternity Decision Tool** should be used to assess whether the parameters are normal and to identify symptoms of pre-eclampsia.
- Use your clinical judgement to escalate where required. If there is a pre-existing diagnosis of pre-eclampsia in this pregnancy have a lower threshold for urgent conveyance.
- Blood pressure of 160/110 mHg or higher may indicate severe pre-eclampsia; consider escalation to senior/critical care as per local policy but do not delay on scene.
- Eclamptic seizures are generally short-lasting (less than 2 minutes); they can be recurrent.

2.1 Prehospital maternity decision tool

- This tool should always be used when attending patients who are pregnant (or suspected pregnant) regardless of gestation or up to 4 weeks post birth/pregnancy loss/termination.
- Use to aid immediate clinical decision making on scene.
- NEWS2 should not be used in this group of patients.
- This tool should be used alongside clinical judgement and other relevant JRCALC guidelines and local guidance/pathways.
- If there is a high concern (red flag), do not ask for remote advice from the maternity service, act on the concern(s) using the table below.

3. Management

3.1 Management of a patient presenting with suspected pre-eclampsia

- Transfer all patients with suspected pre-eclampsia into the nearest hospital with consultant-led obstetric services. Use the prehospital maternity decision tool to ascertain priority of conveyance.
- Administer **Magnesium Sulfate**:
  – If there is history of a recent seizure or for patients presenting with severe pre-eclampsia: BP 160/110 or more with any current associated symptoms:
     – headache (severe and frontal)
     – visual disturbance
     – history of proteinuria
     – epigastric, or RUQ pain
     – twitching or tremor
     – nausea, vomiting
     – confusion
     – rapidly progressing oedema
  – Obtain IV access (LARGE BORE cannula). DO NOT administer fluid boluses because of the risk of provoking pulmonary oedema and kidney damage.
  – Administer loading dose Magnesium Sulfate IV over 15 minutes (see **Magnesium Sulfate**). Consider escalation to senior/critical care as per local policy but **do not delay on scene**.

3.2 Management of a patient presenting with an eclamptic seizure

- Women with seizures from 20 weeks of pregnancy (if the top of the uterus (fundus) is at or above the level of the umbilicus) to 14 days post birth should be treated as if they have eclampsia, **even when there is a history of epilepsy**. If more than 14 days post-partum, refer to **Seizures in Adults** or **Seizures in Children**. Eclamptic seizures may occur without any prior blood pressure concerns or symptoms.
- Where there is history of a recent seizure (reason for call or since call was placed), safe and time critical extrication to the ambulance should be a priority.
- Administer **Magnesium Sulfate**.
- Request senior clinical support as per local procedures/pathways **DO NOT DELAY ON SCENE**. Rapidly convey the patient to hospital to facilitate ongoing treatment.

	High concern (red flag)	Medium concern (amber flag)	Low concern (green flag)	Medium concern (amber flag)	High concern (red flag)
Respiratory Rate (/min)	Below 7	7-8	9-21	22-24	Above 24
SpO₂ (%)	Below 95% Any oxygen requirement	N/A	95-100%	N/A	N/A
Pulse Rate (bpm) during pregnancy and up to 48 hours after birth	Below 63	63-70	71-112	113-121	Above 121
Pulse Rate from 48 hours AFTER birth (bpm)	Below 51	51-57	58-98	99-107	Above 107
Systolic Blood Pressure (mmHg)	Below 94	94-100	101-135	136-144	Above 144
Diastolic Blood Pressure (mmHg)	Below 57	57-61	62-88	89-96	Above 96
Temperature (°C)	Less than 35.7	35.7 - 36.1	36.2-37.2	37.3 - 37.4	Above 37.4

	Low concern (green flag)	Medium concern (amber flag)	High concern (red flag)
Consciousness	Alert	N/A	CVPU (Confusion, Voice, Pain, Unresponsive)
Cardiac symptoms	Nil	N/A	Chest Pain Shortness of Breath Palpitations
Abdominal pain	Nil	N/A	Any pain or contractions 20-37* weeks Constant abdominal pain (any gestation) Uterine scar pain (any gestation)
Symptoms prior to 20 weeks pregnant	Nil	Abdominal pain	Shoulder tip pain One sided abdominal pain Suspected/confirmed ectopic pregnancy
PV blood loss LESS THAN 20 weeks pregnant	Nil	Maternity sanitary pad not fully soaked within 30 minutes	Maternity sanitary pad fully soaked (50mls) within 30 minutes
PV loss MORE THAN 20 weeks pregnant	Sticky, pink, mucous plug (show) more than 37 weeks pregnant Clear fluid over 36+6 weeks	Sticky, pink, mucous plug (show) less than 37 weeks pregnant	Any fresh red bleeding Blood stained amniotic fluid Meconium stained waters (green) Offensive smelling waters Waters broken under 37 weeks
Postnatal PV blood loss (lochia)	Maternity sanitary pad not fully soaked within 30 minutes	N/A	Maternity sanitary pad fully soaked (50mls) within 30 minutes Offensive smelling lochia
Pre-eclampsia/Eclampsia symptoms (MORE THAN 20 weeks gestation)	Nil	Nausea & vomiting Malaise	Severe pain just below ribs Severe headache Problems with vision Sudden oedema to feet/hands/face
Neurological	Asymptomatic	N/A	Active seizure History of recent seizure
Appearance	Looks well	N/A	Looks unwell

*Labour pain 37 weeks and above - refer to Imminent Birth guideline

Additional concerns:
Patient/family/clinician concerns should always be considered as part of the clinical assessment
Language barriers – use interpreting services and convey to hospital for further assessment
If recommended transfer is declined – escalate according to local protocols
Mental capacity concerns – follow local protocols
Safeguarding concerns – follow local protocols

	All green flags	1 amber flag	Any red flag or 2 amber flags
Action required	Consider calling the maternity unit to discuss plan of care. Follow local guidance.	Transport to hospital via ambulance.	Requires time critical assessment in hospital. Minimise time on scene.
Emergency pre-alert	No	Consider	Follow local guidance.
Destination	Follow local guidance.	Follow local guidance.	Follow local guidance.
Ongoing observations	If conveying continue regular observation	Observations every 15 minutes	Observations every 5 minutes

Pre-eclampsia and Eclampsia

TABLE 5.10 – Management if the patient is currently seizing

Immediately:
- Request senior clinical support early as per local guidance.
- Position the patient for safety and comfort. Protect from dangers during the seizure, especially aspiration and head injuries, during the seizure.

Assess

Airway
- Consider an oropharyngeal airway but do not attempt to force an oropharyngeal airway into a convulsing patient if there is trismus or if it is not tolerated. A nasopharyngeal airway can be a useful adjunct. Use caution in patients who may have a basal skull fracture or facial injury.

Breathing
- Administer high-concentration oxygen using a reservoir mask at 15 l/min, until a reliable oximetry measurement can be obtained; clinicians should then aim for an oxygen saturation of 94–98% (or 88–92% if the patient is at risk of hypercapnic respiratory failure, e.g. COPD). Refer to **Oxygen**.

Circulation
- Measure BP as soon as possible.

Blood Glucose Level
- Measure capillary blood glucose and document the result. If glucose is <4 mmol/l, treat according to **Glycaemic Emergencies in Adults and Children**.

Administer Magnesium Sulfate:
- Obtain IV access (LARGE BORE cannula) or IO access. DO NOT administer fluid boluses because of the risk of provoking pulmonary oedema and kidney damage.
- Administer Magnesium Sulfate IV over 5 minutes (refer to **Magnesium Sulfate**)

If the patient is **currently seizing** and Magnesium Sulfate is unavailable or ineffective administer Benzodiazepines (refer to **Midazolam/Diazepam**).

- Monitor clinical observations, repeat every 5 minutes.
- Request senior clinical support as per local procedures/pathways **DO NOT DELAY ON SCENE.** Rapidly convey the patient to hospital to facilitate ongoing treatment.
- Undertake a time critical conveyance to convey urgently to nearest hospital with consultant-led obstetric service. Provide a pre-alert stating "Eclamptic seizure".

KEY POINTS!

Pre-eclampsia and Eclampsia
- Pre-eclampsia should be suspected when there is hypertension and/or reported symptoms detailed in the **Prehospital Maternity Decision Tool** after 20 weeks' gestation and up to 14 days post birth.
- Pre-eclampsia is a multi-organ condition and is associated with poor outcomes for women and their babies.
- Eclamptic seizures may occur without hypertension.
- Women with eclampsia can present after 20 weeks' gestation. They can also present for the first time in the postnatal period, usually within 48 hours following birth.
- Women who experience health inequalities (e.g. black and Asian women, women living in a deprived area) are more likely to develop pre-eclampsia and eclampsia.

Pre-eclampsia and Eclampsia

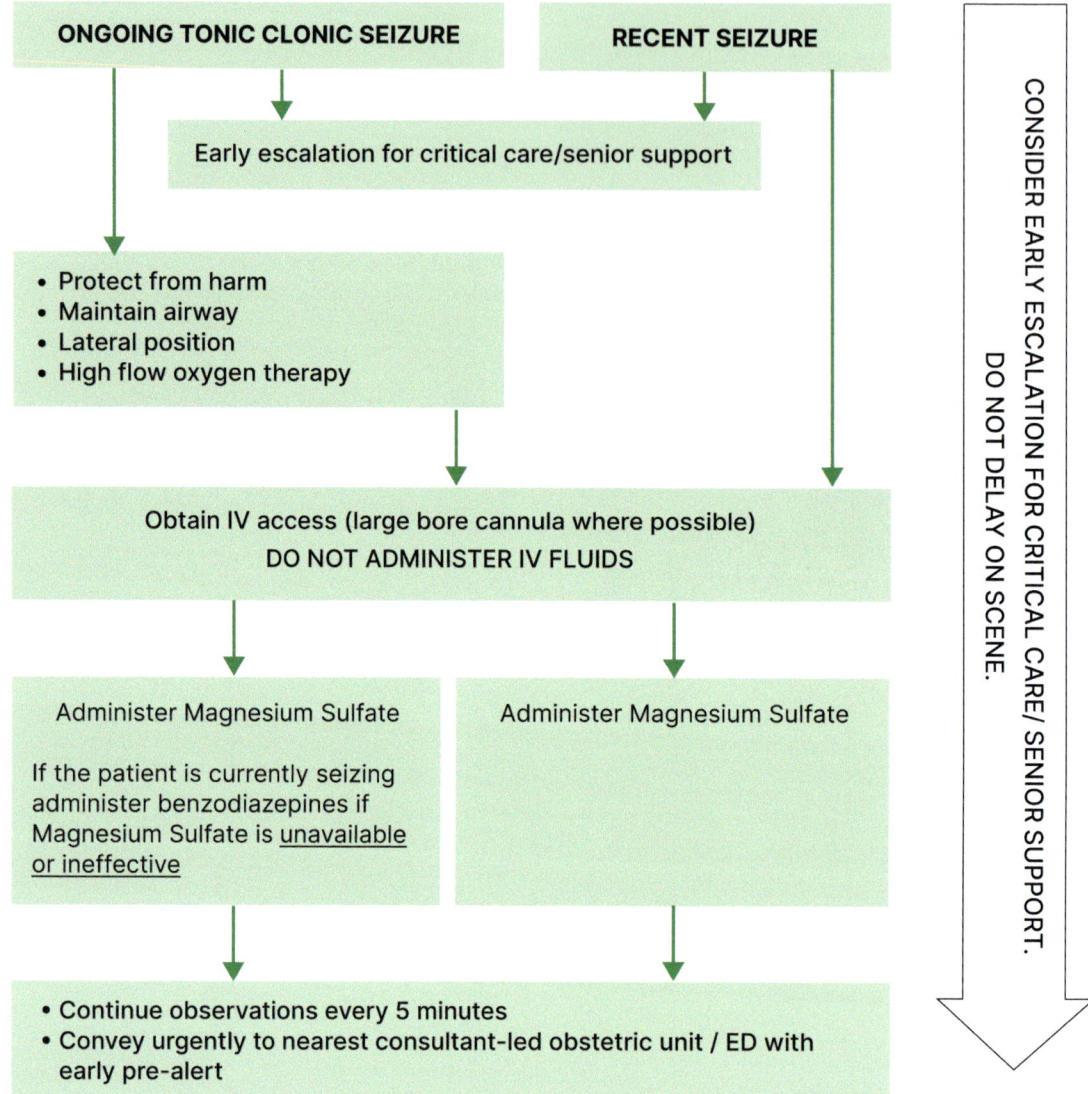

Figure 5.17 – Management of seizures after 20 weeks of pregnancy up to 14 days post-birth (regardless of history of epilepsy)

Further Reading

Risk factors (not exhaustive)

- Health inequalities: Black and Asian women, non-English speakers, limited or no antenatal care in this pregnancy or residing in a deprived area.
- Hypertensive disorder: Pre-pregnancy blood pressure condition (e.g. essential hypertension), or pre-eclampsia/eclampsia in a previous pregnancy.
- Current pregnancy: Receiving investigations or treatment for pre-eclampsia (this may be already be managed in the community), or report of proteinuria in current pregnancy. Taking low-dose aspirin in this pregnancy (prescribed to prevent pre-eclampsia).
- Medical history: Living with a chronic condition or an auto-immune disorder (e.g. diabetes, lupus, kidney disease).
- Multiple pregnancy: Twins or triplets (or more) in this pregnancy.
- Maternal age: Under 20 years old or over 40 years old.
- BMI: Body Mass Index of 35 kg/m² or more.
- Family history: A family history of pre-eclampsia (mother or maternal grandmother).

NB If there are 2 or more of these risk factors together, the risk of pre-eclampsia is significantly higher.

Pre-eclampsia and Eclampsia

Bibliography

1. Ali M, et al. "Haemorrhagic stroke and brain vascular malformations in women: risk factors and clinical features." *The Lancet. Neurology* 2024, 23(6): 625–635.

2. Dhindsa HS, et al. "Recognition and Treatment of Eclampsia on a Rural Scene Call: A Case Study of Coordinated Ground and Air Emergency Medical Services." *Air Medical Journal* 2017, 36(6): 341–343.

3. Docheva N, et al. "Racial differences in healthcare utilization among patients with suspected or diagnosed preeclampsia: A retrospective cohort study." *Pregnancy Hypertension* 2023, 33: 8–16.

4. Gebremedhin AT, et al. "Interpregnancy interval and hypertensive disorders of pregnancy: A population-based cohort study." *Paediatric and perinatal epidemiology* 2021, 35(4): 404–414.

5. Hayes C and Graham Y. "Epilepsy in pregnancy: an emergency care context." *Journal of Paramedic Practice* 2020, 12(4): 1–6.

6. Hutchcraft ML, et al. "A One-Year Cross Sectional Analysis of Emergency Medical Services Utilization and Its Association with Hypertension in Pregnancy." *Prehospital Emergency Care* 2022, 26(6): 838–847.

7. National Institute for Health and Care Excellence (NICE) 2024. Hypertension in pregnancy: Diagnosis and management: Guidance, NICE. Available at: https://www.nice.org.uk/guidance/ng133/chapter/Recommendations#management-of-gestational-hypertension (Accessed: 20 December 2024).

8. Saving lives, improving mothers' care 2024 – lessons learned to inform maternity care from the UK and Ireland confidential enquiries into maternal deaths and morbidity 2020–22: MBRRACE-UK: NPEU (2024) UK. Available at: https://www.npeu.ox.ac.uk/mbrrace-uk/reports/maternal-reports/maternal-report-2020–2022 (Accessed: 20 December 2024).

9. Kayem G et al. "Maternal and obstetric factors associated with delayed postpartum eclampsia: a national study population." Acta *Obstetricia et Gynecologica Scandinavica* 2011, 90(9): 1017–1023. https://doi.org/10.1111/j.1600-0412.2011.01218.x

Shoulder Dystocia

1. Definition

- Shoulder dystocia is a time critical emergency, which occurs when the baby's head has been born but one of the shoulders becomes stuck behind the mother's pubic bone, delaying the birth of the baby's body. Additional manoeuvres are required to release the shoulder that is stuck.

2. Diagnosis/identification

- After the head is born, if the body is not delivered with maternal effort during the next contraction, management for shoulder dystocia should be started.

3. Management of Shoulder Dystocia

a) Note the time that the head is born

b) Consider senior clinical support (do not delay on scene time if emergency conveyance is needed)

c) Prepare for newborn life support (refer to **Newborn Life Support**). Be prepared for post-partum haemorrhage (refer to **Management of Post-partum Haemorrhage (PPH)**).

d) Perform Manoeuvre 1: **McRoberts** (to increase the diameter of the pelvis)

   (i) Ensure the patient is lying **completely flat**; discourage pushing and offer **Nitrous Oxide (Entonox® or Nitronox™)**.

   (ii) Simultaneously hyperflex the thighs towards the maternal abdomen (legs bent at the knees)

   (iii) Keep the legs parallel (do not abduct)

e) Simultaneously, place hands on either side of the baby's head and **apply gentle axial traction** on the baby's head for **up to 30 seconds**.

   (i) Axial traction means **keeping the baby's head in-line with its own spine**. Avoid pulling downwards or twisting the baby's neck at any time.

f) If the baby is not born, perform Manoeuvre 2: **suprapubic pressure** (reduces diameter of the baby's shoulders) whilst the woman remains in the McRoberts position. **Continue to discourage pushing.**

   (i) Using a CPR grip, position hands on the woman's abdomen, just above the maternal pubic bone.

   (ii) Apply **downwards pressure** towards the floor. First use **CONTINUOUS** pressure for **up to 30 seconds**.

   (iii) Simultaneously **apply gentle axial traction**.

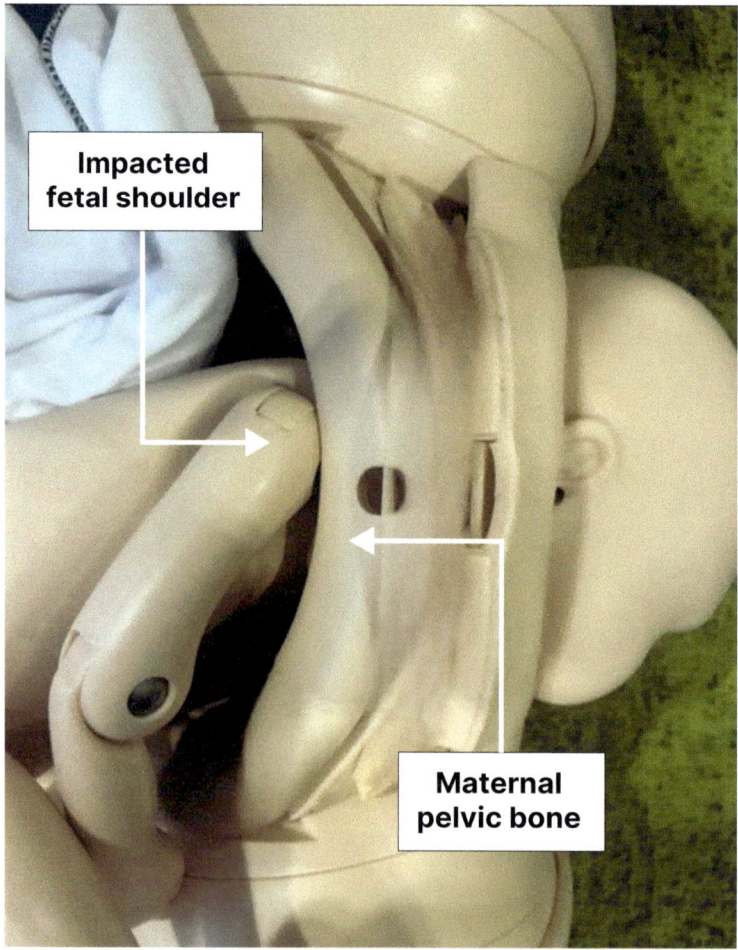

Image of mannequin to show baby's shoulder stuck against maternal pelvic bone and the baby's head out.

Shoulder Dystocia

g) If the baby is not born, perform Manoeuvre 3: **Rocking** suprapubic pressure for **up to 30 seconds** in the **same position** and **direction**. Simultaneously **apply gentle axial traction**.

h) If the baby is not born, change the woman into the **'all fours' position** (increases diameter of pelvis)

   (i) Position the woman on her hands and knees, ensuring the thighs are touching the abdomen with the woman's chest as close to the floor as possible.

   (ii) **Apply gentle axial traction** for **up to 30 seconds**.

i) If the baby is not born, undertake time critical conveyance to nearest consultant led obstetric unit with early pre-alert (Unless local guidance differs).

j) **DO NOT delay on scene for senior clinical support and rendezvous en route if needed**.

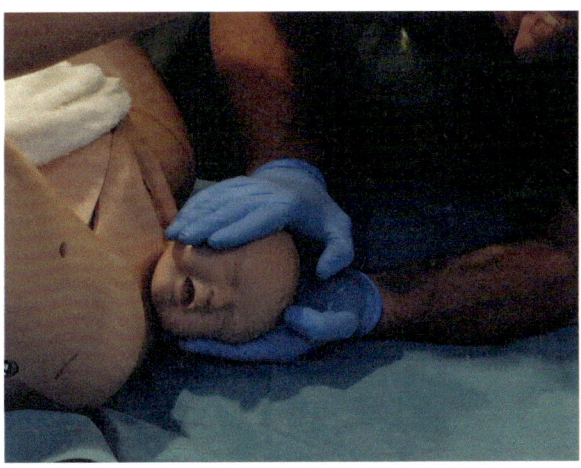

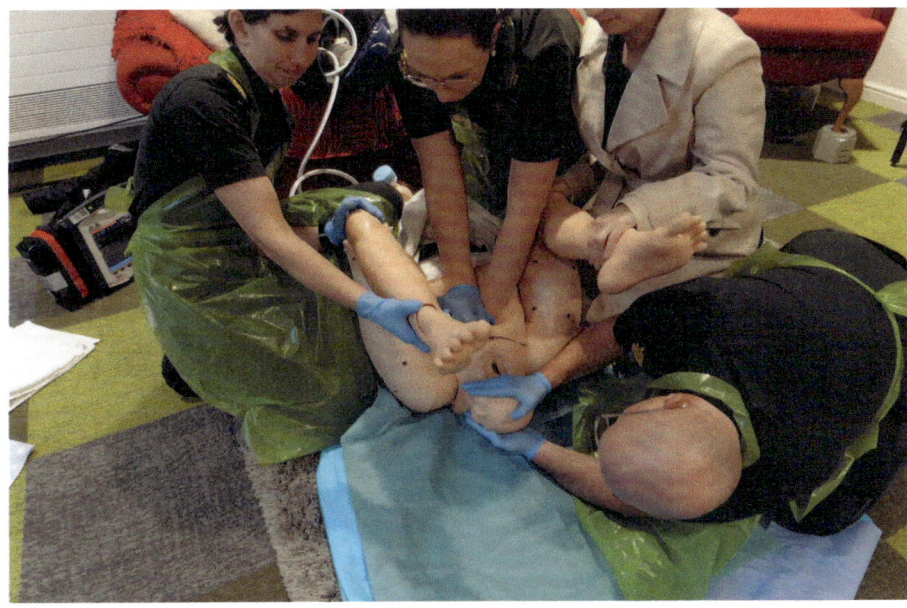

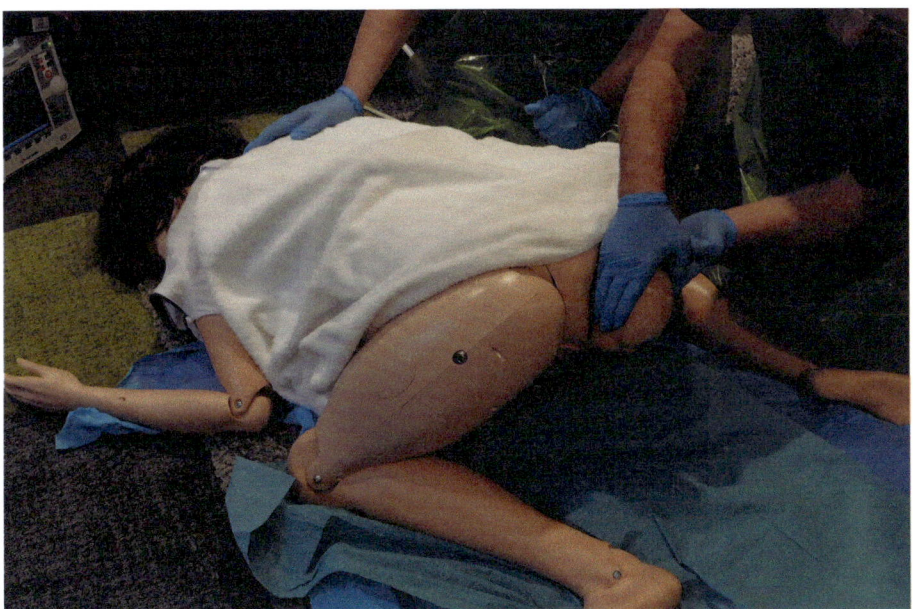

Shoulder Dystocia

4. Management of Shoulder Dystocia Algorithm

```
Head born, body not delivered with maternal
effort during the next contraction
                │
                ▼
     Shoulder Dystocia Declared
                │
                ▼
    • Do you need more help?
    • Prepare for Newborn Life Support
                │
                ▼
    • Discourage pushing
    • Offer Entonox
```

CONTINUOUSLY DISCOURAGE PUSHING — DO YOU NEED MORE HELP?

Lone workers (with NO bystanders/help):

1. **Manoeuvre 1** – Ask the woman to lie completely flat and bring her knees up towards her chest, holding them with her hands. Apply gentle axial traction (up to 30 seconds)
2. **Manoeuvre 4** - Support the woman into All Fours position. Apply gentle axial traction (up to 30 seconds)
3. Alternate between these two manoeuvres until help arrives, then proceed with the algorithm

Multiple people on scene:

Continue algorithm below

Manoeuvre 1 (up to 30 seconds)
McROBERTS
1. Lie completely flat
2. Hyperflex the thighs towards the maternal abdomen, keeping legs parallel
3. Gentle axial traction

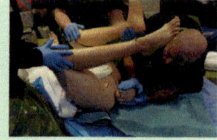

Manoeuvre 2 (up to 30 seconds)
SUPRAPUBIC PRESSURE
1. Continue McRoberts
2. Apply suprapubic pressure: CPR grip, position hands above pubic bone
3. Apply CONTINUOUS downwards pressure towards the floor
4. Gentle axial traction

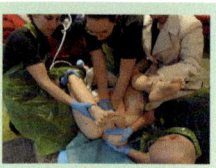

Manoeuvre 3 (up to 30 seconds)
ROCKING SUPRAPUBIC PRESSURE
1. Continue McROBERTS
2. Apply rocking suprapubic pressure
3. Gentle axial traction

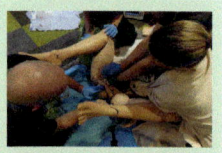

Manoeuvre 4 (up to 30 seconds)
ALL FOURS POSITION
1. Support the woman into all fours position
2. Gentle axial traction

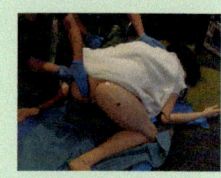

Extrication and Conveyance
1. Walk the woman to the ambulance with a towel between the legs anticipating birth at all times
2. Convey in a lateral position, using a pillow/blanket between the woman's legs
3. Convey urgently to nearest consultant led obstetric unit with early pre-alert

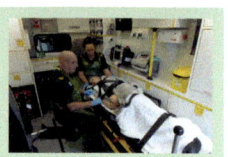

Ambulance clinicians would not be expected to perform any manoeuvres en route to hospital.

Shoulder Dystocia

5. Extrication and Conveyance with Unresolved Shoulder Dystocia

- Encourage the woman to walk to the ambulance, facilitating a sling with a sheet/blanket between the woman's legs whilst she walks.
- Monitor continuously during extrication and conveyance, preparing for birth, should the shoulder release.
- Convey the patient securely in right/left lateral with padding between the woman's knees.
- Convey urgently to nearest consultant led obstetric unit with early pre alert. Refer to 'Appropriate destination for conveyance' in (**Maternity Care**).
- Place a pre-alert as per local procedures "obstetric emergency, shoulder dystocia". Consider requesting maternity staff to meet you at a designated entrance/ambulance maternity arrival point.
- Ambulance clinicians would not be expected to perform any manoeuvres en route to hospital. The woman should be fully secured at all times. If the birth of the baby occurs, the ambulance should be stopped as soon as it is safe to do so, for care to be provided.

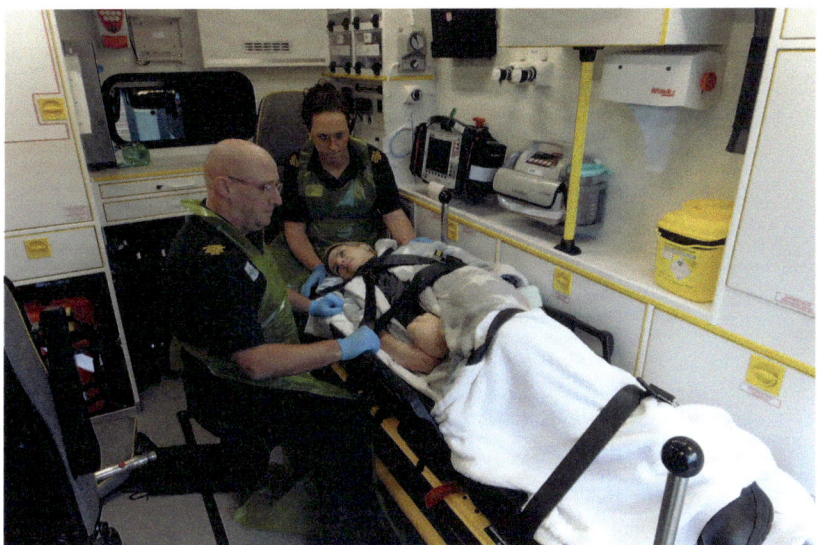

6. Lone Worker

- If on scene alone, attempt Manoeuvres 1 and 4 (McRoberts and all fours) until help arrives:
  - Manoeuvre 1 – Ask the woman to lie completely flat and bring her knees up towards her chest, holding them with her hands. Apply gentle axial traction (up to 30 seconds)
  - Manoeuvre 4 – Support the woman into All Fours position. Apply gentle axial traction (up to 30 seconds)
- Alternate between these two manoeuvres until help arrives.
- Bystanders can be asked to support legs during McRoberts. Gentle axial traction should always be done by a healthcare professional.

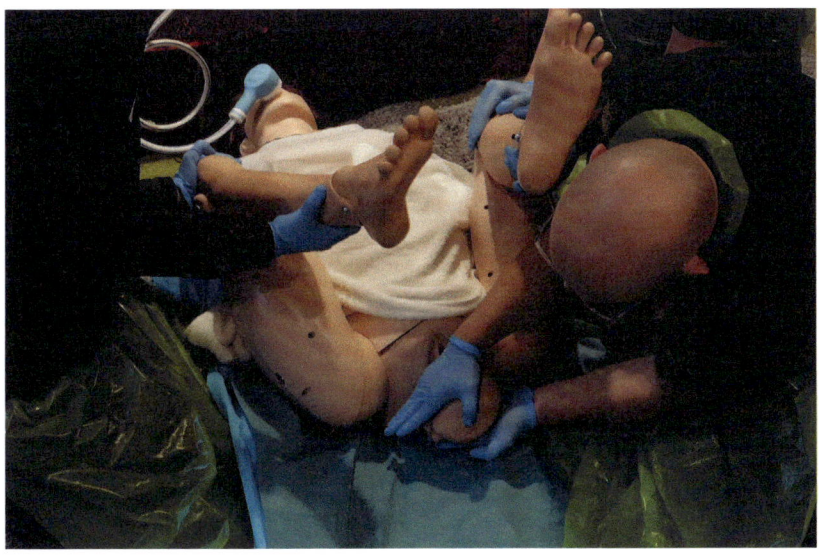

Shoulder Dystocia

> **KEY POINTS!**
>
> **Shoulder Dystocia**
> - McRoberts manoeuvre is a simple, rapid, and effective intervention resolving up to 90% of shoulder dystocia (especially when combined with suprapubic pressure [SPP]).
> - In a correctly positioned McRoberts, the patient must be completely flat, hyperflex the thighs towards the maternal abdomen (legs bent at the knees). Ensure that the legs remain parallel.
> - During gentle axial traction, keep the baby's head in line with its own spine.
> - If each manoeuvre has been carried out once and has failed to release the baby's shoulder, convey urgently to nearest obstetric unit/ED with early pre-alert.
> - Do not delay on scene to await senior clinical support. Consider rendezvous en route.

References

1. RCOG 2012. Shoulder Dystocia. Green-top Guideline No. 42, 2nd edition. Available from: https://www.rcog.org.uk/media/ewgpnmio/gtg_42.pdf

2. Zhang HY, Guo RF, Wu Y, Ling Y. Normal Range of Head-to-body Delivery Interval by Two-step Delivery. *Chin Med J (Engl)* 2016, May 5; 129(9): 1066–71. doi: 10.4103/0366-6999.180522.

Trauma in Pregnancy

1. Introduction

- The management of pregnant women with traumatic injuries requires a special approach.
- Mechanism of injury may indicate possible trauma to enlarged internal organs and structures, especially trauma occurring in the third trimester. For example, trauma to the gravid uterus during domestic violence can be linked to placental abruption (refer to **Imminent Birth**).
- It is important to remember that resuscitation of the mother may facilitate resuscitation of the fetus.

2. Incidence

- In the UK, 5% of maternal deaths are as a result of trauma, with a high proportion related to domestic violence and road traffic collisions.

Mechanism of Injury

- Domestic violence.
- High-energy transfer (especially road traffic accidents).
- Fall from height.

3. Severity and Outcome

- Managing a pregnant woman with major trauma is rare; however, both blunt and penetrating trauma can cause catastrophic haemorrhage.
- Trauma can lead to major placental abruption (separation) with significant hidden blood loss within the uterus and no visible vaginal bleeding abruption (refer to **Imminent Birth**).

4. Pathophysiology

- There are a number of physiological and anatomical changes during pregnancy that may influence the management of the pregnant woman with trauma (refer to **Maternity Care (including Obstetric Emergencies Overview)**).

5. Assessment and Management

TABLE 5.11 – ASSESSMENT and MANAGEMENT of: Trauma in Pregnancy

Assess <C>ABCDE

- Quickly assess the scene and the woman as you approach.
- Undertake a primary survey – specifically assess for:
  - abdominal pain – should be presumed to be significant and may be associated with internal concealed blood loss
  - vaginal blood loss
  - abruption may occur 3–4 days after the initial incident
  - stage of the pregnancy and impact on resuscitation if >20 weeks gestation
  - any medical problems with the pregnancy or relevant previous medical history
  - twins or multiple pregnancy
  - fetal movements (refer to **Maternity Care (including Obstetric Emergencies Overview)**).
- Review the maternity handheld record if available.
- If domestic violence is suspected, consider any other children/adults present who may be at risk (refer to **Safeguarding Adults at Risk** and **Safeguarding Children**).
- Control external catastrophic haemorrhage using direct and indirect pressure or tourniquets where indicated (refer to **Trauma Emergencies in Adults – Overview**).
- Refer to **Maternal Resuscitation** where cardiac/respiratory arrest is identified.
- Open, maintain and protect the airway in accordance with the woman's clinical need.
- Administer high levels of supplemental oxygen and aim for a target saturation within the range of 94–98% (refer to **Oxygen**). Provide assisted ventilation as indicated (refer to **Airway Management**).
- If the woman is unable to position herself (e.g. if she is unconscious), she should be positioned on the left (right side up) by using a spinal board and her airway should be monitored. Where resources allow, the uterus can be manually displaced to the maternal left side (and this must be recorded on the patient record form), as illustrated in Figure 5.1 in **Maternity Care (Including Obstetric Emergencies Overview)**.
- Provide cervical spine protection as necessary (refer to **Spinal Injury and Spinal Cord Injury**).

(continued)

Trauma in Pregnancy

TABLE 5.11 – ASSESSMENT and MANAGEMENT of: Trauma in Pregnancy (continued)

- Manage thoracic injuries (refer to **Thoracic Trauma**). **NB** The management of thoracic injuries is the same as for the non-pregnant woman.
- Insert a minimum of one large bore IV cannula (16G) – do not delay transfer.
- Administer intravascular fluids as indicated to maintain a systolic blood pressure above 90 mmHg (refer to **Intravascular Fluid Therapy in Adults**).
- Undertake a secondary survey <C>ABCDE.

Assess the Woman's Level of Pain

- Pain management (refer to **Pain Management in Adults and Children**). **NB** Administer morphine cautiously if the patient is hypotensive.
- Apply splints as appropriate, for example to pelvis (refer to **Major Pelvic Trauma**) or long bone fractures (refer to **Limb Trauma**).

Assess Blood Glucose

- Measure blood glucose en route to the appropriate facility.
- Nil by mouth.

Assess for Burns and Scalds

- For the management of burns, treat as non-pregnant woman (refer to **Burns and Scalds** and **Intravascular Fluid Therapy in Adults**).

KEY POINTS!

Trauma in Pregnancy

- **All trauma is significant.**
- **If the pregnant woman is found in cardiac arrest or develops cardiac/respiratory arrest en route, commence advanced life support and pre-alert the nearest ED with an obstetric unit.**
- **Resuscitation of the woman may facilitate resuscitation of the fetus.**
- **Compression of the inferior vena cava by the gravid uterus (>20 weeks) is a serious potential complication; manually displace the uterus to the maternal left. Maintain during transfer.**
- **Due to the physiological changes in pregnancy, signs of shock may be slow to appear following trauma, hypotension being an extremely late indication of volume loss. Signs of hypovolaemia during pregnancy are likely to indicate a 35% (class III) blood loss and must be treated aggressively.**
- **Abruption may occur 3–4 days after the initial incident.**
- **If sexual assault or domestic violence is suspected, consideration must be given to potential safeguarding issues and provision made to ensure safety is maintained (refer to Safeguarding Adults at Risk).**

Bibliography

1. Centre for Maternal and Child Enquiries. Saving mothers' lives: reviewing maternal deaths to make motherhood safer: 2006–2008. *BJOG: An International Journal of Obstetrics & Gynaecology* 2011, 118(suppl. 1).
2. Woollard M, Simpson H, Hinshaw K, Wieteska S. Obstetric services. In *Pre-hospital Obstetric Emergency Training*. Oxford: Wiley-Blackwell, 2009: 1–6.
3. Woollard M, Hinshaw K, Simpson H, Wieteska S. Anatomical and physiological changes in pregnancy. In *Pre-hospital Obstetric Emergency Training*. Oxford: Wiley-Blackwell, 2009: 18–27.
4. Woollard M, Hinshaw K, Simpson H, Wieteska S. Structured approach to the obstetric patient. In *Pre-hospital Obstetric Emergency Training*. Oxford: Wiley-Blackwell, 2009: 38–52.
5. Woollard M, Hinshaw K, Simpson H, Wieteska S. Emergencies in late pregnancy. In *Pre-Hospital Obstetric Emergency Training*. Oxford: Wiley-Blackwell, 2009: 62–110.
6. Woollard M, Hinshaw K, Simpson H, Wieteska S. Emergencies after delivery. In *Pre-hospital Obstetric Emergency Training*. Oxford: Wiley-Blackwell, 2009: 111–124.
7. Woollard M, Hinshaw K, Simpson H, Wieteska S. Management of non-obstetric emergencies. In *Pre-hospital Obstetric Emergency Training*. Oxford: Wiley-Blackwell, 2009: 136–165.

Vaginal Bleeding during Pregnancy up to 20 weeks Gestation

1. Introduction

- In a pre-hospital context the most likely causes of bleeding prior to 20 weeks' gestation are suspected miscarriage or ectopic pregnancy (usually <13 weeks). Bleeding may be largely concealed (internal) with ectopic pregnancy.

Unknown or uncertain gestation

- If the top of the uterus (fundus) is under the level of the umbilicus treat the patient as though they are under 20 weeks gestation.

2. Miscarriage

Definition: Miscarriage is defined as the spontaneous loss of pregnancy before the baby reaches 24 weeks gestation. It is estimated 1 in 4 pregnancies will result in miscarriage; this happens most commonly in the first trimester (i.e. <13 weeks).

- Miscarriage is "suspected" if a patient with a positive pregnancy test experiences symptoms as described below.
- Miscarriage is "confirmed" when an ultrasound scan in hospital has confirmed that the pregnancy is definitely not ongoing. At that point, the patient will be offered either surgical management, medical management with medication to help empty the uterus, or may be sent home to wait for their miscarriage to pass. Patients may call emergency services during this time.
- An ambulance clinician can only confirm a miscarriage themselves if they observe a deceased baby delivered, and are aware of a pre-existing scan which rules out the possibility of multiple pregnancy.
- Be aware that when viability is uncertain on an ultrasound scan, a patient will also be sent home to await events. This may result in a miscarriage occurring at home, but in many cases, repeat ultrasound 7 to 10 days later may confirm viability (i.e. a developing baby).

Symptoms associated with miscarriage:

- Bleeding – light or heavy, often with clots and/or jelly-like tissue.
- Pain – central, crampy, suprapubic or backache.
- Signs of pregnancy may be subsiding, e.g. nausea or breast tenderness.

Red flags requiring a time critical transfer to ED (consider a pre-alert):

1. Clinical signs of hypovolaemic shock
2. A maternity pad is soaked within 30 minutes (approximately 50 mls)
3. Total blood loss >500 mls
4. Significant symptoms (including hypotension) without significant external blood loss (may indicate 'cervical shock' due to retained miscarriage tissue lodged in the cervix). Symptomatic bradycardia may arise due to vagal stimulation
5. Any signs/symptoms of ectopic pregnancy (see below)

3. Management

If there are no red flags, then arrange for assessment in ED, by a GP or in an early pregnancy unit according to local arrangements within the next 4 hours.

Management of patients with miscarriage in the presence of excessive bleeding/red flags.

- Refer to **Medical Emergencies in Adults – Overview**.
- In cases of confirmed miscarriage, uterotonics and tranexamic acid can be administered in line with local guidance and scope of practice.

NB Do not give uterotonic drug(s) or tranexamic acid in suspected miscarriage.

Women requiring admission to ED

- Keep the patient nil by mouth.
- Assess and treat hypovolaemic shock with fluids as per **Medical Emergencies in Adults – Overview**.
- Provide pain relief as required (refer to **Pain Management in Adults and Children**).

IV access should only be attempted if it will NOT delay time on scene and there is a clinical need for a cannula.

4. Ectopic Pregnancy

Definition: A pregnancy that is implanted outside the uterus. The majority of ectopic pregnancies implant in the Fallopian tube. Most commonly presents in early pregnancy (<10 weeks gestation).

History which should raise a suspicion of ectopic pregnancy:

- Previous ectopic pregnancy.
- Intra-uterine contraceptive device fitted.
- Pelvic inflammatory disease.
- Sterilisation or reversal of sterilisation or other tubal surgery.
- Subfertility (delay in conceiving).
- Endometriosis.

Common symptoms suggestive of ectopic pregnancy:

- Often presents at around 6–8 weeks gestation, so usually only one period has been missed.
- Crampy lower abdominal or pelvic pain (often lateralised).

Vaginal Bleeding during Pregnancy up to 20 weeks Gestation

- Vaginal bleeding is variable – often light bleeding or brown discharge only.

Other symptoms suggestive of ectopic pregnancy:
- Unexplained dizziness, fainting or syncope.
- Shoulder-tip pain.
- Unusual bowel symptoms (including rectal pressure or pain on defaecation).
- Unusual urinary symptoms.

Signs of possible ectopic pregnancy:
- **May be minimal or absent**
- Pallor
- Tachycardia (>100 bpm)
- Postural (orthostatic) hypotension
- Abdominal distension
- Signs of developing peritonism (i.e. signs suggestive of intraabdominal bleeding):
  – Abdominal tenderness or guarding (commonly, but not always, lateralised)
  – Rebound tenderness (commonly, but not always, lateralised)

Symptoms and signs characteristic of a RUPTURED ectopic pregnancy (i.e. ongoing intra-abdominal bleeding):
- Acute, severe lower abdominal or pelvic pain
- Shoulder tip pain (reflects diaphragmatic irritation by intra-abdominal blood)
- Pallor, clamminess +/- skin coolness
- Tachycardia +/- hypovolaemic shock (SBP <100 mmHg)
- Rigid, tender abdomen +/- guarding
- Rebound tenderness

5. General Management of Pregnancy Loss

- Any baby born before 22 completed weeks of pregnancy should receive comfort care and not survival focussed care (see **Care of the Newborn** guideline).
- For complications associated with therapeutic termination ('abortion'), refer to **Vaginal Bleeding: Gynaecological Causes**.

Emotional care
- Whether loss/termination of pregnancy is planned or unplanned, this can be a profound and complicated emotional experience for the patient and their family. Sensitivity and compassion will be paramount.
- It is important to refer to the baby as a "baby" and not a "fetus" – both when speaking to the patient/family and in documentation.
- Ask the parents if they have a name for the baby and ask if they would like you to use the baby's name.
- Manage a miscarried baby or pregnancy tissue with respect and dignity (see below).
- Unless miscarriage has already been confirmed by hospital or it is obvious that a baby has been passed, explain to the patients/family that you are not able to diagnose or confirm miscarriage in the pre-hospital setting. Explain you will not be able to confirm the gender of the baby.

Practical clinical care during a miscarriage
- Perform primary and secondary surveys as normal.
- Observe for signs of excessive post miscarriage bleeding and manage as stated above.
- Extricate using the quickest, safest means.

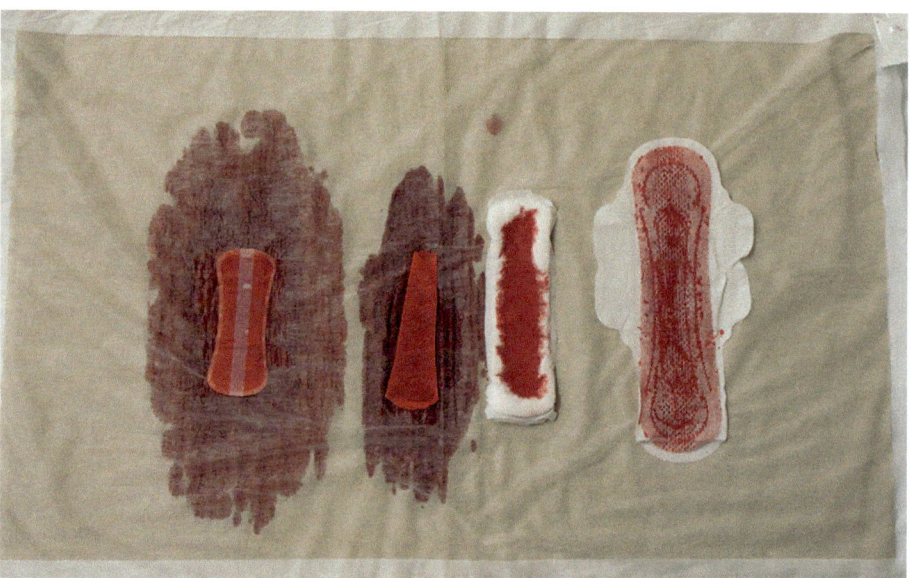

Sanitary pads all showing 50 mls blood

Vaginal Bleeding during Pregnancy up to 20 weeks Gestation

- If the patient is undergoing therapeutic termination (abortion) and has any abnormal observations or excessive bleeding (see above) convey to the nearest ED. Do not transport back to the clinic providing the termination (abortion).

Management of a miscarried baby and pregnancy tissue

- Fetal tissue, including the baby, may be passed by the patient during a miscarriage. The management of pregnancy tissue must follow the principles below to ensure that all staff comply with the Human Tissue Act (2007).
- Miscarried tissue should be handled delicately and treated with respect; this may have profound impact on the patient/family in coming to terms with their loss.
- Products of conception may resemble blood-stained tissue, or resemble a discernible baby with placenta still attached depending on the gestation. If the baby is delivered and the placenta is still in situ, apply clamps and cut the cord. Take extra care not to pull on the cord as it will be very friable.
- Every reasonable effort should be made to obtain products of conception and take them to hospital. This is so that the hospital can weigh and assess the loss, but also because the hospital will need to offer the patient a choice of how they are ultimately disposed of. This includes tissue that may be passed in to the toilet.
- In all cases, inform the woman of what you know has been passed and be clear on what you cannot confirm. Discuss her preferences about management of the pregnancy tissue/her baby.
- Wrap the baby gently in a comfort pad or a soft towel and offer the woman/family members the opportunity to hold the baby; this may be an important part of her grieving process.
- If the patient does not want to see or hold the pregnancy tissue or baby, wrap the baby in a sensitive way using a towel or comfort pad and convey to hospital.
- Document how the pregnancy tissue/baby was conveyed and hand the pregnancy tissue/baby to the nurse or midwife at transfer of care.

KEY POINTS!

Vaginal Bleeding during Pregnancy up to 20 weeks Gestation

- **Symptoms of hypovolaemic shock occur very late in otherwise fit young women; tachycardia may not appear until 30% of circulating volume has been lost, by which stage the patient is very unwell.**
- **Haemorrhage may be revealed (evident vaginal blood loss) or concealed (little or no obvious loss).**
- **In the presence of a CONFIRMED miscarriage, a uterotonic (syntometrine or misoprostol) and intravenous tranexamic acid administration should be considered.**

References

1. NICE. Ectopic pregnancy and miscarriage: diagnosis and initial management (NG126). London: NICE, 2019. Last updated: 23 August 2023. Available from: https://www.nice.org.uk/guidance/ng126/resources.

Vaginal Bleeding during Pregnancy after 20 weeks Gestation

1. Diagnosis

- **ANY** bleeding in pregnancy or suspected pregnancy after 20 weeks of pregnancy reported by the patient or seen by a clinician.
- Bleeding can be **internal** (concealed) as well as **external** (revealed).

Unknown or uncertain gestation

- If the top of the uterus (fundus) is at or above the level of the umbilicus treat the patient as though they are over 20 weeks gestation.

2. Management

- **ANY bleeding after 20 weeks may be life threatening requiring time critical transport to the nearest hospital with an early pre-alert according to local guidelines.**
- Minimise time on scene and expedite transport to hospital. Restrict interventions on scene as much as possible.
- Observations should be taken en route. Do not be reassured by normal observations or bleeding slowing/stopping.
- IV access should only be attempted if it will **NOT** delay time on scene.
- Extricate by the quickest, safest means possible.
- Convey in lateral position.
- Only provide facial oxygen if saturations <94%.
- Assess and treat hypovolaemic shock with fluids as per **Medical Emergencies in Adults**.
- Provide pain relief as required (refer to **Pain Management in Adults and Children**).
- Do not administer any other medicines.
- Keep the patient nil by mouth.

3. Pain

- Any uterine pain or lower back pain prior to 37 weeks should be treated as threatened preterm labour and requires time critical transfer to the nearest hospital with an early pre-alert. Convey according to local guidelines.
- Contraction pain should come and go with regular breaks.
- Constant pain is not normal and must be considered time critical and managed as above. It may be due to placental abruption or a uterine rupture.

4. Causes

(For reference only; management is the same regardless of the cause)

- **Placenta Praevia:** the placenta is implanted near or covering the cervix. This can lead to haemorrhage during the pregnancy or when labour begins. Bleeding is usually painless.
- **Placental Abruption:** the placenta partially or fully detaches from the uterine wall. This can be a result of hypertensive disease or direct trauma to the abdomen (e.g. domestic violence, fall, RTC). Bleeding can be accompanied by constant pain and/or contractions or (rarely) painless. The amount of revealed blood (i.e the amount seen) may not reflect the total blood loss.
- **Uterine rupture:** the uterine scar from previous uterine surgery (e.g. caesarean section) can partially or fully open.
- **Trauma:** this can be a direct cause of bleeding, or trauma can cause placental abruption.
- **Vasa praevia:** this is a rare condition where fetal blood vessels running across of the internal aspect of the cervix rupture. Blood loss is directly from the fetus. Bleeding is usually light, but may be catastrophic as a baby's total blood volume is low (only 85 ml/kg in late pregnancy).

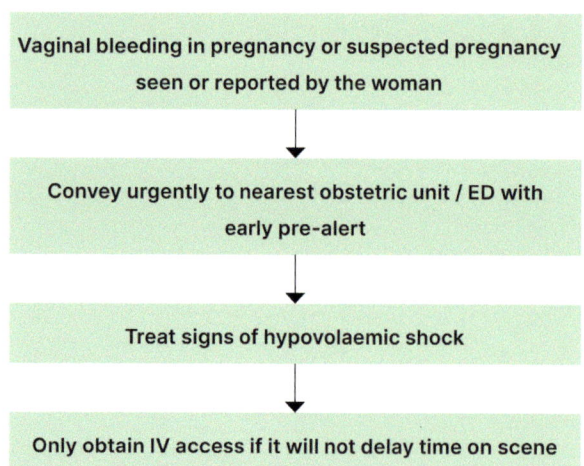

Vaginal Bleeding during Pregnancy after 20 weeks Gestation

KEY POINTS!

Vaginal Bleeding during Pregnancy after 20 weeks Gestation

- All bleeding seen by clinicians or reported by the woman after 20 weeks should be treated as time critical.
- Do not be reassured by normal observations or bleeding slowing/stopping.
- Any bleeding could result in fetal compromise requiring emergency delivery on arrival to hospital. Every minute counts.
- Maternal haemodynamic changes in pregnancy mean that pregnant women may appear well even when a large amount of blood has been lost (for example, tachycardia may not appear until 30% of circulating volume has been lost).
- Bleeding after 20 weeks in the pre-hospital setting is ALWAYS a time critical emergency; in-hospital staff may have reduced level of concern following review of the patient and assessment of fetal wellbeing.

References

1. NICE. Preterm labour and birth (NG25). London: NICE, 2015. Last updated: 02 August 2019.
2. PROMPT. (2017). Course Manual 3rd edition.
3. RCOG. (2011). Green Top Guideline no. 63 Antepartum haemorrhage. https://www.rcog.org.uk/en/guidelinesresearch-services/guidelines/gtg63/ (Updated 2014).
4. RCOG. (2016) Green-top Guideline No. 52 Prevention and Management of Postpartum Haemorrhage. https://www.rcog.org.uk/en/guidelines-researchservices/guidelines/gtg52/

Vaginal Bleeding: Gynaecological Causes

1. Introduction

- A number of conditions can cause vaginal bleeding that is different from normal menstruation. Such conditions may result in a call to the ambulance service, including:
  - excessive menstrual period
  - normal or excessive menstrual period associated with severe abdominal pain
  - following surgical or medical therapeutic termination ('abortion') (**NB** bleeding often continues for up to 10 days after treatment)
  - following gynaecological surgery (e.g. hysterectomy) (**NB** heavy, ongoing bleeding commencing 7–14 days after surgery can indicate pelvic infection requiring antibiotics and may require hospital assessment)
  - colposcopy (**NB** slight bleeding may occur up to 10 days after a colposcopy). A colposcopy is an outpatient test where the cervix is inspected following an abnormal cervical smear. Treatment such as cone biopsy for the abnormal smear may have been undertaken. Heavy bleeding post-colposcopy affects very few women in this situation. Heavy, ongoing bleeding at 7–14 days post-procedure can indicate infection requiring antibiotics and may require hospital assessment
  - gynaecological cancers, either before diagnosis or after treatment (i.e. cervix, uterus or vagina), may present with heavy vaginal bleeding
  - trauma; this can include post-coital tears and may be caused by sexual assault/rape.
- This guideline provides guidance for the assessment and management of gynaecological vaginal bleeding. For causes of bleeding in early or late pregnancy, refer to **Vaginal Bleeding during Pregnancy up to 20 Weeks Gestation**, **Vaginal Bleeding during Pregnancy after 20 Weeks Gestation**, **Management of Post-partum Haemorrhage (PPH)**.

2. Incidence

- Women over 50 years old are more at risk of cancers of the uterus and cervix.

3. Severity and Outcome

- The majority of causes of vaginal bleeding do not compromise the circulation, but blood loss can be alarming.

Sexual Assault

- In sexual assault cases, there may be other injuries.
- When sexual assault is suspected (especially in a child or vulnerable adult), there are clear safeguarding issues (refer to **Safeguarding Children** and **Safeguarding Adults at Risk**).
- It is not the role of the ambulance service to investigate. This is a police matter.
- Remember that the victim of sexual assault has physical forensic evidence on their body and clothing, and represents a 'crime scene' (refer to **Sexual Assault**).

4. Assessment and Management

For the assessment and management of vaginal bleeding, refer to Table 5.12.

TABLE 5.12 – ASSESSMENT and MANAGEMENT of: Vaginal Bleeding

Assess <C>ABCDEF

- Quickly assess the woman and scene as you approach.
- Undertake a primary survey.
- Evaluate whether the woman has any **TIME-CRITICAL** features or any signs of hypovolaemic shock.
- If any **TIME-CRITICAL** features are present, correct **A** and **B** and transport to nearest suitable receiving hospital.
- Provide an alert/information call.

Vaginal Bleeding: Gynaecological Causes

TABLE 5.12 – ASSESSMENT and MANAGEMENT of: Vaginal Bleeding *(continued)*

Assess Blood Loss

- Ask about clots, blood-soaked clothes, bed sheets and number of soaked tampons/towels/pads, and, where necessary, visibly inspect. **NB** Blood under the feet or between toes indicates significant bleeding.
- If **NON-TIME-CRITICAL**, perform a more thorough assessment of the woman with brief secondary survey for lower abdominal tenderness or guarding.
- Measure temperature and consider sepsis (refer to **Sepsis**).
- Check the woman's age:
  - \>50 years – more at risk of cancers of the uterus/cervix
  - <50 years – may be pregnant.
- Obtain IV access – insert a **LARGE BORE (16G)** cannula.
- If there is visible external blood loss >500 ml, refer to **Intravascular Fluid Therapy in Adults** and **Intravascular Fluid Therapy in Children**.

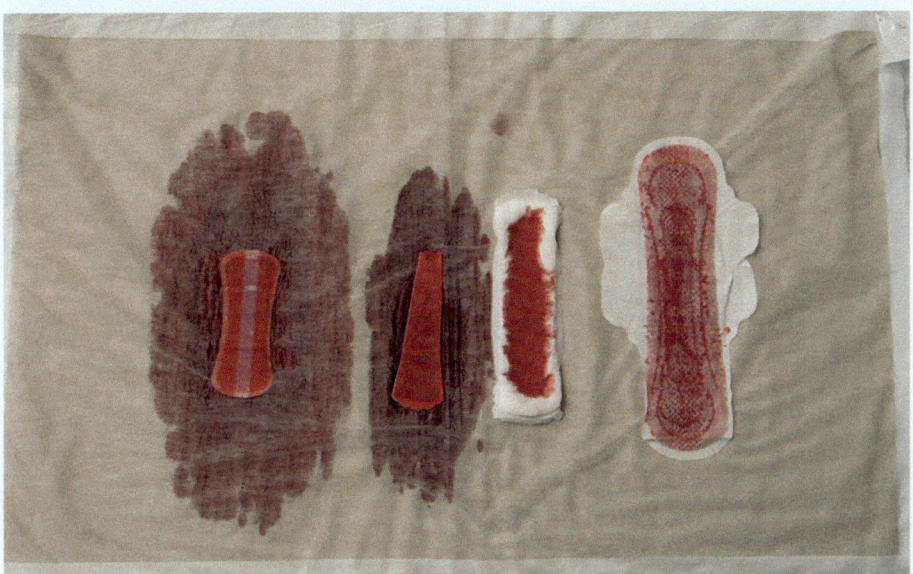

50 ml blood loss on various sanitary towels.

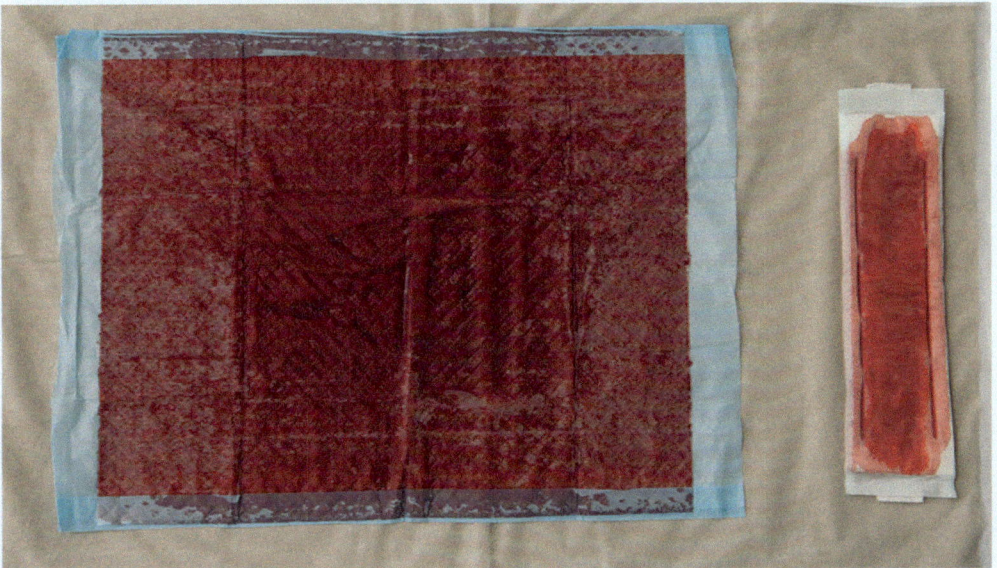

500 ml blood loss on maternity pad and 50 ml on maternity towel.

Monitor SpO$_2$ (94–98%)

- If oxygen (SpO$_2$) <94%, administer O$_2$ to aim for a target saturation within the range of 94–98%.

(continued)

Vaginal Bleeding: Gynaecological Causes

TABLE 5.12 – ASSESSMENT and MANAGEMENT of: Vaginal Bleeding *(continued)*
Assess the Woman's Level of Pain
• Titrate analgesia against pain (refer to **Pain Management in Adults and Children**): – Paracetamol – Entonox – Morphine – **NB** administer cautiously if the patient is hypotensive.
Assess the Woman's Comfort
• Nil by mouth. • Adjust the woman's position as required. • Transfer to further care.

KEY POINTS!

Vaginal Bleeding: Gynaecological Causes

- The majority of vaginal bleeding episodes do not compromise circulation, but blood loss can be alarming.
- Following gynaecological surgical interventions, heavy, ongoing vaginal bleeding commencing 7–14 days post-procedure may indicate underlying infection.
- Assess blood loss; ask about number of soaked tampons/towels/pads and visually inspect.
- Provide analgesia where indicated.
- If you suspect a miscarriage or ectopic pregnancy, refer to **Vaginal Bleeding during Pregnancy up to 20 Weeks Gestation**.

Bibliography

1. Centre for Maternal and Child Enquiries. Saving mothers' lives: reviewing maternal deaths to make motherhood safer: 2006–2008. *BJOG: An International Journal of Obstetrics & Gynaecology* 2011, 118 (suppl. 1).
2. Woollard M, Hinshaw K, Simpson H, Wieteska S. Emergencies in early pregnancy and complications following gynaecological surgery. In *Pre-hospital Obstetric Emergency Training*. Oxford: Wiley-Blackwell, 2009: 53–61.
3. Woollard M, Hinshaw K, Simpson H, Wieteska S. Management of non-obstetric emergencies. In *Pre-hospital Obstetric Emergency Training*. Oxford: Wiley-Blackwell, 2009: 136–165.

6

Special Situations

Atropine for CBRNE

1. Presentation
- Pre-filled syringe containing 1 milligram atropine in 5 ml.
- Pre-filled syringe containing 1 milligram atropine in 10 ml.
- Pre-filled syringe containing 3 milligrams atropine in 10 ml.
- An ampoule containing 600 micrograms in 1 ml.
- Duodote® containing 2.1 milligrams of atropine sulphate.

2. Indications
- Organophosphate (OP) poisoning.
- Adults and children with a clinical diagnosis of poisoning by OP nerve agents, as an adjunct to maintenance of oxygenation.
- Atropine should be administered for confirmed OP poisoning, or where features of OP poisoning develop. Clinical diagnosis of nerve agent poisoning (see below) is suggested by the characteristic features of nerve agent poisoning, associated with a history of possible exposure. Clinical features must include one or more of the following: bronchorrhoea, bronchospasm, severe bradycardia (<40 bpm).

3. Contra-Indications
Hypersensitivity to atropine sulphate or excipients in nerve agent poisoning.

4. Cautions
- There are no other absolute criteria for the exclusion from administration of atropine in the treatment of OP poisoning, as the consequences of not instituting prompt treatment in poisoned patients will usually outweigh the risks associated with treatment. However, caution needs to be administered in the following:
  - Patients with ulcerative colitis.
  - Patients with risk of urinary retention.
  - Patients with glaucoma.
  - Patients with conditions characterised by tachycardia (e.g. thyrotoxicosis, heart failure).
  - Patients with myasthenia gravis.

5. Side Effects
Reactions are mostly dose related and usually reversible, and include:
- Loss of visual accommodation.
- Photophobia.
- Arrhythmias, transient bradycardia followed by tachycardia.
- Palpitations.
- Difficulty in micturition.

6. Additional Information
Toxic doses may cause CNS stimulation manifesting as restlessness, confusion, ataxia, lack of coordination, hallucinations and delirium. In severe intoxication, CNS stimulation may give way to CNS depression, coma, circulatory and respiratory failure and death.

Characteristic Features of Nerve Agent Poisoning
- Miosis, excess secretions (e.g. lacrimation and bronchorrhoea).
- Respiratory difficulty (e.g. bronchospasm or respiratory depression).
- Altered consciousness, convulsions, together with a history of possible exposure.

6.1 Nerve Agent Poisoning
- Atropine must only be administered after the patient is adequately oxygenated.
- In OP poisoning there is no maximum dose and large doses (e.g. 20 milligrams) may be required to achieve atropinisation. Signs of atropinisation include dry skin and mouth and an absence of bradycardia (e.g. heart rate adult ≥80 bpm; heart rate child ≥100 bpm). **NB** DO NOT rely on reversal of pinpoint pupils as a guide to atropinisation.
- Administering large volumes intramuscularly could lead to poor absorption and/or tissue damage; therefore, administer the smallest volume possible and divide where necessary and practicable. Vary the site of injection for repeated doses; appropriate sites include buttock (gluteus maximus), thigh (vastus lateralis), lateral hip (gluteus medius) and upper arm (deltoid).

Atropine for CBRNE

Dosage and Administration

Intravenous 1 milligram in 5 ml

ROUTE: Intravenous/intraosseous/intramuscular (as appropriate).

NAME	AGE	ROUTE	INITIAL DOSE	REPEAT DOSE	DOSE INTERVAL	CONCENTRATION	VOLUME	MAX DOSE
Atropine for CBRNE	≥8 years	IV/IO/IM	2 milligrams	2 milligrams	5 minutes	1 milligram in 5 ml	10 ml	No limit
Atropine for CBRNE	12 months – 7 years	IV/IO/IM	600 micrograms	600 micrograms	5 minutes	1 milligram in 5 ml	3 ml	No limit
Atropine for CBRNE	Birth – <12 months	IV/IO/IM	200 micrograms	200 micrograms	5 minutes	1 milligram in 5 ml	1 ml	No limit

Intravenous 1 milligram in 10 ml

ROUTE: Intravenous/intraosseous/intramuscular (administer the smallest volume possible and divide where necessary and practicable).

NAME	AGE	ROUTE	INITIAL DOSE	REPEAT DOSE	DOSE INTERVAL	CONCENTRATION	VOLUME	MAX DOSE
Atropine for CBRNE	≥8 years	IV/IO/IM	2 milligrams	2 milligrams	5 minutes	1 milligram in 10 ml	20 ml	No limit
Atropine for CBRNE	12 months – 7 years	IV/IO/IM	600 micrograms	600 micrograms	5 minutes	1 milligram in 10 ml	6 ml	No limit
Atropine for CBRNE	Birth – <12 months	IV/IO/IM	200 micrograms	200 micrograms	5 minutes	1 milligram in 10 ml	2 ml	No limit

Atropine for CBRNE

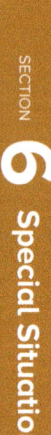

Intravenous 3 milligrams in 10 ml

ROUTE: Intravenous/intraosseous/intramuscular (as appropriate).

NAME	AGE	ROUTE	INITIAL DOSE	REPEAT DOSE	DOSE INTERVAL	CONCENTRATION	VOLUME	MAX DOSE
Atropine for CBRNE	≥8 years	IV/IO/IM	2 milligrams	2 milligrams	5 minutes	3 milligrams in 10 ml	6.7 ml	No limit
Atropine for CBRNE	12 months – 7 years	IV/IO/IM	600 micrograms	600 micrograms	5 minutes	3 milligrams in 10 ml	2 ml	No limit
Atropine for CBRNE	Birth – <12 months	IV/IO/IM	200 micrograms	200 micrograms	5 minutes	3 milligrams in 10 ml	0.6 ml	No limit

Intravenous 600 micrograms in 1 ml

ROUTE: Intravenous/intraosseous/intramuscular.

NAME	AGE	ROUTE	INITIAL DOSE	REPEAT DOSE	DOSE INTERVAL	CONCENTRATION	VOLUME	MAX DOSE
Atropine for CBRNE	≥8 years	IV/IO/IM	2 milligrams	2 milligrams	5 minutes	600 micrograms in 1 ml	3.3 ml	No limit
Atropine for CBRNE	12 months – 7 years	IV/IO/IM	600 micrograms	600 micrograms	5 minutes	600 micrograms in 1 ml	1 ml	No limit
Atropine for CBRNE	Birth – <12 months	IV/IO/IM	200 micrograms	200 micrograms	5 minutes	600 micrograms in 1 ml	0.3 ml	No limit

Chemical Biological Radiological Nuclear (CBRN) Incidents Including Hazardous Materials

1. Introduction

- Chemical, biological, radiological and nuclear (CBRN) incidents require a different approach from other incidents. Priorities include ensuring that the duration of exposure to the hazardous environment or substance is kept to a minimum and that the responders do not themselves become casualties.
- On recognition that an incident may involve CBRN, the Initial Operational Response (IOR) should be implemented, when safe to do so, which aims to quickly reduce people's exposure to a hazardous agent.
- Once the responsible agent(s) have been identified, specific procedures and treatment plans can be instigated.
- Specialist teams such as the Hazardous Area Response Team (HART) and Specialist Operational Response Team (SORT) are trained to work in these environments and should be mobilised as soon as possible.

2. Initial Operational Response (IOR)

- IOR is a quick and effective way of helping people caught up in a CBRN incident.
- The people and area in the vicinity may have become contaminated. The longer the contaminant is in contact with a person (either in the air or on the person), the worse the effects will be. IOR looks to separate the person from the contaminant in the quickest possible time, to reduce the health effects on that person.
- Casualties should be advised to follow the instructions from first responders, who will direct their actions using the Remove, Remove, Remove guidance (see Figure 6.1).
- It also allows non-protected responders to safely help the public before the arrival of specialist CBRN personnel.

3. Recognise, Assess, React

3.1 Recognise

- Recognise the indicators of a hazardous substance incident.
- Information gathering from the initial call by call handlers will form part of the initial recognition of the type of incident first responders will encounter. Key questions that will inform the response include the 5Ws:
  - What is happening? What indicators suggest hazardous substances?
  - Where is it? Are there factors which make this location more attractive as a target or more vulnerable to an attack e.g. A significant event, iconic location, critical national infrastructure or a Publicly Accessible Location (PAL).
  - Why is it suspicious? Has this been found as part of a venue search and why was this search taking place?
  - Who found it? Has anyone else seen it? If this is a member of the public have their details been obtained in order that further information can be obtained if required.
  - When was it found? What time was it found?

3.2 Assess

Visual Indicators
  - Was the offender(s) seen to carry out a deliberate act, where are they now, which direction did they leave in?
  - Any unusual/out of context liquids, powders, vapours, smells or tastes?
  - Any unusual and/or unattended materials, devices or equipment?
  - What are the physical symptoms (disorientation, sweating, irritation, twitching/convulsions, nausea/vomiting, breathing difficulties)?

Physical Symptoms

- Casualties can be an indicator of a hazardous substance incident and should be considered in conjunction with other indicators and signs or symptoms. These may include, but not limited to the physical symptoms of:
  - Disorientation and sweating.
  - Twitching and convulsions.
  - Airway irritation and breathing difficulties.
  - Eye and skin irritation.
  - Nausea and vomiting.

Casualty Assessment Tool

- In some cases, such as industrial incidents, the agent may already be known. In other cases, such as deliberate releases, the agent or agents may only be identified later using specialist equipment.
- Once casualties have been decontaminated, utilise the CBRN CRESS (consciousness, respiration, eyes, secretions, skin) tool (Figure 6.3) to identify what agent a casualty may have been exposed to or what clinical presentation they may have, so the appropriate initial clinical management can be provided. Ensure good communication so that once the agent(s) have been identified, any changes required to the treatment plan can be initiated, including for casualties who have already left the scene.

4. Specific Agents

4.1 Nerve Agent

- The classic presenting features of nerve agent exposure are those for organophosphate poisoning. Organophosphates can be found in pesticides and some herbicides, and agricultural

Chemical Biological Radiological Nuclear (CBRN) Incidents Including Hazardous Materials

Figure 6.1 – Remove, Remove, Remove guidance.

exposure or deliberate self-harm can result in toxicity.

- Where it is suspected or confirmed that a casualty has been poisoned with a nerve agent, the ambulance service's protocol is to administer a nerve agent countermeasure. The DuoDote® auto-injector is the countermeasure of choice and should be administered as per local policy/training. This drug is under Schedule 19 Exemption of the Human Medicines Regulations (2012), and can be administered by any trained member of staff under a local medicines protocol.
- A number of DuoDote® doses are carried on every front-line ambulance vehicle, with additional supplies in mass casualty vehicles (MCVs) and HART supplies.
- Each DuoDote® auto-injector contains 2.1 mg atropine and 600 mg pralidoxime for intramuscular injection into a large muscle group. It is suitable for adults and children over 1 year old but there is current clinical debate around minimum weight or body mass. If considering administration to children, expert advice should be sought from a practicing emergency physician and/or independent prescriber.
- For guidance on initial dose and any subsequent dosing see Table 6.1.
- Those patients with **severe** symptoms (unconsciousness, convulsions, respiratory arrest, severe respiratory distress, cyanosis or bradycardia <40 bpm) should have three doses of DuoDote® administered immediately, ideally into different large muscle groups to maximise absorption.
- Those patients with **moderate** symptoms (not walking, not obeying commands, confusion, excessive secretions, wheeze and incontinence) should have one dose of DuoDote® administered,

Chemical Biological Radiological Nuclear (CBRN) Incidents Including Hazardous Materials

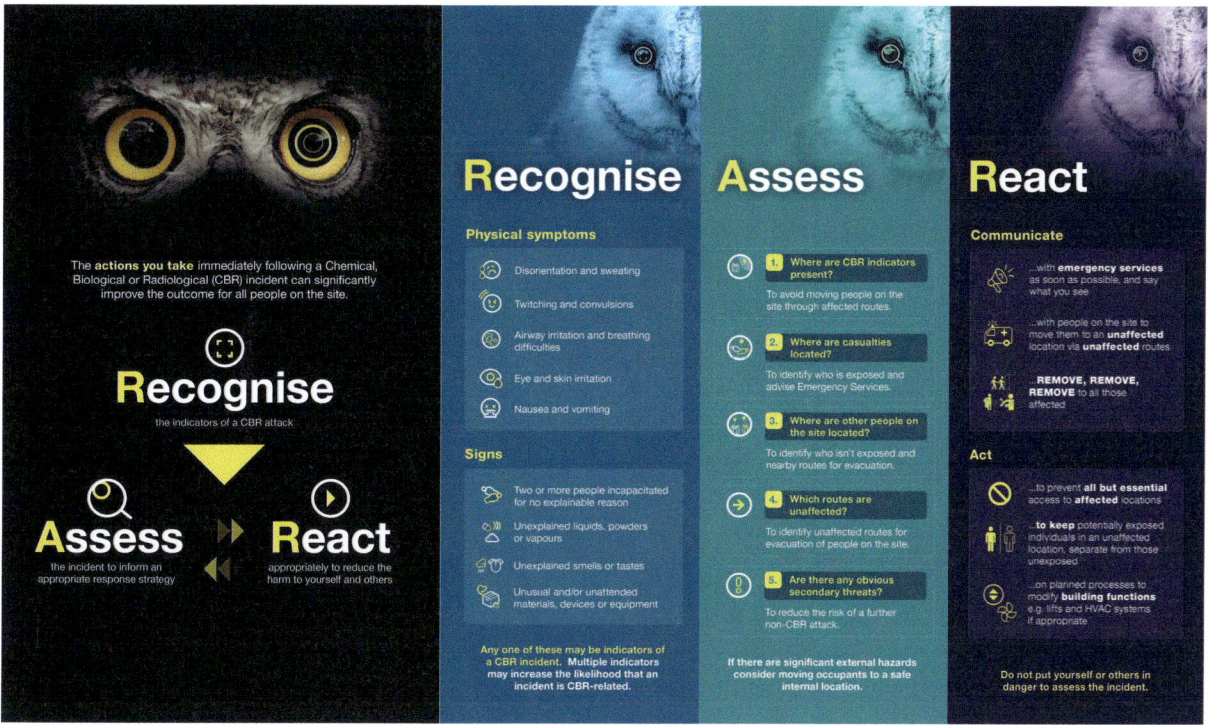

Figure 6.2 – Recognise, Assess, React from the Centre for the Protection of National Infrastructure (CPNI)

with re-assessment every 15 minutes. If symptoms persist, a repeat dose should be given. If severe symptoms develop, administer an additional two doses to reach the total of three doses of DuoDote®.

- For **paediatric** patients, the dosing should be based on age. Those 12 years and over are managed as adults. DuoDote® is contraindicated in those under 1 year of age and atropine should be used instead.

CRESS		NERVE AGENT	CYANIDE	OPIATE (MORPHINE)	ATROPINE	SEPSIS	HEAT STROKE
C	Consciousness	Convulsions	Unconscious/ Convulsions	Reduced → unconscious	Agitated/ Confused	Normal, reduced or altered	Altered
R	Respiration	Increased or reduced → stopped	Increased or stopped	Reduced → stopped	Increased	Increased	Increased
E	Eyes	Pinpoint pupils*	Normal/Large pupils	Pinpoint pupils	Large pupils/ Blurred vision	Normal	Normal/Large pupils
S	Secretions	Increased	Normal	Normal	Dry mouth/ Thirsty	Normal/ Sputum	Normal
S	Skin	Sweaty	Pink → blue	Normal/Blue	Flushed/Dry	Warm → pale Non-blanching rash	Varied
	Other Features	Vomiting Incontinence Slow Pulse Headache	Sudden onset		Fast pulse	Fast pulse Fever (>38.3°C) Bio-syndrome** No radial pulse	High temperature (>38°C)

Figure 6.3 – Casualty assessment tool from the Recognise, Assess, React (RAR) for Chemical, Biological and Radiological (CBR) Incidents CPNI.
IOR Guidance 2023 Link: https://www.jesip.org.uk/wp-content/uploads/2023/04/IOR-2023-Accessible.pdf

Chemical Biological Radiological Nuclear (CBRN) Incidents Including Hazardous Materials

TABLE 6.1 – Dosages of DuoDote®

Age	Initial Dose	Repeat Dose	Maximum Dose
12 years and over (Adult)	1–3 according to severity	1 every 15 minutes	3
8–11 years	1	1 after 15 minutes	2
1–7 years *Obtain advice from an emergency physician or independent prescriber.*	1	N/A	1
Less than 1	Contraindicated. Use atropine (see below).	N/A	N/A

- Once DuoDote® has been administered, if able to do so, gain IV/IO access. Administer high-flow oxygen.
- If seizures are present, administer anticonvulsant diazepam (IV/IO) or midazolam (buccal) in accordance with local protocol.
- In those severely symptomatic patients in whom:
  - the maximum dose of DuoDote® has been reached and they remain severely symptomatic
  - there is no DuoDote® immediately available or
  - DuoDote® is contraindicated due to age

Administer atropine via IV/IO route in accordance with guidance below. If IV/IO access cannot be achieved, IM is acceptable in extremis.

- In organophosphate and nerve agent poisoning, large doses of atropine may be required to adequately reverse the systemic effects (atropinisation), and the patient should be reassessed every 5 minutes with a view to repeat dose. Absence of bradycardia is the most reliable indicator of adequate effect, aiming for a heart rate over 80 bpm for adults and over 100 bpm for children under 12 years of age.
- Ensure the correct dose is administered, as presentations of atropine vary (3 mg in 10 ml, 1 mg in 10 ml, 1 mg in 5 ml and 600 mcg in 1 ml).

Refer to **Atropine for CBRNE**.

TABLE 6.2 – DuoDote® for Non-specialists and Specialists

Non-specialists	Specialists (Hazardous Area Response Team (HART))
• Administer DuoDote® (as per instructions/training) to casualties who are showing signs and symptoms of nerve agent poisoning once they have been decontaminated.	• Will administer DuoDote® to casualties in the hot/warm zone who have nerve agent poisoning.
• Seek expert advice to identify countermeasures for biological agents and all other chemical agents.	• Will seek specialist advice on appropriate countermeasures for casualties exposed to biological and all other chemical agents.
• Use DuoDote® on themselves if they have signs and symptoms of nerve agent poisoning.	

4.2 Cyanide

- Cyanide-containing substances are highly toxic and act at a cellular level by inhibiting the metabolism of oxygen to produce energy. So cellular hypoxia can result despite adequate inspired oxygen levels and SpO_2.
- Cyanide-containing substances can occur in solid (crystalline), liquid or gaseous forms and are used in several industrial processes. Cyanide-containing gases can be formed from burning plastics and are often present in house fires. Poisoning may be due to accidental or intentional exposure.
- Given the highly toxic nature, the onset of symptoms is often very rapid, within 20–30 seconds of exposure to toxic levels, and death can occur within 5–8 minutes. If a patient remains asymptomatic after 15 minutes, significant poisoning is unlikely unless there is ongoing exposure.

Treatment

- This should primarily focus on standard ABC approach, ensuring the safety of staff to prevent exposure. Specific antidotes for cyanide poisoning are available, though several of these are potentially toxic in their own right if administered when cyanide toxicity is not present.

Chemical Biological Radiological Nuclear (CBRN) Incidents Including Hazardous Materials

- Hydroxycobalamin is emerging as the safest effective antidote and is carried by some specialist pre-hospital care teams.
- If there is a suspicion of cyanide toxicity, ensure the safety of responders and seek expert advice urgently.

4.3 Opioids

- The classic features of opioid toxicity (respiratory depression, decreased level of consciousness and pin-point pupils) are well recognised from the administration of morphine as an analgesic and from patients with opiate addiction and a history of misuse.
- The management principles are fundamentally the same, with a focus on maintaining respiration and oxygenation. Synthetic opioids, such as fentanyl and carfentanil, are far more potent than morphine (80–1,000 times the potency of morphine). Therefore, toxic doses may be very small. Due to the potency, the period of respiratory depression may be prolonged, and cardiovascular collapse is more common. This potency often requires a higher dose and increased frequency of naloxone to achieve effective reversal of systemic effects.
- Synthetic opioids may be encountered in illicit drug laboratories (IDL), where those drugs are manufactured and are sometimes used for large animal tranquilisation. They may be absorbed through skin exposure or inhalation of vapour.
- If you suspect significant toxicity from a high-potency synthetic opioid, ensure the safety of responders and seek expert advice on patient management.

4.4 Atropine

- The features of atropine toxicity are classic for anticholinergic toxidrome (symptoms caused by dangerous levels of toxins in the body) and are often seen in accidental and intentional medication overdoses, or exposure to some toxic plants. High temperature leading to hyperpyrexia can result in severe morbidity. The management is principally symptomatic, though specific antidotes are available in hospital. Severe anticholinergic toxicity can result in death. Seek expert advice and convey the patient to an appropriate receiving facility.

For more information regarding CBRN clinical management, visit:

https://narueducationcentre.org.uk/

https://www.gov.uk/government/publications/chemical-biological-radiological-and-nuclear-incidents-recognise-and-respond.

4.5 Corrosive Substances

- There has been a significant increase in both the profile and frequency of serious criminal assaults using acids and other corrosive materials across the UK.
- These cause significant harm to individuals. While the overall number of people impacted by this type of attack remains low, responders are advised to use the Remove, Remove, Remove guidance in the event they attend a victim of such an attack (see Figure 6.3).
- The key management principle for reducing harm from corrosive chemical exposure is irrigation with clean water. This is effective whether the corrosive chemical is strongly acidic or caustic alkali.
- When using high-volume irrigation on large areas of contamination, ensure measures to reduce or minimise the patient becoming hypothermic.
- There is emerging evidence of the benefits of amphoteric solutions, such as Diphoterine©. This is carried by some specialist services within police, fire and ambulance, and is kept in many emergency departments. However, if amphoteric solution is not immediately available, irrigation should NOT be delayed awaiting availability.
- Burns on large body-surface areas, chemical burns or those affecting special areas (eyes, face, hands and genitalia) should be transferred to an appropriate receiving facility in accordance with local guidelines.

TABLE 6.3 – Dos and Don'ts for Corrosive Substances

Do	Don't
Exercise extreme caution if there appear to be multiple patients or an ongoing attack.	**Do not** approach containers or substance spillages.
Wear eye protection and gloves (double glove, nitrile gloves).	**Do not** pull contaminated clothing over the head or remove clothing that is adhering to the skin.
Protect any exposed skin by wearing a jacket to provide a barrier.	
Avoid becoming contaminated.	**Do not** delay on-scene time for patients with large burns or burns to the face, eyes or hands.

(continued)

Chemical Biological Radiological Nuclear (CBRN) Incidents Including Hazardous Materials

TABLE 6.3 – Dos and Don'ts for Corrosive Substances *(continued)*

Advise HART if there are large numbers of patients or extensive contamination.	**Do not** apply any form of occlusive dressing (e.g. clingfilm).
Move to a ventilated area to minimise vapour hazards.	
Request fire and rescue service (FRS) assistance to provide copious amounts of water.	
Irrigate casualties freely with clean water for 20 minutes. Try to ensure any run off does not come into contact with other uncontaminated parts of the body.	
Early and thorough irrigation of the face and eyes is particularly important to minimise the risk of long-term damage.	
Contaminated jewellery should be removed, rinsed and placed in bag/wrapped to avoid skin contact and given back to the patient.	
If possible, get the victim to do as much of the work themselves with direction – this may not always be practicable, but will greatly reduce exposure to first responders.	
Consider mobilising SORT team for decontamination if numbers are higher.	

4.6 Individual Chemical Exposure (ICE)

- Individual Chemical Exposure (ICE) events are frequently characterised by the use of a chemical, a mixture of chemicals or commercially available gases with the intent to self-harm predominantly via ingestion or inhalation.
- These events commonly occur in sealed or partially sealed environments, such as vehicles, residential bathrooms, hotel rooms, other enclosed areas or a bag over the casualty's head where a small amount of gas can quickly reach lethal concentrations. ICE events are usually single casualty or pairs rather than groups.
- Any event involving exposure of an individual to chemicals or other hazardous substances may present a serious risk to the public, emergency services and to other health workers, such as hospital and mortuary staff, who may come into contact with the contaminated individual.
- ICE events are complex in nature and will require multi-agency response; specialist responders (HART) should be requested as a matter of urgency.

TABLE 6.4 – Individual Chemical Exposure for Non-specialists and Specialists

Non-specialists		Specialists
Do	Don't	HART
Be cautious if an ICE incident is suspected, and stay a safe distance from the scene.	**Do not** approach the scene if an ICE incident is suspected or confirmed.	Have appropriate PPE to enter the inner cordon to provide life saving interventions or to perform ROLE.
Call for HART immediately and provide a (M)ETHANE report to control.	**Do not** become exposed to any hazardous substances.	Will provide medical support to partner agencies who are committed to the inner cordon.
Seek specialist advice if required.	**Do not** attempt to perform resuscitation or medical treatment if there are clear signs of the casualties being contaminated. This should only take place if the responder is in appropriate PPE.	

Chemical Biological Radiological Nuclear (CBRN) Incidents Including Hazardous Materials

4.7 Ionising Radiation

There are four main types of ionising radiation:

- alpha
- beta
- gamma and X-rays
- neutrons.

There are two main types of hazards from radioactive material:

- **Radiation Hazard:** Where a solid or contained source is only emitting radiation, this is referred to as a 'radiation hazard'. The radiation travels from the fixed source, through the air, to the human body. The target absorbs the energy from the radiation but is not itself made 'radioactive'. An analogy to this may be the heat emitted by a lit open fireplace.

- **Contamination Hazard:** Contamination is a potential problem with any radioactive material, except electrically generated x-rays (which can be turned off). If a material that contains radioactive isotopes is in a form that is easily dispersed (i.e. dusts, powders, liquids, gases), the radioactive substance can become attached to the exterior of the body or other surfaces by direct contact or airborne dispersion (e.g. dust, spray, mist etc.). It may also enter the body through inhalation, ingestion or through an open cut or wound. In this sense, internal radioactive contamination poses much the same threat as any other chemical toxin or 'hazardous materials exposure'. Once inside the body, alpha- and beta-emitting materials, which are not considered high risk in terms of external radiation, may deliver damaging ionising radiation directly into tissue or travel around the body via normal biological mechanisms. An analogy to this may be the smoke and soot given off by a fire, travelling around the room. The patient will continue to receive a radiation exposure from any inhaled or ingested radioactive material until it is excreted or decays away.

Contamination cannot be destroyed or neutralised like a chemical or biological agent. It can, however, be removed. The aim of decontamination is to move radioactive contamination from the contaminated person or object onto something else, which can then be isolated and disposed of correctly.

It is important for emergency responders to make a distinction between sealed (closed) sources of radioactivity and unsealed (open) sources of radioactivity.

- **Sealed Sources** A sealed source is a radioactive source that is encapsulated into a solid material, usually metal. The encapsulation is intended to prevent the escape of the physical radioactive material, while allowing the radioactive energy to pass through. Because the radioactive source substance is encapsulated or plated onto a surface, sealed sources do not present a contamination hazard under normal conditions; however, they can still present a significant radiation hazard.

- **Unsealed Sources** Unsealed sources consist of powders, liquids or sometimes gases which contain radioactive elements and which could easily be released from their containers through leaks and spillages and dispersed into the environment. The main hazard with unsealed sources is contamination, although there may also be a significant irradiation hazard from the bulk material. Sealed sources may become unsealed in the event of explosion, intense fire or severe damage.

- **Special Form** Some sealed sources are designed to a standard known as 'special form', as defined by transport legislation. To meet it, the source capsule must remain intact after several rigorous tests, which include heating, bending and striking tests. The standard is intended to show that the radioactive material would not be released to form a contamination hazard, even in the event of major damage. It might still present a significant radiation hazard.

4.8 Decontamination

- Those that have been contaminated can be treated by non-specialist staff wearing clinical PPE using strict hygiene protocols. Contamination levels can easily be monitored with appropriate equipment.

Radiation Trefoil

Chemical Biological Radiological Nuclear (CBRN) Incidents Including Hazardous Materials

TABLE 6.5 – Treatment for Contaminated Patients

P1	P2 and P3
Patients with life-threatening injuries should not have their treatment or transfer delayed for decontamination, other than the removal of clothing and personal belongings. (This should be undertaken during IOR.)	Patients should be decontaminated as far as reasonably practicable on scene, before approaching the ambulance for transport.
Any such clothing should be regarded as contaminated waste until proven otherwise, and so should be left in the scene where it can be appropriately removed.	If it is not practicable to decontaminate a patient before transfer to hospital, they may be wrapped in a sheet or blanket to prevent the spread of contamination.
Open wounds should be dressed, and the patient wrapped in sheets or blankets to stop the further spread of contaminant. The face and hands may be cleaned with wipes.	
Specialists (HART) will wear appropriate PPE to deal with non-ambulant patients in the inner cordon. Have detection, identification and monitoring (DIM) equipment to monitor radiation dose and amount of contamination on a casualty.	
SORT will provide clinical decontamination for mass casualties if required.	

4.9 Illicit Drugs Laboratories (IDLs)

- There is a risk in the UK from IDLs, which present many chemical hazards, explosive risk and fire hazards to the emergency services. They are places where illegal drugs have been or are being manufactured.
- Synthetic opioids e.g. Fentanyl Methylamphetamines and their by-products are of concern. Fentanyl represents a significant health risk to responders when manufactured illicitly.
- If you come across or suspect a location to be an IDL, use Table 6.6.

TABLE 6.6 – IDL for Non-specialists and Specialists

Non-specialists		Specialists
Do	**Don't**	**HART**
Evacuate immediately and stay a safe distance away.	**Do not** touch or otherwise disturb the substance.	Will wear appropriate PPE to enter the inner cordon to provide life saving interventions or to perform ROLE.
Provide control with a METHANE report.	**Do not** attempt to perform resuscitation or medical treatment if there are clear signs of the casualty(s) being contaminated. This should only take place if the responder is in appropriate PPE.	Will provide medical support to partner agencies who are committed to the inner cordon.
Seek expert advice.		

KEY POINTS!

CBRN incidents

- Request specialist response as soon as possible.
- Ensure Initial Operational Response (IOR) is followed.
- Follow Recognise, Assess, React (RAR).
- Communicate METHANE.
- If unsure of agent involved, use the CRESS tool.
- Follow specific guidance for known agents.

Major, Complex and High-Risk Incidents

1. Major Incidents

1.1 Initial Actions for a Major Incident

- Each NHS ambulance trust has a major incident plan, which will define key actions that ambulance staff must take if they are faced with a major incident. First and foremost, follow the plan of your service.
- The Cabinet Office Lexicon of civil protection terminology defines a major incident as: "An event or situation with a range of serious consequences which requires special arrangements to be implemented by one or more emergency responder organisation".
- The *Civil Contingencies Act 2004* defines an emergency of this magnitude in the following terms:
  - a. An event or situation which threatens serious damage to human welfare in a place in the United Kingdom.
  - b. An event or situation which threatens serious damage to the environment of a place in the United Kingdom
  - c. War, or terrorism, which threatens serious damage to the security of the United Kingdom.
- An incident which requires a highly technical response, or the utilisation of specialist capabilities could also be termed a **COMPLEX** incident.
- The first clinician on scene at incidents such as these should provide an initial report back to the using the METHANE model, which has been approved for use by each of the emergency services under the Joint Emergency Services Interoperability Programme (JESIP). The METHANE model is described in Figure 6.4.

The major incident standard declarations are:
  - **Major incident alert/standby** – The term used by any member of staff to prefix messages indicating tha an incident with the potential to generate a large number of casualties has or may have occurred.
  - **Major incident confirmed/declared** – The term used by any member of staff to prefix a message to confirm that a major incident has occurred, indicating that the plan should be implemented and a full pre-determined attendance/response is required.
  - **Major incident cancel** – The term used by a commander to cancel a major incident alert.
  - **Ambulance major incident stop** – The term used by a commander to indicate that sufficient ambulance and/or medical resources are available at the scene and that no further assistance is required.
  - **Ambulance major incident scene evacuation complete** – The term used by a ommander to indicate that the treatment and removal of casualties from the scene is complete.
  - **Ambulance major incident stand down** – The term used by a commander to indicate the conclusion of all ambulance service activity in connection with a declared major incident and a return to normal modes of operation.

Your own organisation or healthcare system may have slightly different variations on these standard declarations.

- The early declaration of a major incident ensures that the appropriate resources are activated at the earliest opportunity. These messages should be part of a METHANE report, as outlined in Figure 6.4.
- The next step will usually be to follow the Major Incident Action Cards of your organisation.

1.2 Command and Control

During a larger scale incident, a multi-agency command structure will form. The following information provides an overview of how the ambulance service will integrate in the wider command and control framework.

- There are NHS Standards for ambulance service command, to which local ambulance service plans are aligned. The ambulance service will work closely with other responding agencies using the joint working principles outlined in Figure 6.5.
- Important command decisions will be taken in the multi-agency setting using the joint decision model shown in Figure 6.6.
- Ambulance clinicians may be given a briefing by commanders. They may use the following 'IIMARCH' model, outlined in Figure 6.7.

1.3 Operational Discretion

- The term 'operational discretion' is used within the emergency services to describe decisions made by individuals which may depart from organisational protocol or standard operating procedures.
- Clinicians are used to using their professional discretion to apply clinical practice guidelines to a range of different situations. In the context of complex or major incidents, operational discretion is usually used to describe command decisions
- Emergency plans and procedures are written generically to cover anticipated incidents. However, by their nature, emergencies are often dynamic with unique features.
- When managing an incident, emergency service commanders or responders may need a degree of flexibility to adapt plans and procedures to achieve a desired outcome. This will often be within the context of life saving operations or situations where events are deteriorating despite existing plans and procedures being put in place.

Major, Complex and High-Risk Incidents

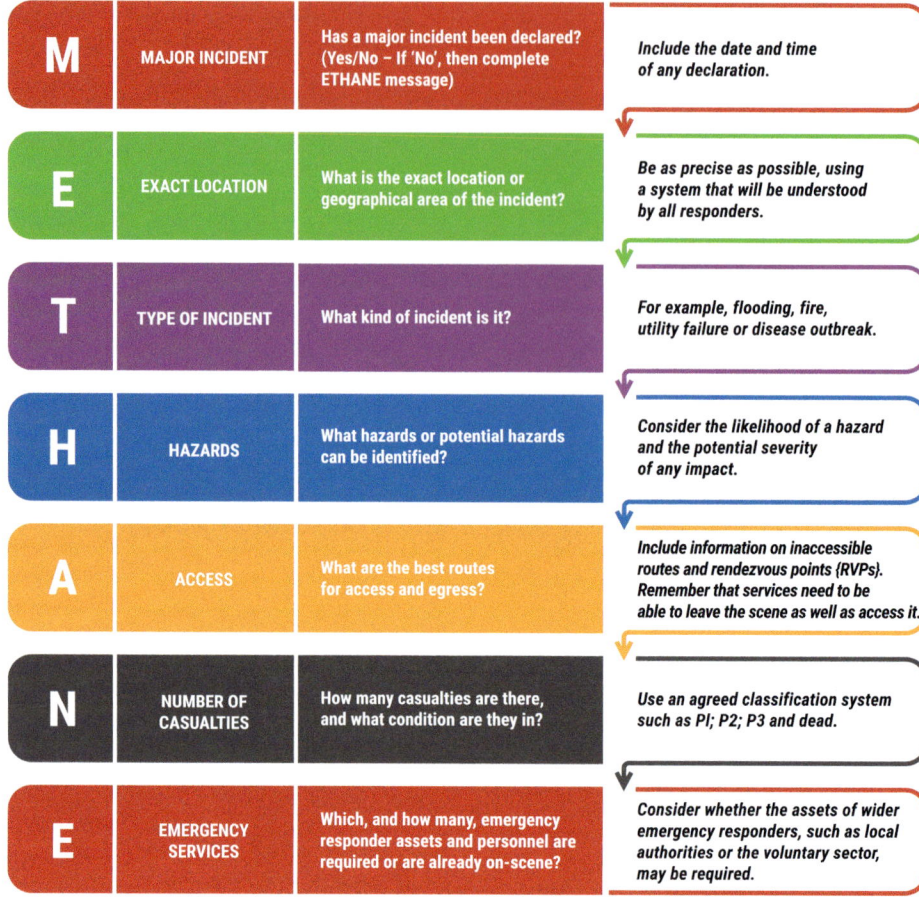

Figure 6.4 – The METHANE report model.

CO-LOCATE
Co-locate with other responders as soon as practicably possible at a single, safe and easily identified location.

COMMUNICATE
Communicate using language which is clear, and free from technical jargon and abbreviations.

CO-ORDINATE
Co-ordinate by agreeing the lead organisation. Identify priorities, resources, capabilities and limitations for an effective response, including the timing of further meetings.

JOINTLY UNDERSTAND RISK
Jointly understand risk by sharing information about the likelihood and potential impact of threats and hazards, to agree appropriate control measures.

SHARED SITUATIONAL AWARENESS
Establish shared situational awareness by using M/ETHANE and the Joint Decision Model.

Figure 6.5 – Joint working principles for the emergency services.

Major, Complex and High-Risk Incidents

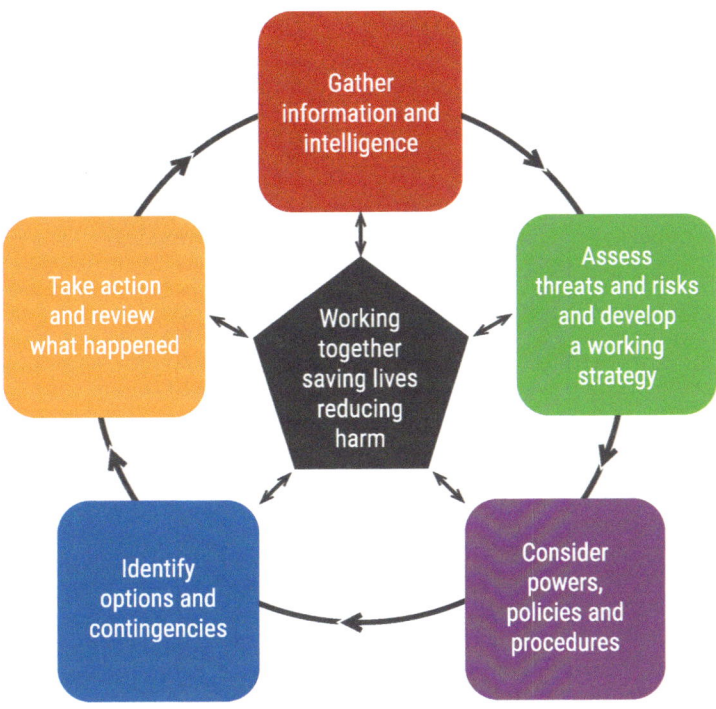

Figure 6.6 – Joint Decision Model (JDM)

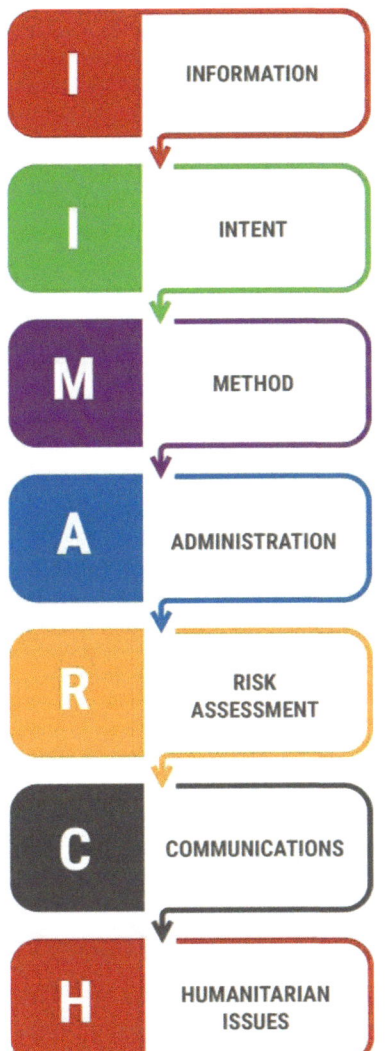

Figure 6.7 – IIMARCH Briefing Tool

- Operational discretion should not be used where existing plans and procedures fit the circumstances. Discretion is not a substitute for gaps in knowledge of what is already covered by existing provisions or what existing capabilities can achieve.

- Organisations plan carefully for emergency incidents. Preparations include risk assessments, training, equipment provisions and operational procedures. Specialist capabilities also provide an increased range of capability options. These things combine to create a safe system of work which the organisation has a duty of care to maintain for its staff. Using discretion to depart from these carefully considered provisions is not without risk. Use of discretion by individuals who are employed professionals within an organisation is, therefore, limited. Any departure from approved plans and procedures will be subject to considerable post incident scrutiny. The use of operational discretion needs to be proportionate and justifiable. The amount of discretion used by an individual and the amount of flexibility exercised should also be in direct proportion to the individual's experience and competence.

- The duty of care balance between providing a safe system of work for responders and taking carefully considered risks to save life or improve clinical outcomes for patients provides an important basis for justifying the use of operational discretion. Refer to **Duty of Care**.

1.4 On-Scene Risk Management

- All ambulance clinicians attending a major or complex incident have a responsibility to

Major, Complex and High-Risk Incidents

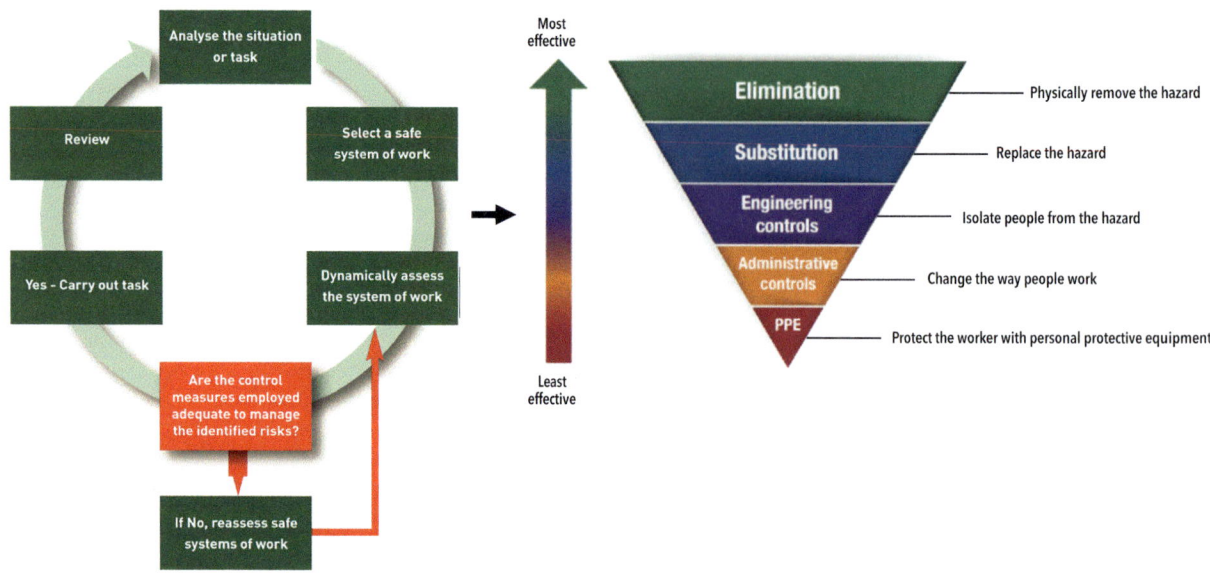

Figure 6.8 – Risk Management Overview.
Source for artwork on right-hand side (hierarchy of control measures) – HSE: L25 – PPE at Work – Guidance on Regulations (4th Ed., 2022), p.10, Figure 1).

support risk management at the scene. Clinicians must ensure that a dynamic risk assessment is undertaken. The situation must be regularly reviewed and any hazards that need to be considered by commanders should be reported, i.e., those hazards that present a risk to patients and responders.

- Figure 6.8 provides an overview of how commanders and responders will approach assessing and then controlling the hazards and risks present at the scene.
- During a complex or major incident, ambulance responders may be assigned specific roles. This will include command roles and operational functions. Key roles are denoted by the nationally specified tabards shown in Figure 6.9.
- National guidance on command and control can be found on the NARU website
- Always refer to your local organisation's plans and procedures.

1.5 Triage

- During the initial stages of an incident with large numbers of casualties, there are unlikely to be enough clinical responders to stay with each casualty and provide treatment. Therefore, Ten Second Triage (TST) shown in Figure 6.11 should be applied to ensure the best for everyone is achieved until such time that resources are sufficient to provide further care.
- Ten Second Triage (TST) is a new primary scene triage tool that has been developed for use by all first responders to any incident with multiple casualties.
- Primary scene triage is used in multiple casualty incidents to identify the most severely injured casualties, prioritise those who need immediate Life-Saving Interventions (LSIs) and to help guide evacuation decisions. It provides a simple framework for an approach to a chaotic scene that will help all responders optimise their ability to move quickly and efficiently from one casualty to the next in order to save as many lives as possible.
- Previously, triage was limited to use only by Ambulance Services in the UK. As of April 2023, in addition to NHS Ambulance Services, other emergency services including Police, Fire and Rescue Services (FRS), Voluntary Aid Agencies and the UK Armed Forces will be able to adopt Ten Second Triage (TST) as the initial triage for any multiple casualty incident. TST should be used to direct casualty treatment and evacuation priorities for any multiple casualty scenario prior to arrival of health care assets or under the guidance of health care assets when present.

There are 4 colour bands available:

White on Red	P1 Priority One
Black on Yellow	P2 Priority Two
White on Green	P3 Priority Three
Black on Silver	Not Breathing

Major, Complex and High-Risk Incidents

COMMAND TABARDS

Tactical Commander (Ambulance Incident Commander)
White lower half with green & white checked shoulders.

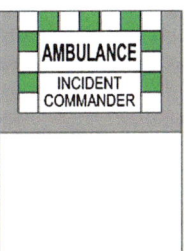

Ambulance Operational Commander and any functional role not individually listed
Saturn yellow lower half and green & white checked shoulders. Insert as per role.

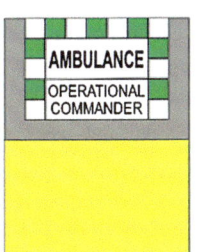

Airwave Tactical Advisor
Green & white check.

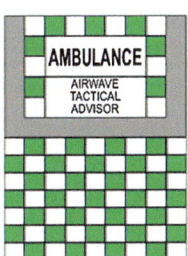

Ambulance Safety Officer (ASO)
Blue lower half with green & white checked shoulders.

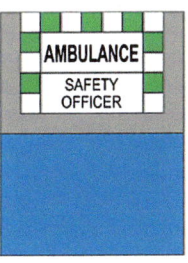

Decontamination Officer
Purple lower half with green & white checked shoulders.

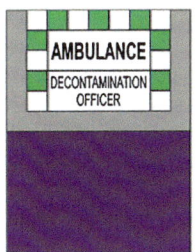

Doctor
Red lower half with green & white checked shoulders.

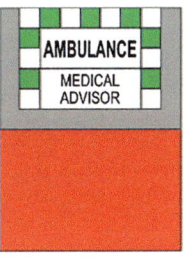

Strategic Advisor, Tactical Advisor or National Inter-Agency Liaison Officer (NILO)
Green lower half with green & white checked shoulders. Insert as per role.

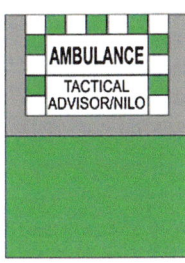

Ambulance Entry Control Officer (ECO)
Green & yellow all over check.

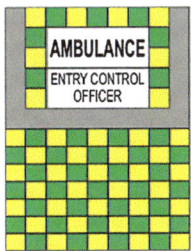

Loggist
Orange lower half and green & white checked shoulders. All orange is any support function.

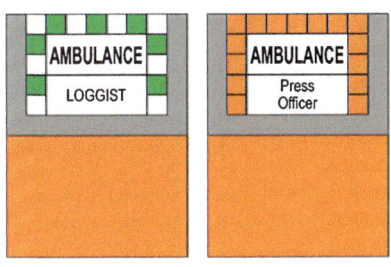

Figure 6.9 – Nationally Agreed Incident Command Tabard.

- A white checked border is used to identify the TST bands (see Figure 6.10), in order to differentiate them from the tagging used for the MITT system (or any other triage system) which have a solid-coloured tag throughout.

- The Major Incident Triage Tool (MITT) has been designed and validated as a unified replacement to the NASMeD Triage Sieve, Triage Sort and Paediatric Triage Tape that can be used by healthcare responders after TST and when sufficient resources allow. It is intended to aid

Major, Complex and High-Risk Incidents

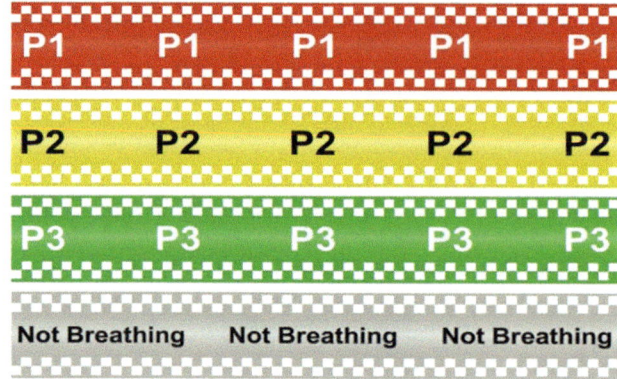

Figure 6.10 – Example of TST bands

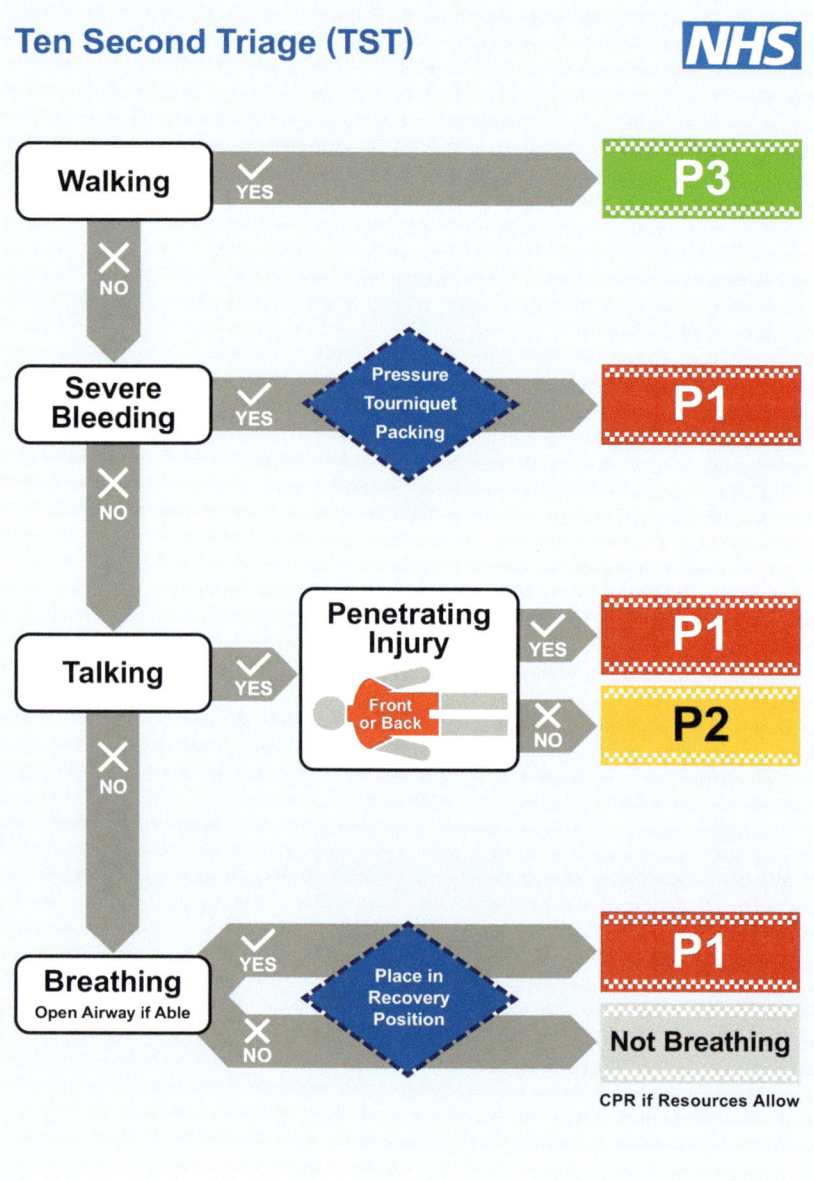

Figure 6.11 – Ten Second Triage Algorithm

Major, Complex and High-Risk Incidents

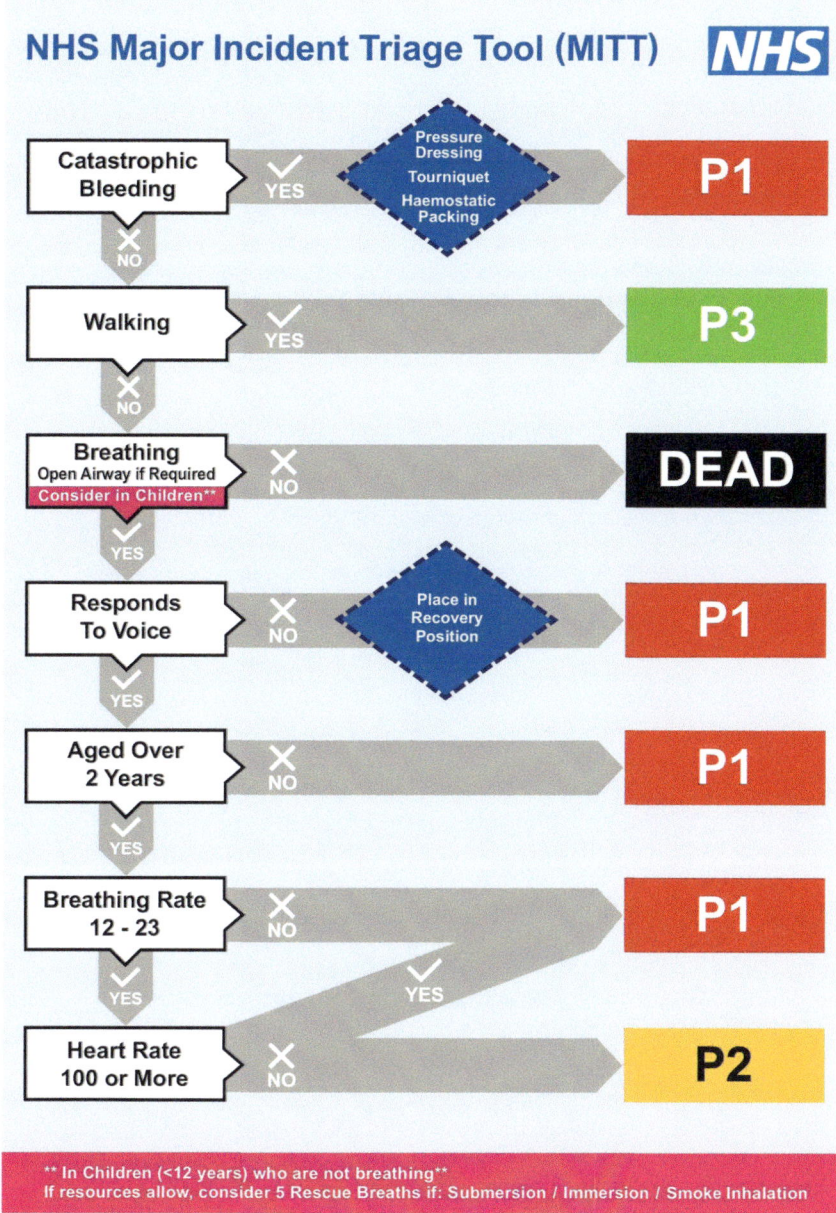

Figure 6.12 – Major Incident Triage Tool Algorithm.

clinical decision making where demand/resourcing precludes senior clinician-led decision making (or if enhanced/critical care is not available).

- The decision to switch to MITT will be made by the on-scene ambulance commander and should only be taken once TST is complete for all casualties that can be accessed. MITT should only be instituted once casualties reach a CCP or CCS rather than being performed on scene.
- Once TST is complete and casualties are being extricated to a CCP or CCS, the main decision for the on-scene ambulance commander will be whether to follow up TST with:
  - 1. Business As Usual (BAU) standard clinical practice
  - 2. MITT

- Some of the factors to consider that will influence this decision include the:
  - Number of patients
  - Number of clinical resources
  - Ability to transport to definitive care.
- Regardless of whether TST is followed by BAU or MITT, the priorities should be:
  - Rapid evacuation of high acuity TST P1 to definitive care
  - Re-triage of Silver tagged "Not Breathing" patients to Dead or viable for resuscitation (P1).
- If MITT is instituted a triage card should be used and TST band left in situ. Casualties triaged with MITT will be marked with a triage tag with a block colour (i.e., without a checked border) to identify

Major, Complex and High-Risk Incidents

the tag as MITT rather than a TST band. It should also have space to write treatment notes as well.

2. Specialist Capabilities

- NHS ambulance services maintain a range of specialist capabilities to support the response to major, complex, and high-risk incidents. These capabilities are interoperable, which means they can be used locally or combined to provide a national response.
- When responding to a major, complex, or high-risk incident, it is essential for ambulance staff to request these specialist services early. They can be easily stood down if not required.
- The interoperable specialist capabilities are summarised in Table 6.7.

TABLE 6.7 – Ambulance Service Interoperable Specialist Capabilities

Core Capability	Tactical Options	
Hazardous Area Response Teams (HART)	**Hazardous Substances** Incidents involving hazardous substances where malicious intent is not suspected or confirmed.	• Working inside the inner cordon • Specialist operational response (SOR) • Industrial accidents • High Consequence Infectious Disease (HCID) • Complex transportation accidents • Individual Chemical Exposure (ICE) incidents.
	Chemical, biological, radiological, nuclear (CBRN) Incidents involving a hazardous substance and the suspicion or confirmation that its release was deliberate with ideological motivation or intent.	• Specialist operational response (SOR) • Component part of wider CBRN capability
	Marauding terrorist attack (MTA) Incidents involving an attacker actively and deliberately seeking out new victims, using one or more identified attack methodologies.	• Support to operations requiring the use of specialist ambulance responders with ballistic PPE • Component part of wider MTA capability
	Safe working at height (SWaH) Patient management where a fall from a distance liable to cause injury could occur. Can be below as well as above ground level.	• Manmade structures • Natural environments

Major, Complex and High-Risk Incidents

TABLE 6.7 – Ambulance Service Interoperable Specialist Capabilities *(continued)*

Core Capability	Tactical Options	
	Confined space A confined space is one which is both enclosed or largely enclosed and has a reasonably foreseeable specified risk to workers of: • explosion • fire • loss of consciousness • asphyxiation • drowning	• Substantially enclosed spaces • Building collapse • Compromised atmospheres • Entrapments
	Unstable terrain Any terrain which poses a heightened risk of injury or entrapment due to its unstable nature.	• Active rubble pile • Rural access/ difficult terrain
	Water operations Inland incidents within 3 m of the water's edge (or at any location where there is a risk of falling into water). Offshore/in a tidal range only alongside other competent agencies.	• Swift water rescue • Urban and rural flooding • Boat operations
	Support to security operations (SSO) To provide immediate medical support during high-risk security operations; including relevant partners engaged in those operations; where there is a significant potential for injury or death to security personnel, the public and other parties.	• Support to police operations • Illicit drug laboratories • VIP close protection support • Pre-planned events as part of wider EPRR response.
Marauding terrorist attack (MTA)	• Working inside a ballistically unsafe area (warm zone) • Siege/stronghold	
Chemical, biological, radiological, nuclear explosives (CBRN)	• Initial Operational Response (IOR) • Specialist Operational Response (SOR) provided by HART & SORT • Interim decontamination of casualties • Full wet or dry decontamination of casualties	
Command and control (C2)	• Strategic command of major and critical incidents • Tactical command of major and critical incidents • Operational command of major and critical incidents • National Interagency Liaison Officers (NILOs) • Advisors (e.g. Medical, Airwave, TacAd, etc.) • Functional roles including loggists	
Mass casualties	• Capabilities to treat large numbers of casualties (e.g. Mass Casualty Vehicles and equipment) • Casualty clearing stations (CCS) • National coordination of patient transfers	

Major, Complex and High-Risk Incidents

3. Security

3.1 UK Threat Levels

- The threat level for the UK from international terrorismis set by the Joint Terrorism Analysis Centre (JTAC). MI5 is responsible for setting the threat level from Northern Irish Related Terrorism in Northern Ireland.
- Determination of threat level is based on available intelligence, terrorist capability, terrorist intentions, and timescale (the likelihood of an attack in the near term).
- Threat levels are designed to give a broad indication of the likelihood of terrorist attack.
  - **LOW** means an attack is unlikely.
  - **MODERATE** means an attack is possible, but not likely.
  - **SUBSTANTIAL** means an attack is likely.
  - **SEVERE** means an attack is highly likely.
  - **CRITICAL** means an attack is highly likely in the near future.

(Source: https://www.mi5.gov.uk/threat-levels)

- When the threat level is changed, particularly to **SEVERE** or **CRITICAL**, ambulance staff should seek specific advice from their own organisations. In general, staff should consider the following safety guidance:
  - Always remain alert to the danger of terrorism and report any information relating to an imminent threat to life or property to the police on 999 or the anti-terrorist hotline: 0800 789 321.
  - To provide information not relating to an imminent threat, contact Mi5 either online via https://www.mi5.gov.uk/contact-usor by telephone, on 0800 111 4645.

3.2 Personal Safety

If there is an increase in threat level or there is a heightened state of security, the following steps will help to ensure personal safety. However, these are also sensible precautions for clinicians to apply at all times:

- Challenge anyone on site who is not visibly displaying ID.
- Know the exits on all sites that are regularly visited or worked at.
- Consider means and routes for leaving the building or site.
- Beware of the surroundings. Look out for any suspicious or unusual behaviour, including unattended bags or packages.
- Vary routines, such as route to work or parking spot.
- Ensure your line manager knows where you are.
- Avoid travelling in uniform.
- Remove ID cards and vehicle car passes when leaving the workplace.
- Avoid drawing unnecessary attention to your occupation outside work.
- Update privacy settings on personal social media accounts so that information is only shared with known people. Never include operational or work information.

For more information regarding the Stay Safe campaign and other safety advice, visit:

https://www.gov.uk/government/publications/stay-safe-film

https://www.gov.uk/government/publications/recognising-the-terrorist-threat

3.3 Protectively Marked Documents

- All information that the government needs to collect, store, process, generate, dispose, or share to deliver services and conduct government business has intrinsic value and requires an appropriate degree of protection.
- Ambulance staff may come across protectively marked documents as part of routine work, especially work that may be associated with emergency preparedness. Failure to appropriately handle these documents (or associated materials) and the information contained within them can have serious consequences, including dismissal and potential criminal liability.
- Security classifications indicate the sensitivity of information and the need to protect it. There are three levels of classification:
  - **OFFICIAL:** The majority of information that is created, processed, sent or received in the public sector and by partner organisations, which could cause no more than moderate damage if compromised and must be defended against a broad range of threat actors with differing capabilities using nuanced protective controls. Official classifications may be accompanied by a descriptor which will mandate special handling requirements. This includes 'Official – Sensitive'. If you receive material with an 'Official – Sensitive' descriptor, you must ensure you handle that material in accordance with the Government Protective Marking Scheme requirements.
  - **SECRET:** Very sensitive information that requires enhanced protective controls, including the use of secure networks on secured dedicated physical infrastructure and appropriately defined and implemented boundary security controls, suitable to defend against highly capable and determined threat actors, whereby a compromise could threaten life (an individual or group), seriously damage the UK's security and/or international relations, its financial security/stability or impede its

Major, Complex and High-Risk Incidents

ability to investigate serious and organised crime.

- **TOP SECRET:** Exceptionally sensitive information assets that directly support or inform the national security of the UK or its allies AND require an extremely high assurance of protection from all threats with the use of secure networks on highly secured dedicated physical infrastructure, and robustly defined and implemented boundary security controls.

(Source: https://www.gov.uk/government/publications/government-security-classifications)

3.4 Unattended and Suspicious Items

- No unattended item should be ignored, but should always be assessed proportionately, considering what can be seen and anything you know about its discovery. For example, in the case of unattended hand luggage, it may be possible to ask if its owner is nearby.

- However, when an item has been hidden from view deliberately, or has visual clues suggesting it may be hazardous – wires, circuit boards, batteries, adhesive tape, liquids, putty-like or unusual substances etc. – or has been found after a suspicious event, an immediate and focused response is required. This will involve telling someone what you have seen and why you think it is suspicious.

- If you believe any unattended item represents a potential risk to life, you must report it as soon as possible and alert those nearby.

- When dealing with suspicious items, the following steps should be taken:
  - Do not touch it.
  - If you are in an owned public space, or a managed building, report it to a member of staff or security, if available. If they are not available, alert the Police via Ambulance Control but do not use your mobile phone within 15 metres of the suspicious item and place yourself out of sight of the item.
  - If you believe there may be a risk to life, move away at least 100 metres from a small item such as a rucksack; at least 200 metres away from a small vehicle or large item, such as a car or a wheelie bin; and at least 400 metres away from a large vehicle, such as a van or lorry.
  - Once at a safe distance, stay behind hard cover (such as concrete or brick) and away from secondary hazards, such as glazed areas or parked vehicles, and do not re-enter the evacuated area until directed it is safe to do so.

Remember: If you think it's suspicious, say something.

(Source: Unattended and suspicious items | ProtectUK)

3.5 Improvised Explosive Device (IED) Threat

- An IED is a bomb which can be made from Homemade Explosives (HME). Although IEDs may be 'home-made', they can still be as powerful as commercial or military explosives, be sophisticated in their design and be very effective.

- IEDs may be delivered using the following methods:

(This list is not exhaustive)
  - 1. Person Borne IED (PBIED)
  - 2. Postal or mail device – often a Victim Operated IED (VOIED)
  - 3. Remote Controlled IED (RCIED)
  - 4. Vehicle Borne IED (VBIED) and Under Vehicle IED (UVIED)

(Source: Attack methodology: Improvised Explosive Devices (IEDs) | ProtectUK)

- Where information and intelligence indicate that a viable explosives threat exists, the use of the JDM and these principles will assist commanders in the appropriate deployment of responders to save lives. All options should be explored to enable the rapid rescue and evacuation of casualties from the affected area.

3.6 Post/Partial IED detonation

- For any "explosion" put in a minimum 100 metre cordon as there may be a remaining explosive hazard. **However, where there are casualties then the situation may be too dynamic to achieve that immediately. The rapid treatment and movement of casualties will remain the priority.**

- Do not touch or move anything you do not have to.

- Move people away from the seat of explosion as quickly as possible (accepting that casualties may make this a slower process).

- Essential personnel may go forward to protect and save life, following a JDM assessment.

- Utilise any available hard cover.

- Spend the minimum amount of time in the area as possible and keep the numbers to the minimum required to achieve the operational effect.

- Consider the need for respiratory protection measures. Dust, smoke, debris and CBRN hazards may be present.

(Source: JESIP *Responding to a Marauding Terrorist Attack: Joint Operating Principles for the Emergency Services* (3rd Ed., 2023))

Major, Complex and High-Risk Incidents

4. Incidents Involving Firearms and Weapons

- The prevalence of criminal or terrorism-related incidents is a significant risk to the public and emergency services personnel. In recent times, Europe, the UK and indeed many other countries have seen numerous actual or attempted attacks on their sovereign soil by non-State actors.
- In the UK, violent criminal attacks, using bladed and other types of weapons, are on the increase. Acts of terror have been conducted with varying degrees of sophistication, ranging from attacks using easily accessible items, such as knives and vehicles, to more complex incidents involving firearms, home-made explosives (HME) and improvised explosive devices (IEDs).
- It may not be obvious to responders (especially those first on scene) that an incident involving weapons has occurred and subsequently that there may still be a potential risk to the public and responders alike.
- Once on scene, incidents with mechanisms of injury (MOI) of penetrating and/or blast injury, particularly those with no apparent explanation, should be attended with caution. If either a criminal or terror-related act has occurred, then the safety of the responder(s) is paramount and unprotected responders should consider withdrawing from the area if they feel that their safety is compromised.
- The Home Office has issued specific advice to the public if they become caught up in an MTA or an active shooter event in the form of the Run, Hide, Tell campaign (Figure 6.13).
- While aspects of the Home Office campaign are applicable to the ambulance service, ambulance responders also owe a duty of care to reported casualties (refer to **Duty of Care**).
- The following guidance should be considered by ambulance personnel involved in an actual or suspected violent or terrorist attack:
  - Withdraw from the scene as quickly as possible. If possible, take casualties and mission-critical medical equipment.
  - Move in a direction away from the actual or perceived threat and avoid running in straight lines.
  - Move from point to point using hard cover as necessary and if available.
  - The distance to withdraw to is situationally dependent and individual judgement should be used.
  - If police and/or security services are present, they may give a specific distance to move to.
  - Safe distances in incidents involving firearms will depend on the type of weapon(s) being used. Some firearms have an effective range of as little as 50 m, while other types of weapon systems may have an effective range of up to 400 m.
  - When explosive devices are suspected to have been used or will be used, the minimum distance will again vary depending on the type and size of the device.
  - Once at a safe distance, responders should seek cover that gives physical protection and protection from view. Cover from ballistic or explosive threats could be a solid structure like a building, for example.

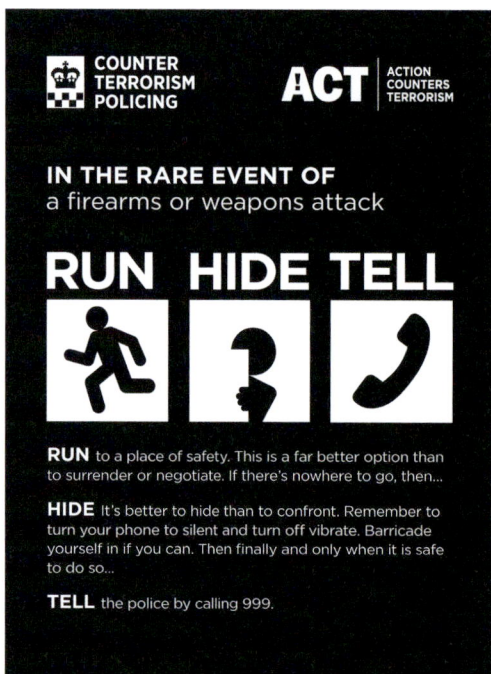

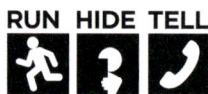

Figure 6.13 – Run, Hide, Tell

(Source: RHT A5 leaflet (protectuk.police.uk))

Major, Complex and High-Risk Incidents

- If physical cover is not achievable, then the responder should look for areas that will provide cover from view, for example a depression in the terrain.
- Once in cover, plan an escape route.
- Avoid isolated or obvious forms of cover, such as lone objects.
- Try to select cover that, while providing protection, also gives maximum fields of view.
- When in cover, scan the area for secondary threats and be prepared to move again if not satisfied with the area selected for cover.
- Stay calm and control breathing. Remain focused.
- Once it is safe to do so, it is imperative that the responders update the situation as soon as practicable using the METHANE reporting method.
- Ask for assistance from the police and the Hazardous Area Response Team (HART) if they are not already present or en route.
- Continue to provide situational updates if practicable and safe to do so.
- Turn the volume down on the communication system and speak quietly. Where possible, use an earpiece.
- Turn other mobile devices to silent (turn OFF any vibrating alert) while still in danger.
- HART units and Specialist Operational Response Teams (SORTs) are specifically trained and equipped with ballistic personal protective equipment (PPE) to operate within a ballistic warm zone while responding to MTAs. HART also provide support to security operations (SSO). For any incidents of criminal attack involving weapons or terrorism, HART should be deployed as a matter of reflex. The deployment of SORT will normally be triggered by information received by the ambulance Emergency Operations Centre (EOC).
- Incidents involving different types of weapons result in different types and severities of injuries.

- For specific guidance on treatment algorithms, refer to **Trauma Emergencies in Adults – Overview**, **Trauma Emergencies in Children – Overview**, **Head Injury** and **Thoracic Trauma**.

5. Water Rescue

- Ambulance responders are frequently called to incidents involving water. Non-specialists should not enter fast-moving water.
- Where patient(s) require lifesaving interventions (refer to the **Submerged Person Tool**), there are steps that can be taken by all ambulance staff prior to specialist teams arriving. Consider the following:
  - Carry out a dynamic risk assessment.
  - Inform the EOC of the situation.
  - Request specialist assistance, including HART assets, as soon as possible.
  - Wear a lifejacket if working within the warm zone (3 m from water's edge).
  - Shout at the patient to swim towards you.
  - If they are unable to do so, throw a safety buoy (or similar) for them to hold on to and pull them to safety.
  - Do not carry out a task that is likely to cause you to enter the water unintentionally and become a casualty yourself.
  - Only enter the water if it is shallow enough and, based on the risk assessment, you are competent to do so (i.e. a shallow pool in a recreational park as opposed to a canal, lake or fast-flowing river).
  - Do not enter flood water without the support of specialist water responders.
- Ideally, non-specialists should not be working within the warm zone without appropriate training, equipment or PPE, but it is recognised that in some low-risk incidents it is unacceptable to delay lifesaving interventions awaiting specialist help. This must be managed appropriately within each trust.
- For specific guidance on treatment algorithms, refer to **Drowning**, **Hypothermia**, or others depending on patient assessment.

6. High-consequence Infectious Disease (HCID)

- Examples of high consequence infectious diseases are:
  - Ebola
  - Lassa fever
  - Marburg virus
  - pandemic influenza
  - other 'category 4' pathogens.
- It is crucial that the correct response to patient(s) with suspected/confirmed infectious disease is achieved to protect all those involved. The need for such a response will usually be pre-planned. Where this is not the case and an infectious disease is suspected, several precautions are needed.
- The patient should be isolated and further advice sought from a Tactical Advisor/NILO and trust protocols followed. Normally, universal precautions will be sufficient to protect ambulance responders. A more thorough history than normal will need to be obtained from the patient. Transfers of high-risk patients are usually completed by specialist HART staff who have access to additional protective equipment. If ambulance responders suspect they may have

Major, Complex and High-Risk Incidents

been exposed (i.e. needlestick injury), report and present for medical treatment immediately.

6.1 Pandemic Flu

- This is the highest-grade risk in the National Risk Register of Civil Emergencies. All ambulance responders should be familiar with their local trust's plans to respond to such patients. Universal precautions are normally appropriate. All ambulance responders should have access to FFP3 masks, or equivalent, and be appropriately fit tested. All ambulance responders are encouraged to receive an annual flu vaccination in order to protect themselves, their families and the public.

7. Transport Incidents

7.1 Rail Incidents

Table 6.8 outlines how to manage rail incidents.

TABLE 6.8 – Management of Rail Incidents

Non-specialists	Specialists (HART)
Do not approach the track without authorisation from the Ambulance Operational Commander (if on scene or via EOC if they are en route) that the power is off and trains stopped as confirmed by Network Rail Route Control.	
Request HART support and provide a METHANE report to control.	Have appropriate PPE and specialist equipment to deal with such an incident.
	Will provide medical support to partner agencies responding to the incident.
Use the mnemonic POWER: • **P**ower off and trains stopped confirmed by authorised person. When in doubt, contact EOC. • **O**ff the tracks unless the patient appears viable. • **W**ear PPE (minimum hi-vis jacket and helmet). • **E**nsure EOC and ambulance commander knows clinicians are entering or leaving trackside. • **R**apidly remove a viable patient and treat in the safest agreed area off the tracks.	
Identify your location at track to Network Rail Control via Ambulance Control (EOC) (use signal; bridge or overhead line support number plates; quarter-mile posts at track side; station or level crossing nearby; electrical substation name plate).	

7.2 Industrial Docks

- Report to the rendezvous point (RVP) to meet dock staff and be taken to the incident. If the activity is close to the water's edge, ensure HART attendance is requested early.
- Many docks contain structures that require staff to work at height or in confined spaces, i.e. ships, ISO containers and cranes. An early request for specialist resources who are equipped, trained and authorised to work in such environments is imperative. Request HART early.
- Local ambulance services may have site-specific plans and arrangements for large dockland areas. For further information, contact the EPRR Department.

7.3 Airports

- Each airport will have a site-specific plan for incidents and emergencies on their site. This will have been developed in conjunction with the emergency services, including ambulance services. When responding to an airport emergency, clinicians will usually be asked to report to a designated RVP, where they will be met and taken airside by airport staff. Identify relevant RVPs in advance. These will be contained in your local plans.
- Each ambulance service will also have a pre-determined attendance (PDA) for such incidents. For further information on airport incidents, contact the EPRR Department.

7.4 Carriageways and Motorways

General guidelines:

- Blue lights and hazard warning lights should be left ON, unless the scene has been secured and a major incident has been declared.
- Ensure hi-vis PPE is worn and a helmet to provide protection from debris and during any extrication.
- Approach from the rear of the incident, if possible, at low speed.
- Identify hazards, consider parking position and identify a safe area of work.

Major, Complex and High-Risk Incidents

- Request police/Highways England if not already present.
- Follow the flow of traffic unless directed otherwise by police or Highways England.
- Do not stop on the non-incident carriageway to gain access to an incident on the opposite side, irrespective of how urgent the situation appears on the affected carriageway or of the distance to the next junction or crossing point.
- In multiple vehicle collisions, it may be necessary to sectorise the scene to promote understanding and aid communication.

Actions on arrival:

- Ensure the road is closed or restricted.
- The first vehicle should park before the incident and additional vehicles should park beyond it, creating a boundary for a safe working area (except on motorways, where all vehicles should park beyond the incident in the obstructed lane).
- Exit the vehicle on the side away from moving traffic.
- Liaise with police, Highways England and the FRS.
- Ascertain the number and location of casualties trapped or injured and report to the control room.
- Ensure an operational commander is appointed to coordinate ambulance resources, and stand back to liaise with other agencies.
- Prioritise extrication and request further resources if required (i.e. HART for additional equipment and capabilities).
- Establish an inner and outer cordon around the scene of operations, if appropriate.
- Keep the working area clear by creating an equipment dump.
- Treat all non-activated SRS devices as live; high-voltage electrical systems should all be treated as live even when the engine is not running.
- Fires in an LPG-powered car will be treated by the FRS as a cylinder incident.

Table 6.9 is used by Agencies to help inform lane closures.

TABLE 6.9 – Lane Closures for Road Incidents

Incident location	Lane closures required
Two-way local roadway	Both lanes
Hard shoulder of the motorway or similar	Hard shoulder and lane 1
Lane 1 of a 3-lane roadway	Hard shoulder, lane 1 and lane 2
Lane 2 of a 3-lane roadway	Lanes 1, 2 and 3
Lane 3 of a 3-lane roadway	Lanes 2 and 3
Across the central reservation	Lanes 2 and 3 of both carriageways

Leaving the incident:

- Do not move any vehicles, especially those providing the fend-off protection before consulting with other emergency services.
- Maintain high visibility when moving away from the incident and re-joining traffic flows. Use warning lights until clear of the incident.

'All lane running':

- Some sections of the motorway may be utilised for 'all- lane running' (Figure 6.14). On these sections, the hard shoulder area may be used for live traffic at certain times. Lanes are then described as 1–4.

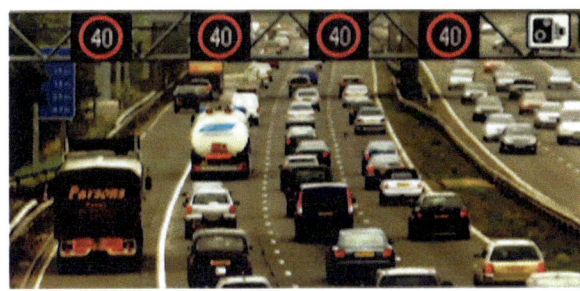

Figure 6.14 — All-lane running.

Bibliography

1. Public Health England. *Chemical, Biological, Radiological and Nuclear Incidents: Recognise and respond*. 2018. Available from: https://www.gov.uk/government/publications/chemical-biological-radiological-and-nuclear-incidents-recognise-and-respond.
2. NHS England. *Clinical guidelines for major incidents and mass casualty events*. 2018. Available from: https://www.england.nhs.uk/publication/clinical-guidelines-for-major-incidents-and-mass-casualty-events/.
3. National Ambulance Resilience Unit. *Compliance & Quality Assurance: National Provisions for Interoperable Capabilities*. 2018. Available from: http://naru.org.uk.

Police Incapacitants

1. Introduction

- The deployment of police incapacitants on individuals and/or groups can lead to conditions requiring pre-hospital care.
- The aim of this guideline is to support clinical decision making for the management of patients following the deployment of:
  - Conducted Energy Devices (CED) previously termed Conducted Electrical Weapons (CEW). Predominantly in the UK, TASER™ products.
  - Irritant Sprays, previously termed incapacitant sprays, i.e. CS/PAVA.
  - Attenuating Energy Projectiles (AEP).
  - Batons.
- Not all patients exposed to police incapacitants will require hospital assessment; however, all patients should undergo a primary survey.
- Carry out a dynamic risk assessment; continually re-assess throughout the incident.

2. Conducted Energy Devices (CED)

CEDs are battery-operated hand-held devices which deliver up to 50,000 volts of electricity at low energy levels (0.1 J), in rapid pulses (~ 5 seconds), via two barbed electrodes. There are three variants of CED produced by TASER™ authorised for use by police forces within the UK. These are TASER™ X2, X26 and T7: the barb design varies according to type (refer to Figure 6.15).

- The barbs are designed to stick into skin or clothes and connect to the device by fine long copper wires, or via two probes directly applied to the skin or clothes.
- Firing the device results in pain and a transient loss of voluntary control of muscles, often causing the patient to fall. These devices are currently in use by all police forces in the United Kingdom.
- Before touching the patient, ensure the wires are disconnected from the device; the wires break easily by cutting with scissors.

There is an increased risk of combustion if a CED is deployed after the deployment of incapacitant sprays or following contact with flammable liquids such as petrol.

Assessment and management

- Most people incapacitated with a CED do not require hospital assessment; however, patients should undergo a primary survey especially assessing for the presence of:
  - Neck and back injuries. (Spinal fractures from muscle contraction have been described elsewhere.)
  - Secondary injuries as a result of the fall.
  - Cardiac symptoms.
  - Acute behavioural disturbance (ABD).
  - Attached electrodes.
- Death and severe injuries are rare, with most injuries associated with falling or probe penetration. Immediate cardiac dysrhythmia is very rare. Occasional cases of stroke, seizure and rhabdomyolysis have been reported.
- For the assessment and management of symptoms, conditions and injuries following deployment of CED, refer to Table 6.10.

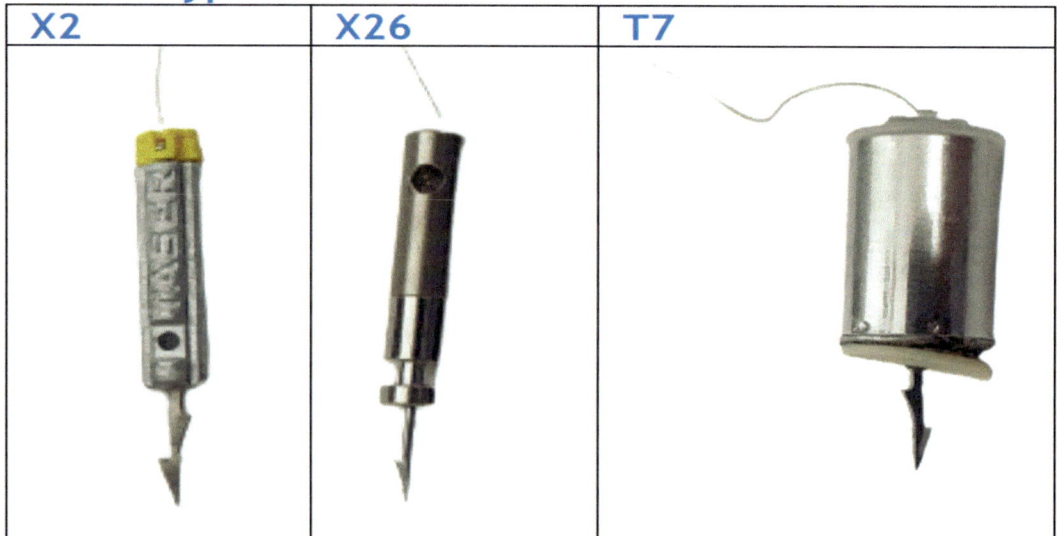

Figure 6.15 – CED (TASER™) barb types. Reproduced with permission from the Faculty of Forensic & Legal Medicines and the FFLM CED Hub https://fflm.ac.uk/cedhub.

Police Incapacitants

TABLE 6.10 – ASSESSMENT and MANAGEMENT: Following the Deployment of a CED

PRIMARY EFFECTS

Pain

Refer to **Pain Management in Adults and Children**.

Electrode Removal

The electrodes vary in length and have a 'fish hook'-type end which is designed to stick to clothes and into the skin. **NB** Although the lengths of the barbs may vary, the management principles remain the same.

Probes very rarely penetrate beyond the dermis.

Electrode removal for Taser™ X2 & X26:

(For removal of the Taser™ T7, a cartridge safety clip is designed to aid removal. This is carried by police officers deploying the device along with instructions into use).

- Slightly stretch the skin around the electrode and pull sharply on the electrode. This usually only causes slight discomfort.
- The electrode is a biohazard and should be placed in a sealed container and may often be retained by the police for evidence. It can be disposed of as clinical waste if directed by the police.
- Clean the area.
- Cover the site with an adhesive dressing.
- Advise tetanus booster within 72 hours if not covered for tetanus. Antibiotics are not routinely required unless the patient is immunocompromised.

NB If the electrode cannot be removed at the first attempt or breaks during attempted removal, leave in situ and transfer to definitive care.

DO NOT attempt to remove the electrodes if they are:

- Attached to skin where blood vessels are close to the skin surface (e.g. neck and groin).
- Attached to one or both eye(s).
- Attached to the face.
- Attached to the genitalia.
- Attached to the mouth or throat or if the electrode has been swallowed.
- Firmly embedded in the scalp.
- Embedded in a joint (e.g. finger).
- Broken.

In these circumstances, cut the wire close to the electrode, leaving approximately 4 cm attached to the electrode, and transfer to definitive care.

Burns

- Superficial burns are likely around the area where the electrode attached to the skin and electricity was delivered.
- Burns may also occur if a CED is deployed after the deployment of incapacitant sprays or following contact with flammable liquids such as petrol.
- Refer to **Pain Management in Adults and Children** and **Burns and Scalds**.

Cardiac Conditions/Symptoms

- Cardiac conditions have been reported following the deployment of a CED, including increases in heart rate, cardiac arrhythmia and sudden cardiac death and cardiac arrest.
- ECGs are not needed for all patients. However, always undertake a 12-lead ECG and monitor blood pressure and oxygen saturation for patients:
  - Complaining of chest pain.
  - With cardiac symptoms (e.g. tachycardia, bradycardia).
  - With significant cardiac history (e.g. angina, arrhythmias or a myocardial infarction).
  - Fitted with pacemakers or cardioverter defibrillator. These patients should be transferred to definitive care for assessment.
- Cardiac arrhythmia: (refer to **Cardiac Arrhythmia and Sudden Cardiac Death** for specific guidance).
- Cardiac arrest: (refer to the appropriate **Resuscitation** guidelines).

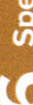

(continued)

Police Incapacitants

TABLE 6.10 – ASSESSMENT and MANAGEMENT: Following the Deployment of a CED *(continued)*

PRIMARY EFFECTS

Convulsions
- The deployment of a CED may elicit a convulsion or epileptic fit, though this is very rare.
- For specific guidance, refer to **Seizures in Adults** and **Seizures in Children**.

Obstetric and Gynaecological Conditions
- Spontaneous miscarriage has been reported following the deployment of CED.
- Refer to the appropriate **Maternity Care** guidelines.
- Any patient who is known to be pregnant and has been subject to CED discharge should be transferred to definitive care for assessment.

Soft Tissue Injury/Injuries
(Contusions, tendon damage, abrasions, dislocations, lacerations, puncture wounds)
- Abrasions, lacerations and puncture wounds:
  - Clean the area with an alcohol/antiseptic wipe.
  - Cover the site with an adhesive dressing.
  - Advise tetanus booster within 72 hours if not covered for tetanus.
- Contusions, damage to ligament and tendons: These injuries should be managed accordingly and transferred to definitive care.
- Puncture wounds around highly vascular areas should be assessed for significant pain, swelling or haematoma. If present, these patients should be transferred to definitive care for assessment.
- Puncture wounds around the neck and chest should be assessed for signs of subcutaneous emphysema. If present, these patients should be transferred to definitive care for assessment.

Head Injury
- Head injuries and loss of consciousness may also result from intracranial penetration of an electrode.
- For specific guidance, refer to **Head Injury** and **Altered Level of Consciousness**.

SECONDARY EFFECTS

Head, Neck and Back Injuries, Contusions, Abrasions and Lacerations
- The powerful muscular contractions caused by the deployment of a CED may result invertebral fractures, usually thoracolumbar.
- The loss of voluntary control of the muscles caused by the deployment of a CED may result in falls, leading to injuries of the head, neck and back, contusions, abrasions, lacerations, ligament and tendon injury, etc.
- For specific guidance, refer to **Head Injury** and **Spinal and Spinal Cord Injury**.

Contusions, abrasions, lacerations, ligament and tendon injury: Manage as per soft tissue injuries above.

COINCIDENTAL EFFECTS

Injuries and Conditions Unrelated to CED Deployment
- Injuries and/or conditions may be sustained or develop that are unrelated to the deployment of a CED, for example as the result of a physical struggle, the consumption of drugs or physical exhaustion.
- Assess and manage coincidental injuries as per condition, cognisant of the effects of drugs, dehydration or exhaustion.

Acute Behavioural Disturbance (ABD)
- A CED may be deployed on people in patients suffering from acute behavioural disturbance (ABD). People in this state may be at a greater risk of collapse, arrhythmias and sudden death. This may be unrelated to deployment of a CED – undertake a **TIME-CRITICAL** transfer and provide an alert/information call.
- For specific guidance, refer to **Acute Behavioural Disturbance**.

Police Incapacitants

3. Irritant Sprays

- Irritant sprays (Peripheral Chemosensory Irritants (PCSIs)) used within UK police forces include:
  - PAVA 'Pepper spray' (oleoresin, capsicum, pelargonic acid, vanillylamide). These are synthetic variants of capsicum products and dissolved in glycol, ethanol and water.
  - CS spray 2-chlorobenzalmalononitrile (O-chlorobenzylidene malononitrile). CS is solid at room temperature and dissolved in methyl isobutyl ketone (MIBK) as a solvent. When the solvent evaporates, the CS particles give their effect.

They have similar actions and the broad principles of management are the same. Severe injury, disability and death are very rare.

Actions

- The sprays cause irritation (burning sensation) when in contact with exposed skin and mucus membranes including eye, nose and mouth and respiratory tract, causing lacrimation (tearing), rhinorrhoea (runny nose), sialorrhoea (drooling), disorientation, dizziness, breathing difficulties, coughing and vomiting.
- The effects are usually short-lived (under 30 minutes), but some can persist for up to 2–6 hours.

Management

- Avoid entering a contaminated or closed environment.
- Avoid exposure to contaminated clothing.
- Wear gloves, apron and eye protection.
- Any irrigation may exacerbate symptoms transiently, and cool saline or water must be used to reduce risk of reactivating the irritant product.

Assessment and management

- Most people exposed to incapacitant sprays do not require hospital assessment.
- For the assessment and management of symptoms and conditions following deployment of incapacitant sprays, refer to Table 6.11.

TABLE 6.11 – ASSESSMENT and MANAGEMENT: Following the Deployment of Incapacitant Sprays

General Symptoms

Lacrimation, rhinorrhoea, sialorrhoea, dizziness, coughing and vomiting.

- Move the patient away from the source of the contamination.
- Expose to fresh air. This can be augmented by fanning.
- Remove contaminated clothing and place into sealed bags to prevent secondary exposure to patient or others.
- Reassure that effects will decrease rapidly after initial exposure.
- For patients with heavy contamination of the skin and eyes, irrigate with tap water.
- If skin symptoms persist for longer than 20 minutes, transfer to further care and consider irrigation with cool tap water.

Eye Symptoms

Lacrimation, blurred vision, stinging eyes, photophobia, blepharospasm, periorbital oedema, corneal injury.

Symptoms will usually resolve within 15–30 minutes.

- Move the patient away from the source of the contamination.
- Expose to fresh air. This can be augmented by fanning.
- Reassure that effects will decrease rapidly after initial exposure.
- Advise the patient not to rub their eyes for 2–3 hours.
- Encourage patient to remove any contact lenses.
- If the patient cannot open their eyes after 30 minutes, transfer to definitive care for assessment.
- If symptoms persist for longer than 60 minutes, consider irrigation with tepid sterile saline.

(continued)

Police Incapacitants

> **TABLE 6.11** – ASSESSMENT and MANAGEMENT: Following the Deployment of Incapacitant Sprays *(continued)*
>
> **Breathing Difficulties**
>
> Shortness of breath and coughing are common and are usually self-limiting.
>
> Bronchospasm and laryngospasm are rare.
>
> - For specific guidance refer to **Dyspnoea**.
> - The majority of symptoms should settle within 15–30 minutes.
> - Those with pre-existing respiratory disease, such as asthma and COPD, are at increased risk of more severe effects.

4. Attenuating Energy Projectiles (AEP)

- Projectiles such as plastic bullets, rubber bullets or bean bags can cause sudden death (after strikes to the head, chest or abdomen), dislocations, fractures, joint damage, ligament and tendon damage, haemorrhage and haematoma, compartment syndrome, blunt intra-abdominal injury (splenic rupture, subcapsular liver/haematoma), blunt thoracic cavity injury (pneumothorax/haemothorax) and penetrating injuries to thorax, abdomen, eye, arm, leg and blood vessels.
- A sudden, single-blow blunt trauma to the front of the chest may on rare occasions lead to cardiac arrest due to the rhythm disturbance; this is the opposite of a pre-cordial thump for witnessed cardiac arrest. Refer to **Resuscitation** guidelines.
- Within police forces in the UK, the most common AEP is a soft-nosed 37 mm projectile. The nose cap has a hollow void to minimise the peak force, with the aim to deliver a high amount of kinetic energy while reducing the potential for life-threatening injury. The use is strictly regulated and restricted to accredited officers (Authorised Firearms Officers and Public Order Officers), and the training states the target area should be below the waist to minimise risk of injury to head, chest and abdomen.

5. Batons

- Baton strikes can cause:
  - dislocations
  - fractures
  - joint, ligament and tendon damage
  - haemorrhage and haematoma
  - compartment syndrome
  - death.
- Baton strikes to limbs will typically cause 'tramline bruising'; this is of no significant concern unless there is evidence of underlying fracture or neuromuscular condition.
- 'Police use of force' guidance within the UK advocates baton strikes avoiding head, neck, chest and groin to minimise the risk of serious and life-threatening injuries.

> **KEY POINTS!**
>
> **Police Incapacitants**
>
> - **Ensure the wires are disconnected from the CED before touching the patient.**
> - **DO NOT remove electrodes in any of the instances listed in Table 6.10.**
> - **Patients may also sustain secondary injuries (e.g. head injuries and fractures following a fall).**
> - **Transfer to definitive care any patient with one or more of the following: cardiac symptoms, neck and back injuries and ABD.**
> - **The symptoms of patients exposed to irritant sprays should settle after exposure to air. If symptoms persist after 20–30 minutes, transfer to definitive care.**

Index

ABBEY pain scale, 66
abdominal aortic aneurysms (AAAs), 195
abdominal pain, 194–203
    assessment and management, 200–202
    causes and symptoms, 194, 195–199
abdominal trauma, 518–520
    assessment and management, 518–520
abuse
    adult, 83–84
    children, 88–90
    mental health, 392–394
acute behavioural disturbance (ABD), 205–213
    assessment and management, 207, 208–211
    definition of, 205
    signs and symptoms, 207
acute cholecystitis, 195–199
acute coronary syndrome (ACS), 214–219
    algorithm, 219
    assessment and management, 215–218
acute heart failure (AHF), 325, 328–329
    dyspnoea, 287–289
acute hypothermia, 345
acute limb ischaemia, 491–493
acute pancreatitis, 195–199
acute pulmonary oedema, 325
acute stroke, 477–478
adrenal crisis, 51, 222
adrenal insufficiency, 221–225
    assessment and management, 223–224
Advance Decision to Refuse Treatment (ADRT), 30, 62, 162
    for left ventricular assist devices, 371
advanced life support, 115–133
    in adults, 115–117
    airway and breathing management, 121–124, 125
    assessment and management, 115
        airway sizes, 121, 123–124
        bag-mask ventilation, 121
        capnography, 122, 123
        supraglottic airways, 121–122
        tracheal intubation, 122
    in children, 117
    defibrillation, 117–121
    mechanical chest compression devices, 124
    reversible causes and specialist circumstances, 126–130
    trauma, 130–133
aggression, mental health, 392–394
agitation, 39, 205, 226–229
    assessment, 226–227
    causes, 226
    head injury and, 552–553
    level of, 226–227
    management, 228
    mental health, 392–394
agonal breathing, 134
agonal rhythm, 166
airway burns, 512, 522
alcohol withdrawal, 232
    seizures and, 439
alcoholic cirrhosis, 302
alcoholic ketoacidosis, 231–232
alcohol-related brain injury, 403
alcohol-related pancreatitis, 231
alcohol-use disorders, 231–234
    assessment and management, 232, 233–234
allergic reactions including anaphylaxis, 236–242
    assessment, 241–242
    management, 238, 241–242
    signs and symptoms, 237
    triggers, 242
altered level of consciousness (ALoC), 243–250
    altered metabolic states, 244

    Glasgow Coma Scale, 249
analgesia, 64–72
anaphylaxis
    asthma in adults and children, 251
    dyspnoea, 287–289
angioedema, 237
anti-fibrinolytic drug, 629
antipyretics, 300
aortic aneurysm, 484–487
aortic dissection, 487, 489–491
arteriovenous fistula haemorrhage, 495–496, 497
asthma
    acute exacerbation, dyspnoea, 287–289
    in adults and children, 251–257
        assessment and management, 252, 253, 254–256, 257
        features of severity, 252
        risk factors, 251
    cardiac arrest and, 129
asylum-seeking children, safeguarding, 94
ATMIST format, 501
    acute behavioural disturbance, 210
    cardiac arrest, 114
atrial fibrillation, 267–270
    falls and, 541
atrial flutter, 267–270
atropine, 666–668
    cardiac arrest, 113
autism, 4
Autistic SPACE, 4–5
autonomic dysreflexia, 11
AVPU scale, 513

bacterial meningitis, 298–299
bag-mask ventilation (BVM), 121
bariatric patients, advanced life support for, 130
basal skull fracture, 551
basic life support (BLS)
    in adult, 134–136
        assessment and management, 134–135
    in children, 137–141
behavioural emergencies, 258–261
    assessment and management, 258, 259–261
behaviours, managing, 46
bilateral tonic-clonic seizures (BTCS), 437–438
biliary colic, 195–199
bimanual compression, 630
blast injury, 518, 587
blood glucose monitors, 306
blood ketone meters, 306, 307
blunt trauma, 518
    cardiac arrest and, 132
    to trunk or limbs, 48
bone fractures, 92
bradycardia, 262
    assessment and management, 262–263, 264
    medical emergencies in children, 188
breaking bad news, 167
breathlessness
    non-pharmacological management of, 38
    oxygen administration, 37
    pharmacological management of, 38
breech birth, 601–605
Brøset Checklist, 227
Brugada syndrome, 265
Buchanan bibs, 146–148
burns and scalds, 93, 522–526
    assessment and management, 523–525
    Lund and Browder chart, 525
    Wallace's Rule of Nines, 525

Index

capacity, defined, 56
capnography, 122, 123
cardiac arrest
    after drowning event, 529
    ambulance services response, 113–114
    chain of survival, 110
    drug therapy, 113
    due to anaphylaxis, 238
    hanging and, 509
    human factors in, team resource management, 110–111
    implantable cardioverter defibrillator for, 352
    intravascular fluid therapy in children, 55
    maternal resuscitation, 632–636
    modifications for, in pregnancy, 635
    out-of-hospital, 110–114
    in pregnancy, 635, 636
cardiac arrhythmia, 262–270
    acute myocardial ischaemia or infarction, 262
    arrhythmias table, 267–270
    bradycardia, 262
    sudden cardiac death, 265
    tachycardia, 263
cardiac rhythm management, 369
cardiac tamponade, 128, 586
cardiogenic shock, 325
cardiomyopathies, 267
cardiopulmonary resuscitation (CPR)
    checklist use, 113
    clinical handover, 114
    end of life care and, 35
cardiovascular disease (CVD), 484
catastrophic haemorrhage
    in adult, 508
    in children, 511, 515
cauda equina syndrome (CES), 11–12, 357, 574–575
cerebral palsy, 12
cervical spondylotic myelopathy (CSM), 357
chemical biological radiological nuclear (CBRN) incidents, 130, 669–676
    atropine, 673
    casualty assessment tool, 669, 671
chemical burns, 522
chest compressions, 369–370
child sexual exploitation/abuse (CSE/CSA), 88–90
childhood stroke, 479
chronic hypothermia, 345
chronic obstructive pulmonary disease (COPD), 271–276
    assessment and management, 272–274, 275
    signs and symptoms, 271
clinical decision making, 45–46
Clinical Frailty Scale (CFS), 176–177, 504, 540, 541
cluster headaches, 321–322
cognitive impairment, pain scales for, 66
communication, 45
    dementia and, 403–404
    difficulties, 79–81
    mental health, 396
community management
    for abdominal pain, 202
congestive cardiac failure (CCF), 325
consent
    domestic abuse, 23–24
    inability to, 77
    maternity care, 591
    patient confidentiality, 76–77
    in pre-hospital care, 22
    public interest and, 77
    to sharing sexual orientation with other health professionals, 6
constipation, 195–199
continuous glucose monitors (CGMs), 306
continuous positive pressure ventilation (CPAP), 331
Conveyance Decision Tool, 554–555
convulsive status epilepticus, 450
cord prolapse, 613–615
coronary thrombosis, 128
corticosteroids, 221
CPR-induced consciousness, 126
CRB-65 score, 292
croup, children, 431–433
    assessment, 432
    management, 432
    referral pathway, 432–433
crowning, 617
crush injury, 562
crush syndrome, 48, 562

Data Protection Act 2018, 74
de novo heart failure, 326
death
    action to be taken after, 166
    after medicine administration, 42
    during major incident, 166
    maternal, 632
de-cannulation, 146–148
decapitation
    in adult, 160
    in children, 169
decomposition/putrefaction
    in adults, 160
    in children, 169
de-escalation techniques, 397
defibrillation, 117–121
dehydration
    examination, 420
    symptoms and signs, 421
delirium, 39, 205, 277–283
    assessment and management, 280–282
    causes, 279
    referral and decision making, 283
    signs and symptoms, 278–279
delirium tremens, 232
dementia, 278, 402–404
depression, 278
    staff health and wellbeing, 106
diabetes insipidus, 12–13
diabetic foot problem, 493–495
diabetic ketoacidosis (DKA), 315–316
    assessment and management, 317
    risk factors for, 316
    risk levels, 307
    signs and symptoms of, 316
diabulimia, 318
diarrhoea, bloody, 419
diazepam
    seizures in adults, 447
    seizures in children, 451
direct death, 632
direct discrimination, 2–3
disability, 3–5
    children, 94
discriminatory abuse, 83–84
disproportionate tachycardia, 298
diverticular disease, 195–199, 303
do not attempt cardiopulmonary resuscitation (DNACPR), 163, 371
domestic abuse, 23–26
    assessment and management, 24–25
domestic violence, 83–84
driving
    diabetes and, 309
    seizures and, 439

Index

drowning, 528–532
    discharge on scene, 532
    submerged person tool, 531
dual sequential defibrillation, 120
DuoDote®, 670
    dosages, 672
duty of care, 27–29, 679
dyspnoea, 285–293
    assessment and management, 287, 290–292

early onset neonatal sepsis, 609–610
eating disorders, 405
eclampsia, 645–648
ectopic pregnancy, 195–199, 657–658
electrical injuries, 522, 534–537
    assessment and management, 534–535, 536
electro-convulsive therapy (ECT), 385
electronic health information, 74
emergency tracheostomy and laryngectomy pre-hospital management, 142–150
    assessment and management, 143, 144, 145
en caul birth, 623–624
end of life care, 30–43
Entonox, 70–72, 623
epiglottitis, 13
    dyspnoea, 287–289
Epilepsy Passport, 450
Equality Act 2010, 2
Escherichia coli 0157:H7 infection, 419
exertional heat stroke, 333
exhaustion hypothermia, 345
expected deaths, 166, 170, 173
external pacing, 120–121
Extra-corporeal membrane oxygenation (ECMO), 126
extremely preterm birth, 609, 621–622

factor V Leiden, 13–14
falls in older adults, 538–548
    assessment and management, 540–543, 545–548
FAST test, for stroke/TIA, 479
febrile convulsions, 301
febrile illness in children, 294–301
    assessment, 295–296
    red flags, 300
febrile seizures, 450
female genital mutilation (FGM), 597–599
    mandatory reporting
        in adults, 85
        in children, 96
fenestrated tracheostomy tube, 146–148
fentanyl, 70–72
financial/material abuse, 83–84
fire service, disclosure of information, 76
1st degree AV nodal block, 267–270
FLACC Scale, 64, 65
flail chest, 583–584
flange, 146–148
flash glucose monitoring, 306
foetal maceration, in newborn, 169
foreign body airway obstruction (FBAO), 151–155
    in adults, 154
    assessment and management, 152
    in children, 154
4AT screening tool, 280–281
fractures, 92, 559
    abuse, 92
    basal skull, 551
    bone, 92
    closed, 559
    neck of femur/hip, 560
    open, 551, 559
    splinting, 561
    types of, 92
    vertebral insufficiency, 357
freebirth, 622–623
functional/dissociative seizures, 437–439

gasping, 112–113
gastritis, 195–199, 302
gastrointestinal bleeding, 232
gastrointestinal (GI) bleeding, 302–305
    assessment and management, 303–304
gender, 5–7
    related conditions, 5
    sexuality and, 8
Glasgow Coma Scale, 249, 506, 516–517, 550–551
    in adults, 183
    in children, 192
glucocorticoid steroid-dependent patients, 221–222
glycaemic emergencies, in adults and children, 306–318
    considerations for patients with diabetes, 306–309
    mental health and, 318
    sick-day rules, 307–308
Gold Standard Framework, 34
Greenstick fracture, 92
Guillain-Barre syndrome, 14
gunshot wounds, 518

haematemesis, 302
haemophilia, 14–15
haemostasis, 47
hanging, 509
harmful drinking, 231
head injury, 49, 550–556
    assessment, 550–551, 556
    in older person, 553
    spinal injury and spinal cord injury, 576
    traumatic brain injury, 553–554
headache, 320–324
    assessment and management, 322–323
    cluster, 321–322
    medication-overuse, 321
    migraine, 320–321
    signs and symptoms, 320
head-up CPR, 124
health inequality, 2
heart failure, 325–332
    assessment and management, 326–330
    signs and symptoms, 327
Heartmate 3, 366
heat exhaustion, 333
heat illness, 401
heat related illness, 333–336
    assessment and management, 335–336
    medications predisposing to, 334
hemicorporectomy
    in adults, 160
    in children, 169
hepatic encephalopathy, 232
hepatitis, 195–199
herpes simplex encephalitis, 298
high risk pregnancy, 616–617
HOT checklist, 132
human factors, 45–46
hyperactive delirium, 278
hypercalcaemia, 32
hyperglycaemia, 313–315
    signs and symptoms of, 316
hyperkalaemia, 126–127
hyperosmolar hyperglycaemic state (HHS), 317–318
hyperthermia, 127–128
hyperventilation syndrome, 338–343

Index

assessment and management, 342
    signs and symptoms, 339
hypoactive delirium, 278
hypoglycaemia, 309–313
    agitation and, 227
    assessment and management, 311–312
    signs and symptoms, 311
hypokalaemia, 126–127
hypostasis
    in adults, 160
    in children, 169
hypothermia, 127, 345–348
    assessment and management, 346–348
    risk factors, 345
hypovolaemia, 126
    LVAD, 370–371
hypovolaemic shock, 54–55
hypoxia, 126
    agitation and, 227

iatrogenic harm, 392–394
ibuprofen, 70–72, 361
immersion, definition of, 528
immersion hypothermia, 345
imminent birth, 601, 616–627
    assessment, 616
    management of, 618, 626
    signs of, 617–618
immobilisation
    cautions/precautions, 575
    of children, 577
    hazards of, 576
    sequence for, 576–577
    for spinal injury, 575–577, 579
    for trauma emergencies in adults, 506
implantable cardioverter defibrillator (ICD), 350–354
    algorithm, 355
    assessment and management, 351, 353–354
incineration
    in adults, 160
    in children, 169
Independent Mental Capacity Advocates (IMCAs), 62
indirect death, 632
indirect discrimination, 3
infant feeding, 620
infection, low back pain and, 357
inflammatory bowel disease, 195–199, 303
inhaled foreign body, 251
inner cannula, 146–148
insulin pumps, 308
intentional poisoning, 412
intestinal obstruction, 195–199
intracerebral haemorrhage (ICH), 478–479
intramuscular administration, site of injection, 40
intravascular fluid therapy
    in adults, 47–52
    in children, 54–55
    for drowning, 530
    for sepsis, 467
ischaemia, in limb trauma, 560
ischaemic bowel, 195–199
ischaemic limbs, 491–493

Kawasaki disease, 16, 298
ketamine, 70–72, 72
knee dislocation, 561
'knee-rolling' exercise, 362, 363
Korsakoff's syndrome, 403

labour, third stage of, 619–620
laryngectomy, 142, 146–148

lasting power of attorney (LPA), 30, 62, 163
leadership skills, 45
learning disability, 4, 79
left bundle branch block (LBBB), 216, 267–270
left ventricular assist devices (LVADs), 365–376
    assessment of, 366, 367
    implantation centres, 376
left ventricular failure (LVF), 325–326
left ventricular systolic dysfunction (LVSD), 325
limb crush injuries, 48
limb threatening injuries, 560–561
limb trauma, 559–567
    assessment and management, 562–567
local anaesthetic blocks, 72
local authorities, disclosure of information, 76
long bone fractures, 513
'long lie,' 540
long QT syndrome, 265–267
low back pain (non-traumatic), 356–363
    assessment and management, 358–360
low BMI, young adults with, fluid therapy for, 51
lower lobe pneumonia, 195–199
lung pump theory, 111

magnesium sulfate, 645
major, complex and high-risk incidents, 677–691
Mallory-Weiss tears, 302
Marfan syndrome, 16
massive cranial and cerebral destruction
    in adult, 160
    in children, 169
massive pulmonary emboli, 425
maternal collapse, 634
maternal death, 632
maternal resuscitation, 632–636
    assessment and management, 636
maternity care (including obstetric emergencies overview), 590–599
    appropriate destination for conveyance, 592
    assessment, 592–594
    at-risk ethnic groups, 596
    concealment, denial and unknown pregnancy, 597
    female genital mutilation, 597–599
    maternal deaths, 596–597
    prehospital maternity decision tool, 594, 595
maternity safeguarding, 95–96
mean arterial pressure, 550
mechanical chest compression devices (mCPR), 124
mechanical restraint, 399
medical emergencies
    in adults, 175–184
        assessment and management, 177–181
        clinical frailty scale, 175
        Glasgow Coma Scale, 183
    in children, 185–193
        assessment and management, 186–191
        modified Glasgow Coma Scale, 192
medical transitioning, 6
MedicAlert® type jewellery, 176
medication-overuse headaches, 321
Medtronic Inc. HVAD, 372
meningitis, 298
meningococcal disease, signs and symptoms, 298–299
meningococcal meningitis and septicaemia, 379–383
    assessment and management, 379–382, 383
    febrile illness, 298
    risk of infection to ambulance personnel, 382
mental capacity, 56, 395
    agitation and, 227
    alcohol-use disorders, 233
    dementia and, 403

Index

Mental Capacity Act 2005, 56–62
mental health
    diabetes and, 318
    equality in, 387–388
    heat illness in, 401
    sepsis, 461
Mental Health Act, 386
    conveyance under, 387
    provisions, 387
mental health presentation, 385–408
    algorithm, 406
    assessment, 388–395
    management, 396
Mental Health Services, 385
Mental State Examination, 389–391
metaphyseal fracture, 92
metastatic spinal cord compression (MSCC), 20–21
    end of life care, 31
    low back pain and, 357
METHANE model, 677, 678
methoxyflurane, 70–72, 271
midazolam
    seizures in adults, 447
    seizures in children, 451, 453
    in traumatic brain injury, 553, 553–554
migraine, 320–321
miscarriage, 657
Modified Glasgow Coma Scale, 517
monomorphic ventricular tachycardia, 267–270
morphine, 37, 70–72, 331
    for heart failure, 331
motor neurone disease, 16–18
mucus plug, 146–148
Multi-Agency Public Protection Arrangements (MAPPAs), 94
multiple sclerosis, 18
multiple small pulmonary emboli, 425
muscular dystrophy, 19
muscular paralysis, electrical injuries, 534
musculoskeletal pain, 356–357
myasthenia gravis, 19–20
myocardial dysfunction, 156
myocardial ischaemia, pain and, 409

naloxone
    in end of life care, 41–42
    in opioid overdose, 129
National Early Warning Score (NEWS2), 80, 462–463
neglect, 392–394
    adults, 83–84
    children, 88–90
neonatal jaundice, 608
neurodiversity, 4
neurological compromise, 192
neutropenic sepsis, 32, 458–459
new dyspnoea, 326
newborn
    care of, 607–612
        assessment and management, 610–611
    life support, 638–644
        algorithm, 642
        assessment and management, 638–642
non-accidental poisoning, 412
non-accidental/deliberate injury, 90
non-binary, 6, 8
non-exertional heat stroke, 333
non-fatal strangulation, 99–101
non-haemorrhagic emergencies, 49–51
non-mobile (non-independent) babies, safeguarding, 91–92
non-traumatic chest pain/discomfort, 409–411
    aneurysm-type pain, 409
    assessment and management, 409–411

indigestion-type pain, 409
muscular-type pain, 409
pleuritic-type pain, 409
Numeric Pain Rating Scale, 65

oblique fracture, 92
oesophageal varices, 302
oesophagitis, 303
older adults
    falls in, 538–548
    head injuries in, 553
    mental health, 395
older children, safeguarding, 93
open fractures, 551
opioid
    in end of life care, 42
    overdose, 41, 129
oral analgesia, 69
oral tranquilisation, 228
organ perfusion, impaired, 48
orthopnoea, 326
outer cannula, 146–148
out-of-hospital cardiac arrest, 110–114
    ambulance services response, 113–114
    chain of survival, 110
    drug therapy, 113
    human factors in, team resource management, 110–111
overdose and poisoning, in adults and children, 412–417
    assessment and management, 413–416, 417
oxygen saturation, in sepsis, 460–461
oxygen therapy, for sepsis, 467
oxygen transport, 47

pacemakers, 120–121
paediatric gastroenteritis, 419–424
    assessment, 419–420, 423
    management, 422
    red flag symptoms, 422
pain
    agitation and, 227
    assessment of, 35, 36, 63, 63–64
    at end of life, 35
    head injury and, 552–553
    non-pharmacological management of, 36, 67
    pharmacological management of, 36, 68
pain management
    in adults and children, 63–72
    pain scales, 64, 65
PAINAD pain scale, 67
paracetamol, 37
    for pain, 70–72
    for sepsis, 468
parenteral analgesia, 69–70
Parkinson's disease, 20
paroxysmal nocturnal dyspnoea (PND), 326
patient confidentiality, 74–77
    anonymisation of information, 75
    best practice, 75
    consent, 76–77
    Data Protection Act 2018, 74
    disclosure of information, 75–76
    electronic information, 74
    information-sharing policy, 75
    NHS Policy, 74
    patient identifiable information, 74–75
    patients' rights of access to personal health records, 75
    protection of patient information, 74
peak expiratory flow rate (PEFR), 253, 254
peer-on-peer exploitation, 88–90
pelvic inflammatory disease, 195–199
pelvic ring disruptions, 569

Index

pelvic trauma, 569–572
    assessment and management, 569–571
penetrating trauma, 518
    cardiac arrest and, 132
    to limbs, 48
    to trunk, 48
peptic ulcer, 195–199, 302
perinatal hypoxia, 607
peripheral vein thrombosis, 425
peritonitis, 195–199
personal protective equipment (PPE), 130
physical abuse
    adults, 83–84
    children, 88–90
physical restraint
    in acute behavioural disturbance, 208–210
    mental health presentations, 399
PINCH ME mnemonic, 279–280
placenta praevia, 660
placental abruption, 660
pleural effusion, dyspnoea and, 287–289
pneumonia, 299, 434
    community acquired, CRB-65 score for, 292
    dyspnoea, 288
    febrile illness in children, 298
    severity assessment, 434
pneumothorax, 287–289
police
    acute behavioural disturbance in, 212
    disclosure of information, 75–76
    report abuse to, 91
police incapacitants, 692–696
    assessment and management, 692
polymorphic ventricular tachycardia, 267–270
post-partum haemorrhage (PPH), 628–631
    bimanual compression, 630
    management, 628, 629–630
post-traumatic stress disorder (PTSD), 106
postural hypotension, falls and, 541–542
predominant peripheral oedema, with/without pulmonary oedema, 325
pre-eclampsia, 645–648
    assessment, 645
    definitions, 645
    management, 645–647, 648
pre-existing hypertensive disease, 47–48
pregnancy
    cardiac arrest and, 129
    electrical injuries, 534
    mental health, 404–405
    multiple, 623
    physiological changes, 591–592
    sepsis and, 459
    trauma in, 655–656
Prehospital Maternity Decision Tool, 645–646
premature ventricular complex (PVC), 267–270
preterm birth, 608–609
preterm labour/birth, 621
Prevent strategy, 85–86
prevention, safeguarding, 82
primary headaches, 320
protection, safeguarding, 82
pulmonary embolism (PE), 425–429
    assessment and management, 426–428, 429
    Wells Criteria, 426
pulmonary thrombosis, 128
pulse, blood pressure *versus*, 47
pulseless electrical activity, 165–166

quinsy (peritonsillar abscess), 434

race, 3
racial differences, acute coronary syndrome and, 214
radicalisation, 392–394
rapid tranquillisation, 211
reactive hypoglycaemia, 311
Recommended Summary Plan for Emergency Care and Treatment (ReSPECT), 30, 164
reduced level of consciousness, 247–249
refractory anaphylaxis, 238, 240
refractory ventricular fibrillation, 120, 166
renal failure
    in end of life care, 42
    intravascular fluid therapy in children, 54
respiratory illness, in children, 430–435
    antibiotics, 433
restraint, 60
    by ambulance staff, 61
    mechanical, 399
return of spontaneous circulation (ROSC), 156–159
    assessment and management, 156–158
rib fractures, 92, 584–585
right bundle branch block (RBBB), 216, 267–270
right ventricular failure (RVF), 326
rigor mortis
    in adults, 160
    in children, 169
ruptured aortic aneurysms, 485–487

safeguarding
    adults at risk, 82–86
        assessment and management, 86
        consent, 84–85
        Prevent, 85–86
        wellbeing, 84
    children, 87–98
        assessment and management, 97
        duty to report to police, 91
        extra-familial harm, 91
        maternity, 95–96
        mobile babies and toddlers, 92–93
        non-mobile (non-independent) babies, 91–92
        older children and adolescents, 93
        parental consent, 95
        recognition of abuse, 90–91
        significant harm, 87–88
        special circumstances, 93–94
    drowning, 532
    mental health, 399
SAVE mnemonic, 228
SBAR (Situation, Background, Assessment, Recommendation), 590–591
SCENE incident management, 500, 511
sciatica, 358
2nd degree AV block Mobitz type I, 267–270
2nd degree AV block Mobitz type II, 267–270
secondary headaches, 320
segmental emboli, with pulmonary infarction, 425
seizures
    in adults, 437–449
        assessment and management, 439–447
        bilateral tonic-clonic seizures, 437–438
        driving, 439
        emergency medical treatment, 447–448
        epileptic seizures, 437
        functional/dissociative seizures, 437–439
        syncope, 439
    in children, 450–455
        assessment, 450–451
        benzodiazepine in, 451
        common cause, 450
        convulsive status epilepticus, 450

Index

febrile seizures, 450
hospital transfer, 452
hypoglycaemia, 451
management, 451–454
self-harm, 392–394, 401
self-neglect, 83–84, 392–394
semi-recumbent position, 602, 603, 604
sepsis, 457–469
assessment, 459
children and, 463–468
definitions, 457
fluid therapy for, 50
management, 467–468
NEWS2, 462–463
prehospital screening tools, 461
signs of, 459–460
women and pregnancy, 459
septic arthritis/osteomyelitis, 298
septicaemia, 379
Serious Crime Act 2015, 91
sexual abuse
adults, 83–84
children, 88–90
defined, 99–101
sexual assault, 99–105
assessment and approach, 101–103
care pathways, 103–104
Sexual Assault Referral Centre (SARC), 103–104
sexual consent, defined, 99–101
sexual orientation, 5–6
sexuality, gender and, 8
shaking injuries, abuse, 92
shock
examination, 420
medical causes of, 54
symptoms and signs, 421
shoulder dystocia, 621, 650–654
definition, 650
diagnosis/identification, 650
management, 650–651, 652
sickle cell disease, 472–476
assessment and management, 473–475
medical emergencies, 472
sinus bradycardia, 267–270
situational awareness, 45
skin colour, 3
skin tone, 3
skin-to-skin care, 607, 620
skull fracture, 92
social prescribing, 385
social transitioning, 6
SOCRATES, 63
speaking valve, 146–148
spinal injury and spinal cord injury, 574–580
assessment and management, 577–578
immobilisation, 575–577, 579
risk factors, 574
spinal metastases, 20–21
spiral fracture, 92
splinting, 561
ST segment elevation myocardial infarction (STEMI), 215, 216
stab wounds, 518
stable angina, features of, 409
staff health and wellbeing, 106–107
trauma emergencies, 509
Steroid Emergency Card, 222
steroid-dependent patients, 223–224
stoma, 146–148
stridor, croup (children), 431
stroke, 477–482
assessment and management, 480–481

FAST test, 479
signs and symptoms, 477–478
ST-segment depression, 216
subacute hypothermia, 345
subarachnoid haemorrhage (SAH), 322, 478–479
subcutaneous administration, site of injection, 40
submersion
definition of, 528
survival and, 530
substance use, 58, 392–394
sudden cardiac death, 249, 265–267
suicide, 392–394, 401–402
superior vena cava compression, 31
Supportive and Palliative Care Indicators Tool (SPICT), 34
supraglottic airways, 121–122
supraventricular tachycardia (SVT), 267–270
implantable cardioverter defibrillator for, 352
surgical emphysema, 587
Surviving Sepsis Campaign, 457

tachycardia, 263
assessment and management, 263, 265
broad complex, 265
children, 188
febrile illness, 297, 298
implantable cardioverter defibrillator for, 352
tachypnoea, 187, 297, 434
TEACH mnemonic, 81
tension pneumothorax, 128, 585–586
tension-type headaches, 321
termination of resuscitation and verification of death
in adults, 160-168
in children, 169–174
thermal burns, 522, 525
thermoregulation, 619
3rd degree (total) AV block, 267–270
thoracic pump theory, 111
thoracic trauma, 581–587
assessment and management, 581–583
thrombin, 629
thrombosis, 128
toddlers, safeguarding, 92–93
torsade de pointes, 267–270
torsion of testis, 195–199
tort of negligence, 27
total body surface area (TBSA), 522
tracheal intubation, 122
traction splint, 561
traffic light system, for assessing paediatric fever, 296–297
transgender, 6, 8
transient ischaemic attack (TIA), 477–482
assessment and management, 480–481
transient loss of consciousness (TLoC), 244–247
transitioning, 6, 8
transverse fracture, 92
trauma
cardiac arrest and, 130–133
in children, 54–55
from electrical injuries, 534
in haemorrhagic emergencies, 48–49
in non-haemorrhagic emergencies, 49
pain and, 64
in pregnancy, 655–656
vaginal bleeding during pregnancy, 660
trauma emergencies
in adults, 500–510
assessment and management, 501–503
ATMIST format, 501
primary survey, 501
SCENE incident management, 500
secondary survey, 501–505, 504–505

Index

in children, 511–517
    airway, 511–512
    analgesia, 516
    'AVPU' scale, 513
    bradycardia, 513
    primary survey, 511
    SCENE, 511
    secondary survey, 516
traumatic brain injury
    management, 551–553
    midazolam in, 553–554
triplets, 623
'tripod' posture, children, 432
12-lead ECG
    for acute coronary syndrome, 215–216
    for falls in older adults, 540–541

UKONS/Macmillan Primary Care Triage Pocket Tool, 32, 33
ultrasound, for cardiac arrest, 129
unexpected death, 166
upper respiratory tract infections (URTIs), 433–434
    assessment, 433
    hydration, 433
    management, 433, 434
urinary tract infection (UTI), 298
urinary tract pathology, 195–199
urticaria, 237
uterine contractions, 616–617
uterine massage, 629
uterine rupture, 660
uterotonic drugs, 629

vaginal bleeding, during pregnancy
    after 20 weeks gestation, 660–661
        causes, 660
        diagnosis, 660
        management, 660
    up to 20 weeks gestation, 657–659
        ectopic pregnancy, 657–658
        management, 657–658
        miscarriage, 657
vaginal bleeding, gynaecological causes, 662–664
    assessment and management, 662–664
vasa praevia, 660
vascular emergencies, 484–497
    aortic aneurysm, 484–487
    aortic dissection, 487, 489–491
    AV fistula haemorrhage, 495–496, 497
    diabetic foot problem, 493–495
    ischaemic limbs, 491–493
vasopressors, for sepsis, 467, 468
venous thromboembolism (VTE), 426
ventricular fibrillation
    fine, 119
    recurrent, 120
    refractory, 120, 166
ventricular tachycardia, implantable cardioverter defibrillator for, 352
verbal calming, 208
verbal de-escalation
    for acute behavioural disturbance, 208
    for agitation, 228
vertebral insufficiency fractures, 357
victimisation, 392–394
violence, 392–394

waterbirth, 621
wellbeing, 84
Wells Criteria, for pulmonary embolism, 426
Wernicke-Korsakoff syndrome, 231
Wong-Baker FACES pain rating scale, 65

young people
    mental health, 395
    witnessing cardiac arrest, 167